Ebersole & Hess'

TOWARD
HEALTHY
AGING

Human Needs & Nursing Response

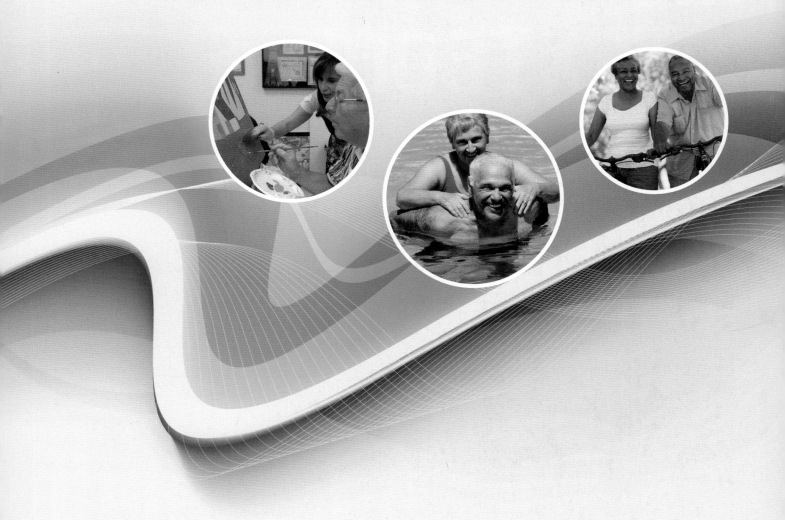

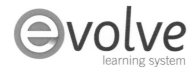
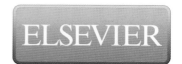
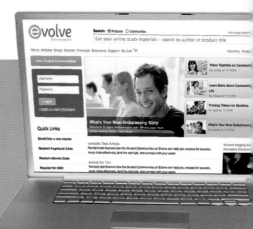

Ebersole & Hess'
TOWARD HEALTHY AGING

Human Needs & Nursing Response

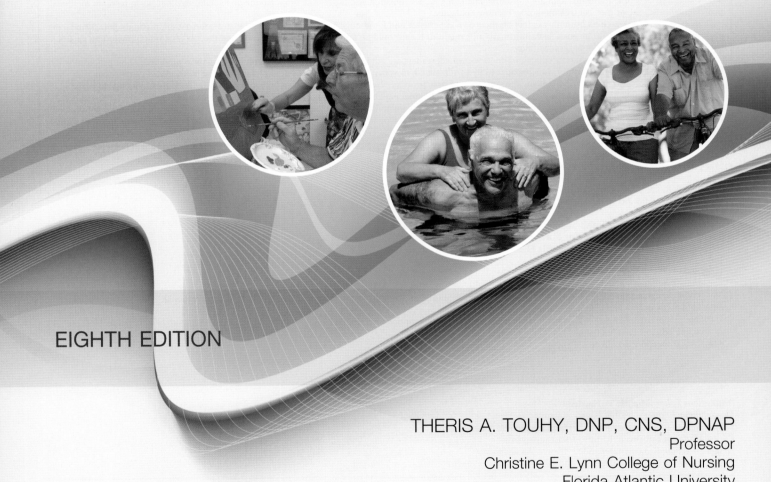

EIGHTH EDITION

THERIS A. TOUHY, DNP, CNS, DPNAP
Professor
Christine E. Lynn College of Nursing
Florida Atlantic University
Boca Raton, Florida

KATHLEEN JETT, PHD, GNP-BC
University of Florida
Gainesville, Florida

ELSEVIER

3251 Riverport Lane
St. Louis, Missouri 63043

EBERSOLE & HESS' TOWARD HEALTHY AGING: HUMAN NEEDS AND NURSING RESPONSE   ISBN: 978-0-323-07316-5

Library of Congress Cataloging-in-Publication Data

Touhy, Theris A.
    Ebersole & Hess' toward healthy aging : human needs & nursing response / Theris A. Touhy, Kathleen Jett.—8th ed.
        p. ; cm.
    Ebersole and Hess' toward healthy aging : human needs & nursing response
    Toward healthy aging : human needs & nursing response
    Rev. ed. of: Toward healthy aging / Priscilla Ebersole ... [et al.]. 7th ed. c2008.
    Includes bibliographical references and index.
    ISBN 978-0-323-07316-5 (hardcover : alk. paper)
    1. Geriatric nursing. 2. Aging. 3. Older persons–Health and hygiene. I. Jett, Kathleen Freudenberger. II. Ebersole, Priscilla. III. Hess, Patricia A., 1938– IV. Toward healthy aging. V. Title. VI. Title: Ebersole and Hess' toward healthy aging : human needs & nursing response. VII. Title: Toward healthy aging : human needs & nursing response.
    [DNLM: 1. Geriatric Nursing. 2. Aged. 3. Aging. 4. Health   Promotion. WY 152]
    RC954.E23 2012
    618.97′0231—dc23

                                                                                              2011019101

Acquisitions Editor: Michele D. Hayden
Developmental Editor: Heather Bays
Publishing Services Manager: Jeff Patterson/Hemamalini Rajendrababu
Project Manager: Bill Drone/Kiruthiga Kasthuriswamy
Design Direction: Kimberly Denando

Cover photo of art program courtesy of Florida Atlantic University (FAU) Memory and Wellness Center "Artful Memories" program.

Printed in China

Last digit is the print number: 9 8 7 6 5 4 3

To my husband Bob, my sons Danial, Andrew, and Peter, and my beautiful daughters-in-law, Amber and Rose and Kathy, for their support of my writing and for loving me always no matter what.

To Colin Keating Touhy and Molly Capps Touhy, my beautiful grandchildren, who make me laugh and remember what is really important in my life.

To all the students who read this book. May your nursing be competent and caring for people from birth to death. I look forward to the many ways each of you will improve the journey toward healthy aging through your competence and compassion.

To all of my students who have embraced gerontological nursing as their specialty and are improving the lives of older people through their practice and teaching

To the wise and wonderful older people who I have been privileged to nurse, and to their caregivers. Thank you for making the words in this book a reality for the elders for whom you care, and for teaching me how to be a gerontological nurse.

Theris A. Touhy

To my husband Steve, who is a source of support through thick and thin. Without his willingness to keep me supplied with food, the long hours sitting in front of the computer and writing would not have been possible. To our four children and four wonderful grandchildren, who always remind me that the best part of life is the time we spend together and that the older we get, the more we have loved and the more adventures we have shared.

Kathleen Jett

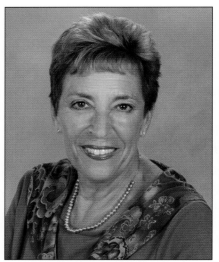

Theris A. Touhy, DNP, CNS, DPNAP, has been a clinical specialist in gerontological nursing and a nurse practitioner for 30 years. Her expertise is in the care of older adults in nursing homes and of those with dementia. The majority of her practice as a clinical nurse specialist and nurse practitioner has been in the long-term care setting. She received her BSN degree from St. Xavier University in Chicago, a master's degree in care of the aged from Northern Illinois University, and a Doctor of Nursing Practice from Case Western Reserve University. Dr. Touhy is a professor in the Christine E. Lynn College of Nursing at Florida Atlantic University, where she has served as Assistant Dean of Undergraduate Programs. She teaches gerontological nursing and long-term, rehabilitation, and palliative care nursing in both the undergraduate, graduate, and doctoral programs. Her research is focused on spirituality in aging and at the end of life, caring for persons with dementia, and caring in nursing homes. Dr. Touhy was the recipient of the Geriatric Faculty Member Award from the John A. Hartford Foundation Institute for Geriatric Nursing in 2003, is a two-time recipient of the Distinguished Teacher of the Year in the Christine E. Lynn College of Nursing at Florida Atlantic University, and was awarded the Marie Haug Award for Excellence in Aging Research and Dr. Touhy was inducted into the national academic of practice in 2007, from Case Western Reserve University. She is co-author with Dr. Kathleen Jett of *Gerontological Nursing and Healthy Aging* and is co-author with Dr. Priscilla Ebersole of *Geriatric Nursing: Growth of a Specialty.*

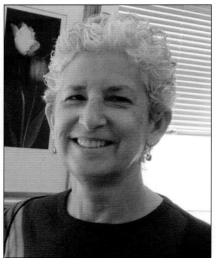

Kathleen Jett, PhD, GNP-BC, has been actively engaged in gerontological nursing for over 30 years. Her clinical experience is broad, from her roots in public health to clinical leadership in long-term care, assisted living and hospice, researcher and teacher, and advanced practice as both a clinical nurse specialist and nurse practitioner. Dr. Jett received her bachelor's, master's, and doctoral degrees from the University of Florida, where she also holds a graduate certificate in gerontology. In 2000 she was selected as a Summer Scholar by the John A. Hartford Foundation—Institute for Geriatric Nursing. In 2004 she completed a Fellowship in Ethno-Geriatrics through the Stanford Geriatric Education Center. Dr. Jett has received several awards, including recognition as an *Inspirational Woman of Pacific Lutheran University* in1998 and 2000 and for her excellence in undergraduate teaching in 2005 and Distinguished Teacher of the year within the Christine E. Lynn College of Nursing at Florida Atlantic University. A board-certified gerontological nurse practitioner, Dr. Jett was inducted into the National Academies of Practice in 2006. The thread that ties all of her work together has been a belief that nurses can make a difference in the lives of older adults. She is currently a research consultant at the College of Nursing at the University of Florida and a nurse practitioner at Oak Hammock, a life-care community associated with the University. In addition to her professional activities, Dr. Jett is actively engaged in the lives of her grandchildren in their multi-generational household in rural High Springs, Florida.

CONTRIBUTOR

Dr. Ellis Quinn Youngkin, PhD, RNC, ARNP
Professor and Associate Dean
Christine E. Lynn College of Nursing;
Women's Health Care Nurse Practitioner
University Student Health Services
Florida Atlantic University
Boca Raton, Florida

CASE STUDIES

Gloria Carr PhD, RN
Assistant Professor
The University of Memphis
Loewenberg School of Nursing
Memphis, Tennessee

INSTRUCTOR'S MANUAL

Cathy L. Hinson Franklin-Griffin, PhD, RN, CHPN
Nurse Educator, RN-BSN Option Program
Winston-Salem State University
Winston-Salem, North Carolina;
Nurse Educator/Faculty Mentor, NCLEX-RN Review Program
Kaplan Education, Inc.
East Territory, USA

POWERPOINT LECTURE SLIDES WITH AUDIENCE RESPONSE SYSTEM QUESTIONS

Valarie S. Grumme, MSN RN CCRN
Clinical Manager MICU/CCU
Memorial Regional Hospital
Hollywood, Florida

REVIEW AND CRITICAL THINKING QUESTIONS

Kathleen Blais, RN, MSN, EdD
Professor Emerita
Florida International University
College of Nursing and Health Sciences
Nursing
Miami, Florida

NCLEX® TEST BANK

Linda Turchin, RN, MSN, CNE
Assistant Professor
School of Nursing and Allied Health Administration
Fairmont State University
Fairmont, West Virginia

REVIEWERS

Kathleen Blais, RN, MSN, EdD
Professor Emerita
Florida International University
College of Nursing and Health Sciences
Nursing
Miami, Florida

Virginia Burggraf, DNS, RN, C, FAAN
Radford University
Radford, Virginia

Sherri Cozzens, MSN, RN
DeAnza College
San Jose, CA

Valerie Gruss, PhD, ANP/GNP-BC
Clinical Assistant Professor
Department of Biobehavioral Health Science
Institute of Health Care Innovation
University of Illinois
Chicago, Illinois

Christy Seckman, DNP, MSN-FNP, RN
Assistant Professor
Goldfarb School of Nursing
Barnes-Jewish College
St. Louis, Missouri

JoAnn Swanson, MSN, RN-BC, ONC
Assistant Professor
School of Nursing
Bellin College
Green Bay, Wisconsin

In 1981, Dr. Priscilla Ebersole and Dr. Patricia Hess published the first edition of *Toward Healthy Aging: Human Needs and Nursing Response,* which has been used in nursing schools across the globe. Their foresight in developing a textbook that focuses on health, wholeness, beauty, and potential in aging has made this book an enduring classic. In 1981, few nurses chose this specialty, few schools of nursing included content related to the care of elders, and the focus of care was on illness and problems. Today, gerontological nursing is a strong and evolving specialty with a solid theoretical base and practice grounded in evidence-based research. Dr. Ebersole and Dr. Hess set the standards for the competencies required for gerontological nursing education and the promotion of health while aging. Many nurses, including us, have been shaped by their words, their wisdom, and their passion for care of elders. Now, 30 years later, it is our privilege to co-author the totally revised and updated eighth edition of this text. We thank these two wonderful pioneers and mentors for the opportunity to build on such a solid foundation. We hope that we have kept the heart and spirit of their work, for that is truly what has inspired us, and so many others, to care for elders with competence and compassion.

We believe that *Toward Healthy Aging* is the most comprehensive gerontological nursing text available. The content ranges from biological, such as the etiology of common chronic conditions and geropharmacology, to caring for persons with dementia, to understanding current evolving issues in care of older adults such as transitional care and evidence based gerontological nursing. *Toward Healthy Aging* is an appropriate text for both undergraduate and graduate students and is an excellent reference for nurses' libraries. This edition makes an ideal supplement to health assessment, medical-surgical, community, and psychiatric and mental health textbooks in programs that do not have a freestanding gerontological nursing course.

Within the covers, the reader will find the latest evidence-based gerontological nursing protocols to be used in providing the highest level of care to adults in settings across the continuum. The content is consistent with the Recommended Baccalaureate Competencies and Curricular Guidelines for the Nursing Care of Older Adults, the Geriatric Nursing Education State of the Science Papers, and the Hartford Institute for Geriatric Nursing Best Practices in Nursing Care to Older Adults. The text has been on the list of recommended reading for the ANCC Advanced Practice Exam for a number of years. New chapters titled Communicating with Older Adults, and Nursing Across the Continuum of Care, add to its value. In addition, this text includes specific strategies to promote healthy aging from a life span approach, case studies and opportunities for critical thinking, and comprehensive resources for further study.

We have been honored to build on the work of Dr. Ebersole and Dr. Hess and to provide a rich, state-of-the-science edition of a classic text. We hope that the readers benefit as much from using it as we did revising it!

Theris A. Touhy
Kathleen Jett

ACKNOWLEDGMENTS

This book would not have been possible without the support and guidance of the staff at Elsevier, especially Heather Bays, Developmental Editor, who listened to all of our suggestions and concerns and understood how important this work was to us and to nursing students. Special thanks also to Shelly Hayden, Managing Editor. We also acknowledge our reviewers, contributors, and previous authors, for without their efforts, this edition would not have been possible. Finally, we acknowledge the past and future readers who, we hope, will provide us with enough feedback to keep us honest in any future writing.

Theris A. Touhy
Kathleen Jett

CONTENTS

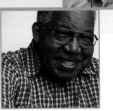

Gerontological Nursing and an Aging Society

Theris A. Touhy

℮volve http://evolve.elsevier.com/Ebersole/TwdHlthAging

A YOUTH SPEAKS

Until my grandmother became ill and needed our help, I really didn't know her well. Now I can look at her in an entirely different light. She is frail and tough, fearful and courageous, demanding and delightful, bitter and humorous, needy and needed. I'm beginning to think that old age is the culmination of all the aspects of living a long life. **Jenine, 28 years old**

A MIDDLE-AGED PERSON SPEAKS

Nursing care of the aged brings one in touch with the most basic and profound questions of human existence: the meanings of life and death; sources of strength and survival skills; beginnings, ending, and reasons for being. It is a commitment to discovery of the self—and of the self I am becoming as I age. **Stephanie, middle-aged faculty**

AN ELDER SPEAKS

I'm 95 years old and have no family or friends that still survive. I wonder if anyone will be there for me when I leave the planet, which will be very soon I am sure. Mothers deliver, but who will deliver me into the hand of God? **Name withheld**

LEARNING OBJECTIVES

On completion of this chapter, the reader will be able to:

1. Specify demographic changes related to the aging experience in the twenty-first century.
2. Understand the many factors that facilitate or hinder the aging process.
3. Recognize the great diversity of older adults.
4. Discuss strategies to prepare an adequate and competent eldercare workforce to meet the needs of the growing numbers of older people.
5. Identify several factors that have influenced the development of gerontological nursing as a specialty practice.
6. Discuss several formal geriatric organizations and their significance to nurses.
7. Compare various gerontological nursing roles and requirements.
8. Discuss nursing research studies on the care of older adults and the role of gerontological nurses in research.

THE STUDY OF AGING

As we look to the future, our society will have more people older than 65 years than ever before in our history. By 2050 one in five Americans will be over the age of 65. This statistic will change the face of aging as we know it now and present many challenges as well as many opportunities for our future. Healthy aging is now an achievable goal for many and it is essential that we have the knowledge and skills to help people of all ages, races, and cultures achieve this goal.

In the past, healthy older men and women frequently eluded the attention of gerontologists. Thus study samples of the elder adults, most likely taken from institutionalized subjects, were often extrapolated to the healthier population. This led to a picture of aging that viewed older people as frail and dependent with little to look forward to in the last years of life. To some extent, that view of aging remains today and is steeped in the myths perpetuated about older adults. Older people are often viewed as ill, lonely, depressed, abandoned by family, a burden to society, just waiting to die. The reality is that the majority of those aged 65 and older regard their health as good or excellent; increasing numbers are extending their active working lives into their 70s and 80s; many have close and meaningful relationships with their families in parent, grandparent and great-grandparent roles; and the number of people living to 100 years of age is projected to grow at more than 20 times the rate of the total population by 2050. The developmental period of elderhood is an essential part of a healthy society and as important as childhood or adulthood (Thomas, 2004). We can expect to spend 40 or more years as older adults, and our preparation for this time in our lives certainly demands attention as well as expert care.

How does one maximize the experience of aging and enrich the years of elderhood regardless of the physical and psychological changes that commonly occur? Nurses have a great responsibility to help shape a world in which older people can thrive and grow, not merely survive. Most nurses care for older people during the course of their careers. In addition, the public will look to nurses to have the knowledge and skills to assist people to age in health. Every older person should expect care provided by nurses with competence in gerontological nursing. Gerontological nursing is not for someone else or only for a specialty group of nurses. Knowledge of aging and gerontological nursing is core knowledge for the profession of nursing (Young, 2003). How nurses move our aging society forward toward the middle of the twenty-first century will determine our character, as we are no greater than the health of America. That is what this textbook is all about.

Words, statistics, and research data can only paint a picture of how aging looks. The most significant learning regarding the intricacies and challenges of aging and survival strategies comes from discussions with elders themselves. They are our role models, and their diversity makes it possible for us to develop a greater understanding of life if we only listen to what they say and that which is unsaid. Many years ago, Irene Burnside (1975), one of the geriatric nursing pioneers, said it beautifully:

> Listen to the aged for they will tell you about living and dying.
>
> Listen to the aged for they will enlighten you about problem-solving, sexuality, grief, sensory deprivation, and survival.
>
> Listen to the aged for they will teach you how to be courageous, loving, and generous.
>
> They are a distinguished faculty without formal classrooms, tenure, sabbaticals. They teach not from books but from long experience in living. p. 1801

GERONTOLOGY

Gerontology is the scientific study of the effects of time on human development, specifically the study of older persons. It is at the opposite end of the spectrum from embryology and often includes several decades before death. Gerontology, by virtue of the Greek origin of the word *geron* (old man), should mean the study of old men, but many more women than men grow old. A large part of the study of aging comes from attending to older adults and the aging person in ourselves and how we perceive our own aging. These approaches are fundamentally important to gerontology. Inquisitions into and curiosity about

aging are as old as curiosity about life and death itself. Much that was thought to have been correct about aging has been shown through research to be half-truth, myth, or supposition. In developing a science and philosophy of aging, one essentially builds on personal experience; ultimately we all do this.

Gerontology began as an inquiry into the characteristics of long-lived people, and we are still intrigued by them. In 1000 BCE, the average life span was 18 years and people who lived to old age were curiosities, stimulating reverence, speculation, and myth. Anecdotal evidence was used in the past to illustrate issues assumed to be universal. Only in the past 50 years have serious and carefully controlled research studies flourished. Theoreticians and researchers most commonly interested in the study of aging are sociologists, psychologists, and biologists. Their conceptual bases underlie their perspectives regarding survival issues. Nursing draws from its own body of knowledge, as well as from all of these disciplines, to describe, monitor, protect, and evaluate the quality of life experienced by the old.

The term *geriatrics* was coined by an American physician, Ignatz Nascher, around 1900 because he recognized that the medical care of older people involved special considerations, much like the field of pediatrics. Nascher authored the first textbook on medical care of the elderly in the United States in 1914 (Nascher, 1914). Aging has been seen as a biomedical problem that must be reversed, eradicated, or held at bay as long as possible. Therefore, the impact of disease, morbidity, and impending death on the quality of life and the experience of aging have provided the impetus for much of the study by gerontologists. In this way, aging has inevitably been seen through the distorted lens of disease. However, we are finally recognizing that aging and disease are separate entities although frequent companions. The trend toward the medicalization of the study of aging has influenced the general public as well. The biomedical view of the "problem" of aging is reinforced on all sides. A shift in the view of aging to one that centers on the potential for health, wholeness, and quality of life, and the significant contributions of older people to society, is increasingly the focus in the research, popular literature, and public portrayals of older people.

How Old Is Old?

An individual ages chronologically, biologically, psychologically, sociologically, and spiritually as a unitary being. A disciplinary rather than a humanistic perspective sometimes makes it appear that these are separate components of existence. There is such overlap that disciplinary lines are no longer appropriate in planning care. Interprofessional approaches and care programs are essential and are rapidly becoming the model method of providing health care to older people.

Chronology is becoming a less significant factor to consider in aging. "Old" is a relative concept based on how one acts and feels physically, mentally, socially, and culturally. One can feel old when competing with younger folk or feel young when they are much healthier or younger looking than age contemporaries. One's *chronological age* (years lived) may or may not correspond to one's *biological age* (age of organ systems), *psychological age* (how old one feels), and *social age* (roles and relationships). In the United States, the chronological age of 65 years is the standard by which one is awarded the status of senior citizen, whether or not it is desired. In 1935, 65 years was chosen as the age at which a person could receive benefits and services under Social Security. As people live and work longer, the eligibility age for Social Security benefits is increasing.

The category of "old" is arbitrary and varies with time, place, cohort, and perception. Because of the great variations between a 65-year-old and an 85-year-old, old age has been further categorized into young-old (ages 65-74), middle-old (ages 75-84), and old-old (85 years and older). From the gerontological nursing perspective, functional age, or the ability to perform activities of daily living (ADLs), is a more essential measure of age than chronological age.

Today's Older People

The parents of the baby boomers, the children of the Great Depression, make up the majority of the present older generation. Some immunizations became available in their childhood, but many parents feared them and most children had all of the "childhood" diseases, such as measles, mumps, chickenpox, and whooping cough. Some had tuberculosis, poliomyelitis, and smallpox. Malnutrition was rampant among the people with socioeconomically deprived. Dental care was neglected. In areas where the water was "soft," lacking minerals, teeth were soft and cavity-prone. "Pigeon chest," a malformation of the rib cage caused by lack of vitamin D, was common. Goiter and myxedema were less common but were present regionally because of unrecognized iodine deficiencies. These problems were identified and almost eradicated before the next generation, the baby boomers, came along.

The survivors in this generation are called the "notch" babies; few in number at birth, even fewer survived childhood, adolescence, and World War II. War and patriotism molded their young adulthood. Most of these elders are fairly sturdy, but their adolescent and young adult lifestyles contributed to many problems that are now evident. The use and abuse of cigarettes and alcohol were considered sophisticated. A double standard prevailed in the expectations of men and women. Exercise was not valued by most because desirable work was steadily becoming less physically strenuous, and physical exertion was still associated with hard work. Remote memories of poverty and deprivation haunted many of them and propelled them into excesses when such were available and affordable. Few gave much thought to their own aging during their middle years because most were preoccupied with providing for their children the things they had missed. Saving for children's college education was a high priority.

Nonagenarians and Centenarians

There is an expanding group of the very old, those now older than 90 years (nonagenarians), who remain mobile and active. They are genetically hardy. These are an extraordinarily select group of individuals who have managed to survive the numerous dangers and diseases of childhood and, with the advancement of medical science, have overcome disorders that would have killed their parents. Some remember the influenza pandemic of 1918 in which numerous young and vital individuals died within a few hours of developing influenza. Many of these present elders, because of the rigorous conditions of survival in their youth, are now living well into their 90s.

This generation raised their families during the depths of the Great Depression. Desperation was prevalent in the country at the time. Few were able to achieve a higher education, and many did not even complete grade school. The bulk of the working population were farmers, agricultural workers, factory workers, miners, and clerks. Unemployment was rampant. Individuals worked very hard for the essentials of existence and felt fortunate if they were employed. Henry Ford became famous for offering wages of $5 a day and producing assembly-line cars that made automobiles available to the common person. These individuals, who are the last to remember traveling by horse and wagon, have also flown across the nation in supersonic jet airplanes. Older people of today have been catapulted through socioscientific periods too numerous to mention. The shifts in human thought, technical capacities, and modes of life that have occurred within the single lifetime of the very old are stunning. These include the agrarian age, the industrial age, the atomic age, the space age, the microelectronic age, and the cyberspace age as we are all connected by the World Wide Web.

This generation has experienced more hardship and more lifestyle disruption and change than any of which we are aware. Federal aid, Social Security, the Works Progress Administration, and numerous other New Deal programs were instituted as survival measures during the depths of the Great Depression. Few of these individuals thought much about old age, and many say they are surprised to have lived so long. These elders rarely throw anything away because every scrap has potential value when one has known early deprivation. Many of them arrived in the United States in early childhood as steerage passengers, emigrating with their parents from Europe.

Centenarians, the "elite-old," are approached with some awe as our society seeks routes to longevity. The number of centenarians in the United States has doubled every decade since 1970, and they are the fastest growing segment of our population. One in 26 Americans can expect to live to be 100 by 2025, compared with only one in 500 in 2000 (Administration on Aging, 2009). There are 221,500 supercentenarians (those older than 110). Many of the "elite-old" are bright and alert and have an unequaled personal history. However, although centenarians appear to be healthy for a longer period of time, almost 50% live in nursing homes. In part this may be due to the absence of living children, siblings, or spouses (Hooyman and Kiyak, 2011).

Most centenarians are female (85%) and come from families in which longevity is common. Although there are fewer male centenarians, they are less likely than women to have significant mental or physical disabilities at that age, and older men who survive to age 90 represent the hardiest segment of their birth cohort (Christensen, 2001; Hooyman and Kiyak, 2011). Persons of color who live to age 85 are "hardier" than their white counterparts (racial crossover effect). Thirty percent of centenarians have no evidence of dementia (Silver et al., 2001). They are often sought for their opinions on the key to longevity. The supposition is that because they have lived so long they know the secrets to learning, growing, and thriving. Various centenarians have recommended such things as a daily highball, hard work, church attendance, healthy diets, or the continuation of sexual activity. Unfortunately, few agree and the myths abound. Lifestyle factors that do seem significant include diet, maintaining proper weight, exercise, avoidance of smoking, social connections, and how well a person handles stress (Mentes, 2006). Researchers all over the world are studying centenarians. Many questions and conflicting findings still exist regarding both the physiological and psychological adaptation of centenarians. Several websites offer a fascinating look at centenarians, including pictures: http://www.adlercentenarians.org/ and http://www.grg.org/calment.html.

The Future Old

A healthier old age seems to be within reach for the population in general and particularly for the segment dubbed "baby boomers." The first wave of baby boomers will turn 65 in 2011, and between 2008 and 2030 this group will swell the ranks of older adults. They are informed and educated, have been alerted to the importance of beginning to prepare early for a good old age, and expect a much higher quality of life as they age than did their elders. More and more of them find that they are caregivers to the older members of their family, sometimes as many as two generations, and have a very personal understanding of the needs of elders. These almost-elders are giving us new perspectives on the aging process. They, and the numerous longitudinal studies of aging now in progress, are changing the concepts of aging and the field of gerontology. Interest is increasing in anti-aging medicine and prolongevity (significant extension of the human life span and/or average life expectancy without lengthening suffering and infirmity). Yet much depends on world economics, and unrest exists among these individuals as they contemplate the possibility of insufficient resources in their final years.

There is no typical baby boomer. Although it has been fashionable to consider the baby boomers en masse, they are extremely diverse, differing by as much as 19 birth years, separated by race, culture, and socioeconomic status. Baby boomers range from well-known figures such as Sir Paul McCartney, Bill Clinton, Stevie Wonder, and Cher to the parents of many students reading this book.

To plan well for their retirement years, we must consider the following:
- Their diversity
- The uncertain political and economic future
- Potential major shifts in lifestyle expectations
- Changing health care delivery and reimbursement systems
- Progress in technology and medical management
- Shifts in values and ethics that will profoundly affect daily life

Articles about menopause proliferate, midlife crises abound, and anxiety about the future is rampant. Will there be income support, adequate retirement, available health care, disability benefits, and all the things the present generation of the old have relied on? The major concerns of baby boomers are health, finances, job security, sending children to college, and caring for parents. They have been called the "sandwich generation," because they try to meet the needs of "boomerang" children (those young adults who repeatedly return home because they cannot generate sufficient incomes to live independently) and elderly parents. Shirley Chater (a nurse and a former director of Social Security) called them the "double whopper" generation. "Triple whopper" is probably more accurate today, because many older people are also the primary caretakers of grandchildren. Gerontologists, marketing strategists, and the age industry are attempting to predict anticipated challenges. Many uncertainties remain about the conditions, status, and benefits baby boomers will experience. Some of the major concerns are based on the shift of lifestyles away from the traditional family. Single parents, blended families, limited parenthood, unmarried parents, and gay and lesbian parents all represent lifestyles that may or may not produce children willing or available to assist parents as they age (see Chapter 22 for further discussion of caregiving roles and responsibilities).

AGING TODAY

A revolution is occurring in gerontological nursing as older adults are gaining full status and recognition in society. The "baby boomer" generation is entering the ranks of the young-old (those 60-74 years old). The old-old and the elite-old (those 90 years and older) are the fastest growing segment of the aging population, as technologic advances have facilitated their survival. Each of these age groups presents with different characteristics, desires, interests, and health concerns. It is important to look at the unique needs of each, rather than to group all older adults together. Just as care of a newborn is different from the care of a 12-year-old, a 60-year-old requires different care than a 90-year-old.

Demographics of Aging

Demography, the statistical study of the size and distribution of populations, is extremely significant in gerontology. The decennial U.S. Census occurs every 10 years, and the 2010 census will be especially important because it will dictate national concerns and policies regarding aging, as well as future directions.

Aging in the United States

The 2010 total population of the United States was 308,745,538. Of these, almost 38 million are older than 65 years, making up 12.6% of the population. Of these, 42.2% are older men and 57.8% are older women. By 2030, almost 1 in 5 Americans (72 million people) will be 65 years or older. The age group 85 years and older is now the fastest growing segment of the U.S. population (Figure 1-1). At present, about 0.0173% of the population are at least 100 years old, compared with 0.1% in 1901 (U.S. Census Bureau, 2012). The total number is expected to increase by more than 400% by 2030. The majority of these centenarians will be women (U.S. Census Bureau, 2010).

Life Expectancy

An American's average life expectancy at birth has trended upward as a result of reduced death rates for children and young adults, new drugs, medical technology, and better disease prevention. Between 1985 and 2005, the death rates for the population aged 65 to 84 dropped, especially for men. For men aged 65 to 74, the death rate has dropped by 32.3% and by 23.5% for men aged 75 to 84. Life expectancy at age 65 increased by only 2.5 years between 1900 and 1960 but has increased by 4.2 years from 1960 to 2007 (Administration on Aging, 2009). In 2010, the life expectancy for infant girls in the United States was 80.8 years, whereas for boys it was 75.7 years. However, among African-Americans, life expectancy was 70.2 years for men and

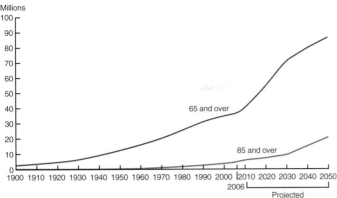

NOTE: Data for 2010–2050 are projections of the population.
Reference population: These data refer to the resident population.
SOURCE: U.S. Census Bureau, Decennial Census, Population Estimates and Projections.

FIGURE 1-1 Population Age 65 and Over and Age 85 and Over; Selected Years 1900-2008 and Projected 2010-2050. (Redrawn from Federal Interagency Forum on Aging-related Statistics: *Older Americans 2010: key indicators of well-being,* Washington DC, 2010, U.S. Government Printing Office.)

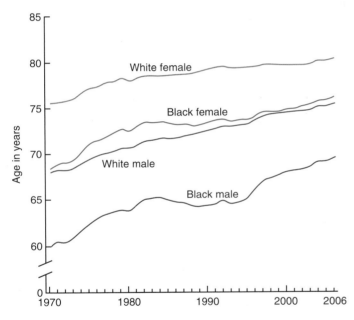

FIGURE 1-2 Life Expectancy, by Race and Sex: United States, 1970-2006. (Redrawn from National Center for Health Statistics, Centers for Disease Control and Prevention, U.S. Department of Health and Human Services: Deaths: final data for 2006, *National Vital Statistics Report* 57[14], April 17, 2009.)

77.2 years for women, evidence of an important health disparity (U.S. Census Bureau, 2010) (Figure 1-2). Hispanics in the United States outlive whites by 2.5 years and blacks by nearly 8 years (CDC, 2010).

A 2008 report comparing the United States with 18 other industrialized countries reported that in 2002-2004, the United States had among the highest death rates from causes amenable to health care of the countries studied. The report attributed the slow decline in U.S. amenable mortality to the increase in the uninsured population (American Medical Association, 2008).

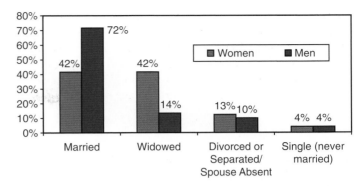

FIGURE 1-3 Marital Status of Persons 65 Years of Age and Older, 2008. (Redrawn from *Administration on Aging, U.S. Department of Health and Human Services:* A profile of older Americans [2009]. Available at http://www.aoa.gov/AoARoot/Aging_Statistics/Profile/index.aspx [accessed November 2010].)

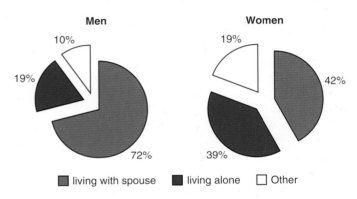

FIGURE 1-4 Living Arrangements of Men and Women 65 Years of Age and Older, 2008. (Redrawn from Administration on Aging, U.S. Department of Health and Human Services: *A profile of older Americans* [2009]. Available at http://www.aoa.gov/AoAroot/Aging_Statistics/Profile/2009/docs/2009profile_508.pdf [accessed November 2010].)

Marital Status

The majority of people over the age of 80 live independently in the community. Older men are more likely to be married than older women, and 42% of all older women are widowed. There are more than four times as many widows as widowers (Figure 1-3). The number of older people who are divorced or separated is increasing and can be expected to rise as the baby boomers age. In the United States, 39% of women and 19% of men over the age of 65 live alone (Figure 1-4).

Living Arrangements

Florida has the highest proportion of people over the age of 65 (17.6%) followed by West Virginia (15.7%), Pennsylvania (15.3%), Maine (15.1%), and Iowa (14.8%). Between 1998 and 2008, the 65 years-and-older population increased 25% or more in Alaska, Nevada, Arizona, Utah, New Mexico, Idaho, Georgia, South Carolina, Colorado, and Delaware (Administration on Aging, 2009) (Figure 1-5). Most persons 65 years of age and older live in metropolitan areas (80.6%) (Administration on Aging, 2009). In the comparatively mobile population of the United States, the experience of aging is greatly influenced by where one lives.

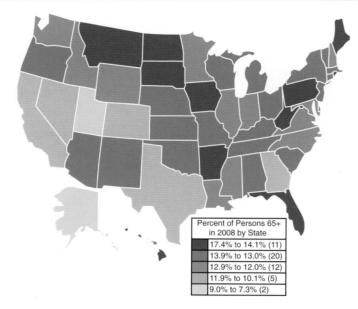

FIGURE 1-5 Persons over 65 Years of Age and Older, by State. (Redrawn from Administration on Aging, U.S. Department of Health and Human Services: *A profile of older Americans: 2009.* Available at http://www.aoa.gov/AoAroot/Aging_Statistics/Profile/2009/docs/2009profile_508.pdf [accessed November 2010].)

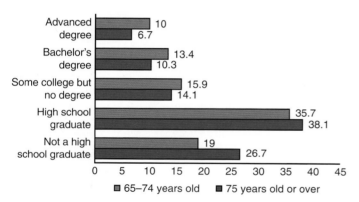

FIGURE 1-6 Education Level of Adults 65 Years of Age and Older: 2008. Data are expressed as percentages. (Data from U.S. Census Bureau: *Current population survey.* http://factfinder.census.gov/servlet/QTTable?_bm=y&-geo_id=01000US&-qr_name=DEC_2000_SF3_U_QTP20&-ds_name=DEC_2000_SF3_U)

Education

The educational level of the older population is increasing (Figure 1-6). Between 1970 and 2008, the percentage of older persons who had completed high school rose from 28% to 77.4%. In 2008, about 20.5% had a bachelor's degree or higher. Completion of high school varies considerably by race and ethnic origin: 82.3% of the white population, 73.9% of Asians and Pacific Islanders, 59.7% of African Americans, and 45.9% of Hispanics. However, the increase in educational levels is also evident within these groups. In 1970, only 30% of older white individuals and 9% of African Americans had completed high school (Administration on Aging, 2009). The baby boomers, and people currently 65 to 69 years of age, are more educated than the current old-old and future generations will continue this educational trend.

Income and Employment

In 2008 households headed by persons 65 and over reported a median income of $44,188. Median income varies as follows by race and culture: $46,527 for non-Hispanic whites, $32,901 for Hispanics, $35,025 for African Americans, and $38,859 for Asians. The percentage of people living below the poverty level was 9.7% in 2008. However, a recent report by the Alliance for Children and Families (2010) notes that 18% of Americans will have experienced poverty by the age of 70, 29% by the age of 80, and 41% by the age of 90. Longer life expectancies, fluctuating economic conditions, and rising health care costs contribute to increasing concerns about poverty in old age in this country.

Gender, racial, and cultural disparities exist. One of every 14 older white individuals was poor in 2008, compared with 20% of older African Americans and 19.3% of Hispanics. Women make up 6 or the 10 older people at risk or already living in poverty (Alliance for Children and Families, 2010). The highest poverty rates were experienced by older Hispanic women (43%) and older African American women (34.7%) who lived alone. Women, particularly culturally and ethnically diverse women, face great challenges as they age. The United States has one of the highest poverty rates for older women among industrialized countries. The problems of aging are largely problems of older women. Factors influencing the poverty status of older women include pay inequity, occupational segregation, caregiving responsibilities, longer life expectancy, rising health care costs, and women's work patterns, all of which reduce pension earnings, public assistance benefits, and personal savings (Hounsell and Riojas, 2006).

An increasing number of people over the age of 65 are remaining in or returning to the workforce. Between 2006 and 2016, the number of people age 55 to 64 who are working is expected to climb by 36.5%. The number of workers over the age of 75 will rise by more than 80% during that time period. By 2016, workers over the age of 65 will account for 6.1% of the total labor force, up sharply from their 2006 rate of 3.6%. Some of this is because of a desire to continue their careers but is more frequently out of economic necessity (Administration on Aging, 2009; Hooyman and Kiyak, 2011) (Figure 1-7).

Diversity of Aging in the United States

Racially and culturally diverse older people make up about 19% of all older Americans. This is projected to increase to

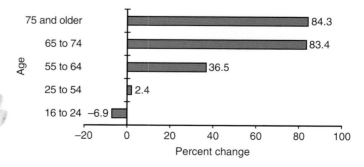

FIGURE 1-7 Projected Percentage Change in Labor Force, by Age: 2006-2016. (Redrawn from U.S. Bureau of Labor Statistics: *Older workers: are there more older people in the workplace?* Available at http://www.bls.gov/spotlight/2008/older_workers/ [accessed November 2010].)

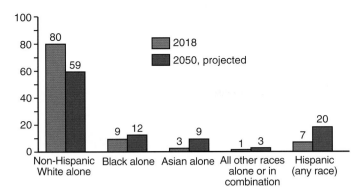

FIGURE 1-8 Population Age 65 Years and Over, by Race and Hispanic Origin: 2008 and Projected 2050. (Redrawn from Federal Interagency Forum on Aging-related Statistics: *Older Americans 2010: key indicators of well-being,* Washington DC, 2010, U.S. Government Printing Office.)

approximately 40% by 2050. Most of this growth in racially and culturally diverse Americans is a result of patterns of immigration and higher fertility rates. The number of African-American elders will increase by 128%; the population of Asian-American elders will increase by 301%; Hispanic-American elders will grow 322%; and Native Americans and Alaska Native elders will increase by about 193%. By 2050, the percentage of the older population that is non-Hispanic white is expected to decline from 84% to 64%. Among all ethnic and racial groups, the Hispanic older population is projected to grow the fastest, from about 2 million in 2000 to more than 13 million by 2050 (Figure 1-8). The fastest growth will occur in those 85 years of age and older. By midcentury, groups that have historically been called minorities will become the majority in most states (Administration on Aging, 2009; Hooyman and Kiyak, 2011).

Although the health status of racial and ethnic groups has improved over the past century, disparities in major health indicators between white and nonwhite groups are growing. Increasing the numbers of health care providers from different cultures and ensuring cultural competence of all providers is essential to meet the needs of a rapidly growing, ethnically diverse elderly population. Chapter 5 discusses gender and cultural issues in aging in more detail.

Global Aging

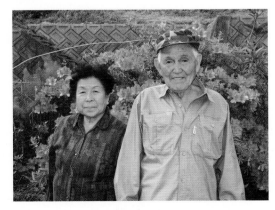

An elder couple in Japan. Courtesy of Mio Oto, PhD, RN, Tokyo Metropolitan Geriatric Hospital and Institute of Gerontology, Human Care Research Team, Tokyo, Japan.

The world population, now totaling more than 6 billion people, is getting older. Projections by the united nations show that by 2050, there will be more people 60 years and older than people younger than 15 years. In fewer than 50 years, one person in five will be older than 60 years. Western Europe and Japan already have more older people than young people, and they will be joined by the rest of Asia in 2040 and the United States shortly thereafter. Asia, Latin America, and Africa are already home to more than two thirds of the world's older people.

Japan (82.6 years), Hong Kong (82.6 years), Hong Kong (82.2), Iceland (81.8 years), and Switzerland (81.7 years) have the longest life expectancy. Of course, these statistics are influenced by the infant mortality rates, which are lowest in Sweden, Iceland, Japan, and Singapore. The United States has a higher infant mortality rate than 28 other countries and ranks 38th in life expectancy at birth (Population Division, Department of Economic and Social Affairs, United Nations, 2009). In 2010, the infant mortality rate in the United States, which has been at the same level for years, dropped about 2% to a record low of 6.59 deaths per 1,000 births. However, the rate for black infants is about twice that of whites (Minino, Xu, Kochanek, 2010).

Experts predict that the number of older people in the developing world will double in the next 20 years. In 2015, 67% of the world's older people will live in developing countries (Figure 1-9). Older people in developed and developing countries face different challenges as they age. James Martin, in an address to the International Federation on Aging in 2006, calls this a century of extremes. In the United States, we are studying regenerative medicine and predicting that people could live to 120 years, whereas in Botswana, life expectancy is 27 years. Around the world, 100 million older people live on $1 or less per day. Poverty, hunger, and lack of access to basic life necessities are all too common in developing countries for people of all ages. Of older people in developing countries, 80% have no regular income, lack of food is a serious cause of ill health, and older widows are among the poorest and most vulnerable groups.

The human immunodeficiency virus (HIV)/acquired immunodeficiency syndrome (AIDS) epidemic has had devastating economic, social, physical, and psychological effects on older women and men, especially in sub-Saharan Africa. Almost 13 million children have lost one or both parents to HIV/AIDS, the vast majority in sub-Saharan Africa. As many as 9 of 10 orphans are cared for by their extended family, mainly the grandparents (see www.helpage.org). As we study how to care for older people, it is important to remember that our view must be expanded to include older people across the globe, who have very different needs. More details on international aging can be found in the International Plan of Action on Ageing (available at http://www.un.org/esa/socdev/ageing/madrid_intlplanaction.html).

Who Will Care for an Aging Society?

America's eldercare workforce is dangerously understaffed and unprepared to care for the growing numbers of older adults. The demand for gerontological nurses and other health

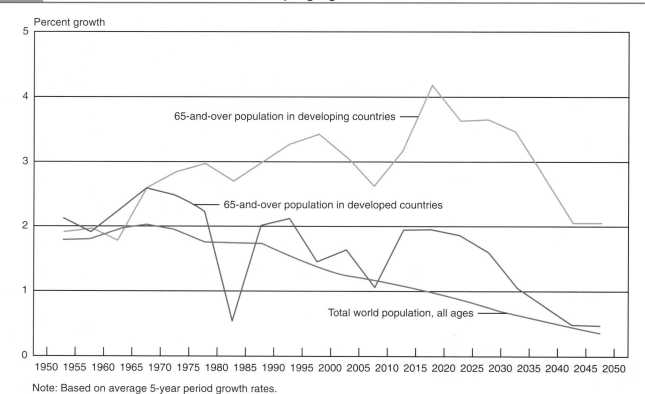

Note: Based on average 5-year period growth rates.

FIGURE 1-9 Average Annual Percent Growth of Older Population in Developed and Developing Countries: 1950 to 2050. (Kinsella K and Wan H: U.S. Census Bureau, International Population Reports, P95/09-1, *An Aging World*: 2008, U.S. Government Printing Office, Washington, DC, 2009.)

professionals, as well as direct care staff, prepared to deliver care in all settings is critical. Older adults are the core consumers of health care, with higher rates of outpatient provider visits, hospitalizations, home care, and long-term care service use than other age groups. Eldercare is projected to be the fastest growing employment sector in the health care industry. In spite of demand, the number of health care workers who are interested and prepared to care for older people remains low (Institute of Medicine, 2008). Less than 1% of registered nurses and only 6% of advanced practice nurses are certified in gerontology (Mezey et al., 2004).

Geriatric medicine faces similar challenges with just 7,128 geriatricians, one for every 2,546 older Americans. By 2030, it is estimated that this number will increase to only 7,750, one for every 4,254 older Americans, far short of the predicted need for 36,000 (Institute of Medicine, 2008). Other professions such as social work have similar shortages.

The Eldercare Workforce Alliance, a group of 28 national organizations representing older adults and the eldercare workforce, including family caregivers, health care professionals, and direct care workers, has begun to address these concerns. Immediate goals of the Alliance are to strengthen the direct care workforce through better training, supervision, and improved compensation; address clinician and faculty shortages through incentives such as loan forgiveness, increased public funding for training, and better compensation; ensure a competent workforce by encouraging agencies and organizations that certify and regulate the eldercare workforce to require demonstrated and continued competence; and redesign health care

delivery by adopting cost-effective care coordination models (www.eldercareworkforce.org/). Improving the competency and adequacy of the eldercare workforce is essential to meet the needs and demands of a burgeoning aging population. "The consequences of inaction will be profound" (American Geriatrics Society, 2005, p. S246).

DEVELOPMENT OF GERONTOLOGICAL NURSING

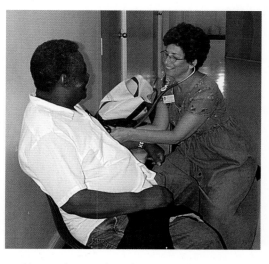

Nurses provide care in a number of settings. (Courtesy Kathleen Jett.)

Efforts to determine the appropriate term for nurses caring for older people have included gerontic nurses, gerontological nurses, and geriatric nurses. None of these terms is restrictive. We presently prefer the term gerontological nurse. *Gerontological* nursing has emerged as a circumscribed area of practice only within the past six decades. Before 1950, gerontological nursing was seen as the application of general principles of nursing to the older adult client with little recognition of this area of medical nursing as a specialty similar to obstetric, pediatric, or surgical nursing. Whereas most specialties in nursing developed from those identified in medicine, this was not the case with gerontological nursing because health care of the older adult was traditionally considered within the domain of general nursing (Davis, 1985). In examining the history of gerontological nursing, one must marvel at the advocacy and perseverance of nurses who have remained deeply committed to the care of older adults despite struggling against insurmountable odds over the years.

The foundation of gerontological nursing as we know it today was built between 30 and 50 years ago, largely by a small cadre of nurse pioneers, many of whom are now gone. The specialty was defined and shaped by these innovative nurses who saw, early on, that older individuals had special needs and required the most subtle, holistic, and complex nursing care. These pioneers presented seminal thoughts and investigated new ideas related to the care of older people; refuted mythical tales and fantasies about aging; and found realities through investigation, clinical observation, practice, and documentation, setting in motion activities that markedly influenced the course of the aging experience. They saw new possibilities and a better future for older people. The wisdom they shared is still relevant today, and we owe them a debt of gratitude for their commitment, compassion, and persistence in establishing the specialty practice. Box 1-1 presents the views of some of the geriatric nursing pioneers, as well as of current leaders, on the practice of gerontological nursing and what draws them

---

BOX 1-1 REFLECTIONS ON GERONTOLOGICAL NURSING FROM GERONTOLOGICAL NURSING PIONEERS AND CURRENT LEADERS IN THE FIELD

Doris Schwartz, Gerontological Nursing Pioneer

"We need to remind ourselves constantly that the purpose of gerontic nursing is to prevent untimely death and needless suffering, always with the focus of doing with as well as doing for, and in every instance to attempt to preserve personhood as long as life continues."

(From interview data collected by Priscilla Ebersole between 1990 and 2001.)

Mary Opal Wolanin, Gerontological Nursing Pioneer

"I believe that one of the most valuable lessons I have learned from those who are older is that I must start with looking inside at my own thinking. I was very guilty of ageism. I believed every myth in the book, was sure that I would never live past my seventieth birthday, and made no plan for my seventies. Probably the most productive years of my career have been since that dreaded birthday and I now realize that it is very difficult, if not impossible, to think of our own aging."

(From interview data collected by Priscilla Ebersole between 1990 and 2001.)

Bernita Steffl, Gerontological Nursing Pioneer

"There is always an interesting person there, sometimes locked in the cage of age. I think I have helped at least a few of my students with this approach, 'You see me as I am now, but I see myself as I've always been and all the things I've been—not just an old lady.'"

(Bernita Steffl) Ebersole P, Touhy T: *Geriatric nursing: growth of a specialty*, New York, 2006, Springer, p. 52)

Terry Fulmer, Dean, College of Nursing, New York University and Co-Director, John A. Hartford Institute for Geriatric Nursing

"I soon realized that in the arena of caring for the aged, I could have an autonomous nursing practice that would make a real difference in medical outcomes. I could practice the full scope of nursing. It gave me a sense of freedom and accomplishment. With older patients, the most important component of care, by far, is nursing care. It's very motivating."

(Ebersole P, Touhy T: *Geriatric nursing: growth of a specialty*, New York, 2006, Springer, p. 129.)

Neville Strumpf, Edith Clemmer Steinbright Professor in Gerontology, University of Pennsylvania, Director of the Hartford Center of Geriatric Nursing Excellence and Center for Gerontological Nursing Science

"My philosophy remains deeply rooted in individual choice, comfort and dignity, especially for frail, older adults. I fervently hope that the future will be characterized by a health care system capable of supporting these values throughout a person's life, and that we shall someday see the routine application of evidence based practice to the care of all older adults, whether they are in the community, a hospital, or the nursing home. We have not yet achieved that dream."

(Ebersole P, Touhy T: *Geriatric nursing: growth of a specialty*, New York, 2006, Springer, p. 145.)

Mathy Mezey, Professor Emerita and Associate Director, The Hartford Institute for Geriatric Nursing, New York University College of Nursing

"Because geriatric nursing especially offers nurses the unique opportunity to dramatically impact people's lives for the better and for the worst, it demands the best that you have to offer. I am very optimistic about the future of geriatric nursing. Increasing numbers of older adults are interested in marching into old age as healthy and involved. Geriatric nursing offers a unique opportunity to help older adults meet these aspirations while at the same time maintaining a commitment to the oldest and frailest in our society."

(Ebersole P, Touhy T: *Geriatric nursing: growth of a specialty*, New York, 2006, Springer, p. 142.)

Jennifer Lingler, PhD, RN, FNP Assistant Professor, School of Nursing, University of Pittsburgh

"When I was in high school, a nurse I knew helped me find a nursing assistant position at the residential care facility where she worked. That experience sparked my interest in older adults that continues today. I realized that caring for frail elders could be incredibly gratifying, and I felt privileged to play a role, however small, in people's lives. At the same time, I became increasingly curious about what it means to age successfully. I questioned why some people seemed to age so gracefully, while others succumbed to physical illness, mental decline, or both. As a Building Academic Geriatric Nursing Capacity (BAGNC) alumnus, I now divide my time serving as a nurse practitioner at a memory disorders clinic, teaching an ethics course in a gerontology program, and conducting research on family caregiving. I am encouraged by the realization that as current students contemplate the array of opportunities before them, seek counsel from trusted mentors, and gain exposure to various clinical populations, the next generation of geriatric nurses will emerge. And, I am confident that in doing so, they will set their own course for affecting change in the lives of society's most vulnerable members."

(Jennifer Lingler as cited in Fagin C, Franklin P: Why choose geriatric nursing? Six nursing scholars tell their stories, *Imprint* September/October, 2005, p. 74.)

to the specialty (Box 1-1). For a comprehensive review of the history of the specialty, including Dr. Ebersole's interviews with geriatric nursing pioneers, the reader is referred to Geriatric Nursing: Growth of a Specialty (Ebersole and Touhy, 2006). Nurses are proud to be the standard bearers of excellence in the care of older people (Table 1-1).

Early History

The origins of gerontological nursing are rooted in England and began with Florence Nightingale as she accepted a position in the Institution for the Care of Sick Gentlewomen in Distressed Circumstances. Nightingale's concern for the frail and sick elderly was continued by Agnes Jones, a wealthy Nightingale-trained nurse, who in 1864 was sent to Liverpool Infirmary, a large Poor Law institution. The care in the institution had been poor, the diet meager, and the nurses often drunk. But Miss Jones, under the tutelage of Nightingale, improved the care dramatically, as well as reduced the costs.

In the United States, almshouses were the destination of destitute older people and were insufferable places with "deplorable conditions, neglect, preventable suffering, contagion, and death from lack of proper medical and nursing care" (Crane, 1907, p. 873). As early as 1906, Lavinia Dock and other early leaders in nursing addressed, in the *American Journal of Nursing* (AJN), the needs of the elderly chronically ill in almshouses. Dock and her colleagues cited the immediate need for trained nurses and pupil education in almshouses, "so that these evils, all of which lie strictly in the sphere of housekeeping and nursing,—two spheres which have always been lauded as women's own—might not occur" (Dock, 1908, p. 523). In 1912 the American Nurses Association (ANA) Board of Directors appointed an Almshouse Committee to continue to oversee nursing in these institutions. World War I distracted them from attention to these needs. But in 1925, the ANA advanced the idea of a specialty in the nursing care of the aged.

With the passage of the Social Security Act of 1935, federal monies were provided for old-age insurance and public assistance for needy older people not covered by insurance. To combat the fear of almshouse placement, Congress stipulated that the Social Security funds could not be used to pay for care in almshouses or other public institutions. This move is thought to have been the genesis of commercial nursing homes. During the next 10 years, many almshouses closed and the number of private boarding homes providing care to elders increased. Because retired and widowed nurses often converted their homes into such living quarters and gave care when their boarders became ill, they can be considered the first geriatric nurses and their homes the first nursing homes.

Two nursing journals in the 1940s described centers of excellence for geriatric care: the Cuyahoga County Nursing Home in Ohio and the Hebrew Home for the Aged in New York. An article in the AJN by Sarah Gelbach (1943) recommended that nurses should have not only an aptitude for working with the elderly but also specific geriatric education. The first textbook on nursing care of the elderly was published by Newton and Anderson in 1950, and the first published nursing research on chronic disease and the elderly (Mack, 1952) appeared in the premier issue of *Nursing Research* in 1952.

In 1962 a focus group was formed to discuss geriatric nursing, and in 1966 a geriatric practice group was convened. However, it was not until 1966 that the ANA formed a Division of Geriatric Nursing. The first geriatric standards were published by the ANA in 1968, and soon after, geriatric nursing certification was offered. Geriatric nursing was the first specialty to establish standards of practice within the ANA. In 1976 the Division of Geriatric Nursing changed its name to the Gerontological Nursing Division to reflect the broad role nurses play in the care of older people. In 1984 the Council on Gerontological Nursing was formed and certification for geriatric nurse practitioners (GNPs) and gerontological clinical nurse specialists (GCNSs) became available. Nursing was the first of the professions to develop standards of gerontological care and the first to provide a certification mechanism to ensure specific professional expertise through credentialing (Ebersole and Touhy, 2006).

Today, nurses can be certified at both the generalist and specialist levels (GNP, GCNS) in gerontological nursing (see http://www.nursecredentialing.org/). The most recent edition of *Scope and Standards of Gerontological Nursing Practice* was published in 2010 and identifies levels of gerontological nursing practice (basic and advanced) and standards of clinical gerontological nursing care and gerontological nursing performance.

Current Initiatives

The most significant influence in enhancing gerontological nursing has been the work of the Hartford Institute for Geriatric Nursing, funded by the John A. Hartford Foundation. Mathy Mezey, EdD, RN, FAAN, directed the institute, located in the College of Nursing at New York University, from its inception in 1996 until 2010 and now serves as an Associate Director. It is the only nurse-led organization in the country seeking to shape the quality of the nation's health care for older Americans by promoting geriatric nursing excellence to both the nursing profession and the larger health care community. Initiatives in nursing education, nursing practice, nursing research, and nursing policy include enhancing geriatrics in nursing education programs through curricular reform and faculty development, the development of nine Centers of Geriatric Nursing Excellence, predoctoral and postdoctoral scholarships for study and research in geriatric nursing, and clinical practice improvement projects to enhance care for older adults (Mackin et al., 2006; Miller et al., 2006; Souder et al., 2006) (see www.hartfordign.org).

Another significant influence on improving care for older adults was the Nurse Competence in Aging (NCA) project, a 5-year initiative created in 2002 through an alliance of the ANA, the American Nurses Credentialing Center (ANCC), and the Hartford Institute for Geriatric Nursing. Funded by Atlantic Philanthropies, through the American Nurses Foundation, the initiative addressed the need to ensure competence in geriatrics among nursing specialty organizations. The initiative provided grant and technical assistance to more than 50 specialty nursing organizations, developed a free web-based comprehensive gerontological nursing resource center (ConsultGeriRN.org) where nurses can access evidence-based information on topics related to the care of older adults (see www.consultgerirn.org),

TABLE 1-1   PROFESSIONALIZATION OF GERONTOLOGICAL NURSING

YEAR	ACHIEVEMENT
1906	First article published in *American Journal of Nursing* (AJN) on care of the elderly
1925	AJN considers geriatric nursing as a possible specialty in nursing
1950	Newton and Anderson publish first geriatric nursing textbook
	Geriatrics becomes a specialization in nursing
1962	American Nurses Association (ANA) forms a national geriatric nursing group
1966	ANA creates the Division of Geriatric Nursing
	First master's program for clinical nurse specialists in geriatric nursing developed by Virginia Stone at Duke University
1970	ANA establishes Standards of Practice for Geriatric Nursing
1974	Certification in geriatric nursing practice offered through the ANA; process implemented by Laurie Gunter and Virginia Stone
1975	*Journal of Gerontological Nursing* published by SLACK; first editor, Edna Stilwell
1976	ANA renames Geriatric Division "Gerontological" to reflect a health promotion emphasis
	ANA publishes *Standards for Gerontological Nursing Practice*; committee chaired by Barbara Allen Davis
	ANA begins certifying geriatric nurse practitioners
	Nursing and the Aged is edited by Irene Burnside and published by McGraw-Hill
1977	First gerontological nursing track funded by the Division of Nursing and established by Sister Rose Therese Bahr at the University of Kansas School of Nursing
1979	*Education for Gerontic Nursing* written by Laurie Gunter and Carmen Estes; suggested curricula for all levels of nursing education
1980	*Geriatric Nursing* first published by AJN; Cynthia Kelly, editor
1983	Florence Cellar Endowed Gerontological Nursing Chair established at Case Western Reserve University, first in the nation; Doreen Norton, first scholar to occupy chair
	National Conference of Gerontological Nurse Practitioners established (now the gerontological advanced practice nurses association)
1984	National Gerontological Nursing Association established
	Division of Gerontological Nursing Practice becomes Council on Gerontological Nursing (councils established for all practice specialties)
1989	ANA certifies gerontological clinical nurse specialists
1992	John A. Hartford Foundation funds a major initiative to improve care of hospitalized older patients: Nurses Improving Care for Healthsystem Elders (NICHE)
1996	John A. Hartford Foundation establishes the Institute for Geriatric Nursing at New York University under the direction of Mathy Mezey
2000	Recommended baccalaureate competencies and curricular guidelines for geriatric nursing care published by the American Association of Colleges of Nursing and the John A. Hartford Foundation Institute for Geriatric Nursing
	The American Academy of Nursing established Building Academic Geriatric Nursing Capacity (BAGNC) in 2000 with support from the John A. Hartford Foundation
2001	Hartford Institute for Geriatric Nursing Coalition of Geriatric Nursing Associations formed
2002	Nurse Competence in Aging (funded by the Atlantic Philanthropies) initiative to improve the quality of health care to older adults by enhancing the geriatric competence of nurses who are members of specialty nursing organizations
2004	*Nurse Practitioner and Clinical Nurse Specialist Competencies for Older Adult Care* published by the American Association of Colleges of Nursing and the Hartford Institute for Geriatric Nursing
2007	Atlantic Philanthropies provides a grant to the American Academy of Nursing of $500,000 to improve care of older adults in nursing homes by improving the clinical skills of professional nurses
	American Association for Long-term Care Nurses formed
2008	Four new Centers of Geriatric Nursing Excellence (CGNEs) are funded by the John A. Hartford Foundation, bringing the total number of centers to nine. Existing centers are at the University of Iowa, University of California San Francisco, Oregon Health Sciences University, University of Arkansas, University of Pennsylvania, Arizona State University, Pennsylvania State University, University of Minnesota, and University of Utah
	Research in Gerontological Nursing is launched by SLACK; editor, Dr. Kitty Buckwalter
	Geriatric Nursing Leadership Academy established by Sigma Theta Tau International with funding from the John A. Hartford Foundation
	John A. Hartford Foundation funds the Geropsychiatric Nursing Collaborative (Universities of Iowa, Arkansas, and Pennsylvania; American Academy of Nursing)
	Institute of Medicine publishes *Retooling for an Aging America: Building the Health Care Workforce* report
2009	*National Consensus Model for APRN Regulation, Licensure, Accreditation, Certification and Education* designates adult-gerontology as one of six population foci for APRNs
	John A. Hartford Foundation funds Phase 2 of the Fostering Geriatrics in Pre-Licensure Nursing Education, a partnership between the Community College of Philadelphia and the National League for Nursing
2010	Adult-gerontology primary care nurse practitioner competencies published by the John A. Hartford Foundation Institute for Geriatric Nursing, the AACN, and National Organization of Nurse Practitioner Faculties (NONPF)
	Sigma Theta Tau's Center for Nursing Excellence established
	ANA publishes Gerontological Nursing: Scope and Standards of Practice
	AACN and Hartford Institute for Geriatric Nursing publishes Recommended Baccalaureate Competencies and Curricular Guidelines for the Nursing Care of Older Adults

ACNP, acute care nurse practitioner; ANP, adult nurse practitioner; APRN, advanced practice registered nurse; FNP, family nurse practitioner; GNP, geriatric nurse practitioner.

Note: For a complete listing of John A. Hartford Foundation funding for geriatric nursing see http://www.hgni.org/091008%20HGNI%20Project%20Descriptions.pdf

and conducted a national gerontological nursing certification outreach (Stierle et al., 2006).

An extension of this work is the Resourcefully Enhancing Aging in Specialty Nursing (REASN) project, funded in 2007 by Atlantic Philanthropies, to extend the involvement of specialty nursing organizations in improving competencies in providing care to older adults. This project focuses on building intensive collaborations with 13 hospital-based specialty associations to create geriatric educational products and resources to ensure the geriatric competencies of their members (see http://hartfordign.org/Resources/specialty_practice/).

In 2008 a $1.6 million grant from the John A. Hartford Foundation was awarded to Sigma Theta Tau International (STTI) to establish the Geriatric Nursing Leadership Academy (GNLA). Working with the Hartford Centers of Geriatric Nursing Excellence, the purpose of the GNLA is to develop the leadership skills of geriatric nurses in positions of influence in a variety of health care settings and to improve the quality of health care for older adults and their families (www. nursingsociety.org/LeadershipInstitute/GeriatricAcademy/ Pages/introduction.aspx).*

GERONTOLOGICAL NURSING EDUCATION

Most nurses will care for older people during the course of their careers regardless of the setting. However, schools of nursing have only begun to include gerontological nursing content in their curricula and most still do not have freestanding courses in the specialty similar to courses in maternal/child or psychiatric nursing. When content is integrated throughout the curriculum, less than 25% of the content is devoted to geriatric care (Berman et al., 2005). "Gerontological nursing content needs to be integrated throughout the curriculum, in addition to a stand-alone course, so that gerontology is valued and viewed as an integral part of nursing care" (Miller et al., 2009, p. 198).

Faculty with expertise in gerontological nursing are scarce; less than 30% of baccalaureate programs have at least one full-time faculty member certified in gerontological nursing (Berman et al., 2005; Mackin et al., 2006). Important resources for faculty education in gerontological nursing include the Geriatric Nursing Education Consortium (GNEC), the Advancing Care Excellence for Seniors (ACES), the Hartford Geriatric Nursing Initiative (HGNI), and the Building Academic Geriatric Nursing Capacity (BAGNC).

The purpose of the GNEC, a national initiative of the American Association of Colleges of Nursing (AACN) with funding from the John A. Hartford Foundation, is to enhance geriatric content in senior-level undergraduate courses. As a result of this project, 808 faculty from 418 schools of nursing from all 50 states have been educated in the fundamentals of geriatric nursing and the use of geriatric curriculum resources. The GNEC educational curriculum and evidence-based modules reflecting the state-of-the-science approach to care for older

adults are available electronically and via Webinars (see http:// www.aacn.nche.edu/gnec.htm).

Advancing Care Excellence for Seniors (ACES), a 3-year grant funded by the John A. Hartford Foundation to foster gerontological nursing education in prelicensure programs, is a collaborative effort between the National League for Nursing (NLN) and the Community College of Philadelphia. ACES provides faculty development materials, teaching tools and strategies, and curricular guidelines, and essential nursing actions to Advance Care Excellence for Seniors (see www.nln.org/ACES and Evolve Resources at http://evolve.elsevier.com/Ebersole/ TwdHlthAging).

The BAGNC initiative includes the Building Geriatric Nursing Capacity Scholars and Fellows Awards Program and the nine Hartford Centers of Geriatric Nursing Excellence. This program, coordinated by the American Academy of Nursing, has stimulated increasing interest in academic geriatric nursing through scholarships and fellowships for research, faculty, and leadership development (see http://www.geriatricnursing.org/ about/about.asp).

The Essentials of Baccalaureate Education for Professional Nursing Practice (AACN, 2008) specifically addresses the importance of geriatric content and structured clinical experiences with older adults across the continuum in the education of students. In 2010, AACN and the Hartford Institute for Geriatric Nursing, New York University, published the *Recommended Baccalaureate Competencies and Curricular Guidelines for the Nursing Care of Older Adults,* a supplement to The Essentials document (See Appendix 1-A). In addition, gerontological nursing competencies for baccalaureate and graduate programs preparing advanced practice nurses in specialties other than gerontological nursing have been developed (see http:// www.aacn.nche.edu/Education/Hartford/resources.htm). Those in the field of nursing education must seriously consider specific minimal requirements in the care of older adults at each level of education to fulfill the responsibility of nurses to the public and the profession and to meet accreditation criteria. All nursing education programs should be "gerontologized" to ensure that graduates are competent enough to meet the needs of an aging population.

GERONTOLOGICAL NURSING ROLES

Gerontological nursing roles encompass every imaginable venue and circumstance. The opportunities are limitless because we are a rapidly aging society. Older adults are the largest consumers of health care services in all settings and the majority of nurses practicing today are caring for geriatric patients (Gebhardt et al., 2009). In acute care facilities, older adults comprise 60% of the medical-surgical patients and 46% of critical care patients. Kagan reminds us that "older adults are the work of hospitals but most nurses practicing in hospitals do not say they specialize in geriatrics ... We, as a profession and a force in an aging society, must make the transformation to understanding care of older adults is acute care nursing" (2008, p. 103).

A gerontological nurse may be a generalist or a specialist. The generalist functions in a variety of settings – hospital, home, subacute and long-term care facilities, community –

---

*For a comprehensive list of websites providing resources for gerontological nurses, see student resources on Evolve at http://evolve. elsevier.com/Ebersole/TwdHlthAging.

providing nursing care to individuals and their families. National certification as a gerontological nurse is a way to enhance the knowledge of nurses who care for older adults and should be encouraged (see http://www.nursecredentialing .org/Documents/Certification/Application/NursingSpecialty/ GerontologicalNurse.aspx).

To prepare nurse generalists, it is important to provide students with nursing practice experiences with elders across the continuum of care. For clinical practice sites, one is not limited to the acute care setting or the nursing home. Creative faculty members consider sites such as retirement homes, assisted living facilities, adult day programs, and senior housing complexes. Experiences with well elders in the community and opportunities to focus on health promotion should be the first experience for students. This will assist them to develop more positive attitudes toward older people, understand the full scope of nursing practice in the specialty, and learn nursing responses to enhance health and wellness. Rehabilitation centers, subacute and skilled nursing facilities, and hospice settings provide opportunities for leadership training, nursing management of complex problems, interdisciplinary teamwork, and research application for more advanced students. Box 1-2 presents a study comparing the nature of nursing work in long-term care (LTC) and the intensive care unit (ICU). Results of the study suggest that ICU nursing work is a biomedically intensive environment, whereas LTC is a nursing intensive environment (Leppa, 2004). (See Chapter 16 for further discussion on practice across the continuum of care.)

The gerontological nursing specialist has advanced preparation at the master's level and performs all of the functions of a generalist but has developed advanced clinical expertise, as well as an understanding of health and social policy and proficiency in planning, implementing, and evaluating health programs. With shortages in nursing faculty prepared in gerontological nursing, there is a critical need for nurses who have master's and doctoral preparation and expertise to care for older adults to assume faculty roles.

One of the most important roles to have emerged in the past several decades is that of the advanced practice gerontological nurse (APGN) as a major service provider. APGNs include geriatric nurse practitioners (GNPs) and gerontological clinical nurse specialists (GCNSs), both prepared at the master's level. The education and training programs arose from evident need, particularly in the long-term care setting. Many GNPs have nursing facility practices managing complex care of frail older adults in collaboration with interprofessional teams.

GNPs serve in geriatric and family practice clinics, long-term care, hospitals, home health care agencies, acute and subacute rehabilitation, continuing care retirement communities, assisted living facilities, hospice, managed care organizations, specialty care clinics (e.g., Alzheimer's, heart failure, diabetes), area agencies on aging, public health departments, schools of nursing, and private practice (see www.gapna.org). There are at present a full range of opportunities to be filled in this growing advanced practice nursing specialty. Practice privileges vary from state to state, but the federal Medicaid and Medicare programs allow for individual provider numbers and direct reimbursement for nationally certified APGNs.

Advanced practice nurses have demonstrated their skill in improving health outcomes and cost-effectiveness. The role of the APGN in skilled nursing facilities is well established, and the positive outcomes for care include increased patient and family satisfaction, decreased costs, less frequent hospitalizations and emergency room visits, and improved quality of care (Bakerjian, 2008). At present, fewer than 6% of all advanced practice nurses are certified as GNPs and GCNSs. These numbers are far short of the current and projected need. Family and adult nurse practitioner programs often attract more students, and

---

BOX 1-2 RESEARCH HIGHLIGHTS

Comparing Long-Term Care Nursing Work with Intensive Care Unit Nursing Work

A pilot study (Leppa, 2004) was done to explore the nature of nursing work in LTC nursing home environments (subacute, Medicare, dementia units) and to compare it with the nature of nursing work in ICU environments, using the Leatt Measure of Nursing Technology (Leatt and Schneck, 1981).* This instrument operationalizes and measures the nature of nursing work in terms of uncertainty (percentage of patients with more than one diagnosis and with complex nursing problems and how much nursing intuition or judgment is required in providing care); variability (percentage of patients with similar health problems in the unit and the variety of nursing techniques used); and instability (percentage of patients requiring frequent observation and care or specialized monitoring and potential emergency situations).

Findings suggest that the nature of work in LTC and ICU environments is comparable in terms of work uncertainty, variability, and instability. Long-term care nursing scores for uncertainty and variability in nursing work were as high as ICU scores. The LTC respondents emphasized the complexity of the medical and psychosocial needs of their patients and families as one theme in the nature of their work. In LTC, nurses must attend to the needs of both individual patients and the wider community. They must grasp how other patients, family members, and nursing staff are affected by the care provided, especially in the dementia units. Respondents discussed the fragility of their patients, the importance of knowing their patterns, and the need for astute observational skills to detect subtle changes that could indicate a change in physiology.

ICU care and LTC require different nursing skills, judgment, and knowledge, but the results of this study suggest that the work of nurses in LTC is as complex and demanding as ICU nursing work and that there are many similarities in terms of uncertainty and nursing judgment, patient variability, and instability. LTC nursing work is performed on multiple levels (individual, family, patient groups, and patient–nursing assistant groups) across the continuum of care (rehabilitation, subacute, custodial, and palliative) and presents a wide variety of opportunities for student learning and professional nursing practice. "The ICU work environment is a biomedically intensive environment and the LTC nursing environment is a nursing intensive environment … highly autonomous and centered on nursing care" (Leppa, 2004, p. 32). Further study is needed to explore the breadth of nursing work in LTC from the perspective of LTC nurses and patients. A better understanding of the complexities of this type of nursing work may help attract more students and nurses to this speciality. LTC nursing work is challenging, highly autonomous, requires specialized knowledge and skills, and should be seen as different, not as "less than" because it does not involve as much medical technology.

ICU, intensive care unit; *LTC,* long-term care.

Data from Leppa CJ: The nature of long-term care nursing work, Journal of Gerontological Nursing 30:26, 2004.
*Leatt P, Schneck R: Nursing subunit technology: a replication, *Administrative Science Quarterly* 26:225, 1981.

many of these graduates go on to practices that include a large number of older adults. Some have had intensive attention in their curricula to gerontological nursing care, but some have not and must learn on the job. The lack of faculty with expertise in gerontological nursing, sparse attention to gerontological nursing in basic nursing programs, and the routing of federal grants for education in medicine and nursing to family practice are some of the reasons for the low numbers of nurses choosing graduate preparation in gerontological nursing.

The national *Consensus Model for APRN Regulation: Licensure, Accreditation, Certification, and Education* (LACE), finalized in 2008, defines advanced practice registered nurses (APRNs) and standardized requirements for each of the four APRN regulatory components included in LACE. Under the Consensus Model for APRN Regulation, APRNs must be educated, certified, and licensed to practice in a role and a population. In addition to the four roles, APRNs are educated and practice in at least one of six population foci: family/individuals across the life span, adult-gerontology, pediatrics, neonatal, women's health/gender-related, or psychiatric-mental health.

The Hartford Institute for Geriatric Nursing, the AACN, and the National Organization of Nurse Practitioner Faculties (NONPF) have published Adult-Gerontology Primary Care Nurse Practitioner Competencies (AACN, 2010). Resources for both faculty and students will also be developed and include gerontology-focused content modules, curricular models, and case studies to provide guidance for the development and implementation of the adult-gerontology primary care NP curriculum.

The Patient Protection and Affordable Care Act, signed into law in March 2010, provides many initiatives that will have a direct impact on gerontological nursing with regard to workforce, education, and practice. It is anticipated that there will be additional federal funding to support advanced education in gerontological nursing, education of faculty, and advanced training for direct care workers employed in long-term care settings (see http://hartfordign.org/policy/healthcare_tips/).

ORGANIZATIONS DEVOTED TO GERONTOLOGY RESEARCH AND PRACTICE

The Gerontological Society of America (GSA) demonstrates the need for interdisciplinary collaboration in research and practice. The divisions of Biological Sciences, Health Sciences, Behavioral and Social Sciences, Social Research, and Policy and Practice include individuals from myriad backgrounds and disciplines who affiliate with a section based on their particular function rather than their educational or professional credentials. Nurses can be found in all sections and occupy important positions as officers and committee chairs in the GSA.

This mingling of the disciplines based on practice interests is also characteristic of the American Society on Aging (ASA). Other interdisciplinary organizations have joined forces to strengthen the field. The Association for Gerontology in Higher Education (AGHE) has partnered with the GSA, and the National Council on Aging (NCOA) is affiliated with the ASA. These organizations and others have encouraged the blending of ideas and functions, furthering our understanding of old age

and of the integration necessary for optimal care. International gerontology associations, such as the International Federation on Aging and the International Association of Gerontology and Geriatrics, also have interdisciplinary membership and offer the opportunity to study aging internationally.

Organizations specific to gerontological nursing include the National Gerontological Nursing Association (NGNA), the Gerontological Advanced Practice Nurses Association (GAPNA), the National Association Directors of Nursing Administration in Long Term Care (NADONA/LTC) (also includes assisted living RNs and LPNs/LVNs as associate members), The American Association for Long-term Care Nursing (AALTCN), and the Canadian Gerontological Nursing Association (CGNA). The CGNA, founded in 1985, addresses the health needs of older Canadians and the nurses who care for them. In 2003, the CGNA formed an alliance with the NGNA to exchange information and share mutual goals and opportunities for the advancement of both groups (Mantle, 2005). In 2001, the Coalition of Geriatric Nursing Organizations (CGNO) was established to improve the health care of older adults across care settings. The CGNO represents more than 28,700 geriatric nurses from 8 national organizations and is supported by the Hartford Institute for Geriatric Nursing and located at New York University College of Nursing (New York, NY).

RESEARCH ON AGING

In the nearly four decades since the institution of Medicare and Medicaid, growth in gerontology as a scientific pursuit has been colossal. Federal and foundation dollars in support of research and research training have attracted many to the field of aging.

Some of the major problems in aging research are that older people, although statistically ranging from 65 to 115 years old, are often grouped into a single category. Studies of older people often include those 50 years old, eligible for certain memberships and discounts based on age deference, and the 104-year-old residing in a nursing home. These are considered a group, although they have few if any similar characteristics. Research and gerontological knowledge are strongly influenced by federal bulletins that are distributed nationwide to indicate the type of research most likely to receive federal funding. These are published in requests for proposals (RFPs). In a very real way, the "alzheimerization" of aging has come about because, since the establishment of the National Institute on Aging (NIA) in 1971, the study of Alzheimer's disease has been awarded the largest share of research dollars for aging. Alzheimer's disease remains a primary area of research concentration, with a considerable focus on etiology, prevention, and medications that may halt or slow progress of the disease. Many gerontologists believe that the amount of funding is inadequate in light of projections concerning the number of older people who will develop Alzheimer's disease (Chapter 19).

The investigators of the Baltimore Longitudinal Studies of the Aged have been collecting data and periodically publishing findings for almost 40 years. These studies were initially restricted to males, but more recently studies of females have been included as well. Several substantial longitudinal studies of older people are now presenting current evidence about elders from several cohorts.

The NIA, the National Institute of Nursing Research, the National Institute of Mental Health, and the Agency for Health Care Research and Quality continue to make significant research contributions to our understanding of older people. The meaning and experience of aging remain elusive, complex, and highly individualistic. Phenomenological studies have the potential to provide some of the richest information about the lived experience of aging. However, in both quantitative and qualitative research, the study of culturally and racially diverse older people is most lacking.

Nursing Research

Gerontological nursing research and practice have evolved to such a point that the best practice standards are being published and distributed widely. Nurses have generated significant research on the care of older adults and have established a solid foundation for the practice of gerontological nursing. Research with older adults receives considerable funding from the National Institute of Nursing Research (NINR), and their website (www.nih.gov/ninr) provides information about results of studies as well as funding opportunities. *Research in Gerontological Nursing,* a new journal edited by Dr. Kitty Buckwalter, published its first issue in 2008. Gerontological nurse researchers publish in many of the journals devoted to gerontology.

Nursing research has significantly affected the quality of life of older people and gains more prominence each decade. Federal funding for gerontological nursing research is increasing and more nurse scholars are studying nursing issues related to older people. Many nursing research studies and evidence-based protocols are featured in this text. Some of the most important nursing studies have investigated methods of caring for individuals with dementia, reducing falls and the use of restraints, pain management, delirium, care transitions, and end-of-life care.

Miller and colleagues (2006) note that little research has been conducted on community-based living alternatives, such as assisted living settings, for older adults. These authors suggest the following research priorities: community and home-care resources for older adults, family caregiving issues (particularly minority elders), research on diverse older populations, and

a shift from the emphasis on illness and disease to the expectation of wellness, even in the presence of chronic illness and functional impairment. Translational research and continued attention to interdisciplinary studies are increasingly important. Gerontological nurse scholars and researchers May Wykle and Ruth Tappen have identified areas in most need of gerontological nursing research (Ebersole and Touhy, 2006) (Box 1-3).

THE POLITICS OF AGING

The actual development of gerontology has probably been more influenced by political expediency than by any other factor, but politics and economics are so intermeshed that they can rarely be untangled. In the United States, the first real interest in aging emerged in the 1930s, when a population of older persons, who were largely impoverished, became demographically significant. Under the Roosevelt administration and the National Recovery Act (NRA) in the mid-1930s, the United States began moving toward a socialistic political control that persists today, although it is often assailed by conservative policymakers. During the 1940s, the study of aging was set aside to devote attention to the more pressing problems of national defense and developments in weaponry. However, interest in aging rose rapidly after World War II.

Today, funding for health and social services is often tied to stringent governmental requirements. The continued shift of funding responsibility from federal agencies to state agencies continues in light of budget deficits. Health care reform and the passage of the Patient Protection and Affordable Care Act have many significant implications for health care for older people (Chapter 16). One of the paradoxes that hinders the delivery of services to older people in the United States is that America is both a capitalistic and a socialistic society, with health care moving rapidly into a highly competitive marketing mode. Therefore life-sustaining services are now designed for profit, although we simultaneously federally subsidize them. See Table 1-2 for a summary of important political developments in the field of aging.

BOX 1-3	FUTURE DIRECTIONS FOR GERONTOLOGICAL NURSING RESEARCH, AS SUGGESTED BY WYKLE AND TAPPEN

- Staffing patterns and the most appropriate mix to improve care outcomes in long-term care settings
- The influence of culture, diversity, and ethnicity on aging
- Health disparities and health literacy
- Factors contributing to successful aging, health promotion, and wellness in the upcoming baby boomer generation
- Retirement decisions of the baby boomers, how they are made and how they are changing from our current knowledge level
- Dementia as a chronic illness and staying well with the disease
- Caregiving, particularly intergenerational
- Values and attitudes of the current generation toward aging and their expectations
- Interventions to assist with the increasing prevalence of drug and alcohol abuse and other mental health problems of the current and future generations of older adults

- Integration of current best practice protocols into settings across the continuum in cost-effective and care-efficient models
- Models of acute care designed to prevent negative outcomes in elders
- Strategies to increase preparation in gerontological nursing and increased recruitment of the brightest and best into gerontological nursing
- Models of interprofessional communication and care
- Health promotion and illness management interventions in the assisted living setting; role of professional nurses and advanced practice nurses in this setting; aging in place
- Development of models for end-of-life care in the home and nursing home

From M.L. Wykle and R.M Tappen as cited in Ebersole P, Touhy T: Geriatric nursing: growth of a specialty, New York, 2006, Springer.

TABLE 1-2	POLITICAL EVENTS INFLUENCING AGING

YEAR	EVENT
1935	Social Security Act signed by Franklin D. Roosevelt
1937	National Institutes of Health established; first of the special institutes to study diseases common to older people
1948	Hospital Construction and Facilities Act (Hill-Burton) provided funds for construction of long-term care facilities
1950	First National Conference on Aging held in Washington DC
1951	Federal Committee on Aging and Geriatrics created to coordinate federal programs for the aging
1956	Special Staff on Aging established within the U.S. Department of Health, Education, and Welfare. Federal Council on Aging replaced Intradepartmental Working Group on Aging
1959	Senate subcommittee authorized to consider problems of the elderly and aging; Federal Council on Aging reconstituted at the cabinet level
1960	First appropriation passed for Section 202, Housing Act of 1959, authorizing direct loans for housing for the elderly
1961	First White House Conference on Aging held in Washington DC. Senate Special Committee on Aging established as advocate for older Americans
1962	Federal Council on Aging became President's Council on Aging
1963	President Kennedy sent Congress the first presidential message on elderly citizens; designated May as Senior Citizens Month. Special Staff on Aging became Office of Aging in HEW's new Welfare Administration
1965	President Johnson signed Older Americans Act, creating Administration on Aging (AOA). Amendments to the Social Security Act established Medicare program
1967	Age Discrimination in Employment Act brightened job outlook for Americans 40 to 65 years old
1971	Second White House Conference on Aging held in Washington DC
	Cabinet-level Domestic Council Committee on Aging created
	ACTION—the federal volunteer agency—established and given responsibility for senior volunteer programs previously administered by the AOA
1972	New act passed establishing a Nutrition Program for the Elderly, to be administered by the AOA. Supplementary Security Income (SSI) enacted
1973	Amendments to Older Americans Act called for state agencies on aging to establish area agencies on aging to plan for comprehensive, coordinated service delivery systems for older people at the local level
	Establishment of a National Clearinghouse on Aging and a Federal Council on the Aging with members appointed by the President
1974	Research on Aging Act established the National Institute on Aging within the National Institutes of Health; Robert N. Butler appointed director
1975	House of Representatives Special Committee on Aging established.
	Amendments to the Older Americans Act, establishing four new priority areas under Title IV:
	a. Transportations
	b. Home Services
	c. Legal Services
	d. Residential Repair and Renovation
1976	Title V of the Older Americans Act received an appropriation for the first time since inception of the act in 1965. Five million dollars was appropriated "to pay part of the cost of acquisition, alteration, or renovation of community facilities that will serve as multipurpose Senior Centers"
1977	Title V refunded at the rate of $20 million annually
1981	Third White House Conference on Aging held in Washington DC.
	Mandatory retirement laws revised
1982	T. Franklin Williams appointed director of the National Institute of Aging
1983	Diagnostic Related Groups (DRGs) instituted by the Health Care Financing Administration to control costs of Medicare
1984	Sexual discrimination in pension benefit payments outlawed by U.S. Supreme Court
1987	Federal nursing home reform Act from the Omnibus reconciliation Act of 1987
1988	Medicare Catastrophic Coverage Act
1989	Medicare Catastrophic Coverage Act repealed
1991	Fourth White House Conference on Aging stalled. AOA funds cut drastically
	Omnibus Budget Reconciliation Act (OBRA) (nursing home reform law)
1992	Proposals from multiple sources for rescue of health care system
1993	National Institute for Nursing Research established as a separate entity
1995	Fourth White House Conference on Aging (WHCoA). Focused on preservation of Medicare, Medicaid, Social Security, and the Older Americans Act (OAA)
1996	Majority of elders moved through Medicare changes to managed care systems
1998	Congress considers privatizing Social Security
2000	National Family Caregiver Support Program
2003	Medicare Prescription Drug, Improvement, and Modernization Act instituted
2005	Medicare payment for preventive benefits expanded
	Continued proposals for privatization of Social Security
	Fifth WHCoA
2010	Patient Protection and Affordable Care Act passed

PROMOTING HEALTHY AGING: IMPLICATIONS FOR GERONTOLOGICAL NURSING

The rapid growth of the older population brings forth opportunities and challenges for the world now and in the future. With the promise of a healthier old age, health care professionals, particularly nurses, will play a significant role in creating systems of care and services that enhance the possibility of healthy aging for people of all races and cultures across the life span. Continued attention must be paid to the recruitment and education of health professionals and direct care staff prepared to care for older people to meet critical shortages that threaten health and safety.

Historically, nurses have always been in the front lines in caring for older adults. They have provided hands-on care, supervision, administration, program development, teaching, and research. To a great extent, nurses are responsible for the rapid advance of gerontology as a profession. Gerontological nursing research has gained wide acceptance in the scientific community and has shown that better care is possible and should be expected. Nurses have been and continue to be the mainstay of care of older adults (Wykle and McDonald, 1997; Mezey and Fulmer, 2002).

The solid foundation built by the geriatric nursing pioneers and the current leaders in the specialty; the commitment of gerontological nurses to "tackle difficult but exceptionally meaningful issues that impact profoundly on the health and quality of life for older adults" (Mezey and Fulmer, 2002, p. M440); the opportunities for decision-making, independent action, and innovation; and the significant contribution of gerontological nursing research to improved patient outcomes and health policy position the specialty for continued growth, recognition, contribution, and value to society. Dare we say that gerontological nursing will be the most needed specialty in nursing as the number of older people continues to increase and the need for our specialized knowledge becomes even more critical in every specialty and every health care setting (Ebersole and Touhy, 2006)?

---

evolve To access your student resources, go to *http://evolve.elsevier.com/Ebersole/TwdHlthAging*

KEY CONCEPTS

- Aging must be studied as a complex phenomenon with bio-psychosocial and spiritual aspects affecting the manner in which an individual ages.
- Each cohort of older people is in some ways distinctly different from others, and individual older persons become more unique the longer they live. Thus one must be careful in attributing any specific characteristics to "old age."
- The serious study of gerontology in the United States is comparatively new, reaching back only about 50 years.
- Although the population as a whole is aging, the greatest categorical increase by group percentage is occurring among those 85 years old and older.
- The significant increases in racially and culturally diverse older adults and existing health care disparities require culturally competent practitioners and researchers.
- The current generation of older people are generally healthier than earlier cohorts and rates of disability are declining or stabilizing. However, cultural and racial disparities exist, and there is growing concern that this trend will be reversed with the obesity epidemic.
- The eldercare workforce is dangerously understaffed and unprepared to care for the growing numbers of older adults.

- Nursing has led the field in gerontology because nurses were the first professionals in the nation to be certified as geriatric specialists.
- Certification assures the public of nurses' commitment to specialized education and qualification for the care of older people.
- Requirements for accreditation of nursing programs should include solid evidence of preparation in the care of older adults.
- Research in gerontological nursing has provided the foundation for improved care of older people.
- Advanced practice nurses have either nurse practitioner qualifications or clinical nurse specialist education. Advanced practice role opportunities for nurses are numerous and are seen as potentially cost-effective in health care delivery while facilitating more holistic health care.
- Political actions and appropriations have had far-reaching influence on the individual experience of aging, chiefly through Medicare, Medicaid, and Social Security.

RESEARCH QUESTIONS

1. What aspects of gerontological nursing roles do nurses find most gratifying?
2. Why do so few students choose gerontological nursing as a field of practice? What factors might encourage more interest in the specialty?
3. What is the actual time in the curriculum of baccalaureate nursing schools spent on content and practice experiences related to the care of older people?
4. At what age or in which circumstances are individuals most likely to begin considering their own aging?
5. What are the most frequently held assumptions related to the experience of aging?
6. How will the aging of the population and the increasing cultural diversity affect nursing practice?
7. What are the concerns of younger people and baby boomers related to aging?
8. What are the most effective interventions across the life span to enhance the possibility of healthy aging?

REFERENCES

Administration on Aging, U.S. Department of Health and Human Services: *A profile of older Americans* (2009). Available at http://www.aoa.gov/AoARoot/Aging_Statistics/Profile/index.aspx (accessed November 2010).

Alliance for Children & Families: *Aging in poverty: a call to action* (2010). http://www.familiesinsociety.org/new/SpecialIssue/AgingInPoverty/AgingInPoverty.pdf (accessed March 10, 2011).

American Association of Colleges of Nursing (AACN): *The essentials of baccalaureate education for professional nursing practice* (2008). Available at http://www.aacn.nche.edu/Education/pdf/BaccEssentials08.pdf (accessed November 2010).

American Association of Colleges of Nursing and the John A. Hartford Foundation, Institute for Geriatric Nursing: *Adult-gerontology primary care nurse practitioner competencies*, March 2010. Available at http://www.aacn.nche.edu/Education/curriculum/adultgeroprimcareNPcomp.pdf (accessed December 2010).

American Association of Colleges of Nursing, Hartford Institute for Geriatric Nursing, New York University College of Nursing: *Recommended baccalaureate competencies and curricular guidelines for the nursing care of older adults: A supplement to The Essentials of Baccalaureate Education for Professional Nursing Practice*, September 2010. Available at http://www.aacn.nche.edu/education/pdf/AACN_Gerocompetencies.pdf (accessed December 2010).

American Geriatrics Society, Task Force on the Future of Geriatric Medicine: *Caring for older Americans: the future of geriatric medicine*, Journal of the American Geriatrics Society 53(Suppl 6):S245, 2005.

American Medical Association (AMA): *AMA health care trends, 2008: health status of the population* (2008). Available at http://www.ama-assn.org/ama1/pub/upload/mm/409/2008-trends-chapt-2.pdf (accessed November 2010).

American Nurses Association: *Gerontological Nursing: Scope and Standards of Practice*, Silver Spring, MD, 2010, Nursesbooks.org.

Bakerjian D: *Care of nursing home residents by advanced practice nurses: a review of the literature*, Research in Gerontological Nursing 1:177, 2008.

Berman A, Mezey M, Kobayashi M, et al: *Gerontological nursing content in baccalaureate programs: comparison of findings from 1997 and 2003*, Journal of Professional Nursing 21:268, 2005.

Burnside IM: *Listen to the aged*, American Journal of Nursing 75:1801, 1975.

Centers for Disease Control and Prevention: *United States Life Tables by Hispanic Origin*, 2010. Available at http://www.cdc.gov/nchs/data/series/sr_02/sr02_152.pdf (accessed December 2010).

Christensen D: *Making sense of centenarians: genes and life style help people live through a century*, Science News Online 159:156, 2001. Available at www.sciencenews.org.

Crane C: *Almshouse nursing: the human need*, American Journal of Nursing 7:872, 1907.

Davis B: *Nursing care of the aged: historical evolution*, Bulletin (American Association for the History of Nursing) 47, 1985.

Dock L: *The crusade for almshouse nursing*, American Journal of Nursing 8:520, 1908.

Ebersole P, Touhy T: *Geriatric nursing: growth of a specialty*, New York, 2006, Springer.

Gelbach S: *Nursing care of the aged*, American Journal of Nursing 43:1112, 1943.

Gebhardt MC, Sims TT, Bates TA: *Enhancing geriatric content in a baccalaureate nursing program*, Nursing Education Perspectives 30:245, 2009.

Hooyman N, Kiyak H: *Social gerontology*, Boston, 2011, Allyn & Bacon.

Hounsell C, Riojas A: *Older women face tarnished 'golden years,'* Aging Today 27:7, 2006.

Institute of Medicine, National Academies: *Retooling for an aging America: building the health care workforce* (2008). Available at http://www.iom.edu/Reports/2008/Retooling-for-an-Aging-America-Building-the-Health-Care-Workforce.aspx (accessed November 2010).

Kagan S: *Moving from achievement to transformation*, Geriatric Nursing 29:102, 2008.

Leatt P, Schneck R: Nursing subunits technology: a replication. *Administration Science Quarterly* 26:225–236, 1981.

Leppa CJ: *The nature of LTC nursing work*, Journal of Gerontological Nursing 30:26, 2004.

Mack M: *Personal adjustment of chronically ill old people under home care*, Nursing Research 1:9, 1952.

Mackin L, Kayser-Jones J, Franklin P, et al: *Successful recruiting into geriatric nursing: the experience of the Hartford Centers of Geriatric Nursing Excellence*, Nursing Outlook 54:197, 2006.

Mantle JH: Personal communication, March 2, 2005.

Mentes J: *On being 100 and healthy*, Journal of gerontological nursing 32(4):6, 2006.

Mezey M, Fulmer T: *The future history of gerontological nursing*, Journals of Gerontology Series A, Biological Sciences and Medical Sciences 57:M438, 2002.

Mezey M, Harrington C, Kluger M: *FOCUS ON: professional responsibility*, American Journal of Nursing 104:71, 2004.

Mezey M, Stierle L, Hubqa G, et al: *Ensuring competence of specialty nurses in acute care of older adults*, Geriatric Nursing 28:9, 2007.

Miller J, Coke L, Moss A, et al: *Reluctant gerontologists: integrating gerontological nursing content into a prelicensure program*, Nurse Educator 34:198, 2009.

Miller L, Beck C, Dowling G, et al: *Building gerontological nursing research capacity: research initiatives of the John A. Hartford Foundation Centers of Geriatric Nursing Excellence*, Nursing Outlook 54:189, 2006.

Nascher I: *Geriatrics*, Philadelphia, 1914, P. Blakiston's Son & Co.

Newton K, Anderson H: *Geriatric Nursing*, St. Louis, 1950, C.V. Mosby.

Population Division, Department of Economic and Social Affairs, United Nations: *World population prospects: the 2008 revision* (2009). Available at http://esa.un.org/unpd/wpp2008/index.htm (accessed November 2010).

Schoeni M, Freedman VA, Martin LG: *Why is late-life disability declining?* Milbank Quarterly 86:47, 2008.

Silver MH, Jilinskaia E, Perls TT: *Cognitive functional status of age-confirmed centenarians in a population-based study*, Journals of Gerontology Series B, Psychological Sciences and Social Sciences 56:P134, 2001.

Souder E, Kagan S, Hansen L, et al: *Innovations in geriatric nursing curricula: experiences from the John A. Hartford Centers of Geriatric Nursing Excellence*, Nursing Outlook 54:219, 2006.

Stierle L, Mezez M, Schumann M, et al: *Professional development: the Nurse Competence in Aging Initiative: encouraging expertise in the care of older adults*, American Journal of Nursing 106:93, 2006.

Thomas W: *What are old people for? How elders will save the world*, St. Louis, MO, 2004, Vanderwyk & Burnham.

U.S. Census Bureau: *2010 census special reports: centenarians* (2012). Available at http://www.census.gov/prod/cen2010/reports/c2010sr–03.pdf (accessed January 2013).

U.S. Census Bureau: *The 2010 statistical abstract* (2010). Available at http://www.census.gov/compendia/statab/ (accessed November 2010).

Wykle M, McDonald P: *The past, present and future of gerontological nursing*. In Klein S, editor: *A national agenda for geriatric education*, New York, 1997, Springer.

Young H: *Challenges and solutions for care of frail older adults*, Online Journal of Issues in Nursing 8:1, 2003.

Recommended Baccalaureate Competencies and Curricular Guidelines for the Nursing Care of Older Adults

Gerontological Nursing Competency Statements

1. Incorporate professional attitudes, values, and expectations about physical and mental aging in the provision of patient-centered care for older adults and their families.
Corresponding to Essential VIII

2. Assess barriers for older adults in receiving, understanding, and giving of information.
Corresponding to Essential IV and IX

3. Use valid and reliable assessment tools to guide nursing practice for older adults.
Corresponding to Essentials IX

4. Assess the living environment as it relates to functional, physical, cognitive, psychological, and social needs of older adults.
Corresponding to Essential IX

5. Intervene to assist older adults and their support network to achieve personal goals, based on the analysis of the living environment and availability of community resources.
Corresponding to Essential VII

6. Identify actual or potential mistreatment (physical, mental, or financial abuse, and/or self-neglect) in older adults and refer appropriately.
Corresponding to Essential V

7. Implement strategies and use online guidelines to prevent and/or identify and manage geriatric syndromes.
Corresponding to Essentials IV and IX

8. Recognize and respect the variations of care, the increased complexity, and the increased use of health care resources inherent in caring for older adults.
Corresponding to Essentials IV and IX

9. Recognize the complex interaction of acute and chronic comorbid physical and mental conditions and associated treatments common to older adults.
Corresponding to Essential IX

10. Compare models of care that promote safe, quality physical and mental health care for older adults such as PACE, NICHE, Guided Care, Culture Change, and Transitional Care Models.
Corresponding to Essential II

11. Facilitate ethical, noncoercive decision-making by older adults and/or families/caregivers for maintaining everyday living, receiving treatment, initiating advance directives, and implementing end-of-life care.
Corresponding to Essential VIII

12. Promote adherence to the evidence-based practice of providing restraint-free care (both physical and chemical restraints).
Corresponding to Essential II

13. Integrate leadership and communication techniques that foster discussion and reflection on the extent to which diversity (among nurses, nurse assistive personnel, therapists, physicians, and patients) has the potential to impact the care of older adults.
Corresponding to Essential VI

14. Facilitate safe and effective transitions across levels of care, including acute, community-based, and long-term care (e.g., home, assisted living, hospice, nursing homes) for older adults and their families.
Corresponding to Essentials IV and IX

15. Plan patient-centered care with consideration for mental and physical health and well-being of informal and formal caregivers of older adults.
Corresponding to Essential IX

16. Advocate for timely and appropriate palliative and hospice care for older adults with physical and cognitive impairments.
Corresponding to Essential IX

17. Implement and monitor strategies to prevent risk and promote quality and safety (e.g., falls, medication mismanagement, pressure ulcers) in the nursing care of older adults with physical and cognitive needs.
Corresponding to Essentials II and IV

18. Use resources/programs to promote functional, physical, and mental wellness in older adults.
Corresponding to Essential VII

19. Integrate relevant theories and concepts included in a liberal education into the delivery of patient-centered care for older adults.
Corresponding to Essential I

From: American Association of Colleges of Nursing, Hartford Institute for Geriatric Nursing, New York University College of Nursing: *Recommended baccalaureate competencies and curricular guidelines for the nursing care of older adults* [a supplement to *The essentials of baccalaureate education for professional nursing practice*] (2010). Available at http://www.aacn.nche.edu/education/pdf/AACN_Gerocompetencies.pdf (accessed December 2010).

evolve   For further resources and guide to using the text to integrate the recommended competencies, see Evolve at *http://evolve.elsevier.com/Ebersole/TwdHlthAging.*

Health and Wellness

Theris A. Touhy

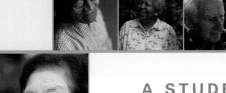

evolve http://evolve.elsevier.com/Ebersole/TwdHlthAging

A STUDENT SPEAKS

I was so surprised when I went to the senior center and saw all those old folks doing tai chi! I feel a bit ashamed that I don't take better care of my body.

Maggie, age 24

AN ELDER SPEAKS

Just a change in perspective! I can choose to be well or ill under all conditions. I think, too often we feel like victims of circumstance. I refuse to be a victim. It is my choice and I have control.

Maria, age 86

LEARNING OBJECTIVES

On completion of this chapter, the reader will be able to:
1. Differentiate between the concepts of health and wellness.
2. Describe the health status of older people.
3. Describe the goals of Healthy People 2020.
4. Discuss the multidimensional nature of wellness.
5. Explain wellness in the context of chronic illness.
6. Identify recommended health promotion and disease prevention strategies for older adults.
7. Describe the role of the nurse in enhancing the health of older people.

In the medical arena, health is considered to be the absence of disease. Conformity to physical and mental capacity norms indicates one's health status. Therefore the more observable the evidence, the more definite the degree of health that can be declared or the diagnosis that can be affixed. Those biological and physiological capacities not considered essential for the performance of *well* activity are less likely to be considered significant.

The emergence of a strong holistic health movement has refocused on a clear definition and operational approach to health and wellness. The holistic approach has long been in existence but has received little attention. Dunn (1961) saw health in a holistic context and defined it as an integrated method of functioning that is oriented toward maximizing the potential of which the individual is capable within the environment in which he or she is functioning. The holistic definition does not limit health to just its physical or mental or even social aspects but, rather, incorporates all of these facets in the total picture. This broader definition of health is particularly important in discussing the health of older people who may have multiple chronic conditions and be considered "ill" when looking through the lens of health-illness models. Consider the following:

Herb is a 70-year-old man with no major health concerns. He works out in the gym daily, runs 2 miles a day, and participates in marathon events. He pays attention to all aspects of his lifestyle, diet, social and family relationships, and spiritual development. Herb can be considered healthy and as someone who has a sense of well-being, a sense of wellness.

Agnes is an 85-year-old woman with diagnoses of hypertension, arthritis, and diabetes. She takes medication for all of these conditions and currently has mobility limitations and is being treated for a diabetic foot ulcer. Agnes continues to live a full life despite her health problems. She does chair exercises daily, follows a therapeutic diet, adheres to her medication routine, and maintains an appropriate body weight. She is a foster grandparent in the local school, maintains a close relationship with her family and friends, has a deep spiritual belief system, and keeps her mind active by reading and doing Sudoku puzzles. She is knowledgeable about her illnesses and strives to prevent complications and maintain her functional ability. Agnes can be considered an older adult in poor health and with disabilities. Yet, she has a sense of well-being, a sense of wellness.

Measurements of a population's health status rely on life expectancy, morbidity, and death tables. These figures provide information about illness but do not reveal the extent to which the living are affected by these conditions. They do not indicate the health status, only the illness. For example, in morbidity tables people who are actually functioning at a high level of wellness are assigned to illness categories. Persons compiling these tables do not consider that the person with health disorders, malignancies, and other conditions may be able to attain and function at a high level of wellness and be a contributing member of the community. The wellness approach is perhaps the most equitable in the evaluation of the older individual's potential for maximal functioning.

WELLNESS

Wellness involves one's whole being—physical, emotional, mental, social, spiritual, and environmental—all of which are vital components. For older people, health also includes the element of physical function. What is considered wellness to the individual must include his or her cultural orientation. Culture cannot be relegated to a subposition under any other health component. It must stand equally so that health care providers can realize and more adequately respond to the significance of culture in the attainment of well-being. Culture affects a person's understanding of health as well as their health behaviors (Chapter 5).

The wellness model refers to health as one aspect in the achievement of wellness. The wellness approach suggests that every person has an optimal level of functioning for each position on the wellness continuum to achieve a good and satisfactory existence (well-being) (Figure 2-1). Even in the presence of chronic illness or multiple disabilities or while dying, movement toward higher level wellness is possible if the emphasis of care is placed on the promotion of well-being in the least restrictive environment, with support and encouragement for the person to find meaning in the situation, whatever it is. The

wellness continuum picks up where the traditional medical model leaves off. Instead of a downward negative trajectory for the health of the older adult, focused on deterioration, the wellness model rises and moves in a positive direction. The individual may reach plateaus in his or her ascension to higher level wellness.

Wellness is not given to a person. Rather, it is a state of being and feeling that one strives to achieve through motivation and health practices. An individual must work hard to achieve wellness just as he or she must work hard to perform competently at a job. In an attempt to meld the broader health/wellness concepts and initiate a more positive approach to the capacities of older people, we offer this working definition for the care of the older individual: *Wellness is the best achievable balance between one's environment, internal and external, and one's emotional, spiritual, social, cultural, and physical processes.*

The wellness model encompasses the idea that health is a consequence of multiple determinants. Health determinants are the range of personal, social, economic, and environmental factors that determine the health status of individuals or populations. These include family, community, income, education, gender, race/ethnicity, place of residence, access to health care, and exposure to toxins, pollutants, and substandard housing. As stated in the Healthy People 2020 recommendations, this approach goes beyond the fundamentals of monitoring health behaviors such as diet and exercise and begins to connect different stages across the life span in terms of physical, emotional, and cognitive development. Health is a consequence of multiple determinants, which operate in nested genetic, biological, behavioral, social, and economic contexts that change as a person develops (Centers for Disease Control and Prevention, 2010a).

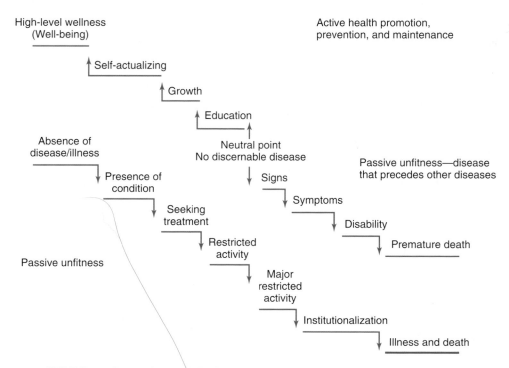

FIGURE 2-1 Comparisons of Wellness/Health and Traditional Medical Continuum.

Dimensions of Wellness

Wellness has been conceptualized as having seven dimensions: physical, emotional, spiritual, intellectual, environmental, occupational, and social. Each dimension, as well as nursing responses to enhance wellness, is discussed in depth in subsequent chapters of this book.

Physical wellness is enhanced through regular physical activity, diet and nutrition, and avoidance of tobacco, drugs, and excessive alcohol consumption. Healthy lifestyles are more influential than genetic factors in helping older people avoid the deterioration traditionally associated with aging. People who are physically active, eat a healthy diet, do not use tobacco, and practice other healthy behaviors reduce their risk of chronic diseases and have half the rate of disability of those who do not. The benefit of these practices extends even to the oldest-old.

Emotional wellness recognizes awareness and acceptance of one's feelings as well as the ability to form interdependent relationships with others based on mutual commitment, trust, and respect. It includes the degree to which one feels positive and enthusiastic about oneself and one's life and the ability to cope effectively with stress. Spiritual wellness recognizes the search for meaning and purpose in our lives and the taking of time to reflect and connect with the universe. Intellectual wellness includes expanding one's knowledge and skills throughout life, discovering new skills and interests, and challenging oneself through creative, stimulating mental activities. Environmental wellness calls for caring for precious resources and creating living spaces and practices that respect and support the environment. Occupational wellness includes doing something that you love, contributing your unique gifts, skills, and talents to work that is personally meaningful and rewarding, and balancing work with leisure time. Social wellness recognizes the importance of staying engaged in meaningful activities and relationship and building a better world for current and future generations (Box 2-1; Hettler, 2010). Environmental wellness calls for caring for precious resources and creating living spaces and practices that respect and support the environment.

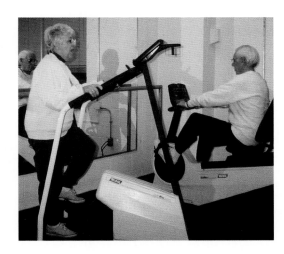

Today's older adult is interested in maintaining strength and endurance. (From Black JM, Hawks JH: *Medical-surgical nursing: clinical management for positive outcomes*, ed 7, St. Louis, 2005, WB Saunders.)

HEALTHY AGING

In a concept analysis of healthy aging (Hansen-Kyle, 2005, p. 52), the following definition emerged: "Healthy aging is the process of slowing down, physically and cognitively, while resiliently adapting and compensating in order to optimally function and participate in all areas of one's life (physical, cognitive, social, and spiritual)." The concept of healthy aging is a multidimensional process and is uniquely defined by each individual. For older adults being healthy is characterized by the way an individual feels in the context of existing illness or disability and the social and/or physical environment. Older adults have described being healthy as having four main components: functional independence, self-care management of illness, positive outlook, and personal growth and social contribution. As one older adult stated: "When you get into your 80s, little pieces of you kind of break off and fall astray … most of us have some little thing going on. And you know, we take care of that. …"

⚕ BOX 2-1   RESEARCH HIGHLIGHTS

Health Practices of Older Adults in Good Health: Engagement Is the Key

A study (Van Leuven, 2010) was performed to investigate the beliefs, values, lifestyles, and health status of adults age 75 and older who identify themselves as healthy. Eighteen older adults (7 men and 11 women) participated in an interview about their health. The mean age of participants was 82.8 years. Eleven lived independently in the community, 5 resided in an assisted living facility, and 2 were residents of a skilled nursing facility. Focus groups were also conducted with staff in medical offices and in assisted living and skilled nursing facilities to obtain their views of factors contributing to healthy aging. The following questions guided the interview with the older adults:

Would you rate your current state of health as excellent, good, fair, or poor? Why did you select this rating?

What does it mean to be healthy as you age?

What activities do you engage in to maintain or improve your health?

What suggestions do you have for others about health in aging?

What suggestions do you have for health care providers about health in aging?

Of the older adult participants, 77.8% perceived their health as good or excellent. Among those who perceived their health as good or excellent, the following emerged as important to health: involvement in managing their own health, staying active and engaged in a variety of community and intergenerational activities, learning to adjust to change and loss, finding a health care provider who balanced care with compassion, and a supportive environment. Staff described a healthy older adult as someone with "spark," who is "feisty" and is still "very vital" despite chronic problems.

Engagement emerged as a crucial factor in successful aging. Assessment of engagement and assistance in supporting engagement is an important nursing role with older adults. Future research needs to examine what interventions are most effective in stimulating social relationships and community involvement among older adults in all settings. Similar to other studies, findings reinforce the idea that health can coexist with disease and is a state of mind that is not reflected in a list of diagnoses.

Data from Van Leuven KA: Health practices of older adults in good health, *Journal of Gerontological Nursing* 36:38, 2010.

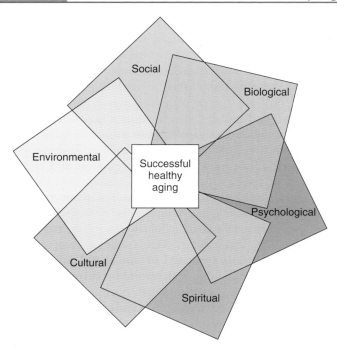

Social

Biological

Environmental

Successful
healthy
aging

Psychological

Cultural

Spiritual

FIGURE 2-2 Healthy Aging. (Developed by Patricia Hess.)

Older adults have been added as a new topic area in HP 2020 with the goal of improving health, function, and quality of life. Emerging issues identified in the health of older adults include efforts to coordinate care, help older adults manage their own care, establish quality measures, identify minimum levels of training for people who care for older adults, and research and analyze appropriate training to equip providers with the tools they need to meet the needs of older adults. Other new additions to HP 2020 that are relevant to the health of older adults include dementias, sleep health, health-related quality of life and well-being, and lesbian, gay, bisexual, and transgender health (see chapters 11, 19, 21, 22). A summary of HP 2020 objectives for older adults is presented in Box 2-3.

Health Status of Older People

Self-reported Health

In 2008, 39% of noninstitutionalized older persons rated their health as excellent or very good (compared with 60.7% for all

(Miller and Iris, 2002, p. 255). The interrelationship of the facets that compose successful healthy aging are similar to the dimensions of wellness (Figure 2-2). Each aspect is like a petal, anchored to the center and overlapping the other petals, each affecting the whole. Alterations in or loss of a petal can change the overall effect or appearance and its wholeness.

The conviction by nurses and other caregivers that older people are individuals with declining health generates responses that include treating the older person as ill and feeble, or potentially so. It is therefore expected by some that attempts to reverse conditions or situations, maintain a level of ability, or institute preventive health measures are useless for older people. Nothing could be further from the truth; all old people are improvable (Bortz, 1991). Historically, the principles of disease prevention and health promotion have not been aggressively applied to the problems of older adults. The focus has been on managing illnesses rather than on reducing risks, maintaining optimal function, and decreasing disability associated with illness.

Healthy aging can no longer be viewed by looking only at older adults. The likelihood of a longer, more functional old age begins in the prenatal period and continues throughout life with health promotion efforts and appropriate clinical care. As Barondess (2008) states: "To a substantial degree, the health of the emergent adult is in the hands of the pediatrician" (p. 147). Exciting research in the field of epigenetics is leading to new understanding of the effect of environmental factors and lifestyle habits such as diet, stress, smoking, and prenatal nutrition on life expectancy for individuals and their children (see http://www.epigenome.org/ for more information). Recommendations for the framework of Healthy People 2020 recognize this and include attention to the effect of early life factors, together with later life factors, on health outcomes. Overarching goals of healthy people 2020 are presented in Box 2-2.

 BOX 2-2   HEALTHY PEOPLE 2020

Overarching Goals

- Attain high-quality, longer lives free of preventable disease, disability, injury, and premature death
- Achieve health equity, eliminate disparities, and improve the health of all groups
- Create social and physical environments that promote good health for all
- Promote quality of life, healthy development, and healthy behaviors across all life stages

From U.S. Department of Health and Human Service, Office of Disease Prevention and Health Promotion: *Healthy People 2020 Framework.* s: *Phase 1 report: recommendations for the framework and format of Healthy People 2020* (2010). Available at http://www.healthypeople.gov (accessed December 2010).

 BOX 2-3   HEALTHY PEOPLE 2020 SUMMARY OF OBJECTIVES

Older Adults

- Increase the proportion of older adults who use the Welcome to Medicare benefit
- Increase the proportion of older adults who are up to date on a core set of clinical preventive services
- Increase the proportion of older adults with one or more chronic health conditions who report confidence in managing their conditions
- Reduce the proportion of older adults who have moderate to severe functional limitations
- Increase the proportion of older adults with reduced physical or cognitive function who engage in light, moderate, or vigorous leisure-time physical activities
- Increase the proportion of the health care workforce with geriatric certification
- Reduce the proportion of noninstitutionalized older adults with disabilities who have an unmet need for long-term services and supports
- Reduce the proportion of unpaid caregivers of older adults who report an unmet need for caregiver support services
- Reduce the rate of emergency department visits due to falls among older adults
- Increase the number of States, the District of Columbia, and Tribes that collect and make publicly available information on the characteristics of victims, perpetrators, and cases of elder abuse, neglect, and exploitation

persons aged 18 and older). There were few differences between the sexes, but ethnically and diverse older people were less likely to rate their health as excellent or very good than were older white people (Figure 2-3).

Disability and Chronic Illness

The current generation of older people is generally healthier than earlier cohorts, and rates of disability are declining or stabilizing (Manton et al., 2008). Future cohorts of older people may be healthier and more functional well into their 80s and 90s. Fries's (1980, 1990) concept of compression of morbidity proposes that premature death will be minimized, and disease and functional decline will be compressed into a period of 3 to 5 years before death. There is some evidence that this is already occurring because major diseases such as arthritis, arteriosclerosis, and respiratory problems now appear 10 to 25 years later than for past cohorts (Fries, 2002; Hooyman and Kiyak, 2011).

However, rates of disability and chronic illness continue to be higher among racially and ethnically diverse older adults and need continued attention (Hooyman and Kiyak, 2011). For example, American Indians and Alaska Natives (AI/AN) "appear to be experiencing expansion of morbidity rather then compression. Among other health needs, more than one in five AI/AN elders have diabetes and this population experience higher rates of physical disability than age-matched White counterparts" (Goins et al, 2010, p. 1340). Further, some research suggests that overweight and obesity in adults aged 60-69, and among younger people, may have the potential to reverse declining disability rates. Obesity among U.S. adults has risen from 11% to 16% in the early 1960s to 28% to 34% in 2000. Levels of obesity are projected to be as high as 45.4% within 20 years (Seeman et al., 2010) (Chapter 14).

The incidence of chronic illness increases with age. More than 80% of people over the age of 70 experience at least one chronic condition and 50% have multiple health problems. Some are relatively minor and do not significantly affect function whereas others can cause pain and disability. Heart disease, hypertension, arthritis, cancer, and diabetes are the most prevalent chronic illnesses in the older adult population. Prevention and management of chronic illness are a priority for all health care professionals and are receiving increased attention in the development of new models of care as well as research. Chapter 15 discusses chronic illness among older adults in more depth.

Causes of Death

Heart disease, stroke, and cancer remain the leading causes of death, although there have been significant declines in death due to heart disease. Stroke fell from the third leading cause of death for the first time in five decades (Minino, Xu, Kochanek, 2010). However, racial disparities continue in stroke incidence, which has decreased significantly among white people but has increased slightly among African Americans (Kleindorfer et al., 2010). In 2007 significant increases occurred for suicide and chronic liver disease and cirrhosis as causes of death. Alzheimer's disease surpassed diabetes as a leading cause of death (Centers for Disease Control and Prevention, 2010b). Genetics plays a part in 9 of the 10 leading causes of death in the United States.

Four preventable risk factors, that is, smoking, high blood pressure, elevated blood glucose, and overweight and obesity, currently reduce life expectancy in the United States by 4.9 years in men and 4.1 years in women (Danaei et al., 2010). Only 3% of the population in the United States follows the basic four healthy habits: no smoking, 30 minutes of moderate intensity exercise 5 days a week, eating five servings of fruit and vegetables per day, and maintaining a normal body weight (Desai et al., 2010). Continued attention to reducing these preventable risk factors is essential to improve the health of the nation as well as to increase life expectancy for all people.

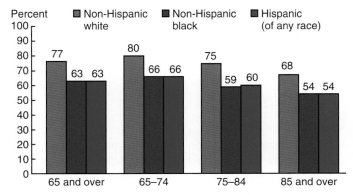

Percent

Non-Hispanic white   Non-Hispanic black   Hispanic (of any race)

NOTE: Data are based on a 3-year average from 2006-2008. See Appendix B for the definition of race and Hispanic origin in the National Health interview Survey.
Reference population: These data refer to the civilian noninstitutionalized population.
SOURCE: Centers for Disease Control and Prevention, National Center for Health Statistics, National Health interview Survey.

FIGURE 2-3 Respondent-reported Good to Excellent Health among the Population 65 and Older by Age Group, Race, and Hispanic Origin: 2006-2008. (Redrawn from Federal Interagency Forum on Aging-related Statistics: *Older Americans 2010: key indicators of well-being*, Washington DC, 2010, U.S. Government Printing Office.)

BOX 2-4 FOCUS ON GENETICS

The 10 leading causes of death in 2010, in order of rank, are presented below:
1. Diseases of the heart*
2. Cancer
3. Stroke
4. Chronic lower respiratory diseases
5. Accidents (unintentional injuries)
6. Alzheimer's disease
7. Diabetes mellitus
8. Influenza and pneumonia
9. Nephritis, nephrotic syndrome, and nephrosis
10. Septicemia

Data from Office of Public Health Genomics, Centers for Disease Control and Prevention, U.S. Department of Health and Human Services: *Genomics and health* (2010). Available at http://www.cdc.gov/nchs/FASTATS/deaths.htm.

BOX 2-5   USE OF CLINICAL PREVENTIVE SERVICES BY RACE AND ETHNICITY

For American Indian/Alaska Native Adults
40% need influenza vaccination
36% need pneumococcal vaccination
35% need colorectal screening
32% need diabetes screening
19% need breast cancer screening

For Asian/Pacific Islander Adults
49% need colorectal cancer screening
47% need diabetes screening
47% need pneumococcal vaccination
35% need influenza vaccination
29% need breast cancer screening

For Black Adults
47% need pneumococcal vaccination
44% need influenza vaccination

37% need colorectal cancer screening
30% need diabetes screening
14% need breast cancer screening

For Hispanic Adults
51% need pneumococcal vaccinations
47% need colorectal cancer screening
38% need influenza vaccination
28% need diabetes screening
16% need breast cancer screening

For White Adults
34% need colorectal screening
31% need diabetes screening
30% need pneumococcal vaccination
29% need influenza vaccination
17% need breast cancer screening

From: Centers for Disease Control and Prevention, Administration on Aging, Agency for Healthcare Research and Quality and Centers for Medicare and Medicaid Services: *Enhancing the use of clinical preventive services among older adults,* Washington DC: AAPP, 2011.
Retrieved March 21, 2011 from http://www.cdc.gov/aging/pdf/Clinical_Preventive_Services_Closing_the_Gap_Report.pdf

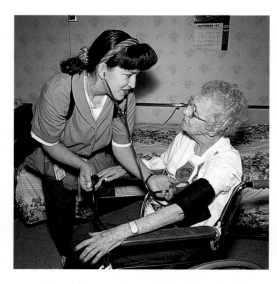

Assessment of the older person's medical and functional states should be performed before beginning an exercise program. (From Lewis SM, Heitkemper MM, Dirksen SR: *Medical-surgical nursing: assessment and management of clinical problems,* ed 7, St. Louis, 2007, Mosby.)

DISEASE PREVENTION AND HEALTH PROMOTION FOR OLDER ADULTS

With increasing life expectancy and numbers of older people, the positive outcomes of health promotion and disease prevention interventions for this age group are receiving significant attention. Older adults and the future aging population are increasingly taking responsibility for their health and adopting healthier lifestyles and habits. "The relationships between health practices, quality of life, and longevity are compelling. A substantial number of health problems in old age can be prevented, or controlled, by changing health behaviors, especially physical activity" (Miller and Iris, 2002, p. 249) (Chapter 12). Yet, too few older adults actively engage in health promotion activities. Robinson and Reinhard (2009) predict that in the next 50 years personalized health information, sometimes based on genetic

analysis, will help target lifelong health promotion and disease prevention. Estimates are that 90% of older Americans never receive routine screening tests for bone density, colon or prostate cancer, or glaucoma and that 60% don't receive routine preventive health services, including screening for high blood pressure or cholesterol (Curry, 2008). Use of clinical preventive services varies by race, ethnicity, level of education, and income. Culturally and racially diverse older adults and those with fewer years of education and lower income are less likely to have recommended preventive services (Box 2-5). Health care providers need to actively promote preventive medicine and a healthy lifestyle for older adults (Morley and Flaherty, 2002). Expanding access to preventive services beyond traditional health care settings to community sites and locations, offering multiple services in one location at convenient times, culturally appropriate education and services, and development of policies and supportive environments that remove barriers and close gaps is essential population (Centers for Disease Control and Prevention. Administration on Aging. Agency for Healthcare Research and Quality and Centers for Medicare and Medicaid Services, 2011).*

Goals

Goals for disease prevention and health promotion in older adults include reducing premature mortality and morbidity (compression of morbidity), maintaining functional independence, and extending life expectancy while maintaining or enhancing the quality of life (Resnick, 2003a).

Primary and Secondary Disease Prevention

Both primary prevention (prevention of disease before it occurs), and secondary prevention (detection of disease at an early stage) are included. Primary prevention activities include healthy lifestyle behaviors such as regular exercise, smoking

---

*Additional resources to assist older people and nurses to obtain information on the health of older people can be found on the Evolve website at http://evolve.elsevier.com/Ebersole/TwdHlthAging.

BOX 2-6 THE HEALTH PROMOTIONS MNEMONIC FOR PRIMARY AND SECONDARY PREVENTION

Hypertension screen
Environmental screen for safety issues
Apnea during sleep screen
Loss of weight
Tetanus vaccination
Hear in a noisy environment
Pain screen and treatment
Resistance and other exercises
Osteoporosis screen
Mood screen (depression)
Occult blood in stool
Testosterone deficiency (andropause)
Influenza and pneumococcal vaccinations
Oral screen for caries and abscesses
Nicotine education (smoking and chewing tobacco)
Sugar screen (diabetes mellitus)

From Morley J, Flaherty J: It's never too late: health promotion and illness prevention in older persons, *Journals of Gerontology Series A, Biological Sciences and Medical Sciences* 57:M338, 2002.

BOX 2-7 MEDICARE COVERAGE FOR DISEASE PREVENTION

- Abdominal aortic aneurysm screening
- Cardiovascular screenings
- Colorectal cancer screening
- Adult immunizations
- Bone mass measurements
- Diabetes screening
- Pap test and clinical breast examination if over 65 years of age with a recent abnormal screening test
- Diabetes supplies
- Diabetes self-management training
- Glaucoma tests for high-risk individuals
- Screening for diabetic retinopathy
- Hearing and balance examinations
- HIV screening for those at risk
- Annual screening mammograms
- Foot examinations and treatment for those with diabetes-related nerve damage and/or those who meet certain criteria
- Medical nutrition therapy (for beneficiaries with diabetes or renal disease)
- Initial preventive physical examination
- Smoking and tobacco use cessation counseling

HIV, human immunodeficiency virus.
From Centers for Medicare & Medicaid Services: *Prevention—general information overview* (2010). Available at http://www.cms.gov/PrevntionGenInfo/ (accessed November 2010); and AARP Public Policy Institute: *Fact sheet: improvements to Medicare's preventive services under health reform* (2010). Available at http://assets.aarp.org/rgcenter/ppi/health-care/fs180-preventive.pdf (accessed November 2010).

cessation, moderate use of alcohol, low-fat diets, stress management, active social engagement, and cognitive stimulation. Box 2-6 presents the HEALTH PROMOTIONS mnemonic as a guide to primary and secondary prevention.

Guidelines

Recommendations for secondary disease prevention include evidence-based screening guidelines developed for older adults from a variety of organizations. These guidelines are continually being evaluated in light of new research findings (Table 2-1). The passage of the Patient Protection and Affordable Health Care Act in 2010 has expanded coverage for preventive services under the Medicare program. The health reform law specifies that any Medicare-covered service recommended with a grade of A or B by the U.S. Preventive Services Task Force (USPSTF) for any indication or population must be fully covered under Medicare with no cost-sharing for the patient. An annual wellness visit and personalized prevention plan is part of the new coverage and includes a health risk assessment; updated medical history; list of current providers providing care; list of prescription medications; height, weight, and blood pressure measurements; a screening schedule for appropriate preventive services over the next 5 to 10 years; and a list of risk factors with treatment options for those risks (see http://www.cms.gov/PreventionGenInfo/ and http://assets.aarp.org/rgcenter/ppi/health-care/fs180-preventive.pdf) (Box 2-7).

In addition, Medicare covers an initial preventive physical examination (IPPE), also known as a Welcome to Medicare examination, during the first 12 months of enrollment in Part B Medicare. Increasing the proportion of older adults who use this benefit is one of the objectives for older people in HP 2020 (U.S. Department of Health and Human Services, 2010). A new government website provides up-to-date information about disease prevention and health promotion for all ages as well as information about prevention benefits under the Patient Protection and Affordable Health Care Act (http://www.healthcare.gov/learn/index.html).

Guidelines must be adapted on the basis of the unique needs of the various age cohorts of older people. An individualized approach with a focus on increasing quality and years of healthy life is necessary.

In general, determining whether an older adult should undergo screening or not depends on several key factors: whether the disease or condition will impact on the quality of life, whether treatment is an acceptable option and what are the implications of delaying treatment. ... Ideally, the goal when working with older adults, is to help them decide on what behaviours will help them achieve their highest level of health and function. (Resnick, 2003a, pp. 48, 54)

Interventions for healthy older adults will differ from those for frail older persons or those at the end of life. However, health promotion activities such as regular exercise, avoidance of smoking and excessive alcohol use, and immunizations are recommended for all older adults.

Influenza and pneumococcal immunization rates among older adults continue to fall below the Healthy People 2010 objectives of 90% coverage among noninstitutionalized people aged 65 and over. More than 30% of older adults are not immunized against pneumonia or influenza. African Americans, Hispanic, American Indian/Alaska Native. and Asian/Pacific Islander older adults have lower immunization rates compared with the rest of the population (Centers for Diseases Control and Prevention, Administration on Aging, Agency for Healthcare Reasearch and Quality and Centers for Medicare and Medicaid Servises, 2011). In an average year, influenza causes approximately 36,000 deaths and 200,000 hospitalizations in the United States. Older adults are at high risk for influenza and pneumonia-related deaths (Trust for America's Health, 2010).

TABLE 2-1   DISEASE PREVENTION AND HEALTH PROMOTION FOR OLDER ADULTS*

Immunizations

Influenza	One dose annually at the beginning of flu season
Pneumovax	Once after 65 yr (may be indicated earlier for at risk persons); booster after 5 yr if initial vaccination was before age 65 or if other risk factors are present
Tetanus, diphtheria, pertussis (Td/Tdap)	Booster every 10 years
Zoster	One dose
Hepatitis A and B	Recommended if other risk factors present (based on medical, occupational, lifestyle, and other indicators)
Measles, mumps, rubella	Recommended if other risk factors present (based on medical, occupational, lifestyle, and other indicators) or if evidence of lack of immunity and significant risk for exposure
Varicella	If evidence of lack of immunity and significant risk for exposure

Screening: All Persons

Blood pressure	Annually if <120/80 mm Hg; more frequently if >120/80 mm Hg and if other risk factors are present (e.g., African American race, diabetes, CHD)
Serum cholesterol	Routine screen in men >35 yr and women >45 yr and treat those at increased risk of CHD. Every 5 yr or more frequently in those at risk
Fecal occult blood and rectal examination	Annually
Flexible sigmoidoscopy or colonoscopy	Every 5-10 yr beginning at age 50 yr and continuing until age 75 yr
Diabetes mellitus screening	Every 3 yr; more frequently if high risk; no upper age limit suggested
Eye examination	Annual visual acuity and glaucoma screening
Obesity	All adults screened for obesity (BMI > 30 kg/m2) and offer counseling and behavioral interventions. no upper age limit suggested
Tobacco	All adults; provide interventions for smoking cessation in those who smoke; no upper age limit suggested
Depression screening	Annually
Dental examination and cleaning	Annually for those with teeth; cleaning every 6 mo, every 2 yr for denture wearers
Hearing test	All persons every 2-5 yr
Digital rectal examination	Annually for men
PSA	Provider should offer to men >50 yr with a life expectancy of at least 10 yr and to 45-yr-old men at higher risk, i.e., those with a first-degree relative diagnosed with prostate cancer at <65 yr and those who are African American (ACS); PSA age 50-70 if average risk and at age 45 yr if African American; recommend against screening for men >75 yr (USPSTF)
Mammogram	Varying recommendations: Every 1-2 yr in women ≥40 with annual CBE; no upper age limit suggested but limited evidence beyond 74 yr (USPSTF, ACS). Continue as long as the woman is in reasonably good health and would be a candidate for treatment (ACS)
Pap smear and pelvic examination	At least every 3 yr, stopping at age 65 if three consecutive negative examinations (USPSTF) or at age 70 yr if previously screened (ACS)

Screening: At-risk Older Adults

Thyroid function, ECG, bone density, mental status assessment, substance abuse screening, urinary incontinence assessment, functional assessment, medication reconciliation, skin cancer assessment, fall risk assessment, elder abuse or neglect assessment, driving safety assessment, ultrasound to screen for abdominal aneurysm (once for men aged 65-75 yr who have ever smoked)

Health Promotion Counseling

Exercise	At least 30 min of moderate-intensity physical activity daily
Nutrition	Adequate intake of vitamins and minerals with attention to calcium and antioxidants
Protective measures	Seatbelts, sunscreen, smoke detectors, fall risk reduction, driving safety, home safety

ACS, American Cancer Society; BMI, body mass index; CBE, clinical breast examination; CHD, coronary heart disease; ECG, electrocardiogram; PSA, prostate-specific antigen; USPSTF, U.S. Preventive Services Task Force.
Data from Agency for Healthcare Research and Quality, U.S. Department of Health and Human Services: *U.S. Preventive Services TaskForce (USPSTF)* (2010). Available at http://www.ahrq.gov/clinic/uspstfix.htm (accessed November 2010); Centers for Disease Control and Prevention, U.S. Department of Health and Human Services: Recommended adult immunization schedule—United States, 2010, *MMWR Weekly* 59(1), 2010; Hall KT, Chyun DA: General screening recommendations for chronic disease and risk factors in older adults, *Try This*, issue 27, 2010; and Miller C: *Nursing for wellness in older adults,* Philadelphia, 2009, Lippincott Williams & Wilkins.
*Based on available 2010 recommendations. Consult clinical guidelines for updated information (http://www.ahrq.gov/)

Cognitive Health

Knowledge about memory and memory changes related to aging is still developing. However, accumulating evidence suggests that there are many strategies to maintain and enhance cognitive health and vitality throughout life. At present, there is not enough evidence to identify which factors or interventions may increase or decrease the risk of developing Alzheimer's disease or other cognitive declines, but attention to brain health remains an important part of overall health promotion activities and should be encouraged (Agency for Healthcare

Research and Quality, 2010) "Modification of risk factors remains a cornerstone for dementia prevention until disease-modifying agents prove efficacious" (Desai et al., 2010, p. 1).

Cognitive health is defined as "the development and preservation of the multidimensional cognitive structure that allows the older adult to maintain social connectedness, an ongoing sense of purpose, and the abilities to function independently, to permit functional recovery from illness or injury, and to cope with residual functional deficits" (Hendrie et al., 2006, p. 12). This view of healthy cognitive aging (healthy brain aging) is comprehensive and proactive and implies that cognitive health is much more than simply a lack of decline with aging (Desai et al., 2010).

Nurses need to educate people of all ages about effective strategies to enhance cognitive health and vitality and to promote cognitive reserve and brain plasticity. Suggested strategies include prevention and management of chronic conditions, maintaining a healthy weight, avoiding excess caloric intake, limiting sodium and fat intake, increasing antioxidant defense by consuming fresh fruits and vegetables, physical activity, participation in mentally stimulating activity, and social engagement (Yevchak et al., 2008; Desai et al., 2010). *The Healthy Brain Initiative: A National Public Health Road Map to Maintaining Cognitive Health* (http://www.cdc.gov/aging/healthybrain/roadmap.htm) and the *Cognitive and Emotional Health Project: The Healthy Brain* (http://trans.nih.gov/cehp/index.htm) are examples of national efforts to promote cognitive health. Figure 2-4 presents a checklist that health care providers can use to promote healthy brain.

1	Counseled regarding smoking cessation	☐
	Comments:	
2	Advised to follow guidelines proposed jointly by the American Heart Association and the American College of Sports Medicine regarding daily physical activity	☐
	Comments:	
3	Counseled regarding healthy nutrition (e.g., Mediterranean diet, DASH [Dietary Approaches to Stop Hypertension] diet)	☐
	Comments:	
4	Counseled regarding the importance of intellectually challenging and creative leisure activities	☐
	Comments:	
5	Counseled regarding strategies to promote emotional resilience and reduce psychological distress and depression (e.g., relaxation exercises, mindfulness-meditation practices)	☐
	Comments:	
6	Advised to maintain an active, socially integrated lifestyle	☐
	Comments:	
7	Discussed strategies to achieve and maintain optimal daily sleep	☐
	Comments:	
8	Provided education about strategies to reduce risk of serious head injury (e.g., wearing seat belts, wearing helmets during contact sports, bicycling, skiing, skateboarding)	☐
	Comments:	
9	Provided education about strategies to reduce exposure to hazardous substances (e.g., wearing protective clothing during the administration of pesticides, fumigants, fertilizers, and defoliants)	☐
	Comments:	
10	Provided education and counseling regarding negative health effects of alcohol consumption more than recommended as safe by the National Institute of Alcoholism and Alcohol Abuse	☐
	Comments:	
11	Provided education about importance of achieving and maintaining healthy weight to promote overall health	☐
	Comments:	
12	Discussed and implemented strategies to achieve optimal blood pressure control	☐
	Comments:	
13	Discussed and implemented strategies to achieve optimal control of dyslipidemia (e.g., high cholesterol)	☐
	Comments:	
14	Discussed and implemented strategies to achieve optimal control of blood sugar/diabetes	☐
	Comments:	
15	Discussed risks and benefits of medications, supplements, herbal remedies, and vitamins to promote brain health	☐
	Comments:	
16	Discussed and implemented secondary prevention of stroke strategies (e.g., daily baby aspirin)	☐
	Comments:	

FIGURE 2-4 Checklist to Promote Healthy Brain Aging: A Guide for Clinicians. (From Desai A, Grossberg G, Chibnall J: Healthy brain aging: a road map, *Clinics in Geriatric Medicine* 26:1, 2010. Courtesy of Center for Healthy Brain Aging, St. Louis University School of Medicine, St. Louis, MO.)

Gerontological nurse researcher Dr. Barbara Resnick has made a significant contribution to our understanding of health among older people, but there is still far too little research on this topic, particularly among racially and culturally diverse older adults. Additional research is also necessary to determine best practice approaches to maintaining and improving the health of older adults in various age cohorts as well as among those who are experiencing physical and cognitive limitations. Although important throughout life, the period of preretirement and retirement may be an opportune time to enhance the focus on health prevention and promotion (Wilson and Palha, 2007). *Promoting Preventive Services for Adults 50-64: Community and Clinical Partnerships* (Centers for Disease Control and Prevention, AARP, American Medical Association, 2009) provides guidelines for disease preventive services for this age group as well as indicators and baseline data at national and state levels to monitor progress and to promote successful strategies (see www.cdc.gov/aging).

PROMOTING HEALTHY AGING: IMPLICATIONS FOR GERONTOLOGICAL NURSING

Gerontological nurses use a holistic approach to enhance wellness in older people. The focus is on maximizing strengths, minimizing limitations, facilitating adaptation, and encouraging growth for all older people. Healthy aging does not mean the absence of disease; rather, it means achieving the highest level of personal wellness no matter the health condition. A broad view of wellness and its dimensions provides nurses with a framework for health promotion in older adults that includes interventions in the physical, emotional, social, intellectual, spiritual, and environmental realms. In essence, healthy aging begins in the prenatal period and continues throughout the life course. The focus of health professionals, as well as the nation, should be on the creation of social and physical environments that enhance the potential of good health for all and promote healthy development and healthy behaviors at every stage of life.

Prevention or postponement of chronic illness may be a realistic goal for many older people or those soon to be old. However, it may not be realistic for older adults who are already experiencing these conditions. In this case, managing chronic illness, preventing unnecessary functional decline, and creating environments and conditions supportive of the highest quality of life are appropriate goals. An important nursing role is to educate older people about the positive outcomes of health promotion and disease prevention activities in reducing premature mortality and morbidity (compression of morbidity), maintaining functional independence, and extending life expectancy while maintaining or enhancing the quality of life (Resnick, 2003a).

Nurses can be very influential in the development of disease prevention and health promotion interventions for older adults in settings across the continuum, and several successful models have been described (Resnick, 2003a,b; Gerson et al., 2004; Galik et al., 2009). Opportunities to achieve the highest possible level of wellness should be available to the active independent older adult in comprehensive and affordable programs in the community (e.g., YMCA, senior centers, retirement communities). For the older person experiencing more limitations as a result of chronic illness, assisted living facilities and skilled nursing facilities should provide opportunities for health promotion and wellness activities (e.g., exercise, health education, cognitive stimulation, opportunities for continued engagement and growth). And, even in acute care and primary care settings, interventions to enhance health and well-being should be as important as management and treatment of illness. The goal is always to promote the highest quality of life no matter the age or condition of the person.

ℯvolve   To access your student resources, go to *http://evolve.elsevier.com/Ebersole/TwdHlthAging*

KEY CONCEPTS

- The "medicalization" of our society has brought about the common belief that the absence of disease is health.
- Wellness is a concept, not a condition. It is human adaptation at the most individually satisfying level in response to existing internal and external conditions.
- With increasing life expectancy and numbers of older people, the positive outcomes of health promotion and disease prevention interventions for this age group are receiving significant attention.
- Preparation for healthy aging begins in the prenatal period and is fostered through social and physical environments that promote healthy development and healthy behaviors at every stage of life.
- Older people rate their health in terms of the ability to function.
- Older adults have been added as a new topic area in HP 2020 with the goal of improving health, function, and quality of life. Goals for disease prevention and health promotion in older adults include reducing premature mortality and morbidity (compression of morbidity), maintaining functional independence, and extending life expectancy while maintaining or enhancing the quality of life.
- Continued attention must be given to racial and cultural disparities in the health of older people.
- Four preventable risk factors—smoking, high blood pressure, elevated blood glucose, and overweight and obesity—currently reduce life expectancy in the United States by 4.9 years in men and 4.1 years in women.
- A nurse with a wellness focus designs interventions to enhance health promotion and disease prevention for older adults across the continuum of care.
- Even in chronic illness and the dying process, an optimal level of wellness and well-being is attainable for each individual.

CASE STUDY   WELLNESS IN LATE LIFE

Rhonda recently celebrated her ninetieth birthday with a large number of family and friends attending from far and near. She said, "That was the best day of my life! I was married three times but none of the weddings were as exciting as this. I have attained what I would never have thought possible when I was 50. Yes, life has been a struggle. One husband died in the Second World War, one was abusive and we were divorced, and the last husband, a wonderful man, developed Alzheimer's and I cared for him for six years. My children sometimes wonder how I have managed to keep such a positive outlook. I believe my purpose in living so long is to be an example of aging well."

Rhonda is frail and thin, and she has advanced osteoarthritis for which she routinely takes ibuprofen and calcium tablets. She does not tolerate dairy products, so she uses lactose-free products. She eats sparingly but likes almost all foods and is concerned about good nutrition. She daily rides the stationary bike in her apartment and last year walked a mile each day but has not regained her full function since a broken hip last June. While she was immobilized, she developed pressure wounds on her heels and coccyx but recently went to a wound center at a nearby hospital and is being treated effectively. She religiously follows the routine. As for religion, she says, "The closer I get to dying, the more I wonder what it is all about but I really just enjoy every day. Of course, I got depressed when I fell and broke my hip and I don't enjoy using the walker when I go out of the apartment but I feel blessed to have so many good people in my life."

Based on the case study, develop a nursing care plan using the following procedure*:

- List Rhonda's comments that provide subjective data.
- List information that provides objective data.

- From these data, identify and state, using accepted format, two nursing diagnoses you determine are most significant to Rhonda at this time. List two of Rhonda's strengths that you have identified from the data.
- Determine and state outcome criteria for each diagnosis. These must reflect some alleviation of the problem identified in the nursing diagnosis and must be stated in concrete and measurable terms.
- Plan and state one or more interventions for each diagnosed problem. Provide specific documentation of the source used to determine the appropriate intervention. Plan at least one intervention that incorporates Rhonda's existing strengths.
- Evaluate the success of the intervention. Interventions must correlate directly with the stated outcome criteria to measure the outcome success.

CRITICAL THINKING QUESTIONS

1. What lifestyle changes might you suggest for Rhonda, and what would be your reason for doing so?
2. Where would you place Rhonda in the continuum of wellness? Explain your reasons for doing so.
3. Construct a definition of health that seems to you to incorporate the essential elements of a holistic perspective.
4. Discuss your thoughts about wellness as it relates to the medical concerns about old age.
5. Define wellness for yourself. What would you want to change in your life to achieve a sense of wellness?
6. Discuss the concept of wellness while dying and your thoughts about this issue.

*Students are advised to refer to their nursing diagnosis text and identify possible or potential problems.

RESEARCH QUESTIONS

1. Do most elders believe there is a state of wellness in spite of physical illness?
2. What do elders believe about the concept of "wellness"?
3. What are the factors that indicate one is in a state of "wellness"?
4. What are the variables that indicate a dying person is in a state of "wellness"?
5. What are the perceptions of younger people about the possibility of healthy aging?
6. How do nurses enhance wellness for older adults in various settings across the continuum?
7. What are the differences in following recommended health promotion and prevention guidelines among older people in different age cohorts?
8. What are the barriers and facilitators to accessing health promotion and disease prevention services among older adults?
9. How do racially and ethnically diverse older adults view healthy aging?

REFERENCES

Agency for Healthcare Research and Quality, U.S. Department of Health and Human Services: Preventing Alzheimer's disease and cognitive decline (2010). U.S. Preventive Services Task Force (USPSTF). Available at http://www.ahrq.gov/downloads/pub/evidence/pdf/alzheimers/alzcog.pdf (accessed November 2010).

American Medical Association: Health status of the population (2008). Available at www.ama-assn.org/go/healthcaretrends (accessed November 2010).

Barondess J: Toward healthy aging: the preservation of health, *Journal of the American Geriatrics Society* 56:145, 2008.

Bortz WM: *We live too short and die too long*, New York, 1991, Bantam Books.

Center for Diseases Control and Prevention, Administration on Aging, Agency for Healthcare Reasearch and Quality Centers for Medicare and Medicaid Services: Enhancing the use of clinical preventive services among older adults, Washington. http://www.cdc.gov/aging/pdf/clinical_preventive_Services_Closing_the_Gap_Report.pdf.

Centers for Disease Control and Prevention, U.S. Department of Health and Human Services: Healthy aging: improving and extending quality of life among older Americans: at a glance 2010 (2010a). Available at http://www.cdc.gov/chronicdisease/resources/publications/AAG/aging.htm (accessed November 2010).

Centers for Disease Control and Prevention, U.S. Department of Health and Human Services: Leading causes of death (2010b). Available at http://www.cdc.gov/nchs/fastats/lcod.htm (accessed November 2010).

Centers for Disease Control and Prevention, AARP, American Medical Association: Promoting preventive services for adults 50-64: community and clinical partnerships (2009). Available at http://www.cdc.gov/aging/ (accessed November 2010).

Curry R: Ageism in healthcare: Time for a change, *Aging Well* 1:16, 2008.

Danaei G, Rimm E, Oza S, et al: The promise of prevention: the effects of four preventable risk factors on national life expectancy disparities by race and county in the United States, *PLoS Medicine* 7:e1000248, 2010. Available at http://www.plosmedicine.org/article/info%3Adoi%2F10.1371%2Fjournal.pmed.1000248 (accessed November 2010).

Desai A, Grossberg G, Chibnall J: Healthy brain aging: a road map, *Clinics in Geriatric Medicine* 26:1, 2010.

Dunn HL: *High-level wellness*, Arlington, VA, 1961, R.W. Beatty.

Fries JF: Aging, natural death, and the compression of morbidity, *New England Journal of Medicine* 303:130, 1980.

Fries JF: The compression of morbidity: near or far? *Milbank Quarterly* 67:208, 1990.

Fries JF: Reducing disability in older age, *JAMA* 288:3164, 2002.

Galik EM, Resnick B, Pretzer-Aboff I: Knowing what makes them tick: motivating cognitively impaired older adults to participate in restorative care, *International Journal of Nursing Practice* 15:48, 2009.

Gerson L, Dorsey C, Berg J, et al: Enhancing self-care in community dwelling older adults, *Geriatric Nursing* 25:272, 2004.

Hansen-Kyle L: A concept analysis of healthy aging, *Nursing Forum* 40:45, 2005.

Hendrie H, Albert M, Butters M, et al: The NIH Cognitive and Emotional Health Project: report of the Critical Evaluation Study Committee, *Alzheimer's & Dementia* 2:12, 2006.

Hettler B; National Wellness Institute: 6 Dimensions of Wellness. Available at http://www.nationalwellness.org/index.php?id_tier=2&id_c=25 (accessed November 2010).

Hooyman N, Kiyak H: *Social gerontology*, ed 9. Boston, 2011, Allyn & Bacon.

Kleindorfer D, Khoury J, Moomaw C, et al: Stroke incidence is decreasing in whites but not in blacks: a population based estimate of temporal trends in stroke incidence from the Greater Cincinnati/Northern Kentucky Stroke Study, *Stroke* 41:1326, 2010.

Manton K, Gu X, Lowrimore G: Cohort changes in active life expectancy in the U.S. elderly population: experience from the 1982-2004 National Long-term Care Survey, *Journals of Gerontology Series B, Psychological Sciences and Social Sciences* 63:S269, 2008.

Miller A, Iris M: Health promotion attitudes and strategies in older adults, *Health Education & Behavior* 29:249, 2002.

Miniño AM, Xu JQ, Kochanek KD: *Deaths: Preliminary Data for 2008*. National Vital Statistics Reports; vol 59 no 2. Hyattsville, MD: National Center for Health Statistics. 2010.

Morley J, Flaherty J: It's never too late: health promotion and illness prevention in older persons, *Journals of Gerontology Series A, Biological Sciences and Medical Sciences* 57:M338, 2002.

Resnick B: Health promotion practices of older adults: testing an individualized approach, *Journal of Clinical Nursing* 12:46, 2003a.

Resnick B: Health promotion practices of older adults: model testing, *Public Health Nursing* 20:2, 2003b.

Robinson K, Reinhard S: Looking ahead in long-term care: the next 50 years, *Nursing Clinics of North America* 44:253, 2009.

Seeman T, Merkin S, Karlamangla A: Disability trends among older Americans: National Health and Nutrition Examination Surveys, 1988-1994 and 1999-2004, *American Journal of Public Health* 100:100, 2010.

Trust for America's Health: Adult immunization: shots to save lives (2010). Available at http://healthyamericans.org (accessed November 2010).

U.S. Department of Health and Human Service, Office of Disease Prevention and Health Promotion: *Healthy People 2020 Framework. s: Phase 1 report: recommendations for the framework and format of Healthy People 2020* (2010). Available at http://www.healthypeople.gov (accessed December 2010).

Wilson D, Palha P: A systematic review of published research articles on health promotion at retirement, *Journal of Nursing Scholarship* 39:330, 2007.

Yevchak A, Loeb S, Fick D: Promoting cognitive health and vitality: a review of clinical implications, *Geriatric Nursing* 29:302, 2008.

Theories of Aging

Kathleen Jett

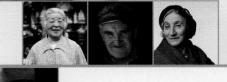

A STUDENT SPEAKS

Until I started learning about the science of the aging process I had no idea how complicated it could be. We seem to have learned so much but still have so much more to learn.

Helena, age 23

AN ELDER SPEAKS

When I was a young girl Einstein was proposing the molecular theory of matter, and we had never heard of DNA or RNA. We only knew of genes in the most rudimentary theoretical sense. Now I hear that scientists believe there is a gene that is controlling my life span. I really hope they find it before I die.

Beatrice, age 72

LEARNING OBJECTIVES

On completion of this chapter, the reader will be able to:

1. Describe the interrelationships between the various biological theories of aging.
2. Compare and contrast theories of programmed aging with error theories of aging.
3. Recommend strategies to promote healthy aging that are consistent with the state of the science of biological theories of aging.
4. Compare and contrast the major psychosocial theories of aging.

5. Use at least one sociological theory of aging to support or refute commonly provided social services for older adults living in the community.
6. Create strategies to foster the highest level of wellness in aging, based on the developmental theories of aging.
7. Explain how personality may influence the lived experience of aging.

Theories are made in an attempt to explain phenomena, to give a sense of order, and to provide a framework from which we can view the world. The theories of aging have been broadly drawn, from cellular changes to physical, to those in the sociological and psychological realms. The extant theories are no longer thought to be in competition with each other. Instead, each offers a view of different and often overlapping aspects of the changes we associate with living a long life.

Although we have not yet come to a conclusion about why or how we age, we do know that aging is influenced by all aspects of personhood, be they biological, psychological, sociocultural, functional, or spiritual. Only when life is considered in its totality can we begin to understand aging. This chapter provides the reader with an overview of several prominent theories of aging. The knowledge provides the context in which gerontological nurses can promote health and render caring.

WHAT IS AGING?

In everyday language, *aging* is most often described in terms of chronology, or by the measurement of time since birth. However, each culture has its own definition of when one becomes recognized as a "senior" or elder or older adult. Some groups define aging in functional terms; that one becomes "old" when one is no longer able to perform one's usual activities (Jett, 2003). Social aging is determined by role, such as retiree or as a wise woman/man of the clan; of status change when a parent becomes a grandparent. Transitions into the status of "senior" are often marked by ritual, such as special celebrations, invitations to join groups such as the American Association of Retired Persons or the qualification for "senior discounts." Although this number is rising, one qualifies for "old age" benefits in the United States at 65 years of age. Physiological aging is a complex process involving every cell in the body. The physical traits by which we identify one as older (e.g., gray hair, wrinkled skin) are referred to as the aging phenotype, that is, an outward expression of one's individual genetic makeup (Carnes et al., 2008).

BIOLOGICAL THEORIES OF AGING

Biological aging, referred to as *senescence,* is an exceedingly complex, genetically regulated, interactive process of change (Ostojić et al., 2009). Whereas there is a growing body of knowledge about the genomics of aging, what triggers the associated changes at the cellular or organ level is still a topic of debate. However, it is commonly believed that the aging phenotype reflects declining functional capacity of the most basic structures in the cells, which in turn affects the functioning of the organism, be it a yeast cell, a mouse, or a human (National Institute of Aging [NIA], 2003). Is the timing of the decline preprogrammed within the cell itself, or is it random? Is there a maximal life span? How important is the lifetime effect of the environment—be it physical (e.g., pollution) psychological, or social (e.g.inequity)? Why do some people age faster than others? (Box 3-1). And perhaps most importantly of all, what is the relationship between aging and illness?

Cellular Functioning

Survival of an organism depends on successful cellular reproduction. The genetic components of each cell, that is, deoxyribonucleic acid (DNA) and ribonucleic acid (RNA), serve as templates for reproduction, ensuring that, theoretically, new cells formed during mitosis are exactly the same as the old cells in form and function. That they will, in fact, be identical with each and every replication.

If this were true, the organism would not change; it would not "age." Instead, the cells become increasingly complex. For example, an infant does not learn to walk or talk until the neurons have adequate myelination, that is, until the myelin sheath is thick enough to facilitate smooth and rapid transmission of impulses. The cells also accumulate damage resulting in errors seen in replication. These changes are made visible in the traits we associate with aging. The association of cellular errors and the aging phenotype is no longer in question (Nomellini et al., 2008). It is the causation and patterns of effect that are in debate and discovery. We do not know for certain if the damage and changes are orderly and predictable, or random and chaotic (Box 3-2).

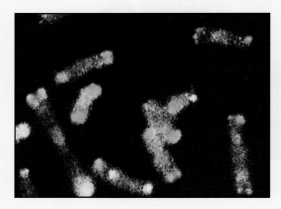
Data from Calado RT: Telomeres and marrow failure, Hematology, the American Society of Hematology Education Program Book 2009:338, 2009; and National Institute of Aging (NIA): Aging under the microscope: a biological quest, NIH Publication No. 02-2756. Bethesda, MD, 2003, U.S. Government Printing Office. Available at www.nia.nih.gov (accessed November 2010).

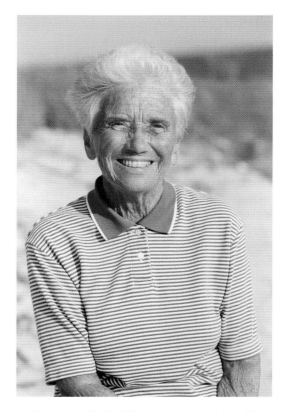

Programmed Aging Theories

Programmed aging theories suggest that aging is the result of predictable cellular death; that the cell and organism have genetically determined life spans referred to as the Hayflick limit or the biological clock (NIA, 2003). Much of the contemporary work on programmed aging has evolved from the groundbreaking work of Hayflick and Moorehead (1981). In a test of their theory, they found that living cells could be preserved indefinitely by keeping them at subzero temperatures. However, when thawed, the cells continued to replicate from the point at which they had been interrupted, and the total number of replications remained constant.

Neuroendocrine Control or Pacemaker Theory

The *neuroendocrine* control or *pacemaker theory* explains aging as a programmed decline in the functioning of the nervous, endocrine, and immune systems (De la Fuente, 2008). It is not that the cells "die"; instead, they lose their ability to reproduce, a process referred to as *replicative senescence.*

Current research centers on the effect of hormones on neuroendocrine functioning, especially dehydroepiandrosterone (DHEA) and melatonin. DHEA is produced by the adrenal glands, and the amount secreted diminishes with time. Adding DHEA to the diets of experimental animals appears to have increased their longevity and bolstered their immune response (Legrain and Girard, 2003; Perrini et al., 2005). Melatonin, produced by the pineal gland, has been found to be a powerful regulator of biological rhythms and antioxidants. Its secretion is also markedly reduced as one ages (Srinivasan et al., 2005). Other hormones under examination in relation to aging are growth factors, estrogen, and testosterone (NIA, 2003).

Immunity Theory

The immune system in the human body is a complex network of cells, tissues, and organs that function separately, but together protect the body from invasion by exogenous substances, such as pathogens. The body maintains homeostasis through the actions of this protective, self-regulatory system, controlled by B lymphocytes (humoral immunity) and T lymphocytes (cellular immunity) (De la Fuente, 2008).

The *immunity theory* presents aging as a programmed accumulation of damage and decline in the function of the immune system, or *immunosenescence.* The damage is the result of oxidative stress (see p. 36). The ability of lymphocytes to withstand oxidative stress appears to be a key factor in the aging phenotype; T lymphocytes show more signs of "aging" than do B lymphocytes (Swain and Nikolich-Zugich, 2009). The T cells are thought to be responsible for hastening the age-related changes caused by autoimmune reactions as the body battles itself. Cellular errors in the immune system have been found to lead to an auto-aggressive phenomenon in which normal cells are misidentified as alien and are destroyed by the body's own immune system. This phenomenon is used to explain the increase in autoimmune disorders as we age (De la Fuente, 2008).

An increasing number of health problems common in later life are being considered in terms of impaired immunosenescence and autoimmunity. Alzheimer's disease, rheumatoid conditions, atherosclerosis, hypertension, and thromboembolism are among those that have been studied in association with immunity and directly linked to related oxidative stress (see (Box 3-3). Of significant importance in the clinical setting is the increased susceptibility to infections, autoimmune disorders, and cancers (Gomez et al., 2008).

Error Theories

The *error theories* propose that the aging phenotype is the result of an accumulation of random errors in the synthesis of cellular DNA and RNA. With each replication, more errors occur until the cells are no longer able to fully function, and the changes become visible.

BOX 3-3   DISEASES AND DISORDERS LINKED TO OXYGEN-DERIVED FREE RADICALS

- Atherosclerosis
  - Heart disease
  - Stroke
- Brain disorders
  - Ischemic brain injury
  - Aluminum toxicity
  - Alzheimer's disease
  - Neurotoxins
- AIDS-associated dementia
- Cancer
- Cardiac myopathy
- Chronic granulomatous disease
- Diabetes mellitus
- Eye disorders
  - Macular degeneration
  - Cataracts
- Inflammatory disorders
- Iron overload
- Lung disorders
- Asbestosis
- Oxygen toxicity
- Emphysema
- Nutritional deficiencies
- Radiation injury
- Reperfusion injury
- Rheumatoid arthritis
- Skin disorders
  - Solar radiation
  - Burns
  - Contact dermatitis
  - Bloom syndrome
- Toxic states
- Xenobiotics (CCl_4, paraquat, cigarette smoke, etc.)
- Metal ions (Ni, Cu, Fe, etc.)
- Amyotrophic lateral sclerosis?
- Huntington's disease?
- Parkinson's disease?

AIDS, acquired immunodeficiency syndrome.
From McCance KL, Huether SE: *Pathophysiology: the biologic basis for disease in adults and children,* ed 6, St. Louis, MO, 2010, Mosby.

Wear-and-Tear Theory

One of the earliest theories of aging, the *wear-and-tear theory,* proposes that cell errors are the result of "wearing out" over time because of continued use. Cells are aggravated by the harmful effects of internal and external stressors, which include pollutants and injurious metabolic by-products, now known as free radicals. These may cause a progressive decline in cellular function or the death of an increasing number of cells. Striated muscle, heart muscle, muscle fibers, nerve cells, and the brain are irreplaceable when destroyed by wear and tear or by mechanical or chemical injury (Carnes et al., 2008). As science advanced so did the understanding of the ideas proposed in the wear-and-tear theory of aging.

Cross-linkage Theory

The *cross-linkage theory* describes aging as the result of accumulated damage from errors associated with cross-linked proteins. For unknown reasons cellular glucose attaches to protein, either by glycosylation or by glycation. Once attached, a chain reaction of bonding or "cross-linking" between the protein and the glucose causing them to become stiff and thick. The newly cross-linked proteins are called *AGEs,* or *advanced glycation end-products* (Eyetsemitan, 2007). Cross-linking is an area of research especially as it applies to wound healing.

Because collagens are the most plentiful proteins in the body, this is where the cross-linking can be seen most easily in the form of stiffened joints and skin. Skin that was once smooth, silky, firm, and soft becomes dry, sags, and is less elastic. Collagen is also a key component of the lungs, arteries, and tendons. Similar changes can be seen there (see Chapter 4). Cross-linking may also cause cholesterol to attach to cell walls, leading to atherosclerosis, and the lens to cloud and stiffen, leading to cataracts.

Substances that may act as cross-linking agents include unsaturated fats and metal ions such as aluminum, zinc, and magnesium. Many medications taken by older adults (e.g., antacids, anticoagulants) contain aluminum and may exacerbate cross-linking, although a causative effect has not yet been clarified (Valko et al., 2005).

Oxidative Stress Theory (Free Radical Theory)

The *free radical* or *oxidative stress theory of aging* has garnered strong support as correlative evidence has accumulated over the last 35 years (Jang and Van Remmen, 2009). Proponents of this theory postulate that the errors are the result of random damage from free radicals. Free radicals are molecules that contain unpaired ions and therefore an extra electrical charge. They exist only momentarily but are highly reactive to molecules in the cell membrane. As the free ion charge latches onto other molecules, damage occurs, especially to the membranes of unsaturated lipids such as mitochondria. Free radicals are natural by-products of the cellular metabolism of oxygen and are always present to some extent. In the immune system they are useful for destroying bacteria and other foreign substances. The accumulation of free radicals is referred to as "oxidative stress" or "oxidative damage." Mitochondrial DNA appears to be most affected by these changes (Figure 3-2) (Gruber et al., 2008).

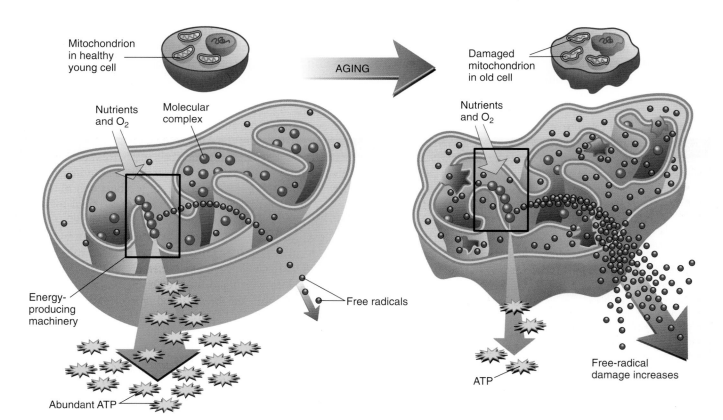

FIGURE 3-2 Mitochondria in young and old cells. ATP, adenosine triphosphate. (From McCance KL, Huether SE: *Pathophysiology: the biologic basis for disease in adults and children,* ed 6, St. Louis, MO, 2010, Mosby.)

BOX 3-4   RESEARCH HIGHLIGHTS

Increasing the Life Span

There is increasing evidence that caloric restriction (CR) of 20% to 60% increases life expectancy in a range of organisms, including rhesus monkeys. CR was also found to reduce the number of disease states common in later life, to decrease brain atrophy, and to increase the "youthfulness" of appearance (Shimokawa et al., 2008; Cox and Mattison, 2009). An interest in the potential effects of CR has given rise to the *CR Society International,* a professional and lay association of persons interested in related research and support for persons who are restricting their diets in hopes of prolonging their lives.

BOX 3-5   PROMOTING HEALTHY AGING CONSISTENT WITH THE BIOLOGICAL THEORIES OF AGING

- Exercise on soft surfaces, using good body mechanics. (Wear-and-tear)
- Avoid skin dryness and joint stiffening. (Cross-link)
- Avoid environmental pollutants and unnecessary radiation. (Oxidative stress)
- Watch for research related to the effect of unsaturated fats and heavy metals on cell health. (Cross-link)
- Watch for research on the use and presence of antioxidants. (Oxidative stress)
- Avoid stress. (Oxidative stress, immunity)
- Minimize the potential for infection: wash hands frequently, undergo immunizations, and avoid those who are ill. (Immunity)

In youth, naturally occurring vitamins, hormones, enzymes, and antioxidants neutralize the free radicals as needed (Valko et al., 2005). In simplistic terms, the oxidative stress theory, first proposed by Harman (1956), advocates that, over time, the production of free radicals increases and the body's ability to remove them decreases (Hornsby, 2010). When the accumulation of damage occurs faster than the cells can repair themselves, the damage significantly impairs function (Grune et al., 2001).

• • •

Although all these theories provide possible clues to aging, they also raise many questions and stimulate continuing research. A unifying theory does not yet exist that explains the mechanics and causes underlying the biological phenomenon of aging, and it is apparent that the theories are no longer distinct. The science of the biology of aging continues to advance at a rapid pace, fueled in large part by the success of the human genome project (Box 3-4). The science of *epigenetics,* or how the genes are influenced by environment, lifestyle, role, and other factors, is an area of intensive research. It is hoped that more research will lead to the discovery of other pathways and key changes in gene expression seen as the aging phenotype.

PROMOTING HEALTHY AGING: IMPLICATIONS FOR GERONTOLOGICAL NURSING

In the application of our growing knowledge of biological aging, it appears reasonable to expect that slowing or reducing cellular damage may have the most potential for promoting healthy aging. Although this is not likely to lead to increased longevity, helping persons identify pollutants in their environments, from those associated with industrial emission to ultraviolet light to second-hand smoke, may decrease the excess burden and consequently harmful effects of oxidative stress. Stress reduction may lead to improved or maintained immunity. As more is learned about the effect of antioxidants and the substances in which they are found, the gerontological nurse can use the knowledge of biological theories of aging to encourage the healthiest diets and judicious use of herbs and dietary supplements (see Chapter 10). With an understanding of potential changes in immunity, the conscientious nurse can take an active role in promoting specific preventive strategies such as the use of immunizations (especially influenza and pneumococcal) and the avoidance of exposure to others with infections (Box 3-5).

PSYCHOSOCIAL AND DEVELOPMENTAL THEORIES OF AGING

Psychosocial and developmental theories of aging attempt to explain and predict the changes in roles and relationships in middle and late life, with an emphasis on adjustment. The majority of these began appearing in the literature in the 1950s and continued to emerge in the 1970s and early 1980s. All had a notable absence of the consideration of culture as an influencing factor consistent with the historical period from which they emerged. While knowledgable, it is of note that these early theoreticians were exclusively white. They gained popularity from what is called "face validity," making sense based on the personal and professional experience of both scientists and clinicians. This set of theories has been descriptive with little variation since they were first proposed. Problems of intersubjectivity of meaning, testability, and empirical adequacy have been persistent. Nonetheless, the psychosocial and developmental theories of aging remain part of the backdrop of how aging is conceptualized.

Role Theory

One of the earliest explanations of how older adults adjust to aging was proposed by Cottrell in 1942. *Role theory* proposes that the ability of an individual to adapt to changing roles over the life course is a predictor of adjustment to personal aging. As individuals evolve through the various stages in life, so do their roles. In successful aging, as one role is completed, another one takes its place that is valued comparatively. For example, the wage-earning work role may be replaced by that of a volunteer or the parent becomes the grandparent. Resistance to role changes or failure to assume new roles indicates poor adjustment to one's own aging.

Age Norms

Role theory may be operationalized in the phenomena of *age norms.* Age norms are socially and culturally constructed expectations of what is deemed as acceptable behavior. They are based on the assumption that chronological age (and gender) implies roles; for example, one may hear, "If only they would act their age," or "You are too old to do/say/behave like that." Age norms may serve as limitations and be expressed in negative stereotypes. Although the beliefs in age-segregated roles are still present, challenges began with the socially controversial but popular television of the 1970s (e.g., *Maude,* 1972-1978) and later in the 1980s (*The Golden Girls,* 1985-1993). In both of these shows, the characters behaved in ways that challenged long-established age norms for white middle- and late-aged women. With the aging of the baby boomers, the popular culture continues to challenge role theory and age norms. Both men and women are assuming roles and engaging in behavior in 2010 that were unimaginable when role theory was first proposed.

Activity Theory

In 1953 Havinghurst and Albrecht first proposed that continued activity was an indicator of successful aging. The focus was on the individual's need to maintain a productive life for it to be a happy one. The theorists saw activity as necessary to maintain life satisfaction and positive self-concept. The productivity of middle life (see Erikson) is thought to be best replaced with equally engaging pursuits in late life (Maddox, 1963). Activity meant that the person is able to "stay young." The theory was based on the assumption that it is better to be active (and young) than inactive and better to be happy than unhappy (Havinghurst, 1972).

Activity theory has continued to enjoy favor as it is still consistent with Western society's emphasis on work, wealth, and productivity. Failure to remain active and productive is viewed by many as signs of failure at any age (Wadensten, 2006).

Disengagement Theory

In contrast, *disengagement theory* proposed that in the natural course of aging the individual does, and should, slowly withdraw from his or her former roles and activities to allow the transfer of power to the younger generations (Cumming and Henry, 1961). The transfer was viewed as necessary for the maintenance of social equilibrium; therefore the elders' withdrawal is seen as successful aging (Wadensten, 2006). The disengagement perspective probably provided the basis for age discrimination, such as occupational practices in which an older employee is replaced with a younger one. Although this practice was covertly accepted in the past, it is now challenged socially and legally. It is now accepted that an elder's withdrawal is not necessarily a good thing for society.

Continuity Theory

According to *continuity theory,* an individual tends to develop and maintain a consistent pattern of behavior, substituting one role for a similar one as the person matures. Late life roles, responsibilities, and activities are a reflection of a continuation of life patterns (Havinghurst et al., 1968). Personality is seen not only to be enduring but also as becoming more entrenched and pronounced as one ages. Personality influences the roles and activities we choose and the level of

BOX 3-6	CONTINUITY FOR HEALTH

Mrs. J. was 75 and had just been diagnosed with advanced breast cancer. She would be staying in the hospital to complete her tests and begin treatment. When asked what would help her cope the most, she was quick to respond. "Every morning of my life I start the day with quiet meditation; this way I can keep everything in perspective and find healing and direction for the day. But since I have been here I have been unable to do this at all. There are always people coming in and out of my room or making noise on the intercom. I just need 20 minutes to myself in peace and calm. Can you make that happen?"

satisfaction drawn from life. Successful aging is associated with one's ability to maintain and continue previous behaviors and roles, or to find suitable replacements (Wadensten, 2006) (Box 3-6).

Age-stratification Theory

According to *age-stratification theory,* social aging can be best understood by considering the individual as a member of an age group, with similarities to others in the group. Age stratification can take a number of different forms, including the conceptualization of "young," "middle-aged," and "old." Alternatively, Thomas's (2004) proposal suggests that "childhood" and "adulthood" are followed by "elderhood." The concept of age stratification is used today in references to "cohort effects."

Modernization Theory

Modernization theory attempts to explain the social changes that have resulted in the devaluing of both the contributions of elders and the elders themselves. Before about 1900 in the United States, materials and political resources were controlled by the older members of society (Achenbaum, 1978). The resources included not only their time, but also their knowledge, traditional skills, and experience. They held power through property ownership, including decision-making related to food distribution. Older women often held important religious and cultural roles of instructing youth and controlling ceremony (Sokolovsky, 1997).

According to the modernization theory, the status and value of elders are lost when their labors are no longer considered useful, kinship networks are dispersed, the information they hold is no longer pertinent to the society in which they live, and the culture in which they live no longer reveres them (Hendricks and Hendricks, 1986). It is proposed that these changes are the result of advancing technology, urbanization, and mass education (Cowgill, 1981).

DEVELOPMENTAL THEORIES OF AGING

Developmental theories presuppose that aging is an ongoing and incremental step-wise progression between birth and death. Like the psychosocial theories, they are widely accepted as accurate descriptions but have not been empirically tested.

Jung's Theory of Personality

Psychologist Carl Jung, a contemporary of Sigmund Freud, proposed a theory of the development of personality throughout life, from childhood to old age (Jung, 1933/1971). He was one of the first psychologists to define the last half of life as having a purpose of its own, quite apart from species survival; distinctly different from early life. "We cannot live the afternoon of life according to the programme of life's morning—for what was great in the morning will be little at evening, and what in the morning was true will at evening have become a lie" (Jung, 1933/1955, p. 108).

According to this theory, a personality is either extroverted, that is, oriented toward the external world, or introverted and oriented to the subjective inner world of the individual. Jung suggested that aging results in a movement from extraversion to introversion. Beginning perhaps at midlife, individuals begin to question their own dreams, values, and priorities. The potential for resultant crisis of emotional upheaval is a step in the process of personality development. With chronological age and personality development, Jung proposed that the person is able to move from a focus on outward achievement to one of acceptance of the self and awareness that both the accomplishments and challenges to a lifetime can be found within oneself. The development of the psyche and the inner person is accompanied by a search for personal meaning and the spiritual self. This personality of late life can easily be compared with Erikson's ego integrity, Maslow's self-actualization, and Tornstam's gerotranscendence, which are described in the following sections.

Erikson

Psychologist Erik Erikson is best known for articulating life as a series of developmental stages. Most students have studied Erikson's *eight-stage* or *task model*. Erikson (1950/1993) theorized a predetermined order of development and specific tasks that were associated with specific periods across the life span. He proposed that successful mastery of one task was necessary for successful movement to the next stage of maturity. Erikson's task of middle age is generativity, or that which establishes oneself and contributes in meaningful ways for the future and future generations. Failure to accomplish this stage results in stagnation. What has been called the "final task" of the stage of late life is that of ego integrity as opposed to despair. Ego integrity, drawing from a Freudian perspective, implies a sense of completeness and cohesion of the self.

In later years, as octogenarians, Erikson and his wife Joan reconsidered his earlier work from the perspective of their own aging and their cohorts (Erikson et al., 1986). They modified their "either/or" stance of the tasks to the recognition of the balance of each of the tasks. That is, within each person there is dialectic, for example, the ego in a simultaneous state of integrity and despair; and the goal is to achieve balance in the two rather than an absolute resolution of despair and replacement with integrity. In 1986 they wrote, "The process of bringing into balance feelings of integrity and despair involves a review of and a coming to terms with the life one has lived thus far" (Erikson et al., 1986, p. 70).

Peck

The work of Robert Peck (1968) can be considered as taking Erikson's final stage to a deeper level. He proposed three discrete tasks that, when achieved, would result in ego integrity or even Maslow's self-actualization. Peck describes three tasks of later life:

Ego differentiation versus work role preoccupation: The person no longer defines herself or himself by life work role but by individual personhood.

Body transcendence versus body preoccupation: The body and changes are accepted as part of life rather than as a source of identity and focus.

Ego transcendence versus ego preoccupation: The person sees oneself as part of a greater whole rather than as an individual requiring special attention.

To achieve integrity using Peck's theoretical model, one must develop the ability to redefine self, to let go of occupational identity, to rise above body discomforts, and to establish meanings that go beyond the scope of self-centeredness.*

Maslow

Another well-known developmental theory with applications to aging is *Maslow's hierarchy of needs* (Maslow, 1954). This combines the bio/psycho/social needs of the individual from the most basic need for food and shelter to the most complex, that of self-actualization, or gerotranscendence. Like Erikson, Abraham Maslow proposed that the higher levels cannot be met without first meeting the lower level needs. In other words, moving toward healthy aging is an evolving and developing process. As basic-level needs are met, the satisfaction of higher level needs is possible, with ever-deepening richness to life, regardless of one's age. Although it has not been tested, this theory may be less culturally biased than others.

Tornstam

In 1989, Swedish sociologist Lars Tornstam proposed what he called the *theory of gerotranscendence* (Tornstam, 1989; Wadensten, 2006, 2007). He draws from disengagement theory and the frameworks of Jung, Erikson, Peck, and Maslow. Aging is viewed as the movement from birth to death and maturation toward wisdom. Aging is an ever-evolving process altering one's view of reality, a sense of spirituality and meaning beyond oneself. In as much, gerotranscendence implies achieving wisdom through personal transformation. As did Peck before him, Tornstam describes the necessity of transcending individual identity, the body, the ego. However, the theory of gerotranscendence goes further; time becomes less important, as do superficial relationships. The spiritual self and the spiritual world take on new meaning; that the drawing inward does not have to be disengagement with the world and can be instead, a time of introspection leading to wisdom.

---

*The reader is reminded that all existing theories were developed from a Eurocentric perspective and may have less usefulness when describing aging within other cultures, especially those that are collective rather than individualistic (see Chapter 5).

PROMOTING HEALTHY AGING: IMPLICATIONS FOR GERONTOLOGICAL NURSING

Psychosocial and developmental theories of aging provide the gerontological nurse with useful information to serve as a backdrop for the development of one's philosophy of care (Box 3-7). Although they have been neither proved nor disproved, they have stood the test of time, as least as they have applied to white elders. They have been used as the rationale for many things, from the creation of senior activity centers to laws regulating employment.

Although different theories will resonate with different nurses, Maslow's hierarchy of needs can be used as an example of how the theories can benefit patients and nurses alike. Application of the theory will lead to better understanding of individuals and their concerns at any particular time and in any particular situation. And, finally, it can serve as a guide to set priorities in nursing interventions to promote healthy aging (Figure 3-3).

The gerontological nurse works to ensure that, first, the basic needs of the older adult are met and realizes that only then are higher levels of wellness possible. The person with dementia may begin to wander or become agitated because of the need to find a toilet, and not knowing where to look. Until the toileting needs are met, the nurse's attempt to comfort or redirect is likely to be ineffective and frustrating. The person who lives alone but is unable to shop or cook will be distressed and perhaps irritable until arrangements can be made for home-delivered meals, either commercially or through a friend or family member.

As basic needs are met, a person will feel safe and secure. The person will likely sleep better and feel more comfortable when interacting with others. While interacting with others, people often begin to meet their needs of belonging. Maslow sees people as social beings with a need to belong to something outside of themselves. These needs are met through memberships in churches, synagogues, mosques, and civic or social organizations and through ties to family and friends. After retirement, a member of a work organization may replace the belonging need with special interest groups. If it is not replaced, there is a risk for isolation and depression. When a person moves to live with a child in a distant city or into an assisted living facility or nursing home, meeting belonging needs can be especially challenging and the nurse may work with the elder to form new alliances and associations. The nurse works to create environments in which meaningful relationships and activities can remain a part of the elder's life.

A person whose basic needs are met, who feels safe and secure, and who has a sense of belonging will also have self-esteem and self-efficacy. In other words, people will accept and honor who they are and will feel that they have some personal power and self-confidence; they will know that they are important as people and that they inherently have value. Self-esteem is not something someone can give to anyone else. It is, however, something that others can negatively influence through ageist attitudes and behavior. For example, any time the nurse assumes that a patient cannot do something, based solely on the person's age, the nurse is being ageist and is actually belittling the individual. Unfortunately, this is commonly seen but can be challenged by the knowledgeable and sensitive gerontological nurse.

Finally, some people reach Maslow's highest level of wellness, that of self-actualization. Self-actualization is seen as people reaching out beyond themselves and finding meaning in their lives and a sense of fulfillment. It is a way to achieve the sense of integrity described by Erikson. It is a way of finding continuity in what otherwise can be seen as a disconnected or fragmented life. And according to Jung, it is a natural state of development.

This may not seem possible for all, but the nurse can foster this in unique and important ways. The author (KJ) was asked to speak to a group in a nursing home about death and dying. To her surprise, the room was not filled with staff, as she had expected, but with the frailest of elders slumped in their wheelchairs. Instead of the usual lecture, she talked about legacies and asked the silent audience, "What do you want people to remember about you? What made your life worthwhile?" Without exception, each member of the audience had something to say, from "I had a beautiful garden" to "I was a good mother" to "I helped design a bridge." Meaning can be found for life everywhere—you just have to ask.

• • •

Many questions about late life development remain unanswered. Do biological differences exist between persons of different races and ethnicities, and how does this influence the aging of the human body? How does aging within a culture affect the individual, family, and community? How do people change in the later years? What is the reason for and purpose of aging? What is one meant to accomplish in the last half of the life span? What are the expected internal and external resources? What is the meaning of this last part of the life span? These are not new questions. There are still many areas of adult development and aging that have been minimally explored and may be the essence of development in maturity and late life.

BOX 3-7 AREAS OF NURSING ASSESSMENT CONSISTENT WITH THE PSYCHOSOCIAL THEORIES OF AGING

- Currently held roles, role satisfaction, and emerging roles (role theory)
- Individual's and family's expectations of age norms and effect on self-esteem (role theory)
- Current level of activity and satisfaction with such (activity theory)
- Effect of changes in health on usual roles and activities (role theory, activity theory)
- Cultural beliefs and expectations related to roles, activity, and both engagement and disengagement related to these (role theory, activity theory, disengagement theory)
- Usual life patterns and personality and attention to any change in these as an indication of a potential problem (continuity theory)
- Knowledge of the historical context of the individual and potential influence on perception and responses (age-stratification theory)
- Opportunities for contributions of knowledge to society (modernization theory)
- Sense of self and self-worth (modernization theory)
- Ability to meet spiritual and existential needs (theory of gerotranscendence)

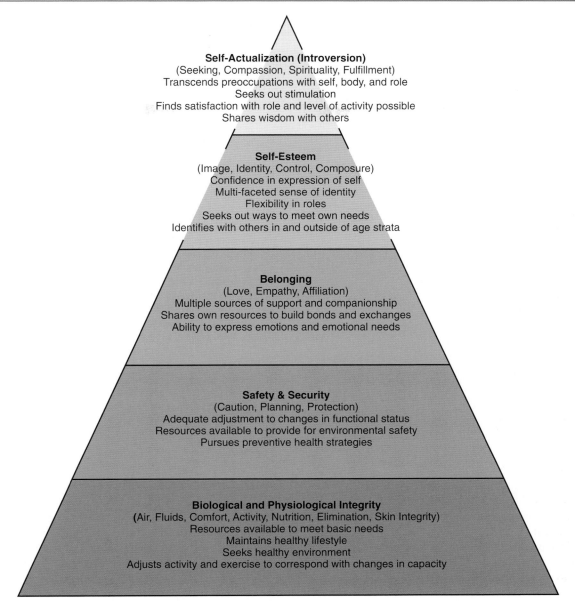

Self-Actualization (Introversion)
(Seeking, Compassion, Spirituality, Fulfillment)
Transcends preoccupations with self, body, and role
Seeks out stimulation
Finds satisfaction with role and level of activity possible
Shares wisdom with others

Self-Esteem
(Image, Identity, Control, Composure)
Confidence in expression of self
Multi-faceted sense of identity
Flexibility in roles
Seeks out ways to meet own needs
Identifies with others in and outside of age strata

Belonging
(Love, Empathy, Affiliation)
Multiple sources of support and companionship
Shares own resources to build bonds and exchanges
Ability to express emotions and emotional needs

Safety & Security
(Caution, Planning, Protection)
Adequate adjustment to changes in functional status
Resources available to provide for environmental safety
Pursues preventive health strategies

Biological and Physiological Integrity
(Air, Fluids, Comfort, Activity, Nutrition, Elimination, Skin Integrity)
Resources available to meet basic needs
Maintains healthy lifestyle
Seeks healthy environment
Adjusts activity and exercise to correspond with changes in capacity

FIGURE 3-3 Maslow's Hierarchy of Needs and Areas of Potential Nursing Assessment and Education Consistent with the Theories of Aging. (Modified from Ebersole P, Hess P, Touhy T, et al: *Gerontological nursing and healthy aging*, ed 2, St. Louis, MO, 2005, Mosby.)

evolve To access your student resources, go to *http://evolve.elsevier.com/Ebersole/TwdHlthAging*

KEY CONCEPTS

- When one is viewed as old is culturally and socially determined.
- When one begins to have features that are identified as "old" is significantly affected by one's genetic make-up and environmental stressors.
- There is no longer one exclusive explanation for aging or for adaptation to aging.
- The biological theories are divided into two groups: programmed and error theories.
- Regardless of the theory, biological aging results in damage within the cell itself, resulting in a decrease in its ability to function or reproduce.
- The increased incidence of many chronic diseases in later life can be explained by the immunity theory.
- A commonality of the biological theories of aging is the effect of oxidative stress occurring at the cellular level.
- The commonality of the developmental theories of aging is the movement or maturing of the individual to higher levels of acceptance of self.

CASE STUDY   ONE WOMAN'S AGING EXPERIENCE

Jennie attained the remarkable age of 100 years the day before Christmas. There were numerous celebrations of her birthday by friends and family. She was delighted and surprised because little had been made of her birthday in previous years. She always explained it away by the fact it was so near Christmas. Aside from joint pains, difficulty in breathing at times (even though she had never smoked), frequent falls, and limited energy, she considered herself healthy, had rarely been ill enough to see a physician, and had only recently begun taking a medication for her heart. Jennie sometimes awoke during the night with urinary urgency and then had difficulty falling asleep again. At those times she would sip a shot of brandy and read until she fell asleep. During the day she wore a protective pad because she tended to leak urine when she coughed or laughed. Jennie had a large network of friends and an attentive family, though she was well acquainted with grief and loss. Her husband of 75 years had died three years before, and she had left her lovely home and beloved dog when she moved into the retirement center at age 97. She was deeply spiritual but not religious in a ritualized sense. Her great-great-granddaughter was majoring in gerontology at the local university and often talked to Jennie about her life and remarkable adaptation in an attempt to find the key to her longevity.

On the basis of this case study, develop a nursing care plan using the following procedure*:

- List Jennie's comments that provide subjective data.
- List information that provides objective data.
- From these data, identify and state, using accepted format, two nursing diagnoses you determine are most significant to Jennie at this time. List two of Jennie's strengths that you have identified from the data.
- Determine and state outcome criteria for each diagnosis. These must reflect some alleviation of the problem identified in the nursing diagnosis and must be stated in concrete and measurable terms.

- Plan and state one or more interventions for each diagnosed problem. Provide specific documentation of the source used to determine the appropriate intervention. Plan at least one intervention that incorporates Jennie's existing strengths.
- Evaluate the success of the intervention. Interventions must correlate directly with the stated outcome criteria to measure the outcome success.

CRITICAL THINKING QUESTIONS

1. Discuss Jennie's physical changes as they relate to the biological theories of aging.
2. Jung talked about elders' movement toward introversion and meaning in late life. Does Jennie fit this pattern?
3. Consider the psychosocial theories of aging and discuss how each would or would not apply to Jennie.
4. Where on Maslow's Hierarchy of Needs would you place Jennie and why?
5. Imagine you are Jennie and discuss with your great-great-granddaughter your thoughts about your own aging.
6. Discuss the meanings and the thoughts triggered by the student's and elder's viewpoints as expressed at the beginning of the chapter. How do these vary from your own experience?
7. Imagine yourself at 90 years old and describe the lifestyle you will have and the factors that you believe account for your long life.
8. Organize a debate in which each individual attempts to convince others of the logic of one particular concept of aging.
9. List and discuss the psychological tasks of aging that you believe will be most difficult for you to accomplish.
10. Describe in a brief essay the characteristics of the oldest person you have known.

*Students are advised to refer to their nursing diagnosis text and identify possible or potential problems.

RESEARCH QUESTIONS

1. What physical changes can be attributed strictly to the aging of an organism?
2. What environmental factors have the potential to affect longevity?
3. What factors in relationships have the potential to contribute to survival?
4. What are the identifiable factors in extreme longevity?
5. What caloric distribution of carbohydrates, proteins, and fats contributes to longevity?

REFERENCES

Achenbaum WA: *Old age in a new land*, Baltimore, 1978, Johns Hopkins Press.

Carnes BA, Staats DO, Sonntag WE: Does senescence give rise to disease? *Mechanisms of Ageing and Development* 129:693, 2008.

Cottrell L: The adjustment of the individual to his age and sex roles, *American Sociological Review* 7:617, 1942.

Cowgill D: Aging and modernization: a revision of the theory. In: Kart C, Manard B, editors: *Aging in America: readings in social gerontology*, Palo Alto, CA, 1981, Mayfield.

Cox LS, Mattison JA: Increasing longevity through caloric restriction or rapamycin feeding in mammals: common mechanisms or common outcomes? *Aging Cell* 8:607, 2009.

Cumming E, Henry W: *Growing old*, New York, 1961, Basic Books.

De la Fuente M: Role of neuroimmunomodulation in aging, *Neuroimmunomodulation* 15:213, 2008.

Erikson EH: *Childhood and society. 1950.* Reprint. New York, 1993, Norton.

Erikson EH, Erikson JH, Kivnick HQ: *Vital involvement in old age: the experience of old age in our time*, New York, 1986, Norton.

Eyetsemitan FE: Perception of aging in different cultures. In: Robinson M, Novelli W, Pearson C, Norris L, editors: *Global health and global aging*, San Francisco, Wiley, 2007, p. 58.

Gomez CR, Nomellini V, Faunce DE, et al: Innate immunity and aging, *Experimental Gerontology* 43:718, 2008.

Gruber J, Schaffer S, Halliwell B: The mitochondrial free radical theory on ageing—where do we stand? *Frontiers in Bioscience* 13:6554, 2008.

Grune T, Shringarpure R, Sitte N, et al: Age-related changes in protein oxidation and proteolysis in mammalian cells, *Journals of Gerontology Series A, Biological Sciences and Medical Sciences* 56:B459, 2001.

Harman D: Aging: a theory based on free radical and radiation chemistry, *Journal of Gerontology* 11:298, 1956.

Havinghurst RJ: *Developmental tasks and education*, New York, 1972, David McKay.

Havinghurst RJ, Albrecht R: *Older people*, New York, 1953, Longmans, Green.

Havinghurst RJ, Neugarten BL, Tobin SS: Disengagement and patterns of aging. In: Neugarten BL, editor: *Middle age and aging*, Chicago, 1968, University of Chicago Press.

Hayflick L, Moorehead PS: The serial cultivation of human diploid cell strains, *Experimental Cell Research* 25:585, 1981.

Hendricks J, Hendricks CD: *Aging in mass society: myths and realities*, Boston, 1986, Little, Brown.

Hornsby PJ: Senescence and life span, *Pflügers Archiv: European Journal of Physiology* 459:291, 2010.

Jang Y, Van Remmen H: The mitochondrial theory of aging: insight from transgenic and knockout mouse models, *Experimental Gerontology* 44:256, 2009.

Jett KF: The meaning of aging and the celebration of years among rural African-American women, *Geriatric Nursing* 24:290, 2003.

Jung CG: *Modern man in search of a soul.* 1933. Reprint (Dell WS, Baynes CF, translators). New York, 1955, Harcourt Harvest.

Jung CG: The stages of life. 1933. Reprint (Hull RFC, translator). In: Campbell J, editor: *The portable Jung,* New York, 1971, Viking Press.

Legrain S, Girard L: Pharmacology and therapeutic effects of dehydroepiandrosterone in older subjects, *Drugs Aging* 20:949, 2003.

Maddox G: Activity and morale: a longitudinal study of selected elderly subjects, *Social Forces* 42:195, 1963.

Maslow A: *Motivation and personality,* New York, 1954, Harper & Row.

National Institute of Aging (NIA): *Aging under the microscope: a biological quest,* NIH Publication No. 02-2756. Bethesda, MD, 2003, U.S. Government Printing Office. Available at www.nia.nih.gov (accessed November 2010).

Nemoto S, Finkel T: Aging and the mystery of Arles, *Science* 429:149, 2004.

Nomellini V, Gomez CR, Kovacs EJ: Aging and impairment of innate immunity, *Contributions to Microbiology* 15:188, 2008.

Ostojić S, Pereza N, Kapović M: A current genetic and epigenetic view on human aging mechanisms, *Collegium Antropologicum* 33:687, 2009.

Peck R: Psychological developments in the second half of life. In Neugarten B, editor: *Middle age and aging,* Chicago, 1968, University of Chicago Press.

Perrini S, Laviola L, Natalicchio A, et al: Associated hormonal declines in aging: DHEAS, *Journal of Endocrinological Investigation* 28:85, 2005.

Shimokawa I, Chiba T, Yamaza H, et al: Longevity genes: insights from calorie restriction and genetic longevity models, *Molecules and Cells* 26:427, 2008.

Sokolovsky F, editor: *The cultural context of aging: worldwide perspectives,* ed 2, Westpoint, CT, 1997, Plenum Press.

Srinivasan V, Maestroni GJ, Cardinali DP, et al: Melatonin, immune function and aging, *Immunity & Ageing* 2:17, 2005.

Swain SL, Nikolich-Zugich J: Key research opportunities in immune system aging, *Journals of Gerontology Series A, Biological Sciences and Medical Sciences* 64:183, 2009.

Thomas WH: *What are old people for: how elders will save the world,* New York, 2004, VanderWyk & Burnham.

Tornstam L: Gero-transcendence: a reformulation of the disengagement theory, *Aging (Milano)* 1:55, 1989.

Valko W, Morris H, Cronin MT: Metals, toxicity and oxidative stress, *Current Medicinal Chemistry* 12:1161, 2005.

Wadensten B: An analysis of the psychosocial theories of ageing and their relevance to practical gerontological nursing in Sweden, *Scandinavian Journal of Caring Sciences* 20:347, 2006.

Wadensten B: The theory of gerotranscendence as applied to gerontological nursing—part 1, *International Journal of Older People Nursing* 2:290, 2007.

Physiological Changes

Kathleen Jett

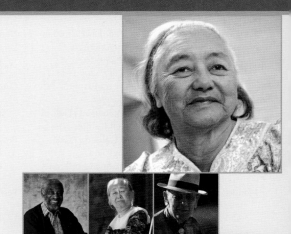

evolve *http://evolve.elsevier.com/Ebersole/TwdHlthAging*

A STUDENT SPEAKS

I always thought that physiologically an older adult was just like a younger one, but they are not! This could be really important when I do things like give medications.
Helen, age 20

AN ELDER SPEAKS

Strange how these things creep up on you. I really was surprised and upset when I first realized it was not the headlights on my car that were dim but only my night vision. Then I remembered other bits of awareness that forced me to recognize that I, that 16-year-old inside me, was experiencing normal changes that go along with getting older.
Sally, age 60

LEARNING OBJECTIVES

On completion of this chapter, the reader will be able to:

1. Identify and discuss the normal age-related changes to the human physiological systems.
2. Begin to differentiate normal changes with aging from potentially pathological conditions.
3. Discuss the implications of the normal age-related changes on the promotion of healthy aging.
4. Identify nursing interventions that promote healthy physiological aging.

Aging is a universal experience that begins at the moment of birth. Aging affects every cell in every organ in the body. However, neither all persons, nor all organs within any one person, age at the same rate. Although questions about the process abound, all agree that the associated physiological changes are cumulative. While a number of the changes that come with normal aging are clinically insignificant, three have important consequences. These are the loss or decrease in compensatory reserve, the progressive loss in the efficiency of the body to repair damaged tissue, and the decreased functioning of the immune system.

Although universal, the aging process is a wholly unique experience. Its variations have both intrinsic and extrinsic origins but are more intertwined than previously thought. It is influenced not only by one's genetic make-up but also by the environment. Extrinsic factors such as smoking and sun exposure will change the appearance of the skin as well as the ability of the cells to remove oxygen from the air.

Physiological changes with aging pick up speed in the 30s. By the 40s the changes begin to become noticeable; more so in the 50s and beyond. Although changes are occurring at the cellular level (see Chapter 3), external signs are the clues by which most people judge someone as "getting older." This external appearance is an expression of one's genetic make-up and epigenetic influence and is referred to as the "aging phenotype."

Several of the normal age-related changes are similar to those seen in the presence of pathological conditions. Differentiating these from those that are expected is sometimes difficult. Many internal changes mimic disease manifestations and might be interpreted as a pathological state in need of medical attention (Box 4-1). On the other hand, normal changes can mask early signs of potentially reversible disease processes, such as when the changes are incorrectly attributed to aging (Box 4-2). It is important for those who care for older adults to carefully explore the changes that do occur rather than immediately categorize them as either pathological or normal. Although normal age-related changes have usually been studied in concert with the most common pathological or disease conditions seen in late life, it is important for the gerontological nurse to be aware that they are not one and the same.

This chapter provides a detailed look at physiological and biological changes in the human body that are associated with

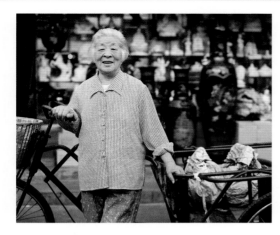

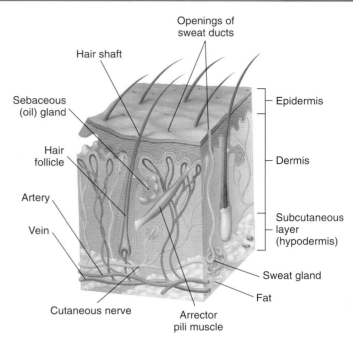

FIGURE 4-1 Structure of the Skin. (From Thibodeau GA, Patton KT: *Anatomy & physiology*, ed 5, St. Louis, MO, 2003, Mosby.)

BOX 4-1	EXAMPLES OF NORMAL AGE CHANGES POTENTIALLY MISINTERPRETED AS INDICATORS OF PATHOLOGY

- Slight delay in reflex response
- Loss of hair on lower extremities
- Decreased spoken word recognition
- Reduced pupillary response (bilateral)
- Decreased color discrimination

BOX 4-2	EXAMPLES OF INDICATORS OF PATHOLOGY POTENTIALLY MISINTERPRETED AS NORMAL AGE CHANGES

- Memory loss
- Incontinence
- Falling
- Sudden confusion
- Constipation

normal healthy aging. The purpose of this chapter is to provide the nurse with the knowledge necessary to begin to differentiate normal changes from potential pathology. In doing so, the nurse will then be better able to analyze his or her assessment findings so that changes that are suggestive of pathology can be addressed in a timely manner. With the identification, the gerontological nurse can facilitate healthy aging and adaptation to life's changes. Nursing implications specific to the promotion of health can be found in boxes throughout the chapter.

THE INTEGUMENT

The integument is the largest organ of the body (Figure 4-1). It provides clues to hereditary, dietary, physical, and emotional conditions and health. The skin serves as a means of communication and enables us to experience touch, warmth, cold, and pain. It protects the internal organs, helps regulate body temperature, serves as an efficient vehicle for the excretion of salts, water, and organic wastes, and stores fat. It helps protect the person from the damage of ultraviolet rays and produces vitamin D. Finally, the integument gives each person his or her unique and changing appearance. The integument is composed of the skin, hair, and nails. The skin is made up of three layers: the epidermis, the dermis, and the underlying subcutaneous layers between the skin and the muscles. The age-related changes in skin, hair, and nails are obvious to others and may be the first things noticed and attributed to "old age."

Skin

Characteristic thinning, dryness, roughness, wrinkles, and lightening are to be expected. These changes may be of clinical significance, such as those altering the absorption of topical medications (see Chapter 9). Extrinsic causes of skin changes include environmental factors such as exposure to pollutants, chemicals, and solar radiation. Sun exposure, in particular, increases the extent and speed of the normal changes in aging skin. An increased incidence of skin cancer is usually the result of a lifetime of solar exposure. An increased number of allergic rashes, irritations, and infections is associated with lessened immunity. Intrinsic changes occur gradually over time and have been tied to the oxidation and cross-link theories of aging (see Chapter 3).

Epidermis

The epidermis, the outer layer of skin, is composed primarily of tough keratinocytes and squamous cells. Melanocytes produce melanin, which gives the skin color. The epidermis is

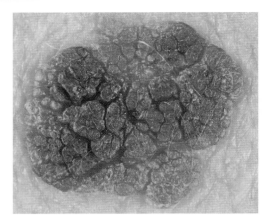

FIGURE 4-2 Seborrheic keratosis in an older adult. (From Habif TP: *Clinical dermatology: a color guide to diagnosis and therapy, ed 5,* St. Louis, 2010, Mosby.)

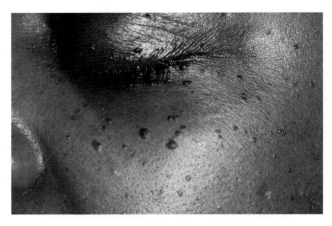

FIGURE 4-3 Dermatosis Papulosa Nigra. (From Neville B, Damm DD, Allen CM, et al: *Oral & maxillofacial pathology,* ed 3, St. Louis, MO, 2009, WB Saunders.)

in a constant state of renewal through regeneration, cornification, and shedding.

The epithelium in a healthy young adult renews itself every 20 days, whereas epithelial renewal in an older adult may take 30% to 50% longer because the keratinocytes become smaller and regeneration slows (Saxon et al., 2010). This has significant implications for the slowed wound healing seen in the older adult.

The number of melanocytes in the epidermis decreases about 10% to 20% per decade, resulting in lightening of the overall skin tone, regardless of original skin color, with a decrease in the amount of protection from ultraviolet rays (Saxon et al., 2010). Pigment spots (freckles and nevi) enlarge with age and can become more numerous with increased exposure to natural and artificial light. Lentigines, referred to as "age spots" or "liver spots," are common in older, lighter skinned persons. They are frequently found on the backs of the hands, wrists, and faces of light-skinned persons older than 50 years.

Thick, brown, raised lesions with a "stuck on" appearance (seborrheic keratosis) are also common (Figure 4-2). They are the most common benign tumors in older, lighter skinned individuals. In one study of 22 residents of the Orthodox Jewish Home for the Aged (Cincinnati, OH), seborrheic keratosis was found in 29.3% of the men and 37.9% of the women (Balin, 2009). Dermatosis papulosa nigra, a variant of keratosis in persons with darker skin, consists of multiple, firm, smooth, dark brown to black flattened papules 1 to 5 cm in diameter (Nowfar-Rad and Fish, 2009). Although they often begin in youth, they increase significantly with age and are clinically insignificant (Figure 4-3).

Dermis

The dermis is a supportive layer of connective tissues that provide stretch, recoil, and tensile strength. It lies just beneath the epidermis and is composed of elastin, collagen, and fat cells. It supports blood vessels; nerves; hair follicles; and sebaceous (oil), eccrine (sweat-moisture), and apocrine (sweat-odor) glands. A thin basement membrane holds the dermis to the epidermis.

The dermis loses about 20% of its thickness with aging (Saxon et al., 2010). The thinness of the dermis is what causes older skin to look more transparent and fragile. Dermal blood vessels are reduced, resulting in skin pallor and cooler skin temperature. Cross-linkage increases (see Chapter 3) and collagen synthesis decreases, causing the skin to "give" less under stress and to tear more easily. Elastin fibers, especially susceptible to cross-linking, thicken and fragment, leading to loss of stretch and resilience and a "sagging" appearance. The effect of changes in collagen and elastin can be found throughout the body, as is discussed below.

Vascular hyperplasia causes more pronounced varicosities, benign cherry angiomas, and venous stars. Skin becomes dryer because of decreases in sebum production, and the risk for cracking and xerosis increases (see Chapter 11).

Hypodermis

Beneath the dermis and above the muscles lies the subcutaneous tissue of the hypodermis. It contains connective tissues, blood vessels, and nerves, but the major component is subcutaneous fat, or adipose tissue. The primary purposes of the fat are to store calories and contribute to thermoregulation. It helps give the body its shape and acts as a shock absorber against trauma. As one ages, lean muscle is slowly replaced by fat tissue in some parts of the body.

Alteration in body weight occurs as lean mass declines and body water is lost with a concomitant higher risk for dehydration (Figure 4-4). Subcutaneous fat seems to "shift" locations with aging. Loss of fat around the orbit of the eye creates a sunken appearance. Landmarks become more prominent, and muscle contours are easily identified. Women older than 45 years begin to see the skinfolds on the back of their hands diminish, even if weight gain is substantial. At the same time, the amount of adipose tissue increases in the abdomen and, for women, in the thighs, even without a change in actual body weight. One study found that women's waist circumference increased up to 5.7 cm in the 6 years surrounding menopause (Sowers et al., 2007).

Thermoregulation. Despite the increase in adiposity, the ability to regulate temperature is diminished by a number of

Proportion of Body Weight Represented by Water

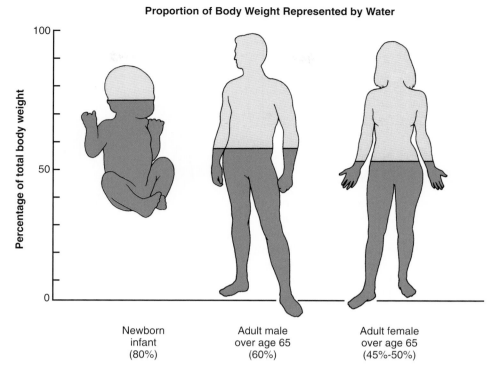

FIGURE 4-4 Changes in Body Water Distribution with Age. (From Thibodeau GA, Patton KT: *Structure & function of the body,* ed 13, St. Louis, MO, 2008, Mosby.)

causes. The risk for hyperthermia is elevated with the reduced efficiency of the eccrine glands. They become fibrotic, and surrounding connective tissue becomes avascular, resulting in a decline in the body's ability to cool itself through perspiration; there is an increased risk for heat exhaustion and heat stroke. There is also an increased risk for hypothermia. As sebaceous glands secrete less oil, moisture evaporates more readily. Windy, dry, cold weather can accelerate loss of body heat by evaporation (Cunningham and Brookbank, 1988).

Hair

Usually the most noticeable age-related changes are hair thinning and graying from diminishing melanocytes. Regardless of gender, 50% of the population older than 50 years has gray or partly gray hair. If originally blond, the hair color may turn shades of yellow or yellow-green.

Changes in hair are sex-based. For men, vertex and frontal and temporal hair loss, or androgenic alopecia, may begin in the late teens or early 20s, and by 60 years of age 80% of men are substantially bald. The amount of hair increases in the ears, nose, and eyebrows (Saxon et al., 2010). Women may experience the same pattern of hair loss as men, but it is less pronounced. Their hair is more likely to become thinner overall and finer. Terminal hair can occur in the face and chin area after menopause with the altered balance of estrogen and androgens. For both men and women, axillary, extremity, and pubic hair diminishes and, in some instances, disappears. Absence of lower extremity hair may be misinterpreted as a sign of peripheral vascular disease. Race, gender, sex-linked genes, and hormonal balance influence the maximal amount of hair that one has and the changes that will occur throughout

life. Persons of Asian descent are less hairy than white individuals, and Native Americans may have little or no body hair (Rossman, 1986).

Diffuse alopecia may occur in both sexes. It can also occur because of iron deficiency, hypothyroidism, autoimmunity, systemic diseases, medications, anabolic steroids, chronic renal failure, hypoproteinemia, or inflammatory skin diseases. Granulomatous disorders, such as sarcoidosis, and inflammatory disorders, such as discoid lupus or lichen planus can cause hair loss because of scarring. Differentiation of normal and pathological causes for hair loss is necessary.

Nails

Due in part to decreased circulation, fingernails and toenails thicken, change shape and color. Nails become more brittle, flat or concave (rather than convex), with longitudinal striations. Nails may yellow or appear grayish with poorly defined or absent lunulae. Pigmented bands may appear in the nails of persons with darker skin tones and must be differentiated from melanoma. Brittle nails with splitting ends or layers commonly occur. The cuticle becomes less thick and wide. Vigorous manipulation of the cuticle, such as in manicures, may lead to slowed nail growth. Although not a normal part of aging, onychogryphosis (thickening and distortion of the nail plate) and the fungal infection onycholysis are common. Vertical ridges (onychorrhexis) may appear as a result of poor nutrition, microtrauma, and disease (Chiu, 2000). Although the nails need more careful attention, this may be less possible because of other changes, such as loss of close vision.

See Box 4-3 for interventions that promote healthy skin and potential implications for gerontological nursing.

BOX 4-3   PROMOTING HEALTHY SKIN

- Avoid excessive exposure to ultraviolet light.
- Keep moisturized.
- Avoid soaps that dry the skin.
- Always use sunscreens.
- Keep well hydrated.
- Protect the skin from injury.

THE MUSCULOSKELETAL SYSTEM

A functioning musculoskeletal system is necessary for the body's movement in space, for gross responses to environmental forces, and for the maintenance of posture. This complex system comprises bones, joints, tendons, ligaments, and muscles. Although none of the age-related changes to the musculoskeletal system are life-threatening, any of them could affect one's ability to function and therefore one's quality of life. Some of the changes are visible to others and have the potential to affect the individual's self-esteem.

Structure and Posture

Changes in stature and posture are two of the obvious outward signs of aging. They occur very gradually and are caused by multiple developmental factors involving skeletal, muscular, subcutaneous, and fat tissue. Vertebral disks become thin as a result of gravity and dehydration, causing a shortening of the trunk. When combined with a slight curving of the cervical vertebra, height is lost; loss of up to 3 inches is not uncommon. The long bones, which are not affected, take on the appearance of disproportionate size. A stooped, slightly forward-bent posture is common and may be accompanied by slightly flexed hips and knees and somewhat flexed arms, bent at the elbows. To maintain eye contact, it may be necessary to tilt the head backward, which makes it appear that the person is jutting forward. Posture and structural changes occur primarily because of age-related bone calcium loss and atrophic cartilage and muscle (Figure 4-5).

Accompanying the changes in posture, shoulder width decreases because of shrinkage of the deltoid muscles and acromion processes. Chest width and pelvis width increase, and abdominal length decreases while its girth increases. An overall picture of a seemingly disproportionate individual may be seen, as if the person needs to be "stretched out a bit."

Bones

Bones are composed of both organic tissue and inorganic products, especially minerals. Bone is a constantly changing tissue. There is ongoing and cyclic resorption (into the bloodstream) and renewal (into the bone) of minerals, especially calcium. With age, resorption is more rapid than renewal (Box 4-4). This results in reduced bone mineral density (BMD). Reduced BMD is four times more common in older women than in men. For women it is directly associated with hormonal changes following menopause, with the most rapid loss in the first 5 to 10 years. Women who are not taking hormone replacement may lose up to 50% of their cortical bone mass by the time they are 70 years old (Crowther-Radulewicz, 2010). In men, reduced BMD is primarily due to prolonged steroid use.

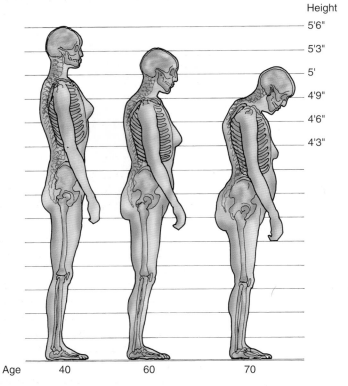

Height
- 5'6"
- 5'3"
- 5'
- 4'9"
- 4'6"
- 4'3"

Age   40   60   70

FIGURE 4-5 Normal Spine at Age 40 Years and Osteoporotic Changes at Ages 60 and 70 Years. These changes can cause a potential loss of as much as 6 to 9 inches in height. Note the exaggerated thoracic and lumbar curves at age 70 years. (From Ignatavicius DD, Workman ML: *Medical-surgical nursing: patient centered collaborative care*, ed 6, Philadelphia, 2010, WB Saunders. Data from Sattin RW, Easley KA, Wolf SL, et al: Reduction in fear of falling through intense tai chi exercise training in older, transitionally frail adults, *Journal of the American Geriatrics Society* 53:1168, 2005.)

BOX 4-4   RESEARCH HIGHLIGHTS

Do We Really Need Extra Vitamin D?

Vitamin D is produced by the skin in response to exposure to sunlight. Researchers have established the importance of adequate levels of vitamin D to minimize bone loss. It has long been known to be essential for calcium homeostasis and bone mineralization, with deficiencies leading to rickets and osteomalacia. It is now known that even less severe insufficiencies may have deleterious effects: an increased risk for autoimmune disorders and a high risk for infection. Low levels have also been observed in association with insulin production, glucose tolerance, cardiovascular risk, and a number of other conditions. Now with new and more available measures of the level of circulating 25-hydroxyvitamin D (25-OHD), less severe insufficiency has been found to be almost endemic and may affect 1 billion persons worldwide. To clarify the question of the need for supplementation, the Institute of Medicine in the United States issued a recommendation in November 2010 of a dietary intake of 600 international units a day for all persons under 70 and 800 for those over 70 years of age.

IOM: *Dietary reference intakes for calcium and vitamin D.* 2010. http://www.iom.edu/~/media/Files/Report%20Files/2010/Dietary-Reference-Intakes-for-Calcium-and-Vitamin-D/Vitamin%20D%20and%20Calcium%202010%20Report%20Brief.pdf

Chambers ES, Hawrylowicz CM: The impact of vitamin D on regulatory T cells. Curr Allergy Asthma Rep, 2010, Nov 23 e pub ahead of print.

Excessive loss of BMD leads to in osteopenia or *osteoporosis* (see Chapter 15). Osteoporosis of the cervical spine results in a C-shaped or kyphotic neck. Resorption of the bone in the mandible leads to poorly fitting dentures and painful sensations when chewing or biting. But by far the most important issue related to osteoporosis is the increased risk for fall-related fractures. See Chapter 12 for a detailed discussion related to falls.

Joints, Tendons, and Ligaments

The joints make movement possible. Tendons and ligaments are bands of connective tissue that bind the bones to each other and allow the joints to articulate. Cartilage is a fibrous tissue that lines the joints and supports specific body parts, such as the ears and nose.

Age-related changes in articular cartilage result from biochemical changes: increases in transglutaminase and possibly calcium pyrophosphates. As the cartilage in the joint dries, it becomes thinner, and results in less fluidity of movement or pain as bone rubs on bone. With progressive loss of cartilage, the common pathological condition of osteoarthritis may develop (see Chapter 15). Cartilage in the nose and ears continues to grow throughout life, leading to a change in facial appearance in late life, especially for men.

Like the skin, ligaments, tendons, and joints show the result of cellular cross-linkage over time. Consequently they become dryer and stiffer, resulting in hardened, more rigid, less flexible movement and predisposing them to tearing. Further weakening occurs with disuse and deconditioning.

Muscles

The three types of muscles are skeletal, smooth, and cardiac. Skeletal muscle is essential for movement, posture, and heat production; much of it is under voluntary control. Smooth muscle, under the control of the autonomic nervous system, is found throughout the body, primarily in the lining of the organs and blood vessels. Cardiac muscle is a special muscle found only in the heart. Muscle mass can continue to build until a person is in his or her 50s. However, between 30% and 40% of the skeletal muscle mass of a 30-year-old may be lost by the time the person is in his or her 90s (Crowther-Radulewicz, 2010).

Age-related changes to muscles are known as *sarcopenia* and are seen almost exclusively in the skeletal muscle. Loss is caused by physical inactivity, a change in the central and peripheral nervous systems, and reduced skeletal protein synthesis.

Suggested nursing interventions to promote healthy aging of bones and muscles can be found in Box 4-5.

BOX 4-5   PROMOTING HEALTHY BONES AND MUSCLES

- Ensure regular intake of vitamin D supplementation and calcium.
- Undergo regular but protected exposure to sunlight.
- Engage in regular weight-bearing exercise (e.g., tai chi).
- Engage in regular flexibility and balance exercises (e.g., yoga).
- For women: consider preventive pharmacotherapeutics.
- Avoid excessive joint strain.

THE CARDIOVASCULAR SYSTEM

The cardiovascular system comprises the blood, the blood vessels, and the heart. The cardiovascular system is responsible for the transport of oxygen and nutrient-rich blood to the organs and the transport of metabolic waste products to the excretory organs. The most relevant age-related changes in this system are myocardial and blood vessel stiffening, decreased β-adrenoceptor responsiveness, impaired autonomic reflex control of the heart rate, left ventricular hypertrophy, and fibrosis (Brashers and McCance, 2010). In health, changes in the cardiovascular system are minimal and have little or no effect on its ability to function except when the need for blood flow is increased as in illness. However, the prevalence of cardiovascular disease, particularly heart disease, is so high that it is sometimes mistaken as normal in later life. Much heart disease is preventable (see Chapter 15).

Heart

Electrocardiographic changes with aging under normal circumstances are minimal. PR, QRS, and QT intervals lengthen slightly. Catecholamines and certain enzymes that influence the force and speed of heart contractions diminish in concentration, resulting in a longer interval between contractions, weakened cardiac force, and a greater energy demand on heart muscle. Lower contractile strength, reduced cardiac output, and reduced enzymatic stimulation together cause the heart to respond to the work demand with less efficient performance and greater energy expenditure than would be required at a younger age (Brashers and McCance, 2010).

Contraction of the older heart is prolonged, most likely because of the slower release of calcium into the myoplasm during systole. These changes are reflected as decreased maximal heart rate, stroke volume, cardiac output, ejection fraction, and oxygen uptake and together are referred to as *reduced cardiac reserve* or *presbycardia*.

Despite these limitations, the healthy older heart is able to sustain adequate function for everyday life. Presbycardia becomes significant only when the person is physically or mentally challenged. It takes longer for the heart to accelerate to meet a sudden demand and longer to return to its resting state. For the gerontological nurse, this means that the increased heart rate one might expect to see when a younger person is in pain, anxious, febrile, or hemorrhaging may not be immediately evident. Instead, the nurse must depend on other signs of distress in the older patient. Similarly, the older heart may not be able to adequately compensate for other physical conditions that impose added cardiac demand, such as infection, anemia, cardiac arrhythmias, surgery, diarrhea, hypoglycemia, malnutrition, or circulatory overload. In these circumstances, the gerontological nurse must be alert to signs of rapid decompensation of both the previously well elder and one who is medically fragile.

Valves

Four valves control the flow of blood in, out, and within the heart. When the competence of a valve is compromised, a small amount of blood may "leak" backward, or regurgitate, during the heart's contraction or relaxation. The sound of the backflow is described as a *murmur* and is graded from 1 (not significant) to 6 (profound and life-threatening). In normal aging, the valves may be thicker and stiffer as a result of lipid deposits and collagen cross-linking, making slight incompetence and mild systolic murmurs an expected finding. Late-life valvular changes may be exacerbated by earlier rheumatic infections and arteriosclerosis. Aortic and mitral valves are the most commonly affected. At least 50% of elders have a grade 1 or 2 systolic murmur. Diastolic murmurs are always indicative of a serious problem in cardiac hemodynamics and are always abnormal.

Conductivity

As a completely unique muscle, the heart alone has the capacity to produce its own stimulation for movement, that is, contraction alternated with relaxation. The stimulation originates in specialized pacemaker cells found in the sinoatrial (SA) node, the atrioventricular (AV) node, and the bundle of His. The bundle of His bifurcates into right and left bundle branches. The beating movement produces "heart sounds," described as S1 and S2, in the healthy heart.

During the third and fourth decades of life, and accelerating in the sixth decade, SA node cells decrease in number. The number of SA cells at age 75 years is only 10% of that which existed at age 20 years (Taffet and Lakatta, 2003). Similarly, the AV node and the bundle of His lose a number of conductive cells into the fourth decade, and the left bundle loses cells between the fifth and seventh decades (Saxon et al., 2010).

Despite these changes in conductivity, the aging heart is able to adapt. This means that the resting rate remains unchanged with age but that the maximal heart rate is achieved with decreased activity. Sinus rates of fewer than 60 beats/minute are common in the elderly and do not necessarily indicate SA node disease. Significant interference with the blood flow to the SA node, either by occlusion or by narrowed arteriosclerotic vessels, can produce arrhythmias in late life as it would at any age. Slight arrhythmias, such as skipped or occasional extra beats, become more common with aging and are probably insignificant.

Blood Vessels

The major blood vessels involved in both the coronary and systemic circulation are the veins and arteries. The coronary arteries produce a rich and dependable blood supply to the heart. The younger heart propels oxygen-rich blood through highly elastic and flexible arteries, which expand and contract depending on the body's need for oxygen. However, several of the same age-related changes seen in the skin and muscles affect the intima of the blood vessels, especially the arteries, resulting in arterial wall stiffening and narrowing.

The most significant age-related change is reduced elasticity. Elastin fibers fray, split, straighten, and fragment. While there is little change in flow to the coronary arteries or the brain, perfusion of other tissues and organs is reduced. Reductions in the perfusion of the liver and kidneys can be significant in relation to medication metabolism (see Chapter 9).

Systolic blood pressure increases with age. Arterial wall stiffening consistently increases and baroreceptor activity decreases, which is thought to be associated with changes in catecholamine levels. Less dramatic changes are found in the veins, although they do become somewhat stretched and the valves

---

BOX 4-6 **PROMOTING A HEALTHY HEART**

- Maintain control of blood pressure at all times.
- Engage in regular exercise.
- Eat a low-fat, low-cholesterol balanced diet.
- Maintain tight control of diabetes.
- Do not smoke, and avoid exposure to smoke.
- Avoid environmental pollutants.
- Practice stress management.
- Minimize sodium intake.
- Maintain ideal body weight.

---

become less efficient. Pooling of blood increases the venous pressure. This means that edema develops more quickly and there is greater risk for deep vein thrombosis, especially in the lower extremities. The normal changes with aging, when combined with long-standing but unknown weakness of the vessels, may become visible as marked varicosities and contribute to the increased rate of stroke and aneurysms in later life.

Key points in promoting a healthy heart can be found in Box 4-6.

THE RESPIRATORY SYSTEM

The respiratory system is the vehicle for ventilation and gas exchange, particularly the transfer of oxygen into and the release of carbon dioxide from the blood. The respiratory structures depend on the musculoskeletal and nervous systems for full function. Like the cardiovascular system, in healthy aging only subtle changes occur in the respiratory system. The changes are seen in every component of each systems, including the lungs, thoracic cage, respiratory muscles, and respiratory centers in the central nervous system, and these changes are mostly insignificant. Specific age-related changes include loss of elastic recoil, stiffening of the chest wall, inefficiency in gas exchange, and increased resistance to air flow (Figure 4-6). Respiratory problems are common but are almost always attributed to exposure to environmental toxins (e.g., pollution, cigarette smoke) rather than the aging process itself (Sheahan and Musialowski, 2001).

As with the cardiovascular system, the biggest change in the aging respiratory system is its lower efficiency, in this case of gas exchange and ability to handle secretions. Under normal conditions this has little or no effect on the performance of customary life activities. However, when an older individual is confronted with a sudden demand for increased oxygen or is exposed to noxious or infectious agents, a respiratory deficit may become evident and can be life-threatening (Table 4-1).

The risk for infection is exacerbated by age-related structural changes in the respiratory system, combined with the diminution of the immune response (see p. 59). For example, the cilia, which normally act as brushes to repel foreign substances or to propel mucus out of the trachea, become less responsive and less effective. This is compounded by a diminished cough reflex. When impairment such as dysarthria, dysphagia, or decreased esophageal motility is superimposed, these normal changes significantly increase the risk for aspiration, aspiration pneumonia, and their sequelae.

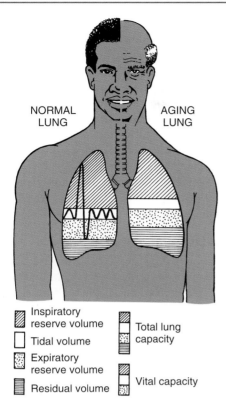

FIGURE 4-6 Changes in Lung Volume with Aging. (From McCance KL, Huether SE: *Pathophysiology: the biologic basis for disease in adults and children,* ed 6, St. Louis, MO, 2010, Mosby.)

TABLE 4-1   AGE-RELATED CHANGES IN THE RESPIRATORY SYSTEM

RESPIRATORY FUNCTION	PHYSIOLOGICAL CHANGES	CLINICAL PRESENTATION
Mechanics of breathing	Increased chest wall compliance Loss of elastic recoil Decreased respiratory muscle mass and strength	Decreased vital capacity Increased reserve volume Decreased expiratory flow rates
Oxygenation	Increased ventilation–perfusion mismatch Decreased cardiac output Decreased mixed venous oxygen Increased physiological dead space Decreased alveolar surface area available for gas exchange Reduced CO_2 diffusion capacity	Decreased PaO_2 Increased A–a oxygen gradient
Control of ventilation	Decreased responsiveness of central and peripheral chemoreceptors to hypoxemia and hypercapnia	Decreased V_t Increased respiratory rate Increased minute ventilation
Lung defense mechanisms	Decreased number of cilia Decreased effectiveness of mucociliary clearance Decreased cough reflex Decreased humoral and cellular immunity Decreased IgA production	Decreased ability to clear secretions Increased susceptibility to infection Increased risk of aspiration
Exercise capacity	Muscle deconditioning Decreased muscle mass Decreased efficiency of respiratory muscles Decreased reserves	Decreased maximal oxygen consumption Breathlessness at low exercise levels
Breathing pattern	Decreased responsiveness to hypoxemia and hypercapnia Change in respiratory mechanics	Increased respiratory rate Decreased V_T Increased minute ventilation

A–a, alveolar–arterial gradient; V_T, tidal volume.
From Meiner S: *Gerontologic nursing,* ed 4, St. Louis, MO, 2011, Mosby; modified from Pierson DJ, Kacmarek RM, editor: *Foundations of respiratory care,* New York, 1992, Churchill Livingstone.

Airways

Nose

With age, especially in men, the nose elongates downward as support of the upper and lower lateral cartilage weakens. The subsequent droop of the end of the nose can restrict airflow at the nasal valve junction. Narrowing of this valve in the presence of minor septal deviations that were not a problem in one's younger years can cause breathing problems in one's later years.

Trachea and Larynx

Stiffening of the larynx and tracheal cartilage occurs as a result of calcification and cross-linking. Voice pitch increases for men and decreases for women, but substantially more so for elders who are in poor health. Breathlessness in speech is the result of air escaping through an incompetent glottis; this is not a normal part of aging.

Chest Wall and Lung

The potential for greater lung expansion exists but cannot be realized because of structural limitations that develop in the thoracic walls. Ossification or rigidity of the costal cartilage and the downward slant of the ribs create a less compliant, more rigid rib cage limiting chest expansion. If skeletal defects such as kyphoscoliosis or arthritic costovertebral joints are present, this situation is exacerbated by further reducing the size of the chest cavity area. Intercostal and accessory muscles and the diaphragm become more compliant, or "floppier," as a consequence of muscle weakness and less effective recoil. Respiratory muscle strength and endurance may decrease by up to 20% by the age of 70 (Sharma and Goodwin, 2006).

The loss of elastin attachment in the alveolar walls causes a collapse of the small airways and uneven alveolar ventilation, trapping air and increasing dead space, decreasing vital capacity, and decreasing expiratory flow (Tockman, 2000). This is heard as an increase in lung resonance with percussion. This reduced efficiency of air expulsion resembles mild emphysema but is considered a normal finding and is referred to as "senile emphysema."

Total lung capacity is not significantly altered but, rather, is redistributed. Residual capacity increases with the diminished inspiratory and expiratory muscle strength of the thorax. Incomplete lung expansion does not provide for inflation of the lung bases and leads to basilar lung collapse and hyperinflation of the lung apices. The auscultation of slight atelectasis is common.

Legend for Figure 4-6:
- Inspiratory reserve volume
- Tidal volume
- Expiratory reserve volume
- Residual volume
- Total lung capacity
- Vital capacity

NORMAL LUNG   AGING LUNG

BOX 4-7 PROMOTING HEALTHY LUNGS

- Obtain pneumonia immunization.
- Obtain annual influenza immunization.
- Avoid exposure to smoke and pollutants.
- Do not smoke.
- Avoid persons with respiratory illnesses.
- Seek prompt treatment of respiratory infections.
- Wash hands frequently.

Greater diaphragmatic motion is needed because of the restriction of the costal structures and the general overall change in muscle strength of the body. The lack of basilar inflation, ineffective cough response, and a less efficient immune system, as noted, pose potential problems, especially for persons who are sedentary, bedridden, or limited in activity or mobility.

Oxygen Exchange

The effectiveness of gas exchange is measured by blood gas analysis and reported as pH, Pco_2, and Po_2. Whereas the pH and Pco_2 do not change with aging, Po_2 declines because of the changes already discussed. The maximal Po_2 possible at sea level can be estimated by multiplying the person's age by 0.3 and subtracting the product from 100. For example, the maximal Po_2 of a 60-year-old is 82 as calculated $(100 - [60 \times 0.3])$, compared with 73 in a 90-year-old $(100 - [90 \times 0.3])$ (Brashers, 2010, p. 1263).

Chemoreceptor function is altered or blunted at the peripheral and central chemoreceptor sites. Compensatory responses to hypercapnia and hypoxia are decreased while perception of dyspnea is intact or even enhanced. This response is independent of mechanical lung changes and is attributed to alterations in the neuromuscular drive to breathe. Compensatory responses may be significantly hindered in situations of stress.

Reliable pulmonary function values that depict normal respiratory function specific to the older adult are difficult to determine. The absence of reliable pulmonary measures requires that the nurse use other methods to assess the person's respiratory ability and needs, such as by increased attention to the respiratory rate and evidence of shortness of breath and cyanosis. Key instructions for older adults in promoting healthy lungs can be found in Box 4-7.

THE RENAL AND UROLOGICAL SYSTEMS

The renal system is responsible for excreting toxins, regulating water and salts, and maintaining the acid–base balance in the blood. The kidneys, the primary organs in the renal system, are highly vascular. They produce the hormone *erythropoietin,* which stimulates the bone marrow to produce red blood cells, and the enzyme *renin,* which helps regulate blood pressure. In aging there are both anatomical and functional changes.

Kidneys

Like other organs, in health the renal system continues to function adequately. The age-related loss of nephrons, kidney mass, and ability to concentrate urine ordinarily leads to little change in the body's ability to regulate its body fluids and the ability to maintain adequate fluid homeostasis under usual circumstances.

The size and function of the kidneys begin to decrease in the fourth decade and are significantly decreased by the middle of the sixth decade; the kidney is 20% to 30% smaller by the end of the eighth decade (Saxon et al., 2010). Kidney mass and weight decrease mainly in the cortical portion, where the reduction in number of glomeruli corresponds to the weight loss of the organ. By the eighth decade, age-related glomerular sclerosis is evident, the cause of which is unknown. Microscopically, the renal tubules develop diverticula in the distal portion of the nephron. In general, these changes pose little threat to well-being unless nephron function is abruptly reduced by an acquired renal disease or a sudden salt or water over load or deficit (Wiggins, 2003).

Glomerular Filtration Rate

One measure of renal function is the glomerular filtration rate (GFR). It is determined by measuring creatinine clearance, that is, the rate at which creatinine is filtered from the blood. The presence of creatinine in the blood is directly related to muscle metabolism. A linear decline in GFR in some persons begins at about age 40 years, at a rate of 0.8 ml/min/1.73 m² per year. Of note, up to one third of older adults do not exhibit a decline in GFR, suggesting that factors other than age may be responsible for altered renal function. The most important implication for any changes in serum creatinine, and therefore GFR, relate to drug metabolism and excretion (Huether, 2010a).

Regardless of the filtration rate, the ability to concentrate urine decreases. This means that the older adult can tolerate neither dehydration nor fluid overload as well as a younger adult. As a result of this reduced efficiency, hyperkalemia is more common. Sudden large changes in pH or fluid load can quickly lead to either hypervolemia or hypovolemia. Hypovolemia can quickly lead to renal insufficiency. These changes in function are especially important to the gerontological nurse when caring for the person who is exposed to changes in the environment, from renal-toxic medications to high temperatures, or for the person who has functional limitations affecting his or her ability to obtain adequate fluids. Such persons should be considered at very high risk for adverse events.

Ureters, Bladder, and Urethra

The ureters, bladder, and urethra are muscular structures that change with aging in the same manner as muscles found elsewhere. Some tone and elasticity are lost. This is most notable in the bladder, where it is accompanied by loss of bladder holding capacity. The first urge to void occurs at a lower bladder volume (150-300 ml) and total bladder capacity decreases to 300 from 600 ml. Weakened contractions during emptying can lead to postvoid residual and increased risk for bladder infections. Changes causing urinary incontinence increase in frequency but should never be considered a normal part of aging.

THE ENDOCRINE SYSTEM

The endocrine system works with the nervous system both to regulate and integrate the body systems and body activities. The endocrine system effects control through the production and secretion of hormones from glands throughout the body. Hormones are responsible for and control reproduction, growth and development, maintenance of homeostasis, response to stress, nutrient balance, cell metabolism, and energy balance. Two key points relative to hormonal control and effects are as follows: (1) a particular hormone may have an effect on many body systems and functions, and (2) one body function may require the coordinated action of many hormones. The primary glands of the endocrine system are the pituitary, thyroid, parathyroid, adrenal, pineal, and thymus. The pancreas, the ovaries, and the testes are not glands, but they contain endocrine tissue. In contrast to the other systems, there are no consistent or predictable changes with aging that affect function, with the exception of the ovaries (Hill, 2006).

Diseases associated with the endocrine system can occur at any age. However, the complex interrelationships between this system and others make it almost impossible to specifically attribute any endocrine disease to the aging process.

Thyroid Gland

The thyroid gland mostly influences the metabolic rate and production of body heat. An increased incidence of hypothyroidism in older adults may be the result of slight atrophy, fibrosis, and inflammation of the thyroid gland (Brashers and Jones, 2010). Diminished thyroxine (T_4) and decreased plasma triiodothyronine (T_3) appear to be age-related. Decreased serum T_3 is likely the result of decreased secretion of thyroid-stimulating hormone (TSH) by the pituitary gland.

Adrenal Glands

The adrenal glands produce glucocorticoids, necessary to regulate electrolytes, especially sodium and potassium. Like the other glands, the adrenal glands become more fibrous with age. Although this does not affect the maintenance of glucocorticoid levels, it does decrease their metabolic clearance rate. The leaner a person is, the less cortisol is used by their body; as the lean-to-fat ratio changes with aging, so might the use of cortisol. Higher cortisol levels may lead to a decrease in cortisol secretion. Although it is not yet known, these changes may affect the circadian patterns of adrenocorticotropic hormone (ACTH) and cortisol secretion. Cortisol is widely used as a biomarker for a number of things but is nonspecific. With continuing research, the implications of the changes in glucocorticoid levels in older adults may become clear (see also Chapter 8).

Endocrine Pancreas

The endocrine pancreas secretes insulin, glucagon, somatostatin, and pancreatic polypeptides. The secretion of these substances does not appear to decrease significantly in later life. However, for reasons unknown, there is a decreased sensitivity to insulin. When combined with increased needs for insulin in obesity, the result is often the development of type 2 diabetes mellitus (T2DM). Older adults have a higher rate of T2DM than any other group, with significant variation by ethnicity and region (see Chapter 15).

THE DIGESTIVE SYSTEM

The digestive system includes the gastrointestinal (GI) tract and accessory organs that aid in the system's purpose of digestion. Few functional changes with aging occur. However, the changes

---

BOX 4-8   PROMOTING HEALTHY DIGESTION

- Practice good oral hygiene.
- Wear properly fitting dentures.
- Seek prompt treatment of dental caries and periodontal disease.
- Eat meals in a relaxed atmosphere.
- Maintain adequate intake of fluids.
- Provide time for response to the gastrocolic reflex.
- Respond promptly to the urge to defecate.
- Eat a balanced diet.
- Avoid prolonged periods of immobility.
- Do not smoke.

---

that do occur can negatively affect comfort, function, and quality of life. In addition, many of the medications commonly prescribed to older adults can interfere with digestion and evacuation. For recommendations on promoting healthy digestions see Box 4-8.

Mouth and Teeth

After years of wear and tear, teeth eventually lose enamel and dentin and then they become more vulnerable to caries (cavities). With osteoporotic bone changes, roots become more brittle and break more easily, with resultant tooth loss. For reasons unknown, the gums also become more susceptible to periodontal disease. Taste buds decline in number and the sense of smell lessens, leading to decreased ability to taste. With less saliva, a very dry mouth (xerostomia) is common. Even in health, when combined, these changes all have the potential to decrease the pleasure and comfort of eating, which could lead to anorexia and subsequent weight loss (see Chapter 14). A number of medications taken for common health problems can quickly exacerbate potential problems, especially xerostomia. When the gerontological nurse administers medications to an older adult or conducts medication education, he or she should warn persons about this potential (see Chapter 12). For recommendations on promoting healthy digestions see Box 4-8.

Esophagus

In youth, food passes quickly through the esophagus to the stomach because of the strong and coordinated contractions of associated muscles, or *peristalsis*. In aging, the contractions increase in frequency but are more disordered with less effective propulsion, known as *presbyesophagus*. The sluggish emptying of the esophagus forces the lower end to dilate and may lead to digestive discomfort. Pathological processes that are seen with increasing frequency in older adults include gastroesophageal reflux disease (GERD) and hiatal hernias.

Stomach

Aging is also associated with decreased gastric motility and volume, and reductions in the secretion of bicarbonate and gastric mucus (Huether, 2010b). The reductions are caused by age-related gastric atrophy that results in hypochlorhydria (insufficient hydrochloric acid). Decreased production of intrinsic factor can lead to pernicious anemia if the stomach is not able to use ingested B_{12} vitamins. The protective alkaline viscous mucus of the stomach is lost because of the increase in stomach pH. This makes the stomach more susceptible to *Helicobacter pylori* infection as well as peptic ulcer disease, particularly with the use of nonsteroidal antiinflammatory drugs. Loss of smooth muscle in the stomach delays emptying time, which may lead to anorexia or weight loss as a result of distention, meal-induced fullness, and premature satiety (Price and Wilson, 2002).

Small Intestine

The small intestine is a muscular tube, five to six meters long, in which nutrients are absorbed from the food contents into the bloodstream. The functional units are the villi, small in-pouchings in the intestinal folds. They also secrete some of the digestive enzymes necessary for digestion and absorption.

Age-related changes include those related to smooth muscle, noted earlier, and those related to the villi, the anatomical structures essential for absorption. The villi become broader and shorter and less functional; blood flow decreases. Proteins, fats, minerals (including calcium), vitamins (especially B_{12}), and carbohydrates (especially lactose) are absorbed more slowly and in lesser amounts (Huether, 2010b).

Large Intestine

The large intestine, about 1.5 meters long, transports food residue, unabsorbed gastric secretions, shed epithelial cells, and bacteria from the small intestine to the rectum for expulsion by defecation. Peristalsis slows somewhat with aging, but not so much that constipation occurs, even though there is a blunted response to rectal filling. Constipation is more often the result of side effects of medications and life habits, immobility, inadequate fluid intake, and lack of response to the gastrocolic reflex (see Chapter 11).

Accessory Organs of Digestion

The accessory organs of the GI tract include the liver, gallbladder, and pancreas. Each contributes in unique ways in the digestive process.

Liver and Gallbladder

The liver is second only to the skin in organ size. It is highly vascular and dependent on blood from both the arterial and venous systems. Among other things, the liver produces bile and bile salts, key ingredients for intestinal emulsion and absorption of fats. The bile is stored in the gallbladder until it is needed during the digestive process. The liver is able to store blood for use as needed and is the primary site for the metabolism of most toxic substances (e.g., medications, alcohol) that enter the bloodstream.

The liver continues to function throughout life, even with the decrease in hepatocyte function and reduced liver mass that occurs with age. The decrease in mass brings with it a concomitant decrease in liver blood flow. This change has a potentially significant effect on drug metabolism (see Chapter 9). Liver regeneration is slowed in later life but not greatly impaired. Alertness for changes in hepatic health is especially important relative to the metabolism of medications and other toxins.

There does not seem to be any specific age-related changes in the gallbladder; however, the incidence of gallstones (cholelithiasis) increases (Huether, 2010b). This is possibly caused by the increased lipogenic composition of bile from biliary cholesterol. A decrease in bile acid synthesis causes a reduction in the hydroxylation of cholesterol. This, in conjunction with the decrease in hepatic extraction of low-density lipoprotein (LDL) cholesterol from the blood, increases the level of serum cholesterol in the older adult.

Exocrine Pancreas

The pancreas functions in both the endocrine and digestive systems. The exocrine pancreas secretes enzymes and alkaline fluids that are essential for digestion. Although with age the pancreas becomes more fibrotic, has increased fatty acid deposits, and atrophies slightly, these changes should not affect function. However, the overall reduction in the volume of pancreatic secretions may explain the decreased tolerance for fatty foods.

THE NERVOUS SYSTEM

The nervous system is the most complex of all and functions both alone and with all the other systems. The nervous system is divided into the central nervous system (CNS) and the peripheral nervous system (PNS). In conjunction with the endocrine system, it is responsible for the maintenance of homeostasis. The nervous system effects and is affected rapidly through the impulses of neurons, the basic nerve cells. The neurons generate electrical and chemical impulses by selectively changing their cell membranes and communicating these changes to other neurons by the release of chemicals known as *neurotransmitters.*

Although many neurophysiological changes occur with aging, they do not occur in all older persons and do not always have the same effect. For example, the presence of neurofibrillary tangles is a classic sign of dementia and is found in the brains of all persons with Alzheimer's disease, but they are found also in the brains of persons without dementia. Although it is difficult to show a true cause and effect of age-related changes in the nervous system, some changes appear to be consistent (Table 4-2). Cognitive changes are discussed in Chapter 19.

The Central Nervous System

The CNS is divided into three functional components: the higher level brain (cerebral cortex), the lower level brain (basal ganglia, thalamus, hypothalamus, cerebellum, and brainstem), and the spinal cord. Each CNS neuron has a body (soma), fingerlike projections (dendrites), and a single axon.

The aging CNS is not well understood. We do know that the number of neurons found in the CNS decreases, with a concomitant decrease in brain weight and size (Figure 4-7). This change in size is seen primarily in the frontal lobe of the cerebral cortex and appears as "atrophy" on neuroimaging. Determining the effects of this loss is ongoing.

Cellular changes include loosening of the dendrite structure in the neuron, the deposition of amyloid and lipofuscin, and the presence of neurofibrillary tangles, senile plaques, and Lewy bodies (Sugarman, 2010). Lipofuscin is a yellow-brown pigment seen in older cells, but its effect is not yet fully known. It may be associated with the disruption of protein synthesis. "Neurofibrillary tangles" describes the physical appearance of the neurons, resulting from changes in neural fiber proteins. Senile

TABLE 4-2	SIGNIFICANT CHANGES IN THE AGING NERVOUS SYSTEM
NEUROLOGICAL COMPONENTS	**CHANGES**
Central Nervous System	
Neurons	Shrinkage in neuron size and gradual decrease in neuron numbers
	Structural changes in dendrites
	Deposit of lipofuscin granules, neuritic plaque, and neurofibrillary bodies within the cytoplasm and neurons
	Loss of myelin and decreased conduction in some nerves, especially peripheral nerves (PNs)
Neurotransmitters	Changes in the precursors necessary for neurotransmitter synthesis
	Changes in receptor sites
	Alteration in the enzymes that synthesize and degrade neurotransmitters
	Significant decreases in neurotransmitters, including acetylcholine (ACh), glutamate, serotonin, dopamine, and γ-aminobutyric acid
Peripheral Nervous System	
Motor	Muscular atrophy—decrease in muscle bulk
	Decrease in electrical conduction
Sensory	Decrease in electrical conduction
	Atrophy of taste buds
	Alteration in olfactory nerve fibers
	Alteration in the nerve cells of the vestibular system of the inner ear, cerebellum, and proprioception
Reflexes	Altered electrical conduction of the nerves, caused by myelin loss
	Altered reflex responses (ankle, superficial reflexes)
Reticular formation	Physiological changes in the reticular activating system (RAS) results in decreased stages 3 and 4 of the sleep cycle
Autonomic Nervous System	
Basal ganglia	Slowing of autonomic nervous system response as a result of structural changes in the basal ganglia

From Meiner S: *Gerontologic nursing,* ed 4, St. Louis, MO, 2011, Mosby.

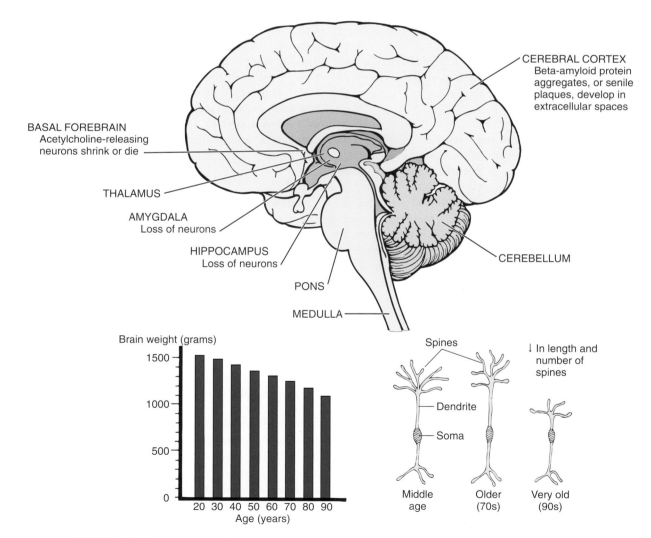

FIGURE 4-7 Changes in the Brain with Aging. (*Top,* From Meiner SE, Lueckenotte AG: *Gerontologic nursing,* ed 3, St. Louis, MO, 2006, Mosby. *Bottom left and right,* modified from Sekoe DJ: Aging brain, aging mind, *Scientific American* 267:133, 1992. Copyright 1992 by Scientific American, Inc. All rights reserved. *Top,* Courtesy Carole Donner, Tucson, AZ.)

plaques represent areas of nerve degeneration that can be found in the interstitial spaces of the cerebral cortex of the older brain. There is some thought that the loss of neurons coupled with the cellular changes is related to the overall slowed responses to sensory stimuli seen in aging (Sugarman, 2010).

Subtle changes in cognitive and motor functioning occur in the very old. Mild memory impairments and difficulties with balance may be seen as normal age-related changes in neurodegeneration and neurochemistry (see Chapter 19). Changes in neurotransmitters occur with the decreasing levels of choline acetyltransferase, serotonin, and catecholamines. Other enzyme such as monoamine oxidase (MAO) increase. Redundancy of brain cells may forestall the effects of these changes, but the exact number of cells required for certain functions is not known.

The Peripheral Nervous System

The PNS is composed of cranial nerves projecting from the brain and spinal nerves in afferent and efferent pathways. The PNS includes the somatic nervous system and the autonomic nervous system (ANS). The somatic nerves include the cranial nerves and others that carry information to and from the brain. The ANS is divided between the parasympathetic and sympathetic nerves. It activates smooth muscle, glands, and cardiac muscle. The ANS works in association with other systems (e.g., endocrine) to maintain homeostatic equilibrium and is controlled to some extent by higher brain centers.

The best overall descriptors of the age-related changes to the PNS are a slowness of functioning and prolonged recovery phases after activation, especially of the ANS.

Proprioception

Proprioception, the awareness of one's position in space, is a combined product of neurological and muscular feedback. Kinesthetic perception enables a person to automatically respond to changes in environmental stimuli. In a younger person, this response is not only automatic but also almost instantaneous and, in many cases, protects the person from accidental injury. For example, a 20-year-old is walking on a smooth surface when suddenly an irregularity in the surface is encountered. The person is likely to trip. However, instead of falling, the body quickly adjusts the center of gravity and continues on—perhaps not even noticing what has happened. This ability decreases as the person ages. Kinesthetic perception becomes less reliable, and falls, with or without injury, are much more likely to occur. Both the level of awareness of the threat to one's position and the speed of response are a function of the age of the neurological system. In addition, conditions such as arthritis, stroke, some cardiac disorders, and damage to the structures of the inner ear may affect peripheral and central mechanisms of stability.

SENSORY CHANGES

Age-related changes to the senses are both structural and neurological.

Smell

Sensitivity to odors increases through adolescence and then declines after age 60 years, with an increasing rate of decline after 80 years (Huether, 2010c). This is attributed to loss of cells in the olfactory bulb of the brain and a decrease in the number of sensory cells in the nasal lining. This change has implications both for appetite and for safety related to reduced ability to smell toxic substances, such as smoke or gas, in the environment.

Taste

A gradual decline in taste perception occurs with aging. The number of fungiform papillae (containing taste buds) on the tongue decreases up to 50% by the age of 50 years (Huether, 2010c). Taste buds atrophy, lose efficiency in relaying flavor, and decline in number. Salivary amylase, an enzyme that facilitates sweet sensations, lessens. Higher concentrations of flavor are required, especially for sodium, although all the primary taste qualities are affected: sweet, salty, bitter, and sour (Horowitz, 2005). However, taste changes alone in the healthy person are modest and not considered significant. The most important potential effect on appetite occurs in combination with any loss of smell as just noted or with special diets, such as low-sodium diets. Changes are accelerated in the presence of dental problems, medications, or smoking.

Touch

Tactile sensitivity decreases (somatesthesia) with age because of skin changes and reduced functioning of some of the most distal sensory neurons. This is particularly striking in the fingertips, palms of the hands, and lower extremities (Meisami, 1995). However, the extent of neuropathy seen in older adults (e.g., with diabetes) makes it difficult to pinpoint tactile changes as a normal part of aging. Normal and pathology-induced changes in somatesthesia are closely tied to those of pain perception.

Sight

Changes in eye structure begin early, are progressive in nature, and are both functional and structural. The structures most affected are the cornea, anterior chamber, lens, ciliary muscles, and retina (Huether, 2010c). All the age-related changes affect visual acuity and accommodation. Although presbyopia (decreased near vision as a result of aging) is first seen between 45 and 55 years of age, 80% of those older than 65 years have fair to adequate far vision past 90 years of age. Nearly 95% of adults older than 65 years wear glasses for close vision (Burke and Laramie, 2000), and 18% also use a magnifying glass for reading and close work. Extraocular changes have both cosmetic and comfort effects. See Box 4-9 for interventions to promote healthy vision in late life.

Extraocular Changes

Like the skin elsewhere, the eyelids lose elasticity and drooping (senile ptosis) may result. In most cases, this is only a cosmetic concern. In extreme cases, it can interfere with vision if the lids sag far enough over the lower lid margin. Spasms of the orbicular muscle may cause the lower lid to turn inward. If it stays this way, it is called *entropion*. With the curling of the lid, the lower lashes also turn inward, causing irritation and scratching of the cornea. Surgery may be needed to prevent permanent injury. Decreases in orbicular muscle strength may result in *ectropion*,

BOX 4-9 PROMOTING HEALTHY VISION

- Protect eyes from ultraviolet light; wear sunglasses when outside.
- Avoid eye strain; use a bright light when needed.
- See health care provider promptly for changes in vision.
- Have yearly dilated eye examination.
- Seek emergency care with any acute-onset visual disturbance.

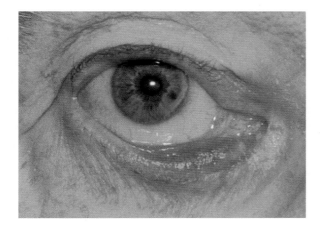

FIGURE 4-8 Ectropion. (From Swartz MH: *Textbook of physical diagnosis: history and examination,* ed 6, Philadelphia, 2009, WB Saunders.)

or an out-turning of the lower lid (Figure 4-8). Without the integrity of the trough of the lower lid, tears run down the cheek instead of bathing the cornea. This, and an inability to close the lid completely, lead to excessively dry eyes (xerophthalmia) and the need for artificial tears. The person also may need to tape the eyes shut during sleep.

A reduction of goblet cells in the conjunctiva is another cause for drying of the eyes in the older adult. Goblet cells produce mucin, which slows the evaporation of tear film, and are essential for eye lubrication and movement (Tumosa, 2000).

Ocular Changes

The cornea is the avascular transparent outer surface of the eye globe that refracts (bends) light rays entering the eye through the pupil. With aging, the cornea becomes flatter, less smooth, and thicker, with the changes noticeable by its lackluster appearance or loss of sparkling transparency. The result is the increased incidence of astigmatism.

The anterior chamber is the space between the cornea and the lens. The edges of the chamber include the canals that control the volume and movement of aqueous fluid within the space. With aging, the chamber decreases slightly in size and volume capacity because of thickening of the lens. Resorption of the intraocular fluid becomes less efficient and may lead to eventual breakdown in the absorption process. If the change is greater, it can lead to increased intraocular pressure and the development of glaucoma (Huether, 2010c).

The iris is a ring of muscles inside the anterior chamber. The iris surrounds the opening into the eye (the pupil), gives the eye color, and regulates the amount of light that reaches the retina. With age the iris becomes paler in color as a result of pigment loss and increases in the density of collagen fibers. A normal

age-related change in the iris is related to other neurological changes—that is, slowed response to sensory stimuli, in this case, to light and dark. Slowness to dilate in dark environments creates moments when elders cannot see where they are going. Because of the slow ability of the pupils to accommodate to changes in light, glare can be a major problem. Glare is not only caused by sunlight but also by the reflection of light on any shiny object, such as headlights or polished floors (Meisami et al., 2002). Persistent pupillary constriction is known as *senile miosis.*

At the edges of the cornea and the iris is a small ring known as the *limbus.* In some older adults, a gray-white ring or partial ring, known as *arcus senilis,* forms 1 to 2 mm inside the limbus. It does not affect vision and is composed of deposits of calcium and cholesterol salts.

The lens, a small, flexible, biconvex, crystal-like structure just behind the iris, is responsible for visual acuity as it adjusts the light entering the pupil and focuses it on the retina. Age-related changes in the lens are probably universal. The constant compression of lens fibers with age, the yellowing effect, and the inefficiency of the aqueous humor, which provides the lens with nutrition, all have a role in altered lens transparency. Lens cells continue to grow but at a slower rate than previously. The lens can no longer focus (refract) close objects effectively, described as decreased accommodation. Changes to the suspensory ligaments, ciliary muscles, and parasympathetic nerves contribute to the decreased accommodation as well. Finally, light scattering increases and color perception decreases. For the person who was myopic (near-sighted) earlier in life, this change may actually improve vision.

Lens opacity (cataracts) begins to develop around the fifth decade of life. The origins are not fully understood, although ultraviolet light contributes, with cross-linkage of collagen creating a more rigid and thickened lens structure.

Intraocular Changes

The vitreous humor, which gives the eye globe its shape and support, loses some of its water and fibrous skeletal support with age. Opacities other than cataracts can be seen by the person as lines, webs, spots, or clusters of dots moving rapidly across the visual field with each movement of the eye. These opacities are called "floaters" and are bits of coalesced vitreous humor that have broken off from the peripheral or central part of the retina. Most are harmless but annoying until they dissipate or one gets used to them. However, if the person sees a shower of these and a flash of light, immediate medical attention is required and is always considered an ocular emergency (Meisami et al., 2002).

The retina, which lines the inside of the eye, has less distinct margins and is duller in appearance than in younger adults. Fidelity of color is less accurate with blues, violets, and greens of the spectrum; light colors such as reds, oranges, and yellows are more easily seen. Color clarity diminishes by 25% in the sixth decade and by 59% in the eighth decade. Some of this difficulty is linked to the yellowing of the lens and impaired transmission of light to the retina, and the fovea may not be as bright. Drusen (yellow-white) spots may appear in the area of the macula. As long as these changes are not accompanied by distortion of objects or a decrease in vision, they are not clinically significant. Finally, the number of rods and associated nerves at the periphery of the retina is reduced, resulting in peripheral vision that is not as discrete or is absent (Tumosa, 2000). Arteries in the back of the eye may show atherosclerosis and slight narrowing. Veins may show indentations (nicking) at the arteriovenous crossings if the person has a long history of hypertension.

Hearing

Like the eye, age-related changes affect both the structure and function of the ear. Up to one third of all persons over age 65 have hearing loss of genetic or environmental origin (Huether, 2010c). The number increases until 40% to 50% of persons over 75 are thought to have hearing loss, affecting slightly more men than women. Hearing loss may be conductive, sensorineural, central, or mixed. It may also be the result of the ototoxicity of a number of medications. Central hearing loss is from lesions somewhere along the central auditory nerve pathways. The most common late-life hearing loss is sensorineural and referred to as *presbycusis*. This is the loss of hearing high-frequency sounds, such as consonants, while lower frequency hearing remains intact. Word discrimination is most affected. People complain that they can "hear but can't understand." For example, "The cat in the hat" may be heard as "e at in e at"—with the brain filling in the missing sounds with mixed success (Table 4-3).

In addition, unilaterally or bilaterally, impairment of the aging otic nerve can cause a condition known as *tinnitus*, a buzzing, clicking, roaring, ringing, or other sound in the ear. It becomes most acute in quiet surroundings. For ways in which the nurse can promote healthy hearing see Box 4-10.

Outer Ear

When observing the external ear, the prominent feature is the auricle, or pinna. With aging, it loses flexibility and becomes

BOX 4-10	PROMOTING HEALTHY HEARING

- Avoid exposure to excessively loud noises.
- Avoid injury with cotton-tipped applicators and other cleaning materials.
- Use assistance devices as appropriate, for example, hearing aids.
- If sudden changes in hearing occur, see health care provider promptly.

longer and wider. The ear lobe (lobule) sags, elongates, and develops wrinkles. The tragus becomes larger in men. Together these changes make the ear appear larger.

The auditory canal behind the tragus narrows, causing inward collapsing. Stiffer and coarser hair lines the ear canal, especially in men. Cerumen glands atrophy. The ear wax becomes thicker and dryer, making it more difficult to remove; cerumen impactions are a substantial cause of conductive hearing loss (see Chapter 6).

Middle Ear

The middle ear begins with the tympanic membrane (eardrum) and ends at the oval window. In between are the ossicles (malleus, incus, and stapes bones). The middle ear is responsible for the mechanical transmission of sound waves from the vibrating eardrum through the bones. With aging, the drum becomes dull, less flexible, somewhat retracted, and gray in appearance. The ossicle joints between the malleus and stapes may calcify, causing joint fixation or reduced vibration of these bones and therefore reduced sound transmission.

Inner Ear

The oval window receives vibrations from the middle ear and transfers them to the bony and membranous labyrinths of the fluid-filled inner ear. Within the inner ear are also the vestibule, cochlea, semicircular canals, and a series of channels in the temporal bone. Fluids within the inner ear transmit vibrations from one organ to another. Movement of the basilar membrane stimulates fine hairs of the organ of Conti within the cochlea. It is from here that nerve impulses are sent to the auditory center of the brain via the auditory nerve. Altered motion of the cochlear ducts may occur in middle age and is considered to be cochlear conductive hearing loss. The role of basilar membrane stiffening as a possible cause of this type of hearing loss is speculated. Changes in the efficiency of the cochlea and hair cells of the organ of Corti are responsible for the impaired transmission of sound waves along the nerve pathways of the brain and resultant sensorineural loss presdycusis.

THE REPRODUCTIVE SYSTEM

The reproductive systems in men and women serve the same physiological purpose—human procreation. Several organs in the system also can be a source of physical pleasure and a means of physical intimacy between persons. Age-related changes are under both nervous and hormonal control. Although both aging men and aging women undergo changes, the changes affect women significantly more than men. Women lose the ability to procreate after the cessation of ovulation and

TABLE 4-3	CHANGES IN HEARING CAUSED BY AGING
CHANGES IN STRUCTURE	**CHANGES IN FUNCTION**
Cochlear hair cell degeneration	Inability to hear high-frequency sounds (presbycusis, sensorineural loss); interferes with understanding speech; hearing may be lost in both ears at different times
Loss of auditory neurons in spiral ganglia of organ of Corti	Inability to hear high-frequency sounds (presbycusis, sensorineural loss); interferes with understanding speech; hearing may be lost in both ears at different times
Degeneration of basilar (cochlear) conductive membrane of cochlea	Inability to hear at all frequencies, but more pronounced at higher frequencies (cochlear conductive loss)
Decreased vascularity of cochlea	Equal loss of hearing at all frequencies (strial loss); inability to disseminate localization of sound
Loss of cortical auditory neurons	Equal loss of hearing at all frequencies (strial loss); inability to disseminate localization of sound

From McCance KL, et al.: *Pathophysiology: the biologic basis for disease in adults and children*, ed 6, 2010, St. Louis, MO, Mosby.

menses (menopause), whereas men remain fertile their entire lives. A discussion of sexuality in late life can be found in Chapter 22.

The Female Reproductive System

Age-related changes to the female reproductive system begin in puberty and continue through menopause. *Perimenopause* is the transition period 5 to 10 years before the cessation of menses. During this time follicular loss slowly accelerates, with up to 90% of women noting variability in the frequency and quality of menstrual flow. The changes may or may not be accompanied by mood lability and vasomotor instability or hot flashes/flushes and night sweats. Ovulation is often variable during perimenopause. *Menopause,* or the cessation of menses, occurs by about 51 years of age for most women and about 2 years earlier for smokers (Deneris and Huether, 2010). Both symptoms and timing depend on a number of factors including genetics, health, lifestyle, and concurrent medications. During this time, reproductive hormone levels fluctuate significantly, especially those of estradiol and estrone. As the level of these two decreases, the body responds with increases in follicle-stimulating hormone (FSH) and luteinizing hormone (LH) in an attempt to compensate.

As menopause signals the end of the reproductive phase of a woman's life, several other age-related changes occur, particularly in the breast tissue and urogenital structures. As ovarian function decreases, the breast tissue involutes. During perimenopause, mammary tissue decreases and again even further at menopause as glandular tissue is replaced with fat and connective tissue.

At the same time, a number of changes in the urogenital structures occur. Outwardly, the labia majora becomes less prominent and pubic hair thins. The ovaries and uterus slowly atrophy, and neither may be palpable. The vagina shortens, narrows, and loses some of its elasticity, typical of aging muscle and skin. Vaginal walls also lose their ability to lubricate quickly, especially if the woman is not sexually active. The vaginal epithelium changes considerably; the pH rises from 4.0-6.0 before menopause to 6.5-8.0 afterward (Deneris and Huether, 2010). The vaginal changes result in the potential for dyspareunia (painful intercourse), trauma during intercourse, and more susceptibility to infection. Menopause is also often accompanied by lowered libido in women; however, the mechanism of this is not known and treatment has been elusive.

The Male Reproductive System

Although the changes in the male reproductive system are not as dramatic as in women, effects of aging begin to be noticed in the 50s. Even in normal, healthy aging, the testes atrophy, lose weight, and soften. The seminiferous tubules thicken, and obstruction caused by sclerosis and fibrosis could occur, decreasing spermatogenic capacity. Although sperm count does not decrease, fertility may be reduced because of the higher number of sperm lacking motility or because of structural abnormalities. Erectile changes are also seen: more stimulation is needed to achieve a full erection, ejaculation is slower and less forceful, and refractory periods are longer (Deneris and Huether, 2010). As with women, alterations in hormone balances may play a part in the age-related changes in men. Testosterone level is reduced in all men but not enough to be considered a true deficiency (andropause) in most.

By the age of 80 years, the prevalence of prostatic enlargement among men approaches 80% (Andriole, 2008). The condition known as *benign prostatic hypertrophy (BPH)* may be related to changes in testosterone levels. The only time BPH is considered a problem is when the enlargement is such that it causes compression of the urethra. As a result, the man may experience urinary retention leading to repeated urinary tract infections and/or overflow incontinence. Depending on the degree and location of enlargement, retrograde ejaculation may occur, reducing fertility. Intervention is pursued only when the symptoms of BPH interfere with the man's quality of life.

THE IMMUNE SYSTEM

The immune system functions to protect the host from invasion by foreign substances and organisms. To do so, it must be able to differentiate self from non-self (Kishiyama, 2006). The immune system includes parts of many of the systems already discussed, and includes white blood cells, bone marrow, thymus, the lymphatic system, and spleen.

The decrease in immune functioning as we age is associated with multiple interrelated factors, including changes in lymphocyte function and relative lymphocyte populations. Late life brings a decrease in T-cell function and cell-mediated response to infectious agents and other foreign substances. The thymus, where T cells mature, decreases in size and volume over time. In older people it may be only 15% of the size it was in mid-life (Rote, 2010).

These changes are referred to as *immunosenescence.* Although their effect is not well understood, there is an increase in immunoglobulins leading to a decrease in innate immunity and more common autoimmune responses. There is a decreased ability to develop adequate immunity after an infection or after an immunization such as that for influenza.

Being alert for signs and symptoms of both infection and autoimmune changes is probably as important as prevention and protection from infection for the older adult (Box 4-11). A number of age-related changes have been described as having implications for the increased risk for infection in the older adult. For example, the skin is thinner and therefore less resistant to bacterial invasion. The reduced number of cilia in the lungs leads to an increased risk for pneumonia. The friability

---

BOX 4-11 IMPLICATIONS FOR NURSES
Prompt Response to Indications of Potential Infection*

- Sudden change in level of continence
- Sudden change in mental status or cognitive abilities
- Increased respirations
- Increased somnolence or agitation
- Unusual pallor

*Elevated white blood cell count, positive chest x-ray, and temperature elevation may be late signs of infection or impending sepsis.

of the urethra increases the risk for urinary tract infections, especially in women. At the same time, as the body is less able to mount a quick offense against infection, the usual responses may not be seen as quickly, for example, elevated white blood cell count (see Chapter 8) or increased temperature.

Early studies by Stengel (1983) found that oral temperature norms in well elders were significantly lower in women older than 80 years than in younger women. Older men consistently had an even lower temperature than women of comparable age. The old-old may have a temperature of 96.8° F with an average range of 95° to 97° F. By tympanic membrane thermometer, the temperature may be 96° F. These findings emphasize the need to carefully evaluate the basal temperature of older adults and recognize that even low-grade fevers (98.6° F) in the elderly may signify serious illness. *Because of this and because of a delayed immune response, a lack of fever (greater than 98.6° F) cannot be used to rule out an infection.*

It can be concluded that complex functions of the body decline more than simple body processes; that coordinated activity, which relies on interacting systems such as nerves, muscles, and glands, has a greater decremental loss than single-system activity; and that a uniform and predictable loss of cell function occurs in all vital organs. Yet most older adults are able to function effectively within the physical dictates of their body and continue to live to a healthy old age, capable of wisdom, judgment, and satisfaction.

Many of the age changes that occur and have been discussed here will be elaborated further in subsequent chapters.

---

evolve   To access your student resources, go to *http://evolve.elsevier.com/Ebersole/TwdHlthAging*

KEY CONCEPTS

- Many age-related changes are observable and measurable over time.
- The rate of aging varies enormously from person to person and from system to system within the same person.
- Individuals normally and gradually lose bone mass and some structural integrity of organs.
- Physical appearance inevitably changes, with a downward shift of skin and tissue integrity brought about by the pressure of gravity over time.
- Lubrication of joints, elasticity, enzymatic processes, and cellular fluids diminish during aging.

- In healthy aging, changes to the heart and lungs do not affect everyday activity. However, these changes can become significant if the body is stressed.
- Immune and endocrine changes are significant in the aging process.
- Because of changes in the immune system there is a greater risk for infection; at the same time there is a delayed response to, and therefore signs and symptoms of, an infection.
- Nervous system acuity and sensory acuity are diminished in aging, and these losses are often compensated for by the use of accoutrements or aids.

CASE STUDY   CHANGES WITH AGING

Mrs. Rodriguez is a 60-year-old Latina who lives with her daughter and family. Her granddaughter Elena has just started nursing school and has become more aware of her grandmother's health. She has noticed the following conditions, which she is afraid are signs of health problems.

Mrs. Rodriguez is complaining about her knees; they are feeling stiffer, especially in the morning. She is having difficulty reading her crossword puzzles and states that the letters are just too small. She hasn't noticed it, but those around her find that they understand them better when they look at her while they are speaking. She is also complaining that she gets out of breath easily, especially when she is climbing the steps to her second-floor room—something she has done without difficulty for years.

Based on the case study, develop a nursing care plan using the following procedure*:

- List Mrs. Rodriguez's comments that provide subjective data.
- List information that provides objective data.
- Separate the data into those changes that are likely to be associated with normal changes with aging and those that may be indicative of a potential health problem.
- From these data, identify and state, using accepted format, two nursing diagnoses you determine are most significant to Mrs. Rodriguez at this time. List two of Mrs. Rodriguez's strengths that you have identified from the data.

- Determine and state outcome criteria for each diagnosis. These must reflect some alleviation of the problem identified in the nursing diagnosis and must be stated in concrete and measurable terms.
- Plan and state one or more interventions for each diagnosed problem. Provide specific documentation of the source used to determine the appropriate intervention. Plan at least one intervention that incorporates Mrs. Rodriguez's existing strengths.

CRITICAL THINKING QUESTIONS

1. As a student, you have already taken a course on the normal changes with aging. Based on what she tells you, develop a care plan to optimize her health in light of the changes she reported.
2. Which of the age-related changes has the potential to have the most effect on one's quality of life?
3. Which of the age-related changes has the most implications for the risk of infection in an older adult?
4. For each system, suggest additional strategies to promote healthy aging in the presence of normal age-related changes to the system.
5. An older patient says to the nurse, "I think the older I get, the more falling apart I am. I seem to be good for nothing!" What response from the nurse will recognize normal changes with aging but foster self-esteem at the same time?

*Students are advised to refer to their nursing diagnosis text and identify possible or potential problems.

RESEARCH QUESTIONS

1. Where do individuals seek knowledge of the aging process?
2. Is chronological age more significant than physiological age in determining functional efficacy?
3. When does one become aware of changes in function that are related to aging? Which change is likely to appear first?

How much influence does environment have on reduced hearing capacity?
4. How do age-related changes differ in males and females?

REFERENCES

Andriole GL, for the Merck Manual for Healthcare Professionals Online Medical Library: *Benign prostatic hypertrophy (BPH)* (2008). Available at http://www.merck.com/mmpe/sec17/ch240/ch240a.html?qt=prostate&alt=sh. Accessed December 2010.

Balin AK, for eMedicine: *Seborrheic keratosis* (2009). Available at http://emedicine.medscape.com/article/1059477-overview. Accessed November 2010.

Burke MA, Laramie JA: *Primary care of the older adult: a multidisciplinary approach*, ed 2, St. Louis, MO, 2000, Mosby.

Brashers VL *Structure and function of the pulmonary system*. In McCance KL, Huether SE, Brashers VL, et al., editors: *Pathophysiology: the biologic basis for disease in adults and children*, ed 6, St. Louis, MO, 2010, Mosby.

Brashers VL, Jones RE: *Mechanisms of hormonal regulation*. In McCance KL, Huether SE, Brashers VL, et al., editors: *Pathophysiology: the biologic basis for disease in adults and children*, ed 6, St. Louis, MO, 2010, Mosby.

Brashers VL, McCance KL: *Structure and function of the cardiovascular system*. In McCance KL, Huether SE, Brashers VL, et al., editors: *Pathophysiology: the biologic basis for disease in adults and children*, ed 6, St. Louis, MO, 2010, Mosby.

Chiu N: *Aging and the skin*. In Beers MH, Berkow R, editors: *The Merck manual of geriatrics*, ed 3, Whitehouse Station, NJ, 2000, Merck Research Laboratories.

Crowther-Radulewicz CL: *Structure and function of the musculoskeletal system*. In McCance KL, Huether SE, Brashers VL, et al., editors: *Pathophysiology: the biologic basis for disease in adults and children*, ed 6, St. Louis, MO, 2010, Mosby.

Cunningham WR, Brookbank JW: *Gerontology: the psychology, biology, and sociology of aging*, New York, 1988, Harper & Row.

Deneris A, Huether SE: *Structure and function of the reproductive systems*. In McCance KL, Huether SE, Brashers VL, et al., editors: *Pathophysiology: the biologic basis for disease in*

adults and children, ed 6, St. Louis, MO, 2010, Mosby.

Hill C: *Endocrine function*. In Meiner SE, Lueckenotte AG: *Gerontologic nursing*, ed 3, St. Louis, MO, 2006, Mosby.

Horowitz M: *Aging and the gastrointestinal tract*. In Beers MH, Berkow R, editors: *The Merck manual of geriatrics*, ed 3, Whitehouse Station, NJ, 2005, Merck Research Laboratories.

Huether SE: *Structure and function of the renal and urologic systems*. In McCance KL, Huether SE, Brashers VL, et al., editors: *Pathophysiology: the biologic basis for disease in adults and children*, ed 6, St. Louis, MO, 2010a, Mosby.

Huether SE: *Structure and function of the digestive system*. In McCance KL, Huether SE, Brashers VL, et al., editors: *Pathophysiology: the biologic basis for disease in adults and children*, ed 6, St. Louis, MO, 2010b, Mosby.

Huether SE: *Pain, temperature regulation, sleep, and sensory function*. In McCance KL, Huether SE, Brashers VL, et al., editors: *Pathophysiology: the biologic basis for disease in adults and children*, ed 6, St. Louis, MO, 2010c, Mosby.

Kishiyama JL: *Disorders of the immune system*. In McPhee SJ, Ganong WF, editors: *Pathophysiology of disease: an introduction to clinical medicine*, ed 5, New York, 2006, McGraw-Hill.

Meisami E: *Aging of the sensory system*. In Timiras PS, editor: *Physiological basis of aging and geriatrics*, ed 2, Boca Raton, FL, 1995, CRC Press.

Meisami E, Brown C, Emerle H: *Sensory systems: normal aging, disorders, and treatments of vision and hearing in humans*. In Timiras PS, editor: *Physiological basis of aging and geriatrics*, ed 3, Boca Raton, FL, 2002, CRC Press.

Nowfar-Rad M, Fish F: *Dermatosis papulosa nigra* (2009). Available at http://emedicine.medscape.com/article/1056854-overview. Accessed May 16, 2010.

Price S, Wilson L: *Pathophysiology: clinical concepts of disease processes*, ed 6, St. Louis, MO, 2002, Mosby.

Rossman I, editor: *Clinical geriatrics*, ed 3, Philadelphia, 1986, Lippincott.

Rote NS: *Adaptive immunity*. In McCance KL, Huether SE, Brashers VL, et al., editors: *Pathophysiology: the biologic basis for disease in adults and children*, ed 6, St. Louis, MO, 2010, Mosby.

Saxon SV, Etten MJ, Perkins EA: *Physical change and aging: a guide for the helping professions*, ed 5, New York, 2010, Springer.

Sharma G, Goodwin J: Effect of aging on respiratory system physiology and immunology, *Clinical Interventions in Aging* 1:253, 2006.

Sheahan SL, Musialowski R: Clinical implications of respiratory system changes in aging, *Journal of Gerontological Nursing* 27:26, 2001.

Sowers M, Zheng H, Tomey K, et al: Changes in body composition in women over 6 years at midlife: ovarian and chronological aging, *Journal of Clinical Endocrinology and Metabolism* 92:895, 2007.

Stengel GB: *Oral temperature in the elderly*, *Gerontologist* 23:306, 1983 (special issue).

Sugarman RA: *Structure and function of the neurologic system*. In McCance KL, Huether SE, Brashers VL, et al., editors: *Pathophysiology: the biologic basis for disease in adults and children*, ed 6, St. Louis, MO, 2010, Mosby.

Taffet GE, Lakatta EG: *Aging of the cardiovascular system*. In: Hazzard WR, Blass JP, Halter JB, et al., editors: *Principles of geriatric medicine and gerontology*, New York, 2003, McGraw-Hill.

Tockman MS: *Aging and the lung*. In Beers MH, Berkow R, editors: *The Merck manual of geriatrics*, ed 3, Whitehouse Station, NJ, 2000, Merck Research Laboratories.

Tumosa N: *Aging and the eye*. In Beers MH, Berkow R, editors: *The Merck manual of geriatrics*, ed 3, Whitehouse Station, NJ, 2000, Merck Research Laboratories.

Wiggins J: *Changes in renal function*. In Hazzard WR, Blass JP, Halter JB, et al., editors: *Principles of geriatric medicine and gerontology*, New York, 2003, McGraw-Hill.

Culture, Gender, and Aging

Kathleen Jett

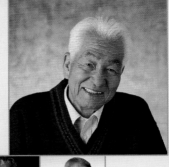

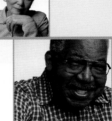

ℯvolve *http://evolve.elsevier.com/Ebersole/TwdHlthAging*

A STUDENT SPEAKS

We are trying to do our work with the patient but her daughter keeps getting in the way and tells us what we can or cannot do. We are just trying to help, but I don't think they appreciate us. I think it would be better if the daughter just goes away.   **Sandy, age 20**

AN ELDER SPEAKS

It seems like I don't fit in anywhere any more. My children do their best, but they have to work and my grandchildren don't have the same respect for me that I had for my grandparents. I know they love me but it is just not the same.   **Yi Liu, age 87**

LEARNING OBJECTIVES

On completion of this chapter, the reader will be able to:

1. Recognize the current knowledge related to health disparities and their potential impact on older adults of color and women.
2. Relate major historical events that have affected each cohort of elders.
3. Compare several different ethnically based approaches to health care.
4. Describe several of the unique circumstances related to gender and aging.
5. Identify personal factors contributing to ethnic and cultural sensitivity.
6. Discuss approaches that facilitate an appreciation of diverse cultural and ethnic experiences.
7. Accurately identify situations in which expert interpretation is necessary.
8. Understand key points of working with interpreters.
9. Formulate a care plan incorporating ethnically sensitive interventions.
10. Develop gerontological nursing interventions geared toward reducing health disparities.

Interest in and attention to culture and gender issues in health care are increasing. This interest is stimulated to a great extent by the realization of a demographic imperative and the recognition of the significant *health disparities and inequities* in the United States. The *demographic imperative* refers to the significant increases in both the total numbers of older adults and the relative proportion of older adults in most countries across the globe. These numbers reflect a "gerontological explosion" of older adults from ethnically distinct groups (Figure 5-1).

Today's nurse is expected to provide competent care to persons with different life experiences, cultural perspectives, values, and styles of communication. Cross-cultural communication is especially important because of the potential health complexity during late life and the likely combination of

generational and cultural differences between the patient and the nurse. The nurse will need to communicate effectively with persons regardless of the languages spoken. In doing so, the nurse may depend on limited verbal exchanges and attend more to facial and body expressions, postures, gestures, and touching. However, these forms of communication, heavily influenced by culture, are easily misunderstood. To skillfully assess and intervene, nurses must develop cultural sensitivity through awareness of their own ethnocentricities. Effective nurses then develop cultural competence through new cultural knowledge about ethnicity, culture, language, and health belief systems and acquire the skills needed to optimize intercultural communication.

This chapter provides an overview of culture, gender, and aging, as well as strategies gerontological nurses can use to best respond to the changing face of elders and, in doing so, help reduce health disparities and promote social justice (see http://www.apha.org/meetings/highlights/Theme.htm). These strategies include increasing cultural sensitivity, knowledge, and skills in working with diverse groups of older adults.

THE GERONTOLOGICAL EXPLOSION

In the United States, the percentage of persons of racial or ethnic groups other than white European has increased

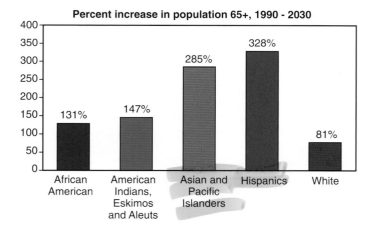

FIGURE 5-1 Percent Increase in U.S. Population Age 65 Years and Older, 1990-2030. (From U.S. Census Bureau, January 2000.)

significantly. It is projected that by 2050 persons from groups that have long been counted as statistical minorities will assume membership in what can be called the *emerging majority*. Although not yet a majority, those persons from minority groups who are at least 65 years of age will increase from 20% to 42%; among those at least 85, the numbers will increase from 15% in 2010 to 33% in 2050 (Vincent and Velkoff, 2010).

When projected to 2050 there will be some significant shifts in the percentage share among all racial and ethnic groups as well as those of mixed race in the ≥65 population. For example, those who report "white alone" will decrease from 87% to 77%; black alone will increase from 9% to 12% between 2010 and 2050 (Vincent and Velkoff, 2010). Other groups will double or triple their current numbers. The greatest period of growth will be between 2010 and 2030. For a group-to-group comparison in growth see Box 5-1 through Box 5-4. It must be noted, however, that these and many of the figures available today are drawn from the U.S. Census, in which persons of color are often underrepresented and those who reside illegally are not included at all. In reality, the number of ethnic elders in the United States may be or will become substantially higher.

Even within the census racial and ethnic categories, there is considerable diversity. The broad terms are useful statistically but are considerably less useful for the gerontological nurse caring for an ethnic elder. One who self-identifies as an "American Indian" is a member of one of more than 500 tribal groups, each with both common and unique cultural features. An elder

---

BOX 5-1   A STATISTICAL PROFILE OF BLACK OLDER AMERICANS AGED 65 YEARS OR MORE

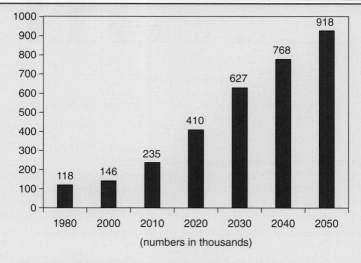

The Older Black Population: Past, Present, and Future.

In 2008:
- There were 3.2 million persons identified as black or African American, or 8.3% of those 65 or older. This number is expected to increase to 11% by 2050.
- Fifty percent lived in eight states: New York, Florida, California, Texas, Georgia, North Carolina, Illinois, and Virginia.
- Sixty percent had completed high school, compared with 9% in 1970.
- The majority of both men (60%) and women (58%) lived with a spouse or another person.

- Households headed by black elders reported a mean income of $35,025, compared with $44,188 for all older households.
- The poverty rate was twice that of all elderly (20% compared with 9.7%). However, this was improved from 48% in 1968.
- Since 1960 the life expectancy has increased by 2.6 years for black men and by 3.6 years for black women, but these increases are still behind that of all elders.

From Administration on Aging: *A statistical profile of black older Americans aged 65+* (2010). Available at http://www.aoa.gov/AoARoot/Aging_Statistics/minority_aging/Facts-on-Black-Elderly-plain_format.aspx. Accessed December 2010.

BOX 5-2   A STATISTICAL PROFILE OF AMERICAN INDIAN AND NATIVE ALASKAN ELDERLY

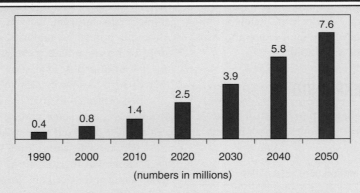

(numbers in millions)

Past, Present, and Future: American Indian and Alaskan Native Persons 65+, 1990-2050 (numbers in thousands).

In 2007:

- Persons identified as American Indian or Native Alaskan (AI/NA) made up 0.6% of the older population; this percentage is expected to grow to 1% by 2050. Part of this growth will be due to the increasing number of persons who, unlike previously, are now identifying themselves as one of these groups.

- The actual number of AI/NA persons 65 or older was 212,605. This included the fewest in New Hampshire (n = 256) and the most in California (n = 29,438).
- Fifty-one percent of all AI/NA elderly lived in six states: California (13.8%), Oklahoma (11.2%), Arizona (9.4%), New Mexico (6.5%), Texas (5.7%), and North Carolina (4.3%).

From Administration on Aging: *A statistical profile of American Indian and Native Alaskan elderly* (2010). Available at http://www.aoa.gov/AoARoot/Aging_Statistics/minority_aging/Facts-on-AINA-Elderly2008-plain_format.aspx. Accessed December 2010.

BOX 5-3   A STATISTICAL PROFILE OF ASIAN OLDER AMERICANS AGED 65 YEARS OR MORE

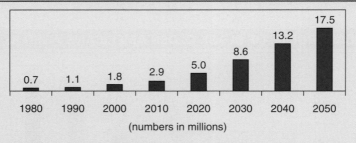

(numbers in millions)

The Older Asian, Hawaiian, and Pacific Islander Population: Past, Present, and Future.

In 2008:

- There were more than 1.3 million persons 65 or older identified as Asian, Hawaiian, or Pacific Islander living in the 50 United States and the District of Columbia.
- At present, they comprise 3.4% of the older population, increasing to 8.6% by 2050.
- Sixty percent lived in three states: California (40.5%), Hawaii (9.6%), and New York (9.2%).
- The number of Asian older persons who had a bachelor's degree or higher (32%) was more than 50% higher than for the overall older population.

- The majority of both men (92%) and women (80%) lived with a spouse or another person.
- Households headed by an Asian elder reported a mean income of $48,859 compared with $44,188 for all older households.
- The poverty rate for Asian elderly was slightly greater than the overall rate (12.1% compared with 9.7%), with the rate for women somewhat more than that for men (12.8% compared with 11.1%).

From Administration on Aging: *A statistical profile of Asian older Americans aged 65+* (2010). Available at http://www.aoa.gov/AoARoot/Aging_Statistics/minority_aging/Facts-on-API-Elderly2008-plain_format.aspx. Accessed December 2010.

who self-identifies as Asian/Pacific Islander is from one of more than a dozen countries that rim the Pacific Ocean and speaks one (or more) of more than 1000 languages or dialects. Persons classified as black Americans are usually assumed to identify themselves as African American, although an increasing number are from any one of the Caribbean Islands, each with a distinct culture and, in some cases, language.

Adding to the diversity in the United States is the number of persons emigrating from other countries; the rate at which this number is growing exceeds that of the native born. Although access to the United States varies with global politics, older adults are continually being reunited with their adult offspring, whom they assist with homemaking and care for younger children in the family as they are cared for themselves. It is

BOX 5-4   A STATISTICAL PROFILE OF HISPANIC OLDER AMERICANS AGED 65 YEARS OR MORE

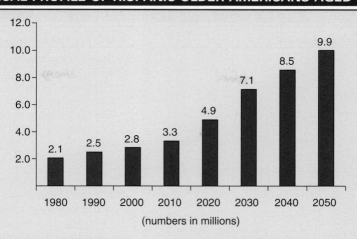

The Older Hispanic Population: Past, Present, and Future.

In 2008:
- The Hispanic older population was 2.7 million, or 6.8% of all persons 65 and older. This number is expected to grow to 17.5 million by 2050, or 19.8% of all elders.
- Seventy percent resided in four states: California (27%), Texas (19%), Florida (16%), and New York (9%).
- Although there has been improvement, there continue to be significant differences in the educational attainment of Hispanic elders. In 2008 only 46% had finished high school, and 9% held a bachelor's degree or higher (compared with 77% and 21% for the total older population).

- The percentage of Hispanic older men and women living alone (15% and 26%, respectively) was lower than the overall rate, and the percentage of those living with other relatives was almost twice the overall rate.
- Households headed by Hispanic elders reported a mean annual income of $33,418 compared with $46,720 for non-Hispanic white households.
- Hispanic elders were twice as likely as non-Hispanic white elderly to live in poverty (19.3% compared with 7.6%).

From Administration on Aging: *A statistical profile of Hispanic older Americans aged 65+* (2010). Available at http://www.aoa.gov/AoARoot/Aging_ Statistics/minority_aging/Facts-on-Hispanic-Elderly.aspx. Accessed December 2010.

becoming increasingly common for communities to provide and support senior centers with activities and meals reflective of their diverse participants. The diversity of values, beliefs, languages, and historic life experiences of elders today challenges nurses to gain new awareness, knowledge, and skills to provide culturally and linguistically appropriate care. Nurses practicing in those areas with the most diversity (California, New York, and Texas) are highly likely to care for persons from a variety of backgrounds in the same day and a culture other than their own (Administration on Aging, 2010).

HEALTH DISPARITIES AND OLDER ADULTS

The document *Healthy People* has served as a guide for the promotion of health and the prevention of disease and disability since it was first published in 1979 and updated in 2000. It is in the process of revision in 2010 (U.S. Department of Health and Human Services [USDHHS], 2009a). In the past, one of the goals was to decrease health disparities. At present one of the new overarching goals goes much further: "Achieve health equity, eliminate disparities, and improve the health of all groups" (USDHHS, 2009b) (Box 5-5). This goal and its associated objectives have significant implications for the consideration of culture, gender, and aging and for the practice of gerontological nursing. Addressing health disparities begins with providing culturally competent and proficient care.

BOX 5-5   HEALTHY PEOPLE 2020
Overarching Goals

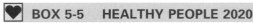

- Attain high-quality, longer lives free of preventable disease, disability, injury, and premature death.
- Achieve health equity, eliminate disparities, and improve the health of all groups.
- Create social and physical environments that promote good health for all.
- Promote quality of life, healthy development, and healthy behaviors across all life stages.

From U.S. Department of Health and Human Services: Healthy people 2020 framework (2009b). Available at http://www.healthypeople.gov/hp2020/Objectives/framework.aspx. Accessed December 2010.

Health Disparities

The term *health disparity* refers both to differences in the state of health and in health outcomes between groups of persons. An associated term is *health inequity,* which refers to the excess burden of illness, or the difference between the expected incidence and prevalence and that which actually occurs in excess, in a comparison population group. Those found to be especially vulnerable to health disparities and inequities include older women, men and women of color, and the poor. Among older poor adults, women of all races and ethnicities predominate.

| TABLE 5-1 | BLACKS COMPARED WITH WHITES ON MEASURES OF QUALITY AND ACCESS FOR MOST CURRENT DATA YEAR: SPECIFIC MEASURES, 2009* | |

TOPIC	BETTER THAN WHITES	WORSE THAN WHITES
Cancer		Colorectal cancer diagnosed at advanced stage
		Adults age 50 and over who report they ever received a colonoscopy, sigmoidoscopy, proctoscopy, or fecal occult blood test
		Colorectal cancer deaths per 100,000 population
		Breast cancer diagnosed at advanced stage
		Cancer deaths per 100,000 female population due to breast cancer
Heart disease	Deaths per 1000 admissions with acute myocardial infarction as principal diagnosis, age 18 and over	
	Hospital patients who received recommended care for heart failure	
HIV and AIDS		New AIDS cases per 100,000 population age 13 and over
Respiratory diseases		Adults age 65 and over who ever received pneumococcal vaccination
		Hospital patients with pneumonia who received recommended care
Functional status preservation and rehabilitation		Female Medicare beneficiaries age 65 and over who reported ever being screened for osteoporosis
Supportive and palliative care	Long-stay nursing home residents who were physically restrained	High-risk long-stay nursing home residents with pressure sores
		Short-stay nursing home residents with pressure sores
		Home health care patients who were admitted to the hospital
Timeliness		Emergency department visits in which patients left without being seen
Access	People without a usual source of care due to a financial or insurance reason	People who have a usual primary care provider

AIDS, acquired immunodeficiency syndrome; HIV, human immunodeficiency virus.
*Modified for those most relevant to older adults.
From Agency for Healthcare Quality and Research: Priority populations: older adults. In: *National healthcare quality report, 2009.* Available at http://www.ahrq.gov/qual/nhdr09/Chap4.htm. Accessed December 2010.

In 2002 the Institute of Medicine (Washington DC) prepared an analysis of the state of the science on health disparities. It began with the acknowledgment that persons of color had difficulty accessing the same care as their white counterparts. The researchers were to determine the state of care while controlling for access issues.

The result of the study was that, even when controlling for unequal access, health care treatment in and of itself was unequal (Smedley et al., 2002). The barriers to quality care were found to be wide, ranging from those related to geographical location to age, gender, race, ethnicity, and sexual orientation. Disparities were consistently found across a wide range of disease areas and clinical services. Among the findings were the following:

- Disparities were found even when clinical factors, such as stage of disease presentation, comorbidities, age, and severity of disease, were taken into account.
- Disparities were found across a range of clinical settings, including public and private hospitals and teaching and non-teaching hospitals.
- Disparities in care were associated with higher mortality among minorities.

In the years since then, the Agency for Healthcare Research and Quality (Rockville, MD) has produced national healthcare quality reports and national healthcare disparities reports to track the prevailing trends in health care quality and access for vulnerable populations, including the elderly and those from minority populations. Each year another aspect of care is highlighted. Most of the information available consists of comparisons between the white and black populations. There is still inadequate data available about other groups, e.g., Native Alaskans for an adequate assessment of their health care status

(Table 5-1 and Figure 5-2). None-the-less older adults of color have been described as facing "double jeopardy" for health disparities because of two risk factors for vulnerability (age and ethnicity). For black women, the risk becomes "triple jeopardy," and poverty adds a fourth factor.

Cultural Proficiency

To address health disparities and inequities, it is necessary not just to become competent but to become culturally proficient health care providers and organizations, that is, able to move smoothly between the world of the nurse and the world of the patient (and in this case, the world of the elder). Nurses should become aware of and understand the considerable problems that many older women in general, and men and women from ethnically distinct groups, encounter in the pursuit and receipt of health care and the considerable disparities in health outcomes. Through this awareness, more compassionate and relevant care can be provided.

By increasing awareness, nurses learn of their personal biases, prejudices, attitudes, and behaviors toward persons different from themselves in age, gender, sexual orientation, social class, economic situations, and many other factors. Through increased knowledge, nurses can better assess the strengths and challenges of the older adult and know when and how to effectively intervene to support rather than hinder cultural strengths. Skills in cultural competence include putting cultural knowledge to use in assessment, communication, negotiation, and intervention.

Cultural Awareness

The development of cultural proficiency begins with increased awareness of our own beliefs and attitudes and those commonly seen in the community at large and in the community of health

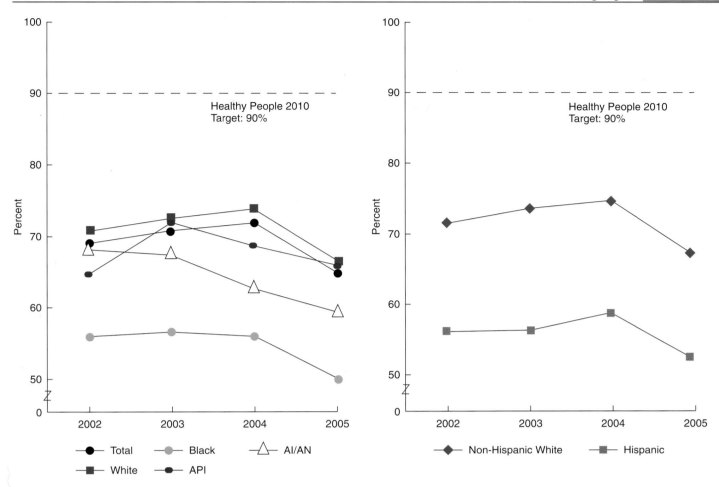

FIGURE 5-2 Medicare Beneficiaries Age 65 and Over Who Had an Influenza Vaccination in the Last Winter, by Race and Ethnicity, 2002-2005. AI/AN, American Indian or Alaska Native; API, Asian or Pacific Islander. (From Agency for Healthcare Quality and Research: Older adults: prevention, influenza vaccination. In: *National healthcare quality report, 2009.* Available at http://www.ahrq.gov/qual/nhdr09/Chap4d.htm#older_ adults. Accessed December 2010.)

BOX 5-6   MOVING TOWARD CULTURAL SENSITIVITY AND HEALTHY AGING

- Become familiar with your own cultural perspectives, including beliefs about disease etiology, treatments, and factors leading to outcomes.
- Examine your personal and professional behavior for signs of bias and the use of negative stereotypes.
- Remain open to viewpoints and behaviors that are different from your expectations.
- Appreciate the inherent worth of all persons from all groups.
- Develop the skill of listening to both nonverbal and verbal communication.
- Develop sensitivity to the clues given by others, indicating the paradigm from which they face illness and aging.
- Learn to negotiate, rather than impose, strategies to promote healthy aging consistent with the beliefs of the persons to whom we provide care.

---

care (Box 5-6). Increased awareness requires openness and self-reflection. Consider the following:

A gerontological nurse responded to a call from an older patient's room. For some unknown reason, he repeatedly and without comment dropped his watch on the floor while talking to the nurse. She calmly picked it up, handed it back to him, and continued talking. During one of the droppings, an aide walked in the room, picked up the watch, and attempted to hand it back to him. The patient immediately started yelling and cursing at the aide for attempting to steal his watch. When telling this story, the nurse thought the whole situation odd, but not too remarkable. It was not until she learned about subtle racism in health care settings that she realized the more harmful, racist behavior of the man—he was white, and so was she; the aide was black.

If the nurse is white, it is realizing that whiteness alone often means special privilege and freedoms. Older adults of color may not have had the same advantages or experiences as the nurse (McIntosh, 1989). Cultural awareness means recognizing the presence of the "isms" (e.g., racism, social classism, ageism) and how these have the potential to impact not only health care but also the quality of life for older adults (Smedley et al., 2002). Awareness includes considering how the nurse feels about gender. For example, is sexuality accepted in the same way in older men as in older women?

An awareness of one's thoughts and feelings about others who are culturally different from oneself is necessary. These thoughts and feelings can be hidden from oneself but may be evident to clients. To be aware of these thoughts and feelings about others, one can begin to share or write down personal memories of those first experiences of cultural differences. Questions such as "When did I first provide care for someone I thought was different from me? How did I feel? How did I act? How did they react to me providing them with care?" are a good starting point for the process of cultural self-discovery.

Cultural awareness has several levels. The first is the self-level, requiring self-understanding of one's experiences and values. The second level involves the ability to work with and build relationships with a member from another cultural group. The third level is the recognition of factors beyond culture, such as health, safety, and poverty, that affect members of a cultural group. On the fourth level, it is important to understand how one's own community history affects how others are viewed. On the last level, one must be able to step outside of cultural bias and accept that other cultures have different ways of perceiving the world that are equal to our own.

Cultural Knowledge

Cross-cultural knowledge can minimize frustration and cultural conflict among older adult patients, nurses, and other health care providers. It will allow the nurse to more appropriately and effectively improve client health outcomes. However, cultural knowledge should never yield to assumptions—only an avenue of essential communication—about the beliefs and practices that are unique to those persons living within a culture, a family, and a community.

Cultural knowledge is both what the nurse brings to the caring situation and what the nurse learns about older adults, their families, their communities, their behaviors, and their expectations. Essential knowledge includes the elder's way of life (ways of thinking, believing, and acting). This knowledge is obtained formally or informally through the professional experience of nursing and caring. Over time, the nurse builds up a reservoir of information about the beliefs of his or her clients and how they behave.

Some nurses prefer to use what can be called an "encyclopedic" approach to details of a particular culture or ethnic group, such as proper name usage, greeting, eye contact, gender roles, foods, and beliefs about relevant topics (e.g., the meaning of aging, the appropriate expression of pain, death practices, caregiving). Another approach involves increasing knowledge with more global application to nursing care and the ethnic elder rather than specific details about any one culture group.

Definitions of Terms. Cultural knowledge includes the appropriate use of terms, especially race, culture, and ethnicity. Often used interchangeably, each actually has a separate meaning. *Race* is defined in terms of phenotype as expressed in traits, such as eye color, facial structure, hair texture, and especially skin tones. In a genomic analysis of persons identified as member of a racial group there is little difference. The term "race" is best used as a proxy for geographic origins and lineage with implications for pharmacogenomics more than anything else (see Chapter 9). However, the relative usefulness of race is diminishing because of widespread mixing of the gene pool, making it increasingly uncommon for any one person to be genetically homogeneous (Gelfand, 2003). Acknowledgment of this heterogeneity was demonstrated

when a new racial category of "mixed" was added to the 2000 U.S. Census forms.

Culture is the shared and learned beliefs, expectations, and behaviors of a group of people. Style of dress, food preferences, language, and social behavior are reflections of culture. Culture guides thinking, decision-making, and action. Beliefs about aging may be relatively consistent within one culture group (Jett, 2003). Cultural beliefs about aging are often portrayed in the media, both in print and on the screen. For example, the 2005 movie *In Her Shoes* portrays a number of white stereotypes about aging, both positive and negative. A particular characteristic of culture is that it is transmitted from one member to another through a process called *enculturation*. Culture provides directions for individuals as they interact with family and friends within the same group. Culture allows members of the group to predict each other's behavior and respond in ways that are considered appropriate (Spector, 2008).

Acculturation is the process by which a person from a minority or marginalized culture adopts that of the dominant or majority culture in which they find themselves. There has been much concern about aging immigrants and how culture facilitates or hinders the adjustments needed in late life in the United States. Pierce and colleagues (1978/1979) and Spector (2008) wrote that various types of acculturation were more critical to functional adaptation than others. For example, outward adaptation that incorporates language, dress, and behavior was seen as superficially important. On a deeper level, traditional personal value orientations, including concepts of time, and personal relationships to others and nature, were more likely to remain in the original cultural context. These have been a source of conflict between parents and children when caregiving is needed. The parents may expect the children to provide all the care that is needed. The more acculturated children may feel significant conflict as their "American" lives do not reflect or support their filial duties.

Ethnicity refers to a culture group with which one self-identifies. Persons from a specific ethnic group may share common nationality, migratory status, race, language or dialect, or religion. Traditions, symbols, literature, folklore, food preferences, and dress are often expressions of ethnicity. Persons from a specific ethnic group may not share a common race. For example, persons who identify themselves as "Hispanic" may be from any race and from any one of a number of countries. However, most Hispanic persons share the Catholic religion and the Spanish language. It is more accurate to ask an elder to self-identify ethnicity rather than make assumptions.

Orientation to Time. The concept and use of time is culturally constructed and has significant implications in the use of health care. Time orientation has long been theoretically recognized but often overlooked as a factor influencing the use of health care, especially preventive practices (Lukwago et al., 2001). Older adults are more likely to use the orientation of their culture of origin, which may contrast significantly with that of the health care system in the United States.

A future time orientation is consistent with that of Western medicine. Prevention today is important because of its effect on future health. One who is ill today can make an appointment for the "next available" opening. In other words, the health problem can "wait" until an office appointment with a health care provider tomorrow—the problem will still be there and the delay will not necessarily affect the outcome. This also means that health screenings today are believed to be valuable in that they may detect a potential problem today for treatment or prevention of future development at a later time—days, weeks, or years ahead.

In contrast to those with a future time orientation are those with past or present time orientations. Persons oriented to the present experience a problem now, and treatment is believed to be needed at the time the problem is perceived and may not be needed in the future. The outcome is seen as current and not future. Preventive actions are not consistent with this approach.

Persons oriented to the past view the health of the present as dependent on the actions of the past, either in a past life or earlier in this life, or on events or circumstances experienced by one's ancestors. Dishonoring ancestors by failure to perform certain rituals may result in illness. Illness today may be a punishment for past deeds.

Conflicts between the future-oriented Westernized world of the nurse and those with past or present orientations are not hard to imagine. Such elders are likely to be labeled as *noncompliant* for failure to keep appointments or for failure to participate in preventive measures, such as a turning schedule for a bed-bound patient or immunizations. Members of present-oriented groups are often accused by the media of overusing hospital emergency departments, when in fact it may be the only option available for today's treatment what are viewed as today's problems.

The nurse can, however, listen closely to the elder and find out which orientation has the most value for him or her and find ways to work with it rather than expect (often unsuccessfully) the person to conform. In this way we are reaching out beyond our ethnocentrism to improve the quality of gerontological nursing care.

Orientation to Family and Self. Another useful concept in caring for ethnic elders is orientation to family and self. White Americans of European descent tend to highly value autonomy and individuality, with identity bound first to oneself. Rathbone-McCune, in a large, classic study (1982), found that European American elders would go to great lengths and live with significant discomfort rather than ask for help. To seek or receive help was considered a sign of weakness and dependence, to be avoided at all costs. The reliance on the individual is institutionalized in the passing of the Patient Self-Determination Act of 1990, in which the rights and responsibilities of the individual to participate in all decisions regarding his or her health are articulated.

This orientation is in sharp contrast to that of a collectivist, or the belief in familism (Lukwago et al., 2001; Scharlach et al., 2006). The identity of a member of a collectivist culture is drawn from family ties (broadly defined) rather than individual accomplishments. The "family" is more important than the individual, and decisions are made by a group and for the benefit of the group rather than the individual. Within family groups, the exchange of help and resources is both expected and commonplace. This orientation applies to most groups other than European Americans. The cultural belief of familism is particularly significant as it relates to expectations for elder care

and health-related decision-making. Jett (2002) found that help-seeking and help-giving among frail, elderly African American women were common experiences. The receipt of help was considered a sign of the love of others, and a reflection of the status of the elder. The greater the affection of others, the higher the level of help received, and that "good things will come to you" if the recipient lived a good life (Jett, 2002, p. 384). On the surface, the Health Insurance Portability and Accountability Act (HIPAA) rules established to protect the privacy of the individual are in direct conflict with this cultural pattern. When a nurse who values individuality provides care for an elder who has a collectivist perspective or vice versa, the potential for cultural conflict exists, illustrated by the following scenario:

> An older Filipino woman is seen in her home by a Euro-American public health nurse and found to have a blood pressure of 210/100 mm Hg and a blood sugar level of 380 mg/dl. The nurse insists on calling the patient's nurse practitioner and arranging immediate transportation to an acute care hospital. The woman insists that she must wait until her son-in-law and daughter get out of work so she and the nurse can discuss it with them before any action be taken. The daughter and her husband will decide where and when she will go for treatment. She is concerned about the welfare of the family and wants to ensure that income is not lost by leaving work early. The family also jointly decides if they can afford a provider's visit and a possible hospitalization. The nurse's main concern is the health of the individual elder, and the elder's concern is her family. The nurse is operating from the value that says an individual is independent and responsible for personal health care decisions, inconsistent with that of the elder.

Intensity of Relationships. Another concept that has implications for working with elders in cross-cultural situations is "context," which refers to the characteristics of relationships and behaviors toward others (Hall, 1977, 1990). The context is loosely divided into high and low and refers to the intensity of the interactions, including expressions of emotion and relationship with the nurse. When caring for the *high-context* elder, he or she will inquire about the nurse's health, family, or work. In return, the caring nurse first is expected to return the same and appear genuinely interested in the person, and secondarily address health care needs. Body language is more important than spoken words; it conveys the intended message. The quality of the relationship between the nurse and the person is more important than, perhaps, the needs of the person. The majority of cultures across the globe are high context in nature.

In sharp contrast are low-context relationships and behaviors, which are prevalent in the culture of Western medicine and nursing drawing from northern European roots. *Low-context* health care encounters are task-oriented, and the relationship between the patient and provider may be of little significance. For example, Mrs. Gomez is not the 82-year-old immigrant from Mexico, mother of seven and grandmother of 30; instead, she is the "fractured hip in room 203." For the person who is low context, small talk may be considered a waste of time. A direct approach is expected, with a literal message such as "Just tell me what is wrong with me!" Nonverbal communication is of little to no significance. The culturally competent nurse is skilled enough to assess the patterns of those cared for and to move between the contexts to provide the highest quality of caring.

Cohort Effect. Each of us shares historical experiences with others, often those of the same age, ethnic background, or country of origin. These shared experiences provide the context in which we age, known as the "cohort effect." For example, men in many parts of the world born between 1920 and 1930 were very likely to have been active participants in World War II. In comparison, men born between 1940 and 1950 in the United States were likely to have been involved in the Vietnam conflict. Those participants in the more recent wars in the Middle East range in age, but form a cohort by a sharing of the experience. All of these represent very different experiences; it is not surprising that persons in each of these cohorts have different world perspectives and different health problems. Likewise, most white women born between 1920 and 1930 were raised with what are known as *traditional values and roles* and may have either never worked outside the home or been limited to lower paying "women's work," such as domestic services, teaching, and nursing (most black women were already working as domestics or in agriculture). In contrast, women born between 1930 and 1940 experienced pressure to work outside the home and also had considerably more opportunities, partly as the result of the feminist revolution of the 1960s. For some ethnic elders it may be more appropriate to think in terms of existential time; before and after the Jim Crow era for African-American elders in the rural south, or before and after the Mariel boatlift of 1980 for Cuban Americans.

Beliefs about Health, Illness, and Treatment. Fundamental cultural knowledge is that of beliefs about health, illness, and treatment. Older adults have lifelong experiences with illness of self, family, and others within their ethnic groups. The significance they attach to illness symptoms and their reactions to these are related to the outcomes they have experienced or observed in the past. The diversity of the population has brought the strong potential for a clash of health belief systems, language, and attitudes about health and illness between the care provider and the elder. Many of the beliefs and practices do not fit into the traditional format of health care as most care providers know it, that is, a Western biomedical paradigm. Other belief paradigms include magico-religious and naturalistic/holistic.

Biomedical. The biomedical, scientific, or Western medical paradigm espouses the belief that disease is the result of abnormalities in structure and function of body organs and systems. It is the dominant model used by those educated in Western health care. The objective term *disease* is used by care providers, and *illness* is a subjective term to describe symptoms of discomfort or sickness. A personal state of illness has distinct social dimensions. Assessment and diagnosis are directed at identifying the pathogen or process causing the abnormality and removing or destroying the cause or at least repairing or modifying the problem through treatment. Clinicians use what is referred to as the *scientific method*, as well as laboratory and other procedures, to treat the disease or disease process. Preventive strategies are those in which pathogens, chemicals, activities, and dietary agents known to cause malfunction are avoided.

Magico-religious. In the magico-religious theory of illness and disease causation, both are caused by the actions of a higher power, for example God, gods, or supernatural forces or agents such as ghosts, ancestors, or evil spirits (Winkelman, 2009). Health is viewed as a blessing or reward of God and illness as a punishment for a breach of rules, breaking a taboo, or displeasing or failing to please the source of power. Beliefs that illness and disease are attributed to the wrath of God are prevalent among members of the Holiness, Pentecostal, and Fundamentalist Baptist churches. Examples of magical causes of illness are voodoo, especially among persons from the Caribbean; root work among southern African Americans; hexing among Mexican Americans and African Americans; and Gaba among Filipino Americans. Practitioners of magico-religious rituals are most often cultural healers such as the shaman, curandero(a), espirita, etc. Treatments may consist of or include religious practices such as praying, meditating, fasting, wearing amulets, burning candles, and establishing family altars. Such practices may be used both curatively and preventively. Another preventive strategy is to ensure that one maintains good relationships with others (Samovar et al., 2010).

Significant conflict with nurses may result when a patient refuses biomedical treatments because to do so may be viewed as a sign of disrespect for God or as challenging God's will. Although this approach is more common in certain groups, most of us believe in this approach to some extent. How many nurses and their older patients have prayed to a higher power that health be restored or maintained? This belief system can be traced back to the ancient Egyptians, thousands of years ago, and persists in whole or in part in many groups. Current practices included in this group are the "laying on of hands" and prayer circles. It is not uncommon to hear an older adult pray for a cure or to lament "What did I do to cause this?"

Naturalistic or holistic. The naturalistic or holistic health belief system is based on the concept of balance and stems from the ancient civilizations of China, India, and Greece (Young and Koopsen, 2005). Many people throughout the world view health as a sign of balance—of the right amount of exercise, food, sleep, evacuation, interpersonal relationships, or geophysical and metaphysical forces in the universe, such as chi. Disturbances in this balance result in disharmony and subsequent illness. Diagnosis requires the determination of the type of imbalance. A common manifestation of this theoretical approach is in the yin and yang of ancient China and in the hot/cold theory common throughout the world. The naturalistic system practiced in India and some of its neighboring countries is known as *ayurvedic medicine*. It is often applied along with practices of Western medicine.

Yin and yang is an ancient Chinese concept that has been used continuously for more than 5000 years. Health is viewed as a state of perfect balance between the yin and the yang, dark and light, male and female. When one is in balance, a feeling of inner and outer peace is experienced. Illness represents an imbalance of yin and yang. Balance may be restored by herbs, acupuncture, acupressure, or controlled deep-breathing exercises.

In the hot/cold theory illness is classified as either hot or cold and believed to be the result of an excess of heat or cold that has entered the body and caused an imbalance. Hot and cold are generally metaphorical, although at times temperature is an aspect. Various foods, medicines, environmental conditions, emotions, and body conditions, such as menstruation and pregnancy, may possess the characteristics of either hot or cold (Spector, 2008). Diagnosis requires identifying the disease as either hot or cold. Remedies are similarly divided. The opposite element is used for treatment, for example, if the disease is the result of excess hot, treatment will be with something that has cold properties, and vice versa. The treatments may take the form of herbs, food, dietary restrictions, or medications from Western medicine that have hot and cold properties, such as antibiotics, massage, poultices, and other therapies.

Obstacles to Cultural Knowledge

Gerontological nurses providing culturally proficient care help promote health equity through awareness of and sensitivity to both overt and covert barriers to cultural knowledge. Among these barriers are ethnocentrism, stereotyping, and other "isms." As a result of any of these, we may see cultural conflict in the nursing situation. Conflict can occur any time a person interacts with another whose beliefs, values, customs, languages, and behavior patterns differ from their own. For example, an immigrant Korean nurse is instructed to ambulate an 80-year-old patient. He says that he is tired and wants to remain in bed. The nurse does not insist. The European American nurse manager reprimands the immigrant Korean nurse for not ambulating the patient as ordered and the patient for not getting out of bed. The immigrant Korean nurse says to another Korean nurse: "Those Americans do not respect their elders; they talk to them as if they were children."

In the traditional Korean culture, men are the decision-makers and older adults are revered. The European American nurse complains to a colleague that "those Asian nurses allow men to run all over them."

Ethnocentrism

In the responses of both nurses in the previous section, each denigrated the other's culturally prescribed behavior to underscore that his or her own cultural response was "correct." These are examples of what is known as *ethnocentrism,* or the belief that one's own ethnic group is superior to that of another's. In health care, we have a unique culture and usually expect patients to adapt to us. We expect them to be on time for appointments, to follow our instructions, and to listen to what we say and then do what we tell them to do. If we are caring for elders in an institutional setting, we expect them to agree with, for example, the frequency of prescribed bathing, eating (and timing of this), and sleep and rest cycles. The better acculturated an elder is to the culture of the institution and nurse, the less the potential for conflict. The elder will eat the meals provided, even if the food does not look or taste like what she has always eaten. A non–English-speaking resident will accommodate the staff, with or without the help of an interpreter.

Stereotyping

Although cultural knowledge is helpful and essential, it should be applied cautiously. *Stereotyping* is the application of limited knowledge about one person with specific characteristics to other persons with the same general characteristics and, in doing so, limits the recognition of the heterogeneity of any group. Relying on knowledge of a positive stereotype can be useful as a starting point in understanding but can also be used to limit understanding of the uniqueness of the individual and to impose unrealistic expectations. For example, a common stereotype about older African Americans may be that the church is a source of support. If the nurse simply assumes this to be true, it could have a negative outcome, such as fewer referrals for other forms of support (e.g., home-delivered meals). On the other hand, this stereotype can be used to shortcut the assessment. In discussing discharge plans with an African American elder, the nurse may say, "Is your church one of the resources you will be able to depend on when you return home?"

Cultural Skills

Promoting healthy aging and providing the highest quality of care for elders from all culture groups require not only awareness and knowledge but also the ability to apply both with a new or refined set of skills. In doing so, the self-esteem of the elder is enhanced. The appropriate use of communication and language is a foundational skill and intimately tied to the concept of the self. The self is continuously constructed and inextricably bound up with the linguistic categories available in a given culture (Berman, 1991). Communication is an issue not only of language but also of idiom, style, jargon, voice tone, inflection, and body language. We can conceive of ourselves only within the language we know. To make each contact with others fully meaningful, shared communication is essential.

Communication also means listening carefully to the person, especially for his or her perception of the situation, and attending not just to the words but also to the nonverbal communication and the meaning behind the stories. Listen to the elder's perception of the situation, desired goals, and ideas for treatment. Cultural skills include the ability of nurses to explain their perceptions clearly and without judgment, acknowledging that both similarities and differences exist between their perceptions and goals and those of their patients. The application of these skills plays an essential part in assessment, in future encounters, and in the development of the plan of care.

Unspoken Communication. Communication begins long before a word is spoken. In many cultures the unspoken message may be as or more important than what is heard. For persons with dementia, from any culture, this is especially true.

The handshake. A handshake is the customary and expected greeting in what is called "mainstream [European] America." A firm handshake is thought to be a sign of good character and strength. Yet this is not always the case. To an American Indian elder, a firm or vigorous handshake may be interpreted as a sign of aggression. Their handshake may instead be more of a passing of the hand with a light touch as a sign of respect rather than of weakness. In the Muslim culture, cross-gender physical contact (including handshakes) may be considered highly inappropriate or even forbidden. Before the nurse makes physical contact with an elder of any culture, he or she should ask the person's permission or follow his or her lead, such as an outstretched hand.

Eye contact. Making eye contact during verbal communication is another highly valued behavior in the mainstream American culture. Direct eye contact is taught to be a sign of being honest, trustworthy, and straightforward. Nursing students are taught to establish and to maintain eye contact when interacting with patients, but this behavior may be misinterpreted by older adults of other cultural groups. The less-acculturated ethnic elder may avoid eye contact, not as a sign of deceit but as a sign of respect. A more traditional American Indian elder may not allow the nurse to make eye contact, moving his or her eyes slowly from the floor to the ceiling and around the room. Direct eye contact is considered disrespectful in most Asian cultures. Looking one directly in the eye implies equality. Older adults may avoid eye contact with physicians and nurses if health professionals are viewed as authority figures. In some cultures, direct eye contact between men and women is considered a sexual advance. The gerontological nurse can follow the lead of the elder by being open to eye contact but not forcing this type of contact in any way or use it to assign value.

The use of silence. The value, use, and interpretation of silence also vary markedly from one culture to another. In general, Eastern cultures value silence over the use of words; in Western cultures, the opposite is true. For older adults of many Eastern cultural groups, especially those in which the Confucian philosophy is embraced, silence is a sign of respect for the wisdom and expertise of the speaker. Silence is expected of young family members and of family members who have less authority. In traditional Japanese and Chinese families, silence during a conversation may indicate the speaker is giving the listener time to ponder what has been said before moving on to another idea. In Native American cultures, it is believed that one learns self-control, courage, patience, and dignity from remaining silent. Silence during a conversation may signify that the listener is reflecting on what the speaker has just verbalized. French, Spanish, and older adult immigrants from the former Soviet Union may interpret silence as a sign of agreement (Tripp-Reimer and Lauer, 1987; Purnell and Paulanka, 2003).

Spoken Communication. Unspoken communication is usually accompanied by a spoken component. If both the nurse and the elder speak the same language, communication is facilitated, although attention to cross-cultural factors is not precluded. However, when different languages are spoken, interpretation and sometimes translation are needed for optimal care. *Translation* is the exchange of one written language for another, such as in the translation of patient education materials. *Interpretation,* on the other hand, is the processing of language from one spoken language to another in a manner that preserves the meaning and tone of the original language without adding or deleting anything. The job of the interpreter is to work with two different linguistic codes in a way that will produce equivalent messages (Haffner, 1992). The interpreter tells the elder what the nurse has said and the nurse what the elder has said without adding meaning or opinion.

An interpreter is needed any time the nurse and the elder speak different languages, when the elder has limited English proficiency, or when cultural tradition prevents the elder from speaking directly to the nurse. The more complex the decision-making, the more important are the interpreter and his or her skills. These circumstances are many, such as when discussions are needed about the treatment plan for a new condition, the options for treatment, advanced care planning, or even preparation for care after discharge from a health care institution.

BOX 5-7   GUIDELINES FOR WORKING WITH INTERPRETERS

- Before an interview or session with a client, meet with the interpreter to explain the purpose of the session.
- Encourage the interpreter to meet with the client before the session to identify the educational level and attitudes toward health and health care and to determine the depth and type of information and explanation needed.
- Look and speak directly to the client, not the interpreter.
- Be patient. Interpreted interviews take more time because long, explanatory phrases often are needed.
- Use short units of speech. Long, involved sentences or complex discussions create confusion.
- Use simple language. Avoid technical terms, professional jargon, slang, abbreviations, abstractions, metaphors, and idiomatic expressions.
- Encourage interpretation of the client's own words rather than paraphrased professional jargon to get a better sense of the client's ideas and emotional state.
- Encourage the interpreter to avoid inserting his or her own ideas and to avoid omitting information.
- Listen to the client and watch nonverbal communication (facial expression, voice intonation, body movement) to learn about emotions regarding a specific topic.
- Clarify the client's understanding and the accuracy of the interpretation by asking the client to tell you in his or her own words what he or she understands, facilitated by the interpreter.

Modified from Lipson JG, Dibble SL, Minarik PA, editors: *Culture and nursing care: a pocket guide,* San Francisco, 1996, UCSF School of Nursing Press.

It is ideal to engage interpreters who are trained in medical interpretation and who are of the same sex, social status, and, in some cases, age as the elder. Unfortunately, too often children or even grandchildren are called on to act as interpreters. When they are not available, secretaries or housekeepers are asked to fill this role. When doing so, the nurse must realize that either the interpreter or the elder may "edit" his or her comments because of cultural restrictions about the content, that is, what is or is not appropriate to speak about to parent, child, or stranger. At other times "interpreter lines" via the phone or computer are used. If this is the only option possible, the nurse must expect that the information obtained is limited at best and that misunderstandings are likely. To maximize the potential quality when working with an interpreter, the nurse first introduces herself or himself to the client and the interpreter and sets down guidelines for the interview. Sentences should be short, employing the active tense, and metaphors should be avoided because they may be impossible to convert from one language to another. The nurse asks the interpreter to say exactly what is being said, to use the first person, and to direct all conversation to the client.

For more information on working with interpreters, see Box 5-7 and refer to the detailed guidelines and protocols available from Enslein and colleagues at the University of Iowa (Enslein et al., 2001, 2002).

GENDER

Gender, which refers to the personal, cultural meaning of biological differences, is fundamental to personal identity and is the primary way in which experiences are organized. Gender incorporates those and other, less measurable characteristics that are the result of a coalescence of cohort, culture, and genetics. Environmental influences, social expectations, and early socialization, as well as innate capacities, all seem to fall within the purview of these three categories.

Consideration of aging from a cultural perspective provides rich context for providing the highest quality gerontological care. When adding knowledge about gender issues, our perspectives can broaden and our sensitivities deepen. Gender studies in general have become increasingly popular.

The goals of a gender-focused research center include such aims as the following:

- Basic and clinical research related to gender-specific needs and characteristics
- Developing and testing gender-specific therapeutic strategies
- Providing gender-appropriate health recommendations
- Disseminating research findings that promote understanding of gender-specific issues

However, to identify the relevance of gender is exceedingly difficult and requires a breadth of perspective. In the past two decades we have moved from simply describing biological differences to emphasizing the shaping of gender roles by socialization patterns, and we are now in a phase of describing gender in terms of social structure and cultural patterns.

From a demographic perspective, gender differences can be quite remarkable, from life expectancy to social support. Women usually live longer than men and are much more likely to live alone after widowhood. Men who survive their wives often remarry and live alone significantly less often than women. However, women usually have larger social networks outside the work environment than do men, which could potentially reduce social isolation after the death of a spouse or companion (Aday et al., 2006). And gender-related health problems emerge: women increasingly confront osteoporosis and breast and uterine cancer, whereas men are vulnerable to prostate enlargement and prostatic cancer. Heart disease is the primary cause of death for both men and women, yet women are treated less aggressively than are men.

Older Women

Older women are the fastest growing segment of the population, especially among those older than 85 years. Older women are also more likely than men to be widowed or divorced and to live alone (See Chapter 1).

Social Status

The social status of women varies by culture and is quite different from that of their male counterparts. For the gerontological nurse, the variations have implications that might be overlooked. Women who live alone are more likely to be white and never married; they have probably never had children or have outlived their children, or have outlived their husbands (Hooyman and Kiyak, 2011). If they live with others, it probably will be, first, a spouse or partner and, second, a daughter. Only rarely do white women live with other relatives, but this is much more common for women of color. Whereas most women in European-American groups hold a lower status compared with men, older women of color often hold elevated social status,

respected for both their age and their contributions to the family, community, and church or religious community. Women, in sharp contrast to men, often have an extended social support network made up of not only family but also friends and neighbors. This network may be especially strong among older lesbian women who, over a lifetime, have created tight fictive kin groups.

Economic Status

Overall, older women are at a significant economic disadvantage. This has implications in many ways, from the ability to purchase transportation and to see health care providers, to the ability to pay for health care and to have the opportunities to live in safe and well-maintained "healthy" homes. Of those who are older than 65 years and considered poor, 75% are women. The older a woman is, the more likely she is to be poor (this has been called the "feminization of poverty"). Income and marital status are connected, with most widowed and never-married women having the lowest incomes of all (see Chapter 1).

To be eligible for Social Security, one has to have worked at least 40 quarters based on an income of at least $1090 per quarter. However, the amount of benefit is calculated on an average of the best 35 years of employment (U.S. Social Security Administration, 2010). If someone has worked less than 35 years, the non–income-producing years are counted as zero income and are still included in the calculation. For women, this is usually particularly relevant because of discontinuous employment as a result of interruptions with childbirth and other caregiving responsibilities. The continuing low wages for women (compared with men) exacerbate the problem. Women, on average, continue to earn approximately 77% of that of men in the same positions and professions, which again is ultimately reflected in their Social Security income (Department of labor, 2008).

Another structural problem facing women is pension laws. Although no longer allowed in large organizations, smaller companies are still permitted to have their pension "survivor benefit" optional without survivor consent. This means that the wage earner may opt to receive higher pension payments while living with no or little continuation to his or her survivor. And for the small companies, notification is not required. This means that the survivor benefit can be declined without informing the potential survivor, most likely a woman (Box 5-8).

Health Status

Women live longer than their male cohorts, and are also subject to a greater number of chronic diseases (Figures 5-3 and 5-4). Rather than cause death, these health conditions are more likely

---

BOX 5-8   LEFT ALONE

While the author worked as a hospice nurse, she cared for a couple during the husband's very long and difficult death. There was concern about the wife's health as a 24-hour caregiver with no children and no nearby relatives. Their income was very limited, but she thought it was adequate to pay their bills and maintain their small home in a rural, isolated community, although her husband "handled all of those things." After his death, she found that he had opted for a "no survivor benefit" pension. She was almost immediately profoundly impoverished and in danger of becoming homeless with few options.

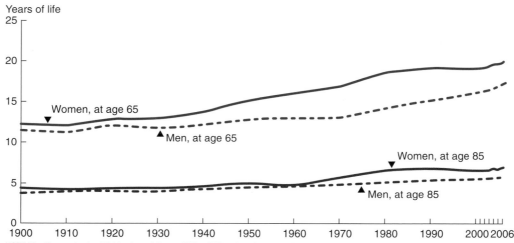

NOTE: The life expectancies (LEs) for decennial years 1910 to 1990 are based on decennial census data and deaths for a 3-year period around the census year. The LEs for decennial year 1900 are based on deaths from 1900 to 1902. LEs for years prior to 1930 are based on the death registration area only. The death registration area increased from 10 states and the District of Columbia in 1900 to the coterminous United States in 1933. LEs for 2000–2006 are based on a newly revised methodology that uses vital statistics death rates for ages under 66 and modeled probabilities of death for ages 66 to 100 based on blended vital statistics and Medicare probabilities of dying and may differ from figures previously published.
Reference population: These data refer to the resident population.
SOURCE: Centers for Disease Control and Prevention, National Center for Health Statistics, National Vital Statistics System.

FIGURE 5-3 Life Expectancy at Ages 65 and 85, by Sex, Selected Years 1900-2006. (Redrawn from Federal Interagency Forum on Aging-Related Statistics: *Older Americans 2010: Key indicators of well-being*, Washington DC, 2010, U.S. Government Printing Office.)

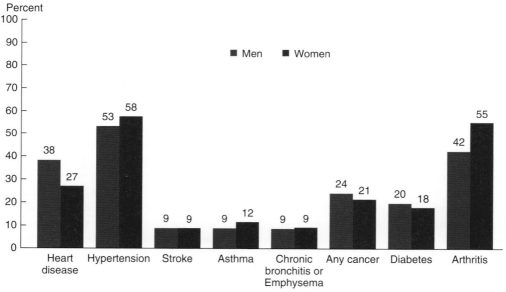

NOTE: Data are based on a 2-year average from 2007–2008. See Appendix B for the definition of race and Hispanic origin in the National Health Interview Survey.
Reference population: These data refer to the civilian noninstitutionalized population.
SOURCE: Centers for Disease Control and Prevention, National Center for Health Statistics, National Health Interview Survey.

FIGURE 5-4 Chronic Health Conditions among the U.S. Population Age 65 and Over, by Sex, 2007-2008. (Redrawn from Federal Interagency Forum on Aging-related Statistics: *Older Americans 2010: key indicators of well-being*, Washington DC, 2010, U.S. Government Printing Office.)

to lead to problems with everyday activities and functioning (those things one needs to do to get through the day) (Figure 5-5). Because of the number of illnesses, women take more prescription medications, for which they may not be able to pay. If poor, women—especially women of color—are more likely to receive a lower quality of care or do not get care because of costs.

Many areas of health specific to women (e.g., breast health, menopause) and as they affect women (e.g., osteoporosis, heart disease) are slowly receiving more attention (Helzner et al., 2005; O'Dell and McGee, 2006; Watson et al., 2006). Before the 1990s, almost all research that was later applied to women (e.g.,

the safety of synthetic estrogen) was actually conducted on men. The "Women's Health Initiative" was the first major wide-range project to enroll women to study women's health issues. Since it began recruiting participants in 1991, the knowledge about women's health has grown in ways formerly thought impossible. Among other things the study has already revolutionized what we thought we knew about the effect and safety of hormone replacement therapy (HRT) (http://www.nhlbi.nih.gov/whi/index.html).

Yet the quality and receipt of health care depend largely on access through health insurance. If an older woman (especially

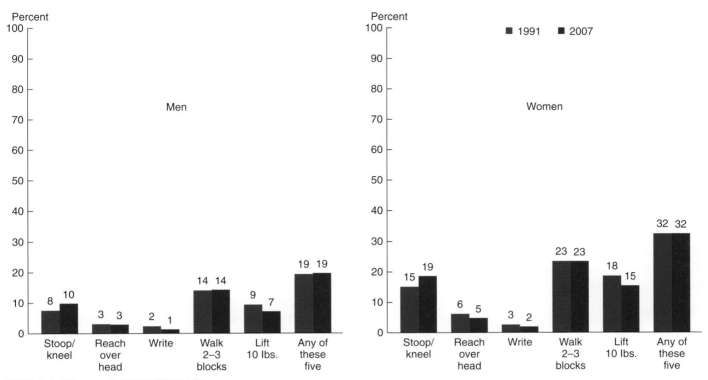

NOTE: Rates for 1991 are age adjusted to the 2007 population.
Reference population: These data refer to Medicare enrollees.
SOURCE: Centers for Medicare and Medicaid Services, Medicare Current Beneficiary Survey.

FIGURE 5-5 Percentage of Medicare Enrollees Age 65 and Over Who Are Unable to Perform Certain Physical Functions, by Sex, 1991 and 2007. (Redrawn from Federal Interagency Forum on Aging-related Statistics: *Older Americans 2010: key indicators of well-being*, Washington DC, 2010, U.S. Government Printing Office.)

one who is divorced or widowed) is not yet 65 years of age (when she may qualify for Medicare), does not have insurance, and becomes ill, she is in serious trouble. Women are more likely to be working for employers who do not provide health benefits, for example, in many nursing homes, domestic services, and small businesses. If insurance is available, she may not earn enough to purchase the plan, but her income may be too high to qualify for Medicaid. Helping women (and men) who lose insurance through divorce has been attempted. "Conversion" laws require that one's former spouse (either deceased or divorced) continue to provide access to insurance for up to three years after the death or divorce—although the premium may be prohibitive.

Despite the difficulties of aging for women, maturity brings new opportunities for many. They may find caregiving responsibilities rewarding. Or, with children grown, they have free time for the first time in their lives and go back to school, develop new interests, become athletes or gardeners, or mentor others.

Older Men

When considering men and aging, there is an interesting paradox. Until the past 10 to 15 years, the majority of research was done with groups composed entirely or primarily of men. Yet most of the literature on aging, when gender specific, is about older women, because they make up the majority of the population 65 years of age and older.

It is easy to make assumptions about the social and economic status of older men, especially in contrast to older women, as noted earlier. The differences in health status, especially when combined with racial and ethnic differences, bear closer examination and will become more interesting in the coming years. For example, men used to predominate among those with lung cancer, a fact greatly influenced by their occupational exposure to toxins and smoking. Now lung cancer is the leading type of cancer death for both men and women. The number of women with chronic obstructive pulmonary disease (COPD) is also increasing because of increased cigarette smoking. Men die younger than women, with black men having the shortest life span of all (see Chapter 1). Yet our understanding of all these phenomena is still limited.

The primary focus on older men has been in specific health issues that are theirs alone (Philpot and Morley, 2000). Benign prostatic hypertrophy is now recognized as affecting most men at some time in their lives. Erectile dysfunction (ED) may be receiving the most attention because of the increase in pharmacological interventions now possible and the openness of ED discussion in the media. Prostate cancer is now recognized as particularly important among African-American men because of its higher prevalence and death rate when compared with all other men (National Cancer Institute, 2010). Lastly, men have joined women in their fight against the aging process, with the rising popularity of hair implants, hair color "designed for men," and other cosmetic surgery and treatments.

Several questions arise when discussing gender issues related to aging, including the following:

- Why, if older women have so many disadvantages, do they survive longer and seemingly maintain morale, in spite of being old, poor, and alone?

- Why is it so difficult for men to seek medical help before life-threatening conditions occur?
- What effect will the baby boomers have on gender parity or disparity?

PROMOTING HEALTHY AGING: IMPLICATIONS FOR GERONTOLOGICAL NURSING

To fully understand another culture or gender, one must enter into an unknown conceptual world in which time, space, religion, tradition, and wellness are expressed through a unique language that conveys these formulations about the nature of the world and humanity. Cultural consistency is a component of many features of the nurse–patient interaction: communication, space, time, socialization, environment, and biology. Collectively, the personal uniqueness is established.

Assessment

Contact between elders and gerontological nurses often begins with assessment. During that time, the nurse and the elder have an opportunity to come to know each other. Listening is the key to assessment, as the nurse tries to understand the situation and the person. One must also remember that great generational cohort and cultural differences may exist between practitioner and client.

A number of "cultural assessment" tools have been created to detail an individual's beliefs and practices in very specific and comprehensive ways. Because of the complexity already inherent in the assessment of an older adult, adding an additional tool may be too burdensome for both the elder and the nurse. Instead of using a specific tool, the nurse can use cultural knowledge and sensitivity to watch for nuances of behavioral patterns throughout any patient or resident encounter (Box 5-9). The Explanatory Model, developed by Kleinman and associates (1978) and Pfeifferling (1981) has helped nurses and other health care professionals obtain relevant information in a culturally sensitive manner. An adaptation of this model appears in Chapter 7 (Box 7-1). It can serve as a guide for needed information and should not be viewed as a rigid tool.

Key information in the assessment is the determination of the health belief paradigm discussed earlier. Most people (nurses and patients alike) ascribe to more than one belief system, combining Western biomedical approaches with those that may be considered more traditional. To optimize the healthy aging of a person who depends on the nurse for intervention and caring, the nurse should learn to be sensitive to the possibility that the person may hold one or more of these beliefs. Significant conflict with nurses may result when a patient refuses biomedical treatments because the patient believes that accepting the treatment is a sign of disrespect for God (as challenging God's will) or because he or she does not believe the treatment will restore balance. Learning more about the person's beliefs regarding disease causation and effective treatment will allow the nurse to work between the cultures of medicine and the person to promote better health.

However, information about beliefs alone is inadequate. Nursing concerns must focus on overall health care for persons by assisting them to gain access to needed services through ascertaining the affordability, efficacy, accessibility, and availability of information, as well as drawing upon past experiences and developing a level of trust (Box 5-10).

BOX 5-9   A CULTURALLY COMPETENT PATIENT ENCOUNTER

Determination of:
- Preferred cultural, ethnic, and racial identity
- Expectations concerning dress and formality of the encounter
- Expectations concerning use of names, titles, addressing the patient and the nurse
- Preferred language
- Level of health and reading literacy and availability of assistance if needed
- Past personal and ethnic experience with the Western health care model
- Level of acculturation, adherence to traditional approaches, openness to new approaches
- Immigration experience and confidentiality of the health care encounter
- Factors influencing decision-making: who, how, when, what

BOX 5-10   THE TUSKEGEE EXPERIMENT

Among some African Americans today there remains mistrust of receiving care from white health care providers, especially those from large organizations or those conducting research. This distrust at some level will continue until the memory of the infamous "Tuskegee Experiment" fades. In an effort to study the "natural history of syphilis" in 1932, nearly 600 black men from Macon County, Mississippi, were recruited to participate in a study conducted jointly be the Public Health Service and the Tuskegee Institute. Almost 400 of them had documented syphilis and were told they were being treated for "bad blood" but were never treated for syphilis, even when penicillin was found to be an effective treatment. They were neither offered the treatment nor informed of the need for it. Ethical concerns were not raised until 1968, and the study was closed down in 1972. In 1997 President Clinton apologized on behalf of the nation, and not long afterward strict rules on the conduct of research were created. The last participant died on January 16, 2004. The last widow died on January 27, 2009.

For more information, see http://www.cdc.gov/tuskegee/timeline.htm.

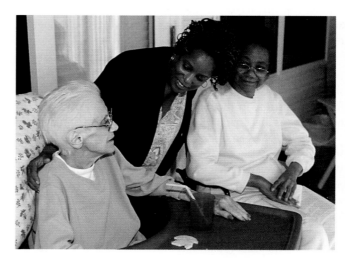

Nurses are caring for more elders from multiple ethnicities. From Lewis SM et al: Medical-surgical nursing: assessment and management of clinical problems, ed 6, St. Louis, 2004, Mosby.

Designing Interventions

Promoting healthy aging in cross-cultural settings includes the ability to develop a plan of action that considers the perspective of both the elder/family and the nurse/health care system and to negotiate an outcome that is mutually acceptable. Skillful cross-cultural nursing means developing a sense of mutual respect between the nurse and the elder. It is working "with" the client rather than "on" the client.

The LEARN Model

The LEARN model (Berlin and Fowkes, 1983) uses the perspective shown in the explanatory model and expands it to the person–nurse interaction. The LEARN model is a useful tool in guiding the nurse in the clinical setting while interacting with elders of any ethnicity. Through it, the nurse will increase his or her cultural sensitivity and, in doing so, will be instrumental in providing more culturally competent care, thus helping reduce health disparities.

> **L** Listen carefully to what the elder is saying. Attend to not just the words but to the nonverbal communication and the meaning behind the stories. Listen to the elder's perception of the situation, the desired goals and ideas for treatment.
>
> **E** Explain your perception of the situation and the problems.
>
> **A** Acknowledge and discuss both the similarities and the differences between your perceptions and goals and those of the elder.
>
> **R** Recommend a plan of action that takes both perspectives into account.
>
> **N** Negotiate a plan that is mutually acceptable.

Given the necessary data, the nurse can use this information to negotiate a clear understanding of problems and solutions with the person or the identified support figure in his or her life. Once an understanding is reached, the nurse may need to include consultation or collaboration with traditional or alternative healers if the elder believes they are important. Locate priests, monks, rabbis, ministers, or indigenous healers if their presence is desired or believed to be helpful. When alternative healing methods are used, respect them as judiciously as those you may be implementing. A sense of caring is conveyed in these gestures of personal recognition. Unbiased caring can surmount cultural differences.

Models of Cross-cultural Care

Ethnic elders can also be found in senior centers, especially those that have introduced culturally appropriate food and activities. The ultimate model for elder services reflective of cultural relativism has been and continues to be the On Lok PACE (Program of All-inclusive Care for the Elderly) Program in San Francisco. Originally designed to meet the home care needs of Chinese and Italian immigrants, it now has the capacity to provide every level of short- and long-term care, as well as residential options, to all older adults. Services are provided in the language of the elder and in the manner that optimizes each person's cultural heritage (Institute on Aging, 2010). Nurses can learn from the work of On Lok and other programs to enhance the care and encourage the health of ethnic elders.

Modifications of existing long-term care services to enhance the well-being of ethnic elders may include the following:

1. Ensuring that the resident has access to professional interpreter services if needed
2. Developing programs that reflect the diversity of the residents and the staff
3. Considering monocultural facilities or units where population demographics warrant
4. Employing staff who reflect the diversity of residents or clients

INTEGRATING CONCEPTS

Promoting healthy aging in the care of ethnic elders frequently provides the gerontological nurse with new challenges while also presenting the opportunity to learn from new perspectives. Unfortunately, poverty is very common in many households of persons of color or of women living alone, and meeting basic needs, especially food and health care, may be difficult. Unless they are political refugees, older immigrants who have never worked in the United States will not qualify for Medicare and may not qualify for Medicaid. The nurse must be sensitive to this possibility without making assumptions or stereotyping. The nurse can assess the components of biological integrity and, if necessary, facilitate the elder or family obtaining whatever supports (e.g., food stamps, home-delivered meals) that are possible and appropriate.

Whereas some ethnic elders have been in the United States most of their lives or their move to the United States was not traumatic, many others have experienced horrific events in their home country or during their immigration process and may hold a unique regard for safety and security. The staff of a Jewish nursing home complained that it was particularly difficult getting some of the residents with dementia to shower. It was some time before they realized that a number of their residents were Holocaust survivors. As the residents' dementia progressed, they were no longer able to distinguish the difference between a shower for hygiene and the fear of "going to the showers" (i.e., to the gas chamber) in the concentration camps of their youths (G. Weissman, personal communication, April 21, 2003).

A sense of belonging for the ethnic elder may be closely tied to self-esteem. Cultural and sexual identity may be one of the major elements of self-concept and a key to self-esteem, and increasingly so as a person becomes more mentally or physically frail. Often ethnic elders are closely tied to family and community and, in some cases, religious communities. Estrangement from their country of origin may be ameliorated if they live in homogeneous communities and may be exacerbated if they live in social isolation or away from persons with similar backgrounds. The monoethnic community (e.g., barrio, Nihonmachi, Chinatown) serves as a buffer and a means of strengthening cohesiveness for elders and others of various cultural groups. Within the community, members are protected from discrimination and the strange language and customs of the society outside.

Family, religion, community, and history are important reference points for self-worth and identity for any individual or ethnic group. Familial supports are variable among groups, social classes, and subcultures, yet the nuclear or extended family is the chief avenue of transmitting cultural values, beliefs, customs, and practices. The family provides orientation, stability, and sanctuary. In a simplistic sense we may say that Asians value familial piety; Hispanics, the extended family (*compadres* translates to *coparents*); African Americans, extended or fictive kin supports; and Native Americans, a system of kinship and line of descent.

Spirituality or religiosity plays a major role in defining many cultures. Religion may function as a consistent experience that affords psychic support in the individual's life. In many black communities, religion is a pervasive force and the place to instill self-determination toward change (Hooyman and Kiyak, 2011). The Issei seek religious tradition in the face of aging and death (Kitano, 1969). Padilla and Ruiz (1976) note that Hispanics tend to seek Spanish-speaking clergy rather than mental health professionals when they have emotional problems. There is a toolkit for improving services provided to diverse communities through the Administration on Aging. This can be downloaded free from http://www.aoa.gov/AoARoot/AoA_Programs/Tools_Resources/DOCS/AoA_DiversityToolkit_full.pdf.

Changes are threatening the historical role of the elder and the traditional family across the globe. Economic independence and mobility of the younger members of the family are chipping away at the insulation afforded by the community. Intergenerational discontinuities of assimilation create a communication gap between the young and the old. Often the elderly are not proficient in the language of the dominant culture, and the younger members may not retain the language of their parents. This may cause isolation and estrangement between the oldest and youngest generations. Members of ethnic minorities are extremely vulnerable in old age. They experience double jeopardy since they may be devalued because of age and ethnicity in their new countries, quite different from their countries of origin. Attitudes and economic inequality also contribute to their problems.

Throughout this chapter older adults are viewed, individually and collectively, as they have been defined and developed by the influence of their time and place in history, their gender, and distinctive group practices and beliefs that have served as the foundation for the self-system. The study of the uniqueness and individuality of each surviving elder is one of the most complex and intriguing opportunities of our day. Realistically, it will be almost impossible to become familiar with the whole range of clinically relevant cultural differences of older adults one may encounter, but to attempt to provide care holistically and sensitively is the most challenging opportunity leading to personal growth for both the nurse and the person receiving care.

---

evolve   To access your student resources, go to *http://evolve.elsevier.com/Ebersole/TwdHlthAging*

KEY CONCEPTS

- Population diversity is rapidly increasing and will continue to do so for many years. This suggests that nurses will be caring for a greater number of minority elders than they have in the past.
- Recent research has revealed significant and persistent disparities and inequities in the outcomes of health for persons from minority groups, with the members of these groups bearing the burden of morbidity and mortality in most areas.
- Nurses can contribute to the reduction of health disparities and the promotion of social justice through increasing their own cultural awareness, knowledge, and skills.
- Cultural proficiency and sensitivity require awareness of issues related to culture, race, gender, sexual orientation, social class, and economic situations.
- Ethnicity is a complex phenomenon encompassing language, traditions, symbols, and folklore expressed as identity.
- Culture is a complex concept reflecting the interrelationship of many components. It includes shared beliefs, expectations, and behaviors.
- Stereotyping can negate the fact that significant heterogeneity exists within cultural groups.

- Health beliefs of various groups emerge from three general belief systems: biomedical, magico-religious, and naturalistic. Elders may adhere to one or more of these systems.
- Gender affects values, perceptions, and the approach to health care assessment and treatment.
- Two cultural patterns that have great potential for conflict between the elder and the health care system are orientation to time and orientation to family and self.
- Effective cross-cultural care to elders includes skills related to language, both verbal and nonverbal.
- The more complex the decision-making, the more important the quality of communication. For those with limited English proficiency, expert interpretation is needed whenever serious decisions are needed. For example, end-of-life care or treatment changes.
- The use of family, children, or support staff as interpreters is not recommended and may result in censored interpretation because of rules of cultural etiquette unknown to the nurse.
- The LEARN model provides a useful framework for working with ethnic elders.

CASE STUDY   WHERE DO I BELONG? WHO AM I?

Georgia thought she was a misfit. She had always thought this. She felt that she was born in the wrong time and most of the time was in the wrong place. She was born in China in 1920, the child of missionary parents. Her parents had built and managed a school for orphaned children in Shanghai. There were many problems and uprisings in China, and when she was 15, the political situation and threat of war were so intense that her parents were asked to leave the school and return to the United States. They were then sent to an Appalachian mining village to manage a small school and clinic. Having grown to adolescence in China, she felt more Chinese than English. She had a difficult adjustment in the poverty-stricken rural mining village in Appalachia, so unlike where she had been. In a few years, her parents sent her to a private religious college, attended mainly by the children of the affluent elders of her church. She married a young army officer, and they were immediately sent to France. Her life from then on seemed to consist of nothing but moves as she followed her husband about. She was grateful that she had never had children; as she said, "My life has always seemed so unsettled, I don't think I could have provided any stability for children." As she aged, she developed crippling arthritis, and her husband provided much of her care. When she was widowed at 80, she almost immediately entered a nursing home. There she found that most of the staff were Filipino and talked among themselves in Tagalog. Again, she felt out of step with the prevailing culture in which she found herself. She became very difficult to get along with, and the staff members were at their wits' end trying to please her. You recently went to work as director of nursing in the facility where Georgia is. How will you help her and the staff maximize their life satisfactions?

On the basis of this case study, develop a nursing care plan using the following procedure*:

- List Georgia's comments that provide subjective data.
- List information that provides objective data.
- From these data, identify and state, using accepted format, two nursing diagnoses you determine are most significant to Georgia at this time. List two of Georgia's strengths that you have identified from the data.

- Determine and state outcome criteria for each diagnosis. These must reflect some alleviation of the problem identified in the nursing diagnosis and must be stated in concrete and measurable terms.
- Plan and state one or more culturally relevant interventions for each diagnosed problem. Provide specific documentation of the source used to determine the appropriate intervention. Plan at least one intervention that incorporates Georgia's existing strengths.
- Evaluate the success of the intervention. Interventions must correlate directly with the stated outcome criteria to measure the outcome success.

CRITICAL THINKING QUESTIONS

1. Define the terms *culture, ethnicity, ethnocentricity, cultural sensitivity,* and *cultural competence.*
2. Identify several personal values or beliefs that are derived from your ethnic and cultural roots.
3. Relate major historical events that have affected your birth cohort, and explain in what way your cohort has been affected.
4. Discuss several different ethnically based approaches to health care.
5. Describe characteristics that you believe are specific to your gender.
6. Construct a cultural genogram, and discuss your roots.
7. Discuss ways in which you have learned to appreciate cultural and ethnic differences.
8. Privately list your stereotypes and "ethnocentrisms" for various ethnic groups, and explore the basis of these beliefs (taught, fear, experience, lack of knowledge). Then consider what can be done to be more culturally sensitive and competent.
9. Select a food or particular behavior and examine differences in custom that arise from ethnic/cultural interpretations.
10. Describe the advocacy role of nurses who care for ethnic elderly.
11. Formulate a care plan incorporating ethnically sensitive interventions.
12. Plan strategies to provide care that is culturally sensitive and acceptable to Georgia without losing focus on the individual's own aging experience.

*Students are advised to refer to their nursing diagnosis text and identify possible or potential problems.

RESEARCH QUESTIONS

1. What are the chief difficulties in providing nursing care for individuals from a different background from one's own?
2. What are the factors that identify a group as an ethnic minority?
3. What are the enduring cohort differences that are unlikely to change throughout life?
4. What are the outcomes of an integrated cultural approach versus a separate-course approach in a curriculum?
5. Why, if older women have so many disadvantages, do they survive longer and seemingly maintain morale in spite of being old, poor, and alone?
6. Why is it so difficult for men to seek medical help before life-threatening conditions occur?
7. What effect will the baby boomers have on gender parity or disparity?

REFERENCES

Aday RH, Kehoe GC, Farney LA: Impact of senior center friendships on aging women who live alone, *Journal of Women and Aging* 18:57, 2006.

Administration on Aging, U.S. Department of Health and Human Services: *Minority aging: statistical profiles* (2010). Available at http://www.aoa.gov/AoARoot/Aging_Statistics/minority_aging/Index.aspx. Accessed December 2010.

Berlin E, Fowkes W: A teaching framework for cross-cultural health care: application in family practice, *Western Journal of Medicine* 139:934, 1983.

Berman HJ: From the pages of my life, *Generations* 15:33, 1991.

Department of Labor: *Women's earnings as a percentage of men's, 1997-2007,* October 29, 2008. http://www.bls.gov/opub/ted/2008/oct/wk4/art03.htm. Accessed December 2010.

Enslein J, Tripp-Reimer T, Kelley LS, et al: *Evidence-based protocol: interpreter facilitation for persons with limited English proficiency,* Iowa City, IA, 2001, University of Iowa, Gerontological Nursing Interventions Research Center, Research dissemination core, 2001.

Enslein J, Tripp-Reimer T, Kelley LS, et al: Evidence-based protocol: interpreter facilitation for individuals with limited English proficiency, *Journal of Gerontological Nursing* 28:5, 2002.

Gelfand D: *Aging and ethnicity: knowledge and service,* ed 2, New York, 2003, Springer.

Haffner L: Translation is not enough: interpreting in a medical setting, *Western Journal of Medicine* 157:255, 1992.

Hall ET: *Beyond culture,* Garden City, NY, 1977, Anchor Press.

Hall ET: *Understanding cultural differences,* Yarmouth, ME, 1990, Intercultural Press.

Helzner EP, Cauley JA, Pratt SR, et al: Race and sex differences in age-related hearing loss: the health, aging and body composition study, *Journal of the American Geriatrics Society* 53:2119, 2005.

Hooyman N, Kiyak HA: *Social gerontology*, ed 8, Boston, 2011, Allyn & Bacon.

Institute on Aging (IOA): *On Lok Lifeways: a PACE program provided by IOA* (2010). Available at http://www.ioaging.org/services/onlok_senior_health_services_sf.html. Accessed December 2010.

Jett KF: Making the connection: seeking and receiving help by elderly African Americans, *Qualitative Health Research* 12:373, 2002.

Jett KF: The meaning of aging and the celebration of years among rural African American women, *Geriatric Nursing* 24:290, 2003.

Kitano H: *Japanese Americans*, Englewood Cliffs, NJ, 1969, Prentice-Hall.

Kleinman A, Eisenberg L, Good B: Culture, illness, and care: clinical lessons from anthropologic and cross-cultural research, *Annals of Internal Medicine* 88:251, 1978.

Lukwago S, Kreuter MW, Bucholtz DC, et al: Development and validation of brief scales to measure collectivism, religiosity, racial pride, and time orientation in urban African American women, *Family & Community Health* 24:63, 2001.

McIntosh P: *White privilege: unpacking the invisible knapsack* (1989). Working paper #189. Wellesley College Center for Research on Women. http://people.ucsc.edu/~marches/PDFs/White%20Privilege%20Unpacking%20the%20Invisible%20Knapsack,%20McIntosh.PDF

National Cancer Institute, National Institutes of Health: *SEER Stat Fact Sheets: Prostate* (2010). Surveillance Epidemiology and End Results Program. Available at http://seer.cancer.gov/statfacts/html/prost.html#incidence-mortality. Accessed December 2010.

O'Dell KK, McGee S: Acupuncture for urgency in women over 50: what is the evidence? *Urologic Nursing* 26:23, 2006.

Padilla A, Ruiz R: *Prejudice and discrimination*. In Hernandez CA, Haug MJ, Wagner NN, editors: *Chicanos: social and psychological perspectives*, ed 2, St Louis, 1976, Mosby.

Pfeifferling JH: *A cultural prescription for mediocentrism*. In Eisenberg L, Kleinman A, editors: *The relevance of social science for medicine*, Boston, 1981, Reidel.

Philpot CD, Morley JE: Health issues unique to the aging man, *Geriatric Nursing* 21:234, 2000.

Pierce R, Clark M, Kaufman S: Generation and ethnic identity: a typological analysis, *International Journal of Aging and Human Development* 9:19, 1978/1979.

Purnell LD, Paulanka BJ: *Transcultural health care: a culturally competent approach*, ed 2, Philadelphia, 2003, F.A. Davis.

Rathbone-McCune E: *Isolated elders: health and social intervention*, Rockville, MD, 1982, Aspen.

Samovar LA, Porter RE, McDaniel ER: *Communicating between cultures*, Boston, 2010, Wadsworth.

Scharlach AE, Kellam R, Ong N, et al: Cultural attitudes and caregiver service use: lessons from focus groups with racially and ethnically diverse family caregivers, *Journal of Gerontological Social Work* 47:133, 2006.

Smedley B, Stith AY, Nelson AR, editors: *Unequal treatment: confronting racial and ethnic disparities in health care (2002)*. Institute of Medicine of the National Academies. Washington DC, 2002, National Academy Press.

Spector RE: *Cultural diversity in health and illness*, ed 7, Upper Saddle River, NJ, 2008, Prentice Hall Health.

Tripp-Reimer T, Lauer GM: *Ethnicity and families with chronic illness*. In Wright LM, Leahy M, editors: *Families and chronic illness*, Springhouse, PA, 1987, Springhouse.

U.S. Department of Health and Human Services (USDHHS): *Developing healthy people 2020: the road ahead* (2009a). Available at http://www.healthypeople.gov/hp2020/default.asp. Accessed December 2010.

U.S. Department of Health and Human Services (USDHHS): *Healthy people 2020 framework* (2009b). Available at http://www.healthypeople.gov/hp2020/objectives/framework.aspx. Accessed December 2010.

U.S. Social Security Administration: *Your retirement benefit: how is it figured* (2010). SSA Publication No. 05-10070. Available at http://www.socialsecurity.gov/pubs/10070.html. Accessed December 2010.

Vincent GK, Velkoff VA; for the Economics and Statistics Administration, U.S. Department of Commerce: *Current population reports: the next four decades: the older population in the United States 2010-2050* (2010). Available at http://www.census.gov/prod/2010pubs/p25-1138.pdf. Accessed December 2010.

Watson J, Xue Q, Semba RD, et al: Serum antioxidants, inflammation and total mortality in women, *American Journal of Epidemiology* 163:18, 2006.

Winkelman MJ: Shaman and other "majico-relious" healers: a cross-cultural study of their origins, nature and social transformations, *Ethos* 18:308, 1990; first published online October 28, 2009.

Young C, Koopsen C: *Spirituality, health and healing*, Thorofare, NJ, 2005, SLACK.

Communicating with Older Adults

Theris A. Touhy

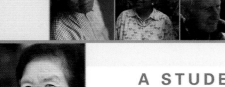

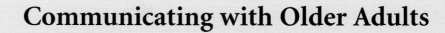
evolve http://evolve.elsevier.com/Ebersole/TwdHlthAging

A STUDENT SPEAKS

During the years I worked as a food server I grew accustomed to waiting on older people. They can't always read the menu, they complain that the lighting in the restaurant is too low, they like their dinner experience to be slower, they can't find their silver when they need it, the soup is never hot enough and the cup of coffee is never full enough. They would yell at me because they could not hear me. It used to make me mad, but now I understand they are just real people experiencing growing old. Yes, they may have problems like losing some of their senses and other physical changes, but in actuality they are the same as me.

Debbie, age 27

AN ELDER SPEAKS

One of the great frustrations is the matter of eyesight. One can get used to large print and hope for black letters on white paper but why do modern publishers seem to prefer the shiny, slick off-white paper and pale ink in minuscule print? And, my new prescription glasses have not restored my ability to cut my own toenails without danger of wounding myself. I find myself wishing for some treatment for incipient cataracts. Please, researchers, let's get rid of this scourge of the elderly.

Lyn, age 85

LEARNING OBJECTIVES

On completion of this chapter, the reader will be able to:

1. Describe the importance of communication to the lives of older adults.
2. Discuss how ageist attitudes affect communication with older adults.
3. Discuss diseases of the eye and ear that may occur in older adults
4. Describe the importance of screening, health education, and treatment of eye diseases to prevent unnecessary vision loss

5. Identify effective communication strategies for older adults with speech, language, hearing, vision, and cognitive impairment.
6. Describe interventions that facilitate communication individually and in groups.
7. Understand the significance of the life story.
8. Discuss the modalities of reminiscence and life review.
9. Understand how health literacy affects communication and learning and design interventions to enhance understanding.

Communication is the single most important capacity of human beings, the ability that gives us a special place in the animal kingdom. Little is more dehumanizing than the inability to communicate effectively and engage in social interaction with others. The need to communicate, to be listened to, and to be heard does not change with age or impairment. Meaningful communication and active engagement with society contributes to healthy aging and improves an older adult's chances of living longer, responding better to health care interventions, and maintaining optimal function (Rowe and Kahn, 1998;

Williams, 2006; Williams et al., 2008; Herman and Williams, 2009; Levy, 2009; Levy et al., 2009a,b; VanLeuven, 2010).

For some older people, opportunities for social interaction may be more limited as a result of loss of family and friends, illnesses and hearing, vision, and cognitive impairment. The ageist attitudes of the public, as well as health professionals, also present barriers to communicating effectively with older people. Good communication skills are the basis for accurate assessment, care planning, and the development of therapeutic relationships between the nurse and the older person.

This chapter discusses the effect of health professionals' attitudes toward aging on their communication with older people; communication skills essential to therapeutic interaction with older adults; diseases of the eye and ear; screening, health education and treatment of eye diseases to prevent unnecessary vision loss; adaptation of communication for older adults with vision and hearing impairments, inadequate health literacy, speech or language disorders, and cognitive impairment. The significance of the life story, reminiscence, and life review, and communication with groups of elders, are also included in this chapter.

AGEISM AND COMMUNICATION

Beliefs in myths and stereotypes about older adults and ageist attitudes can interfere with the ability to communicate effectively. For example, if the nurse believes that all older people have memory problems, or are unable to learn or process information, he or she will be less likely to engage in conversation, provide appropriate health information, or treat the person with respect and dignity. Ageism, a term coined by Robert Butler (1969), the first director of the National Institute on Aging (Bethesda, MD), is the systematic stereotyping of, and discrimination against, people because they are old, just as racism and sexism accomplish this with skin color and gender. Ageism will affect us all if we live long enough. Although ageism is found cross-culturally, it is essentially prevalent in the United States where aging is viewed with depression, fear, and anxiety (International Longevity Center, 2006).

Ageist attitudes, as well as myths and stereotypes about aging, can be detrimental to older people. On the other hand, holding a positive self-perception of aging can contribute to a longer life span. The survival advantage of a more positive self-perception of aging can add 7.5 years to the life span and contributes more to added years of life than low body mass index, no smoking history, and exercise (Levy et al., 2002). While older people, collectively, have often been seen in negative terms, a most striking change in attitudes toward aging has occurred in the past 25 years. Undoubtedly, this will continue to change as the baby boomers reach retirement age. The impact of media presentation is enormous, and it is gratifying to see robust images of aging; fewer older people are portrayed as victims or as those to be pitied, shunned, or ridiculed by virtue of achieving old age.

Ageism affects health professionals as well and, with few exceptions, studies of attitudes of health professional students toward aging reflect negative views. Examples of the effect of ageism include the few number of students who choose to work in the field of aging, and the lack of education of health professionals in the care of older people, even though the majority of their patients are older adults. It is important for nurses who care for older people to be aware of their own attitudes and beliefs about aging and the effect of these attitudes on communication and care provision. Enhancing one's interpersonal communication skills is the foundation for therapeutic interactions with older adults.

Elderspeak

Elderspeak is a form of ageism in which younger people alter their speech, based on the assumption that all older people

---

BOX 6-1	CHARACTERISTICS OF ELDERSPEAK

- Using a singsong voice, changing pitch and tone, and exaggerating words
- Using short and simple sentences
- Speaking more slowly
- Using limited vocabulary
- Repeating or paraphrasing what has just been said
- Using pet names (diminutives) such as "honey" or "dear" or "grandma"
- Using collective pronouns such as "we"—for instance, "Would we like to take a bath now?"
- Using statements that sound like questions

Modified from: Williams K, Kemper S, Hummert L: Enhancing communication with older adults: overcoming elderspeak, *Journal of Gerontological Nursing* 30:17, 2004; and Williams K: Improving outcomes of nursing home interactions, *Research in Nursing and Health* 29:121, 2006.

have difficulty understanding and comprehending (Touhy and Williams, 2008). It is especially common in communication between health care professionals and older adults in hospitals and nursing homes, but occurs in non–healthcare settings as well (Williams et al., 2003, 2004, 2008; Williams, 2006; Williams and Tappen, 2008; Herman and Williams, 2009). Elderspeak is similar to "baby talk," which is often used to talk to very young children (Box 6-1).

Nurses may not be aware that they are using elderspeak, but research has shown that use of this form of speech is patronizing and conveys messages of dependence, incompetence, and control (Williams, 2006; Williams et al., 2008). Some features of elderspeak (speaking more slowly, repeating, or paraphrasing) may be beneficial in communication with older people with dementia, and further research is needed. Other examples of communication that conveys ageist attitudes are ignoring the older person and talking to family and friends as if the person were not present, and limiting interaction to task-focused communication only (Touhy and Williams, 2008).

THERAPEUTIC COMMUNICATION WITH OLDER ADULTS

Basic communication strategies that apply to all situations in nursing, such as attentive listening, authentic presence, nonjudgmental attitude, cultural competence, clarifying, giving information, seeking validation of understanding, keeping focus, and using open-ended questions, are all applicable in communicating with older adults. Basically, elders may need more time to give information or answer questions simply because they have a larger life experience to draw from. Sorting through thoughts requires intervals of silence, and therefore listening carefully without rushing the elder is important. Word retrieval may be slower, particularly for nouns and names.

Open-ended questions are useful but difficult for some elders. Those who wish to please, especially when feeling vulnerable or somewhat dependent, may wonder what it is you want to hear rather than what it is they would like to say. Communication that is most productive will initially focus on the issue of major concern to the elder, regardless of the priority of the nursing assessment. When using closed questioning to obtain specific information, be aware that the elder may feel on the spot and thus the appropriate information may not be immediately forthcoming. This is especially true when asking questions to determine mental status. The elder may develop a mental block because of anxiety or feel threatened if questions are asked in a quizzing or demeaning manner. Older people may be reluctant to disclose information for fear of the consequences. For example, if they are having problems remembering things or are experiencing frequent falls, sharing this information may mean that they might have to leave their home and move to a more protective setting.

When communicating with individuals in a bed or wheelchair, position yourself at their level rather than talking over a side rail or standing above them. Pay attention to their gaze, gestures, and body language, and the pitch, volume, and tone of their voice to help you understand what they are trying to communicate. Thoughts unstated are often as important as those that are verbalized. You may ask, "What are you thinking about right now?" Clarification is essential to ensure that you and the elder have the same framework of understanding.

Many generational, cultural, and regional differences in speech patterns and idioms exist. Frequently seek validation of whatever you think you heard. If you tend to speak quickly, particularly if your accent is different from the elder's, try to slow down and give the person time to process what you are saying.

COMMUNICATING WITH OLDER ADULTS WITH SENSORY IMPAIRMENTS

Sensory impairments, such as hearing and vision deficits, place older people at risk for communication difficulties. We rely on our senses to perceive the environment and to enjoy the pleasures of life. Gerontological nurses need to have special knowledge and skills to promote effective communication with older people who have these deficits. This section describes adaptations to enhance communication with elders with hearing and vision impairments.

Hearing Impairment

Although both vision and hearing impairment significantly affect all aspects of life, Oliver Sacks (1989), in his book *Seeing Voices,* presents a view that blindness may in fact be less serious than loss of hearing. Hearing loss interferes with communication with others and the interactional input that is so necessary to stimulate and validate. One elderly man said that a great annoyance of hearing loss is in the subtle aspects of living with a partner, who most probably has a hearing loss as well. "You must often repeat what you say, and in lovemaking, whispering sweet words becomes a gesture for yourself alone." Helen Keller was most profound in her expression: "Never to see the face of a loved one nor to witness a summer sunset is indeed a handicap. But I can touch a face and feel the warmth of the sun. But to be deprived of hearing the song of the first spring robin and the laughter of children provides me with a long and dreadful sadness" (Keller, 1902).

Hearing loss is the third most prevalent chronic condition in older Americans and the foremost communicative disorder of older adults. The prevalence of hearing loss is 90% in those older than 80 years. Hearing loss is a common condition in

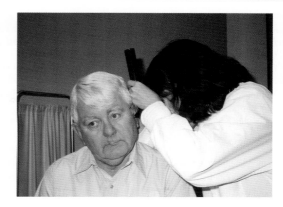

Proper Technique for an Otoscopic Examination. (From Ignatavicius DD, Workman ML: *Medical-surgical nursing: patient-centered collaborative care,* ed 6, St. Louis, MO, 2010, WB Saunders.)

middle-aged adults as well. Estimates are that 20.6% of adults aged 48 to 59 years have impaired hearing. A recent study suggests that cardiovascular disease risk factors may be important correlates of age-related auditory dysfunction. Hearing loss may not be an inevitable part of aging and if detected early, it may be a preventable chronic disease because the same healthy lifestyle changes that improve cardiovascular health may also prevent or delay hearing loss (University of Wisconsin School of Medicine and Public Health, 2011). In all age groups, men are more likely than women to be hearing-impaired.

Hearing loss diminishes quality of life and is associated with multiple negative outcomes including decreased function, miscommunication, depression, falls, loss of self-esteem, safety risks, and cognitive decline (Wallhagen and Pettengill, 2008). Hearing impairment increases feelings of isolation and may cause older adults to become suspicious or distrustful or to display feelings of paranoia. Because older persons with a hearing loss may not understand or respond appropriately to conversation, they may be inappropriately diagnosed with dementia. Older people may be initially unaware of hearing loss because of the gradual manner in which it develops (Box 6-2). The Better Hearing Institute (Washington DC) provides an online hearing test for older adults who want to check their own hearing (see http://www.betterhearing.org/hearing_loss/online_hearing_test/index.cfm).

Hearing impairment is underdiagnosed and undertreated in older people. Although screening for hearing impairment and

BOX 6-2 DO I HAVE A HEARING PROBLEM?
• Do I have a problem hearing on the telephone?
• Do I have trouble hearing when there is noise in the background?
• Is it hard for to me to follow a conversation when two or more people talk at once?
• Do I have to strain to understand a conversation?
• Do many people I talk to seem to mumble (or not speak clearly)?
• Do I misunderstand what others are saying and respond inappropriately?
• Do I have trouble understanding the speech of women and children?
• Do people complain that I turn the TV volume up too high?
• Do I hear a ringing, roaring, or hissing sound a lot?
• Do some sounds seem too loud?

From National Institute on Deafness and Other Communication Disorders: *Hearing loss and older adults* (2010). Available at http://www.nidcd.nih.gov/health/hearing/older.html. Accessed December 2010.

BOX 6-3 RESEARCH HIGHLIGHTS

Hearing Impairment: Significant but Underassessed in Primary Care Settings

A study (Wallhagen and Pettengill, 2008) explored whether primary care providers ever screened older adults for or asked about hearing loss and what effects the lack of inquiry or follow-up may have had on the older adults and their communication partners.

Ninety-one older adults (over 60 years of age) with currently untreated hearing impairment were recruited from 19 different sites—clinics or centers that performed hearing evaluations or provided seminars on hearing loss. Interviews, assessment of subjective hearing impairment based on the Hearing Handicap Inventory for the Elderly (HHIE); subjective rating of the emotional and social impact of hearing loss; and audiograms were used in the study to assess hearing and related interventions.

Of the participants, 85% reported that their primary care provider had never asked about their hearing or provided screening for hearing loss. In fact, 33% had mild hearing loss and 58% had moderate hearing loss. If the provider did ask about hearing loss, the participants were the ones to bring it up in order to obtain a referral for hearing evaluation. Samples of the narrative data revealed how several providers discounted the importance of hearing loss, and other narratives demonstrated the detrimental effects of unrecognized hearing loss on the individuals affected and their communication partners.

Hearing loss is an overlooked geriatric syndrome—a gap in assessment that can have significant negative consequences. Authors recommend that nurses take a leadership role in making hearing assessment a regular part of nursing evaluation and providing educational information and referrals as appropriate. The HHIE-S is an easy-to-administer screening instrument. A single-item, self-report question about hearing such as "Do you have a hearing problem now?" or "Would you say you have any hearing difficulty?" would be useful in suggesting a referral for additional testing.

Data from Wallhagen M, Pettengill E: Hearing impairment significant but underassessed in primary care settings, *Journal of Gerontological Nursing* 34:36, 2008.

appropriate treatment are considered an essential part of primary care for older adults, it is rarely done. A single question—Do you feel you have a hearing loss?—has been shown to have reasonable sensitivity and specificity for hearing impairment (Schumm et al., 2009). Findings of a study performed in 2008 (Box 6-3) suggest that hearing loss is "an overlooked geriatric syndrome in primary care settings—an assessment gap that can have significant negative consequences" (Wallhagen and Pettengill, 2008, p. 41).

The screening rate for hearing impairment among older adults is estimated to be as low as 12.9%, and only about 20% of persons with hearing impairments receive hearing aids (Ham et al., 2007; Wallhagen and Pettengill, 2008). Factors associated with lack of hearing aid use include cost, perceived lack of benefit, and denial of hearing loss. Wallhagen (2009) also suggests that the perceived stigma associated with hearing loss and use of hearing aids is another factor that should be examined. The cost of hearing aids is not covered under Medicare and other health plans, but screening for hearing loss is recommended as part of the comprehensive physical for older adults joining Medicare for the first time (Chapter 2).

Types of Hearing Loss

The two major forms of hearing loss are conductive and sensorineural. *Sensorineural hearing loss* results from damage to any part of the inner ear or the neural pathways to the brain. *Presbycusis* is a form of sensorineural hearing loss that is related to aging. It is the most common form of hearing loss in the United States. Presbycusis is a bilateral and symmetrical sensorineural hearing loss that also affects the ability to understand speech.

Changes in the middle and inner ear make many elders intolerant of loud noises and incapable of distinguishing among some of the sibilant consonants such as *z, s, sh, f, p, k, t,* and *g.* People often raise their voice when speaking to a hearing-impaired person. When this happens, more consonants drop out of speech, making hearing even more difficult. Without consonants, the high-frequency–pitched language becomes disjointed and misunderstood.

Older people with presbycusis have difficulty filtering out background noise and often complain of difficulty understanding women's and children's speech and conversations in large groups. The condition progressively worsens with age. The environment is teeming with distracting sounds and noises, such as traffic, television, appliances, crowds, and noisy restaurants and shopping malls. Institutions in which older adults may be patients are also noisy, with many distracting sounds that make communication difficult for sensory and cognitively impaired older adults—intercoms or pagers, clattering equipment, meal and medication carts, and "canned music."

Use of rapid speech when conversing with an older adult with a hearing impairment will make sounds garbled and unintelligible, and even though the problem is related to presbycusis, it is one that is easily remedied. To gain a better understanding of hearing loss, take the Unfair Hearing Test (Sight & Hearing Association, St. Paul, MN), available at http://www.sightandhearing.org/products/knownoise.asp. Sensorineural hearing loss is treated with hearing aids and, in some cases, cochlear implants.

Conductive hearing loss usually involves abnormalities of the external and middle ear that reduce the ability of sound to be transmitted to the middle ear. Otosclerosis, infection, perforated eardrum, fluid in the middle ear, or cerumen accumulations cause conductive hearing loss. Cerumen impaction is the most common and easily corrected of all interferences in the hearing of older people. Cerumen impaction has been found to occur in 33% of nursing home residents (Hersh, 2010).

Cerumen interferes with the conduction of sound through air in the eardrum. The reduction in the number and activity of cerumen-producing glands results in a tendency toward cerumen impaction. Long-standing impactions become hard, dry, and dark brown. Individuals at particular risk of impaction are African Americans, individuals who wear hearing aids, and older men with large amounts of ear canal tragi (hairs in the ear) that tend to become entangled with the cerumen. When hearing loss is suspected, or a person with existing hearing loss experiences increasing difficulty, it is important first to check for cerumen impaction as a possible cause. If cerumen removal is indicated, it may be removed through irrigation, cerumenolytic products, or manual extraction (Hersh, 2010). Box 6-4 presents a protocol for cerumen removal.

BOX 6-4 PROTOCOL FOR CERUMEN REMOVAL

- Assess for ear pain, traumas, abnormalities, drainage, surgeries, or perforations. These or any other unusual findings should be referred to an otolaryngologist.
- When aural examination reveals cerumen impaction with no other abnormalities, the nurse may irrigate for cerumen removal, using the following techniques.

Note: Do not use a water pick for cerumen removal because water pressure is too high and may damage the ear.

1. Carefully clip and remove hairs in the ear canal.
2. Instill a softening agent such as slightly warm mineral oil 0.5 to 1 ml twice daily or ear drops such as Cerumenex, Debrox, or Murine ear drops for several days until wax becomes softened. Allergic reactions to Cerumenex have been noted if used for longer than 24 hours.
3. Protect clothing and linens from drainage of oil or wax by placing a small cotton ball in each external ear canal.
4. When irrigating the ear, use a hand-held bulb syringe, 2- to 4-ounce plastic syringe, or otologic syringe (20- to 50-ml syringe equipped with an Angiocath rather than a needle) with emesis basin under the ear to catch drainage; tip the client's head to the side being drained.
5. Use a solution of 3 ounces of 3% hydrogen peroxide in a quart of water warmed to 98° to 100° F; if the client is sensitive to hydrogen peroxide, use sterile normal saline.
6. Place towels around the client's neck; empty the emesis basin frequently, observing for residue from the ear; keep the client dry and comfortable; do not inject air into the client's ear or use high pressure when injecting fluid.
7. If the cerumen is not successfully washed out, begin the process again of instilling a softening agent for several days.

Tinnitus

Tinnitus is defined as the perception of sound in one or both ears or in the head when no external sound is present. It is often referred to as "ringing in the ears" but may also manifest as buzzing, hissing, whistling, cricket chirping, bells, roaring, clicking, pulsating, humming, or swishing sounds. The sounds may be constant or intermittent and are more acute at night or in quiet surroundings. The most common type is high-pitched tinnitus with sensorineural loss; less common is low-pitched tinnitus with conduction loss such as is seen in Meniere's disease.

Tinnitus generally increases over time. It is a condition that afflicts many older people and can interfere with hearing, as well as become extremely irritating. It is estimated to occur in nearly 11% of elders with presbycusis. Approximately 50 million people in the United States have tinnitus and about 2 million are so seriously debilitated that they cannot function on a "normal," day to day basis The incidence of tinnitus peaks between ages 65 and 74 and is higher in men than in women; in men, the incidence seems to decrease after this age. Tinnitus is a growing problem for America's military personnel and is the leading cause of service-connected disability of veterans returning from Iraq or Afganistan (American Tinnitus Association, 2010).

The exact physiological cause or causes of tinnitus are not known but there are several likely factors that are known to trigger or worsen tinnitus. Exposure to loud noises is the leading cause of tinnitus and the exposure can damage and destroy cilia in the inner ear. Once damaged, they cannot be renewed or replaced. See http://www.ata.org/for-patients/at-risk#Loud for a video of ways to mitigate noise exposure. Other possible causes of tinnitus include head and neck trauma, certain types of tumors, cerumen build-up, jaw misalignment, cardiovascular disease, and ototoxicity from medications. More than 200 prescription and nonprescription medications list tinnitus as a potential side effect, aspirin being the most common.

Assessment

Tinnitus may be described as pulsatile (matching the beating of the heart) or nonpulsatile (unilateral, asymmetric, or symmetric). Tinnitus may be subjective (audible only to the person) or objective (audible to the examiner). Subjective tinnitus is more common. Objective tinnitus is rare and is frequently due to a vascular or neuromuscular condition. The mechanisms of tinnitus are unknown but have been thought to be analogous to cross-talk on telephone wires, phantom limb pain, or transmission of vascular sounds such as bruits. A simulation of the sounds of tinnitus can be found at http://www.sens.com/helps/demo02/helps_d02_demo_check_2.htm.

Interventions

Some persons with tinnitus will never find the cause; for others the problem may arbitrarily disappear. Hearing aids can be prescribed to amplify environmental sounds to obscure tinnitus, and there is a device that combines the features of a masker and a hearing aid, which emits a competitive but pleasant sound that distracts from head noise. Therapeutic modes of treating tinnitus include transtympanal electrostimulation, iontophoresis, biofeedback, tinnitus masking with alternative sound production (white noise), dental treatment, cochlear implants, and hearing aids. Some have found hypnosis, cognitive behavioral therapy, acupuncture, chiropractic, naturopathic, allergy, or drug treatment to be effective.

Nursing actions include discussions with the client regarding times when the noises are most irritating and having the person keep a diary to identify patterns. There is some evidence that caffeine, alcohol, cigarettes, stress, and fatigue may exacerbate the problem. Assess medications for possibly contributing to the problem. Discuss lifestyle changes and alternative methods that some have found effective. Also, refer clients to the American Tinnitus Association for research updates, education, and support groups.

Interventions to Enhance Hearing
Hearing Aids

A hearing aid is a personal amplifying system that includes a microphone, an amplifier, and a loudspeaker. There are numerous types of hearing aids. The behind-the-ear hearing aid looks like a shrimp and fits around and behind the ear. It is less commonly used now than the small, in-the-ear aid, which fits in the concha of the ear (Figure 6-1). The appearance and effectiveness of hearing aids have greatly improved, and many can be programmed to meet specific needs. Most individuals can obtain some hearing enhancement with a hearing aid.

Although hearing aids generally improve hearing by about 50%, they do not correct hearing deficits. It is important that hearing-impaired elders understand that the goal of hearing aid

thousand dollars, depending on the technology. Batteries are changed every 1 to 2 weeks, adding to overall costs. The cost of hearing aids is not usually covered by health insurance or Medicare.

It is important for nurses in hospitals and nursing homes to be knowledgeable about the care and maintenance of hearing aids. Many older people experience unnecessary communication problems when in the hospital or nursing home because their hearing aids are not inserted and working properly, or are lost. Box 6-5 presents suggestions for the use and care of hearing aids.

Cochlear Implants

Cochlear implants are increasingly being used for older adults who are profoundly deaf as a result of sensorineural hearing loss. A cochlear implant is a small, complex electronic device that consists of an external portion that sits behind the ear and a second portion that is surgically placed under the skin (Figure 6-2). Unlike hearing aids that magnify sounds, the cochlear implant bypasses damaged portions of the ear and directly stimulates the auditory nerve. Hearing through a cochlear implant is different from normal hearing and takes time to learn or relearn. For persons whose hearing loss is so severe that amplification is of little or no benefit, the cochlear implant is a safe and effective method of auditory rehabilitation. Most insurance plans cover the cochlear implant procedure. The transplant carries some risk because the surgery destroys any residual hearing that remains. Therefore, cochlear implant users can never revert to using a hearing aid. Individuals with cochlear implants need to be advised not to undergo magnetic resonance imaging (MRI), and the U.S. Food and Drug Administration advises such individuals "not to even be close to a MRI unit

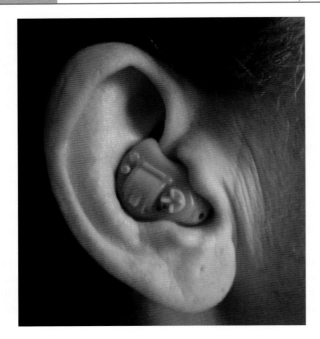

FIGURE 6-1 An In-the-ear Hearing Aid. (Courtesy Kathleen Jett.)

use is to improve communication and quality of life, not to restore normal hearing.

Hearing aids necessitate a period of adjustment and training in correct use. In most states, the purchase of a hearing aid comes with a 30-day trial during which the purchase price is totally refundable. The investment in a good hearing aid is considerable, and a good fit is critical. Before a hearing aid can be purchased, medical clearance must be obtained from a physician. Hearing aids can range in price from about $500 to several

---

BOX 6-5   THE USE AND CARE OF HEARING AIDS

HEARING AID USE
- Initially, wear the aid for 15 to 20 minutes per day.
- Gradually increase the wearing time to 10 to 12 hours.
- Be patient and realize that the process of adaptation is difficult but ultimately will be rewarding.
- Make sure your fingers are dry and clean before handling hearing aids. Use a soft dry cloth to wipe your hearing aids.
- Each day, remove any earwax that has built up on the hearing aids. Use a soft brush to clean difficult-to-reach areas.
- Insert the aid with the canal portion pointing into the ear; press and twist until snug.
- Turn the aid slowly to one-third to one-half volume.
- A whistling sound indicates incorrect ear-mold insertion or that the aid is in the wrong ear.
- Adjust the volume to a level for talking at a distance of 1 yard.
- Do not wear the aid when using a hair dryer or when swimming or taking a shower or bath.
- Note that fine particles of hair spray or make-up can obstruct the microphone component of the hearing aid.

CARE OF THE HEARING AID
- Insert and remove your hearing aid over a soft surface. When inserting or removing the battery, work over a table or countertop or soft surface.
- Insert the battery when the hearing aid is turned off.

- Store the hearing aid in a marked container in a safe place when not in use; remove the batteries.
- Batteries last 1 week with daily wearing of 10 to 12 hours.
- Common problems include a switch that is turned off, a clogged ear mold, a dislodged battery, and twisted tubing between the ear mold and aid.
- Ear molds need replacement every 2 or 3 years.
- Check the ear molds for rough spots that will irritate the ear.
- If sound is not loud enough, check for the following: Need new battery? Sound channel blocked? Aid turned off? Volume set too low? Battery door not closed? Hearing aid loose?
- Check the battery by turning the hearing aid on, turning up the volume, cupping your hand over the ear mold, and listening. A constant whistling sound indicates that the battery is functioning. A weak sound may indicate that the battery is losing power and needs replacement.

REMOVING THE HEARING AID
- Turn the hearing aid off and lower the volume. The on/off switch may be marked by an O (off), M (microphone), T (telephone), or TM (telephone/ microphone). If the aid is not turned off, the batteries will continue to run.
- Remove the ear mold by rotating it slightly forward and then pulling outward.
- Remove the battery if the hearing aid will not be used for several days. This will prevent corrosion from battery leakage.
- Store in a safe place, away from heat and moisture, to prevent loss or damage.

Adams-Wendling L, Pimple C: Evidence-based guideline: nursing management of hearing impairment in nursing facility residents, *Journal of Gerontological Nursing* 34:9, 2008.

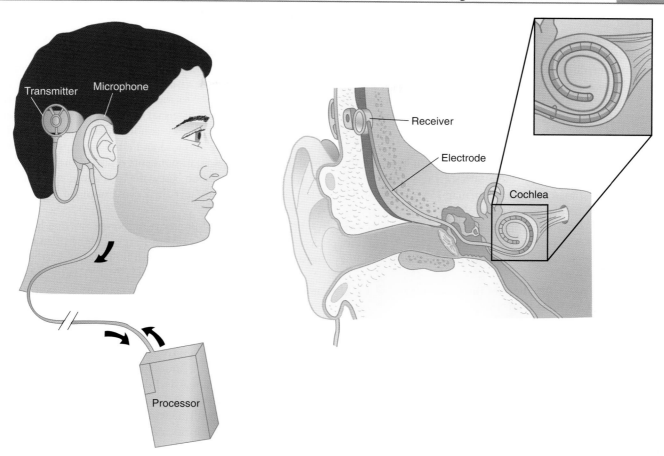

FIGURE 6-2 Cochlear Implant. (From Black JM, Hawks JH: *Medical-surgical nursing: clinical management for positive outcomes,* ed 8, St. Louis, MO, 2009, WB Saunders.)

since it may dislodge the implant or demagnetize its internal magnet" (Wallhagen et al., 2006, p. 47).

Assistive Listening and Adaptive Devices

Assistive listening devices (also called personal listening systems) should be considered as an adjunct to hearing aids or used in place of hearing aids for people with hearing impairment. These devices are available commercially and can be used to enhance face-to-face communication and to better understand speech in large rooms such as theaters, to use the telephone, and to listen to television. Examples of assistive listening and adaptive devices include text messaging devices for telephones and closed-caption television, now required on all televisions with screens 13 inches and larger. Alerting devices, such as vibrating alarm clocks that shake the bed or activate a flashing light, and sound lamps that respond with lights to sounds, such as doorbells and telephones, are also available. Assistive devices, such as personal amplifiers, that amplify sound and send it to the user's ears through earphones, clips, or headphones, are helpful in health care situations in which accurate communication and privacy are essential.

Any facility that receives financial aid from Medicare is required by the Americans with Disabilities Act to provide equal access to public accommodations. This includes access to sign language interpreters, telecommunication devices for the deaf (TDDs), and flashing alarm systems. Nurses working in these facilities should be able to obtain appropriate devices to improve communication with hearing-impaired individuals.

PROMOTING HEALTHY AGING: IMPLICATIONS FOR GERONTOLOGICAL NURSING

Hearing impairment is common among older adults and significantly affects communication, function, safety, and quality of life. Inadequate communication with older adults with hearing impairment can also lead to misdiagnosis and affect adherence to a medical regimen. The gerontological nurse must be able to assess hearing ability and use appropriate communication skills and devices to help older adults minimize or even avoid problems. The Hartford Institute for Geriatric Nursing (New York, NY) *Try This* series provides guidelines for hearing screening (see http://consultgerirn.org/uploads/File/trythis/try_this_12.pdf). An evidence-based guideline for nursing management of hearing impairment in nursing facility residents is also available (Adams-Wendling and Pimple, 2008). Box 6-6 presents communication strategies for elders with hearing impairment.

Vision Impairment

Blindness and visual impairment are among the 10 most common causes of disability in the United States and are associated with shorter life expectancy and lower quality of life. Visual impairment (low vision) is generally defined as a Snellen chart reading of worse than 20/40 but better then 20/200. Legal blindness is defined as a reading equal to or worse than 20/200.

For older adults, visual problems have a negative impact on quality of life, equivalent to that of life-threatening conditions such as heart disease and cancer. The leading causes of visual impairment are diseases that are common in older adults: age-related macular degeneration (AMD), cataract, glaucoma, diabetic retinopathy, and optic nerve atrophy. Vision loss is becoming a major public health problem and is projected to increase substantially with the aging of the population (National Eye Institute, 2010a).

Vision loss from eye disease is a global concern, particularly in the developing countries, where 90% of the world's blind individuals live. Estimates are that more than 75% of the world's blindness is preventable or treatable. Vision 2020 is a global initiative for the elimination of avoidable blindness, launched jointly by the World Health Organization (WHO) and the International Agency for the Prevention of Blindness (http://v2020.org/default.asp).

Older adults represent the vast majority of the visually impaired population. More than two-thirds of those with visual impairment are over age 65. Although there are no gender differences in the prevalence of vision problems in older adults, there are more visually impaired women than men because, on average, women live longer than men. Racial and cultural disparities in vision impairment are significant. African Americans are twice as likely to be visually impaired than are white individuals of comparable socioeconomic status, and Hispanics also have a higher risk of visual complications than the white population. A recent survey conducted in the United States reported that among all racial and ethnic groups participating in the survey, Hispanic respondents reported the lowest access to eye health information, knew the least about eye health, and were the least likely to have their eyes examined (National Eye Institute, 2008).

Estimates of visual impairment among nursing home residents range anywhere from 3 to 15 times higher than for adults of the same age living in the community (Owsley et al., 2007). A study examining the effect of visual impairment among nursing home residents with Alzheimer's disease reported that one in three were not using or did not have glasses that were strong enough to correct their vision. They had either lost their glasses or broken them, had prescriptions that were no longer adequate, or were too cognitively impaired to ask for help (Koch et al., 2005). Routine eye care is sorely lacking in nursing homes and is related to functional decline, decreased quality of life, and depression (Owsley et al., 2007).

Because visual impairment affects most daily activities, such as driving, reading, maneuvering safely, dressing, cooking, and social activities, assessing the effect of vision changes on functional abilities, safety, and quality of life is most important. Decreased vision has also been found to be a significant risk factor for falls. Results of one study (Rogers and Langa, 2010) suggested that untreated poor vision is associated with cognitive decline, particularly Alzheimer's disease. Certain signs and behaviors of visual problems that should alert the nurse to action are noted in Box 6-7.

BOX 6-6　COMMUNICATION STRATEGIES FOR ELDERS WITH HEARING IMPAIRMENT

- Never assume hearing loss is from age until other causes are ruled out (infection, cerumen buildup).
- Inappropriate responses, inattentiveness, and apathy may be symptoms of a hearing loss.
- Face the individual, standing or sitting at the same level, and don't turn away to face a computer when speaking.
- Gain the individual's attention before beginning to speak. Look directly at the person at eye level before starting to speak.
- Determine whether hearing is better in one ear than the other, and position yourself appropriately.
- If a hearing aid is used, make sure it is in place and that the batteries are functioning.
- Ask the patient or family what helps the person to hear best.
- Keep your hands away from your mouth and project your voice by controlled diaphragmatic breathing.
- Do not turn away while speaking.
- Avoid conversations in which the speaker's face is in glare or darkness; orient the light on the speaker's face.
- Careful articulation and moderate speed of speech are helpful.
- Lower your tone of voice, use a moderate speed of speech, and articulate clearly.
- Label the chart, note on the intercom button, and inform all caregivers that the patient has a hearing impairment.
- Use nonverbal approaches: gestures, demonstrations, visual aids, and written materials.
- Pause between sentences or phrases to confirm understanding.
- Restate with different words when you are not understood.
- When changing topics, preface the change by stating the topic.
- Reduce background noise (e.g., turn off television, close door).
- Use assistive listening devices such as a personal amplifier.
- Verify that the information being given has been clearly understood. Be aware that the person may agree to everything and appear to understand what you have said even when he or she did not hear you (listener bluffing).
- Share resources for the hearing-impaired and refer as appropriate.

From Adams-Wendling L, Pimple C: Evidence-based guideline: nursing management of hearing impairment in nursing facility residents, *Journal of Gerontological Nursing* 34:9, 2008.

BOX 6-7　SIGNS AND BEHAVIORS THAT MAY INDICATE VISION PROBLEMS

INDIVIDUAL MAY REPORT:

- Pain in eyes
- Difficulty seeing in darkened area
- Double vision/distorted vision
- Migraine headaches coupled with blurred vision
- Flashes of light
- Halos surrounding lights
- Difficulty driving at night
- Falls or injuries

HEALTH CARE STAFF MAY NOTICE:

- Getting lost
- Bumping into objects
- Straining to read or no reading
- Stumbling/falling
- Spilling food on clothing
- Social withdrawal
- Less eye contact
- Placid facial expression
- TV viewing at close range
- Decreased sense of balance
- Mismatched clothes

A new program focused on vision and aging has been developed by The National Eye Health Education Program (NEHEP) of the National Eye Institute. The program provides health professionals with evidence-based tools and resources that can be used in community settings to educate older adults about eye health and maintaining healthy vision (www.nei.nih.gov/SeeWellToolkit). The program emphasizes the importance of annual dilated eye examinations for anyone over 50 years of age and stresses that eye diseases often have no warning signs or symptoms, so early detection is essential. Clearly, prevention and treatment of eye diseases is an important priority for nurses and other health care professionals.

Diseases of the Eye

Glaucoma

Glaucoma is a leading cause of blindness and visual impairment in the United States, affecting as many as 2.2 million people. An additional 2 million are unaware they have the disease. There are no symptoms of glaucoma in the early stages of the disease. Types of glaucoma include: congenital glaucoma, primary open-angle glaucoma, low tension or normal tension glaucoma, secondary glaucoma (complication of other medical conditions), and acute angle-closure glaucoma, which is an emergency. The etiology of glaucoma is variable and often unknown. However, when the natural fluids of the eye are blocked by ciliary muscle rigidity and the buildup of pressure, damage to the optic nerve occurs. Glaucoma can be bilateral, but it more commonly occurs in one eye.

Open-angle glaucoma accounts for about 80% of cases and is asymptomatic until very late in the disease, when there is a noticeable loss in visual fields. However, if detected early, glaucoma can usually be controlled and serious vision loss prevented. Signs of glaucoma can include headaches, poor vision in dim lighting, increased sensitivity to glare, "tired eyes," impaired peripheral vision, a fixed and dilated pupil, and frequent changes in prescriptions for corrective lenses. Figure 6-3, A shows normal vision and Figure 6-3 B illustrates the effects of glaucoma on vision.

An acute attack of angle-closure glaucoma is characterized by a rapid rise in intraocular pressure (IOP) accompanied by redness and pain in and around the eye, severe headache, nausea and vomiting, and blurring of vision. It occurs when the path of the aqueous humor is blocked and intraocular pressure builds up to more than 50 mm Hg. If untreated, blindness can occur in two days. An iridectomy, however, can ease pressure. Many drugs with anticholinergic properties including antihistamines, stimulants, vasodilators, clonidine, and sympathomimetics, are particularly dangerous for patients predisposed to angle-closure glaucoma. Older people with glaucoma should be counseled to review all medications, both over-the-counter and prescribed, with their primary care provider.

Low tension or normal tension glaucoma is a type of glaucoma that also occurs in older adults. In this type, intraocular pressure is within normal range but there is damage to the optic nerve and narrowing of the visual fields. The cause is unknown, but risk factors include a family history of any kind of glaucoma, Japanese ancestry, and cardiovascular disease. Management consists of the same medications and surgical interventions that are used for chronic glaucoma (Glaucoma Research Foundation, 2008).

A family history of glaucoma, as well as diabetes, steroid use, and past eye injuries have been noted as risk factors for the development of glaucoma. Age is the single most important predictor of glaucoma, and older women are affected twice as frequently as older men. Among African Americans, glaucoma is the leading cause of blindness. African Americans develop glaucoma at younger ages, and the incidence of the disease is five times more common in African Americans than in whites and fifteen times more likely to cause blindness. Factors contributing to this increased incidence include earlier onset of the disease as compared with other races, later detection of the disease, and economic and social barriers to treatment (National Eye Institute, 2010b).

Screening and Treatment

Adults over the age of 65 should have annual eye examinations, and those with medication-controlled glaucoma should be examined at least every 6 months. Annual screening is also recommended for African Americans and other individuals with a family history of glaucoma who are older than 40. A dilated eye examination and tonometry are necessary to diagnose glaucoma. These procedures can be performed by a primary care provider, optometrist, or a nurse practitioner, who will then refer the person to an ophthalmologist if glaucoma is suspected. Medicare pays for annual screening for glaucoma but only in high-risk patients.

Management of glaucoma involves medications (oral or topical eye drops) to decrease IOP and/or laser trabeculoplasty. Medications lower eye pressure either by decreasing the amount of aqueous fluid produced within the eye or by improving the flow through the drainage angle. Beta blockers are the first-line therapy for glaucoma, and the patient may need combinations of several types of eye drops. When caring for older adults in the hospital or long-term care settings, it is important to obtain a past medical history to determine if the person has glaucoma and to ensure that eye drops are given according to the person's treatment regimen. Without the eye drops, eye pressure can rise and cause an acute exacerbation of glaucoma (Capezuti et al., 2008). Usually medications can control glaucoma, but laser surgery treatments (trabeculoplasty) may be recommended for some types of glaucoma. Surgery is usually recommended only if necessary to prevent further damage to the optic nerve.

Cataracts

Cataracts are a prevalent disorder among older adults caused by oxidative damage to lens protein and fatty deposits (lipofuscin) in the ocular lens. By age 80, more than half of all Americans either have a cataract or have had cataract surgery. When lens opacity reduces visual acuity to 20/30 or less in the central axis of vision, it is considered a cataract. Cataracts are categorized according to their location within the lens and are usually bilateral. They are virtually universal in the very old but may be only minimally visible, particularly in individuals with pale irises.

Cataracts are recognized by the clouding of the ordinarily clear ocular lens; the red reflex may be absent or may appear as a black area. The cardinal sign of cataracts is the appearance of halos around objects as light is diffused. Other common

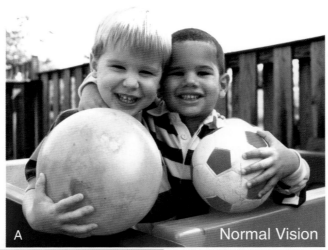

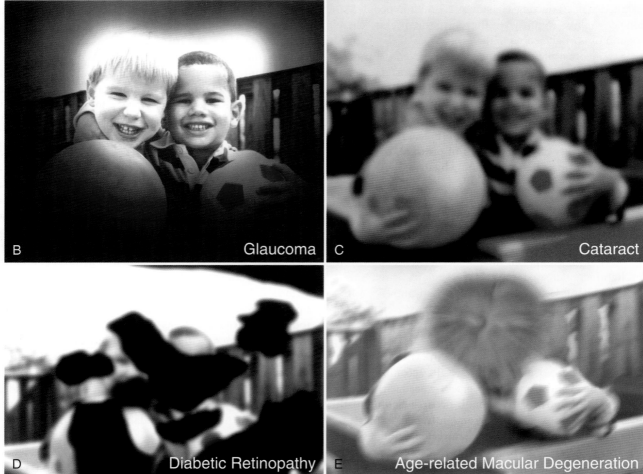

FIGURE 6-3 **A,** Normal vision. **B,** Simulated vision with glaucoma. **C,** Simulated vision with cataracts. **D,** Simulated vision with diabetic retinopahy. **E,** Simulated loss of vision with age-related macular degeneration (AMD). (From National Eye Institute, National Institutes of Health, 2010.)

symptoms include blurring, decreased perception of light and color (giving a yellow tint to most things), and sensitivity to glare. Figure 6-3, C illustrates the effects of a cataract on vision.

The most common causes of cataracts are heredity and advancing age. They may occur more frequently and at earlier ages in individuals who have been exposed to excessive sunlight,

have poor dietary habits, diabetes, hypertension, kidney disease, eye trauma, or history of alcohol intake and tobacco use. Cataracts are more likely to occur after glaucoma surgery or other types of eye surgery. There is some evidence that a high dietary intake of lutein and zeaxanthin, compounds found in yellow or dark leafy vegetables, as well as intake of vitamin E from food and supplements, appears to lower the risk of cataracts in women. Further research is indicated (Moeller et al, 2008).

When visual acuity decreases to 20/50 and the cataract affects safety or quality of life, surgery is recommended. Cataract surgery is the most common surgical procedure performed in the United States. Most often, cataract surgery involves only local anesthesia and is one of the most successful surgical procedures, with 95% of patients reporting excellent vision after surgery. The surgery involves removal of the lens and placement of a plastic intraocular lens (IOL). If the plastic lens is not inserted, the patient may wear a contact lens or glasses. This is not commonly done because the older adult may have difficulty placing and removing the contact lens, and the glasses would be very thick. Cataract surgery is performed with local anesthesia on an outpatient basis, and the procedure has greatly improved with advances in surgical techniques.

Nursing interventions when caring for the person experiencing cataract surgery include preparing the individual for significant changes in vision and adaptation to light and insuring that the individual has received adequate counseling regarding realistic postsurgical expectations. Postsurgical teaching includes covering the need to avoid heavy lifting, straining, and bending at the waist. Eye drops may be prescribed to aid healing and prevent infection. If the person has bilateral cataracts, surgery is performed first on one eye with the second surgery on the other eye a month or so later to ensure healing.

Although race is not a factor in cataract formation, racial disparities exist in cataract surgery in the United States, with African-American Medicare recipients only 60% as likely as whites to undergo cataract surgery (Miller, 2008; Wilson and Eezzuduemhoi, 2005). Cataracts are of even greater concern in Africa and Asia and account for at least half of the blindness in those countries despite the well known technology that can restore vision at an extremely low cost. Recommendations from Vision 2020 include reducing the backlog of the cataract-blind by increased training of ophthalmic personnel, strengthening of the health care infrastructure, and provision of needed surgical supplies in these countries (www.who.int/ncd/vision2020_actionplan/documents/V2020priorities.pdf2004).

Unfortunately, cataracts and other related eye diseases such as maculopathy, diabetic retinopathy, or glaucoma often occur simultaneously, which complicates the management of each. Individuals who have had cataract surgery are less likely to be effectively treated with surgery for glaucoma.

Diabetic Retinopathy

Diabetes has become an epidemic in the United States (Chapter 15). Diabetic eye disease is a complication of diabetes and a leading cause of blindness. Diabetic retinopathy is a disease of the retinal microvasculature characterized by increased vessel permeability. Blood and lipid leakage leads to macular edema and hard exudates (composed of lipids). In advanced disease, new fragile blood vessels form that hemorrhage easily. Because of the vascular and cellular changes accompanying diabetes, there is often rapid worsening of other pathologic vision conditions as well (Figure 6-3, D).

There are no symptoms in the early stages of diabetic retinopathy. Estimates are that 40.8% of adults aged 40 and older with diabetes have diabetic retinopathy, and the incidence increases with age. Most diabetic patients will develop diabetic retinopathy within 20 years of diagnosis. Prevalence rates for diabetes and diabetic retinopathy are higher among racially and culturally diverse individuals and among American Indian and Alaska Native populations (National Eye Institute, 2010c).

Screening and Treatment There is little to no evidence of retinopathy until 3 to 5 years or more after the onset of diabetes. Early signs are seen in the funduscopic examination and include microaneurysms, flame-shaped hemorrhages, cotton wool spots, hard exudates, and dilated capillaries. Constant, strict control of blood glucose, cholesterol, and blood pressure and laser photocoagulation treatments can halt progression of the disease. Laser treatment can reduce vision loss in 50% of patients. Annual dilated funduscopic examination of the eye is recommended beginning 5 years after diagnosis of diabetes type 1 and at the time of diagnosis of diabetes type 2.

Macular Degeneration

Age-related macular degeneration (AMD) is the leading cause of vision loss in Americans 60 years and older. The prevalence of AMD increases drastically with age, with more than 15% of white women over the age of 80 having the disease. Whites and Asian Americans are more likely to lose vision from AMD than African Americans. With the number of affected older adults projected to increase over the next 20 years, AMD has been called a growing epidemic (National Eye Institute, 2010d).

AMD is a degenerative eye disease that affects the macula, the central part of the eye responsible for clear central vision. The disease causes the progressive loss of central vision, leaving only peripheral vision intact. Early signs of AMD include blurred vision, difficulty reading and driving, increased need for bright light, colors that appear dim or gray, and an awareness of a blurry spot in the middle of vision. Figure 6-3, E illustrates the effects of AMD on vision.

AMD results from systemic changes in circulation, accumulation of cellular waste products, tissue atrophy, and growth of abnormal blood vessels in the choroid layer beneath the retina. Fibrous scarring disrupts nourishment of photoreceptor cells, causing their death and loss of central vision. The greatest risk factor for AMD is age. Although etiology is unknown, risk factors are thought to include genetic predisposition, smoking, obesity, family history, and excessive sunlight exposure.

There are two forms of macular degeneration, the "dry" form and the "wet" form. Dry AMD accounts for the majority of cases and rarely causes severe visual impairment, but can lead to the more aggressive wet AMD. Dry AMD generally affects both eyes, but vision can be lost on one eye while the other eye seems unaffected. Dry AMD has three stages, which may occur in one or both eyes. As dry AMD gets worse, the individual may see a blurred spot in the center of vision. One of the most common early signs is drusen. Drusen are yellow deposits under the retina and are often found in people over the age of 60. The relationship between drusen and AMD is not clear, but an increase in the size or number of drusen increases the risk of developing either advanced AMD or wet AMD (National Eye Institute, 2010d).

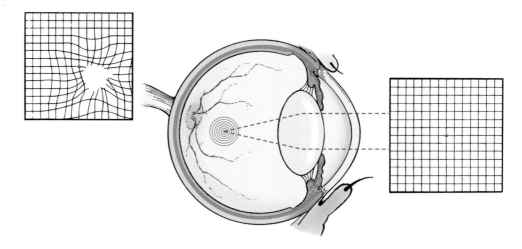

FIGURE 6-4 Macular degeneration: distortion of center vision, normal peripheral vision. (Illustration by Harriet R. Greenfied, Newton, Mass.)

Wet AMD occurs when abnormal blood vessels behind the retina start to grow under the macula. These new blood vessels are fragile and often leak blood and fluid, which raise the macula from its normal place at the back of the eye. With wet AMD, the severe loss of central vision can be rapid, and many people will be legally blind within two years of diagnosis. Peripheral vision usually remains normal, but the person will have difficulty seeing at a distance or doing detailed work such as sewing or reading. Faces may begin to blur, and it become harder to distinguish colors. An early sign may be distortion that causes edges or lines to appear wavy.

An Amsler grid is used to determine clarity of central vision (Figure 6-4). A perception of wavy lines is diagnostic of beginning macular degeneration, and vision loss can occur in days. In the advanced forms, the person may begin to see dark or empty spaces that block the center of vision. People with AMD are usually taught to test their eyes daily using the Amsler grid so that they will be aware of any changes.

Patients in the early stage of the disease may attribute their vision problems to normal aging or cataracts. Early diagnosis is the key, and individuals over the age of 40 should have a dilated eye examination at least every 2 years. The National Eye Institute's Age-Related Eye Disease Study (AREDS) (www.nei.nih. gov/) found that a high-dose formulation of antioxidants and zinc significantly reduces the risk of advanced AMD and associated vision loss. Individuals with intermediate AMD in one or both eyes or advanced AMD (wet form) in one eye but not the other should consider taking the formulation (National Eye Institute, 2010d).

Treatment of wet AMD includes photodynamic therapy (PDT), laser photocoagulation (LPC), and anti-VEGF therapy. LPC uses a laser to destroy the fragile, leaky blood vessels, but it may also destroy healthy tissue and some vision so it is used in only a small number of people with wet AMD. Lucentis and Avastin (anti-vascular endothelial growth factor (VEGF) therapy), are biological drugs that are the most common form of treatment in advanced AMD. Abnormally high levels of a specific growth factor occur in eyes with wet AMD, which promote the growth of abnormal blood vessels. Anti-VEGF

therapy blocks the effect of the growth factor. These drugs are injected into the eye as often as once a month and can help slow vision loss from AMD, and in some cases can improve sight. Photodynamic therapy involves the injection of the drug verteporfin into the arm followed by shining a light into the eye for about 90 seconds. The activated drug destroys the new blood vessels and leads to a lower rate of vision decline but does not stop vision loss or restore vision (National Eye Institute, 2010d).

Detached Retina

This condition can develop in persons with cataracts or recent cataract surgery or trauma, or can occur spontaneously. It manifests as a curtain coming down over the person's line of vision. It necessitates immediate emergency treatment.

Dry Eye

Dry eye is not a disease of the eye but is a frequent complaint among older people. Tear production normally diminishes as we age. The condition is termed keratoconjunctivitis sicca. It occurs most commonly in women after menopause. There may be age-related changes in the mucin-secreting cells necessary for surface wetting, in the lacrimal glands, or in the meibomian glands that secrete surface oil, and all of these may occur at the same time. The older person will describe a dry, scratchy feeling in mild cases (xerophthalmia). There may be marked discomfort and decreased mucus production in severe situations.

Medications can cause dry eye, especially antihistamines, diuretics, beta blockers, and some sleeping pills. The problem is diagnosed by an ophthalmologist using a Schirmer tear test, in which filter paper strips are placed under the lower eyelid to measure the rate of tear production. A common treatment is artificial tears, but dry eyes may be sensitive to them because of preservatives, which can be irritating. The ophthalmologist may close the tear duct channel either temporarily or permanently. Other management methods include keeping the house air moist with humidifiers, avoiding wind and hair dryers, and the use of artificial tear ointments at bedtime. Vitamin A deficiency can be a cause of dry eye, and vitamin A ointments are available for treatment. Sjögren's syndrome, which can occur in older

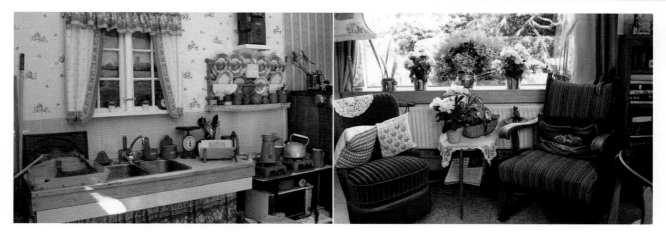

FIGURE 6-5   A, Reminiscence kitchen (Højdevang Sogns Plejejem, Copenhagen, Denmark); **B,** Sitting room (Højdevang Sogns Plejejem). (Photos courtesy Christine Williams, PhD, RN.)

people, is a cell-mediated autoimmune disease whose manifestations include decreased lacrimal gland activity. Systemic manifestations of the autoimmune disease include Raynaud's phenomenon, polyarthritis, interstitial pneumonitis, vasculitis, psychiatric manifestations, and loss of exocrine functions.

Interventions to Enhance Vision

General principles in caring for the older adult with visual impairment include the following: use warm incandescent lighting; increase intensity of lighting; control glare by using shades and blinds; suggest yellow or amber lenses to decrease glare; suggest sunglasses that block all ultraviolet light; select colors with good contrast and intensity; and recommend reading materials that have large, dark, evenly spaced printing.

Use of Contrasting Colors

Color contrasts are used to facilitate location of items. Sharply contrasting colors assist the partially sighted. For instance, a bright towel is much easier to locate than a white towel hanging on a beige wall. When choosing color, it is best to use primary colors at the top end of the spectrum rather than those at the bottom. If you think of the colors of the rainbow, it is more likely that people will see reds and oranges better than blues and greens. Figure 6-5 illustrates the use of color in a nursing home.

Low-vision Assistive Devices

Technology advances in the past decade have produced some low-vision devices that may be used successfully in the care of the visually impaired elder. Persons with severe visual impairment may qualify for disability and financial and social services assistance through government and private programs including vision rehabilitation programs. An array of low-vision assistive devices are now available, including insulin delivery systems, talking clocks and watches, large-print books, magnifiers, telescopes (handheld or mounted on eyeglasses), electronic magnification through closed circuit television or computer software, and software that converts text into artificial voice output. Because individual needs are unique, it is recommended that before investing in vision aids, the client consult with a low-vision center or low-vision specialist. See Resources available at http://evolve.elsevier.com/Ebersole/TwdHlthAging.

Communicating through Touch

A significant amount of vestibular stimulation, information, and sensual gratification comes about through touching. Touch is used for awareness and protective responses. Touch intensifies bonding and defines boundaries of self. Those who have visual and hearing impairments often compensate by cultivating the sense of touch to a high degree. Touch is often lacking in the older person's environment and can contribute to a diminishing sensorium.

Although it varies in individuals, it is thought that touch sensitivity diminishes with aging. Many of these losses are caused by disease processes such as diabetes mellitus. Changes in the sense of touch predispose older people to skin damage, particularly to the development of pressure ulcers. Loss of sensitivity to hot or cold, or thermal sensitivity, predisposes older people to burns and hyperthermia, or to frostbite and hypothermia. Degenerative changes in Meissner's corpuscles in the hands and feet result in diminished sensitivity of the palms and soles. This may cause a decrease in reaction time when stepping on a sharp object or touching a burner on the stove.

Less obvious is the deprivation of tactile senses. Introducing texture (e.g., textured upholstery, soft blanket) into the older adult's environment can enhance tactile input and contribute to safety. The use of caring, expressive touch by nurses is important (Chapter 21).

PROMOTING HEALTHY AGING: IMPLICATIONS FOR GERONTOLOGICAL NURSES

Vision impairment is common among older adults in connection with aging changes and eye diseases and can significantly affect communication, functional ability, safety, and quality of life. To promote healthy aging and quality of life, nurses who care for elders in all settings can improve outcomes for visually impaired elders by assessing for vision changes, adapting the environment to enhance vision and safety, communicating appropriately, and providing appropriate health teaching and referrals for prevention and treatment. Suggestions for

BOX 6-8 STRATEGIES FOR COMMUNICATING WITH ELDERS WITH VISUAL IMPAIRMENT

- Make sure you have the person's attention before you start talking.
- Always speak promptly and clearly identify yourself and others with you. State when you are leaving to make sure the person is aware of your departure.
- Get down to the person's level and face them when speaking.
- Speak normally but not from a distance; do not raise or lower your voice and continue to use gestures if that is natural to your communication.
- When others are present, address the visually impaired person by prefacing remarks with his or her name or a light touch on the arm.
- Use the analogy of a clock face to help locate objects (e.g., describe positions of food on a plate in relation to clock positions, such as meat at 3 o'clock, dessert at 6 o'clock).
- Ensure adequate lighting on your face and eliminate glare.
- For paint, furniture, and pictures, select colors with rich intensity (red, orange).
- Use large, dark, evenly spaced printing and enlarged font size.
- Use contrast in printed material (e.g., black marker on white paper).
- Do not change the room arrangement or the arrangement of personal items without explanation.
- Use some means to identify patients who are visually impaired, and include visual impairment in the plan of care.
- Screen for vision loss, and recommend annual eye examinations for older people.
- If the person is institutionalized, label glasses and have a spare pair if possible.
- Be aware of low-vision assistive devices, such as talking watches and talking books, and facilitate access to these resources
- If the person is blind, offer your arm while walking. Pause before stairs or curbs and alert the person. When seating the person, place his or her hand on the back of the chair. Always let the person know his or her position in relation to objects. Never play with or distract a seeing-eye dog.

communicating effectively with older adults with vision impairment are presented in Box 6-8.

COMMUNICATING WITH OLDER ADULTS WITH NEUROLOGICAL DISORDERS

Three major categories of impaired verbal communication arise from neurological disturbances: (1) reception, (2) perception, and (3) articulation. Reception is impaired by anxiety or is related to a specific disorder, hearing deficits, and altered levels of consciousness. Perception is distorted by stroke, dementia, and delirium. Articulation is hampered by mechanical difficulties such as dysarthria, respiratory disease, destruction of the larynx, and cerebral infarction with neuromuscular effects. Specific difficulties include the following:

- *Anomia:* Word retrieval difficulties during spontaneous speech and naming tasks.
- *Aphasia:* Aphasia is an acquired communication disorder that impairs a person's ability to process language, but does not affect intelligence. Aphasia impairs the ability to speak and understand others, and most people with aphasia experience difficulty in reading and writing. It results from damage to the side of the brain dominant for language. For most people, this is the left side. Aphasia usually occurs

suddenly and often results from a stroke or head injury, but it can also develop slowly because of a brain tumor, an infection, or dementia.

- *Dysarthria:* Impairment in the ability to articulate words as the result of damage to the central or peripheral nervous system that affects the speech mechanism.

Aphasia

The most commonly occurring language disorder after a cerebral vascular accident is aphasia. Cerebral vascular accidents are discussed in Chapter 15. Aphasia, in varying degrees, affects a person's ability to communicate in one or more ways, including speaking, understanding, reading, writing, and gesturing. Depending on the type and severity of the aphasia, there may be little or no speech, speech that is fragmented or broken, or speech that is fluent but empty in content. Broca's area and Wernicke's area in the cerebral cortex are integral to the expression and understanding of language. The National Aphasia Association categorizes the two major types of aphasia as fluent and nonfluent. The following is a description of several types of aphasia that the nurse may encounter with older adults:

Fluent aphasia is the result of a lesion in the superior temporal gyrus, an area adjacent to the primary auditory cortex (Wernicke's area). This type is also known as sensory, posterior, or Wernicke's aphasia. In this form of aphasia the ability to grasp the meaning of spoken words is chiefly impaired, whereas the ease of producing connected speech is not much affected. Therefore Wernicke's aphasia is referred to as a "fluent aphasia." However, speech is far from normal. Sentences do not hang together and irrelevant words intrude— sometimes to the point of jargon, in severe cases. Reading and writing are often severely impaired. Persons with fluent aphasia speak easily with many long runs of words, but the content does not make sense. There are word-finding problems and errors of word and sound substitution. These persons also have difficulty understanding spoken language and may be unaware of their speech difficulties.

Nonfluent aphasia typically involves damage to the posteroinferior portions of the dominant frontal lobe (Broca's area). This type is also called motor, anterior, or Broca's aphasia. In this form of aphasia, speech output is severely reduced and is limited mainly to short utterances of less than four words. Vocabulary access is limited and the formation of sounds by persons with Broca's aphasia is often laborious and clumsy. The person may understand speech relatively well and be able to read, but be limited in writing. Broca's aphasia is often referred to as a "nonfluent aphasia" because of the halting and effortful quality of speech.

Mixed nonfluent aphasia applies to patients who have sparse and effortful speech, resembling severe Broca's aphasia. However, unlike persons with Broca's aphasia, they remain limited in their comprehension of speech and do not read or write beyond an elementary level.

Verbal apraxia or apraxia of speech is a motor speech disorder that affects the ability to plan and sequence voluntary muscle movements. The muscles of speech are not paralyzed; instead there is a disruption in the brain's transmission of signals to the muscles. When thinking about what to say, the person may be unable to speak at all or may struggle to say words. In contrast, the person may be able to say many words or sentences correctly when not thinking about the words. Apraxia frequently occurs with aphasia.

Anomic aphasia is associated with lesions of the dominant temporoparietal regions of the brain, although no single locus has been identified. Persons with anomic aphasia understand and speak readily but may have severe word-finding difficulty. They may be unable to remember crucial content words. This is a frequent form of aphasia characterized by the inability to name objects. The individual struggles to come forth with the correct noun and often becomes frustrated at his or her inability to do so.

Global aphasia is the result of large left hemisphere lesions and affects most of the language areas of the brain. Persons with global aphasia cannot understand words or speak intelligibly. They may use meaningless syllables repetitiously.

In addition to the foregoing syndromes that are seen repeatedly by speech clinicians, there are many other possible combinations of deficits that do not exactly fit into these categories. Some of the components of a complex aphasia syndrome may also occur in isolation. This may be the case for disorders of reading (alexia) or disorders affecting both reading and writing (alexia and agraphia), following a stroke. Severe impairments of calculation often accompany aphasia, yet in some instances patients retain excellent calculation in spite of the loss of language (National Aphasia Association, 2010; www.aphasia.org).

A speech–language pathologist (SLP) should be consulted for each type of aphasia to develop appropriate rehabilitative plans as soon as the individual is physiologically stabilized. SLPs bring expertise in all types of communication disorders and are an essential part of the interdisciplinary team. The SLP can identify the areas of language that remain relatively unimpaired and can capitalize on the remaining strengths. Much can be done in aggressive speech-retraining programs to regain intelligible conversational ability. For those who do not regain meaningful speech, assistive and augmentative communication devices can be most helpful. Happ and Paull (2008) note the importance of consulting with the SLP in acute and critical care settings, as well as in rehabilitation and long-term care, and describe a program to improve communication with ICU patients who are unable to speak.

Alternative and Augmentative Speech Aids

Alternative or augmentative systems are frequently used, and communication tools exist for every type of language disability. These can be low tech or high tech. An example of a low-tech system would be an alphabet or picture board that the individual uses to point to letters to spell out messages or to point to pictures of common objects and situations. High-tech systems include electronic boards and computers. Studies have shown that computer-assisted therapy can help people with aphasia improve speech. An example is speech therapy software that displays a word or picture, speaks the word (using prerecorded human speech), records the user speaking it, and plays back the user's speech.

For individuals with hemiplegic or paraplegic conditions, electronic devices and computers can be voice-activated or have specially designed switches that can be activated by just one finger or by slight contact with the ear, nose, or chin. In addition to speech therapy, some experimental studies indicate that drugs may help improve aphasia in the acute phase of stroke and assist after the acute situation and in chronic aphasia.

PROMOTING HEALTHY AGING: IMPLICATIONS FOR GERONTOLOGICAL NURSING

Nurses are responsible for accurately observing and recording the speech and word recognition patterns of the patient and for consistently implementing the recommendations of the SLP. Communication with the older adult experiencing aphasia can be frustrating for both the affected person and the nurse as they struggle to understand each other. It is important to remember that in most cases of aphasia, the person retains normal intellectual ability. Therefore communication must always occur at an adult level but with special modifications.

Hearing and vision losses can further contribute to communication difficulties for older adults with aphasia. Sensitivity and patience are essential to promote effective communication. In hospitals and nursing homes, it is most helpful if staff caring for the person remain consistent so that they can come to know and understand the needs of the person and communicate these to others. It is exhausting for the person to have to continually try to communicate needs and desires to an array of different people. Plans of care should include specific communication strategies that are helpful for the individual person so that all staff, as well as families and significant others, know the most effective way to enhance communication. Suggestions for communicating with patients with aphasia are presented in Box 6-9.

Dysarthria

Dysarthria is a speech disorder caused by a weakness or incoordination of the speech muscles. It occurs as a result of central or peripheral neuromuscular disorders that interfere with the clarity of speech and pronunciation. Dysarthria is second in incidence only to aphasia as a communication disorder of older adults and may be the result of stroke, head injury, Parkinson's disease, multiple sclerosis, and other neurological conditions. Dysarthria is characterized by weakness, slow movement, and a lack of coordination of the muscles associated with speech. Speech may be slow, jerky, slurred, quiet, lacking in expression, and difficult to understand. It may involve several mechanisms of speech, such as respiration, phonation, resonance, articulation, and prosody (the meter, or rhythm of speech). A weakness or lack of coordination in any one of the systems can result in dysarthria. If the respiratory system is weak, then speech may be too quiet and be produced one word at a time. If the laryngeal system is weak, speech may be breathy, quiet, and slow. If the articulatory system is affected, speech may sound slurred and be slow and labored.

Treatment of dysarthria depends on the cause, the type, and the severity of the symptoms. An SLP works with the individual to improve communication abilities. Therapy for dysarthria focuses on maximizing the function of all systems. In progressive neurological disease it is important to begin treatment early

---

BOX 6-9   COMMUNICATING WITH INDIVIDUALS EXPERIENCING APHASIA

- Explain situations, treatments, and anything else that is pertinent to the person. Treat the person as an adult, and avoid patronizing and childish phrases. Talk as if the person understands.
- Be patient, and allow plenty of time to communicate in a quiet environment.
- Speak slowly, ask one question at a time, and wait for a response. Repeat and rephrase as needed.
- Create an environment in which the person is encouraged to make decisions, offer comments, and communicate thoughts and desires.
- Ask questions in a way that can be answered with a nod or the blink of an eye; if the person cannot verbally respond, instruct him or her in nonverbal responses.
- Be honest with the person. Let him or her know if you cannot quite understand what he or she is telling you but that you will keep trying.
- When you have not understood what the person said, it helps to repeat the part that you did not understand as a question so that the person only has to repeat the part that you did not understand. For example, if you hear "I would like an XX," rather than saying pardon and getting a repetition that may sound the same, try asking "You would like a …?"
- Speak of things familiar to and of interest to the person.
- Use visual cues, objects, pictures, gestures, and touch as well as words. Have paper and pencil available so you can write down key words or even sketch a picture.
- If the person has fluent aphasia, listen and watch for the bits of information that emerge from the words, facial expressions, and gestures. Ignore the nonwords.
- Encourage all speech. Allow the person to try to complete his or her thoughts and to struggle with words. Avoid being too quick to guess what the person is trying to express.
- Use augmentative communication devices, such as a picture board. These are useful to "fill in" answers to requests such as "I need" or "I want." The person merely points to the appropriate picture.
- Try to keep staff caring for the person with aphasia consistent, and make the care plan specific to the most helpful communication techniques.

BOX 6-10   TIPS FOR THE PERSON WITH DYSARTHRIA

- Explain to people that you have difficulty with your speech.
- Try to limit conversations when you feel tired.
- Speak slowly and loudly and in a quiet place.
- Pace out one word at a time while speaking.
- Take a deep breath before speaking so that there is enough breath for speech.
- Speak out as soon as you breathe out to make full use of the breaths.
- Open the mouth more when speaking; exaggerate tongue movements.
- Make sure you are sitting or standing in an upright posture. This will improve your breathing and speech.
- If you become frustrated, try to use other methods, such as pointing, gesturing, or writing, or take a rest and try again later.
- Practice facial exercises (blowing kisses, frowning, smiling), and massage your facial muscles.

Adapted from Dysarthria and copying with dysarthria. Available at www.rcslt.org and www.asha.org. Accessed December 2010.

BOX 6-11   TIPS FOR COMMUNICATING WITH INDIVIDUALS EXPERIENCING DYSARTHRIA

- Pay attention to the speaker; watch the speaker as he or she talks.
- Allow more time for conversation, and conduct conversations in a quiet place.
- Be honest, and let the speaker know when you have difficulty understanding.
- If speech is difficult to understand, repeat back what the person has said to make sure you understand.
- Repeat the part of the message you did understand so that the speaker does not have to repeat the entire message.
- Remember that dysarthria does not affect a person's intelligence.
- Check with the person for ways in which you can help, such as guessing or finishing sentences or writing.

Adapted from Dysarthria and copying with dysarthria. Available at www.rcslt.org and www.asha.org. Accessed December 2010.

---

and continue throughout the course of the disease, with the goal of maintaining speech as long as possible.

The gerontological nurse needs to be familiar with techniques that facilitate communication with persons with dysarthria as well as strategies that can be taught to the person to improve communication. Boxes 6-10 and 6-11 present suggestions for the person with dysarthria and the listener to improve communication.

The nurse may encounter older people in the acute or long-term phase of an illness that affects communication. Although early intensive rehabilitation efforts are the most effective, all older adults with communication deficits should have access to state-of-the-art techniques and devices that enhance communication, a basic human need. In addition to being knowledgeable about appropriate communication techniques, it is important for the nurse to be aware of equipment and resources available to the person with aphasia or dysarthria so that hope can be offered. Teaching families and significant others effective communication strategies is also an important nursing role. Several resources for people with aphasia and dysarthria are presented at http://evolve.elsevier.com/Ebersole/TwdHlthAging.

COMMUNICATING WITH OLDER ADULTS WITH COGNITIVE IMPAIRMENT

The experience of losing cognitive and expressive abilities is both frightening and frustrating. One type of cognitive impairment that affects memory, speech, and communication is dementia (Chapter 19). Older adults experiencing dementia have difficulty expressing their personhood in ways easily understood by others. However, the need to communicate and the need to be treated as a person remain despite memory and communication impairments. No group of patients is more in need of supportive relationships with skilled, caring health care providers. People with cognitive and communication impairments "depend on their relationship with and trust of others to provide emotional support, solve problems, and coordinate complex activities" (Buckwalter et al., 1995, p. 15).

Communication with elders experiencing cognitive impairment requires special skills and patience. "Caregivers are subject to frustration and anxiety when their attempts to communicate with the person who has cognitive limitations are unsuccessful" (Williams and Tappen, 2008, p. 92). Dementia affects both receptive and expressive communication components and alters the way people speak. Early in the disease, word finding is difficult (anomia), and remembering the exact facts of a conversation is challenging. The following quotes, in the words of older adults with dementia, illustrate:

> "I'm aware that I'm losing larger and larger chunks of memory...I lose one word and then I can't come up with the rest of the sentence. I just stop talking and people think something is really wrong with me. For awhile, I'll search for a word and I can see it walking away from me. It just gets littler and littler. It always comes back, but at the wrong time. You just can't be spontaneous" (Snyder, 2001, pp. 8, 11, 16)

> "There are a range of things you want to say over and over because I think it was a word that was important to say and I'll forget...I hope that what I am saying makes sense" (Hain et al., 2010).

People with dementia often use nonsensical or "made-up" words such as calling an electric razor a "whisker grinder." Automatic language skills (e.g., hello) are retained for the longest time. The person may wander from the topic of conversation and bring up seemingly unrelated topics. The person with dementia may fail to pick up on humor or sarcasm or abstract ideas in conversation. Nonverbal and behavioral responses become especially important as a way of communication as verbal skills become more limited. As the disease progresses, verbal output may become less frequent although the grammar and sounds of the language being spoken remain relatively intact.

Williams and Tappen (2008) remind us that even in the later stages of dementia, the person may understand more than you realize and still needs opportunities for interaction and caring communication, both verbal and nonverbal. Often, health care providers do not communicate with older adults with cognitive impairment, or they limit communication only to task-focused topics.

To effectively communicate with a person experiencing cognitive impairment, it is essential to believe that the person is trying to communicate something. It is just as essential for nurses to believe that what the person is trying to communicate is important enough to make the effort to understand. The best thing we can do is to treat everything the person says, however jumbled it may seem, as important and an attempt to tell us something. It is our responsibility as professionals to know how to understand and respond. The person with cognitive impairment cannot change his or her communication; we must change ours (Box 6-12).

Classic research conducted by Ruth Tappen of Florida Atlantic University (Boca Raton, FL) and colleagues (Tappen et al., 1997, 1999) provided insight into communication strategies that were helpful in creating and maintaining a therapeutic relationship with people in the moderate to later stages of dementia. In these studies, conversations between 23 participants in the middle and late stages of Alzheimer's disease were analyzed to clarify what type of communication techniques

---

BOX 6-12   COMMUNICATING EFFECTIVELY WITH PERSONS WITH DEMENTIA

Envision a tennis game: the caregiver is like the tennis coach, and whenever the coach plays the ball, he or she seems to be able to put the ball where the person on the other side of the net can return it. The coach also returns the ball in such a way as to keep the rally going; he or she does not return it to score a point or win the match, but rather returns the ball so that the other player is able to reach it and, with encouragement, hit it back over the net again. Similarly, in our communication with people with dementia, our conversation and words must be put into play in such a way such that the person can respond effectively and share thoughts and feelings.

Source: Kitwood T: *Dementia reconsidered: the person comes first,* Bristol, PA, 1999, Open University Press.

were helpful in creating and maintaining a therapeutic relationship. Interviewers were told to "avoid frequent correction of the individual, encourage the individual to engage in conversation, attempt to make the conversation as meaningful as possible, and to assume that any attempt at communication had some meaning to it, however difficult it was to ascertain that meaning" (Tappen et al., 1997, p. 250). Findings were compared with recommendations in the literature, and specific communication strategies were developed. More than 80% of the participants' responses were relevant in the context of the conversation. The research challenged some of the commonly held beliefs about communication with persons with cognitive impairment, for example, avoiding the use of open-ended questions and keeping communication focused only on simple topics, task-oriented topics, and questions that can be answered with *yes* or *no*.

Findings of this study provided suggestions for specific communication strategies effective in various nursing situations as well as hope for nurses to establish meaningful relationships that nurture the personhood of people with cognitive impairments (Box 6-13). Communication strategies differ depending on the purpose of communication (e.g., performing activities of daily living [ADLs], encouraging expression of feelings). "Approaches to communication must be adapted not only to the person's ability to understand but to the purpose of the interaction. What is appropriate for assessment may be a barrier to conversation that is designed to facilitate expression of concerns and feelings" (Williams and Tappen, 2008, p. 93). The Hartford Institute for Geriatric Nursing *Try This* series (http://consultgerirn.org/uploads/File/trythis/try_this_d7.pdf) provides an evidence-based practice guide for communicating with hospitalized older adults with dementia.

In the past, structured programs of reality orientation (RO) (orienting the person to the day, date, time, year, weather, upcoming holidays) were often used in long-term care facilities and chronic psychiatric units as a way to stimulate interaction and enhance memory. This intervention is still often noted as being of benefit to persons with dementia. However, it has been found that structured RO may place unrealistic expectations on persons with middle- to late-stage dementia and may be distressing when they cannot remember these things. Families, and professional caregivers, can often be heard asking people with dementia to name relatives, state their birth year, and remember other current facts. One can imagine how

BOX 6-13   FOUR USEFUL STRATEGIES FOR COMMUNICATING WITH INDIVIDUALS EXPERIENCING COGNITIVE IMPAIRMENT

SIMPLIFICATION STRATEGIES

Simplification strategies are useful with ADLs:
- Give one-step directions.
- Speak slowly.
- Allow time for response.
- Reduce distractions.
- Interact with one person at a time.
- Give clues and cues as to what you want the person to do. Use gestures or pantomime to demonstrate what it is you want the person to do—for example, put the chair in front of the person, point to it, pat the seat, and say, "Sit here."

FACILITATION STRATEGIES

Facilitation strategies are useful in encouraging expression of thoughts and feelings:
- Establish commonalities.
- Share self.
- Allow the person to choose subjects to discuss.
- Speak as if to an equal.
- Use broad openings, such as "How are you today?"
- Employ appropriate use of humor.
- Follow the person's lead.

COMPREHENSION STRATEGIES

Comprehension strategies are useful in assisting with understanding of communication:
- Identify time confusion (*in what time frame is the person operating at the moment?*).
- Find the theme (*what connection is there between apparently disparate topics?*). Recognize an important theme, such as fear, loss, or happiness.

- Recognize the hidden meanings (*what did the person mean to say?*).

SUPPORTIVE STRATEGIES

Supportive strategies are useful in encouraging continued communication and supporting personhood:
- Introduce yourself, and explain why you are there. Reach out to shake hands, and note the response to touch.
- If the person does not want to talk, go away and return later. Do not push or force.
- Sit closely, and face the person at eye level.
- Limit corrections.
- Use multiple ways of communicating (gestures, touch).
- Search for meaning.
- Know the person's past life history as well as daily life experiences and events.
- Remember there is a person behind the disease.
- Recognize feelings, and respond.
- Treat the person with respect and dignity.
- Show interest through body posture, facial expression, nodding, and eye contact. Assume a pleasant, relaxed attitude.
- Attend to vision and hearing losses.
- Do not try to bring the person to the present or use reality orientation. Go to where the person is, and enjoy the conversation.
- When leaving, thank the person for his or her time and attention as well as information.
- Remember that the quality, not the content or quantity, of the interaction is basic to therapeutic communication.

ADLs, activities of daily living.

upsetting and demoralizing this might be to a person unable to remember.

Students reading this book may liken the feeling to being told they are taking a pop quiz on content not yet assigned for study, and that this will constitute their final course grade. An often-told story in gerontological nursing is about a researcher who was visiting a nursing home daily to administer the Mini-Mental State Examination (MMSE) to residents with dementia as part of her study. One morning, one of the residents hurried to the nursing station; she was quite agitated and frantically kept asking, "What day is today?" The nurse asked her why she was so upset about the day and she responded, "It's not me, but there is a young woman who comes in every day asking that question and I want to help her out."

This is not to say that we should not orient the person to daily activities, time of day, and other important events, but it should be offered without the expectation that they will remember. Caregivers can provide orienting information as part of general conversation (e.g., "It's quite warm for December 10, but it will be a beautiful day for our lunch date"). Rather than structured RO, a better approach is to go where the person is in their world rather than trying to bring them into yours. Identifying with elements of the individual's past and helping them and their caregivers appreciate the connections and feelings are more therapeutic approaches. Validation therapy, developed by Naomi Feil in the 1980s, involves following the person's lead and responding to feelings expressed rather than interrupting to supply factual data.

Deborah Hoffmann, in her wonderful film *Complaints of a Dutiful Daughter*, chronicles her mother's journey through Alzheimer's disease and humorously describes her frustration with trying to keep her mother oriented and in the present. When her mother thought Deborah was one of her sorority sisters from college and talked to her about all the good times they had, she would correct her mother and remind her that she was her daughter and did not go to college with her. After many such conversations and corrections, she finally realized that it was okay if her mother thought she was one of the sorority girls—it made her mother happy to talk about good times and they could laugh and reminiscence together.

PROMOTING HEALTHY AGING: IMPLICATIONS FOR GERONTOLOGICAL NURSING

Care and communication that respect and value the dignity and worth of every person nursed, including those with cognitive impairment, and use of research-based communication techniques, will enhance communication and personhood. "Gerontological nurses who are sensitive to communication and interaction patterns can assist both formal and informal caregivers in using more personal verbal and nonverbal communication strategies that are humanizing and show respect for the person. Similarly, they can monitor and try to change object-oriented communication approaches, which are not only insensitive and dehumanizing, but also often lead to diminished self-image and angry, agitated responses on the part of the patient with cognitive impairment" (Buckwalter et al., 1995, p. 15).

THE LIFE STORY

Older people bring us complex stories derived from long years of living. In caring for older adults, listening to life stories is an important component of communication. The life story can tell us a great deal about the person and is an important part of the assessment process. Stories provide important information about etiology, diagnosis, treatment, prognosis, and experience of living with an illness from the patient's point of view. Listening to memories and life stories requires time and patience and a belief that the story and the person are valuable and meaningful. A memory is an incredible gift given to the nurse, a sharing of a part of oneself when one may have little else to give. The more personal memories are saved for persons who will patiently wait for their unveiling and who will treasure them. Stories are important, as Robert Coles states (1989, p. 7): "The people who come to see us bring us their stories. They hope they tell them well enough so that we understand the truth of their lives. They hope we know how to interpret their stories correctly."

The life story as constructed through reminiscing, journaling, life review, or guided autobiography has held great fascination for gerontologists in the last quarter-century. The universal appeal of the life story as a vehicle of culture, a demonstration of caring and generational continuity, and an easily stimulated activity has held allure for many professionals. The most exciting aspect of working with older adults is being a part of the emergence of the life story: the shifting and blending patterns. When we are young, it is important for our emotional health and growth to look forward and plan for the future. As one ages, it becomes more important to look back, talk over experiences, review and make sense of it all, and end with a feeling of satisfaction with the life lived. This is important work and the major developmental task of older adulthood that Erik Erikson called *ego integrity versus despair*. Ego integrity is achieved when the person has accepted both the triumphs and disappointments of life and is at peace and satisfied with the life lived (Erikson, 1963).

Reminiscing

Reminiscing is an umbrella term that can include any recall of the past. Reminiscing occurs from childhood onward, particularly at life's junctures and transitions. Reminiscing cultivates a sense of security through recounting of comforting memories, belonging through sharing, and self-esteem through confirmation of uniqueness. Robert Butler (2002) pointed out that 50 years ago, reminiscing was thought to be a sign of senility or what we now call Alzheimer's disease. Older people who talked about the past and told the same stories again and again were said to be boring and living in the past. From Butler's seminal research (1963), we now know that reminiscence is the most important psychological task of older people.

For the nurse, reminiscing is a therapeutic intervention important in assessment and understanding. The work of several gerontological nursing leaders, including Irene Burnside,

Priscilla Ebersole, and Barbara Haight, has contributed to the body of knowledge about reminiscence and its importance in nursing. The International Institute for Reminiscence and Life Review (University of Wisconsin, Superior, WI), an interdisciplinary organization bringing together participants to study reminiscence and life review, is another valuable resource for nurses and members of other disciplines involved in research or practice.

Reminiscence can have many goals. It not only provides a pleasurable experience that improves quality of life, but also increases socialization and connectedness with others, provides cognitive stimulation, improves communication, and can significantly decrease depression scores (Haight and Burnside, 1993; Grabowski et al., 2010). The process of reminiscence can occur in individual conversations with older people, be structured as in a nursing history, or can occur in a group where each person shares his or her memories and listens to others sharing theirs. Group work is discussed later in this chapter.

Reminiscence and life story have entered the computer age through the use of digital storytelling. Digital storytelling is another medium that can be used with older people to record their stories and memories in a format that can be shared with others. The digital story is a first-person narrative created by combining recorded voice, still and moving images, and music or other sounds. A study producing personalized multimedia biographies for individuals with cognitive impairment reported that the biography stimulated reminiscence, brought mostly joy but occasionally moments of sadness, aided family members in remembering and better understanding their loved ones, and stimulated social interactions with family members and formal caregivers (Damianakis et al., 2010). Buron (2010) presents a lovely format for person-centered life history collages for use in a nursing home. There are many resources available for those interested in digital storytelling and community centers and educational institutions, as well as the Internet, provide instruction on this medium (http://www.storycenter.org/about.html; http://digitalstorytelling.coe.uh.edu/; http://milehighstories.com/?page_id=21).

The nurse can learn much about a resident's history, communication style, relationships, coping mechanisms, strengths, fears, affect, and adaptive capacity by listening thoughtfully as the life story is constructed. Box 6-14 provides some suggestions for encouraging reminiscence.

Life Review

Robert Butler (1963) first noted and brought to public attention the review process that normally occurs in the older person as the realization of his or her approaching death creates a resurgence of unresolved conflicts. Butler called this process *life review*. Life review occurs quite naturally for many persons during periods of crisis and transition. However, Butler (2002) noted that in old age, the process of putting one's life in order increases in intensity and emphasis. Life review occurs most frequently as an internal review of memories, an intensely private, soul-searching activity.

Life review is considered more of a formal therapy technique than reminiscence and takes a person through his or her life in a structured and chronological order. Life review therapy (Butler and Lewis, 1983), guided autobiography (Birren and

BOX 6-14   SUGGESTIONS FOR ENCOURAGING REMINISCENCE

- Listen without correction or criticism. Older adults are presenting their version of their reality; our version belongs to another generation.
- Encourage older adults to cover various ages and stages. Use questions such as "What was it like growing up on that farm?" "What did teenagers do for fun when you were young?" "What was WWII like for you?"
- Be patient with repetition. Sometimes people need to tell the same story often to come to terms with the experience, especially if it was meaningful to them. If they have a memory loss, it may be the only story they can remember, and it is important for them to be able to share it with others.
- Be attuned to signs of depression in conversation (dwelling on sad topics) or changes in physical status or behavior, and provide appropriate assessment and intervention.
- If a topic arises that the person does not want to discuss, change to another topic.
- If individuals are reluctant to share because they don't feel their life was interesting, reassure them that everyone's life is valuable and interesting and tell them how important their memories are to you and others.
- Keep in mind that reminiscing is not an orderly process. One memory triggers another in a way that may not seem related; it is not important to keep things in order or verify accuracy.
- Keep the conversation focused on the person reminiscing, but do not hesitate to share some of your own memories that relate to the situation being discussed. Participate as equals, and enjoy each other's contributions.
- Listen actively, maintain eye contact, and do not interrupt.
- Respond positively and give feedback by making caring, appropriate comments that encourage the person to continue.
- Use props and triggers such as photographs, memorabilia (e.g., a childhood toy or antique), short stories or poems about the past, and favorite foods.
- Use open-ended questions to encourage reminiscing. If working with a group, you can prepare questions ahead of time, or you can ask the group members to pick a topic that interests them. One question or topic may be enough for an entire group session. Consider using questions such as the following:

  How did your parents meet?
  What do you remember most about your mother? father? grandmother? grandfather?
  What are some of your favorite memories from childhood?
  What was the first house you remember?
  What were your favorite foods as a child?
  Did you have a pet as a child?
  Tell us about your first job.
  How did you celebrate birthdays or other holidays?
  If you were married, tell us about your wedding day.
  What was your greatest accomplishment or joy in your life?
  What advice did your parents give you? What advice did you give your children? What advice would you give to young people today?

Deutchman, 1991), and structured life review (Haight and Webster, 2002) are psychotherapeutic techniques based on the concept of life review.

Gerontological nurses participate with older adults in both reminiscence and life review, and it is important to acquire the skills to be effective in achieving the purposes of both. Life review may be especially important for older people experiencing depressive symptoms and those facing death (Pott et al., 2010). The Hospice Foundation of America provides *A Guide for Recalling and Telling Your Life Story* (http://store.hospicefoundation.org/home.php?cat=5) that nurses and families may find helpful.

Life review should occur not only when we are old or facing death but also frequently throughout our lives. This process can assist us to examine where we are in life and change our course or set new goals. Butler (2002) commented that one might avoid the overwhelming feelings of despair that may surface when there is no time left to make changes if life review had been conducted throughout one's lives.

PROMOTING HEALTHY AGING: IMPLICATIONS FOR GERONTOLOGICAL NURSING

One of the greatest privileges of nursing elders is to accompany them in the final journey of life. As each person confronts mortality, there is a need to integrate events and then to transcend the self. The human experience, the person's contributions, and the poignant anecdotes within the life story bind generations together, validate the uniqueness of each brief journey in this level of awareness, and provide the assurance that one will not be forgotten. When the nurse takes the time to listen to an older person share memories and life stories, it communicates respect and valuing of the individual and provides important data for assessment and coming to know the person. What more can one ask at the end of life than to know that who one is, and what one has accomplished holds personal meaning and meaning for others as well? This is the essence of life's final tasks—achieving ego integrity and self-actualization.

COMMUNICATING WITH GROUPS OF OLDER ADULTS

Group work with older adults has been used extensively in institutional settings to meet myriad needs in an economical manner. Nurses have led groups of older people for a variety of therapeutic reasons. Expert gerontological nurses, such as Irene Burnside and Priscilla Ebersole, have extensively discussed advantages of group work for both older people and group leaders and have provided in-depth guidelines for conducting groups. Box 6-15 presents some of the benefits of group work.

Many groups can be managed effectively by staff with clear goals and guidance and training. Volunteers, nursing assistants, students, and recreation staff can be taught to conduct many types of groups, but groups with a psychotherapy focus require a trained and skilled leader. Perese, Simon and Ryan (2008) and Heliker (2009) provide excellent suggestions for group reminiscence therapy and story-sharing interventions. Some basic considerations for group work are presented in this chapter, but nurses interested in working with groups of older people should consult a text on group work for more in-depth information.

Groups can be implemented in many settings, including adult day health programs, retirement communities, assisted living facilities, nutrition sites, and nursing homes. Examples of groups include reminiscence groups, psychoeducational groups, caregiver support groups, and groups for people with memory impairment or other conditions such as Parkinson's disease or stroke. Groups can be organized to meet any level of human need; some meet multiple needs.

BOX 6-15   BENEFITS OF GROUP WORK WITH ELDERS

- Group experiences provide older adults with an opportunity to try new roles—those of teacher, expert, storyteller, or even clown.
- Groups may improve communication skills for lonely, shy, or withdrawn older people as well as those with communication disorders or memory impairment.
- Groups provide peer support and opportunities to share common experiences, and they may foster the development of warm friendships that endure long after the group has ended.
- The group may be of interest to other residents, staff, and relatives and may improve satisfaction and morale. Staff, in particular, may come to see their patients in a different light—not just as persons needing care but as persons.
- Active listening and interest in what older people have to say may improve self-esteem and help them feel like worthwhile persons whose wisdom is valued.
- Group work offers the opportunity for leaders to be creative and use many modalities, such as music, art, dance, poetry, exercise, and current events.
- Groups provide an opportunity for the leader to assess the person's mood, cognitive abilities, and functional level on a weekly basis.

Adapted from Burnside IM: Group work with older persons, *Journal of Gerontological Nursing* 20:43, 1994.

BOX 6-16   SPECIAL CONSIDERATIONS IN GROUP WORK WITH ELDERS

- The leader must pay special attention to sensory losses and compensate for vision and hearing loss.
- Pacing is different, and group leaders must slow down in both physical and psychological actions.
- Group members often need assistance or transportation to the group, and adequate time must be allowed for assembling the members and assisting them to return to their homes or rooms.
- Time of day a group is scheduled is important. Meeting time should not conflict with bathing and eating schedules, and evening groups may not be good for older people, who may be tired by then. For community-based older people, transportation logistics may become complicated in the evening.
- A warm and friendly climate of acceptance of each member and showing appreciation and enjoyment of the group and each member's contribution are all important. As a result of ageist attitudes in society, older people's wisdom and contributions are not often valued, making them feel useless or a bother.
- Older adults may need more stimulation and be less self-motivating. (This is, of course, not true of self-help and senior activist groups such as the Gray Panthers.)
- Groups generally should include people with similar levels of cognitive ability. Mixing very intact elders with those who have memory and communication impairments calls for special skills. Burnside* suggests that in groups of people with varying abilities, alert persons tend to ask, "Will I become like them?" whereas the people with memory and communication impairments may become anxious when they are aware that they cannot perform as well as the other members.
- Many older people likely to be in need of groups may be depressed or have experienced a number of losses (health, friends, spouse). Discussion of losses and sad feelings can be difficult for group leaders. A leader prone to depression would not be appropriate.
- Leaders must be prepared for some members to become ill, deteriorate, and die. Plans regarding recognition of missing members will need to be clear. The following, which occurred during a reminiscence group conducted by one of the authors (T.T.), illustrates this: "As I arrived at the nursing home for the weekly reminiscence group meeting, I was told by the nursing home staff that one of our members had died. One of the members had been a priest so we asked him to say a prayer for our deceased group member. He did so beautifully, and the group was grateful. The next week, to our surprise, the supposedly deceased member showed up for the group (she had been in the hospital). We didn't know how to handle the situation, but the other members came to our rescue by saying, 'Father's prayers really worked this time.'" Older people's wisdom and humor can teach us a lot.
- Leaders are continually confronted with their own aging and attitudes toward it. Coleaders are ideal and can support each other. It is important to share thoughts and feelings, recapitulate group sessions, and modify approaches as needed. If leading the group alone, locate someone with expertise in group work with elders who can discuss with you the group experiences and provide support and direction. Students generally should work in pairs and will need supervision. Skills in developing and implementing groups for older adults improve with experience. Burnside* reminds us that "all new group leaders should have guidance from an experienced leader to help them weather the difficult times" (p. 43).

*Burnside I: Group work with older persons, *Journal of Gerontological Nursing* 20:43, 1994.

Group Structure and Special Considerations

Implementing a group intervention follows a thorough assessment of environment, needs, and the potential for various group strategies. Major decisions regarding goals will influence the strategy selected. For instance, several older people with diabetes in an acute care setting may need health care teaching regarding diabetes. The nurse sees the major goal as education and restoring order (or control) in each individual's lifestyle. The strategy best suited for that would be motivational or educational. A group of people experiencing early-stage Alzheimer's disease may benefit from a support group to express feelings or a group that teaches memory-enhancing strategies. Successful group work depends on organization, attention to details, agency support, assessment and consideration of the older person's needs and status, and caring, sensitive, and skillful leadership.

Group work with older people is different from that with younger age groups; and there are some unique aspects that require special skills and training and an extraordinary commitment on the part of the leader. Although these unique aspects may not apply to all types of groups of older adults, some strategies are presented in Box 6-16.

Reminiscing and Storytelling with Individuals Experiencing Cognitive Impairment

Cognitive impairment does not necessarily preclude older adults from participating in reminiscence or storytelling groups. Research suggests that communication skills training that involves memory book and life review activities with those who have dementia and their families can (1) increase the quantity and quality of communication between care recipients and caregivers, (2) lower caregiver stress and burden, and (3) reduce behavioral problems (Damianakis et al., 2010). Opportunities for telling the life story, enjoying memories, and achieving ego integrity and self-actualization should not be denied to individuals on the basis of their cognitive status. Modifications must be made according to the cognitive abilities of the person, and although individual life review from a psychotherapeutic approach is not an appropriate modality, individuals with mild to moderate memory impairment can enjoy and benefit from group work focused on reminiscence and storytelling.

When the nurse is working with a group of cognitively impaired older adults, the emphasis in reminiscence groups is on sharing memories, however they may be expressed, rather than specific recall of events. There should be no pressure to answer questions such as "Where were you born?" or "What was your first job?" Rather, discussions may center on jobs people had and places they have lived. Additional props, such as music, pictures, and familiar objects (e.g., an American flag, an old coffee grinder), can prompt many recollections and sharing.

The leader of a group with participants who have memory problems must be more active. Many resources are available to guide these groups, including books such as *I Remember When* (Thorsheim and Roberts, 2000), that offer numerous ways to adapt the reminiscing process for those with cognitive impairment. StoryCorps Memory Loss Initiative (www.storycorps.net/special-initiatives/mli) is an innovative program featuring the stories of people with memory loss. Other helpful resources can be found on Evolve at http://evolve.elsevier.com/Ebersole/TwdHlthAging.

The TimeSlips program (Bastings, 2003, 2006; Fritsch et al., 2009) is an evidence-based innovation, cited by the Agency for Healthcare Research and Quality (Rockville, MD; www.innovations.ahrq.gov), that uses storytelling to enhance the lives of people with cognitive impairment. Positive outcomes associated with the program include enhanced verbal skills and provider reports of positive behavioral changes, increased communication, and sociability, and less confusion. TimeSlips is a beneficial and cost-effective therapeutic intervention that can be used in many settings.

Group members, looking at a picture, are encouraged to create a story about the picture. The pictures can be fantastical and funny, such as from greeting cards, or more nostalgic, such as Norman Rockwell paintings. All contributions are encouraged and welcomed, there are no right or wrong answers, and everything that the individuals say is included in the story and written down by the scribe. Stories are read back to the participants during the session, using their names to identify their contributions. At the beginning of each session, the story from the last session is read to the participants. Care is taken to compliment each member for his or her contribution to the wonderful story. The stories that emerge are full of humor and creativity and often include discussions of memories and reminiscing.

One of the authors (T.T.) has used the storytelling modality extensively with mild to moderately impaired older people with great success as part of a research study on the effect of therapeutic activities for persons with memory loss. Qualitative responses from group participants and families indicated their enjoyment with the process. At the end of the 16-week group, the stories are bound into a book and given to the participants with a picture of the group and each member's name listed. Many of the participants and their families have commented on the pride they feel at their "book" and have even shared them with grandchildren and great-grandchildren. In work by Bastings (2003), some of the stories were presented as a play.

HEALTH LITERACY AND COMMUNICATION

Health literacy is defined as the degree to which individuals have the capacity to obtain, process, and understand basic health information and services needed to make appropriate health decisions (Kobylarz et al., 2010). Limited health literacy has been linked to increased health disparities, poor health outcomes, inadequate preventive care, increased use of health care services, higher risk of mortality for older adults, and several health care safety issues, including medical and medication errors. Improving health literacy for all Americans has been identified as one of the 20 necessary actions to improve health care quality on a national scale (Agency for Healthcare Research and Quality, 2011: Centers for Disease Control and Prevention [CDC], 2009.)

Health literacy is more than the ability to read and write and includes the ability to listen, follow directions, complete forms, perform basic math calculations, and interact with health professionals and health care settings. Educational level cannot be relied on as an indicator of literacy skills for medical information. Health literacy is "approximately five grade levels lower than the last school year completed" (Hayes, 2000, p. 7). Many health education materials, as well as information on the Internet, are written at reading levels above the recommended fifth-grade reading level.

Being health literate "involves a multitude of cognitive processes that are challenging for any one at any age" (Speros, 2009). Nearly nine of 10 adults do not have the level of proficiency in health literacy skills necessary to successfully navigate the health care system. Older adults are disproportionately affected by inadequate health literacy. Chronic illness and sensory impairments further contribute to challenges related to communication and understanding. Among adult age groups, those aged 65 and older have the smallest proportion of persons with proficient health literacy skills. This group also has the highest proportion of persons with health literacy defined as "below basic." More than half of individuals over the age of 65 years are at the below-basic level (CDC, 2009; Kobylarz et al., 2010) (Figure 6-6).

Older adults are a heterogeneous group in their characteristics and literacy skills, and therefore strategies to enhance their understanding of health information need to be individualized. Individuals residing in urban areas, those with poor education or low income, and people for whom English is a second

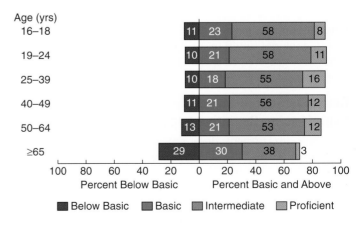

FIGURE 6-6 Health Literacy Skills of U.S. Adults, by Age Group, 2003. (From Kutner M, Greenberg E, Jin Y, et al: *The health literacy of America's adults: results from the 2003 National Assessment of Adult Literacy.* Publication no. 2006-483. Washington DC, 2006, U.S. Department of Education, National Center for Education Statistics.)

language are more likely to perform at lower levels of literacy. Other factors influencing health literacy include the person's basic literacy skills and situations encountered in the health care system as well as the cultural competence and communication skills of health professionals.

Improving Health Literacy for Older Adults (CDC, 2009) provides health professionals with information related to health literacy and strategies for communicating effectively. Resources for assisting health professionals in constructing low-literacy materials for use with older adults are found on Evolve at http://evolve.elsevier.com/Ebersole/TwdHlthAging.

LEARNING IN LATE LIFE

Basic intelligence remains unchanged with increasing years, and older adults should be provided with opportunities for continued learning. Adapting communication and teaching to enhance understanding requires knowledge of learning in late life and effective teaching-learning strategies with older adults. Geragogy is the application of the principles of adult learning theory to teaching interventions for older adults.

The older adult demands that teaching situations be relevant; new learning must relate to what the person already knows and should emphasize concrete and practical information. Aging may present barriers to learning, such as hearing and vision losses and cognitive impairment. Moreover, the process of aging may accentuate other challenges that had already been factors in a person's life, such as cultural and cohort variations and education. Many older adults may have special learning needs based on educational deprivation in their early years and consequent anxiety about formalized learning.

Attention to literacy level and cultural variations is important to enhance learning and the usefulness of what is learned. Mood is extremely important in terms of what individuals (young and old) will recall. In other words, when we attempt to measure recall of events that may have occurred in a crisis situation or an anxiety state, recall will be impaired. This is significant for health care professionals who give information to older adults who are ill or upset, particularly at times of crisis such as hospital discharge. They are not likely to remember the information provided, which contributes to problematic transitions (Chapter 16). Box 6-17 presents strategies to enhance the learning of older adults.

Opportunities for older adults to learn are available in many formal and informal modes: self-teaching, college attendance, participation in seminars and conferences, public television programs, CDs, Internet courses, and countless others. In most universities, older people are taking classes of all types. Fees are usually lower for individuals older than 60 years, and elders may choose to work toward a degree or audit classes for enrichment and enjoyment. The Elderhostel program is an example of a program designed for older people that combines continued learning with travel (www.elderhostel.org).

Older adults comprise the fastest growing population using computers and the Internet. According to data from the Pew Research Center's Internet and American Life Project, 92% of adults aged 50-64 years and 89% of those 65 years and over send and receive emails (Pew Research Center, 2010). Older adults also comprise the fastest growing group using

---

BOX 6-17 GUIDING OLDER ADULT LEARNERS

- Make sure the client is ready to learn before trying to teach. Watch for cues that would indicate that the client is preoccupied or too anxious to comprehend the material.
- Be sensitive to cultural, language, and other differences among the older adults you serve.
- Provide adequate time for learning, and use self-pacing techniques.
- Create a shame-free environment where older adults feel free to ask questions and stay informed.
- Provide regular positive feedback.
- Avoid distractions, and present one idea at a time.
- Present pertinent, specific, practical, and individualized information. Emphasize concrete rather than abstract material.
- Use past experience; connect new learning to what has already been learned.
- Use written material to supplement verbal instruction. Use a list format, a low-literacy level, and large readable font (e.g., Arial, 14 to 16 points).
- Use high contrast on visuals and handout materials (e.g., black print on white paper).
- Consider using Braille and audiotaped information whenever necessary.
- Pay attention to reading ability; use tools other than printed material such as drawings, pictures, and discussion.
- Use bullets or lists to highlight pertinent information.
- Sit facing the client so he or she can watch your lip movements and facial expressions.
- Speak slowly.
- Keep the pitch of your voice low; older people can hear low sounds better than high-frequency sounds.
- Encourage the learner to develop various mediators or mnemonic devices (e.g., visual images, rhymes, acronyms, self-designed coding schemes).
- Use shorter, more frequent sessions with appropriate breaks; pay attention to fatigue and physical discomfort.

Modified from: SPRY Foundation: *Bridging principles of older adult learning: reconnaissance phase final report,* SPRY Foundation, 1999, Washington DC; and Hayes K: Designing written medication instructions: effective ways to help older adults self-medicate, *Journal of Gerontological Nursing* 32:5, 2005.

---

social-networking sites such as Facebook. More than any other age group, older adults perceive the Internet as a valuable resource to help them connect to loved ones and more easily obtain information.

AARP and other organizations such as CyberSeniors provide basic computer and Internet training for older people. Although there has been little research on the use of computers among nursing home residents or among those with dementia, the technology has great potential to meet psychosocial needs for family contact, enjoyment, and stimulation (Tak et al., 2007).

PROMOTING HEALTHY AGING: IMPLICATIONS FOR GERONTOLOGICAL NURSING

Throughout this chapter we have tried to convey the potential for honest and hopeful communication regardless of the impairment the elder may be experiencing. Communicating with older people calls for special skills, patience, and respect. We must break through the barriers and continue to reach toward the humanity of the individual with the belief that communication is the most vital service we offer. This is the heart of nursing. Skilled, sensitive, and caring individual and group communication strategies with older adults are essential to meeting needs and are the basis for therapeutic nursing relationships. Just as all people have the need to communicate and have their basic needs met, they also have the right to experiences that are meaningful and fulfilling. Age, language impairment, or mental status do not change these needs.

Creation of care environments that are rich with pleasant experiences—a good cup of coffee, a meal shared with friends, a sunrise, beautiful music, learning something interesting, or sharing experiences from the life one has lived—is as important as getting enough to eat. Our nursing care with older people experiencing cognitive and communication impairments must be more than keeping their bodies alive, safe, and clean, or preventing injury. The unique contribution that nursing brings to the care of people is the intimate, personal knowing of the person behind the disease and the creation of relationships and environments of care that support, validate, and celebrate the person as someone of value and worth (Touhy, 2004). Within this framework, gerontological nurses assist in the meeting of needs at all levels.

evolve   To access your student resources, go to *http://evolve.elsevier.com/Ebersole/TwdHlthAging*

KEY CONCEPTS

- Communication is a basic need regardless of age or communication or cognitive impairment.
- The sensory apparatus all lose some degree of acuity in the aging process; hearing is the most prevalent loss. The nurse needs to adapt communication to enhance sensory input and enhance communication.
- Group work can meet many needs and is satisfying and rewarding for both the older adult and the group leader.
- In a rapidly changing society, the shared life histories of elders provide a sense of continuity among the generations.
- The life history of an individual is a story to be developed and treasured. This is particularly important toward the end of life.
- Gerontological nursing responses related to communication are focused mainly on using therapeutic communication techniques, providing necessary information, encouraging individuals to express personal interests and preferences and, when function is impeded, ensuring that basic needs are recognized by all, and met to the greatest extent possible.
- Older adults are disproportionately affected by inadequate health literacy and nurses must ensure that health information is provided in an appropriate manner to ensure understanding.

CASE STUDY   HEARING IMPAIRMENT

Sonya is a 66-year-old high school nurse/consultant. She retired from the Army Nurse Corps with an officer's rank after serving 20 years, much of it in the Korean conflict with heavy exposure to shelling in the early part of her career. She became aware of hearing loss at about age 45, and by age 55 years it had become severe. While in the service she had considerable assistance from noncommissioned personnel and functioned well. When she entered civilian life, it became more difficult for her to manage but she was unwilling to admit to others her major hearing deficit. During those years she simply attempted to cover it as much as possible, and some of her coworkers thought she was rather obtuse; others suspected her deafness. When she took the position with the school district, she was involved with three high schools, numerous faculty members, and students, and interpersonal communication was a major aspect of her position. When she was evaluated at the end of the first year, it was pointed out that feedback indicated she was inattentive. She did then admit her hearing problem and was advised to get hearing aids. She said, "I've known several people over the years who have hearing aids, and none of them were really satisfied with them. I guess that is why I have not gotten them before now." She complied but, after a few weeks, rarely wore them. The personnel officer of the school board, after hearing several more complaints of inappropriate communication, told her she must wear the hearing aids if she wished to continue in her position. Sonya knew that hearing aids were essential, not only for communication but also for safety—she had almost been hit by a car while walking because she simply did not hear it coming. Yet she did not want to go back to the audiology clinic, because they did not seem to know what they were doing, and each time she saw someone, the person gave her different information. She tried three different types of aids that seemed of little help. She lost confidence in her ear, nose, and throat specialist because he had been unable to help her resolve the ringing in her ears. Now her school district had contracted with a health maintenance organization, and she was not even sure which health care provider she should see.

On the basis of the case study, develop a nursing care plan using the following procedure*:

- List Sonya's comments that provide subjective data.
- List information that provides objective data.
- From these data identify and state, using accepted format, two nursing diagnoses you determine are most significant to Sonya at this time. List two of Sonya's strengths that you have identified from data.
- Determine and state outcome criteria for each diagnosis. These must reflect some alleviation of the problem identified in the nursing diagnosis and must be stated in concrete and measurable terms.
- Plan and state one or more interventions for each diagnosed problem. Provide specific documentation of the source used to determine the appropriate intervention. Plan at least one intervention that incorporates Sonya's existing strengths.
- Evaluate the success of the intervention. Interventions must correlate directly with the stated outcome criteria to measure the outcome success.

Continued

CASE STUDY—CONT'D

CRITICAL THINKING QUESTIONS

1. What are some of the possible reasons Sonya suffered severe hearing loss at so young an age?
2. Discuss the stigma of hearing loss and hearing aids.
3. Obtain a "hearing aid loaner." Instruct students to wear it for several hours and report their reactions in writing. List difficulties experienced.
4. How would you advise Sonya if you were her nurse/friend?
5. Discuss the various kinds of hearing aids and how they differ.
6. Discuss reasons Sonya may have discontinued wearing her hearing aids.
7. What might you suggest that would be helpful in adapting to wearing a hearing aid?
8. What are some of the options you would discuss with Sonya?
9. Which of the various sensory/perceptual changes of aging would you find most difficult to cope with?
10. Discuss the meanings and the thoughts triggered by the student's and elder's viewpoints expressed at the beginning of the chapter. How do these vary from your own experience?

*Students are advised to refer to their nursing diagnosis text and identify possible or potential problems.

RESEARCH QUESTIONS

1. What are the attitudes of nursing students toward older people and those who work in the field of aging?
2. Are there particular care settings and activities in which elderspeak is more prevalent?
3. What do older people think is helpful in enhancing communication with the hearing and vision impaired?
4. What are the major concerns of nurses related to communicating with a person with aphasia and what strategies do they find helpful in enhancing communication?
5. What benefits do older people experience in sharing their life story?
6. What are effective strategies for reminiscence and storytelling for older adults with cognitive impairment?
7. What are effective evaluation measures to measure understanding of health information?

REFERENCES

Adams-Wendling L, Pimple C: Evidence-based guideline: nursing management of hearing impairment in nursing facility residents, *Journal of Gerontological Nursing* 34:9, 2008.

Agency for Healthcare Research and Quality: Health literacy interventions and outcomes: an updated systematic review. March 2011. Available at http://www.ahrq.gov/clinic/epcsums/litupsum.pdf. Accessed April 2011.

American Tinnitus Association: ATA's top 10 most frequently asked questions, Available at www.ata.org. Accessed December 29, 2010.

Bastings A: Reading the story behind the story: context and content in stories by people with dementia, *Generations* 27:25, 2003.

Bastings A: Arts in dementia care: "This is not the end ... it's the end of this chapter," *Generations* 30:16, 2006.

Birren JE, Deutchman DE: *Guiding autobiography groups for older adults: exploring the fabric of life*, Baltimore, 1991, Johns Hopkins University Press.

Buckwalter KC, Gerdner LA, Hall GR, et al: Shining through: the humor and individuality of persons with Alzheimer's disease, *Journal of Gerontological Nursing* 21:11, 1995.

Buron B: Life history collages: effects on nursing home staff caring for residents with dementia, *Jour Gerontol Nurs* 36(12):38-48, 2010.

Butler R: The life review: an interpretation of reminiscence in the aged, *Psychiatry* 26:65, 1963.

Butler R: Age-ism: another form of bigotry, *The Gerontologist* 9:243, 1969.

Butler R: Age, death and life review (2002). Available at www.hospicefoundation.org. Accessed December 2010.

Butler R, Lewis M: *Aging and mental health: positive psychosocial approaches*, ed 3, St. Louis, MO, 1983, Mosby.

Capezuti J, Swicker D, Mezey M, Fulmer T, editors: *Evidence-based geriatric nursing protocols for best practice*, New York, 2008, Springer.

Centers for Disease Control and Prevention (CDC): *Improving health literacy for older adults: expert panel report 2009*. Atlanta, GA, U.S. Department of Health and Human Services, 2009.

Coles R: *The call of stories*, Boston, 1989, Houghton Mifflin.

Damianakis T, Crete-Nishihata M, Smith K, et al: The psychosocial impacts of multimedia biographies on persons with cognitive impairments, *The Gerontologist* 50:23, 2010).

Erikson EH: *Childhood and society*, ed 2, New York, 1963, WW Norton.

Fritsch T, Kwak J, Grant S, et al: Impact of TimeSlips, a creative expression intervention program, on nursing home staff and residents with dementia and their caregivers, *The Gerontologist* 49:117, 2009.

Glaucoma Research Foundation: Are you at risk for glaucoma (2008). Available at www.glaucoma.org. Accessed March 2008.

Grabowski D, Aschbrenner K, Tome V, et al: Quality of mental health care for nursing home residents: a literature review, *Medical Care Research and Review* 67:627, 2010. Available at http://mcr.sagepub.com/content/early/2010/03/11/1077558710362538. Accessed December 2010.

Haight B, Burnside IM: Reminiscence and life review: explaining the differences, *Archives of Psychiatric Nursing* 7:91, 1993.

Haight B, Webster J: *Critical advances in reminiscence work: from theory to application*, New York, 2002, Springer.

Hain D, Touhy T, Sparks M, Engstrom G: Hearing the whole story: assessment and interventions for individuals and couples living with early stage dementia. Unpublished manuscript.

Ham R, Sloane P, Warshaw G, et al: *Primary care geriatrics*, ed 5, St. Louis, MO, 2007, Mosby.

Happ M, Paull B: Silence is not golden, *Geriatric Nursing* 29:166, 2008.

Hayes K: Literacy for health information of adult patients and caregivers in the rural emergency department, *Clinical Excellence for Nurse Practitioners* 4:35, 2000.

Heliker D: Enhancing relationships in long-term care through story-sharing, *Jour Gerontol Nurs* 35(6):43-49, 2009.

Herman R, Williams K: Elderspeak's influence on resistiveness to care: focus on behavioral events, *American Journal of Alzheimer's Disease and Other Dementias* 24:417, 2009.

Hersh S: Cerumen: insights and management, *Annals of Long-term Care* 18:39, 2010.

International Longevity Center, Anti-Ageism Taskforce: *Ageism in America*, New York, 2006, Open Society Institute. Available at http://openlibrary.org/books/OL16396171M/Ageism_in_America. Accessed December 2010.

Keller H: *The story of my life*, Garden City, NY, 1902, Doubleday.

Kobylarz F, Pomidor A, Pleasant A: Health literacy as a tool to improve the public understanding of Alzheimer's disease, *Annals of Long-term Care* 18:34, 2010.

Koch J, Datta G, Makhdoom S, et al: Unmet visual needs of Alzheimer's patients in long-term care facilities, *Journal of the American Medical Directors Association* 6:233, 2005.

Levy B: Stereotype embodiment: a psychological approach to aging, *Current Directions in Psychological Science* 18:332, 2009.

Levy B, Slade M, Kunkel S, et al: Longevity increased by positive perceptions of aging,

Journal of Personality and Social Psychology 83:261, 2002.

Levy BR, Zonderman A, Slade M, et al: Age stereotypes held earlier in life predict cardiovascular events in later life, *Psychological Science* 20:296, 2009a.

Levy BR, Leifheit-Limson E: The stereotype-matching effect: greater influence on functioning when age stereotypes correspond to outcomes, *Psychology and Aging* 24:230, 2009b.

Miller C: *Nursing for wellness in older adults*, ed 5, Philadelphia, 2008, Wolters Kluwer/Lippincott Williams & Wilkins.

Moeller S, Taylor A, Tucker A et al: Associations between age-related nuclear cataract and lutein and zeaxanthin in the diet and serum in the carotenoids in the Age-Related Eye Disease Study (CAREDS), an ancillary study of the Women's Health Initiative, *Arch Opthalmol* 126(3)354-364, 2008.

National Aphasia Association: What is aphasia? (2010). Available at http://www.aphasia.org. Accessed December 2010.

National Eye Institute, National Institutes of Health: Survey of public knowledge, attitudes, and practices related to eye health and disease (2008). Available at www.nei.nih.gov/news/pressreleases/031308.asp#. Accessed December 2010.

National Eye Institute, National Institutes of Health: Vision loss from age will increase as Americans age (2010a). Available at http://www.nei.nih.gov/news/pressreleases/041204.asp. Accessed December 2010.

National Eye Institute, National Institutes of Health: About glaucoma (2010b). Available at http://www.nei.nih.gov/health/glaucoma/glaucoma_facts.asp. Accessed December 2010.

National Eye Institute: Diabetic Eye Disease (2010c). Available at www.nei.nih.gov/nehep/programs/diabeticeyedisease/goals.asp. Accessed December 2010.

National Eye Institute: Facts about macular degeneration, (2010d). Available at www.nei.nih.gov/health/maculardegen/armd_facts.asp. Accessed December 2010.

Owsley C, Ball K, McGwin G, et al: Effect of refractive error correction on health-related quality of life and depression in older nursing home residents, *Archives of Ophthalmology* 125:1471, 2007.

Pew Research Center: Older adults and social media (2010). Available at http://www.pewinternet.org/Reports/2010/Older-Adults-and-Social-Media.aspx. Accessed December 2010.

Perese E, Simon M, Ryan E: Promoting positive student clinical experiences with older adults through the use of group reminiscence therapy, *Jour Gerontol Nurs* 34(12), 2008.

Pott A, Bahlmeijer E, Onrust S, et al: The impact of life review on depression in older adults: a randomized controlled trial, *International Psychogeriatrics* 22:572, 2010.

Rogers M, Langa K: Untreated poor vision: a contributing factor to late-life dementia, *American Journal of Epidemiology* 171:728, 2010.

Rowe JW, Kahn RL: *Successful aging*, New York, 1998, Pantheon-Random House.

Sacks O: *Seeing voices: a journey into the world of the deaf*, Berkeley, 1989, University of California Press.

Schumm L, McClintock M, Williams S, et al: Assessment of sensory function in the National Social Life, Health, and Aging Project, *Journals of Gerontology Series B, Psychological Sciences and Social Sciences* 64(Suppl 1):i76, 2009.

Snyder L: The lived experience of Alzheimer's—understanding the feeling and subjective accounts of persons with the disease, *Alzheimer's Care Quarterly* 2:8, 2001.

Speros C: More than words: promoting health literacy in older adults, *The Online Journal of Issues in Nursing* 14(3), 2009.

Tak S, Beck C, McMahon E: Computer and Internet access for long-term care residents, *Journal of Gerontological Nursing* 33:32, 2007.

Tappen RM, Williams-Burgess C, Edelstein J, et al: Communicating with individuals with Alzheimer's disease: examination of recommended strategies, *Archives of Psychiatric Nursing* 11:249, 1997.

Tappen RM, Williams C, Fishman S, et al: Persistence of self in advanced Alzheimer's disease, *Image—the Journal of Nursing Scholarship* 31:121, 1999.

Thorsheim H, Roberts B: *I remember when: activity ideas to help people reminisce*, Forest Knolls, CA, 2000, Elder Books.

Touhy T, Williams C: Communicating with older adults. In: Williams C, editor: *Therapeutic interaction in nursing*, ed 2, Boston, 2008, Jones and Bartlett.

Touhy TA: Dementia, personhood, and nursing: learning from a nursing situation, *Nursing Science Quarterly* 17:43, 2004.

University of Wisconsin School of Medicine and Public Health: Hearing lose common in middle age, but could be preventable, February 21, 2011. Available at http://www.med.wise.edu/news-events/news/hearing-loss-common-in-middle-age-but-could-be-preventable/30654. Accessed April 2011.

VanLeuven KA: Health practices of older adults in good health: engagement is the key, *Journal of Gerontological Nursing* 36:38, 2010.

Wallhagen M: The stigma of hearing loss, *The Gerontologist* 50:66, 2009.

Wallhagen M, Pettengill E: Hearing impairment significant but underassessed in primary care settings, *Journal of Gerontological Nursing* 34:36, 2008.

Wallhagen M, Pettengill E, Whiteside M: Sensory impairment in older adults. 1. Hearing loss, *American Journal of Nursing* 106:40, 2006.

Williams C, Tappen R: Communicating with cognitively impaired persons. In Williams C, editor: *Therapeutic interaction in nursing*, ed 2, Boston, 2008, Jones and Bartlett.

Williams K: Improving outcomes of nursing home interactions, *Research in Nursing and Health* 29:121, 2006.

Williams K, Kemper S, Hummert L: Improving nursing home communication: an intervention to reduce elderspeak, *Gerontologist* 43:242, 2003.

Williams K, Kemper S, Hummert L: Enhancing communication with older adults: overcoming elderspeak, *Journal of Gerontological Nursing* 30:17, 2004.

Williams K, Herman R, Gajewski B, et al: Elderspeak communication: impact on dementia care, *American Journal of Alzheimer's Disease and Other Dementias* 24:11, 2008.

Wilson MR, Eezzuduemhoi DR: Opthalmologic disorders in minority populations, *Med Clin North Am* 89(4):795-804, 2005.

Health Assessment

Kathleen Jett

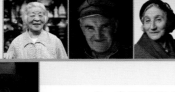

evolve *http://evolve.elsevier.com/Ebersole/TwdHlthAging*

A STUDENT SPEAKS

It takes so long to get a health history from an older person, they have so many stories. I now know to listen carefully and I will find out what I need to know. After all, most of them have had their health problem longer than I have been alive!

Michelle, age 20

AN ELDER SPEAKS

Whenever I go to one of my doctors I feel like they are rushing through and never really give me a good examination. Then I had an appointment with a nurse practitioner who specialized in us older folks. I couldn't believe the difference. I not only felt listened to but I also felt like I got the best exam I have had in a long time. I am sure it will help me get better!

Henry at age 76

LEARNING OBJECTIVES

On completion of this chapter, the reader will be able to:

1. List the essential components of the comprehensive health assessment of an older adult.

2. Discuss the advantages and disadvantages of the use of standardized tools in the gerontological assessment.

3. Describe the purpose of the inclusion of functional assessment when caring for an older adult.

In the promotion of healthy aging, gerontological nurses conduct skilled and detailed assessments of and with the persons who entrust themselves to their care. The process of assessment of older adults is strikingly different from that of younger adults in that it is more detailed even when problem-oriented. If a complete and comprehensive assessment is needed, this is usually performed by a number of members of the health care team, led by the nurse. A comprehensive assessment requires not only physical data but also an integration of the biological, cultural, psychosocial, and functional aspects of the person. Inquiries into physiological and anatomical function, growth and development, family relationships, group involvement, and religious and occupational pursuits are included.

Assessment of the older adult requires special abilities of the nurse: to listen patiently, to allow for pauses, to ask questions that are not often asked, to observe minute details, to obtain data from all available sources, and to recognize normal changes associated with late life that might be considered abnormal in one who is younger (see Chapter 4). In gerontological nursing, assessment takes more time than it does with younger adults

because of the increased medical and social complexities of living longer. The quality and speed of the assessment are an art born of experience. Novice nurses should neither be expected nor expect themselves to do this proficiently but should expect to see both their skills and the amount of information obtained increase over time. According to Benner (1984), assessment is a task for the expert. However, an expert is not always available. By using both a high degree of sensitivity, knowledge of normal changes with aging, and appropriate assessment tools, reasonably reliable data may be obtained by nurses at all skill levels.

The assessment provides information critical to the development of a plan of care that can enhance personal health status, decrease the potential for or the severity of chronic conditions, and encourage self-efficacy and empowerment for self-care. The nurse can consider the results of assessment as a snapshot of an individual's health status at the time it is completed. Periodic assessment of physical, functional, social, and mental status in health and illness allows for comparison with a baseline and for that which nursing care can be planned or adjusted. Health assessment is a complex process that requires entire textbooks to address in detail. In this chapter we provide an overview of parts of the assessment and discussion of tools that are particularly unique or helpful in caring for the older adult.

THE HEALTH HISTORY

The initiation of the health history marks the beginning of the nurse–client relationship and the assessment process. The health history is collected either in written format or verbally in a face-to-face interview or in combination. The history may be given by the person or through a proxy, with the person's consent. If the elder has limited English proficiency, a knowledgeable interpreter is needed and the interview will generally take approximately double the amount of time.

Any health history form or interview should include a patient profile, a past medical history, a review of symptoms and systems, a medication history (prescribed, over-the-counter, "home remedies," and herbals and dietary supplements), and a social history. The health history also includes the self- or proxy-report of functional status. The social history of the older adult should include the current living arrangements, economic resources to deal with current health issues, amount of family and friend support if needed, and the types of community resources available if needed or used. It should also include the identification of those who are involved in health care decision-making and state of advanced care planning. For those who are very old, a family history is only relevant secondary to the social history.

To meet the needs of our increasingly diverse population of elders, the use of questions related to the explanatory model (Kleinman, 1980) is recommended to complement the standard health history, making it applicable to everyone (Box 7-1). The responses will better enable the nurse to understand the elder and plan culturally appropriate and effective interventions.

A comprehensive assessment includes psychological parameters such as cognitive and emotional well-being; caregiver stress or burden; the individual's self-perception of health; and patterns of health and health care, education, family structure, plans for retirement, and living environment. For those living at home, a home safety assessment is important. Areas or problems not frequently addressed by the care provider or mentioned by the elder but that should be addressed are sexual dysfunction, depression, incontinence, alcoholism, hearing loss, and memory loss or confusion (Ham, 2002).

PHYSICAL ASSESSMENT

The health history is followed by the physical assessment or examination at that time or at a time in the near future. Although the manual techniques of the examination do not differ significantly from those used with younger persons, knowledge of the normal changes with aging is essential for the appropriate analysis of the data obtained. When assessing persons from ethnically distinct groups, is it also necessary to be aware of cultural rules of etiquette and taboos that influence the examination (Box 7-2) (see also Chapter 5).

Because of the complex interrelationship among the parts of the complete assessment process, the use of a model or tools may be helpful. The website of the Hartford Institute for

---

BOX 7-1   THE EXPLANATORY MODEL FOR CULTURALLY SENSITIVE ASSESSMENT

1. How would you describe the problem that has brought you here? (What do you call your problem; does it have a name?)
   a. Who is involved in your decision-making about health concerns?
2. How long have you had this problem?
   a. When do you think it started?
   b. What do you think started it?
   c. Do you know anyone else with it?
   d. Tell me what happened to that person when dealing with this problem.
3. What do you think is wrong with you?
   a. How severe is it?
   b. How long do you think it will last?
4. Why do you think this happened to you?
   a. Why has it happened to the involved part?
   b. What do you fear most about your sickness?
5. What are the chief problems your sickness has caused you?
6. What do you think will help clear up this problem? (What treatment should you receive and what are the most important results you hope to receive?)
   a. If specific tests, medications are listed, ask what they are and do.
7. Apart from me, who else do you think can make you feel better?
   a. Are there therapies that make you feel better that I do not know? (Maybe in another discipline?)

Modified from Kleinman A: *Patient and healers in the context of culture: an exploration of the borderland between anthropology, medicine, and psychiatry*, Berkeley, CA, 1980, University of California Press; Pfeifferling JH: A cultural prescription for mediocentrism. In Eisenberg L, Kleinman A, editors: *The relevance of social science for medicine*, Boston, 1981, Reidel.

BOX 7-2   KEY POINTS TO CONSIDER IN OBSERVING CULTURAL RULES AND ETIQUETTE

- Social organization and expectations (e.g., roles of family members and friends)
- Communication style, especially in the health care setting
- Use of personal space and eye contact
- General health orientation related to time (past, present, future)
- Appropriate wording of greetings
- Appropriate use of names
- Appropriateness of touch, especially between genders

Geriatric Nursing (New York, NY; http://hartfordign.org) provides a compilation of key tools used in assessment in their *Try This* series. New evidence-based protocols are regularly added. The tools and directions for their use can be viewed at http://hartfordign.org. This site is a portal to a wealth of information, especially for assessing a number of specific conditions or situations, such as fall risk or restraint use.

Two tools for a basic overall assessment of older adults and those who are medically vulnerable are SPICES and FANCAPES. They use a framework with an emphasis on function at the most basic level and the extent to which assistance is necessary. When alterations are found then further assessment in that particular area is indicated (Montgomery et al., 2008). The acronym *FANCAPES* stands for Fluids, Aeration, Nutrition, Communication, Activity, Pain, Elimination, and Socialization

and social skills. *SPICES* is the mnemonic for Sleep disorders, Problems with eating or feeding, Incontinence, Confusion, Evidence of falls, and Skin breakdown. Both can be used in all settings, may be used in part or total (depending on the need), and are easily adaptable to the functional pattern grouping if nursing diagnoses are used.

Fancapes

Fluids

Evaluation of fluids requires an assessment of the client's state of hydration and those physiological, situational, and mental factors that contribute to the maintenance of adequate hydration. Attention is directed to the ability of the person to obtain adequate fluids independently, to express thirst, to swallow effectively, and to evaluate medications that affect intake and output.

Aeration

Aeration refers to the adequacy of oxygen exchange. Observations include respiratory rate and depth at rest and during activity; talking, walking, and situations requiring added exertion; and the presence or absence of edema in the extremities or abdomen. At a minimum, breath sounds should be evaluated and medications reviewed to evaluate their effects on aeration. A determination of oxygen saturation level is essential any time that respiratory compromise is suspected, such as the potential of pneumonia.

Nutrition

Nutrition assessment includes mechanical and psychological factors in addition to the type and amount of food consumed; ability to bite, chew, and swallow; fit of dentures and condition of the gums and teeth. Alterations in diet related to culture, medical restrictions, available economic resources, and living conditions should be included. If a special diet is needed, it is necessary to know and work with the person who prepares meals if other than the elder. Visual and neurological impairment, which might interfere with the person's ability to prepare a meal or feed him- or herself, should be noted. Functional or economic status may interfere with obtaining groceries or foods for special diets.

Communication

Communication includes sending and receiving verbal and nonverbal information. Assessment of communicative ability includes the determination of sight and sound acuity; voice quality; and adequate function of the tongue, teeth, pharynx, and larynx. Appraisals of the person's ability to read, write, and understand the spoken language of the nurse should be ascertained. This is an important issue, since an undetected limitation of these skills can lead to erroneous conclusions or to the patient's inability to follow directions. Determination of both literacy and health literacy is necessary.

Activity

Although the ability to ambulate is a major component in activity assessment, activity includes more than movement or exercise. The nurse assesses the person's ability to eat, toilet, dress, and groom; to prepare meals; to use the telephone; and to move about with or without assistive devices. Coordination and balance, finger dexterity, grip strength, and other abilities necessary in daily life should also be assessed.

Pain

Physical, mental, and spiritual pain is considered. The presence and absence of pressure and discomfort are key aspects of pain assessment. Information about recent losses or visible symptoms of anxiety may help identify persons in pain. The manner by which a client customarily attains relief from pain or discomfort will provide further information.

Elimination

Bladder and bowel elimination are assessed and include evidence of urinary dribbling or incontinence, use of protective garments or devices. and medications that affect voiding and intestinal peristalsis. The nurse and patient will need to find words that they both understand when talking about bowel and bladder functioning. The words used in health care, such as "stooling" or "voiding," should be avoided unless it is known that they are understood.

Social Skills

Assessment of socialization and social skills includes the individual's ability to negotiate in society, to give and receive love and friendship, and to feel self-worth. Assessment focuses on the individual's ability to deal with loss and to interact with other people in give-and-take situations.

Spices

The Fulmer SPICES has been used widely with older adults as an overall assessment tool regardless of health status or setting (Wallace and Fulmer, 2007). The acronym *SPICES* refers to six common geriatric syndromes of the elderly that require nursing interventions: Sleep disorders, Problems with eating or feeding, Incontinence, Confusion, Evidence of falls, and Skin breakdown. Like with FANCAPES, anything that indicates a problem in one of the categories warns the nurse that more in-depth assessment is needed. It is a system for alerting the nurse to the most common problems that interfere with the health and well-being of older adults, particularly those who have one or more medical conditions.

Functional Assessment

Whereas the emphasis of FANCAPES and SPICES is on physical parameters and those associated with geriatric syndromes, a full functional assessment is broader. It encompasses the evaluation of a person's ability to carry out basic tasks for self-care and tasks needed to support independent living. A thorough functional assessment will help the gerontological nurse work toward healthy aging by accomplishing the following:

- Identifying the specific areas in which help is needed or not needed
- Identifying changes in abilities from one period of time to another
- Determining the need for specific service(s)
- Providing information that may be useful in assessing the safety of a particular living situation

Numerous tools are available that describe, screen, assess, monitor, and predict functional ability. The major tools used in functional assessment determine the individual's ability to perform the tasks needed for self-care (i.e., those needed to maintain one's health), referred to as *activities of daily living (ADLs)*, and, separately, those tasks needed for independent living (i.e., those needed to maintain one's home), referred to as *instrumental activities of daily living* (IADLs). ADLs and IADLs are universal needs; how these needs are met is socially and culturally constructed.

The majority of tools do not break down a task (e.g., eating) into its component parts, such as picking up a spoon or cup or swallowing water; eating is seen as a total task when a person may be able to perform one part and not the other. Most of the tools result in a score of some kind—a rating of the person's ability to do the task alone, to need assistance, or to not be able to perform the task at all. These categories are intended to be mutually exclusive. The ratings are done by self-report, proxy, or observer. It should be noted that research has found that self-reports usually overestimate, and proxies underestimate, abilities to perform activities of daily living. The tools are beneficial in their ability to serve the purposes just noted. However, most are not sensitive to small changes and can be used only as part of a holistic assessment.

The FAST (Functional Assessment Staging) tool for Alzheimer's disease was designed by Barry Reisberg in 1988. It has been found to be a reliable and valid measurement for the evaluation and staging of functional decline in persons with Alzheimer's disease (Sclan and Reisberg, 1992). The tool uses ordinal ranking of seven stages beginning with what is referred to as a "normal adult" to one with "severe dementia." This can be used to plan care and work with the individual and family to prepare for future needs. Varitions of this tool can be easily found on the internet.

Activities of Daily Living

What have become know as activities of daily living (ADLs) were first classified as such in 1963 by Sidney Katz and colleagues. These include bathing, dressing, toileting, continence, transferring (refers to ambulation as well), and feeding. Two of these tasks (dressing [including grooming], and bathing) require higher cognitive function than the others.

Katz Index

The Katz Index (Katz et al., 1963) has served as a basic framework for most of the measures of ADLs since that time (Figure 7-1). There are several versions of the Katz Index. One is based on a three-point scale and allows one to score client

	Independence (1 point) NO supervision, direction, or personal assistance	Dependence (0 points) WITH supervision, direction, personal assistance, or total care
BATHING Points:_____	(1 point) Bathes self completely or needs help in bathing only a single part of the body such as the back, genital area, or disabled extremity.	(0 points) Needs help with bathing more than one part of the body, getting in or out of the tub or shower. Requires total bathing.
DRESSING Points:_____	(1 point) Gets clothes from closets and drawers and puts on clothes and outer garments complete with fasteners. May have help tying shoes.	(0 points) Needs help with dressing self or needs to be completely dressed.
TOILETING Points:_____	(1 point) Goes to toilet, gets on and off the toilet, arranges clothes, cleans genital area without help.	(0 points) Needs help transferring to the toilet, cleaning self, or uses bedpan or commode.
TRANSFERRING Points:_____	(1 point) Moves in and out of bed or chair unassisted. Mechanical transferring aids are acceptable.	(0 points) Needs help in moving from bed to chair or requires a complete transfer.
CONTINENCE Points:_____	(1 point) Exercises complete self-control over urination and defecation.	(0 points) Is partially or totally incontinent of bowel or bladder.
FEEDING Points:_____	(1 point) Gets food from plate into mouth without help. Preparation of food may be done by another person.	(0 points) Needs partial or total help with feeding or requires parenteral feeding.

TOTAL POINTS: _____   6 = High (patient independent)   0 = Low (patient very dependent)

FIGURE 7-1 Katz Index of Independence in Activities of Daily Living. (From Katz S, Downs TD, Cash HR, et al: Progress in development of the index of ADL, *Gerontologist* 10:20, 1970.)

performance abilities as independent, assistive, dependent, or unable to perform. Another version of the tool assigns 1 point to each ADL that can be completed independently and a zero (0) if it cannot. Scores will range from a maximum of 6 (totally independent) to 0 (totally dependent). A score of 4 indicates moderate impairment, whereas 2 or less indicates severe impairment (see Figure 7-1). This scoring puts equal weight on all activities, and the determination of a cutoff score is completely arbitrary. Despite these limitations, the tool is useful because it creates a common language about functioning for all caregivers involved in planning overall care and discharge.

Barthel Index and Functional Independence Measure

The Barthel Index (BI; Mahoney and Barthel, 1965) and the Functional Independence Measure (FIM) are the two tools most commonly used in the rehabilitation setting to assess a person's need for assistance with ADLs. The data are used for both inpatient and postdischarge planning relative to the amount of physical assistance required. In some studies the BI and FIM were found to be comparable (Sangha et al., 2005). In others the FIM was deemed preferable (Kidd et al., 1995). The BI has proved easy to use and especially useful as a method of documenting improvement of a patient's ability. The BI ranks functional status as either independent or dependent and then allows for further classification of "independent" as intact or limited, and of "dependent" as needing a helper or unable to do the activity at all. Instruction is needed in the use and scoring of this tool before using it. The FIM is widely used and the most comprehensive functional assessment tool for rehabilitation settings. It includes measures of ADL, mobility, cognition, and social functioning. It has been widely tested and rates 18 ADLs on a seven-point scale from independent to dependent. The items are sorted into 13 motor items and 5 cognitive items. The tool is highly sensitive but complex and requires training to use accurately and to obtain interrater reliability. Ordinarily the tool is completed by the joint efforts of the multi-disciplinary team and used for both planning and evaluation of progress. Use of this instrument can be requested from the Uniform Data System for Medical Rehabilitation (www.udsmr.org).

Instrumental Activities of Daily Living

The instrumental activities of daily living (IADLs) are tasks needed for independent living, such as cleaning, yard work, shopping, and money management. The successful performance of IADLs requires a higher level of cognitive and physical functioning than do the ADLs. For persons with dementia, the progressive loss of the ability to perform IADLs begins with those that require the highest cognitive functions, such as handling finances and shopping. The original scoring tool for IADLs was developed by Lawton and Brody (1969). Both the original tool and the subsequent iterations again use the self-report, proxy, and observed formats with the three levels of functioning (independent, assisted, and unable to perform). The pros and cons of using these are the same as for the measures of ADLs.

The ADLs and IADLs can also be measured on the basis of performance or demonstration of such. These tools overcome the problems associated with self-report and proxy report and yield more objective measurement of functional status. They take longer to conduct but are more likely to be reliable. One such tool is the "Timed Get-Up-and-Go" test, which is used widely, usually in association with fall risk determination. A protocol for the use of this instrument can be found easily with a web search for the title.

Function and Cognition

When assessing both functional status and cognitive abilities, slightly different tools are indicated. The Blessed Dementia Scale is a 22-item tool that incorporates aspects of ADLs, IADLs, memory, recalling events, and finding one's way outdoors (Blessed et al., 1968). The higher the score, the greater the degree of dementia assessed. The Clinical Dementia Rating (Morris, 1993) and the Global Deterioration Scale (Reisberg et al., 1982) also assess both functional and cognitive abilities and are used to stage dementia including those with mild cognitive impairment (MCI). The Deterioration Scale and several other tools have been found sensitive enough to show therapeutic changes, such as those related to medication adjustments (Reisberg, 2007). Determining the functional and cognitive stage of the dementia can allow the nurse to provide considerable anticipatory teaching to both the family and other caregivers.

SCREENING ASSESSMENT OF COGNITION AND MOOD

Older adults are at great risk for impairments in mental capacity. Cognitive ability is easily threatened by any disturbance in health or homeostasis which can rapidly lead to delirium. Altered mental status may be the first sign of anything from a heart attack to a urinary tract infection. In a general assessment it is helpful to have baseline measures of cognition and mood. However, this is especially important if there are any indications of potential problems. For those with potential problems, any screening may be particularly stressful and necessitate providing an environment and relationship of trust to achieve the most accurate data and produce the least amount of stress or embarrassment. Such screening may be described to the person as similar to auscultation of the heart to "see how it is doing." Like most other assessments these are best administered when the person is comfortable, rested, and free of pain. Gerontological nursing requires skills in basic assessment of mental status, especially cognition and mood, and sensitivity to subtle changes that may indicate a reversible health problem. Positive findings indicate a need for more in-depth evaluations (see Chapters 18 and 19).

Mental Status Examination
Mini-Mental State Examination

The Mini-Mental State Examination (MMSE), the tool most often used in the assessment of mental status, was created by Folstein and colleagues (1975). It is a 30-item instrument that is used to screen for and monitor cognitive function (Wattmo et al., 2010). It remains a useful tool for gross screening of dementia (Mitchell and Malladi, 2010). It tests orientation, short-term memory and attention, calculation ability, language, and construction. Construction may be a proxy measure for

---

MMSE-2 Sample Items

Orientation to Time
"What day is today?"

Naming
"What is this?" [Point to eye.]

Repetition
"Now I am going to ask you to repeat what I say. Ready?
It is a lovely, sunny day but too warm. Now you say that."
[*Wait for examinee response and record response
verbatim. Repeat up to one time.*]

FIGURE 7-2 Mini-Mental State Examination-2. If using this tool, it is recommended that the original instructions found in this chapter be reviewed, especially for persons with visual or manual limitations. The score must be adjusted for low education levels. It is not standardized for non–English-speaking persons. (Reproduced by special permission of the publisher, Psychological Assessment Resources (PAR), Inc., 16204 North Florida Avenue, Lutz, FL 33549, from the Mini-Mental State Examination, by Marshal F. Folstein, MD and Susan E. Folstein, MD, Copyright 1975, 1998, 2001 and the Mini-Mental State Examination-2, Copyright 2010 by Mini Mental LLC, Inc. Published 2001, 2010 by Psychological Assessment Resources, Inc. Further reproduction is prohibited without permission of PAR, Inc. The MMSE-2 can be purchased from PAR, Inc. by calling (813) 968-3003.)

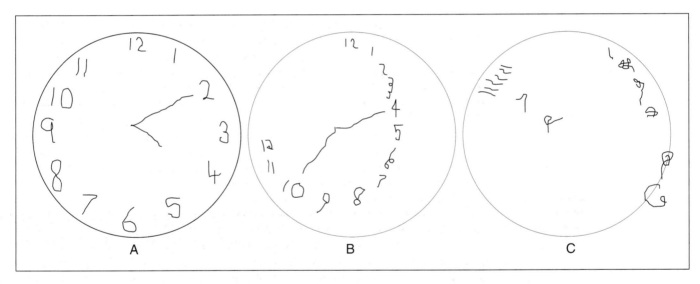

FIGURE 7-3 Examples of Results of a Clock Drawing Test. **A,** Unimpaired; **B** and **C,** impaired. (From Stern TA, Rosenbaum JF, Fava M, et al: *Massachusetts General Hospital comprehensive clinical psychiatry,* ed 1, St. Louis, MO, 2008, Mosby.)

executive function (Figure 7-2). To ensure reliability, it must be administered correctly each time it is used. It cannot be given to persons who cannot see or write or who are not proficient in English. A score of 30 suggests no impairment and a score of 26 or less suggests potential dementia; however, adjustments are needed for educational level. It is more useful for ruling out dementia than for diagnosis. It has little utility for screening for MCI (Mitchell, 2009).

Clock Drawing Test

The Clock Drawing Test is reported to be second only to the MMSE in use across the world (Aprahamian et al., 2010). Although it is useful for the screening and diagnosis of

dementia, it cannot be used to identify those with MCI (Ehreke et al., 2010). The Clock Drawing Test assesses executive function and has been in use since 1992 (Shulman, 2000). Some level of manual dexterity and visual acuity is required and therefore not appropriate for use with individuals who are blind or who have severe arthritis, Parkinson's disease, or stroke that affects their dominant hand. While reading fluency is not necessary, number fluency is. A person is presented with a piece of paper with a circle drawn on it. He or she is then asked to draw the face of a clock and then have the hands indicate 3:45 or 11:10 or a similar time (Figure 7-3). Scoring is based on both the position of the numbers and the position of the hands (Box 7-3). This tool does not establish criteria for dementia, but does

BOX 7-3   CLOCK DRAWING TEST

INSTRUCTIONS

1. Provide the person with a piece of plain white paper with a circle drawn on it, usually about 5 inches in diameter.
2. Ask the person to draw numbers in the circle so that it looks like a clock, and then to put the hands in the circle to read "10 after 11."

SCORING*

WHAT IS DRAWN	POINTS SCORED
Draws closed circle	1 point
Places numbers in correct position	1 point
Includes all 12 correct numbers	1 point
Places hands in correct position	1 point

INTERPRETATIONS

- Errors such as grossly distorted contour or extraneous markings are rarely produced by cognitively intact persons.
- Clinical judgment must be applied, but a low score indicates the need for further evaluation.

*See the website of the Iowa Geriatric Education Center (University of Iowa, Iowa City, IA): https://www.healthcare.uiowa.edu/igec/tools/cognitive/clockDrawing.pdf. Accessed December 2010.

test for constructional apraxia, an early indicator of dementia (Evans, 2008). For details of scoring see the website of the Iowa Geriatric Education Center (University of Iowa, Iowa City, IA) (https://www.healthcare.uiowa.edu/igec/tools/cognitive/clockDrawing.pdf).

Mini-Cog

Historically the MMSE has been the standard tool for screening of mental status/cognitive status. However, the Mini-Cog has been found to be equivalent to the MMSE, less biased, easier to administer, and possibly more sensitive to dementia (Evans, 2008). Although the Mini-Cog was developed some time ago, it is now receiving attention as a cognitive tool that is useful in primary care settings (Mitchell and Malladi, 2010). It assesses short-term memory and executive function. Although it does require the ability to hear, hold a pencil, and write numbers, it is brief and highly sensitive and specific for dementia. To administer the Mini-Cog the three-item recall of the MMSE is combined with the Clock Drawing Test (Box 7-4).

BOX 7-4   THE MINI-COG

1. Say three unrelated words, say each word clearly, about 1 second each.
2. Ask the person to repeat these, (following the instructions in the MMSE*).
3. The person is asked to draw a clock as in the Clock Drawing Test.
4. The person is asked to recall the three words from step 1.

Scoring: Points are awarded for recalled words first. None remembered: dementia likely; all three remembered: dementia unlikely; recall of one or two words upon considering the results of the clock drawing: normal (all numbers and hands correct) or abnormal (any errors).

MMSE, Mini-Mental State Examination.

*If the person is unable to repeat the three words, this is suggestive of impaired cognition, and proceeding with the Mini-Cog is not appropriate. For more information, see Doerflinger C: How to try this: the Mini-Cog, *American Journal of Nursing* 107:62, 2007.

Assessment of Mood

Additional screening tools are necessary to assess mood. This is especially important because of the high rate of depression among older adults; it may be a side effect of a medication or highly associated with some health conditions such as stroke or Parkinson's disease. Persons with untreated or undertreated depression are more functionally impaired and will have prolonged hospitalizations and nursing home stays, lowered quality of life, increased morbidity overall, and reduced longevity. Persons with depression may appear as if they have dementia, and many persons with dementia are also depressed. The interconnection between the two calls for skill and sensitivity on the part of the nurse to ensure that elders receive the most appropriate and effective care possible. Although several tools have been used (e.g., the Beck Depression Inventory [Beck, 1987] or the Zung Depression Scale [Zung, 1965]), the one that is used most often is the Geriatric Depression Scale. The Depression Scale of the Cornell for epidiological studies designed for research; it is now seen in clinical assessments. The Cornell Scale is an observational tool specifically applied to those persons with dementia.

Geriatric Depression Scale

The Geriatric Depression Scale (GDS), developed by Yesavage and colleagues (1983), is a 30-item tool developed specifically for screening older adults and has been tested extensively in a number of settings. Both 15- and 5-item shortened versions are now available (Table 7-1). The GDS is also available in Spanish (Ortiz and Romero, 2008). The GDS has been extremely successful in identifying depression in older adults because it deemphasizes physical complaints, libido, and appetite (Lach et al., 2010). Byrd (2005) notes that one drawback of the shortened versions is that they do not include a question on suicidal

TABLE 7-1   GERIATRIC DEPRESSION SCALE (SHORT FORM)

Are you basically satisfied with your life?	Yes	No*
Have you dropped many of your activities and interests?	Yes*	No
Do you feel that your life is empty?	Yes*	No
Do you often get bored?	Yes*	No
Are you in good spirits most of the time?	Yes	No*
Are you afraid that something bad is going to happen to you?	Yes*	No
Do you feel happy most of the time?	Yes	No*
Do you often feel helpless?	Yes*	No
Do you prefer to stay at home, rather than going out and doing new things?	Yes*	No
Do you feel you have more problems with memory than most?	Yes*	No
Do you think it is wonderful to be alive?	Yes	No*
Do you feel pretty worthless the way you are now?	Yes*	No
Do you feel full of energy?	Yes	No*
Do you feel that your situation is hopeless?	Yes*	No
Do you think that most people are better off than you?	Yes*	No

*Each answer indicated by an asterisk counts as one point. Scores between 5 and 9 suggest depression; scores above 9 generally indicate depression.

From Yesavage J, Brink TL, Rose TL, et al: Development and validation of a Geriatric Depression Screening Scale: a preliminary report, *Journal of Psychiatric Research* 17:37, 1982-1983.

BOX 7-5	CENTER FOR EPIDEMIOLOGIC STUDIES DEPRESSION SCALE

INSTRUCTIONS FOR QUESTIONS

Below is a list of the ways you might have felt or behaved. Please tell me how often you have felt this way during the past week.

Rarely or none of the time (less than 1 day)
Some or a little of the time (1-2 days)
Occasionally or a moderate amount of time (3-4 days)
Most or all of the time (5-7 days)

During the Past Week:

1. I was bothered by things that usually don't bother me.
2. I did not feel like eating; my appetite was poor.
3. I felt that I could not shake off the blues even with help from my family or friends.
4. I felt that I was just as good as other people.
5. I had trouble keeping my mind on what I was doing.
6. I felt depressed.
7. I felt that everything I did was an effort.
8. I felt hopeful about the future.
9. I thought my life had been a failure.
10. I felt fearful.
11. My sleep was restless.
12. I was happy.
13. I talked less than usual.
14. I felt lonely.
15. People were unfriendly.
16. I enjoyed life.
17. I had crying spells.
18. I felt sad.
19. I felt that people dislike me.
20. I could not get "going."

From Radloff LS: The CES-D Scale: a self-report depression scale for research in the general population, *Applied Psychological Measurement* 1:385, 1977.

intent or thoughts. See the website of ConsultGeriRN.org (http://consultgerirn.org/topics/depression/want_to_know_more), the geriatric clinical nursing website of the Hartford Institute for Geriatric Nursing, for more information.

Center for Epidemiologic Studies Depression Scale

The Center for Epidemiologic Studies Depression Scale (CES-D) (Box 7-5) was developed for use in studies of depression in community samples and is frequently used in research. The CES-D seems to provide the most consistently accurate results, particularly with nonwhite older adults, and has been reported to be significantly better than the GDS for both black and white individuals, with higher specificity and sensitivity. The original CES-D contains 20 items, but a shortened, 10-item version has been reported to be a valid screening measure (Heller et al., 2010).

Cornell Scale for Depression in Dementia

The Cornell Scale for Depression in Dementia (CSD-D) was designed to identify major depressive disorders in persons who may have dementia. As some persons with dementia are able to participate in health screening, the person is first interviewed followed by a proxy, that is, someone who is familiar with the person on a day-to-day basis. The interview results can usually be corroborated by skilled observation. Each item is introduced

with "I am going to ask you questions about you/how your relative has been feeling during the past week. I am interested in changes you have noticed and the duration of these changes." There are ample sources for this tool available on the Internet with a simple search for "Cornell Scale."

COMPREHENSIVE GERIATRIC ASSESSMENT

In some cases an integrated approach is used rather than a collection of separate tools. The most well known is the classic Older Americans Resources and Services (OARS), developed by Pfeiffer (1979) and colleagues at Duke University (Durham, NC). The Comprehensive Assessment and Referral Evaluation (CARE) tool was designed for assessment of functional status and mental health (Gurland et al., 1977). These and other tools were considered in the development of the Minimum Data Set (MDS), used in skilled nursing facilities during which time the resident is covered by Medicare. In the home care setting, the Outcomes and Assessment Information Set (OASIS), a computerized assessment tool, is universally used at this time. All these tools are quite comprehensive and therefore quite lengthy. Once completed, they serve as a resource for a detailed plan of care.

The Minimum Data Set

The Minimum Data Set (MDS), a product of the Centers for Medicare and Medicaid, is a comprehensive assessment used in the nursing home setting as a mean to not only plan and monitor care, but in aggregate use, to describe the care in the long-term care setting at large. Recently revised, the MDS 3.0 includes evidence-based measures for pain, cognition, delirium and depression and requires that the facilities use other expert tools of their choice for other aspects of the assessment (Augustine and Capitosti, 2010) (Box 7-6). In a significant change from its previous version, resident interviews are part of five sections of the document. Giving the residents an opportunity to express their own voices revealed that past assessments underestimated depressed mood and pain significantly. In a national trial the 3.0 version was found to be highly accurate, clinical relevant, efficient and improved the detection of clinical problems (Saliba

BOX 7-6	COMPONENTS OF THE MINIMUM DATA SET 3.0

Hearing, Speech and Vision
Cognitive patterns (includes cognitive skills for daily decision making)
Mood
Behavior, including response to care
Preference (level of importance) for Customary Routine and Activities
Activities of Daily Living and Mobility
Bowel and Bladder
Active Disease Diagnoses
Health Conditions, e.g., pain, shortness of breath, history of falls
Swallowing and Nutrition
Oral and Dental Status
Skin conditions
Medications
Special Treatments and procedures, e.g., chemotherapy, oxygen, dialysis, immunization status
Restraints
Participation in assessment and goal setting

and Buchanan, 2008). The data contained within the MDS are also used (in the form of RUGS) to determine the reimbursement that the facility will receive for any particular patient stay under the prospective payment system (Shephard, 2010). A multi-disciplinary tool, parts are completed by different members of the team (e.g., physical therapy, social work, nursing, etc.) but its completion requires the coordination and signature of a registered nurse. The MDS is completed at scheduled times beginning at admission.

Older Americans Resources and Services

The OARS assessment tool is designed so that each component can be used individually. This enables it to be added to or integrated into self-designed tools. It was designed to evaluate ability, disability, and the capacity level at which the person is able to function. Five dimensions are considered for assessment: social resources, economic resources, mental health, physical health, and ADLs. Each component uses a quantitative rating scale: 1, excellent; 2, good; 3, mildly impaired; 4, moderately impaired; 5, severely impaired; and 6, completely impaired. At the conclusion of the assessment, a cumulative impairment score (CIS) is established, which can range from the most fit (score 6) to total disability (score, 30). This aids in establishing the degree of need. Information considered in each domain includes the material in the following sections.

Social Resources

The Social Resources dimension of the OARS evaluates the social skills and the ability to negotiate and make friends (the number of times friends are seen, the number of telephone conversations). In the assessment interview, is the person able to ask for things from friends, family, and strangers? Is a caregiver (or caregivers) available if needed? Who are they, and how long are they available? Does the elder belong to any social network or group, such as a special interest or church synagogue, ashram, temple or other religious community group?

Economic Resources

Data about monthly income and sources (Social Security, Supplemental Security Income, pensions, income generated from capital) are needed to determine the adequacy of income compared with the cost of living and food, shelter, clothing, medications, and small luxury items. This information can provide insight into the elder's relative standard of living and point out areas of need that might be alleviated by the use of additional resources.

Mental Health

Consideration is given to intellectual function, the presence or absence of psychiatric symptoms, and the amount of enjoyment and interaction the person gets from life.

Physical Health

The Physical Health dimension includes the diagnosis of major and common diseases of the type of prescribed and over-the-counter medications the person is taking, and the person's perception of his or her health status. Excellent physical health includes participation in regular vigorous activity, such as walking, dancing, or biking, at least twice each week. Seriously impaired physical health is determined by the presence of one or more illnesses or disabilities that are severely painful or life-threatening or that require extensive care.

Activities of Daily Living

The ADLs included in the OARS are walking, getting into and out of bed, bathing, combing hair, shaving, dressing, eating, and getting to the bathroom on time by oneself. The IADLs measured include tasks such as dialing the telephone, driving a car, hanging up clothes, obtaining groceries, and taking medications and having correct knowledge of their dosages.

PROMOTING HEALTHY AGING: IMPLICATIONS FOR GERONTOLOGICAL NURSING

Whether the nurse is working with a standardized instrument or creating a new one, the goal of assessment is always to assist the patient in improving his or her quality of life. The nurse is expected to collect data that are the most accurate and to do so in the most efficient yet caring manner possible. The use of tools serves as a way to organize the collected data necessary for assessment and to be able to compare data obtained at various times. Each tool has strengths and weaknesses, as does each completed assessment. A number of factors complicate assessment of the older adult. These include the difficulty of differentiating the effects of aging from those originating from disease, the coexistence of multiple diseases, the underreporting of symptoms by older adults, atypical presentation or nonspecific presentation of illness, and the increase in iatrogenic illnesses.

Overdiagnosis or underdiagnosis occurs when the normal age changes are not considered; these include both physical changes and biochemical changes. Underdiagnosis is far more common in the care of the elderly. Many symptoms or complaints are ascribed to normal aging rather than to a disease entity that may be developing. Difficulty in assessing the older adult with multiple chronic conditions is also a challenge. Symptoms of one condition can exacerbate or mask symptoms of another. The gerontological nurse is challenged to provide the highest level of excellence in the assessment of the elderly without burdening the person in the process.

KEY CONCEPTS

- Assessment of the physical, cognitive, psychosocial, and environmental status is essential to meeting the specific needs of the older adult and implementing appropriate interventions.
- Whether the data for an assessment tool are collected by self-report, by report-by-proxy, or through nurse observation will affect the quality and quantity of the data.
- Knowledge of how to use a particular gerontological assessment tool is needed to accurately administer it.
- Comorbidity of many older adults complicates obtaining and interpreting assessment data.

CASE STUDY   A COMPREHENSIVE ASSESSMENT

Eighty-year-old Mrs. Hernandez is newly admitted to your acute care hospital unit. She is there for observation and testing after a witnessed syncopal episode. She lives with her 90-year-old husband, who has mild dementia, and her 60-year-old daughter. Her daughter admits to you that neither of her parents has been doing well and that the doctors "just haven't been able to figure it out." You know that Mrs. Hernandez will be receiving both neurological and cardiac testing. However, as a gerontological nurse you also know that she and her family may benefit most from a comprehensive evaluation. The decision of which assessments to do is within the scope of practice for nurses at your facility.

On the basis of the case study, develop a nursing care plan using the following procedure*:

- List Mrs. Hernandez's comments that provide subjective data.
- List information that provides objective data.
- From these data, identify and state, using accepted format, two nursing diagnoses you determine are most significant to Mrs. Hernandez at this time.
- List two of Mrs. Hernandez's strengths that you have identified from the data.
- Determine and state outcome criteria for each diagnosis. These must reflect some alleviation of the problem identified in the nursing diagnosis and must be stated in concrete and measurable terms.
- Plan and state one or more interventions for each diagnosed problem. Provide specific documentation of the source used to determine the appropriate intervention. Plan at least one intervention that incorporates Mrs. Hernandez's existing strengths.
- Evaluate the success of the intervention. Interventions must correlate directly with the stated outcome criteria to measure the outcome success.

CRITICAL THINKING QUESTIONS

1. What is your reason for selecting the type of assessment you will do, and what is the reason for your ranking?
2. Of the assessment tools that are available to you, which will be the most reasonable to perform within the limitations of an acute care setting?
3. How would any of your answers to the preceding questions change in a skilled nursing facility? Assisted living facility? In the home setting?
4. If you cannot do a complete head-to-toe examination and detailed history, list the parts you will do in order of priority.

*Students are advised to refer to their nursing diagnosis text and identify possible or potential problems.

RESEARCH QUESTIONS

1. What is the importance of measuring ADLs and IADLs in older adults?
2. For each ADL, develop a plan of interventions that you would institute to compensate for ADL deficits and that would still foster an elder's independence as much as is realistic.
3. What makes an assessment tool effective?
4. What tool or tools would be most appropriate for assessing an elder in the community, in the hospital, in long-term care, or in day care? Give your rationale for the choices.

REFERENCES

Augustine N, Capitosti S: The Road ahead: Be prepared for a new direction in providing care. *Advances in Long-Term Care Management.* http://long-term-care.advanceweb.com/Archives/Article-Archives/The-Road-Ahead.aspx. Accessed June 21, 2010.

Aprahamian I, Martinelli JE, Neri AL, et al: The accuracy of the Clock Drawing Test compared to that of standard screening tests for Alzheimer's disease: results from a study of Brazilian elderly with heterogeneous educational backgrounds, *International Psychogeriatrics* 22:64, 2010.

Beck AT: *Beck Depression Inventory: manual,* San Antonio, TX, 1987, Psychological Corporation.

Benner P: *From novice to expert,* Menlo Park, CA, 1984, Addison-Wesley.

Blessed G, Tomlinson BE, Roth M: The association between qualitative measures of dementia and of senile change in the cerebral grey matter of elderly subjects, *British Journal of Psychiatry* 114:797, 1968.

Byrd E: Nursing assessment and treatment of depressive disorders of late life. In Mellilo K, Houde S, editors: *Geropsychiatric and mental health nursing,* Sudbury, MA, 2005, Jones and Bartlett.

Ehreke L, Luppa M, König HH, et al: The Clock Drawing Test a screening tool for the diagnosis of mild cognitive impairment? A systematic review, *International Psychogeriatrics* 22:56, 2010.

Evans LK: Complex care needs in older adults with common cognitive disorders. Section A: Assessment and management of dementia (2008). White paper supported by Hartford Geriatric Institute, American Association of Colleges of Nursing (AACN) and Geriatric Nursing Education Consortium (GNEC). Available at http://hartfordign.org/uploads/File/gnec_state_of_science_papers/gnec_dementia.pdf. Accessed December 2010.

Folstein MF, Folstein SE, McHugh PR: Mini-Mental State: a practical method for grading the cognitive state of patients for the clinician, *Journal of Psychiatric Research* 12:189, 1975.

Gurland B, Kuriansky J, Sharpe L, et al: The Comprehensive Assessment and Referral Evaluation (CARE)—rationale, development and reliability, *International Journal of Aging and Human Development* 8:9, 1977-1978.

Ham RJ: Assessment. In Ham RJ, Sloane PD, Warshaw GA, et al, editors: *Primary care geriatrics: a case-based approach,* ed 4, St. Louis, MO, 2002, Mosby.

Heller K, Viken R, Swindle R: Screening for depression in African American and Caucasian older women, *Aging & Mental Health* 14:339, 2010.

Katz S, Ford AB, Moskowitz RW, et al: Studies of illness in the aged: the index of ADL: a standardized measure of biological and psychosocial function, *JAMA* 185:914, 1963.

Kidd D, Stewart G, Baldry J, et al: The Functional Independence Measure: a comparative validity and reliability study, *Disability and Rehabilitation* 17:10, 1995.

Kleinman A: *Patient and healers in the context of culture: an exploration of the borderland between anthropology, medicine, and psychiatry*, Berkeley, CA, 1980, University of California Press.

Lach H, Chang Y, Edwards D: Can older adults accurately report depression using brief forms? *Journal of Gerontological Nursing* 36:30, 2010.

Lawton MP, Brody EM: Assessment of older people: self-maintaining and instrumental activities of daily living, *Gerontologist* 9:179, 1969.

Mahoney FI, Barthel DW: Functional evaluation: the Barthel Index, *Maryland State Medical Journal* 14:61, 1965.

Mitchell AJ: A meta-analysis of the accuracy of the Mini-Mental Status Examination in the detection of dementia and mild cognitive impairment, *Journal of Psychiatric Research* 43:411, 2009.

Mitchell AJ, Malladi S: Screening and case finding tools for the detection of dementia. 1. Evidence-based meta-analysis of multidomain tests, *American Journal of Geriatric Psychiatry* 18:759, 2010.

Montgomery J, Mitty E, Flores S: Resident condition change: should I call 911? *Geriatric Nursing* 29:159, 2008.

Morris JC: The Clinical Dementia Rating (CDR): current version and scoring rules, *Neurology* 43:2412, 1993.

Ortiz I, Romero L: Cultural implications for assessment and treatment of depression in Hispanic elderly individuals, *Annals of Long-term Care* 16:45, 2008.

Pfeiffer E: *Physical and mental assessment—OARS.* Presented at the 25th annual meeting of the Western Gerontological Society, San Francisco, April 28, 1979.

Reisberg B: Functional Assessment Staging (FAST), *Psychopharmacology Bulletin* 24:653, 1988.

Reisberg B: Global measures: Utility in defining and measuring treatment response in dementia, *International Psychogeriatrics* 19:421, 2007.

Reisberg B, Ferris SH, de Leon MJ, et al: The Global Deterioration Scale for assessment of primary progressive dementia, *American Journal of Psychiatry* 139:1136, 1982.

Saliba D, Buchanan J: *Development and validation of a revised nursing home assessment tool: MDS 3.0.* The RAND Corporation, April 2008.

Sangha H, Lipson D, Foley N, et al: A comparison of the Barthel Index and the Functional Independence Measure as outcome measures in stroke rehabilitation: patterns of disability scale usage in clinical trials, *International Journal of Rehabilitation Research* 28:135, 2005.

Sclan SG, Reisberg B: Functional Assessment Staging (FAST) in Alzheimer's disease: reliability, validity, and ordinality, *International Psychogeriatrics* 4:55, 1992.

Shephard R: MDS 3.0 Are you ready? ADVANCE for Health Information Profesionals. http://health-information.advanceweb.com/Features/Article-3/MDS-30-Are-You-Ready.aspx. Accessed February 17, 2010.

Shulman KI: Clock drawing: is it the ideal cognitive screening test? *International Journal of Geriatric Psychiatry* 15:545, 2000.

Wallace M, Fulmer T: Fulmer SPICES: an overall assessment tool for older adults (revised). *Try This* series. New York, Hartford Institute for Geriatric Nursing, 2007. Available at http://consultgerirn.org/uploads/File/trythis/try_this_1.pdf. Accessed December 2010.

Wattmo C, Wallin AK, Londos E, et al: Long-term outcome and predictive models of activity of daily living in Alzheimer disease with cholinesterase inhibitor treatment, *Alzheimer Disease and Associated Disorders* (Sept 16, 2010 e pub ahead of print PMID 20847636.)

Yesavage JA, Brink TL, Rose TL, et al: Development and validation of a Geriatric Depression Screening Scale: a preliminary report, *Journal of Psychiatric Research* 17:37, 1982-1983.

Zung WW: A self-rating depression scale, *Archives of General Psychiatry* 12:63, 1965.

Kathleen Jett

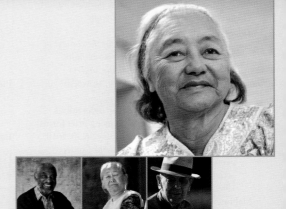

evolve http://evolve.elsevier.com/Ebersole/TwdHlthAging

A STUDENT SPEAKS

I always thought that as people got older, their blood sugars went up a little and that was OK. Now I realize that an elevation in fasting glucose means a problem regardless of one's age.   **Susan, age 20**

AN ELDER SPEAKS

Every time I turn around somebody wants my blood. They say that they need to "watch me closely" but I am not sure what that has to do with my blood. What if they take too much and it causes me to get sick?   **Sung Ye, age 92**

LEARNING OBJECTIVES

On completion of this chapter, the reader will be able to:

1. Identify the laboratory values that increase or decrease with normal aging.
2. Understand the implications and deviations of key abnormal laboratory values in the older adult.
3. Define cautions the nurse should take when interpreting laboratory values in the older adult.
4. Discuss strategies that can be used to maximize the quality of laboratory testing.
5. Discuss the key laboratory tests used to monitor common health problems.

The nurse's knowledge related to laboratory values and diagnostics tests takes on special meaning when working with older adults. The older a person is, the more difficult is the interpretation of findings and the more important are the nurse's skills. These skills include basic interpretation and those required to obtain or supervise specimen collection, to the timing of the procedure and awareness of influences on the results. For nurses working in long-term care settings, knowledge of interpretation is especially important to ensure that the persons with abnormalities in their laboratory results are treated promptly and appropriately. Advanced practice nurses are responsible for diagnostic and prescriptive responses to these results.

Laboratory findings are often reported in relationship to a range of normalized values or reference ranges referred to as "normal limits" within specific parameters. Most laboratory findings and their meanings are the same for older and younger adults. However, deviations from the norm are much more likely to occur and therefore special diligence is needed. Understanding laboratory values in older adults is complicated by the number of concurrent chronic diseases and medications, which

cloud the interpretation. We must take the knowledge of normal changes and consider the person in terms of his or her unique health status and needs.

HEMATOLOGICAL TESTING

Hematological testing refers to that which is associated with the blood and lymph and their component parts. Blood is composed of red blood cells, white blood cells, and cell fragments called *platelets*. Together the cells float in a fluid matrix called plasma. Although several age-related hematological changes occur mainly because of changes in the bone marrow, few of these are clinically significant (Freedman, 2009-2010a). However, a number of disorders commonly seen in later life are diagnosed or monitored through hematological testing. Several conditions also affect the results, such as dehydration, inadequate nutrition, infections, and inflammation.

Several laboratory tests are used to measure and diagnose hematological health. The hemogram includes counts of platelets, white blood cells, and red blood cells, as well as the calculation of a hematocrit and indices. A complete blood count (CBC) is a hemogram plus a differential count. One of the basic laboratory measures that reflect hematopoietic functioning is iron studies. The erythrocyte sedimentation rate uses red blood cells in the measurement of systemic inflammation.

Red Blood Cell Count

The primary function of red blood cells (RBCs, erythrocytes) is to transport molecules of hemoglobin, which in turn transports and exchanges oxygen and carbon dioxide throughout the body. Because the erythrocytes have no nucleus of their own, they cannot reproduce. With the red blood cell's average life span of 120 days, the body is in constant need of replenishment. Red blood cells are produced primarily by the bone marrow, the tissue found inside the spaces of the long bones. There is no indication that there is a change in RBCs in aging; however, the speed at which new blood cells can be produced in late life is reduced (*decreased marrow reserve*). This becomes a potential problem with a loss of blood such as after phlebotomy or frank bleeding. Recovery from the loss takes much longer, increasing the risk of falling, delirium, and other geriatric syndromes. Older adults are up to six times more likely to develop anemia, because of the combination of common diseases and medications taken. The prevalence of anemia is in the 8% to 22% range in older adults, depending on age and concurrent conditions; and is most often normocytic with multifactorial causes, or an anemia of chronic disease (Auerhahn et al., 2007). The categorization of an anemia involves multiple measurements and interpretation and includes the components described in this section, as well as the calculated cell indices of mean corpuscular volume (MCV), mean corpuscular hemoglobin (MCH), and red blood cell distribution width (RDW). A detailed discussion of these indices is beyond the scope of this chapter.

Hemoglobin and Hematocrit

Laboratory results including hemoglobin and hematocrit are commonly reviewed. Hemoglobin is the main component of the red blood cell. It is a conjugated protein whose main function is to transport oxygen from the lungs to the tissues, and carbon dioxide from the tissues to the lungs. It contains iron and the red pigment porphyrin. The iron combines easily with both oxygen and carbon dioxide. Each saturated gram of hemoglobin carries 1.39 mL of oxygen. It is the hemoglobin concentration, not the red blood cell count, that is used as an indicator for anemia. A hemoglobin level equal to or less than 5 g/dL, or more than 20 g/dL, is considered a "critical value," that is, the person is in extreme jeopardy and requires urgent intervention (Pagana and Pagana, 2010). Anemia is usually diagnosed in a man with a hemoglobin of less than 13 g/dL or in a woman with less than 12 g/dL. Levels of less than 13.3 and 12.6 respectively have been associated with a higher risk for death (Hardin, 2010; Zakai, et al., 2005).

The term *hematocrit* means "to separate blood." It is the *relative percentage* of packed RBCs to the plasma in blood, after the two have been separated (often referred to as "spun down"). Although they measure different aspects of the RBCs, the hematocrit and hemoglobin are comparative numbers, with the hemoglobin approximately one third of the hematocrit. For example, a person with a hemoglobin level of 12 g/dL will have

a hematocrit of approximately 36%. Critical values are less than 15% or more than 60% (Pagana and Pagana, 2010). Although the hematocrit is a marker of levels of anemia, it is not a good measure of overall blood volume. Elevations in hematocrit and hemoglobin may be the result of a pathological process but are more often an early sign of hypovolemia from malnutrition, dehydration, or severe diarrhea. The volume depletion must be corrected before an accurate interpretation can be done.

White Blood Cells

White blood cells (WBCs), or leukocytes, are divided primarily into two types—granulocytes (neutrophils, basophils, and eosinophils) and agranulocytes (monocytes and lymphocytes). They are found mainly in the interstitial fluid until they are needed and then travel to the site of invasion or infection. The number of WBCs is regulated largely by the endocrine system and by the need for a particular type of cell (Table 8-1). Each cell has a life span of 13 to 20 days, after which it is destroyed in the lymphatic system and excreted in feces. They are produced by the bone marrow and thymus and are stored in the lymph nodes, spleen, and tonsils. The average adult has 5000 to 10,000 WBCs/mm^3. A major concern in the elderly is WBC elevations, often caused by bacteremia. A WBC count of less than 2500 or more than 30,000/mm^3 is considered critical (Pagana and Pagana, 2010).

Bacteremia in the older population is a common cause for hospitalization, causing sepsis and septic shock and carrying a high mortality rate. In younger adults, the presence of infection or inflammation is commonly manifested as an elevated temperature, lymph node enlargement, and increase in total WBC count. However, in the older adult, these signs may be absent or not seen until the person is quite ill or septic. Rather than an increase in total lymphocytes, only immature neutrophils (bands) may be increased, called *bandemia* or a *left shift*. This lack of or delayed response reflects a diminished ability to respond to the intrusion of foreign substances, consistent with the immunity theory of aging (see Chapter 3). This change has significant implications for the gerontological nurse. Waiting for the "usual signs" of infection in an older adult may result in his or her death. Instead, the nurse must be alert for more subtle signs of illness such as new-onset or increased confusion, falling, or incontinence and respond to these changes earlier rather than later.

Exacerbating an already potentially dangerous situation is the frequency at which leukocytopenia is seen in older adults; it is caused by common medical conditions and commonly

TABLE 8-1	FUNCTIONS OF THE TYPES OF WHITE BLOOD CELLS
CELL TYPE	**CELL FUNCTION**
Neutrophils	Stimulated by pyogenic infections, to fight bacteria
Eosinophils	Stimulated by allergic responses, to fight antigens and parasites
Basophils	Stimulated by the presence of allergens; transport histamine
Lymphocytes	Stimulated by the presences of viral infections
Monocytes	Stimulated by severe infections including viral, parasitic, and rickettsial

Data from Pagana KD, Pagana TJ: *Mosby's manual of diagnostic and laboratory tests*, ed 4, St. Louis, MO, 2010, Mosby.

prescribed medications, for example, some antibiotics, anticonvulsants, antihistamines, analgesics, sulfonamides, and diuretics. On the other hand, increases in leukocytes may be a side effect of several drugs including allopurinol, aspirin, heparin, and steroids (Pagana and Pagana, 2010).

Neutrophils are produced in 7 to 14 days in the bone marrow and are in circulation for about 6 hours. They fight infections by phagocytizing bacteria. *Neutrophilia,* or increased neutrophils, may be an indicator of infections, connective tissue diseases such as rheumatoid arthritis, malignancies, use of medications such as corticosteroids, trauma, and metabolic conditions such as gout, uremia, thyrotoxicosis, and lactic acidosis (Pagana and Pagana, 2010). All are common conditions in late life.

Lymphocytes are divided into two types: T cells and B cells. T cells are produced by the thymus and are active in cell-mediated immunity; B cells are produced in the bone marrow and are involved in the production of antibodies (humoral immunity). In adulthood, 80% of lymphocytes are T cells, with a slight decrease in T cells and increase in B cells with aging. T-cell activity is especially important in late life, due in part to the naturally occurring immunosenescence (Chapter 3), especially depressed T-cell responses and T-cell–macrophage interactions (Auerhahn et al., 2007). Measurement of T cells is included in the monitoring of the health status and treatment response of persons infected with human immunodeficiency virus (HIV) or who have acquired immunodeficiency syndrome (AIDS). Together with neutrophils, lymphocytes make up 75% to 90% of all white blood cells (Pagana and Pagana, 2010).

Monocytes are the largest of the leukocytes. When matured they become macrophages and help defend the body against foreign substances, or what the body believes are foreign substances. The macrophages migrate to a site in the body where they can remove microorganisms, dead RBCs, and foreign debris through the physiological process of phagocytosis.

Eosinophils are involved in allergic reactions. They ingest antigen–antibody complexes induced by IgE-mediated reactions to attack allergens and parasites. High eosinophil counts are found in people with type I allergies such as hay fever and asthma. Eosinophils are involved in the mucosal immune response, which is known to diminish in late life (Freedman, 2009-2010a,b). Increased eosinophils in a peripheral blood smear may also be caused by infections such as tuberculosis or pulmonary fungal infections, rheumatoid arthritis, ulcerative colitis, regional enteritis, seasonal allergic rhinitis, atopic dermatitis, solid tumor cancers, and various lymphomas and leukemias (Pagana and Pagana, 2010).

Basophils transport histamine, a factor in immune and antiinflammatory responses, and heparin. Like eosinophils, they play a role in allergic reactions. They are not involved in bacterial or viral infections.

Platelets

Platelets are small, irregular particles known as thrombocytes, an essential ingredient in clotting. They are formed in the bone marrow, the lungs, and the spleen and are released when a blood vessel is injured. As they arrive at the site of injury, they become "sticky," forming a plug at the site to stop the bleeding and to help trigger what is known as the clotting cascade (Thibodeau

and Patton, 2003). Although the platelet count does not change with aging, the concentrations of a large number of coagulation enzymes increase (factors VII and VIII and fibrinogen). This and other developments indicate the possibility of hypercoagulability. However, at the same time, older adults are more likely to have blood diatheses resulting in unexplained bruising, nosebleeds, excess bleeding with surgery, and so on. If any of these signs are present, platelet counts and coagulation studies should be done. Counts of 150,000 to 400,000/mm^3 are considered normal. Counts less than 100,000/mm^3 are a cause for concern and considered thrombocytopenia; spontaneous hemorrhage may occur when the count falls below 20,000/mm^3; at 40,000/mm^3 spontaneous bleeding is uncommon but prolonged bleeding can occur with trauma or surgery (Auerhahn et al., 2007). *Thrombocythemia* indicates a platelet count greater than 1 million/mm^3; bleeding still may occur due to abnormal functioning. The gerontological nurse caring for frail elders is expected to monitor patients for risk for bleeding, including understanding the meaning of their patients' laboratory findings. For frail elders, such as those in long-term care facilities, thrombocytopenia can quickly lead to death should bleeding occur, such as from the gastrointestinal system or from a subdural hematoma occurring after a fall.

COMMON DIAGNOSTIC TESTING

Measures of Inflammation

Erythrocyte Sedimentation Rate

The *erythrocyte sedimentation rate* (ESR), also referred to as the "sed rate," is the rate at which an RBC falls to the bottom of saline solution or plasma in a set period of time. It is a proxy measure for the degree of inflammation, infection, necrosis, infarction, or advanced neoplasm. It may be slightly elevated (10 to 20 mm/h) in normal, healthy older adults, most likely due to the prevalence of chronic disease (Miller, 2009-2010). A more than minimal elevation indicates elevated serum proteins and inflammatory activity. The ESR is highly nonspecific and cannot be used for the diagnosis of any one disorder. However, it may be useful for monitoring several diseases and their treatments, especially inflammatory conditions such as polymyalgia rheumatica, temporal arteritis, or rheumatoid arthritis (Moore, 2006; Kreiner et al., 2010). If a person of any age has an unexplained rise in ESR, further assessment is indicated.

C-reactive Protein

C-reactive protein (CRP) is produced by the liver during the acute phase of inflammation or in the course of various diseases. Although originally used to determine cardiac events, it has been found a useful indicator for other forms of inflammation as well, such as after injury, surgery, or in the presence of infection. Tests of both CRP and ESR together are currently used, especially for the evaluation of an acute myocardial infarction (AMI). However, in a study of 5777 patients, Colombet and colleagues (2010) concluded that the joint measurement of ESR and CRP was not necessary; the ESR was misleading in a group of patients. The authors recommended that priority be given to the CRP measurement when inflammation is suspected. In another study of 163 persons, the CRP was found to be helpful in diagnosing septic joints, whereas the ESR was not (Ernst et al., 2010). The CRP was also found useful for predicting the risk for coronary heart disease among intermediate-risk subjects (Helfand et al., 2009). There is now a high-sensitivity assay for CRP (hs-CRP), which has increased the accuracy of the measurement even at low levels. While it too is variable and two measurements are needed, it still may be a stronger predictor of cardiovascular events than cholesterol (Pagana and Pagana, 2010).

Iron Studies

Anemia is the condition in which there is a reduced number of red blood cells and consequentially a reduced capacity for the transport of oxygen and carbon dioxide. Although not a normal change with aging, anemia is a common pathological finding in older adults, especially in the postoperative period and in those with long-standing chronic disease or renal insufficiency. In older adults the signs and symptoms are easily confused with other disorders, making diagnosis difficult or delayed. One of the first signs of anemia may be fatigue, which may be confused with a side effect of a medication or falsely attributed to normal aging. Progressive anemia that is untreated or not responsive to treatment will result in the person's death. The advanced practice gerontological nurse must be able to diagnose and treat anemia. The gerontological nurse should be able to recognize the potential for anemia and to monitor its treatment.

Although a number of types of anemia exist, the most common in late life are anemia of chronic disease and inflammation, blood loss anemia, and that associated with protein-energy malnutrition. Diagnostic testing for anemia begins with what are referred to as "iron studies." Iron studies include iron, ferritin, total iron-binding capacity (TIBC), and transferrin measures. Any of these alone is an inadequate measure because of the complexity of their interrelationships. In the presence of reduced hemoglobin, additional tests measuring folic acid and vitamin B_{12} may also be indicated.

Iron

The primary source of iron is through the consumption of iron-containing foods such as dark-green, leafy vegetables and red meats. The iron is transported by the plasma protein *transferrin* into bone marrow for storage and for use later in the production of hemoglobin. The serum concentration of iron is determined by a combination of its absorption and storage, as well as the breakdown and synthesis of hemoglobin. The iron in hemoglobin is necessary not only for the transportation of oxygen and carbon dioxide but also for controlling protein synthesis in the mitochondria, essential for generating energy in the cells (Freedman and Sutin, 2002). Serum iron (Fe) is reported as micrograms per deciliter (μg/dL). The TIBC measures the combination of the amount of iron and the amount of transferrin available in the blood serum. *Ferritin* is a complex molecule made up of ferric hydroxide and a protein, and its measurement reflects body iron stores.

Adequate stores of iron are necessary to maintain health. The body is then able to respond quickly to the demand for increased oxygen and energy and to replenish iron lost through bleeding.

Vitamins

Mild vitamin deficiencies are common in later life and should be considered any time there is cognitive impairment, delayed wound healing, or anemia. Those at highest risk are persons who may have protein-calorie malnutrition. Short-term under-nutrition is associated with B and C vitamin deficiencies. For those with longer durations, the deficiencies may also include A, E, B_{12}, and K (Johnson, 2009-2010). Vitamin D deficiencies are now being found in both apparently healthy and ill adults. Because of the higher risk for and more serious effects from vitamin deficiencies, general supplementation is often recommended.

B Vitamins

The two B vitamins that are especially important to hematological health are folic acid and B_{12}, two of the eight B vitamins in the B-complex. *Folic acid* is formed by bacteria in the intestines; it is necessary for the normal functioning of both RBCs and WBCs, and for deoxyribonucleic acid (DNA) synthesis (Nicoll et al., 2004). It is stored in the liver and can be found in eggs, milk, leafy vegetables, yeast, liver, and fruit. Decreases in folic acid may indicate protein-energy malnutrition, several types of anemia, and liver and renal disease. It is more common among persons with chronic alcohol abuse. Although folic acid levels do not decrease in healthy aging, the nurse must be alert for signs of actual or potential nutritional deficits. Folic acid is usually measured in conjunction with that of vitamin B_{12} levels.

Vitamin B_{12} (cyanocobalamin) is a water-soluble vitamin required for the normal development of RBCs, neurological function, and DNA synthesis. If untreated, vitamin B_{12} deficiency is ultimately fatal. Vitamin B_{12} is found in products such as eggs, fish, shellfish, and meat, half of which may be bioavailable. It is first extracted from food by gastric acid and pepsin in the stomach. In the intestine B_{12} binds with intrinsic factor for absorption and entry into the circulation. Vitamin B_{12} deficiencies resulting in megaloblastic (pernicious) anemia have been attributed solely to lack of intrinsic factor (Box 8-1). More recently a milder form of B_{12} deficiency has been identified and may be caused by normal and common age-related changes in

---

BOX 8-1 LABORATORY TESTING AND VITAMIN B_{12}

Laboratory testing with the following findings indicate a Vitamin B_{12} deficiency:

Serum cobalamin level < 200 pg/mL
   With clinical signs or symptoms and/or related hematological abnormalities
OR
Serum cobalamin level < 200 pg/mL
   On two different occasions
OR
Serum cobalamin level < 200 pg/mL
   With total serum homocysteine level > 13 μmol/L in the absence of renal failure or deficiencies in folate or B_6
OR
Low serum holotranscobalamin levels <35 pmol/L

Adapted from Cadogan MP: Functional implications of vitamin B_{12} deficiency, *Journal of Gerontological Nursing* 36:16, 2010.

the stomach wherein B_{12} is not released from food. This type may apply to 60% to 70% of the cases of vitamin B_{12} deficiency in later life (Cadogan, 2010).

Clinical manifestations of B_{12} deficiencies include elevated homocysteine levels, glossitis, increased lactate dehydrogenase (LDH) levels, paresthesias of the feet and hands, and vibratory and proprioception disturbances. Ataxias will also occur without treatment. Cerebral manifestations include memory impairment, change in taste and smell, irritability, and somnolence. Tests of B_{12} and folate are now part of the standard workup for dementia (Sink and Yaffee, 2004). Testing for a B_{12} deficiency is indicated when there is unexplained neurological or functional decline.

Vitamin D

Vitamin D deficiencies have been found to be common. Aging skin combined with decreased exposure to sunlight result in a reduction of the conversion of 7-dehydrocholesterol to vitamin D_3 (cholecalciferol) by ultraviolet light. In turn, the vitamin D deficiency reduces the absorption of calcium into bone. It has been demonstrated that in response to the lowered levels of calcium, the secretion of parathyroid hormone increases, triggering increased bone resorption. Ensuring adequate intake of calcium and vitamin D is essential for healthy aging.

Vitamin D levels are measured in the blood, using 25-hydroxyvitamin D_2 and 25-hydroxyvitamin D_3 to determine total 25-hydroxyvitamin D levels. A level of 20 ng/mL indicates a deficiency, 20 to 30 ng/mL an insufficiency, and greater than 30 ng/mL a sufficiency (optimal). There is a considerable amount of research currently underway examining the effect and implications of the wide scale deficiencies of Vitamin D that have been observed (Planton, Meyer, Eolund, 2011).

BLOOD CHEMISTRY STUDIES

Blood chemistry studies include an assortment of laboratory tests that are used to identify and measure circulating elements and particles in the plasma and blood: glucose, proteins, amino acids, nutritive materials, excretion products, hormones, enzymes, vitamins, and minerals. Some of these are used for screening and others for monitoring specific health problems or treatments. Some tests are individually selected, but many are done in "panels" or grouped in clusters with a variety of names, including "Chem-7" or "BMP" (basic metabolic panel) or "SMA-16" or "CMP" (complete metabolic panel), among others. The nurse must become familiar with the names and test components used by the laboratory that provides services to her or his patients (Box 8-2).

Hormones: Thyroxin

In the older man and postmenopausal woman, the hormones that receive the most attention are those related to the thyroid gland: triiodothyronine (T_3), thyroxine (T_4), and thyroid-stimulating hormone (TSH). Although changes in thyroid function are not a normal part of aging, the incidence of disturbances, especially hypothyroidism, is seen with increasing frequency. However, some of the deviations are the result of other, nonthyroid conditions. Screening for thyroid disease is a component of the primary health care of older adults, especially

BOX 8-2	EFFECTS OF AGING ON LABORATORY VALUES
INCREASED WITH AGE	**DECREASED WITH AGE**
Alkaline phosphatase	Calcium, serum
Cholesterol, serum	Creatinine kinase, serum
Clotting factors, VII and VIII	Creatinine clearance*
Copper, serum	Dehydroepiandrosterone (DHEA)
Ferritin, serum	1,25-Dihydroxycholecalciferol, serum
Glucose, serum (postprandial)	Estrogen, serum
	Growth hormone
Interleukin-6 (IL-6)	Insulin-like growth factor I (IGF-I)
Norepinephrine, serum	Interleukin-I (IL-I)
Parathyroid hormone	Iron, serum (minimally)
Prostate-specific antigen (PSA)	Phosphorus, serum
Triglycerides, serum	Selenium, serum
Uric acid, serum	Testosterone, serum
	Thiamin, serum
	γ-Tocopherol (vitamin E), plasma
	Triiodothyronine (T3)
	Vitamin B6, serum
	Vitamin B12, serum
	Vitamin C, plasma
	Zinc, serum

*Serum creatinine may be normal, even though creatinine clearance is decreased with age, because creatinine production decreases with age. From Beers MH, Berkow R (eds): The Merch manual of geriatrics, 3e, white house station, NJ, 2000, Merck & co., Inc.

women and persons with depression, anxiety, dementia, or cardiac arrhythmias. A fully functioning thyroid gland (or its replacement) is necessary to maintain life. TSH is produced by the pituitary to stimulate the thyroid to produce T_3, which in turn is converted to T_4.

Although all of the previously mentioned hormones are commonly included in a thyroid panel, the serum free T_4 and TSH levels are the most important for the initial diagnosis. If the person has a goiter, a thyroid scan with technetium may be necessary (Brashers and Jones, 2010). In most cases, treatment (especially thyroid replacement) can be monitored easily on the basis of TSH alone.

Hypothyroidism is the most common disturbance seen in older adults, affecting only 1% of the younger population and 5% of those over 60 (Fitzgerald, 2010) (see Chapter 15). The most common causes are autoimmune thyroiditis, prior radioiodine treatment, and subtotal thyroidectomy. Hypothyroidism can also be iatrogenic, from provider-prescribed thyroid replacement that is not adequately monitored. Hypothyroidism is diagnosed by the clinical picture combined with laboratory findings, especially markedly elevated TSH and reduced total and free T_4 (Table 8-2). However, the accuracy of the laboratory findings is easily affected by concurrent environmental conditions and drug intake, making an accurate diagnosis somewhat difficult (Table 8-3).

Hypothyroidism is seen alone and in a combination with other autoimmune and cardiac conditions. In subclinical hypothyroidism, diagnosis is made on the basis of clinical assessment alone. There is an age-associated decrease in the ability of the body to convert T_4 to T_3 (so that it can be used). The subsequent lack of T_3 will cause the pituitary to increase the production of TSH, indicators of hypothyroidism.

TABLE 8-2   INTERPRETING THYROID TESTING RESULTS

TSH	FREE T₄	CAUSE	RESPONSE
Increased (>10 mU/L)	Low	Clinical hypothyroidism Inadequate replacement therapy	Usually requires treatment
	Normal	Subclinical hypothyroidism	Treatment depends on presence of signs and symptoms
	High	Hypothalamic/pituitary disorder	Referral to an endocrinologist for further testing
Decreased (<0.1 mU/L)	Low	Euthyroid sick syndrome Hypothalamic/pituitary disorder	Referral to an endocrinologist for further testing
	Normal	Subclinical thyrotoxicosis T₃ thyrotoxicosis (if T₃ is elevated)	Referral to an endocrinologist for monitoring
	High	Clinical thyrotoxicosis Excessive replacement therapy	Referral to an endocrinologist for further testing and treatment Adjust dosage and retest

T_3, triiodothyronine; T_4, thyroxine; TSH, thyroid-stimulating hormone.
Adapted from Fitzgerald PA: Endocrine disorders. In McPhee SJ, Papadakis MA, editors: *Current medical diagnosis and treatment 2010*, New York, 2010, McGraw-Hill.

TABLE 8-3   FACTORS AFFECTING LABORATORY TESTING OF THYROID FUNCTIONING

TEST	INCREASED RESULT	DEPRESSED RESULT
TSH	Potassium iodide and lithium	Severe illness, aspirin, dopamine, heparin, and steroids
T_3	Estrogen and methadone	Anabolic steroids, androgens, phenytoin, propranolol, reserpine, and salicylates
T_4	Estrogen, methadone, and clofibrate	Anabolic steroids, androgens, lithium, phenytoin, and propranolol

T_3, triiodothyronine; T_4, thyroxine; TSH, thyroid-stimulating hormone.
Modified from Pagana KD, Pagana TJ: *Manual of diagnostic and laboratory tests*, ed 4, St. Louis, MO, 2010, Mosby.

Hyperthyroidism, or thyrotoxicosis, is significantly less common in older adults. Its prevalence in community-living elders is thought to be 1% to 3% and is more common in women (Gambert and Miller, 2004). It is usually caused by multinodular and uninodular toxic goiter rather than the Graves' disease that is seen in younger adults. Hyperthyroidism can also be caused by iodine-containing substances, such as the antiarrhythmic amiodarone (Cordarone) (Fitzgerald, 2010). Hyperthyroidism is diagnosed on the basis of low or normal serum T_4 and low TSH. Finally, like hypothyroidism, hyperthyroidism can be iatrogenic, or from inadequately monitoring thyroid replacement. Special caution must be used for chronic use of L-thyroxin doses greater than 0.15 mg/day. The nurse is in a key position to monitor the thyroid function of the patient by ensuring timely and appropriate laboratory testing of TSH.

TABLE 8-4   SIGNS AND SYMPTOMS OF DISTURBANCES IN SODIUM LEVELS

	HYPONATREMIA	HYPERNATREMIA
Signs	Plasma Na^+ ≤130 mmol/L (approximately)	Plasma Na^+ ≥150 mmol/L (approximately)
	Drop in BP (in hypovolemia)	Poor skin turgor
	Tachycardia (in hypovolemia)	Dry mucous membranes
Symptoms	Mental status changes	Mental status changes

BP, blood pressure.
Data from Brashers VL, Jones RE: Mechanisms in hormone regulation. In McCance KL, Huether SE, Brashers VL, et al, editors: *Pathophysiology: the biological basis for disease in adults and children*, ed 6, St. Louis, MO, 2010, Mosby.

Electrolytes

Electrolytes are inorganic substances that maintain a complex balance between intracellular and extracellular environments. They regulate hydration and blood pH, and are critical for nerve and muscle function. For example, if there is an imbalance of calcium, sodium, and potassium, muscle weakness or contractions may occur. Their blood levels are reported as solitary measurements or as a part of panels, such as the Chem-7 or the SMA-12 or -16 noted earlier.

A minor electrolyte imbalance may have little effect in a younger adult but may have significantly deleterious results in an older adult, especially one who is medically fragile. When an imbalance is found, an adjustment or addition of a medication (e.g., potassium), an increase or decrease in the fluid intake, or transferring the patient from one setting to another may be needed (e.g., home to hospital, nursing home to hospital, general unit to intensive care unit). Dehydration is the most common cause of electrolyte imbalance in the elderly, especially for those residing in long-term care facilities (Mentes, 2006). The signs and symptoms of an imbalance in the older adult include weakness, fatigue, immobility, or delirium. As these are also seen in a number of other conditions, laboratory testing is required for a definitive diagnosis and the initiation of an appropriate plan of care.

The most common electrolytes of concern in gerontological care include sodium and chloride, potassium, calcium and phosphorus, and glucose.

Sodium and Chloride

The test for sodium (Na^+), measured in circulating blood, is a proxy index of hydration. Sodium is necessary for the maintenance of blood pressure, the transmission of nerve impulses, and the regulation of body fluids into and out of the cells (Cho, 2010) (Table 8-4). The movement of fluids affects blood volume and is tied to thirst. Sodium balance is influenced by renal filtration and blood flow, cardiac output, and glomerular filtration rate (GFR). Laboratory sodium levels indicate the balance between ingested sodium and that which is excreted by the kidneys. Changes in sodium (Na^+) are always accompanied by changes in chloride (Cl^-) because they are predominantly found in combinations as sodium chloride.

A high prevalence of hyponatremia (≤ 130 mmol/L) has been found in long-term care facilities (Auerhahn et al., 2007). Hyponatremia can be divided into three types: decreased extracellular fluid (ECF) volume (diarrhea, renal salt-losing circumstances, etc.), increased ECF volume (e.g., heart failure), or normal ECF from syndrome of inappropriate antidiuretic hormone secretion— with the latter the most common in older adults (Auerhahn et al., 2007). Hyponatremia is usually asymptomatic until the plasma sodium concentration drops below 130 mEq/L, and is usually accompanied by decreased osmolality (<280 mOsm/kg) (Cho, 2010). At this concentration CNS symptoms appear and can become quickly significant, leading to seizures and coma secondary to brain edema. Slow replacement is necessary. Mental status changes and other CNS effects can be seen with levels equal to or less than 125 to 130 mEq/L. Hypovolemic hyponatremia is always accompanied by a significant drop in postural blood pressure and tachycardia as the body attempts to compensate. In the most severe cases, hyponatremia can result in a high rate of morbidity and mortality. Hyponatremia is one of the more common causes of delirium in older adults.

Hypernatremia is an elevation of plasma sodium (>145 mEq/L) and is accompanied by hyperosomolality. It is most often caused by free water loss or dehydration, common among ill older adults in hospital and long-term care facilities. The prevalence in this group is up to 30% with a mortality rate of 42% (Beck, 2004). Low body weight is a risk factor. The mortality rate for this is 40% in hospitalized elders, especially if it occurs quickly and is severe (>158 mEq/L). When sodium levels are more than 155 mEq/L, mental status changes should be expected and carry a poor prognosis in older adults. Signs include lethargy, irritability, and weakness. Severe hypernatremia (>158 mEq/L) is associated with delirium, coma, and seizures (Cho, 2010).

Potassium

Potassium (K^+) is an electrolyte found primarily within the cells themselves. It is essential in maintaining cell osmolality, muscle functioning, and transmitting nerve impulses and is a key component in the maintenance of the acid–base balance. Serum potassium levels decrease as lean body mass decreases. As loss of lean body mass is a normal change of aging, the potassium level bears close watching.

Hypokalemia ($K^+ < 3.5$ mEq/L) is associated with cardiac arrhythmias and may cause glucose intolerance and renal tubular dysfunction. Mild hypokalemia is asymptomatic. Potassium levels less than 2.5 mEq/L are critical and produce muscle weakness, cramping, confusion, fatigue, paralytic ileus, atrial and ventricular ectopy and tachycardia, fibrillation, and sudden death (Pagana and Pagana, 2010). The electrocardiogram (ECG) will demonstrate a characteristic response to hypokalemia.

BOX 8-3	SIGNS AND SYMPTOMS OF DISTURBANCES IN POTASSIUM LEVELS
HYPOKALEMIA	**HYPERKALEMIA**
Generalized muscle weakness	Impaired muscle activity
Fatigue	Weakness
Muscle cramps	Muscle pain/cramps
Constipation	Increased GI motility
Ileus	Bradycardia
Flaccid paralysis	Cardiac arrest
Hyporeflexia	ECG changes:
Hypercapnia	P wave flattened
Tetany	T wave large, peaked
ECG changes:	QRS broad
QT interval prolonged	Biphasic QRS-T complex
T wave flattened or depressed	
ST segment depressed	

ECG, electrocardiogram; GI, gastrointestinal.
For additional information, see Cho KC: Fluid and electrolyte disorders. In: McPhee SJ, Papadakis MA, editors: CURRENT medical diagnosis and treatment *2010*, New York, 2010, McGraw-Hill.

Chronic hypokalemia may lead to significant renal tubular dysfunction.

Hyperkalemia ($K^+ > 5$ mEq/L) usually occurs only in persons with advanced kidney disease, but is also associated with acidosis and inadequate monitoring of potassium-sparing medications such as angiotensin-converting enzyme (ACE) inhibitors. It can also be the result of excessive supplementation for potassium for persons taking potassium-wasting drugs such as loop diuretics (e.g., furosemide [Lasix]). The signs and symptoms of a disturbance in potassium levels may not be evident until it is critical (Box 8-3). Hyperkalemia may be asymptomatic until cardiac toxicity occurs (Cho, 2010).

Calcium and Phosphorus

The measurement of serum calcium is used to determine parathyroid function and calcium metabolism. Calcium (Ca^{2+}) is essential for bone strength, blood clotting, nerve conduction, muscle functioning, and enzymatic activity. Only about 1% of the body's calcium is found in the blood; the remainder is stored in the bones and teeth. The serum level is maintained by release or resorption of bone calcium, depending on the body's needs. Because the serum levels do not change with aging but calcium metabolism does, the result is decreased bone stores. When a significant amount of the stores is lost, osteoporosis is diagnosed.

About half of the serum calcium is bound to proteins, especially albumin, an indicator of nutritional status. Therefore, a low albumin level will be accompanied by artificially low serum calcium. Because of the high rate of malnutrition, this is especially common in medically fragile persons, such as those residing in skilled nursing facilities (Harris and Fraser, 2004). The measurement of serum calcium must be adjusted to determine the actual serum calcium, using a standard formula (add 0.8 mg/dL to the total calcium concentration for each 1-g/dL decrease in albumin below its normal concentration of 4 g/dL).

When the person has true hypocalcemia (serum concentration <8.5 mg/dL), hypoparathyroidism is the most common cause; other causes are vitamin D deficiency, acute pancreatitis, or malignancy. In the older adult hypocalcemia is further exacerbated by the frequency of chronically poor intake and decreased gastrointestinal absorption (Huether, 2010). True hypercalcemia (>12 mg/dL) is most often caused by hyperparathyroidism or a malignancy; it can also be the result of vitamin A or D intoxication, hyperthyroidism, or immobilization. Mild hypercalcemia is asymptomatic and not easily detected. Primary hyperparathyroidism is determined by laboratory assay. Either may be the side effect of a number of medications (Box 8-4).

Calcium levels are inversely related to phosphorus levels—an excess serum level of one causes the kidneys to excrete the other. Phosphorus is a mineral found mostly in the bones and in combination with calcium, with the rest found within the cells. It is required for the generation of bony tissue and functions in the metabolism of glucose and lipids. Phosphorus levels are slightly decreased and worsened with long-term use of antacids.

Glucose

Glucose is the sugar most commonly used by the body for energy. For optimal functioning, the levels of fasting glucose in the body must be maintained between about 70 and 110 mg/dL (depending on the laboratory). Although the required levels do not change with aging, the signs and symptoms of persons with elevations or reductions may change. For many older adults, even slight hypoglycemia can result in confused and depressed CNS activity. At the same time, there is increased glucose tolerance; the typical signs of polydipsia and polyuria may be absent. The diagnostic criteria for altered glucose metabolism are based on either fasting or random blood glucose levels under a variety of conditions (Box 8-5). In older adults, the fasting blood glucose levels are in the higher normal range and it takes longer to return to normal levels after a glucose challenge or after eating. These changes appear to be most likely related to a decrease in the insulin sensitivity of the tissues. As the renal threshold for glucose changes, it can be detected in the urine at lower levels.

Laboratory testing of blood glucose or plasma glucose provides "snapshot" information about the glucose level. For more accurate measurement and monitoring of glucose the glycosylated hemoglobin A1c is used. About 7% of the hemoglobin in the RBCs can combine with glucose through the process of glycosylation. The glucose attachment is not easily reversible and therefore stays for the life of the RBC, approximately 120 days and provides a good estimate of the average blood glucose. In nondiabetics 4% to 5.9% is the normal range; <7% indicates good diabetic control, 8% to 9% fair control, and >9% poor control (Pagana and Pagana, 2010). While it is commonly used, the Hemoglobin A1c is not yet a standard for the diagnosis of diabetes. It is used for monitoring.

The nurse is often responsible for ensuring the quality of the collection of laboratory specimens. In relation to glucose testing, it is important that interpretation of findings is within the context of time since meals or snacks.

Uric Acid

Uric acid is a naturally occurring end product of purine metabolism. It is usually measured in serum chemistry studies but is also found in the urine. Two thirds of the amount normally produced is excreted by the kidneys and the rest via the stool. Elevations in uric acid levels (>7.5 mg/dL) are found when there is either overproduction or underexcretion. Measurement of uric acid levels is indicated in the evaluation of renal failure or leukemia, or, most often, in the diagnosis or treatment of gout or kidney stones. Hyperuricemia (>13 mg/dL) indicates a high risk for kidney stones (Hellmann and Imboden, 2010). A number of conditions and situations can result in increased uric acid levels, including binge alcohol drinking; medications, especially thiazide diuretics; surgery; or acute medical illness. The levels also increase slightly with age and vary between men and women (Pagana and Pagana, 2010).

Prostate-specific Antigen

The primary screening tools for prostate cancer have been the digital rectal examination (DRE) and prostate-specific antigen (PSA). PSA is more sensitive than the DRE; however, it can be elevated by a number of conditions, making the use of it as a screening measure for prostate cancer questionable. A cutoff point of 4.0 ng/mL detects many cases of cancer, as would a lower cutoff. However, the high number of "false positives" led to considerable controversy over the usefulness of this test. At this time it is recommended only for men more than 75 years of age and for those at high risk (U.S. Preventive Services Task Force, 2010). Changes in repeated PSAs over time are more meaningful, with increases of >5% to 8% indicating the need for further evaluation (Miller, 2009-2010).

LABORATORY TESTING FOR CARDIAC HEALTH

Heart disease remains the primary cause of death for all persons. As a result, the gerontological nurse must be knowledgeable about the most common laboratory testing related to cardiac function. These include measures performed after acute cardiac events and those used in the determination of cardiac health and health risk.

Acute Cardiac Events

Older adults who appear to have acute and unexpected changes that may be related to an ischemic event need immediate transportation to an emergency department for evaluation. Once there, initial testing for an acute cardiac event or acute myocardial infarction (AMI) will include an ECG and determination of cardiac enzymes or tissue markers. In addition to measurement of hs-CRP and ESR discussed earlier, creatinine kinase and troponin measurements are used.

Creatinine Kinase

The cardiac enzyme creatinine kinase (CK) is present in various parts of the body and in several forms (called isoenzymes). The isoenzyme CK-MB is associated with cardiac tissue, and laboratory values for CK-MB are used in the diagnosis of AMI, myocardial muscle injury, unstable angina, shock, malignant hyperthermia, myopathies, and myocarditis (Pagana and Pagana, 2010). The CK-MB level rises 3 to 6 hours after an AMI occurs. It peaks at 12 to 24 hours (unless the infarction extends) and returns to normal after 12 to 48 hours; therefore it is not a useful measure after that period of time. A number of drugs commonly used by the elderly, including anticoagulants, aspirin, dexamethasone, furosemide, captopril, colchicine, alcohol, lovastatin, lidocaine, propranolol, and morphine, can cause false CK-MB elevations. For the best diagnosis, CK-MB is used as a comparative measure with troponin.

Troponin

Troponin I and troponin T are cardiac-specific biomarkers for cardiac disease and are used in the evaluation of patients suspected of an acute ischemic event or AMI. They have become the "gold standard" for diagnosis of heart injury. They become elevated as early as 3 hours after an event. Troponin I remains elevated for 7 to 10 days and troponin T remains elevated for 10 to 14 days. The normal level of troponin I is less than 0.03 ng/mL and that for troponin T is less than 0.2 ng/mL (Pagana and Pagana, 2010).

Monitoring Cardiovascular Risk and Health

Increasing attention has been given to three biochemical markers that are believed to have value in the detection of heart disease or in the assessment for risk of cardiovascular disease. These are C-reactive protein (hs-CRP), homocysteine, and brain natriuretic peptide (BNP). Tests for lipids have become increasingly important for both determining health risk and monitoring treatment.

Homocysteine

Homocysteine is a naturally occurring amino acid that is produced in the metabolism of proteins. It appears to promote the progression of atherosclerosis. When elevated it is an important predictor of coronary, cerebral, and peripheral vascular disease. It is also elevated with vitamin B_{12} and folate deficiencies and has been used to monitor malnutrition. A person with an elevation has a five times greater risk for stroke, dementia, and Alzheimer's disease; and a risk factor for osteoporotic fractures. Normal findings range from 4 to 14 μmol/L. Traditional laboratory testing has improved with the development of an enzyme immunoassay.

Brain Natriuretic Peptide

Brain natriuretic peptide (BNP) is a neuroendocrine peptide secreted by the ventricles of the heart in response to excessive stretching and pressure. BNP levels are determined to identify and stratify persons with congestive heart failure, and are implicated in the pathophysiology of hypertension and atherosclerosis as well. Depending on the laboratory, BNP is measured as BNP, pro-BNP, or NT-pro-BNP (Pagana and Pagana, 2010).

Lipids

Dyslipidemia indicates a health risk regardless of one's age and is a major predictor of coronary heart disease. Control of lipids has been found to be significantly important for persons of any age. Laboratory testing for lipids is usually done as a "lipid panel" and includes both cholesterol and triglycerides. It is done both as a health screen and for monitoring the response to treatment, usually with lipid-lowering medications and/or diet. For the most accurate results, the person should have fasted 12 to 15 hours before the test.

Cholesterol. Cholesterol is a sterol compound used by the body to stabilize cell membranes. It is metabolized in the liver, where it is combined with low-density lipoprotein (LDL), high-density lipoprotein (HDL), and very low–density lipoprotein (VLDL). Men's cholesterol levels slowly increase from puberty until about age 60 years. Then it appears to stabilize, only to rise again after age 80 years. The cholesterol levels of women are relatively stable until menopause, at which time they begin to rise. A "total cholesterol" reading, such as those often done at health fairs, is the measurement of overall cholesterol in the blood; it is almost as accurate as serum cholesterol but of little diagnostic value alone. The lipid panel provides total cholesterol as well as the LDL-C and HDL-C breakdown (Table 8-5). As the cholesterol level changes throughout the day and is influenced by position (lying down, etc.), at least two measurements should be averaged.

Many drugs affect cholesterol levels (Box 8-6). An unexplained low serum cholesterol level (≤200 mg/dL) is indicative of several conditions including malnutrition and requires further evaluation (Pagana and Pagana, 2010). A total cholesterol level below 160 mg/dL in a frail elder is a risk factor for

TABLE 8-5   INTERPRETING LIPID PANELS

TOTAL CHOLESTEROL		LDL–CHOLESTEROL		HDL–CHOLESTEROL		TRIGLYCERIDES	
VALUE	INTERPRETATION	VALUE	INTERPRETATION	VALUE	INTERPRETATION	VALUE	INTERPRETATION
<200	Desirable	<100	Optimal	<40	Low	<150	Normal
200-239	Borderline high	100-128	Near optimal	>60	High	150-199	Borderline high
≥240	High	130-159	Borderline high			200-499	High
		160-189	High			>500	Very high
		≥190	Very high				

Data from Grundy S, Cleeman JI, Merz CN, et al; National Heart, Lung, and Blood Institute; American College of Cardiology Foundation; American Heart Association: Implications of recent clinical trials for the National Cholesterol Education Program Adult Treatment Panel III guidelines, Circulation 110:227, 2004.

BOX 8-6   EXAMPLES OF DRUGS THAT AFFECT SERUM CHOLESTEROL LEVELS

INCREASE
- β-Adrenergic blocking agents
- Corticosteroids
- Phenytoin
- Sulfonamides
- Thiazides
- Vitamin D

DECREASE
- Allopurinol
- Captopril
- Chlorpropamide
- Clofibrate
- Colchicine
- Lovastatin
- Niacin
- Nitrates

BOX 8-7   NORMAL FINDINGS: *PROTEINS*

Total protein: 6.4-8.3 g/dL
Globulin: 2.3-3.4 g/dL
Prealbumin: 15-36 mg/dL

From Pagana KD, Pagana TJ: *Mosby's manual of diagnostic and laboratory tests*, ed 4, St. Louis, MO, 2010, Mosby.

increased mortality (Johnson, 2002). Triglycerides are the primary lipids found in the blood and are bound to a protein. They are produced in the liver and circulated in the blood. Excess blood levels are deposited into fatty tissue. Triglycerides peak at midlife. Abnormally low triglyceride levels are suggestive of malnutrition or hyperthyroidism. Reasons for elevated levels include chronic renal failure and poorly controlled diabetes. Severely elevated triglyceride levels (>2000 mg/dL) are a strong risk factor for pancreatitis (Gambert and Miller, 2004).

TESTING FOR BODY PROTEINS

Total Protein

Body proteins are measured by determining the amount of albumin and globulin in the serum. Serum albumin is a measure of nutritional status. Globulins are important in the functioning of antibodies and in the maintenance of osmotic pressure.

Serum Albumin

Serum albumin and globulin are used most often as measures of nutritional status but are also used to diagnose and monitor cancer, protein-wasting states, immune disorders and liver function (Pagana and Pagana, 2010). Although they are commonly ordered, they are neither sensitive nor specific for

nutritional health and a slight decrease is a normal change of aging. Corticosteroids, insulin, phenazopyridine, and progesterone increase protein levels. Dehydration will show a deceptive increase in albumin levels. Albumin levels decrease with overhydration, liver and renal disease, malabsorption, and changes from an upright position to a supine position during the blood draw (Pagana and Pagana, 2010). The half-life of albumin is about three weeks, so changes are not quickly apparent except in sudden and acutely severe conditions. However, albumin levels are most useful as an indicator of the severity of illness and the risk of mortality. Prealbumin (transthyretin) has a half-life of only two to three days and is therefore a more sensitive marker for change. A low prealbumin level can confirm poor nutritional status and serve as a monitor for active treatment (Box 8-7).

LABORATORY TESTS OF RENAL HEALTH

Renal function decreases substantially with age, but in most cases the body is able to compensate adequately, and there are only slight changes in laboratory findings. Still, the results are expected to be within the normal limits for adults. However, laboratory findings may be unreliable in those with reduced lean body mass, excessive dietary intake of protein, alterations in metabolism, and strenuous physical activity before measurement. Because of the frequency of health problems and medications that further affect renal health, measuring and monitoring renal functioning are particularly important to the older adult and the gerontological nurse. The early signs of kidney disease are asymptomatic urinalysis abnormalities: hematuria, proteinuria, pyuria, and casts. Further indicators are elevated blood urea nitrogen or creatinine.

Blood Urea Nitrogen

Urea is the end product of protein metabolism. A concentration greater than 100 mg/dL is a critical value and indicates serious renal dysfunction. The serum chemistry test for blood urea nitrogen (BUN) is used as a gross measurement for renal functioning and the glomerular filtration rate (GFR). Blood levels are directly affected by liver and kidney health. Protein intake affects BUN, and many drugs increase the levels. Changes over time in the BUN level may be more important than any one laboratory result, especially in the assessment of renal insufficiency or renal failure. *Azotemia* is an elevation of BUN. Prerenal azotemia refers to elevations before blood gets to the kidneys; causes include shock, dehydration, congestive heart failure, and excessive protein catabolism such as in starvation. Normal findings for adults are 10 to 20 mg/dL (Pagana and Pagana, 2010).

Creatinine

Creatinine is a by-product of the breakdown of muscle creatinine phosphate that is normally produced in energy metabolism; its level is highly dependent on muscle mass. As long as muscle mass remains the same, the serum creatinine should be constant. It is most specifically used to diagnose and monitor impaired renal function. Therefore the reduced muscle mass of normal aging will result in a decreased creatinine level. Although the measurement of creatinine is a more accurate reflection of renal health than BUN, it also can overestimate renal function in the elderly. As part of a collection of tests within the "renal function panel," the BUN/creatinine ratio is a good indicator of the GFR.

However, because of the number of things that can alter the BUN/creatinine level (and therefore the measurement of creatinine clearance), another test, one for cystatin C, may become more common to assess renal function (Pagana and Pagana, 2010).

The Cockcroft-Gault equation is still used to estimate creatinine clearance (CrCl), using the serum creatinine value and the person's age. Although it somewhat overestimates renal function in the elderly, it is frequently used by clinicians in estimating doses when prescribing drugs for elders with probable diminished renal function (Pagana and Pagana, 2010). It has replaced the 24-hour urine collection for creatinine clearance, which is difficult to do, especially in frail elders. The formula for men is as follows:

$$[(140 - age) \times (weight\ in\ kg)] \div (72 \times serum\ creatinine)$$

In women, because of their smaller muscle mass, the value is multiplied by 0.85 or 85%.

Although the calculated creatinine clearance is a good measure of the glomerular filtration rate, it must be considered within the context of the person's lean body mass, especially in persons who are very small or seriously ill. It is especially important to calculate and monitor creatinine clearance in the administration of potentially nephrotoxic medications such as allopurinol, aminoglycosides, ACE inhibitors, and nonsteroidal antiinflammatory drugs (NSAIDs) (Beck, 2004).

MONITORING FOR THERAPEUTIC BLOOD LEVELS

The monitoring of medications with narrow therapeutic windows is especially important in later life. At levels that are

TABLE 8-6	PREFERRED INTERNATIONAL NORMALIZED RATIO ACCORDING TO INDICATION FOR ANTICOAGULATION
INDICATION	**PREFERRED INR**
Deep-vein thrombosis prophylaxis	1.5-2.0
Orthopedic surgery	2.0-3.0
Deep-vein thrombosis	2.0-3.0
Atrial fibrillation	2.0-3.0
Pulmonary embolism	2.5-3.5
Prosthetic valve prophylaxis	3.0-4.0

INR, international normalized ratio.
From Pagana KD, Pagana TJ: *Manual of diagnostic and laboratory tests*, ed 4, St. Louis, MO, 2010, Mosby.

too low, the effect of medications may be negligible and at levels that are too high, they may become toxic and result in adverse drug events. Although this applies to several antibiotics in use (e.g., vancomycin), this discussion is restricted to medications most commonly prescribed to older adults.

Anticoagulants

Anticoagulation therapy has become a mainstay treatment of atrial fibrillation and in stroke prevention (e.g., after surgery). Any person who is taking warfarin (Coumadin) or heparin must have their coagulation time monitored because of the narrow therapeutic window and variation in timing needed, depending on the purpose of the anticoagulation (Table 8-6). Prothrombin, produced by the liver, is a key component in blood clotting. For the body to produce prothrombin, it must have adequate intake and absorption of vitamin K. In clotting, prothrombin is converted to thrombin as the first part of the coagulation cascade. The prothrombin time (PT) is the most sensitive measure of deficiencies in vitamin K–dependent clotting factors II, VII, IX, and X affected by warfarin use.

The PT is not sensitive to fibrinogen deficiencies and heparin (Nicoll et al., 2004). For persons who are receiving the anticoagulant *heparin*, the partial prothrombin time (PTT) is used to monitor coagulation status and drug dosage.

The PT is among those tests that the gerontological nurse will see done most often and one of the most important ones relating to the immediate needs of the patient. In the past, precise coagulation monitoring was difficult because of variation of test results between laboratories; interpretations were fraught with errors or inconsistencies in calculation from laboratory to laboratory. Today the PT is evaluated by a set international normalized ratio (INR), providing significantly greater reliability. Too high an INR may result in severe and life-threatening bleeding. A PT of 20 seconds (INR > 5.5) is considered a panic level, one that requires immediate intervention. Causes include inadequate monitoring, liver disease, vitamin K deficiencies, bile duct obstruction, and salicylate intoxication. It also may be increased with the concomitant use of such drugs as allopurinol, cholestyramine, clofibrate, and sulfonamides (Pagana and Pagana, 2010). Too low an INR removes the preventive action of the therapy and suggests a hypercoagulation state.

Antiarrhythmics: Digoxin

Digoxin (Lanoxin) is a drug that is commonly used to control ventricular response to chronic atrial fibrillation. It is initiated slowly and carefully to prevent too rapid a reduction in heart rate. Once the patient's dose is stabilized, the nurse monitors the effect of the medication by measuring the heart rate before drug administration and by observing for signs of adverse effects. Monitoring includes periodic determination of blood levels. The normal therapeutic range is 0.9 to 2.0 ng/mL with toxicity occurring at levels above 3.0 ng/mL. However, because of the normal changes with aging that affect pharmacokinetics, toxicity may be evident at levels below 3.0 ng/mL. In many cases there is clinical evidence or suspicions of toxicity regardless of the blood level and should be treated accordingly. In some cases providers depend on clinical assessment rather than the traditional "digoxin level annually." A dose of 0.125 mg may be quite effective for older adults. The nurse can use the blood level only as a general guide, and it must be combined with the clinical presentation (including heart rate) of the person being treated.

Thyroid Hormones

See Hormones on pp. 122-123.

URINE STUDIES

Urine is the end-product of metabolism and contains potentially harmful products or other products that have exceeded the body's threshold of usefulness. If the kidneys are working well and a urine level of a compound is elevated, there should be a corresponding elevation in the blood. However, if the kidney is diseased, urine levels may be deceptively low. The most common urine test in the everyday care of older adults is a urinalysis.

The urinalysis is done both macroscopically by the nurse at the bedside and microscopically in the laboratory. In healthy aging, the findings do not differ by age, but abnormalities are frequently found because of the high rate of diabetes, renal insufficiency, subclinical bacteriuria, urinary tract infections, and proteinuria. Hematuria always requires further evaluation.

The specimen, either from a clean catch or catheterization, should be tested or sent to the laboratory immediately. It may be refrigerated for up to two hours if absolutely necessary. But any specimen that has not been properly stored or tested promptly should be disposed of and a new one obtained. The cleaner and fresher the specimen, the more accurate is the analysis.

The point-of-service (bedside) analysis by the nurse begins with an observation of the specimen for color, odor, and clarity. Colorless urine may be the result of high fluid intake or recent caffeine intake. Dark urine often is the result of dehydration or the presence of microscopic blood or bacteria. Clarity is hindered by the presence of phosphate crystals after a high-protein meal or the presence of a large number of bacteria. A strong or foul odor is suggestive of either a state of dehydration (concentrated urine) or bacteriuria.

The bedside analysis usually concludes with what is called a "urine dip," that is, individual measures compared with a standard. Although the bedside analysis is often used, because of the high rate of false negatives and false positives it should be used only as a screening tool and combined with the clinical assessment of the person. The remainder of the obtained sample is usually sent to the laboratory for microscopic analysis. Both the laboratory and the bedside analyses will measure the urine specific gravity, pH, and the presence of urine protein, glucose, ketones, blood, bilirubin, nitrates, and leukocytes.

The specific gravity is a measure of the adequacy of the renal concentrative mechanism; it measures hydration. Specific gravity in the adult is normally between 1.005 and 1.030. These values decrease with aging because of the 33% to 50% decline in the number of nephrons, which impairs the ability of the kidney to concentrate urine. Nephron function is measured by the glomerular filtration rate (GFR), which is calculated on the basis of creatinine clearance.

The urine pH indicates its acid–base balance. An alkaline pH is usually caused by bacteria (which may indicate a urinary tract infection), a diet high in citrus fruits and vegetables, or the intake of sodium bicarbonates. Acidic urine occurs with starvation, dehydration, and diets high in meats and cranberries.

Protein is measured both with a dipstick and standard urinalysis, as well as by 24-hour urine collection. The dipstick method is limited to the detection of albumin at levels of almost 30 mg/dL, translating into a considerably high rate of proteinuria and always indicating a need for further evaluation of renal function. Proteinuria is defined as an albumin level greater than 150 mg/dL in a 24-hour period.

Ascorbic acid and aspirin can cause false-negative results for glucose. Ketones may be positive in high-protein diets, "crash" diets, or starvation.

Nitrates and/or leukocytes are often found in the presence of infection. A urinalysis suggestive of the presence of bacteria indicates the need for further testing, most often a culture of the urine, and a subsequent testing of sensitivity of the bacteria to antibiotics. This is often ordered as a "U/A [or urine analysis] C & S [culture and sensitivity] as indicated." However, because of the potential lethality of any infection in ill older adults, empiric clinical evidence of a potential infection may require treatment before the three or four days needed for testing results.

IMPLICATIONS FOR THE NURSE IN THE LONG-TERM CARE SETTING

Laboratory tests and regular screening tests are commonly employed when caring for a resident of a nursing home. Protocols for establishing routine laboratory testing procedures for long-term care vary widely from one institution to the next and from one laboratory to the next. Gerontological nurses advocate good resident care by requesting laboratory tests and developing protocols to comply with recommended minimal standards for screening and monitoring laboratory tests for elderly residents in long-term care institutions.

In summary, collecting and monitoring laboratory values are important nursing responsibilities. This can be particularly important for the gerontological nurse because some laboratory values change slightly with aging and the older person may be more sensitive to changes in homeostasis. The variance of values at both ends of the laboratory range could be misinterpreted as abnormal or questionable when they are within the normal range for that gender and age group. We may find eventually that the "normal ranges" in the population, older than 65 years are different from those of the younger population, but this has not yet been determined.

Laboratory values are helpful tools in understanding clinical signs and symptoms, although clinical decisions based on laboratory values alone are not enough for treatment of the whole person. Abnormal laboratory results trigger comprehensive patient assessments, obtaining information about clinical signs and symptoms, patient history, and psychosocial and physical examination. The nurse combines this information with the interpretation of laboratory values to establish the most appropriate care in collaboration with the person's nurse practitioner or physician. The nurse practitioner quickly and accurately interprets the findings and translates these into the medical plan of care.

evolve To access your student resources, go to *http://evolve.elsevier.com/Ebersole/TwdHlthAging*

KEY CONCEPTS

- In most laboratory measures, there is little difference in the results between a younger adult and an older adult.
- Because of more limited reserves, the older adult is often more sensitive to slight variations in biological parameters.
- The laboratory criteria used in the diagnosis of diabetes and thyroid disease do not differ according to age.
- The nurse is often responsible for the initial interpretation of laboratory results. The nurse cannot depend entirely on laboratory values when considering the possibility of medication toxicity.
- The nurse may be responsible for the accurate and appropriate collection of laboratory specimens.
- Medications and chronic disorders complicate the measurement of laboratory values in elders because most elders are taking several medications at any given time that may interact to alter the reliability of laboratory measurements.

CASE STUDY   EVALUATING LABORATORY RESULTS

An 84-year-old white male, Mr. Jones, is being admitted to the nursing home where you work. He has a history of heart disease, hypertension, diabetes, constipation, and anemia of chronic disease. You find that he denies any fever, chest pain, numbness or tingling, leg swelling, or palpitations. His diabetes has been under fairly good control while at home, but he has difficulty telling you how much insulin he has been taking. His skin is slightly warm to the touch. He is lethargic, but you notice that he also has some muscle twitching. He has an order to have blood tests done today, including a CBC and a complete metabolic panel. You request it and get the following results later in the evening. Medications include lisinopril, 20 mg/day; Lasix, 40 mg/day; potassium, 5 mEq/day; insulin 30/70, 12 units every morning; laxative as needed; multivitamin daily.

	RESULT	NORMAL RANGE
SODIUM	135 mEq/L	136-148 mEq/L
POTASSIUM	5.8 mEq/L	3.5-5.3 mEq/L
CHLORIDE	110 mEq/L	97-108 mEq/L
GLUCOSE	60 mg/dL	70-110 mg/dL
BUN	25 mg/dL	10-20 mg/dL
CREATININE	1.8 mg/dL	0.6-1.2 mg/dL
ALBUMIN	2.4 g/dL	3.5-5.8 g/dL
WBCS	7000/mm^3	5000-10,000/mm^3
RBCS	$4.0 \times 10^6/\mu L$	$4.4\text{-}5.8 \times 10^6/\mu L$
HGB	10.2 g/dL	14-18 g/dL
HCT	30.6%	39%-48%

On the basis of the case study, develop a nursing care plan using the following procedure*:

- List Mr. Jones's comments that provide subjective data.
- List information that provides objective data.
- From these data, identify and state, using accepted format, two nursing diagnoses you determine are most significant to Mr. Jones at this time. List two of Mr. Jones's strengths that you have identified from the data.
- Determine and state outcome criteria for each diagnosis. These must reflect some alleviation of the problem identified in the nursing diagnosis and must be stated in concrete and measurable terms.
- Plan and state one or more interventions for each diagnosed problem. Provide specific documentation of the source used to determine the appropriate intervention. Plan at least one intervention that incorporates Mr. Jones's existing strengths.
- Evaluate the success of the intervention. Interventions must correlate directly with the stated outcome criteria to measure the outcome success.

CRITICAL THINKING QUESTIONS

1. Which of the laboratory findings are not within normal limits?
2. Are there any deviations in the results that are consistent with normal aging? If so, which ones and why?
3. Are there any deviations in laboratory results that would be expected in persons with prolonged chronic illness, like Mr. Jones? If so, what are they and why are they expected?
4. Which of the above deviations from normal are potentially the most dangerous for Mr. Jones at this time? If so, why?
5. Could any of the abnormal blood tests be related to his medications?
6. Are there any results that need prompt referral to Mr. Jones's primary care provider? If so, which one(s)?

*Students are advised to refer to their nursing diagnosis text and identify possible or potential problems.

RESEARCH QUESTIONS

1. In what way does food and alcohol intake affect the accuracy of laboratory test results?

2. Summarize laboratory values that are considered "critical" and require some type of immediate response.

REFERENCES

Auerhahn C, Capazuti E, Flaherty E, et al., editors: *Geriatric nursing review syllabus: a core curriculum in advanced practice nursing*, ed 2, New York, 2007, American Geriatrics Society.

Beck LH: Renal systems, fluid and electrolytes. In Landefeld CS, Palmer RM, Johnson MA, et al., editors: *Current geriatric diagnosis and treatment*, New York, 2004, McGraw-Hill.

Brashers VL, Jones RE: Mechanisms in hormone regulation. In McCance KL, Huether SE, Brashers VL, et al, editors: *Pathophysiology: the biological basis for disease in adults and children*, ed 6, St. Louis, MO, 2010, Mosby.

Cadogan MP: Functional implications of vitamin B_{12} deficiency, *Journal of Gerontological Nursing* 36:16, 2010.

Cho KC: Fluid and electrolyte disorders (Chapter 21). In McPhee SJ, Papadakis MA, editors: *CURRENT medical diagnosis and treatment 2010*, New York, 2010, McGraw-Hill.

Colombet I, Pouchot J, Kronz V, et al: Agreement between erythrocyte sedimentation rate and C-reactive protein in hospital practice, *The American Journal of Medicine* 123:863.e7, 2010.

Ernst AA, Weiss SJ, Tracy LA, et al: Usefulness of CRP and ESR in predicting septic joints, *Southern Medical Journal* 103:522, 2010.

Fitzgerald PA: Endocrine disorders. In McPhee SJ, Papadakis MA, editors: *CURRENT medical diagnosis and treatment 2010*, New York, 2010, McGraw-Hill.

Freedman ML: Aging and the blood (Chapter 68). In Beers MH, Jones TV, editors: *The Merck manual of geriatrics*, ed 3, Whitehouse Station, NJ, 2009-2010a, Merck Research Laboratories.

Freedman ML: The anemias (Chapter 69). In Beers MH, Jones TV, editors: *The Merck manual of geriatrics*, ed 3, Whitehouse Station, NJ, 2009-2010b, Merck Research Laboratories.

Freedman ML, Sutin DG: Blood disorders and their management. In Tallis RC, Fillit HM, editors: *Brocklehurst's textbook of geriatric medicine and gerontology*, ed 6, Edinburgh, 2002, Churchill Livingstone.

Gambert SR, Miller M: Endocrine disorders. In Landefeld CS, Palmer RM, Johnson MA, et al., editors: *Current geriatric diagnosis and treatment*, New York, 2004, McGraw-Hill.

Hardin S: Anemia of chronic disease, older adults, and Medicare. *JGN* 36(10): 3-4, 2010.

Harris CL, Fraser C: Malnutrition in the institutionalized elderly: the effects on wound healing, *Ostomy/Wound Management* 50:54, 2004.

Helfand M, Buckley D, Fleming C, et al: *Screening for intermediate risk factors for coronary heart disease*. AHRQ Report 10-05141EF-1. Rockville, MD, 2009, Agency for Healthcare Research and Quality. Available at http://www.ncbi.nlm.nih.gov/books/NBK35208/. Accessed December 2010.

Hellmann DB, Imboden JB: Musculoskeletal disorders (Chapter 20). In McPhee SJ, Papadakis MA, editors: *CURRENT medical diagnosis and treatment 2010*, New York, 2010, McGraw-Hill.

Huether SE: The cellular environment: fluids, electrolytes, acids and bases (Chapter 3). In McCance KL, Huether SE, Brashers VL, et al., editors: *Pathophysiology: the biological basis for disease in adults and children*, ed 6, St. Louis, MO, 2010, Mosby.

Johnson LE: Nutrition. In Ham RS, Sloane PD, Warshaw GA, et al., editors: *Primary care geriatrics*, ed 4, St. Louis, MO, 2002, Mosby.

Johnson LE: Vitamin and trace mineral disorders (Chapter 60). In Beers MH, Jones T: *The Merck manual of geriatrics*, ed 3, Whitehouse Station, NJ, 2009-2010, Merck Research Laboratories.

Kreiner F, Langberg H, Galbo H: Increased muscle interstitial levels of inflammatory cytokines in polymyalgia rheumatica, *Arthritis and Rheumatism* 62:3768, 2010.

Mentes J: A typology of caps and oral rehydration: problems exhibited by frail nursing home residents, *Journal of Gerontological Nursing* 32:13, 2006.

Miller DK: Laboratory values (Appendix 1). In Beers MH, Jones, T: *The Merck manual of geriatrics*, ed 3, Whitehouse Station, NJ, 2009-2010, Merck Research Laboratories.

Moore SA: Laboratory and diagnostic tests. In Meiner SE, Lueckenotte AG, editors: *Gerontologic nursing*, ed 3, St. Louis, MO, 2006, Mosby.

Nicoll D, McPhee SJ, Pignone M, editors: *Pocket guide to diagnostic tests*, ed 4, New York, 2004, McGraw-Hill.

Pagana KD, Pagana TJ: *Mosby's manual of diagnostic and laboratory tests*, ed 4, St. Louis, MO, 2010, Mosby.

Sink KM, Yaffee K: Cognitive impairment and dementia. In Landefeld CS, Palmer RM, Johnson MA, et al., editors: *Current geriatric diagnosis and treatment*, New York, 2004, McGraw-Hill.

Thibodeau GA, Patton KT: *Structure and function of the body*, ed 12, St. Louis, MO, 2003, Mosby.

U.S. Preventive Services Task Force: *The guide to clinical preventive services (2010-2011): recommendations of the U.S. Preventive Services Task Force*. AHRQ Publication No. 09-IP006. Rockville, MD, 2010, Agency for Healthcare Research and Quality.

Zakai NA, Katz R, Hirsch C, et al.: A prospective study of anemia status, hemoglobin concentrations and mortality in an elderly cohort: The Cardiovascular Health Study. *Archiv Int Med* 165, 2214-2220, 2005.

Geropharmacology

Kathleen Jett

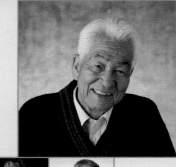

*Special thanks to Gregory Gulick, MD, who contributed to
this chapter in a previous edition.*

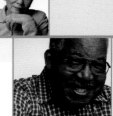

evolve *http://evolve.elsevier.com/Ebersole/TwdHlthAging*

A STUDENT SPEAKS

*Whenever I see patients in the clinic I try to think very carefully before adding any medications, but since most of them have
so many things going on with them, I sometimes wonder where I can start!*   **Helen, age 32, gerontological nurse
practitioner student**

AN ELDER SPEAKS

*Every time I go to the clinic I get another prescription. It just doesn't seem like I should need to take so many, so sometimes
I don't.*   *Annie, age 72*

LEARNING OBJECTIVES

On completion of this chapter, the reader will be able to:
1. Describe the pharmacokinetic changes that occur as a result of normal changes with aging.
2. Describe potential problems associated with drug therapy in late life.
3. Identify medications that are more commonly used in late life.
4. Describe medications and side effects of those more commonly used as psychotherapeutic agents.
5. Identify inappropriate drug use and its application in gerontological nursing.
6. Identify the early signs of adverse drug reactions and strategies to prevent these.
7. Discuss barriers to medication adherence in elders.
8. Discuss the role of the health care professional in assisting elders with adherence to medication regimens.
9. Develop a nursing plan to promote safe medication practices and prevent drug toxicity.

In the United States, persons 65 years of age and older are the largest users of prescription and over-the-counter (OTC) medications. Although making up only about 12% of the population, they consume about one third of all prescriptions drugs and one half of those available OTC (Beyth and Shorr, 2007). The majority (94%) regularly takes prescription medications, 46% take OTCs, and 53% take dietary supplements such as herbs (Qato et al., 2008). Although the statistics vary from study to study, the increase in number of medications with the number of years lived, and chronic conditions acquired, is consistent. The most commonly prescribed and used drugs in the ambulatory older population are cardiovascular drugs, diuretics, nonopioid analgesics, anticoagulants, and antiepileptics (Field et al., 2004). Gastrointestinal preparations and analgesics are the most-used OTC medications, followed by cough products, eye washes, and vitamins. According to a report of the

Agency for Healthcare Research and Quality, Medicare beneficiaries spent about $82 billion in 2007 on medications, one fourth of this or about $19 billion, on those for cholesterol and diabetes (Agency for Healthcare Quality Research, 2010).

Pharmacological interventions can both enhance and endanger the quality and quantity of life. When medications are used inappropriately, they contribute to both morbidity and mortality in this population. Unfortunately, even when drugs are used appropriately, there are times that they may adversely affect the elder's health and well-being. Older adults are at greater risk for polypharmacy, adverse drug events, and inappropriate drug use than are younger adults. The reasons for this are many and include increases in chronic disease and varying levels of geriatric skills of health care providers. When used with caution and care, pharmacological interventions can be used alongside nonpharmacological approaches to maximize healthy aging.

This chapter reviews the basics of pharmacokinetics and pharmacodynamics relevant to geropharmacology. Several issues are addressed with special attention to the use of psychotropic medications.

PHARMACOKINETICS

Pharmacokinetics is the study of the movement and action of a drug in the body. Pharmacokinetics determines the concentration of drugs in the body, which in turn determines effect. The concentration of the drug at different times depends on how the drug is taken into the body (absorption), where the drug is dispersed (distribution), how the drug is broken down (metabolism), and how the body gets rid of the drug (excretion). It is important for the gerontological nurse to understand how pharmacokinetics may differ in an older adult (Figure 9-1).

Absorption

For a drug to be effective, it must be absorbed into the bloodstream. The amount of time between the administration of the drug and its absorption depends on a number of factors, including the route of administration, bioavailability, and the amount of drug that passes through the absorbing surfaces in the body. The most common routes of administration are intravenous, oral, enteral, parenteral, transdermal, and rectal. The drug is delivered immediately to the bloodstream with intravenous administration and quickly via the parenteral, transdermal, and rectal routes. Orally and enterally administered drugs are absorbed the most slowly and primarily in the small intestine.

Drugs given orally pass through the mouth and esophagus and enter the stomach. Most solid oral drug dosage forms (e.g., tablets, capsules, powders, pills) are designed to dissolve in the

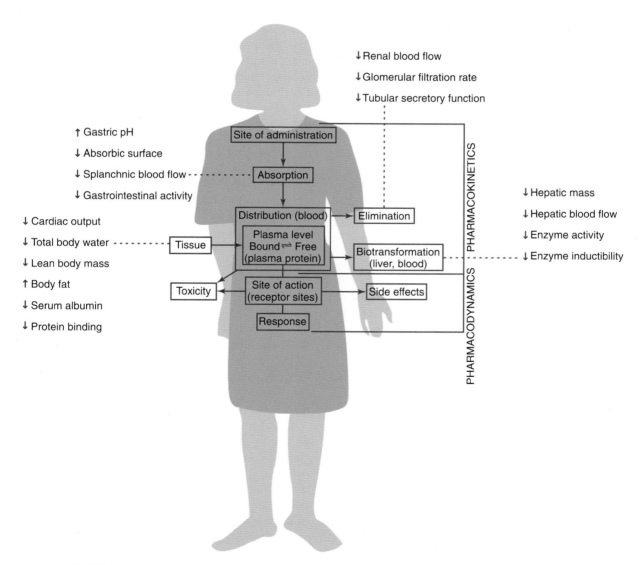

FIGURE 9-1 Physiological Age Changes and the Pharmacokinetics and Pharmacodynamics of Drug Use. (Data from Kane RL, Abrass ID, Ouslander JG: *Essentials of clinical geriatrics,* New York, 1984, McGraw-Hill; Lamy PP: Hazards of drug use in the elderly: common sense measures to reduce them, *Postgraduate Medicine* 76:50, 1984; Montamat SC, Cusack BJ, Vestal RE: Management of drug therapy in the elderly, *New England Journal of Medicine* 321:303, 1989; Roberts J, Tumer N: Pharmacodynamic basis for altered drug action in the elderly, *Clinics in Geriatric Medicine* 4:127, 1988; Vestal RE, Dawson GW: Pharmacology and aging. In Finch CE, Schneider EL, editors: *Handbook of biology and aging,* New York, 1985, Van Nostrand Reinhold.)

stomach. Drugs given enterally (via tube) are intended for an oral administration route but mechanically bypass the mouth and potentially the stomach and duodenum. Many factors affect the rate at which a medication is dissolved. These factors include the amount of liquid in the stomach, the type of coating the tablet has, the extent of tablet compression used in making the tablet, the presence of expanders in the tablet, the solubility of the drug in the acid environment of the stomach, and the rate of peristalsis. Liquid drug dosage forms for oral use come as solutions, suspensions, tinctures, and elixirs. The presence of food in the stomach may or may not delay absorption.

There does not seem to be conclusive evidence that absorption in older adults is changed appreciably. However, we do know that diminished salivary secretion and esophageal motility may interfere with swallowing some medications, which could in turn lead to erosions if adequate fluids are not taken with the medications (Gore and Mouzon, 2006). Decreased gastric acid, common in the elderly, will retard the action of acid-dependent drugs. Delayed stomach emptying may diminish or negate the effectiveness of short-lived drugs that could become inactivated before reaching the small intestine. Some enteric-coated medications, such as enteric-coated aspirin, which are specifically meant to bypass stomach acidity, may be delayed so long in older adults that their action begins in the stomach and may produce undesirable effects, such as gastric irritation or nausea.

Once a drug has been administered orally (or enterally), it may be absorbed directly into the bloodstream from the stomach (e.g., alcohol), but usually passes dissolved into the duodenum or small intestine. The small intestine has a large surface area and is efficient at absorption. Slowed intestinal motility, frequently seen with aging, can increase the contact time and increase drug effect because of prolonged absorption, significantly increasing the risk for adverse reactions or unpredictable effects.

The drug passes from the small intestine into the network of veins surrounding it, known as the *portal system,* and into the liver, where it may undergo metabolism (see below). Drugs that are extensively metabolized as they pass through the liver are said to have a large *first-pass effect.* Drugs with a significant first-pass effect usually require much larger oral doses than the same drug given by injection. In normal aging, both liver mass and blood flow are significantly decreased, resulting in reductions in the metabolism rate with potential but unknown implications for the older adult.

With sublingual and rectal administration, the drug is absorbed through the mucous membrane directly into the systemic circulation. Drying of the mouth, a common side effect of many of the medications taken by older adults, may reduce or delay buccal absorption. Rectal administration may be useful when the patient cannot tolerate oral medications.

Nurses working with older adults are usually familiar with the transdermal drug delivery system (TDDS) because of its long use for the topical application of nitroglycerin; the drug was dispersed in an oil-based cream, placed on a piece of paper (measured by the centimeter), and taped to the skin. The system has developed significantly and is now used for many fat-soluble drugs, usually a medication-impregnated patch (e.g., estrogen, clonidine, nicotine, fentanyl, nitroglycerin). This route overcomes any first-pass problems, is more convenient, acceptable, and reliable than other routes, especially in the outpatient setting and for some persons with cognitive disorders. Ideally the TDDS provides for a more constant rate of drug administration and eliminates concern about gastrointestinal absorption variation, gastrointestinal intolerance, and drug interaction. It is indicated when a slow, timed-release delivery into the tissue and ultimately the bloodstream is desired. The skin must be intact, the patch must remain in place for the designated amount of time, and the previous patch must be removed before a new one is applied. For the elder who is either underweight or overweight, dosing may be unreliable. The characteristic thinning, dryness, and roughness of older skin also may affect absorption of the intended dose. The risk for an allergic reaction to the patch is increased with the normal immune changes with aging.

Distribution

The systemic circulation transports a drug throughout the body to receptors on the cells of the target organ, where a therapeutic effect is initiated. The organs of high blood flow (e.g., brain, kidneys, lungs, liver) rapidly receive the highest concentrations. Distribution to organs of lower blood flow (e.g., skin, muscles, fat) generally occurs more slowly and results in lower concentrations of the drug in these tissues. Circulatory disease, such as peripheral vascular disease, can affect drug distribution.

Lipophilic (fat-soluble) drugs pass through capillary membranes more easily than do hydrophilic (water-soluble) drugs, resulting in more rapid tissue distribution and a greater volume of distribution. Lipophilic drugs concentrate in adipose tissue to a greater extent than in the vasculature or other tissues. As adipose tissue nearly doubles in healthy older men and increases by one half in older women, the risk for accumulation and potentially fatal overdoses is increased. Drugs that are highly lipid soluble are stored in the fatty tissue, thus extending and possibly increasing the drug effect, depending on the level of adiposity (Masoro and Austed, 2003). In contrast, decreased body water in normal aging leads to higher serum levels of water-soluble drugs, such as digoxin, ethanol, and aminoglycosides. This can result in a higher relative volume of lipophilic drugs (e.g., diazepam, lorazepam) and a decreased *relative* volume of hydrophilic drugs (e.g., cimetidine, morphine) (Burchum, 2011).

Distribution also depends on the availability of plasma protein in the form of lipoproteins, globulins, and especially albumin. Some drugs are bound to protein for distribution. Normally, a predictable percentage of the absorbed drug is inactivated as it is bound to the protein. The remaining free drug is available in the bloodstream for therapeutic effect when an effective concentration is reached in the plasma.

The healthy elder shows either no or only an insignificant change in plasma binding proteins. However, albumin may be significantly reduced in those with malnutrition, an acute illness, or a long-standing chronic condition, common among those in need of skilled care at home or in long-term care settings. Unpredictable concentrations of drug are especially dangerous in those with narrow therapeutic windows such as salicylates, lorazepam, diazepam, chlorpromazine, phenobarbital, or haloperidol. Basic drugs (e.g., lidocaine, propranolol) will show increased protein binding and less effect, and acidic drugs (e.g., warfarin, phenytoin) will show decreased protein binding and greater effect because of decreased plasma albumin (Burchum, 2011). This is especially relevant to nurses working with medically fragile elders, such as in the acute care setting.

Metabolism

Some drugs exert their therapeutic effect in their absorbed form, whereas others must be metabolized first. Metabolism is the process wherein the chemical structure of the drug is converted to a *metabolite* that is more easily used and excreted. This process is called biotransformation. A drug will continue to exert a therapeutic effect as long as it remains either in its original state or as an active metabolite or metabolites. Active metabolites retain the ability to have a therapeutic effect and have the same or more chance of adverse effects as the original structure. For example, the metabolites of acetaminophen (Tylenol) can cause liver damage with doses above 4 g in 24 hours; extra strength tablets are commonly used at doses of 1 gram per tablet. The duration of drug action is determined by the metabolic rate and is measured in terms of half-life, that is, the length of time 50% of the drug/metabolites is/are active.

Metabolism occurs in two phases—*phase I* (oxidative) and *phase II* (conjugative). Conjugation reactions primarily convert drugs and their metabolites to glucuronides. Glucuronides are very hydrophilic and are more readily excreted in the urine or bile. The oxidative metabolizing enzymes are known as the *cytochrome P450 (CYP450) monooxygenase system.* The human CYP450 system is composed of about 50 isoforms (e.g., CYP3A3/4), each of which can perform a specific chemical reaction (Wilkinson, 2001). These isoforms metabolize the parent compound by adding or subtracting a part of the drug molecule (e.g., adding an oxygen atom or subtracting a methyl group), thereby changing the molecule into a more hydrophilic (polar) compound. Eight to ten of these isoforms are responsible for the majority of all drug metabolism.

Several of the metabolizing enzymes (CYP450 isoforms) show genetic differences. It has been found that people from different global regions tend to metabolize at different levels of efficiency: there are poor metabolizers, normal metabolizers, rapid metabolizers, and ultrarapid metabolizers (Box 9-1). Although differences in metabolism are important with any class of drugs, they are of particular note in relation to psychotropic and pain medications addressed elsewhere in this chapter.

Because of the high level of variability in metabolism from individual to individual, it is difficult to ascribe decreased drug-metabolizing capability to increased age. Studies have shown no decrease in either conjugative metabolism or CYP450 system function as a result of age. However, with aging, liver activity, mass, and volume and blood flow are diminished, with resultant decreases in hepatic exposure. Drugs that do not undergo significant first-pass metabolism are not affected by the aging liver, but those that undergo extensive first-pass metabolism may exhibit decreased metabolism, increased bioavailability, and a decreased rate of biotransformation (Beyth and Shorr, 2007).

Excretion

Drugs and their metabolites are excreted in sweat, saliva, and other secretions but primarily through the kidneys. They are

BOX 9-1   FOCUS ON GENETICS

Drug Metabolism

As knowledge of the genome explodes, so does our ability to consider the possibility of what has come to be called "personalized medicine." Included in this is consideration of someday selecting medications and formulations consistent with the metabolic enzymes specific to the individual, which should optimize therapeutic effect while minimizing or eliminating any untoward effects. *Cytochrome P450* refers to a group of enzymes found primarily in the liver and responsible for the metabolism and excretion of the majority of drugs. Four phenotypic categories of persons relative to the speed of P450 metabolism have been identified. Someone who is a "poor" or "slow" metabolizer will excrete more slowly and therefore can achieve the same therapeutic effect with a low dose of a medication compared with the high dose needed by a "rapid" or even "ultrarapid" metabolizer. Among persons from the regions of northern Europe, 5% to 10% are poor metabolizers. This contrasts with persons from parts of Asia and Africa, among whom only 1% are poor metabolizers.

Data from Tiwari AK, Souza RP, Müller DJ: Pharmacogenetics of anxiolytic drugs, *Journal of Neural Transmission* 116:667, 2009.

excreted either unchanged or as metabolites. A few drugs are eliminated through the lungs, as unreabsorbed metabolites in bile and feces, or in breast milk. Very small amounts of drugs and metabolites can also be found in hair, sweat, saliva, tears, and semen.

Renal drug excretion occurs when the drug passes through the kidneys; it involves glomerular filtration, active tubular secretion, and passive tubular reabsorption. Glomerular filtration depends on both the rate and the extent of protein binding of the drug. The process involves passive filtration, and only unbound drugs are filtered. Because kidney function declines in many older persons, so does the ability to excrete or eliminate drugs in a timely manner. The glomerular filtration rate, renal plasma flow, tubular function, and reabsorptive capacity decline. The significantly decreased glomerular filtration rate leads to prolongation of the half-life of drugs eliminated through the renal system, resulting in more opportunities for accumulation and potential toxicity or other adverse events. Although renal function cannot be estimated on the basis of the serum creatinine level, it can be approximated by calculating creatinine clearance. There are a number of online ways to calculate creatinine clearance (e.g., see Chapter 8 or http://www.nephron.com/cgi-bin/CGSIdefault.cgi). The doses of many drugs eliminated through the renal system are based on the patient's measured or estimated creatinine clearance. Reductions in dosages for drugs eliminated through the renal system (e.g., allopurinol, vancomycin) are needed when the creatinine clearance is reduced (see also Chapter 4).

PHARMACODYNAMICS

Pharmacodynamics refers to the physiological interactions between a drug and the body, specifically, the chemical compounds introduced into the body and receptors on the cell membrane. Receptors are generally specifically configured cellular proteins that, because of their shape and ionic charge, bind to specific chemicals in the medications. The receptor protein has a specific shape that fits the chemical molecule, like a glove

BOX 9-2	POTENTIAL ANTICHOLINERGIC EFFECTS

- Constipation
- Dry mouth
- Blurred vision
- Dizziness
- Urinary retention
- Confusion

to a hand, with complementary ionic charges. When the chemical binds to the receptor, the therapeutic effect is initiated (e.g., nerve conduction and enzyme inhibition).

Drugs are usually similar in configuration to chemicals occurring naturally in the body, such that they bind to the same receptor sites. When a drug binds to the receptor sites, it may initiate the same physiological action as the natural chemical (agonist) or it may simply occupy the receptor sites and, in doing so, block the ability of the body chemical's usual physiological process (antagonist) depending on desired therapeutic effect. Although the drugs are designed to bind to specific receptor sites for specific purposes, usually they will attach to various other types of receptors as well. The physiological effects that occur as a result of binding to the unplanned types may produce unwanted side effects.

The older a person gets, the more likely he or she will have altered and unreliable pharmacodynamics. Although it is not always possible to explain or predict the alteration, several are known. Those of special note in the elderly are related to drugs with anticholinergic side effects (Box 9-2), which significantly increase the risk for accidental injury and associated with geriatric syndromes. Baroreceptor reflex responses decrease with age. This causes increased susceptibility to positional changes (orthostatic hypotension) and volume changes (dehydration). Age-related increases in sympathetic nervous system activity occur as a result of decreased myocardial sensitivity to catecholamines (e.g., norepinephrine, epinephrine) (Hämmerlein et al., 1998). A decreased responsiveness of the α-adrenergic system results in decreased sensitivity to β-agonists and β-antagonists (β-blockers). Because of the decreased effectiveness of β-blockers and increased sensitivity to diuretics, thiazide diuretics and not β-blockers are recommended for first-line treatment of hypertension in the elderly (Beyth and Shorr, 2007).

ISSUES IN MEDICATION USE

Polypharmacy

Polypharmacy has been defined in many ways: as simply the use of multiple medications, or as the use of multiple medications for the same problem (Planton and Edlund, 2010). Either way, it is extremely common among older adults and a source of potential morbidity and mortality. Steinman and Hanlon (2010) reported that nearly 20% of community-living adults at least 65 years of age took 10 or more medications, and this number is significantly higher among those living in long-term care settings. In a study of 1002 disabled older women living in the community, 60% were taking at least 5 different medications and almost 12% were taking at least 10, when OTCs and

prescription medications were combined (Crentsil et al., 2010). Simple polypharmacy may be necessary if the patient has multiple chronic conditions, even if the provider is following evidence-based guidelines, and especially when no "double-dipping" of medications is possible. Or it may occur unintentionally, especially if an existing drug regimen is not considered when new prescriptions are given, or any number of the thousands of OTC preparations and supplements are added to those prescribed. Polypharmacy is exacerbated by the combination of a high use of specialists and a reluctance of prescribers to discontinue potentially unnecessary drugs that have been prescribed by someone else; therefore treatments are continued longer than necessary (Randall and Bruno, 2006). When communication between patients, nurses, and other health care providers and caregivers becomes fragmented the risk for duplicative medications, inappropriate medications, potentially unsafe dosages, and potentially preventable interactions is accentuated. The two major concerns with polypharmacy are the increased risk for drug interactions and the increased risk for adverse events.

Drug Interactions

The more medications a person takes, either prescribed or OTC, the greater the possibility that one or more of them will interact with each other, a dietary supplement, or other herbal preparation. The more chronic conditions one has, the more likely that a medication for one condition will affect the body in such a way as to influence the other. When two or more medications are given at the same time or closely together, the drugs may potentiate one another (i.e., when given together the drugs have stronger effects than when given alone) or antagonize each other (i.e., when given together one or more of the drugs become ineffective).

Drug–Supplement Interactions

As the popularity of medicinal herbs and other dietary supplements rises, so does the risk for interaction with prescribed medications and other treatments. Although much remains unknown, new knowledge is added almost daily from which the gerontological nurse bases her or his practice. For example, although St. John's wort has been found to have some therapeutic effect on mild to moderate depression, it also may decrease digoxin levels (Scott and Elmer, 2002). Taking warfarin (Coumadin) at the same time as *Ginkgo biloba* may artificially increase the international normalized ratio (INR) and lead to inappropriate and potentially dangerous dosing (Valli and Giardina, 2002).

These interactions represent only a small fraction of the many real and potential nutritional supplement–drug interactions. Because of inadequate labeling requirements, drug interactions may not be listed on the product labels of these supplements. Patients, prescribers, and nurses administering medications need to be aware of the potential interactions of the herbal preparation or nutritional supplement used to the extent possible (Table 9-1) (see also Chapter 10).

Drug–Food Interactions

Foods may interact with drugs, producing increased, decreased, or variable effects. Foods can bind to drugs, affecting their

TABLE 9-1	POTENTIAL INTERACTIONS BETWEEN HERBS AND CONVENTIONAL DRUGS*	
HERB	**CONVENTIONAL DRUG**	**COMMENTS**
Ginkgo leaf	Acetylsalicylic acid Rofecoxib Warfarin Trazodone	Ginkgo combined with acetylsalicylic acid,[†] rofecoxib,[†] or warfarin[†] has been associated with bleeding reactions; ginkgo alone has also been associated with bleeding (case reports). Coma was reported in a patient with Alzheimer's disease who took ginkgo leaf with trazodone[†]
Hawthorn leaf or flower	Digitalis glycosides	Because hawthorn may exert digitalis-like inotropic effects, it is prudent to monitor persons taking this herb in addition to digitalis glycosides closely
St. John's wort	5-Aminolevulinic acid Amitriptyline Cyclosporine Digoxin Indinavir Midazolam Nevirapine Paroxetine Phenprocoumon Sertraline Simvastatin Tacrolimus Theophylline Warfarin	A phototoxic reaction occurred in a patient simultaneously exposed to 5-aminolevulinic acid and St. John's wort[†]; in clinical studies, pretreatment with St. John's wort decreased the area under the curve for amitriptyline (and its active metabolite nortriptyline), digoxin, indinavir, midazolam, phenprocoumon, and the active metabolite of simvastatin (simvastatin hydroxy acid)[‡]; case reports have associated St. John's wort with reduced levels of cyclosporine (sometimes with transplant rejection), tacrolimus,[†] and theophylline[†]; with increased oral clearance of nevirapine; and with reduced effects of phenprocoumon[†] and warfarin; lethargy and grogginess were reported in a patient taking St. John's wort and paroxetine,[†] and the serotonin syndrome has been reported in users of sertraline (case reports); St. John's wort alone has been associated with serotonin syndrome-like events (case reports)
Asian ginseng root	Phenelzine	Mania has been reported in a patient taking ginseng and phenelzine[†]; Asian ginseng alone has also been associated with mania[†]
	Warfarin	A patient taking ginseng and warfarin had a decreased international normalized ratio[†]
Garlic bulb	Ritonavir	Two brief case reports describe gastrointestinal toxic effects in patients taking garlic and ritonavir
	Saquinavir	In a clinical study, the area under the curve for saquinavir decreased by 51% in patients taking garlic for 20 days; it returned to 65% of baseline after a 10-d washout period
	Warfarin	A brief case report described an increased clotting time in two patients taking warfarin and garlic; garlic alone has also been associated with bleeding (case reports)
Kava rhizome	Alprazolam, cimetidine, terazosin	Lethargy and disorientation were reported in a patient receiving this triple-drug regimen[†]
Yohimbe bark	Centrally active antihypertensive agents	Yohimbine (a major alkaloid in yohimbe bark) may antagonize guanabenz and the methyldopa metabolite through its α_2-adrenoceptor antagonistic properties
	Tricyclic antidepressants	In clinical studies, tricyclic antidepressants increased the sensitivity to the autonomic and central adverse effects of yohimbine

*The full version of this table is available from the National Auxiliary Publications Service (NAPS). (See NAPS document no. 05609 for 33 pages of supplementary material. To order, contact NAPS, c/o Microfiche Publications, 248 Hempstead Turnpike, West Hempstead, NY 11552.) Interactions associated with multiple herb therapies are not included. Case reports do not always provide adequate evidence that the remedy in question was labeled correctly. As a result, it is possible that some of the interactions reported for a specific herb were actually due to a different, unidentified botanical or to another adulterant or contaminant.

[†]A single case was reported without reference to previous cases.

[‡]With the exception of phenprocoumon, these drugs are all substrates for cytochrome P450 3A, P-glycoprotein, or both.

From de Smet PA: Herbal remedies, *New England Journal of Medicine* 347:2048, 2002.

absorption. For example, calcium in dairy products will bind levothyroxine, tetracycline, and ciprofloxacin, greatly decreasing their absorption; lovastatin absorption is increased by a high-fat, low-fiber meal. Grapefruit juice contains substances that inhibit CYP3A4-mediated metabolism in the gut (Byrd and Luther, 2010). Blood levels of amiodarone, lovastatin, simvastatin, and buspirone are greatly increased when the drugs are taken on the same day as grapefruit (Greenblatt et al., 2001). Certain foods antagonize the therapeutic action of a drug. The vitamin K in leafy green vegetables antagonizes the anticoagulant effects of warfarin (Burchum, 2011) (Table 9-2). It is recommended that patients taking warfarin ingest a consistent amount of greens to avoid variations in coagulability. Spironolactone, prescribed for end-stage heart failure, increases potassium (K^+) reabsorption by the renal tubule. If a patient ingests a diet high in potassium (e.g., KCl salt substitute, molasses, oranges, bananas) while taking spironolactone or other potassium-sparing agents, toxic K^+ levels can quickly occur.

Drug–Drug Interactions

The polypharmacy that may be a necessary part of health care in later life makes the risk for drug–drug interactions particularly common. These may occur at any time from preparation to excretion. For example, persons who cannot swallow after a stroke may receive all feedings and medications enterally. Medications intended for oral administration must be put in soluble form for passage through the tube without clogging and yet also remain in their original form. When several medications are crushed, mixed together, and then dissolved in water for

TABLE 9-2 COMMON DRUG–FOOD INTERACTIONS IN OLDER ADULTS

FOOD	DRUG	POTENTIAL EFFECT
Caffeine	Theophylline	Increased potential for toxicity
Fatty food	Griseofulvin	Increased absorption of drug
Blue cheese	Penicillin	Antagonistic action
Fiber	Digoxin	Absorption of drug into fiber, reducing drug action
Vitamin K foods: cabbage, greens, egg yolk, fish, rice	Warfarin	Decreased effect of drug, inhibiting anticoagulation
Food	Many antibiotics	Reduced absorption rate of drug
Mineral oil	Oil-soluble vitamins	Fat-soluble vitamins dissolve in oil; deficiency possible
Tyramine foods: aged cheese, wines, pickled herring, chocolate	Monoamine oxidase (MAO) inhibitors (phenelzine [Nardil], tranylcypromine [Parnate]), St. John's wort	May precipitate hypertensive crisis
Vitamin B_6 supplements	Levodopa-carbidopa	Reverses antiparkinsonian effect
Grapefruit juice	Cisapride, calcium channel blockers, quinidine	Altered metabolism and elimination can increase concentration of drug
Citrus juice	Calcium channel blockers	Gastric reflux exacerbated

From Meiner SE: *Gerontologic Nursing*, ed 3, St. Louis, MO, 2011, Mosby.

⚠ SAFETY ALERT

Safe Administration of Medications through Enteral Feeding Tubes

Persons who receive their medications via the enteral route are at high risk for medication errors. To administer them safely is a time-consuming process that requires detailed knowledge of the medications (and their formulation) and the skills to prepare them appropriately. Most often this preparation occurs at the bedside, further increasing the risk for errors. The outcomes of these errors include the following: occluded tube, reduced drug effect, drug toxicity, patient harm, patient death. The three most common errors are incompatible route, improper preparation, and improper administration (Box 9-3).

---

administration, a new product is created and drug–drug interactions may have already begun.

Altered absorption can occur when one drug binds another drug in the small intestine to form a nonabsorbable compound (e.g., tetracycline and calcium carbonate, or ciprofloxacin and iron compounds). Several drugs may compete to simultaneously bind and occupy the receptor sites needed by the other drug, creating varied bioavailability of one or both of the drugs. Interference with enzyme activity may alter metabolism and cause drug deficiencies or toxicities. Antispasmodic drugs slow gastric and intestinal motility. In some instances this drug action may be useful, but when other medications are involved,

BOX 9-3 ADMINISTRATION OF MEDICATIONS THROUGH ENTERAL FEEDING TUBES: THE THREE MOST COMMON ERRORS

1. *Incompatible route:* Medications must be appropriate for the oral route for immediate action and crushable. All products intended for slow or extended release are not crushable as they are intended for only partial dissolution in the stomach; administration may lead to an excessive dose. Watch for extensions such as: CD, CR, ER, LA, SA, SE, TD, TR, XL, and XR as warnings for noncrushable drugs (this list is not inclusive). See the "do-not-crush" lists available from the pharmacy or online (http://www.ismp.org/Tools/DoNotCrush.pdf).
2. *Improper preparation:* Medications administered via an enteral feeding tube must be in a liquid or semiliquid form in order to pass through the tube and not adhere to the lining of the tube. Each medication should be dissolved individually in a product that will not change the product* and will not clog the tube. Watch for oral suspensions and tincture; drug remaining on tubing means reduced dose administered.
3. *Improper administration:* Be sure to know where the distal end of the tube is resting. A drug that requires partial absorption in the stomach cannot be used when it will be administered directly into the duodenum or jejunum. Do not combine with feeding unless directions are to "administer with food."

When more than one tablet is crushed or capsule opened and mixed together before administration, a new "product" has been prepared and may not have the same effect as the two products taken separately. Find "compatibility information" from pharmacists to determine which medications may be mixed in this way.

*See Medication Safety Alert at http://www.ismp.org/Newsletters/acutecare/articles/20100506.asp for more information.

it is necessary to consider the potential problem of drug absorption.

Altered distribution may be caused by displacement of one drug from its receptor site by another drug, or by binding to plasma albumin or α_1-acid glycoprotein. Altered distribution is a common cause of adverse drug reactions in older adults and is especially important to the older adult in the situation of lowered albumin levels, which is common among the chronically ill frail elders often residing in long-term care facilities (Beyth and Shorr, 2007).

Altered metabolism can occur when one drug increases (inducts) or decreases (inhibits) the metabolism of another drug (Hartshorn and Tatro, 2003). Drugs may induce or inhibit the specific CYP450 isoenzymes responsible for metabolizing another drug. One drug may inhibit the metabolism of another drug if they are both substrates for the same metabolic pathway. Tables listing medications affected by those that have an effect on the CYP450 enzymes are available in most references on pharmacotherapeutics.

Altered excretion can occur when one drug changes the urinary pH such that another drug is either reabsorbed or excreted to a greater extent (e.g., sodium bicarbonate raises urinary pH, resulting in greater reabsorption of amphetamine and thereby prolonging its half-life) (Hartshorn and Tatro, 2003). Another mechanism may involve one drug increasing or decreasing active transport in the renal tubules (e.g., probenecid decreases the active transport of penicillin, thereby prolonging its half-life) (Hartshorn and Tatro, 2003).

Pharmacodynamic drug interactions include the additive pharmacological effects of two or more similar drugs (e.g., additive CNS effects of sedative–hypnotic drugs or anticholinergic drugs used simultaneously) (Hartshorn and Tatro, 2003). In pharmacodynamic interactions, one drug alters the patient's response to another drug without changing the pharmacokinetic properties. This can be especially dangerous for older adults when two or more drugs with the same effect are additive; that is, together they are more potent than they are separately.

Adverse Drug Reactions

Adverse drug reactions (ADRs) occur when there is a noxious response to a drug. ADRs range from a minor annoyance to death and are a common cause of hospitalization, especially for persons more than 80 years of age (Zwicker and Fulmer, 2008). The medication categories associated with the most preventable ADRs are well known to gerontological nurses; they include cardiovascular agents, diuretics, nonopioid analgesics, hypoglycemics, and anticoagulants, especially the latter. Those most serious side effects are associated with cardiovascular and psychotropic agents and others with narrow therapeutic windows or are renally excreted (Beyth and Shorr, 2007).

Sometimes an ADR can be predicted from the pharmacological action of the drug, such as bone marrow suppression from chemotherapeutic agents or bleeding from anticoagulants. At other times they are unpredictable, such as in an allergic reaction to antibiotics. Allergic reactions become more common in the older adults as the immune system changes. It is reasonable to assume that many ADRs in older adults go unrecognized because of their nonspecific nature, similarity to some of the subtle changes with aging and the vague signs and symptoms of many of the chronic conditions common in later life.

Many of the reactions are deemed serious, may even be fatal, and most of them are preventable (Hanlon et al., 2006; Zwicker and Fulmer, 2008). When a response reaches the level of harm it is referred to as an *adverse drug event (ADE)*, many of which must be reported to the U.S. Food and Drug Administration or other regulatory body. ADEs can result from the administration of a single drug, or from the interaction of multiple drugs as discussed previously. Although the reporting of ADEs had been limited to prescribed substances, this has now been expanded to include any other products such as dietary supplements for which health-related claims are made. Most reporting is voluntary; however, reporting ADEs and product quality problems contributes to the protection of the public from harm.

Although ADRs and ADEs continue to occur, there has been considerable progress in the development of strategies to reduce their likelihood, especially in the recognition of age-related pharmacokinetic and pharmacodynamic changes in later life. We now know that in many cases an older adult should be prescribed lower dosages of several of the drugs commonly needed, especially when starting a drug regimen. To minimize the likelihood of an ADR, the dose can be slowly increased until it safely reaches a therapeutic level. A common adage related to drug dosing in older adults is, "Start low, go slow, but go." There has also been a recognition that the risk of ADEs is so high with

some drugs that they are simply not recommended for use in persons with any risk factors at all.

The "Do Not Use" List

The appropriate use of medications in the older adult means that such products are used only as needed, at the dose necessary to achieve the desired effects, and in a manner in which the risks and benefits have been considered within the greater context of the person's life, health, lifestyle, and values. As early as 1994, Willcox and colleagues identified 20 drugs that were frequently prescribed to older adults but had questionable risk-to-benefit ratios, especially controversial cardiovascular agents such as propranolol, methyldopa, and reserpine. Since that time, Beers (1997) and others have continued to identify drugs that have higher than usual risk when used in older adults. These have now been transferred to a "do not use" list for residents in nursing facilities, otherwise known as the "Beers list." When one is prescribed without documentation of the overwhelming benefit of its use, it can be considered a form of drug misuse by the prescribing practitioner.

PSYCHOACTIVE DRUGS

The gerontological nurse, especially one working in a long-term care setting, is likely to care for older adults who are receiving psychoactive drugs, especially for the treatment of depression, anxiety, and bipolar disorder. A small group of elders in the community and a growing number of those residing in long-term care facilities are also being treated for a psychosis. As noted previously, drugs with psychoactive properties have a higher than usual risk for adverse events and must be prescribed, administered, and monitored with care. Although some (especially the anxiolytics) are intended for short-term use, most will be needed on an ongoing basis as with other chronic health conditions. The nurse works with the individual to ensure that appropriate biomarkers are measured and to identify the behavioral marker against which the medication's effectiveness is measured (e.g. days of sadness, quality of sleep, ability to enjoy social activities).

Antidepressants

Selective serotonin reuptake inhibitors (SSRIs) have been found to be highly effective antidepressants. SSRIs are the drugs of choice for first-line use in older adults. Most older adults are sensitive to the SSRIs and may find significant relief from depression at low doses (Box 9-4). Most have also been found to be useful for anxiety, and in some cases obsessive-compulsive disorder and posttraumatic stress disorder as well (Ravindran and Stein, 2010). Many are now available in both tablet and oral concentrate form for easier use. Side effects are manageable and usually resolve over time; most cause initial problems with nausea, dry mouth, or sedation. If sexual dysfunction occurs, it will resolve only with discontinuation, therefore if the person is or plans to become sexually active a different drug may be needed.

For those who do not respond to an adequate trial of SSRIs there is another group of antidepressants that combine the inhibition of both serotonin and norepinephrine (SNRIs) (e.g.,venlafaxine[Effexor], bupropion [Wellbutrin], trazodone).

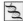

Personalized Medicine

Personalized medicine will include the ability to prescribe the right drugs for the right person; a significant advantage in geriatrics when polypharmacy is already a problem. Two classes of drugs commonly prescribed for anxiety disorders are benzodiazepines and antidepressants. Although benzodiazepines have comparable effects on many persons their use is discouraged in older adults. Antidepressants may be highly effective and with fewer side effects, but show considerably greater variability and no effect in up to one third of patients. The efficacy in any one person appears to be related in part to the length of the allele of the serotonin transporter (5-HTT) gene, with a better response seen in those with longer alleles. As genetics testing makes its way into the clinical setting, there will be more opportunities to improve the efficacy of treatment, while reducing the number of medications prescribed and the potential for adverse drug events.

Data from Tiwari AK, Souza RP, Muller DJ: Pharmacogenetics of anxiolytic drugs, *Journal of Neural Transmission* 116:667, 2009.

These also may be preferred by those who are engaged in or who anticipate sexual activity as they are less likely to have sexual side effects. In the context of reducing polypharmacy, Wellbutrin also reduces nicotine dependency, and trazodone is sedating—for the person who has difficulty getting to or staying asleep. Since the development of the SSRIs and SNRIs, the older monoamine oxidase (MAO) inhibitors and tricyclic antidepressants are no longer indicated in most cases. Moreover, the U.S. Food and Drug Administration has warned that neither SNRIs nor SSRIs should be combined with MAO inhibitors, to avoid the possibility of a potentially life-threatening condition known as serotonin syndrome. Although it sometimes takes time to find the most optimal dose, the nurse can help the elder monitor target symptoms and advocate for continued dose adjustments or changes of medication until relief is obtained.

Anxiolytic Agents

Drugs developed to treat anxiety are referred to as *anxiolytics* or *antianxiety agents*. These agents include the benzodiazepines and buspirone (BuSpar). The SSRIs noted previously were not developed as anxiolytics but have also been found to serve this purpose as well (Ravindran and Stein, 2010). People often self-medicate with antihistamines, especially diphenhydramine (Benadryl), for anxiety and sleep; this is not recommended because of their significant anticholinergic effects that increase the risk for falls or confusion. The decision to treat anxiety pharmacologically is based on the degree to which the anxiety interferes with the person's ability to function and subjective feelings of discomfort.

Benzodiazepines are highly effective anxiolytic and hypnotic agents. They are popular because of their quick sedating effects for the person who is experiencing acute anxiety, such as a new resident in a long-term care facility. However, their side effects include drowsiness, dizziness, ataxia, mild cognitive deficits, and memory impairment (Box 9-5). Signs of toxicity include excessive sedation, unsteady gait, confusion, disorientation, cognitive impairment, memory impairment, agitation, and wandering. Because these symptoms resemble dementia, persons can easily be misdiagnosed once the benzodiazepines have been taken. Almost all have long half-lives and when combined with the normal changes in aging, profound sedation and toxicity are

Mr. Jones was a 260-lb, 75-year-old man who was admitted to an orthopedic ward for a procedure. Because of the man's high level of anxiety about being in the hospital, he was given a total of 20 mg of diazepam (Valium) over a 12-hour period. The following day the man wandered out of the unit and was not seen again until he came to the emergency department with sore feet, 5 days later. He had been wandering the streets with no idea of where he was or how he got there. Valium has been associated with delirium and anterograde amnesia. The half-life of Valium in a younger person is about 37 hours, but in an older adult this may be extended up to 82 hours, with potentially dangerous problems of accumulation.

Data from Buffum J: Unpublished observations, 2003.

TABLE 9-3	COMPARISON OF COMMON BENZODIAZEPINES BY HALF-LIFE	
TRADE NAME	**GENERIC NAME**	**HALF-LIFE (h)***
Valium	Diazepam	20-70
Ativan	Lorazepam	10-20
Klonopin	Clonazepam	18-50
Xanax	Alprazolam	11-15

*Note that the half-life in a healthy older adult may be double the time indicated, depending on age-related changes in the glomerular filtration rate.
From Shorr RI: *Drugs for the geriatric patient,* St. Louis, MO, 2007, WB Saunders.

significant risks (Table 9-3). All are Schedule IV controlled substances and fall under the Omnibus Budget Reconciliation Act (OBRA) regulations in long-term care facilities. If necessary, they should be used for the shortest time possible.

Buspirone (BuSpar) is a nonbenzodiazepine alternative. The mechanism of action is unknown, but it is thought to bind serotonin and dopamine receptors in the CNS, leading to decreased anxiety. Although a side effect is dizziness, this is often dose related and resolves with time. Buspirone is not addicting and may have an additive effect when combined with some of the SSRIs, so lower doses can be used. No effect is felt by the patient or observed by the nurse for 5 to 7 days, and the drug may be inappropriately discontinued for apparent lack of effect. Further research about the clinical usefulness of this drug is needed (Mokhber et al., 2010; Ravindran and Stein, 2010).

Mood Stabilizers

Mood stabilizers include the group of agents used for the treatment of bipolar disorders. Lithium was the first in this category to be approved, but today anticonvulsant medications are used more often, especially valproic acid (Depakene, Depokote) and lamotrigine (Lamictal).

The nurse who is caring for a patient with a bipolar disorder or for one who is taking a mood stabilizer should seek guidance from the person's psychiatrist or psychiatric nurse practitioner regarding specific strategies to enhance the person's quality of life and safe drug administration. The nurse should also be proactive in ensuring that serum concentrations are monitored as appropriate. If the patient is taking lithium, close monitoring by nurses is especially important. Lithium interacts with several other medications and foods. For example, a low-salt diet will elevate the lithium level and a high-salt diet will decrease it. Likewise, thiazide diuretics and nonsteroidal antiinflammatory drugs (NSAIDs) will elevate the serum lithium level. Side effects include confusion, disorientation, and memory loss; flattening of T waves on the electrocardiogram; polyuria and polydipsia; nausea, vomiting, and diarrhea; fine resting tremor; benign goiter; and ataxia.

Antipsychotics

Antipsychotics are tranquilizing medications used primarily to treat psychoses and off-label as mood stabilizers for bipolar disorder. The first such drugs to be produced (in the 1950s) are now referred to as "typical antipsychotics" and the newer, second-generation drugs (developed since the 1990s) are referred to as "atypicals." Their mechanism of action centers on blocking dopamine receptor pathways in the brain. Antipsychotics are often ranked in relation to their side effects, especially sedation, hypotension, and extrapyramidal (and anticholinergic) properties. Antipsychotics also affect the hypothalamic and thermoregulatory pathways. Other side effects include neuroleptic malignant syndrome and movement disorders.

Neuroleptic Malignant Syndrome (NMS)

NMS is a rare but life-threatening neurological emergency which most often presents as an adverse reaction to neuroleptic or antipsychotic drugs. The most typical symptoms are fever (>100.4 degrees), muscle rigidity, autonomic instability (e.g. labile BP, tachycardia) and altered mental status. Common signs are elevated white blood cell count and creatine phosphokinase (CPK). Onset is rapid and unless treated appropriately and quickly, can cause death. The drugs most associated with NMS are the high potency neuroleptics such as haloperidol but others have been implicated, such as chlorpromazine (Compazine) and promethazine (Phenergan). While it occurs most often in the first 2 weeks of the initiation of treatment it must also be considered whenever a dose is increased. NMS is also seen if anti-Parkinson's medications are stopped abruptly. In most instances the person is hospitalized in an intensive care unit while being treated. The immediate response is to recognize that what is being seen may be an adverse reaction, stop the offending medication and promptly and safely cool the patient. Factors which increase the risk for NMS in persons taking any potentially offending drugs include increased ambient temperature, dehydration and extreme agitation.

Movement Disorders

While neuroleptic malignant syndrome is not commonly seen in older adults taking antipsychotics; the more significant potential side effects are movement disorders, also referred to as *extrapyramidal syndrome (EPS)*. These include acute dystonia, akathisia, parkinsonian symptoms, and tardive dyskinesia. Although these side effects are much more common with the typical antipsychotics, they can occur with the atypicals as well. A health care provider should be notified at any time such symptoms or signs are seen. Many are potentially life-threatening. In most cases the offending medication must be stopped immediately, with implications for the potential need for hospitalization.

Acute Dystonia. An acute dystonic reaction is an abnormal involuntary movement consisting of a slow and continuous muscular contraction or spasm. Involuntary muscular contractions of the mouth, jaw, face, and neck are common. The jaw may lock (trismus), the tongue may roll back and block the throat, the neck may arch backward (opisthotonos), or the eyes may close. In an oculogyric crisis, the eyes are fixed in one position. Often this creates a feeling of needing to look up constantly without the ability to make the eyes come down. The reaction may occur hours or days after initiating a drug or after a dose increase. The reaction may last minutes to hours.

Akathisia. Akathisia is a compulsion to be in motion, a sense of restlessness, being unable to be still, having an unrelenting desire to move, and feeling "like crawling out of my skin." The patient is seen pacing, fidgeting, and markedly restless. Often this symptom is mistaken for worsening psychosis instead of the adverse drug reaction that it is. It may occur at any time during therapy.

Parkinsonian Symptoms. The use of antipsychotics may cause a collection of symptoms that mimic Parkinson's disease. A bilateral tremor (as opposed to a unilateral tremor in true Parkinson's), bradykinesia, and rigidity may be seen, which may progress to the inability to move. The patient may have an inflexible facial expression and appear bored and apathetic and be mistakenly diagnosed as depressed. More common with the higher potency antipsychotics, parkinsonian symptoms may occur within weeks to months of initiation of antipsychotic therapy.

Tardive Dyskinesia. When antipsychotics have been used continuously for at least three to six months, patients are at risk for the development of the irreversible movement disorder called tardive dyskinesia (TD). Both low- and high-potency agents are implicated (Bullock and Saharan, 2002; Goldberg, 2002). TD symptoms usually appear first as wormlike movements of the tongue; other facial movements include grimacing, blinking, and frowning. Slow, maintained, involuntary, twisting movements of the limbs, trunk, neck, face, and eyes (involuntary eye closure) have been reported. No treatment reverses the effect of TD. Therefore it is essential that the nurse be attentive for early detection so that the health care provider can make prompt changes to the psychotropic regimen.

Response to treatment is the most important consideration when gerontological patients are taking psychotropics. Subjective patient comments about feelings and symptoms and objective observations about the patient's behavior are important data for evaluating the effectiveness of a drug. When used appropriately and cautiously antipsychotics can provide a person with relief from what may be frightening and distressing symptoms. Inappropriate use of antipsychotic medications may mask a reversible cause for the psychosis, such as infection, dehydration, fever, electrolyte imbalance, an adverse drug effect, or a sudden change in the environment (Bullock and Saharan, 2002). Because of the seriousness and frequency of the side effects they are prescribed at the lowest dose possible and the patient is monitored closely.

PROMOTING HEALTHY AGING: IMPLICATIONS FOR GERONTOLOGICAL NURSING

The gerontological nurse is a key person in ensuring that the medication used is appropriate, effective, and as safe as possible. The knowledgeable nurse is alert for potential drug interactions and for signs or symptoms of adverse drug effects. The nurse promotes the actions necessary to prevent drugs from becoming toxic and to treat toxicity promptly should it occur (Table 9-4). Nurses in the long-term care setting are responsible for monitoring the overall health of the residents, including fluid and dietary intake, and for being alert to the need for laboratory tests and other measures to ensure correct medication dosage. They are responsible for prompt attention to changes in the patient's or resident's condition that are either the result of the medication regimen or affected by the regimen, such as potassium level. The nurse is often the person to initiate assessment of medication use, evaluate outcomes, and provide the teaching necessary for safe drug use and self-administration. In all settings, a vital nursing function is to educate patients and to ensure that they understand the purpose and side effects of the medications and to assist the patient and family in adapting the medication regimen to functional ability and lifestyle.

Assessment

The initial step in ensuring that drug use is safe and effective is to conduct a comprehensive drug assessment. Although in some settings a clinical pharmacist interviews patients about their medication history, more often it is completed through the combined efforts of the licensed nurse and the health care provider (e.g., a physician or a nurse practitioner).

The "gold standard" of assessment is a medicine history with a "brown bag approach," in which the person is asked to bring in a bag all medications he or she is taking, including OTCs, herbals, and other dietary supplements. As each product container is removed from the bag, the necessary information can be obtained. To determine possible misunderstandings or misuse, it is best to ask the person how he or she actually takes the medicine rather than to depend on how the label is written. Through this assessment, the nurse can learn of discrepancies between the prescribed dosage and the actual dosage, potential interactions, and potential or actual ADRs. The basics of the comprehensive drug assessment are the same as for younger adults; see Box 9-6 for details of the information needed in a comprehensive medication that are particularly important for older adults.

The nurse's analysis of the assessment data is centered on identifying unnecessary or inappropriate medications, establishing safe usage, determining the patient's self-medication management ability, monitoring the effect of current medications and other products (e.g., herbals), and evaluating effectiveness of any education provided (Box 9-7). Ideally, the nurse should know what resources are available for teaching about medications, such as the clinical pharmacist. The nurse is well situated to coordinate care, learn about the patient's goals, learn what the patient needs for understanding his or her

TABLE 9-4   TOXIC CHARACTERISTICS OF SPECIFIC DRUGS PRESCRIBED FOR THE ELDERLY

DRUG(S)	SIGNS AND SYMPTOMS

Benzodiazepines
    Diazepam (Valium)
    Lorazepam (Ativan)
	Ataxia, restlessness, confusion, depression, anticholinergic effect

Cimetidine (Tagamet)	Confusion, depression
Digitalis (digoxin)	Confusion, headache, anorexia, vomiting, arrhythmias, blurred vision or visual changes (halos, frost on objects, color blindness), paresthesia
Furosemide (Lasix)	Electrolyte imbalance, hepatic changes, pancreatitis, leukopenia, thrombocytopenia
Gentamicin (Garamycin)	Ototoxicity (impaired hearing and/or balance), nephrotoxicity
Levodopa (L-dopa)	Muscle and eye twitching, disorientation, asterixis, hallucinations, dyskinetic movements, grimacing, depression, delirium, ataxia
Lithium (Eskalith, Lithane)	Confusion, diarrhea, drowsiness, anorexia, slurred speech, tremors, blurred vision, unsteadiness, polyuria, seizures, muscle weakness

Nonsteroidal antiinflammatory drugs (NSAIDs)
    Ibuprofen (Advil, Motrin, Nuprin, Rufen)
    Indomethacin (Indocin)
    Fenoprofen (Nalfon)
	Photosensitivity, fluid retention, anemia, nephrotoxicity, visual changes, bleeding

Phenylbutazone (Butazolidin)
    Piroxicam (Feldene)
    Sulindac (Clinoril)
    Tolmetin (Tolectin)
	Confusion in addition to all other signs and symptoms for NSAIDs

Phenothiazines	Tachycardia, arrhythmias, dyspnea, hyperthermia, postural hypotension, restlessness, anticholinergic effects
Phenytoin (Dilantin)	Ataxia, slurred speech, confusion, nystagmus, diplopia, nausea, vomiting
Procainamide (Pronestyl, Procan, Promine)	Arrhythmias, depression, hypotension, SLE syndrome, dyspnea, skin rash, nausea, vomiting
Ranitidine (Zantac)	Liver dysfunction, blood dyscrasias

Sulfonylureas—first generation
    Chlorpropamide (Diabinese)
    Tolbutamide (Orinase)
	Hypoglycemia, hepatic changes, heart failure, bone marrow depression, jaundice

Theophylline (Theo-Dur, Elixophyllin, Slo-Bid)	Anorexia, nausea, vomiting, gastrointestinal bleeding, tachycardia, arrhythmias, irritability, insomnia, seizures, muscle twitching
Tricyclic antidepressants amitriptyline (Elavil, Endep), doxepin (Sinequan, Adapin), imipramine (Tofranil)	Confusion, arrhythmias, seizures, agitation, tachycardia, jaundice, hallucinations, postural hypotension, anticholinergic effects

SLE, systemic lupus erythematosus.
Data from Semla TP, Beizer JL, Higbee MD: *Geriatric dosage handbook,* ed 12, Cleveland, OH, 2007, Lexi-Comp.

BOX 9-6 COMPONENTS OF A MEDICATION ASSESSMENT WITH SPECIAL EMPHASIS FOR OLDER ADULTS*

- Ability to pay for prescription medications
- Ability to obtain medications and refills
- Persons involved in decision-making regarding medication use
- Drugs obtained from others
- Recently discontinued drugs or "leftover" prescriptions
- Strategies used to remember when to take drugs
- Recent drug blood levels as appropriate
- Recent measurement of liver and kidney functioning
- Ability to remove packaging, manipulate medication, and store supply

*In addition to the standard comprehensive medication assessment, that is, number of drugs, reasons taken, and so on. See any standard pharmacology text.

BOX 9-7 ANALYSIS OF ASSESSMENT FINDINGS RELATED TO MEDICATION USE

1. Is the drug working to improve the patient's symptoms?
   a. What are the therapeutic effects of the drug? (What symptoms are targeted?)
   b. What is the time frame for the therapeutic effects?
   c. Have the appropriate drug and dose been prescribed?
   d. Has the appropriate time been tried for therapeutic effects?
2. Is the drug harming the patient?
   a. What physiological changes are occurring?
   b. What laboratory values are changing?
   c. What mental status changes are occurring?
   d. What functional changes are occurring?
   e. Is the patient experiencing side effects?
   f. Is the drug interacting with any other medication?
3. Does the patient understand the following?
   a. Why he or she is taking the drug
   b. How the drug is supposed to be taken
   c. How to identify side effects and drug interactions
   d. How to reduce or manage side effects
   e. Limitations imposed by taking the drug (e.g., sedative effects)

BOX 9-8 KNOWING WHO YOU ARE TALKING TO

M. François came to the clinic as a new patient with uncontrolled hypertension. The nurse practitioner, through an interpreter, spent a lot of time with him explaining to him how to take his medications, what they were for, and so on. He and his caregiver sat quietly and appeared to understand. When he returned a month later his blood pressure was still out of control. There was a different person with him who asked all of the questions that were addressed at the first appointment. On further inquiry it was determined that the person who brought M. François the first time was just a neighbor helping out and not involved in his day-to-day life at all! His niece who "takes care of things" had been unavailable during the previous appointment and was now available to him and for the appointment.

medications, and arrange for follow-up care to determine the outcome of medication teaching.

Education

Patient education is the most common intervention used to promote medication adherence. Because of the complex needs of the older patient, education can be particularly challenging. The following tips may be helpful when the goal of the nurse is to promote healthy aging related to medication use:

Key persons: Find out who, if anyone, manages the person's medications, helps the person, or assists with decision-making; and with the elder's permission, make sure that the helper is present when any teaching is done (Box 9-8).

Environment: Minimize distraction, and avoid competing with television or others demanding the patient's time; make sure the person is comfortable and is not hungry, thirsty, tired, too warm or too cold, in pain, or in need of the toilet.

Timing: Provide the teaching during the best time of the day for the person, when he or she is most engaged and energetic. Keep the education sessions short and succinct.

Communication: Ensure that you will be understood. Make sure the elders have their glasses or hearing aids on if they are used. Use simple and direct language, and avoid medical or nursing jargon (e.g., "intake"). Speak clearly, facing the person and with light on your face, at head level. Use formal language (e.g., Mr. Jones) unless you have permission to do otherwise. Do not touch the patient unless he or she gives you indications that it is acceptable to do so (e.g., patient lays his or her hand on yours). If the person is blind, Braille instructions may be available from the pharmacy. If the person has limited language proficiency in the country in which care is delivered, a trained medical interpreter is needed.

Reinforce teaching: Although there is a wide array of teaching tools and medication reminders available on the market today, many older adults continue to use the strategies they have developed over the years to remember to take their medications. These may be as simple as a commercially available storage box or turning a bottle upside down once it has been taken for the day, or as intense as having a family member or friend call the person at designated times. Encourage the person to use techniques which have worked in the past or develop new strategies to ensure correct and timely medication use when needed.

SAFE MEDICATION USE

A safe, optimal, and feasible drug plan is one to which the patient can adhere (Box 9-9). Nursing interventions include those that minimize polypharmacy and adverse drug reactions and promote adherence to drugs regimens that promote healthy aging or comfort while dying (Box 9-10). The responsibility of the nurse caring for frail elders takes on new meaning because of the physical and social vulnerability and medical complexity common in late life; drug interactions are more likely and adverse reactions more lethal.

There have been multitudes of studies conducted on interventions to increase adherence to drug regimens. The perfect, one-size-fits-all approach has not yet been found; however, multimodal approaches appear to be the most effective. Education is supported by written or graphic material and further supported by frequent feedback. The "brown bag" approach is used *each* time the person is seen and not just during periodic

BOX 9-9   EVIDENCE-BASED PRINCIPLES FOR REDUCING ADVERSE DRUG EVENTS

By paying attention to the following principles for prescribing and monitoring medications for older adults, one might also reduce the risk for adverse drug events:
- Give the lowest dose possible.
- Discontinue unnecessary therapy.
- Attempt nondrug approaches first.
- Give the safest drug possible.
- Assess renal function.
- Always consider the risk-to-benefit ratio when adding drugs.
- Assess for new interactions with any new prescription.
- Avoid the prescribing cascade, i.e., new medications without consideration of those to be discontinued.
- Avoid inappropriate medications.

Adapted from Zwicker D, Fulmer T: *MEDICATION—Nursing standard of practice protocol: reducing adverse drug events* (2008). Available at http://consultgerirn.org/topics/medication/want_to_know_more#Wrap. Accessed December 2010. See also relevant practice guidelines: Bergman-Evans B: *Improving medication management for older adult clients* [Level I]. NGC Guideline # 003993. Iowa City, IA, 2004, University of Iowa Gerontological Nursing Interventions Research Center, Research Dissemination Core. Available at www.guideline.gov. Accessed December 2010. Health Care Association of New Jersey (HCANJ): *Medication management guideline.* NGC Guideline # 004951. Hamilton, NJ, 2006, Health Care Association of New Jersey. Available at www.guideline.gov. Accessed December 2010. *Note:* Geared for posthospital institutions for adult patients.

BOX 9-10   THE RIGHT MEDICATION

The task for the clinician is not to determine whether too many or too few medications are being taken, but to determine whether the patient is taking the right medications—tailored to the patient's individual circumstances, including his or her constellation of comorbidities, goals of care, preferences, and ability to adhere to medications.

From Steinman MA, Hanlon JT: Managing medications in clinically complex elders: "There's got to be a happy medium," *JAMA* 304:1592, 2010.

encounters with health care providers. When working with older populations these approaches must further consider sensory limitations, such as low visual and auditory acuity, and attend to the potential involvement of the caregiver in the education process.

Safe drug use requires attention to the potential for misuse, including overuse, underuse, erratic use, and contraindicated use, and can otherwise be referred to as nonadherence as well. Misuse by patients may be unintentional, such as with misunderstanding, or purposeful, such as with trying to make a prescription last longer because of cost, or believing that it is not appropriate for the believed cause of illness (Gould and Mitty, 2010). A person may have considerable difficulty adhering to a medication regimen that is inconsistent with his or her established life pattern. For example, the individual cannot follow the instruction to take medication three times per day with meals if he or she eats only two meals each day. In late life adherence is made significantly more complicated by the

TABLE 9-5   EXAMPLES OF CHANGES WITH AGING THAT MAY INTERFERE WITH MEDICATION SELF-ADMINISTRATION

CHANGE IN AGING	CONSEQUENCE
Sensory	
Decreased visual acuity	Greater difficulty in reading instructions
Decreased sensation	Greater difficulty in manipulating medications
Decreased salivation	Greater difficulty in swallowing
Mechanical	
Decreased fine motor coordination	Greater difficulty in manipulating medications and packaging
Stiffening of large joints	Greater difficulty in self-administering medications

complexity of a medication regimen combined with difficulties with self-administration due to normal changes with aging (Table 9-5).

All medications have indications, side effects, interactions, and individual patient reactions. The nurse must determine whether side effects are minimal and tolerable or serious (Table 9-6). Asking the patient produces subjective data; and observing the patient's interactions, behavior, mood, emotional responses, and daily habits provides objective data. From this compilation of data, patient problems can be delineated, nursing diagnoses developed, outcome criteria planned, and interventions initiated.

Lastly, the gerontological nurse is to monitor and evaluate the prescribed treatments for both side effects and efficacy (Planton and Edlund, 2010). Monitoring and evaluating involve making astute observations and documenting those observations, noting changes in physical and functional status (e.g., vital signs, performance of activities of daily living, sleeping, eating, hydrating, eliminating) and mental status (e.g., attention and level of alertness, memory, orientation, behavior, mood, emotional display and affect, content and characteristics of interactions). Monitoring also means ensuring that blood levels are measured as they are needed, such as regular thyroid-stimulating hormone (TSH) levels for all persons taking thyroid replacement, INRs for all persons taking warfarin, or periodic hemoglobin A_{1c} levels for all persons with diabetes (see Chapter 8). Care of a patient also means that the nurses promptly communicate their findings of potential problems to the patient's nurse practitioner or physician. Accurate monitoring requires that the nurse have information about the treatments and medications that are administered.

Medications occupy a central place in the lives of many older persons: cost, acceptability, interactions, untoward side effects, and the need to schedule medications appropriately all combine to create many difficulties. Although nurses, with the exception of advanced practice nurses, do not prescribe medications, we believe that a full understanding of medications is needed by nurses working with elders.

TABLE 9-6   DETERMINING WHETHER A DRUG IS WORKING: MONITORING PARAMETERS AND COMMON SIDE EFFECTS OF GENERAL DRUG CATEGORIES

CLASS OF DRUG	MONITORING ACTIVITY	COMMON SIDE EFFECTS
Antibiotics and antivirals	Improvement of infection: symptom reduction Takes complete prescription	Change in normal flora: yeast infections in mouth or vagina, diarrhea
Antihyperlipidemics	Lipid profile (specific drug is matched to lipid profile) Observation for lifestyle changes (exercise, smoking cessation), dietary alterations (decreased fat intake, elimination of trans-fat products), gradual improvement in low-density lipoprotein (LDL) and high-density lipoprotein (HDL) levels, see change within 2-4 wk Monitor liver function and blood glucose	Statins: Muscle weakness, aches Niacin: Muscle weakness, aches; flushing; elevations in blood glucose or signs/symptoms of elevation
Cardiac medications	Measurement of heart rate and rhythm	Mental status change, visual changes Bradycardia Fever, chills
Anticoagulants	Clotting times (international normalized ratio [INR], prothrombin time)	Bleeding, bruising, blood in stool
Anticonvulsants	Blood levels Seizure activity	Sedation Mental status changes
Antihypertensives	Measurement of blood pressure CNS effects Intake and output Weight	Diuretics/ACE: postural hypotension, bradycardia, hyper/hypokalemia β-Blockers: bradycardia, hypotension, chest pain, constipation, diarrhea, nausea, mental status changes (insomnia, confusion, depression, lethargy)
Antihyperglycemics	Hemoglobin A1c	Hypoglycemia
Antineoplastics	Cancer activity Bone marrow suppression, laboratory values (e.g., white blood cell [WBC] count)	Nausea, vomiting, diarrhea, signs of infection, hair loss, fatigue
Antihistaminics	Relief from allergy symptoms such as rhinitis	Drowsiness, blurred vision, confusion
Antiarthritics	Relief from arthritis symptoms such as pain and inflammation	Gastrointestinal (GI) problems, depression, personality disturbance, irritability, toxic psychoses
Antiparkinsonians	Improved functional status Less visible immobility; improved mobility	Nausea, hypotension, dyskinesia, agitation, restlessness, insomnia
Analgesics	Improved symptoms of pain and inflammation	Nonsteroidal antiinflammatory drugs (NSAIDs): GI distress Opiates: Constipation, sedation, confusion, decreased respiration

From Semla TP, Beizer JL, Higbee MD: *Geriatric dosage handbook,* ed 12, Cleveland, OH, 2007, Lexi-Comp.

▮ KEY CONCEPTS

- The therapeutic goal of pharmacological intervention is to reduce the targeted symptoms without undesirable side effects.
- One must be alert at all times for drug–drug, drug–herb, and drug–food interactions; whereas some are known and anticipated, others are unique.
- Polypharmacy significantly increases the risk of drug interactions and adverse events.
- Any time there is a change in the patient it is reasonable to first consider the possibility of a drug effect.
- Drug misuse may be triggered by prescriber practices, individual self-medication, physiological idiosyncrasies, altered biodegradability, nutritional and fluid states, and inadequate assessment before prescribing.
- Nurses must investigate drugs immediately if a change in mental status is observed in an individual who is normally alert and aware. Many drugs have the potential to cause temporary cognitive impairment.
- One cannot comply with a prescription or treatment when incompatibilities interfere with the practicalities of life or are distressful to the individual's well-being or when actual misinformation or disability prevents compliance.
- The advances made since the 1990s in the development of psychoactive drugs has led to healthier aging for many older adults.

- The side effects of psychotropic medications vary significantly; thus these medications must be selected with care when prescribed for the older adult.
- The response of the elder to treatment with psychotropic medications should show reduced distress, clearer thinking, and more appropriate behavior.
- It is always expected that pharmacological approaches augment rather than replace nonpharmacological approaches.
- Older adults are particularly vulnerable to developing movement disorders (extrapyramidal symptoms, parkinsonian symptoms, akathisia, dystonias) with the use of antipsychotics.
- The Health Care Financing Administration and the congressional Omnibus Budget Reconciliation Act (OBRA) have severely restricted the use of psychotropic drugs for the elderly unless they are truly needed for specific disorders and to maintain or improve function. Then they must be carefully monitored.
- Any time a behavior change is noted in a person, reversible causes must be sought and treated before psychotropic medications are used.
- Antidepressant medications must be tailored to the elder, with careful observation for side effects.

CASE STUDY   AT RISK FOR AN ADVERSE EVENT

Rose was a 78-year-old woman who lived alone in a large city. She had been widowed for 10 years. Her children were grown, and all were successful. She was very proud of them because she and her husband had emigrated to the United States when the children were small and had worked very hard to establish and maintain a home. She had had only a few years of primary education and still clung to many of her "old country" ways. She spoke a mixture of English and her native language, and her children were somewhat embarrassed by her. They thought she was somewhat of a hypochondriac because she constantly complained to them about various aches and pains, her knees that "gave out," her "sugar" and "water" problems, and her heart palpitations. She had been diagnosed with mild diabetes and congestive heart failure. She was a devout Catholic and attended mass each morning. Her treks to church events, to the senior center at church, and to her various physicians (internist; orthopedic, cardiac, and ophthalmic specialists) constituted her social life. One day the recreation director at the senior center noticed her pulling a paper bag of medication bottles from her purse. She sat down to talk with Rose about them and soon realized that Rose had only a vague idea of what most of them were for and tended to take them whenever she felt she needed them.

On the basis of the case study, develop a nursing care plan using the following procedure*:
- List Rose's comments that provide subjective data.
- List information that provides objective data.
- From these data, identify and state, using accepted format, two nursing diagnoses you determine are most significant to Rose at this time.

- List two of Rose's strengths that you have identified from data.
- Determine and state outcome criteria for each diagnosis. These must reflect some alleviation of the problem identified in the nursing diagnosis and must be stated in concrete and measurable terms.
- Plan and state one or more interventions for each diagnosed problem. Provide specific documentation of the source used to determine the appropriate intervention. Plan at least one intervention that incorporates Rose's existing strengths.
- Evaluate the success of intervention. Interventions must correlate directly with the stated outcome criteria to measure the outcome success.

CRITICAL THINKING QUESTIONS
1. When you are given a prescription for medication, what do you ask about it?
2. As a nurse visiting the center for a 6-week student assignment, how would you begin to help Rose?
3. What factors about Rose's probable medication misuse would be most alarming to you?
4. What aspect of Rose's situation related to medications do you think are common among elders?
5. Who should be responsible for teaching and monitoring medication use in Rose's case? In any case?

*Students are advised to refer to their nursing diagnosis text and identify possible or potential problems.

▌ RESEARCH QUESTIONS

1. Do you think most elders seek adequate information about their medications before taking them?
2. Where would you obtain sufficient drug information for persons with limited English proficiency (LEP)?
3. What symptoms do elders self-treat with OTC and herbal medicines?
4. What are nursing roles in preventing adverse events in elders?
5. Among the following three teaching strategies, which works the best: computer-assisted medication teaching, telephone teaching, and in-person medication teaching?
6. Mrs. J., a patient of yours in a long-term care setting, is calling out repeatedly for a nurse; other patients are complaining, and you simply cannot be available for long periods to quiet her. Considering the setting and the OBRA guidelines, what would you do to manage the situation?

REFERENCES

Agency for Healthcare Quality Research: Cholesterol and diabetes lead drug spending for the elderly (2010). Available at http://www.ahrq.gov/news/nn/nn031010.htm. Accessed December 2010.

Beers M: Explicit criteria for determining potentially inappropriate medication use by the elderly, *Archives of Internal Medicine* 157:1531, 1997.

Beyth RJ, Shorr RI: Medication use. In Shorr RI, Hoth AB, Rawls N, editors: *Drugs for the geriatric patient*, St. Louis, MO, 2007, WB Saunders.

Bullock R, Saharan A: Atypical antipsychotics: experience and use in the elderly, *International Journal of Clinical Practice* 56:515, 2002.

Burchum JLR: Pharmacologic management. In Meiner S, editor: *Gerontologic nursing*, ed 4, St. Louis, MO, 2011, Elsevier.

Byrd L, Luther C: Cytochrome P450: drug metabolism—why it's so important, *Geriatric Nursing* 31:385-387, 2010.

Crentsil V, Ricks MO, Xue QL, et al: A pharmacoepidemiologic study of community-dwelling, disabled older women: factors associated with medication use, *American Journal of Geriatric Pharmacotherapy* 8:215, 2010.

Field TS, Gurwitz JH, Harrold LR, et al: Risk factors for adverse drug events among older adults in the ambulatory setting, *Journal of the American Geriatrics Society* 52:1349, 2004.

Goldberg RJ: Tardive dyskinesia in elderly patients: an update, *Journal of the American Medical Directors Association* 3:152, 2002.

Gore VF, Mouzon M: Polypharmacy in older adults: front line strategies, *Advance for Nurse Practitioners* 14:49, 2006.

Gould E, Mitty E: Medication adherence is a partnership, medication compliance is not, *Geriatric Nursing* 31:290, 2010.

Greenblatt DJ, Patki KC, von Moltke LL, et al: Drug interactions with grapefruit juice: an update, *Journal of Clinical Psychopharmacology* 21:357, 2001.

Hämmerlein A, Derendorf H, Lowenthal DT: Pharmacokinetic and pharmacodynamic changes in the elderly: clinical implications, *Clinical Pharmacokinetics* 35:49, 1998.

Hanlon JT, Pieper CF, Hajjar ER, et al: Incidence and predictors of all and preventable adverse drug reactions in frail elderly persons after hospital stay, *Journals of Gerontology Series A, Biological Sciences and Medical Sciences* 61:511, 2006.

Hartshorn E, Tatro D: Principles of drug interaction. In Tatro DS, Hebel SK, Riley MR, et al, *Drug interaction facts 2003*, St. Louis, MO, 2003, Facts and Comparisons.

Masoro EJ, Austed SN, editors: *Handbook of biology and aging*, ed 5, San Diego, CA, 2003, Academic Press.

Mokhber N, Azarpazhooh MR, Khajehdaluee M, et al: Randomized single-blind trial of sertraline and buspirone for treatment of elderly patients with generalized anxiety disorder, *Psychiatry and Clinical Neurosciences* 64:128, 2010.

Planton J, Edlund BJ: Strategies for reducing polypharmacy in older adults, *Journal of Gerontological Nursing* 36:8, 2010.

Qato DM, Alexander GC, Conti RM, et al: Use of prescription and over-the-counter medications and dietary supplements among older adults in the United States, *JAMA* 300:2867, 2008.

Randall RL, Bruno SM: Can polypharmacy reduction efforts in an ambulatory setting be successful? *Clinical Geriatrics* 14:33, 2006.

Ravindran LN, Stein MB: The pharmacologic treatment of anxiety disorders: a review of progress, *Journal of Clinical Psychiatry* 71:839, 2010.

Scott GN, Elmer GW: Update on natural product–drug interactions, *American Journal of Health-System Pharmacy* 59:339, 2002.

Steinman MA, Hanlon JT: Managing medications in clinically complex elders: "There's got to be a happy medium," *JAMA* 304:1592, 2010.

Valli G, Giardina EG: Benefits, adverse effects and drug interactions of herbal therapies with cardiovascular effects, *Journal of the American College of Cardiology* 39:1083, 2002.

Wilkinson G: Pharmacokinetics. In Hardman J, Limbird LE, Gilman AG, editors: *Goodman and Gilman's the pharmacological basis of therapeutics*, ed 10, New York, 2001, McGraw-Hill.

Willcox SM, Himmelstein DU, Woolhandler S: Inappropriate drug prescribing for the community-dwelling elderly, *JAMA* 272:292, 1994.

Zwicker D, Fulmer T: Medication nursing standard of practice protocol: reducing adverse drug events (2008). Available at http://consultgerirn.org/topics/medication/want_to_know_more#Wrap. Accessed December 2010.

The Use of Herbs and Supplements

Ellis Quinn Youngkin

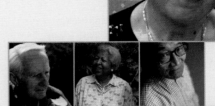

eVolve *http://evolve.elsevier.com/Ebersole/TwdHlthAging*

A STUDENT SPEAKS

I had no idea how many different things people take. Older people have so many remedies! All sorts of teas and leaves for all of their conditions, I wonder if they work.
Helena, age 18

AN ELDER SPEAKS

I would like to take the medicines that the nurse practitioner gives me but I can't always afford them, so I ask my friend what I should do because she knows a lot about teas and other treatments. They really help sometimes and maybe that is all I need!
Jean-Marie, age 65

LEARNING OBJECTIVES

On completion of this chapter, the reader will be able to:

1. Identify the legal standards that affect herb and supplement use.
2. Describe the altered effects of herbs and supplements on the older adult.
3. Discuss the information that older adults should know about the use of select herbs and supplements.
4. Discuss the role of the gerontological nurse when assisting the older adult who uses herbs and supplements.
5. Describe the effects of select commonly used herbs and supplements on the older adult.
6. Develop a nursing care plan to prevent adverse reactions related to herb or supplement use.
7. Identify the important aspects of client education related to the use of herbs and supplements with the older adult.
8. Describe the effects of herbal supplements on the older adult with chronic disease.
9. Describe the effects of herbal supplements on the older adult who is experiencing altered health conditions.

USE OF HERBS AND SUPPLEMENTS IN THE UNITED STATES

Herbs and other supplements have been used by humans for thousands of years to treat illness, but during most of the past century in the United States, they took a back seat to the burgeoning increase in prescription and over-the-counter (OTC) products available. The use of herbs and supplements resurged in the 1990s, and they now make up one of the largest groups of alternative pharmaceuticals used by millions of Americans, especially those 65 years of age or older (Yoon and Schaffer, 2006; Bardia et al., 2007; Cheung et al., 2007; R. Nahin et al., 2009). The 2007 National Health Interview Survey (NHIS) estimated that about 38% of American adults use these and other forms of complementary and alternative medicine (CAM),

spending $33.9 billion (no prescription coverage) for those CAM services and products and $14.8 billion for nonvitamin–nonmineral natural products (R.L. Nahin et al., 2009).

Several popular examples of nonherbal supplements used by older adults are melatonin for sleep; coenzyme Q10, sometimes advised for cardiac strengthening; glucosamine for painful, arthritic joints; and saw palmetto for prostatic hypertrophy. Herbs are considered dietary supplements. Yeh and colleagues (2006) reported on the 2002 National Health Interview Survey that examined the use of complementary and alternative medicine (CAM) for cardiovascular disease. The most common CAM therapies used were herbal and mind–body therapies. Echinacea, garlic, ginseng, *Ginkgo biloba*, and glucosamine with or without chondroitin were the herbs/supplements used most often. Wold and colleagues (2005), studying medication and supplement records of men and women ages 60 to 99 years, found glucosamine to be the most frequently used supplement with ginkgo, chondroitin, and garlic following. Women favored over time such supplements as black cohosh, evening primrose, flaxseed oil, chondroitin, ginkgo, glucosamine, grape seed extract, hawthorn, and St. John's wort. Men were partial to α-lipoic acid, ginkgo, and grape seed extract.

Weng and associates (2004), surveying 318 people in a retirement community, found that 20% of both men and women used herbal supplements, and most (97%) used vitamin and mineral supplements. More than half said that they received information related to supplement use from physicians or nurses. In most studies, women are the majority responders. Cheung and colleagues (2007) found that 62.9% of 445 community-dwelling older adults used CAM—28.3% used megavitamins and 20.7% used herbals. Yoon and Horne (2001), studying for one year community-dwelling women 65 years of age and older, found that more than 40% used an average of 2.5 herbs; 85% of these herbal remedies were used continually. In addition, the study noted that these women used an average of 3.2 prescribed medications and 3.8 OTC supplements and medications. Typically, the women did not tell their health care providers about the use of such alternative therapies. This finding has been supported by other research (Cheung et al., 2007). A large national survey found that 49% of older adults taking herbs never reported them to the provider (Bruno and Ellis, 2005), and 50% were found in another. Persons over 50 years of age may be more likely than younger persons to share information about their use of supplements with their providers (Durante et al., 2001; Israel and Youngkin, 2005).

In a study of older persons with a mean age of 84.8 years who lived in assisted living facilities in the states of Oregon and Washington, 84.4% were using self-prescribed OTC medications and dietary supplements (Lam and Bradley, 2006). Nutritional supplements (vitamins and minerals) were used by 32%, gastrointestinal products by 17%, products to relieve pain by 16.3%, and herbal products by 14.4%. Other products used included topicals and cough and cold drugs. For 51% of the participants, what we call "misuse" occurred through duplication of the active ingredients, the occurrence of drug–illness–food interactions, and inappropriate use. Most thought the products were helping them.

In a study of the perceptions of older users and nonusers of herbal supplements, many believed that they are derived from harmless "natural" plants or substances and therefore were not concerned about, or aware of, any dangers (Snyder et al., 2009). A small 2009 study of older persons' use of herbal supplements found that 55% used herbal supplements, and that 95% of these as well as 75% of nonusers generally believed them to be safe because they could be bought OTC in many places and were natural (Snyder et al., 2009). Those who used herbal supplements perceived supplements to be safe and were not as satisfied with their medical care as those who did not use herbal supplements (Shahrokh et al., 2005).

Herbs and supplements are likely to be used by persons in all ethnic groups. Of 130 older adults (mean age, 71.4 yr) living along the United States–Mexico border, 38.5% were taking five or more drugs (prescription and dietary supplements) daily;

31.5% were at risk for drug interactions (Loya et al., 2009). Zeilmann and associates (2003) studied white Hispanic and non-Hispanic adults 65 years of age and older and reported 49% herb use within the past year.

A 1999 to 2000 National Health and Nutrition Examination Survey assessed the prevalence of dietary supplement use (Radimer et al., 2004). Non-Hispanic white, older, normal-to-underweight women with more education were found to use supplements more than any other racial/ethnic, age, or gender groups. Yoon (2006) found no differences in reported herb use between white American and African-American women 65 years of age and older. There was a significant association between the number of herbs and number of nonprescribed medications used, and their use seemed intended to be complementary to, rather than a replacement for, prescribed therapies. A study of 95 urban older African Americans' use of CAM found that 29.5% used herbs and home remedies (Ryder et al., 2008). Although most subjects in this study (77.3%) disclosed their use of herbs/home remedies to their health care providers, the researchers nonetheless urged providers to probe for persons' use of alternative therapies (Ryder et al., 2008).

The increasing use of herbs and supplements by older adults is related to their hopes of preventing illness, promoting and maintaining health, treating a particular health problem, or replacing some currently missing dietary component (Eskin, 2001; Yoon and Horne, 2001; Yoon et al., 2004; Bruno and Ellis, 2005; Cheung et al., 2007). Elders with chronic conditions and symptoms of a health problem are more likely to use supplements and herbs in addition to their traditional therapies (Stupay and Sivertsen, 2000; Cheung et al., 2007; Ryder et al., 2008). People perceive that such products will give them more control of their health and bodies. Gerontological nurses must anticipate that older persons may use a variety of alternative therapies, including herbs and supplements, in addition to prescribed and OTC drugs. The nurse has a significant obligation to ask the right questions and obtain specific information related to use—reason, form, frequency, duration, dose, any side/adverse effects, plans for continuing, and communication with providers about use.

Standards in Manufacturing

Before 1962 all herbs were regarded as medications. In 1962 the U.S. Food and Drug Administration (FDA) required that all products considered "medications" be evaluated for safety and efficacy, yielding standardization between manufacturers of the same product. The role of the FDA also expanded to that of monitor. In response, herbal manufacturers declared their products as "food" and therefore not subject to FDA regulations (Youngkin and Israel, 1996). In 1994 some regulation was placed over herbs through the Dietary Supplement Health and Education Act (DSHEA), and they were reclassified as "dietary supplements."

By regulation, herbs and other supplements may not be labeled for prevention, treatment, or cure of a health condition of any kind unless the claim has been substantiated by research and recognized by the FDA. Of all the identified herbs, only a handful are FDA approved, such as aloe, psyllium, capsicum, witch hazel, cascara, senna, and slippery elm. Nevertheless, any herb may be hazardous if improperly used, and all adverse events must be reported to the FDA. Only then it will be investigated for possible removal from the market (Allen and Bell, 2002).

Because herbs are not typically under the protection of patent laws, companies have been less inclined to participate in clinical trials to determine their effectiveness, although the market for herbs and supplements is growing so fast that some companies now are conducting more scientific study of their safety and efficacy. However, the lack of consistency among the methods different companies use to produce herbal products makes analytical analyses of them difficult (Allen and Bell, 2002). Despite the fact that few dietary supplements are FDA approved, not every such product is unsafe or ineffective for use (Israel and Youngkin, 2005).

The World Health Organization (WHO, Geneva, Switzerland) and regulatory agencies of individual countries across the world are answering the call for safety and efficacy information based on scientific evaluation (Blumenthal et al., 2000; Israel and Youngkin, 2005). Increasing and valuable scientific information is available to consumers from numerous sources, such as from the National Center for Complementary and Alternative Medicine (NCCAM, Bethesda, MD); however, more systematic scientific trials and reviews are needed.

Thus the consumer must be alert to possible adverse effects and risks from use. Risks include the product containing the wrong parts of the herb, containing no or so little active ingredient that it is ineffective, or being adulterated with one or more unaccounted-for substances that may be dangerous. Mixed herbal supplement therapies, such as some weight loss products, can cause hazardous effects on blood pressure and heart rate and rhythm and can be particularly risky because actually determining what the product contains may be difficult. For example, bitter orange (*Citrus aurantium*) was used to replace ephedra in many weight loss products after its removal from the general market by the FDA in 2004, but bitter orange has synephrine (epinephrine-like) effects that can lead to cardiac arrest and ventricular fibrillation, and thus is unsafe for use (Swanson, 2006).

Nurses must maintain current knowledge about herbs and other supplements so that when they assess older persons about their drug and substance intake, potential and actual harmful effects may be recognized. Consideration of each product's intended use, dose, possible adverse effects, and possible interactions with other substances based on the person's health or illness conditions is required. Many manufacturers today have heeded the call to standardize the production and labeling of herbs and supplements. Honest marketing and the independent testing of products for purity are occurring. Nurses should urge their clients to be wary and to purchase products only from reputable distributors.

HERB FORMS

Different parts of an herb may have uses and actions that are unrelated. The bulb of the garlic plant contains the active essence, whereas the leaf of chamomile is used (Israel and Youngkin, 2005). Herbs are manufactured in several forms; most popular are capsules, extracts, oils, tablets, salves, teas,

and tinctures. Efficacy varies depending on the form of the herb that is used and how it is prepared. An *extract* is a fluid or solid form of the herb that is concentrated. It is made by mixing the crude herb with alcohol, water, or some other solvent that is then distilled or evaporated (Libster, 2002; Skidmore-Roth, 2005). Oils are found in two forms. *Essential oils* are aromatic, volatile, and can be derived from various parts of the fresh plant. To be therapeutic, they are usually diluted. *Infused oils,* on the other hand, are developed when the volatile oil of one herb is mixed with that of another. Herbal oils are often used in massage therapy or aromatherapy (Libster, 2002; Skidmore-Roth, 2005).

When an herb is soaked in water, alcohol, vinegar, or glycerin for a specific time and the liquid is then strained to dispose of the plant remains, a *tincture* is formed. The liquid is used therapeutically at a concentration of 1:5 or 1:10 (Libster, 2002; Skidmore-Roth, 2005). A *salve* is a type of ointment—a semi-solid substance that is used topically. Salves and ointments can be purchased or prepared by "simmering two tablespoons of the herb in 220 grams of a petroleum-based jelly for about ten minutes" (Eliopoulos, 1999, p. 103) or by using herb-infused oil or plain oil with drops of the essential oil or some other wax base and the essential oil (Libster, 2002).

Teas

The consumer should know that teas are both foods and herbs, are not regulated, may be highly concentrated if grown at home, and may be mixed with other substances—a good reason to always check labels. Tea is consumed by millions around the world, second only to water, and newly reported research indicates that some teas may have very positive effects, especially related to cardiovascular disease. Researchers found that drinking three cups of green tea daily was associated with a decreased mortality risk (Kuriyama et al., 2006). Women and nonsmokers seemed to benefit the most from green tea. Animal studies suggest that green tea antioxidants may offer eye tissue protection (Chu et al., 2010); antioxidants in tea and raspberry juice may decrease plaque formation and help decrease the risk of atherosclerosis (Rouanet et al., 2009); and tea alone may lower serum cholesterol levels (Singh et al., 2009). Drinking green tea has also been associated with a decreased risk of some cancers, such as prostate cancer in men and breast and stomach cancers in women (Boehm et al., 2009; Inoue et al., 2009; Shrubsole et al., 2009). Consuming more than four cups of tea daily was associated with a reduced risk of type 2 diabetes in adults (Huxley et al., 2009), and drinking more than four cups of green tea daily was associated with a reduced risk of depression in adults 70 years of age and older (Niu et al., 2009) and in breast cancer survivors (Chen et al., 2010). The consumer needs to remember that tea is generally safe but in excess may be harmful. For instance, senna leaf tea may cause serious fluid and electrolyte imbalance effects if used in excess and for a prolonged period (Israel and Youngkin, 2005). Consumption of more than the recommended amounts of certain teas may cause illness and possible death. For example, comfrey tea has been linked with serious liver disease (Youngkin and Israel, 1996), and drinking very hot tea too fast is associated with an increased risk of esophageal cancer (Islami et al., 2009).

SELECT COMMONLY USED TEAS, HERBS, AND SUPPLEMENTS

Chamomile

Chamomile (*Matricaria recutita* or *Chamomilla recutita*), also known as *German chamomile* or *Hungarian chamomile,*) is usually taken in tea form (Jellin, 1995-2011a). Its many uses include as an antiinflammatory and antispasmodic (said to relax smooth muscle), and to relieve gastrointestinal upset, sleep disorders, and anxiety (Israel and Youngkin, 2005; Natural Standard [a], 2010). Srivastava and associates (2009) found that chamomile extract operates similarly to a nonsteroidal antiinflammatory. A University of Pennsylvania study showed that chamomile use was associated with a reduction in anxiety symptoms as compared with a placebo (Amsterdam et al., 2009). When combined with several other herbs, including peppermint leaf, this type of chamomile is associated with improvement in dyspepsia (acid reflux, pain in the epigastrium, nausea, cramping, vomiting). However, chamomile use has mixed, less clear, and inadequate scientific evidence of value (Basch and Ulbricht, 2005; Natural Standard [a], 2010). In large doses it may cause gastrointestinal (GI) upset, and contact dermatitis and hypersensitivity reactions have been reported. It should be used cautiously with persons who report allergies to ragweed, asters, or chrysanthemums, as life-threatening allergic reactions are reported (Natural Standard [a], 2010). Use with benzodiazepines and other sedative-causing drugs is not advised, and it may inhibit some cytochrome P450 substrates. Taking it with warfain may increase warfarin's effect and increase the risk of bleeding. Chamomile capsules or tablets taken alone are in divided oral doses of 400 to 1600 mg daily or, if used as a tea, one to four cups daily made from tea bags is suggested (Basch and Ulbricht, 2005; Natural Standard [a], 2010).

Echinacea

Echinacea (*Echinacea angustifolia, E. purpurea, E. pallida),* also known as *Sampson root* and *purple coneflower,* is used for the prevention and treatment of upper respiratory infections. The *E. purpurea* variety is suggested as best for upper respiratory infection therapy (Natural Standard [b], 2010). Annual U.S. sales reported by Jellin (1995-2011b) were about $20 million, second only to garlic. Study results indicate that echinacea decreases the risk of developing the common cold and decreases the duration of a cold by at least 1 day (Shah et al., 2007; Natural Standard [b], 2010). Using the purple coneflower extract when a cold first begins and before symptoms become "full-blown" reduced the incidence of colds by 58% and the duration by 1.4 to 1.9 days (Kerr, 2006; Natural Standard: News [b], 2010). Jellin (1995-2010b) indicates modest improvement with the use of this herb at the start of symptoms; Natural Standard: News [a] (2010) and Natural Standard [b] (2010) indicate mixed scientific findings for prevention and treatment.

Echinacea seems to have immune-stimulant qualities but significant benefits are unclear (Natural Standard [b], 2010). Some adverse reactions including fever, sore throat, allergic reactions, diarrhea, nausea and vomiting, and abdominal pain have been reported, but side effects for most (if the drug is taken as directed and indicated) are few (Jellin, 1995-2011b); Natural

Standard [b], 2010). Persons allergic to daisy family plants or who have human immunodeficiency virus/acquired immunodeficiency syndrome (HIV/AIDS) or an autoimmune disease should use this herb with caution. It may interfere with the clearance of drugs eliminated by CYP3A or CYP1A2 in the liver (Gorski et al., 2004). Combining echinacea with acetaminophen and other drugs or herbs that could cause liver damage is discouraged because it may cause liver inflammation (Natural Standard [b], 2010). It is available commercially as capsules, tea, juice, extract, and tincture. If taken in capsule form, 500 to 1000 mg orally for five to seven days is used commonly in research (Natural Standard [b], 2010). Consumed as a tea, the dose ranges from 0.3 to 1 g (Scorza, 2002; Israel and Youngkin, 2005). In tablet form, it is advised three times daily and should contain 6.78 mg of the crude extract when the herb content equals 95% (Jellin, 1995-2011b). Begun at the first sign of a cold or flu, it is taken up to 10 days and should not be continued longer than the package directions advise (Basch and Ulbricht, 2005; Israel and Youngkin, 2005; Jellin, 1995-2011b).

Garlic

Garlic (*Allium sativum* bulb), known by names such as *clove garlic* and *camphor of the poor,* is thought to protect against stroke and atherosclerosis. Composed of more than 200 chemicals, a sulfur called *allicin* is thought to be garlic's primary active health ingredient (Anonymous, 2006). When the garlic clove is crushed, chewed, or chopped, allicin is released. Benefits of garlic are reported to be many, but scientific evidence is mixed (Basch and Ulbricht, 2005; Jellin, 1995-2011c; Natural Standard [c], 2010). Use is associated with decreased blood clots. It has been shown to reduce low-density lipoprotein (LDL) cholesterol, but its impact on high-density lipoprotein (HDL) cholesterol is not clear (Basch and Ulbricht, 2005; Natural Standard [c], 2010). Two meta-analyses showed that garlic use reduces blood pressure in persons with hypertension (Ried et al., 2008; Reinhart et al., 2008). Garlic may have some anticancer activity, particularly gastrointestinal (Anonymous, 2006; Natural Standard [c], 2010), and has been associated with lowered blood glucose in animal studies but unclear results in humans (Natural Standard [c], 2010). Possible adverse reactions include allergic reactions (sometimes severe), increased flatulence, bleeding if taken with drugs or supplements with anticoagulant properties or specific heart drugs, and upper GI irritation with nausea and heartburn, the latter of concern in persons with ulcers or acid reflux (Anonymous, 2006; Natural Standard [c], 2010; Tachjian et al., 2010). Some drugs metabolized by the CYP450 system in the liver may be altered by garlic, and topical garlic preparations can cause skin irritation (Scorza, 2002; Natural Standard [c], 2010). There is no standard dose or accepted standard for which form is best—oil, powder, deodorized extract, or whole clove (Anonymous, 2006; Natural Standard [c], 2010). One suggested dose is dehydrated, noncoated powder, 600 to 900 mg divided into three doses daily (Natural Standard [c], 2010).

Ginkgo biloba

Ginkgo (*Ginkgo biloba* leaf abstract), also known as *maidenhair tree, fossil tree,* and *wonder of the world,* comes from the oldest living tree species (Waddell et al., 2001; Jellin, 1995-2011d). It is prepared in capsule, extract, tablet, and tea form. The usual dose varies depending on its purpose and administered in two or three oral divided doses (Jellin, 1995-2011d; Natural Standard [d], 2010). EGb 761 is the active ingredient (Anonymous, 2003). Many studies, often very small, have examined ginkgo use for innumerable problems ranging from vertigo, tinnitus, macular degeneration, depression, altitude sickness, to acute hemorrhoids but adequate scientific evidence to support its use for such concerns is unclear and inconsistent (Natural Standard [d], 2010).

It is widely believed that ginkgo has positive cognitive events, including attributions that it can be used to treat dementia. Researchers studying data from multiple clinical trials of healthy subjects to learn whether *Ginkgo biloba* improves cognitive functioning found no scientific evidence to support use in healthy subjects for any reason related to cognitive function (Canter and Ernst, 2007). A large randomized, double-blind, placebo-controlled clinical trial—the Ginkgo Evaluation of Memory (GEM) Study—was conducted over 6.1 years (2000 to 2008) with more than 3000 seniors ages 73 to 96 years in many academic medical centers with funding from the National Center for Complementary and Alternative Medicine (R. Nahin et al., 2009; NCCAM [a], 2010). GEM Study data analysis of ginkgo versus placebo also found no scientific evidence that ginkgo impacted cognitive impairment, memory, attention, language, visual–spatial ability, and executive functions or reduced prevalence of dementia and Alzheimer's disease. Blood pressure was not different between ginkgo and placebo users nor did heart attack, stroke, or mortality occurrences differ (NCCAM [b], 2010). A positive finding from a small component of the GEM Study is that peripheral arterial disease (PAD) improved in the ginkgo versus placebo users (R. Nahin et al., 2009; NCCAM [c], 2010). A Cochrane Database review (Birks and Grimley Evans, 2009) also countered the previously described findings, noting that there is no predictable, reliable evidence that is clinically significant of the herb benefiting persons with cognitive decline or dementia. In this review, the herb seemed safe without excess side effects when compared with placebo.

Use of ginkgo is generally tolerated well in research trials (comparable to placebo). However, ginkgo is implicated as causing dangerous interactions with heart medications (Tachjian et al., 2010). One of the more serious side effects of ginkgo use is bleeding (Natural Standard [d], 2010). Persons taking drugs that increase bleeding risk or who have bleeding disorders should take ginkgo with caution and with provider oversight, and report any abnormal response such as bleeding, bruising, dizziness, headache, and blurred vision (Kuhn, 2002). Pre-surgery, ginkgo needs to be stopped according to surgeon directions, generally at least one week or more before the surgery to prevent excessive bleeding during and after surgery. Many other herbs increase the risk of bleeding, such as *Panax ginseng*, ginger, and garlic (Kuhn, 2002; Natural Standard [d], 2010).

Some of the reported side effects of ginkgo include GI upset, headache, hypersensitivity, palpitations, dizziness, muscle weakness, and constipation (Israel and Youngkin, 2005; Jellin, 1995-2011d; Natural Standard [d], 2010). Possible significant interaction effects of ginkgo are reported with certain prescribed drugs (e.g., warfarin, heparin, monoamine oxidase [MAO] inhibitors), OTC drugs (e.g., aspirin, NSAIDs), herbs

(e.g., St. John's wort), supplement drugs (melatonin), to name only a few, and some health conditions are worsened by its use. Ginkgo seeds can be toxic, and consumption may lower the seizure threshold (Allen and Bell, 2002; Jellin, 1995-2011d; Natural Standard [d], 2010). Nurses must carefully assess persons taking ginkgo for complications.

Ginseng

American Ginseng (a Chinese perennial herb), and variations such as Asian ginseng, Chinese ginseng, and Korean ginseng, may be of special interest to older adults. It has had numerous applications over thousands of years' use, but is best known for its use to improve well-being and help with stress adaptation, although research results are mixed (Jellin, 1995-2011e; Natural Standard [e], 2010). Ginseng may benefit persons with heart disorders by reducing LDL cholesterol, lower blood sugar levels in type 2 diabetes, and enhance the immune system, but more research is needed in these areas (Basch and Ulbricht, 2005; Jellin, 1995-2011e; Natural Standard [e], 2010). Research support for the belief that ginseng is possibly effective in improving mood in postmenopausal women and some cognitive functions (such as abstract thinking, math skills, and how quickly one reacts) is not strong; it is not effective in improving memory as a single-use product (Natural Standard [e], 2010). It is associated with improvement in erectile dysfunction in some men (Hong et al., 2002; Natural Standard [e], 2010). For all applications, more controlled studies are recommended.

Ginseng root provides the most active constituents, ginsenosides or panaxosides, but contains other constituents that may also play a role (Jellin, 1995-2011e). The most common preparations are capsules, extracts, teas, and tinctures. Dosages vary with the type of ginseng, the preparation, frequency of consumption, and strength of dose. For example, 100 to 200 mg of standardized ginseng extract (4% ginsenosides) in capsule form taken orally once or twice daily for up to 12 weeks is reported (Natural Standard [e], 2010). Side effects are many (Box 10-1). Persons with hypertension, cardiac problems, or diabetes must use ginseng with significant caution. Ginseng can increase blood pressure (Tachjian et al., 2010) and may interact with other medications and products (Table 10-1). Persons who have had strokes may have increased bleeding if they take ginseng and blood-thinning medications at the same time (Lee et al.,

---

BOX 10-1   POTENTIAL SIDE EFFECTS OF GINSENG OF SIGNIFICANCE FOR OLDER ADULTS

- Tachycardia
- Hypertension
- Hypotension
- Edema
- Diarrhea
- Mania (for persons with bipolar illness)

Data from Jellin J editor; Natural Medicines Comprehensive Database (2011). Available at www.naturaldatabase.com. Accessed December 2010; Natural Standard: The Authority on Integrative Medicine: Gingko, 2009, Available at http://www.naturalstandard.com. Accessed December 2010; Tachjian A, Maria V, Jahangir A: Use of herbal products and potential interactions in patients with cardiovascular diseases, *Journal of the American College of Cardiology* 55:515, 2010.

TABLE 10-1   SELECT HERB–MEDICATION INTERACTIONS*

HERB	MEDICATION	COMPLICATION	NURSING ACTION
Garlic	Any anticoagulant or antiplatelet drug such as warfarin sodium	Risk of bleeding may increase	Advise person not to take without provider approval
	Anticlot drugs such as streptokinase		
	Aspirin, other NSAIDs		
	Antihypertensives	Increased hypotensive effect	Advise provider approval with use
	Antivirals, such as ritonavir	Altered drug effect	Advise against use
	Antimetabolites such as cyclosporine	Risk of less effective response	Advise against use
	Insulin or oral hypoglycemic agent such as pioglitazone or tolbutamide	Serum glucose control may improve; less antidiabetic drug needed	Monitor blood glucose levels
Ginkgo	Aspirin, other NSAIDs	Risk of bleeding may occur	Teach person not to take without approval of provider
	Heparin sodium, warfarin sodium, any anticoagulant		
	Antiplatelet drugs such as ticlopidine		
	Antidiabetic drugs: insulin, oral DMT2 drugs such as metformin	May alter blood glucose levels	Monitor blood glucose closely
	Antidepressants, MAOIs, SSRIs	May cause abnormal response or decrease effectiveness	Advise not to take with these drugs
	Antihypertensives	May cause increased effect	Monitor blood pressure
	Antiseizure drugs	Risk for seizure if history of seizure	Advise against use
Ginseng	Insulin and oral antidiabetic drugs	Blood glucose levels may be altered	Monitor blood glucose levels closely
	Anticoagulant and antiplatelet drugs	May increase bleeding	Advise use with caution and provider oversight
	Aspirin and other NSAIDs		
	MAOIs such as isocarboxazid	Headaches, tremors, mania	Advise against use
	Antihypertensives, cardiac drugs such as calcium channel blockers	May alter effects of drug	Advise against use unless provider monitors closely
	Immunosuppressants	May interfere with action	Advise against use
	Stimulants	May cause additive effect	Advise against use
	Fenugreek	Decreased blood glucose	Monitor closely
Green tea	Warfarin sodium	May alter anticoagulant effects	Advise against use
	Stimulants	May cause additive effect	Advise to use with care
Hawthorn	Digoxin	May cause a loss of potassium, leading to drug toxicity	Monitor blood levels
	β-Blockers and other drugs lowering blood pressure and improving blood flow	May be additive in effects	Monitor blood pressure meticulously; advise that this concern holds true for erectile dysfunction drugs also
Red yeast rice	Fibrate drugs; other cholesterol drugs	May cause additive effects	Avoid concomitant use
	Drugs for diabetes management	May alter blood sugar levels	Monitor blood sugar carefully
	Anticoagulants, antiplatelet drugs, NSAIDs	May increase risk of bleeding	Warn patient and monitor carefully
St. John's wort	Triptans such as sumatriptan, zolmitriptan	May increase risks of serotonergic adverse effects, serotonin syndrome, cerebral vasoconstriction	Advise against use
	HMG-CoA reductase inhibitors	May decrease plasma concentrations of these drugs	Monitor levels of lipids
	MAOIs	May cause similar effects as with use with any SSRI	Advise against use
	Digoxin	Decreases the effects of the drug	Advise against use
	Alprazolam	May decrease effect of drug	Advise against use
	Amitriptyline	May decrease effect of drug	Advise against use
	Ketoprofen	Photosensitivity	Advise sun block use
	Tramadol and some SSRIs	May increase risk of serotonin syndrome	Advise against use
	Olanzapine	May cause serotonin syndrome	Advise against use
	Paroxetine	Sedative–hypnotic intoxication	Advise against use
	Theophylline	Increases metabolism; decreases drug blood level	Monitor drug effects
	Albuterol		
	Warfarin	May decrease anticoagulant effect	Advise against use
	Amlodipine	Lowers efficacy of calcium channel	Advise against use
	Estrogen or progesterone	May decrease effect of hormones	Advise that this effect may occur
	Protease inhibitors or nonnucleoside reverse transcriptase inhibitors in HIV/AIDS treatment; antivirals	May alter drug effects	FDA advises avoidance of this herb for patients taking these drugs

AIDS, acquired immunodeficiency syndrome; DMT2, diabetes mellitus type 2; FDA, U.S. Food and Drug Administration; HIV, human immunodeficiency virus; HMG-CoA, 3-hydroxy-3-methylglutaryl coenzyme-A; MAOIs, monoamine oxidase inhibitors; NSAIDs, nonsteroidal antiinflammatory drugs; SSRIs, selective serotonin reuptake inhibitors.

*The interactions listed represent only a few of the possible herb–drug interactions. Use of herbs that interfere with metabolism of drugs by the liver's cytochrome P450 enzyme system should be avoided or monitored closely by the provider. Any herb has the potential for untoward effects.

Adapted from Basch E, Ulbricht C: *Natural standard herb & supplement handbook: the clinical bottom line,* St. Louis, MO, 2005, Mosby; Jellin J, editor; Natural Medicines Comprehensive Database (2006). Available at www.naturaldatabase.com. Accessed December 2010; *NDH pocket guide to drug interactions,* Philadelphia, 2002, Lippincott, Williams & Wilkins; Natural Standard: The Authority on Integrative Medicine. Available at http://www.naturalstandard.com. Accessed December 2010; Wilson BA, Shannon MT, Stang CL *Nurses drug guide,* Upper Saddle River, NJ, 2004, Pearson Prentice Hall; Yoon SL, Schaffer SD: Herbal, prescribed, and over-the-counter drug use in older women: prevalence of drug interactions, *Geriatric Nursing* 27:118, 2006.

2008). Allergic reactions are reported in people allergic to plants in the Araliaceae family.

American ginseng and Siberian ginseng are two distinct types of ginseng not to be confused with *Panax ginseng*. American ginseng is said to decrease blood glucose levels in type 2 diabetes and also may help decrease the risk of upper respiratory infections, such as cold or flu, in older adults. Siberian ginseng may be helpful in decreasing herpes virus type 2 infections. There is not enough evidence to support its use for improving memory, feelings of well-being, hyperlipidemia, arrhythmias, or stroke outcomes, as some resources suggest. Further controlled studies are needed for all such applications. Ginseng might be easily misunderstood and misused, including *Panax pseudoginseng,* for which no reliable information exists concerning its main reported effectiveness to stop bleeding.

Glucosamine Sulfate

Glucosamine sulfate, also known as *chitosamine,* is used primarily for osteoarthritis (OA) of the knees (Natural Standard [f], 2010) and is commonly used (Jellin, 1995-2011f). Glucosamine sulfate is thought to help reduce pain and improve function with OA of the knee. It is used frequently in combination with glucosamine hydrochloride and chondroitin sulfate for joint pain, but the results of the Glucosamine/Chondroitin Arthritis Intervention Trial (GAIT) found that neither of these drugs, either alone or together, was more effective than placebo, except in one small subgroup with moderate-to-severe pain that had a 20% improvement in pain (Clegg et al., 2006; Bruyere and Reginster, 2007). More recently, Bruyere and Reginster, as well as Fox and Stephens (2009), found that glucosamine *sulfate* and chondroitin sulfate do have some effectiveness in reducing OA symptoms.

Two newer products—Primarine and Relamine—may have some ability to improve symptoms when used with glucosamine sulfate and chondroitin sulfate, but more study is needed (Fox and Stephens, 2009). The nurse might advise that glucosamine sulfate with chondroitin sulfate may be an option for mild to moderate OA pain, but no alternative has been effective with severe OA that is long-standing. Use does not appear to slow OA progression (Natural Standard: News [c], 2009). A prescription form of chondroitin used in Europe may offer some effect against progression (Natural Standard: News [d], 2009). Natural Standard: News [e] (2008) notes that glucosamine sulfate is not effective for hip OA. The nurse should warn of interaction effects with multiple drug or herb/supplement use (prescribed or OTC—particularly blood sugar control drugs and drugs that cause bleeding) (Burks, 2005; Natural Standard [f], 2010). Glucosamine sulfate is usually prepared in capsule, tablet, or liquid form. The dose varies, but the usual dose is 1500 mg daily in one dose or in divided doses (500 mg three times daily) (Jellin, 1995-2011f; Natural Standard [f], 2010). GI upset, insomnia, headache, and skin reactions have been reported. In general, the drug is well tolerated by older adults. Persons with diabetes, asthma, or shellfish allergy should use glucosamine with caution.

Hawthorn

Hawthorn (*Crataegus monogyna, Crataegus laevigata*) may have a positive effect for people with congestive heart failure and coronary circulation, particularly chronic heart failure (Jellin, 1995-2011g; Pittler et al., 2008; Natural Standard [g], 2010). Hawthorn may work by increasing cardiac output, and it also is said to have effects as an antispasmodic, diuretic, sedative, and anxiety reducer (Jellin, 1995-2011g). A 2008 review of randomized, double-blind, and placebo-controlled trials indicated that benefits were significant for hawthorn use as an adjunctive therapy in chronic heart failure (Pittler et al., 2008). However, it may interact with cardiovascular drugs, such as antihypertensives, causing hypotension and limiting its use, and can alter blood sugar levels (Allen and Bell, 2002; Jellin, 1995-2011g; Natural Standard [g], 2010). This drug had mild to moderate, although generally infrequent, reported adverse events from clinical research trials (Daniele et al., 2006). It seems fairly safe when used for short term use, no more than 16 weeks, and requires provider oversight (Jellin, 1995-2011g). Vertigo and dizziness are the most common adverse effects and are of particular concern in the elderly, who have an increased incidence of serious falls. GI upset, allergic response with rash, palpitations, fatigue, and sweating are among the less common side effects. Although used as an extract or tea, it is often taken as a capsule. The standard dose varies for heart failure, but 60 mg three times daily or 80 mg twice per day are common. Some trials use higher doses (Natural Standard [g], 2010).

Red Yeast Rice

Red yeast rice, gaining popularity in Western medicine, has always had strong support in Eastern medicine as a drug to lower low-density lipoprotein cholesterol (LDL-C), especially in individuals with dyslipidemia who cannot tolerate statins (Becker et al., 2008, 2009). Becker and colleagues (2008, 2009) studied 74 and 62 persons, respectively, with high cholesterol levels. The 2008 study found an equal drop in LDL-C between the group taking a statin and the group assigned to combine lifestyle changes with red yeast rice and fish oil consumption. In the second study, Becker and colleagues found that persons taking red yeast rice, who had dyslipidemia and had stopped taking one or more prescribed statins because of myalgias, had significantly lower total cholesterol and LDL-C levels after 12 weeks than those receiving a placebo. Both groups were participating in a lifestyle change program, consuming a Mediterranean-type diet and participated in exercise and relaxation activities. The FDA does warn that the public should buy red yeast products from respected sources, and avoid purchases through the Internet because these products may be adulterated (U.S. Food and Drug Administration, 2007). Additional studies have supported the prior research showing red yeast rice to be tolerated well and its use resulted in similar LDL-C reductions as certain statin drugs in statin-intolerant persons (Halbert et al., 2010; Venero et al., 2010). Persons need to know the potential side effects of red yeast rice, similar to those of lovastatin, such as muscle pain, kidney damage, heartburn, bloating and gas, dizziness, and asthma (Natural Standard [h], 2010). The usual dose is 1200 mg of concentrated red yeast rice powder capsules taken twice daily with food (Natural Standard [h], 2010).

St. John's Wort

St. John's wort (SJW; *Hypericum perforatum*) has many names, such as *demon chaser* and *goatweed*. SJW is most often used to treat mild or moderate depression, although it is used by some without clear evidential support for a large variety of ills such as seasonal affective disorder, anxiety, pain relief, and premenstrual syndrome (Ernst, 2002; Lawvere and Mahoney, 2005; Jellin, 1995-2011h; van der Watt et al., 2008; Ravindran et al., 2009; Natural Standard [i], 2010). Previously, on the basis of major clinical trials, SJW was found to be ineffective for major depression (Sego, 2006; Shelton, 2009). However, other research suggests it may be superior to placebo and as effective as commonly used antidepressants (Linde et al., 2008; NCCAM [d], 2010). The concern of many experts is that if it is not effective, its use could endanger the individual with severe depression, increasing the risk of suicide by delaying the person from seeking appropriate traditional health care.

SJW in recommended doses is considered relatively well tolerated for one to three months, and more recently for one year in one study (Brattstrom, 2009; Natural Standard [i], 2010). Common side effects occur in one to three patients and are less often than with usual antidepressant drugs. Such side effects include photosensitivity, dermatitis, GI upset, restlessness, anxiety, headache, dry mouth, and possible sexual dysfunction (Jellin, 1995-2011h; Natural Standard [i], 2010). Hypomania with bipolar disorder has been reported, as well as suicidal and homicidal thoughts. Other cytochrome P450 enzyme inducers, such as certain other drugs, red wine, broccoli, and cigarette smoke, should be used cautiously with SJW as it may increase serum levels of the other substances (Natural Standard [i], 2010). The list of possible drug–drug, drug–herb/ supplement, herb–disease, and anesthesia interactions is long, which is the primary reason for caution with SJW use and provider oversight. SJW is contraindicated with other antidepressants, especially selective serotonin reuptake inhibitors (SSRIs) (Israel and Youngkin, 2005; Natural Standard [i], 2010) (see Chapter 9).

Individuals taking any antidepressant should wait at least two weeks after discontinuing its use before beginning SJW, as serious adverse effects may occur. Sun exposure avoidance is advised because of possible photosensitivity. When taking this herb, people should be warned not to take medications containing monoamines, such as medications for nasal decongestants, hay fever, and asthma, because this combination may cause hypertension (Waddell et al., 2001). The gerontological nurse must be familiar with these concerns in counseling the older patient. Although clinical trials have used higher doses, the usual dose is 300-mg capsules three times daily or 450 mg twice per day (Israel and Youngkin, 2005; Natural Standard [i], 2010). It may take up to six weeks for SJW to reach its full effect; it should be discontinued slowly (Stupay and Sivertsen, 2000; Jellin, 1995-2011h).

Saw Palmetto

Saw palmetto, a fruit-bearing palm tree known as *Serenoa repens,* grows wild in the southern United States and is said to offer mild to modest symptom improvement for persons with benign prostatic hyperplasia (BPH) (Israel and Youngkin, 2005; Jellin, 1995-2011i; Natural Standard [j], 2010). The herb's effects are thought to exert some estrogenic effects and to inhibit 5-α-reductase and androgen receptors (Natural Standard [j],

2010). BPH symptoms, commonly seen in the elderly, include urinary frequency, dysuria, urgency, hesitancy, and nocturia. Natural Standard [j] (2010) and Dedhia and McVary (2008) note that research trials suggest that saw palmetto is effective in improving symptoms of BPH. Other studies show mixed results in outcomes for BPH symptoms, and thus it may not be as effective as the prescription medication *finasteride,* as promoted in the past. Bent and colleagues (2006) found that saw palmetto did not improve BPH in men who had moderate to severe symptoms, and a Cochrane Database review noted that the herb's actions were not better than placebo for urinary symptoms (Tacklind et al., 2009). The saw palmetto essential oils used for treating mild BPH are in many standardized products today. Although considered not to cause serious toxicity and generally without reported drug interactions, the herb is associated with some mild side effects, such as dizziness, fatigue, rhinitis, decreased libido, headache, and GI upset, and there could be possible adverse reactions not yet seen (Avins et al., 2008; Agbabiaka et al., 2009). Saw palmetto may prolong bleeding time, so use with anticoagulant/antiplatelet drugs, supplements, or herbs is advised with caution and under supervision (Natural Standard [j], 2010). The herb must not be taken with drugs used for the treatment of BPH or prostate cancer, or with any drug or herb/supplement that can affect male sex hormones or that can increase bleeding (Natural Standard [j], 2010). Dosing of 160 mg two times per day or 320 mg once per day is advised (Jellin, 1995-2011i; Natural Standard [j], 2010). Table 10-2 lists select commonly used herbs and supplements and their recommended dosages.

USE OF HERBS AND SUPPLEMENTS FOR SELECT CONDITIONS

Hypertension

A number of herbs, minerals, and supplements may have some positive effect in lowering blood pressure, but will need more research study to support their use in treatment. Some of these are coenzyme Q10, garlic, green tea, hawthorn, melatonin, and magnesium (Natural Standard [k], 2010). Hawthorn has been used to treat hypertension for many years. A British study found that people with diabetes type 2 who were taking medications for the diabetes had a significant reduction in diastolic blood pressure when randomized to take hawthorn (Walker et al., 2006). However, if a person adds hawthorn while already taking β-blockers or calcium channel blockers, it may precipitate dangerous hypotension (Jellin, 1995-2011i). Because therapeutic levels are not established, overtreatment and undertreatment can occur when hawthorn alone is used. Caution is urged when erectile dysfunction drugs are used concomitantly with hawthorn because hypotension may result (Hong et al., 2002). Research shows that dietary calcium in enriched low-fat dairy products taken three times daily may lower blood pressure in moderate hypertension (Natural Standard [k], 2010). Health care providers are urged to provide up-to-date information about the use of any such substance when counseling patients who have hypertension (Edwards et al., 2005). For more information, see the previous sections on garlic and hawthorn in this chapter.

TABLE 10-2	SELECT COMMONLY USED HERBS AND RECOMMENDED DOSAGES*	
HERB/ SUPPLEMENT	**FORM**	**RECOMMENDED DOSAGE**
Chamomile	Capsule or tablet	400-1600 mg in divided doses
	Fluid extract	1-4 mL three times daily
	Tea	One to four cups from tea bags daily
	Tincture	15 mL three to four times daily
Echinacea	Capsule	500 mg-1 g three times per day
	Tea	2 tsp steeped in one cup of boiling water for 10-15 min
	Tincture	0.75-1.5 mL two to five times per day, gargle, and then swallow
	Extract	300-800 mg two or three times per day for up to 6 mo
Garlic	Capsule or tablet	600-1200 mg daily, divided into three doses
	Extract	4 mL daily
	Fresh	4 g daily
	Oil	2-5 mg daily
	Tincture	2-4 mL three times daily
Ginkgo	Capsule or tablet	80-240 mg two or three times daily
	Extract	80 mg three times daily
Ginseng	Capsule or tablet	100-200 mg one or two times daily
	Extract	1-2 mL daily
	Tincture	5-10 mL daily
Glucosamine	Capsule or tablet	500 mg three times daily or 1.5 g once daily
Hawthorn	Extract LI 132	100-300 mg three times daily
	Extract WS 1442	60 mg three times daily or 80 mg twice daily
Red yeast rice	Capsule	1200 mg of concentrated powder twice daily with food
St. John's wort	Capsule	300 mg three times daily (maintenance, 300-600 mg daily)
Saw palmetto	Capsule	160 mg one or two times daily

*Readers are advised to follow the most up-to-date dosage and duration-of-use recommendations from expert sources for any herb or supplement. No proven effective dose is available.

Adapted from Basch E, Ulbricht C: *Natural standard herb & supplement handbook: the clinical bottom line,* St. Louis, MO, 2005, Mosby; Mosby; Jellin J editor: Natural Medicines Comprehensive Database (2006). Available at www.naturaldatabase.com. Accessed December 2010. Natural Standard: The Authority on Integrative Medicine. Available at http://www.naturalstandard.com. Accessed December 2010. Skidmore-Roth L: *Mosby's handbook of herbs and natural supplements,* St. Louis, MO, 2005, Mosby.

Human Immunodeficiency Virus–related Symptoms

The number of persons entering late life who are already infected with HIV is increasing. Many have been using a number of alternative therapies, including herbs, to address their symptoms. Eller and colleagues (2005) found that herbal therapies were among the self-care strategies used by 92% of subjects studied in relation to symptoms of depression and HIV. Of concern is the potential that some herbal products may alter the metabolic action of antiretroviral drugs used in treatment (Walubo, 2007; Ladenheim et al., 2008). For example, SJW is commonly used for depression, but research indicates it may lower the blood level of antiretroviral medications when taken together (Natural Standard [l], 2010). Some studies discuss the use of herbal medicines with HIV/AIDS patients for possible

antiviral benefits (Natural Standard [l], 2010), and others in Thailand and Africa indicate significant improvement in health overall and quality of life, suggesting a need for further study (Tshibangu et al., 2004; Sugimoto et al., 2005).

Gastrointestinal Disorders

Elders with GI problems are likely to use alternative therapies, including herbs (Tillisch, 2006). One example of use is for irritable bowel syndrome (IBS). The Chinese have used herbal therapies for thousands of years to treat IBS. A search of the literature by Liu and colleagues (2006) found that 75 random trials for IBS had been done and that IBS was improved by some of the herbal therapies. Psyllium (*Plantago ovata* and *P. ispaghula*), well known to assist the older person with constipation, is used as a bulk laxative (Natural Standard [m], 2010). It may assist with IBS, although results are conflicting (Basch and Ulbricht, 2005). Calcium is approved by the FDA and scientifically well supported for use in reducing gastric acidity, and probiotic products help control harmful organisms in the gut, such as *Helicobacter pylori* (Natural Standard [m], 2010). There is good evidence that cranberry may decrease *H. pylori* in the stomach, and peppermint oil may offer antispasmodic effects in IBS. Also, see the previous section on chamomile in this chapter for use with GI problems. Chronic alcohol-induced and fulminant hepatitis have both been positively affected by the use of milk thistle (Basch and Ulbricht, 2005; Jellin, 1995-2011j). Comfrey, kava kava, and chaparral are examples of herbs that may be toxic to the gastrointestinal system (Jellin, 1995-2011k).

Cancer

In the United States, many herbs have the potential to be used in the treatment of cancer but none has met the goals for use in Western biomedicine. Patients with cancer often use alternative therapies in self-care. Some of the herbs that need more scientific study for helping patients with cancer include milk thistle and garlic (Williams et al., 2006; Natural Standard [n], 2010). Calcium, garlic, ginkgo, and psyllium are possibly helpful for decreasing colorectal and gastric cancer risk (Jellin, 1995-2011k; Natural Standard [n], 2010).

Some evidence indicates that coffee consumption and greater lung cancer risk are associated, but it is difficult to be sure in the presence of concurrent smoking, which is known to cause lung cancer (Tang et al., 2009, 2010). Drinking green tea has been said to help prevent cancer, but evidence is conflicting and insufficient (Boehm et al., 2009). No significant association between drinking coffee with or without caffeine or tea and breast cancer risk is evident (Ganmaa et al., 2008). Claims are often made that a substance or an herb will "cure" or help the patient with cancer, even though no data support such claims. Clients and their families may become desperate in an effort to "do something" to help. Gerontological nurses must be sensitive to this situation and work with all concerned to provide the most appropriate care possible.

Alzheimer's Disease

Kales and colleagues (2004) found that among 82 elderly veterans with dementia and depression, nearly one fifth of the veterans and their caretakers used herbs and supplements. Ginkgo is often used by older persons with dementia because it increases blood supply to the brain. There is some scientific support for modest improvement in Alzheimer's and dementia symptoms, but the GEM Study (NCCAM [a], 2010), discussed in the earlier section on *Ginkgo biloba*, found no scientific evidence to support the use of this herb to prevent or treat Alzheimer's disease. In an Iranian double-blind, randomized, placebo-controlled trial, sage *(Salvia officinalis)* significantly improved cognitive outcomes as measured by the cognitive subscale of the Alzheimer's Disease Assessment Scale and on the Clinical Dementia Rating Scale in 42 adults ages 65 to 80 years with mild to moderate Alzheimer's disease (Akhondzadeh et al., 2003). Further study is advised in the use of sage with dementia and Alzheimer's disease (Natural Standard [o], 2010). According to William Thies, chief medical and scientific officer of the Alzheimer's Association (Chicago, IL), moderate to heavy physical activity levels, drinking tea one to four times per day, and not being deficient in vitamin D have all been associated with reducing brain decline risk (Marcus, 2010a). Also, more studies are suggested to support and clarify the use of melatonin for sleep benefits and lemon balm for agitation with patients with Alzheimer's disease or dementia, as well as the use of caffeine for protection against cognitive decline (Marcus, 2010a; Natural Standard [o], 2010).

Diabetes

Herbal approaches to diabetes management were in place before the discovery of insulin in 1921. Hundreds of different plants affect blood glucose, and many are still in use. Fenugreek *(Trigonella foenum-graecum)*, a seed powder, when consumed as a cup of tea three times daily or taken orally in a capsule, can induce a hypoglycemic response (Basch and Ulbricht, 2005; Jellin, 1995-2011L), but it can cause diarrhea and flatulence and may increase anticoagulant activity of other drugs the person is taking. Research indicates that every additional daily cup consumed significantly decreases the risk of diabetes, and comparable amounts of decaffeinated coffee and tea result in similar decreases (Huxley et al., 2009). Oba and colleagues (2010) suggest that the protection from coffee may be present regardless of caffeine effect. However, J.D. Lane, a professor at Duke Medical Center (Durham, NC), advises that drinking that much coffee a day may amplify problems with blood sugar in individuals with diabetes (Marcus, 2010b). A number of possible adverse effects may occur with increased caffeine intake, including headache, insomnia, anxiety and nervousness, hypertension, and heart rhythm disturbance. Cinnamon is another herb that has been linked with lowering blood glucose, but scientific evidence is mixed (Jellin, 1995-2011m; Pham et al., 2007; Baker et al., 2008; Kirkham et al., 2009; Natural Standard [p], 2010). Other herbs or supplements linked with some scientific evidence of lowering blood glucose are chromium, ginseng, gymnema, and stevia (Natural Standard [p], 2010). Numerous other substances are said to have unclear or conflicting scientific evidence for lowering blood sugar, such as astragalus, bilberry, black or green tea, chromium, red yeast rice, honey, and even the parasitic vine kudzu, but the evidence is not sufficient to support that these are effective in treating or reducing the development of diabetes type 2 (Jellin, 1995-2011n; Natural Standard [p], 2010). Some supplements do not

help or may even be harmful, such as selenium, fish oil, or coenzyme Q10, particularly if the patient stops taking prescribed medications for diabetes (Natural Standard [p], 2010). If any herb or supplement is used by the patient for diabetes management, the nurse needs to urge careful and regular evaluation by a health care professional, as well as blood glucose monitoring and indicated prescribed medication dose adjustments.

HERB AND SUPPLEMENT INTERACTIONS WITH STANDARDIZED DRUGS

A major issue in the use of herbs and other supplements is the risk for interactions. This is of particular concern because of the number of medications already taken by elders (prescription, OTC, herbal, and nonherbal supplements). A 22-month study of more than 3000 U.S. adults, ages 75 years or older, found that almost 2250 of the study subjects combined at least one prescription drug with one dietary supplement daily, and approximately 10% to 33% combined up to five prescription drugs and five supplements daily (R. Nahin et al., 2009). Many herb and supplement products do interact with prescription or OTC medications, foods, and/or other herbs and supplements (see also Chapter 9). This chapter addresses only select herb–drug interactions especially relevant to older adults because of the extensive nature of such interaction issues.

The more herbs, supplements, and other drugs that the person is taking, the more likely it is that an interaction will occur (see Chapter 9) (Kuhn, 2002). Yoon and Schaffer (2006) reviewed the interaction prevalence of drugs reported in a study of 58 women who were 65 years of age and older. Nearly 75% of them took herbs, prescription drugs, and/or OTC drugs that could interact at a moderate- or high-risk level. Of the total interactions, 63% involved NSAIDs. The authors found this worrisome, because older adults are at risk for bleeding even when NSAIDs are taken properly.

Persons taking medications that have a narrow therapeutic index should be especially discouraged from using herbal remedies. The interaction may cause alterations in absorption, distribution, or metabolism. For example, aloe and rhubarb have been found to bind to medications such as digoxin or warfarin, reducing their effectiveness by limiting their absorption. In these cases, the drug should be taken at least one hour before the herb. Herbs that are more likely to cause a distribution-type interaction may increase the possibility of adverse effects. Metabolism-type interactions may increase or decrease the effectiveness of a medication, depending on the herb and the medication. St. John's wort (SJW) has significant interactions with many conventional drugs that may decrease the drug's concentration by inducing cytochrome P450s (CYPs) and P-glycoprotein, the major drug transporter, and lead to adverse reactions (Zhou and Lai, 2008; Izzo and Ernst, 2009).

Examples of a few herb–drug interactions that may cause or have the potential to cause adverse effects include the following:

- Meadowsweet and black willow together may interact with warfarin and carbamazepine.
- Black licorice can decrease corticosteroid action.

- St. John's wort decreases plasma concentrations or increases clearance of many drugs including alprazolam, amitriptyline, atorvastatin, digoxin, erythromycin, simvastatin, verapamil, and warfarin.
- *Ginkgo biloba* decreases plasma concentrations of omeprazole, ritonavir, and tolbutamide; it can unpredictably interact negatively with antiepileptics, aspirin, diuretics, and ibuprofen, and in some instances has an additive effect when taken with warfarin.
- Echinacea may increase the concentration of caffeine by interfering with its clearance (Kuhn, 2002; Izzo and Ernst, 2009).

Bone (2008) notes that extreme concerns about *Ginkgo biloba* potentiating anticoagulant or antiplatelet effects are not well supported by clinical trials or case reports. However, nurses must still warn patients of potential effects if they take ginkgo.

Because the content of active herb or herbs in products by different manufacturers varies considerably, the therapeutic outcome and potential for herb–drug interactions varies greatly. Table 10-1 lists the interactions between some commonly used herbs and select medications. Complications and nursing actions that can promote healthy aging are also listed.

TABLE 10-3	SELECT HERBS AND THE PERIOPERATIVE PATIENT	
HERB	**PERIOPERATIVE ISSUE**	**PREOPERATIVE DISCONTINUATION**
Echinacea	Allergic reactions; decreased effectiveness of immunosuppressants	No time advised in data; advise discussing with surgeon or anesthesiologist
Garlic	Potential for increased bleeding	1 to 2 weeks before surgery
Ginkgo	Potential for increased bleeding	2 weeks before surgery
Ginseng	Hypoglycemia; potential for increased bleeding	1 to 2 weeks before surgery
St. John's wort	Potential for increased sedation with anesthetics	5 days before surgery*

*Clients taking St. John's wort for depression must be advised not to stop herb abruptly and to discuss with a physician when to stop before surgery. A washout period of three weeks may be needed.
Adapted from Basch E, Ulbricht C: *Natural standard herb & supplement handbook: the clinical bottom line,* St. Louis, MO, 2005, Mosby; Jellin J, editor: Natural Medicines Comprehensive Database (2006). Available at www.naturaldatabase.com. Accessed December 2010. Norred CL, Brinker F: Potential coagulation effects of preoperative complementary and alternative medicines, *Alternative Therapies in Health and Medicine* 7:58, 2001.

PROMOTING HEALTHY AGING: IMPLICATIONS FOR GERONTOLOGICAL NURSING

The gerontological nurse can promote healthy aging in several ways among persons who use or may use herbs and other supplements.

This begins with creating a safe and nonjudgmental relationship wherein an elder feels comfortable describing his or her use and understanding of these products. If a person is reticent, the nurse may encourage sharing this information for safety's sake (Canter and Ernst, 2005; Cheung et al., 2007). Any verbal or nonverbal action from the provider that may block this openness may lead to a potentially dangerous lack of assessment data.

Once this conversation has begun, both the nurse and the elder can begin to evaluate the existing knowledge about and safety in the use of the substance. This includes not only the name of the herb/supplement, but knowledge of its potential side effects and interactions. It is helpful to know what the person hopes to accomplish by using the herb/supplement. Reinforcing the positive effects and reviewing the cost of using the product may assist him or her to relax and open additional lines of communication. The conversation is a useful venue for teaching about the safe use of herbs and other supplements.

Perioperative Assessment

Including herbs and supplements in the perioperative or emergency surgery assessment is of vital importance. The reader is advised to see the article by Messina (2006) for risks associated with the use of 10 herbs by the patient who is to have surgery. As discussed, hypertension, excessive and prolonged bleeding, and the increased chance for interactions between the herb and other drugs are discussed. Herbs that can affect bleeding and clotting time, such as garlic, ginger, ginkgo, and ginseng, should

be especially noted and reported to the surgical team. Many older adults are electing aesthetic surgery today, and these patients must also be assessed carefully preoperatively (Rowe and Baker, 2009). Several select herbs and their perioperative effects are listed in Table 10-3. The American Society of Anesthesiologists suggests all herbal products be stopped two to three weeks before surgery (Kaye et al., 2004). This should be done with provider monitoring if the herb's discontinuation may potentially cause a serious problem.

Interventions

When planning care, the nurse should know that the use of alternative therapies is common, especially among those who are foreign-born or who have lived in ethnically isolated communities. The main reasons given for the use of alternative therapies by elders from areas outside the country of service (especially the United States and Canada) are (1) dissatisfaction with traditional medicine (too impersonal, too high-tech, not effective, produces adverse effects, too costly); (2) the need for more autonomy and control in one's own health care; and (3) incongruence with the elder's concept of health and illness (philosophy derived from cultural beliefs) (Spector, 2000). In many cultures it is expected that family members are included in the planning and decision-making process (O'Hara and Zhan, 1994; St. Hill et al., 2003).

If the elder is using an herb or supplement in an inappropriate manner, the goal is to discontinue use or to use only the advised dosage for a specific condition. This can be done by providing needed information and asking the individual to consider the correct use of the product. The person may be willing to show the specific herb or supplement to the health care professional and discuss safer and better ways to use it. Whatever the selected strategy, the assistance of the family or a close friend could prove to be invaluable (Stupay and Sivertsen, 2000).

If it is unclear whether the herb is beneficial or harmful to the elder, it is the health care professional's responsibility to inform the person about this (Stupay and Sivertsen, 2000). The health care professional may also observe the placebo effect with persons who are taking herbs and supplements. That is, the taking of the product, and not the action of the herb or supplement itself, may produce a positive effect on the person. In this instance, if the herb or supplement causes no harm, it may be continued. However, the safe or unsafe use of a certain herb or supplement in a particular person is often difficult to determine and a placebo effect impossible to measure.

Important interventions of the gerontological nurse in the promotion of healthy aging include education; checking for side effects, adverse reactions, and interactions among herbs, supplements, medications, foods, and the illness; and urging discontinuance of possibly harmful products. Remaining sensitive to the person's situation is essential. Whether it is a need for additional information about a particular herb or supplement or assessment for side effects and interactions, the nurse must be alert for opportunities to intervene on the elder's behalf. In instances in which an adverse reaction or harmful interaction is suspected, the person must be urged to stop taking the herb or supplement and to see his or her prescribing health care provider or seek emergency help promptly. Teaching about side effects and interaction possibilities in realistic and understandable ways may be the most useful intervention.

Education

Scientific data and information about the safe use of herbs must be provided in the context of the person's age and particular learning needs. Follow-up is essential. "Natural" on the label does not mean that it is healthy for every person, and clients may switch from one harmful product to another without talking with their health care provider (Stupay and Sivertsen, 2000). The provider must seek out the best client motivation factors for the use of herbs or supplements to provide significant help.

Several additional issues do need to be addressed with persons who are taking herbs and supplements:

- Elders should be helped to understand the importance of reporting the use of all herbs and supplements to their health care provider. They should be encouraged to speak with the nurse or their health care provider before beginning an herb or supplement for the first time. The emphasis is on the fact that herbs and supplements are still drugs.
- Regarding product safety: (1) There is no standardization among manufacturers, so the amount of active ingredient per dose among brands is inconsistent; (2) herbs and supplements should be purchased from reputable sources; (3) herbs are available in different forms, making accurate dosing difficult; (4) research on both the untoward effects and the benefits of most herbs and supplements is inadequate, making recommendations about specific herbs and supplements difficult; and (5) persons who have allergies to certain plants may have allergies to herbs in the same plant family.
- If side effects occur within an hour or two of taking the supplement, the supplement should be discontinued immediately. If the side effects continue or worsen, the person should report them to the health care provider or go to the nearest emergency department. Because older adults may react differently to supplements, health care providers may need to prescribe less than the recommended dose. Herbs and supplements taken with other such products may cause unpredictable effects (Stupay and Sivertsen, 2000).
- A fact for nurses today is that many older persons do take herbs and supplements along with prescribed and OTC medications. Thus the approach with the person must be open and encouraging for effective assessment, evaluation of risks, appropriate teaching–learning applications, intervention, and monitoring. The gerontological nurse today must be knowledgeable and continue to seek out the latest information about herbs, supplements, OTC medications, prescribed medications, and interactions.

Lastly, the nurse has a responsibility for maintaining a sound knowledge base, as well as having readily available sources of changing current data, regarding the treatments used by the patient, including those both prescribed and used in self-care. At the same time making recommendations for or against the use of herbs and supplements may be considered a form of "prescribing" in some settings, such as long-term and acute care. The nurse is cautioned to be aware of both organizational policies and state nurse practice regulations (Moquin et al., 2009).

evolve To access your student resources, go to *http://evolve.elsevier.com/Ebersole/TwdHlthAging*

▌ KEY CONCEPTS

- Older adults who are diagnosed with chronic conditions are more likely to take herbs and other supplements.
- Many individuals continue their biomedical therapies in addition to herb and supplement therapies.
- The renewed interest in herbal therapies is based in part on the focus on prevention. Herbs are often used by individuals who want to be more involved in their own health care or who are unable to afford prescription medications.
- The U.S. government has no standards in place to control the quality of herbs or herbal products or other supplements.

- Nurses and other health care providers should always ask about the use of herbs and supplements when conducting a health interview.
- Nurses and other health care providers should teach persons to ask about the concurrent use of herbs, supplements, and medications, both prescribed and OTC.
- Patients should be told to stop the herbal treatments for the prescribed period of time before scheduled surgery and should be told why.

CASE STUDY   COMMON USE OF HERBS AND SUPPLEMENTS

Anna is an 80-year-old woman of French descent who lives with her 83-year-old husband in the suburbs of a large city. They have been married for 57 years and have two grown children, six grandchildren, and five great-grandchildren. Anna is very proud of all of them. Anna taught high school English for 20 years but was raised with many of the "old country" traditions, speaking French for most of her formative years. As part of her background, she would rather use herbs and "home treatments" than prescribed "pills." She has been diagnosed with hypertension, diabetes mellitus, and arthritis. She often complains of symptoms that are related to these chronic conditions, but she refuses to consistently follow her diet or take any prescribed medications. Anna attends mass daily and, with her husband, takes part in community activities. While accompanying her husband on a visit to his health care provider, she mentions the use of herbal supplements. After some discussion, the nurse realizes that Anna has little information about herbal supplements and has some incorrect assumptions about them.

On the basis of the case study, develop a nursing care plan using the following procedure*:

- List Anna's comments that provide subjective data.
- List information that provides objective data.

- From these data, identify key aspects of education specific for Anna.
- Plan and state one or more interventions for each identified problem. Provide specific documentation of the source used to determine the appropriate intervention.
- Plan at least one intervention that incorporates Anna's existing strengths.
- Evaluate the success of the intervention. Interventions must correlate directly with the stated outcome criteria to measure the outcome success.

CRITICAL THINKING QUESTIONS

1. How would you begin your discussion with Anna regarding her knowledge of herbal supplements?
2. What information would you be especially interested in obtaining regarding herbal supplements and each of Anna's medical diagnoses?
3. How would you prepare Anna should she need surgery?
4. Prepare a teaching plan for Anna to include the effective use of herbal supplements.

*Students are advised to refer to their nursing diagnosis text and identify possible or potential problems.

RESEARCH QUESTIONS

1. Interview a member of your health care community who recommends the use of herbs and/or supplements along with traditional strategies. How does this individual decide which herbs or supplements to use with each client? How does he or she ensure standardization among products?
2. Tour a local health food store. Read the labels of the more commonly used herbal supplements. Do the labels list the information you expected? How would you make sure that your clients have the necessary information?
3. Visit a senior citizen center. Talk with members about their use of herbal supplements. Keep track of the more commonly used herbs and the reasons for their use. How did the older adults find out about the herbal action?

4. Are older adults aware of possible negative effects of herbs and supplements?
5. What questions do older adults ask before taking an herbal or nonherbal supplement?
6. What information do older adults need before considering taking an herbal or nonherbal supplement?
7. What are the rewards (positive factors) versus the costs (negative factors) of using herbal and nonherbal supplements?
8. What strategies should health care providers use to bridge the gap between herb/supplement remedies and traditional health care?
9. Why do older adults choose to use herbs and supplements?

REFERENCES

Agbabiaka TB, Pittler MH, Wider B, Ernst E: *Serenoa repens* (saw palmetto): a systematic review of adverse events, *Drug Safety* 32:637, 2009.

Akhondzadeh S, Noroozian M, Mohammadi M, et al: *Salvia officinalis* extract in the treatment of patients with mild to moderate Alzheimer's disease: a double blind, randomized and placebo-controlled trial, *Journal of Clinical Pharmacy and Therapeutics* 28:53, 2003.

Allen D, Bell J: Herbal medicine and the transplant patient, *Nephrology Nursing Journal* 29:269, 2002.

Amsterdam JD, Li Y, Soeller I, et al: A randomized, double-blind, placebo-controlled trial of oral *Matricaria recutita* (chamomile) extract therapy for generalized anxiety disorder, *Journal of Clinical Psychopharmacology* 29:378, 2009.

Anonymous: EGb 761, *Ginkgo biloba* extract, Ginkor, *Drugs in R&D* 4:188, 2003.

Anonymous: Garlic: allicin wonderland? *University of California, Berkeley Wellness Letter* 23:1, 2006. Available at http://www.

wellnessletter.com/html/ds/dsGarlicPills.php. Accessed December 2010.

Avins AL, Bent S, Staccone S, et al: A detailed safety assessment of a saw palmetto extract, *Complementary Therapies in Medicine* 16:147, 2008.

Baker WL, Gutierrez-Williams G, White CM, et al: Effect of cinnamon on glucose control and lipid parameters, *Diabetes Care* 31:41, 2008.

Bardia A, Nisley NL, Zimmerman MB, et al: Use of herbs among adults based on evidence-based indications: findings from the National Health Interview Survey, *Mayo Clinic Proceedings* 82:561, 2007.

Basch E, Ulbricht C: *Natural standard herb & supplement handbook: the clinical bottom line*, St. Louis, MO, 2005, Mosby.

Becker DJ, Gordon RY, Morris PB, et al: Simvastin vs therapeutic lifestyle changes and supplements: randomized primary prevention trial, *Mayo Clinic Proceedings* 83:758, 2008.

Becker DJ, Gordon RY, Halbert SC, et al: Red yeast rice for dyslipidemia in statin-intolerant

patients: a randomized trial, *Annals of Internal Medicine* 150:830, 2009.

Bent S, Kane C, Shinohara, K, et al: Saw palmetto for benign prostatic hyperplasia, *New England Journal of Medicine* 354:557, 2006.

Birks J, Grimley Evans J: *Ginkgo biloba* for cognitive impairment and dementia, *Cochrane Database of Systematic Reviews* 1:CD003120, 2009.

Blumenthal M, Goldberg A, Brinckmann J: *Herbal medicine: expanded commission E monographs*, Newton, MA, 2000, Integrative Medicine Communications.

Boehm K, Borrelli F, Ernst E, et al: Green tea (*Camellia sinensis*) for the prevention of cancer, *Cochrane Database of Systematic Reviews* 3:CD005004, 2009.

Bone KM: Potential interaction of *Ginkgo biloba* leaf with antiplatelet or anticoagulant drugs: What is the evidence? *Molecular Nutrition and Food Research* 52:764, 2008.

Brattstrom A: Long-term effects of St. John's wort (*Hypericum perforatum*) treatment: a 1-year safety study in mild to moderate depression, *Phytomedicine* 16:277, 2009.

Bruno JJ, Ellis JJ: Herbal use among U.S. elderly: 2002 National Health Interview Survey, *Annals of Pharmacotherapy* 39:643, 2005.

Bruyere O, Reginster JY: Glucosamine and chondroitin sulfate as the therapeutic agents for knee and hip osteoarthritis, *Drugs & Aging* 24:573, 2007.

Burks K: Osteoarthritis in older adults: current treatments, *Journal of Gerontological Nursing* 31:11, 2005.

Canter PH, Ernst E: Herbal supplement use by persons aged over 50 years in Britain: frequently used herbs, concomitant use of herbs, nutritional supplements and prescription drugs, rate of informing doctors and potential for negative interactions, *Drugs & Aging* 21:597, 2005.

Canter PH, Ernst E: *Ginkgo biloba* is not a smart drug: an updated systematic review of randomized clinical trials testing the nootropic effects of *G. biloba* extracts in healthy people, *Human Psychopharmacology* 22:265, 2007.

Chen X, Lu W, Zheng Y, et al: Exercise, tea consumption, and depression among breast cancer survivors, *Journal of Clinical Oncology* 28:991, 2010.

Cheung CK, Wyman JF, Halcon LL: Use of complementary and alternative therapies in community-dwelling older adults, *Journal of Alternative and Complementary Medicine* 13:997, 2007.

Chu KO, Chan KP, Wang CC, et al: Green tea catechins and their oxidative protection in the rat eye, *Journal of Agricultural and Food Chemistry* 58:1523, 2010.

Clegg DO, Reda DJ, Harris CL, et al: Glucosamine, chondroitin sulfate, and the two in combination for painful knee osteoarthritis, *New England Journal of Medicine* 354:795, 2006.

Daniele C, Mazzanti G, Pittler MH, et al: Adverse-event profile of *Crataegus* spp.: a systematic review, *Drug Safety* 29:523, 2006.

Dedhia RC, McVary KT: Phytotherapy for lower urinary tract symptoms secondary to benign prostatic hyperplasia, *Journal of Urology* 179:2119, 2008.

Durante KM, Whitmore B, Jones CA, et al: Use of vitamins, minerals and herbs: a survey of patients attending family practice clinics, *Clinical and Investigative Medicine* 24:242, 2001.

Edwards Q, Colquist S, Maradiegue A: What's cooking with garlic: is this complementary and alterative medicine for hypertension? *Journal of the American Academy of Nurse Practitioners* 17:381, 2005.

Eliopoulos C: *Integrating conventional and alternative therapies: holistic care for chronic conditions*, St. Louis, MO, 1999, Mosby.

Eller LS, Corless I, Bunch EH, et al: Self-care strategies for depressive symptoms in people with HIV disease, *Journal of Advanced Nursing* 51:119, 2005.

Ernst E: The risk–benefit profile of commonly used herbal therapies: ginkgo, St. John's wort,

ginseng, echinacea, saw palmetto, and kava, *Annals of Internal Medicine* 136:42, 2002.

Eskin SB: *Dietary supplements and older consumers. Data Digest # 66*, Washington DC, 2001, AARP Public Policy Institute. Available at http://assets.aarp.org/rgcenter/consume/dd66_diet.pdf. Accessed December 2010.

Fox BA, Stephens MM: Glucosamine/chondroitin/primorine combination therapy for osteoarthritis, *Drugs Today* 45:21, 2009.

Ganmaa D, Willett WC, Li TY, et al: Coffee, tea, caffeine and risk of breast cancer: a 22-year follow-up, *International Journal of Cancer* 122:2071, 2008.

Gorski JC, Huang SM, Pinto A, et al: The effect of echinacea (*Echinacea purpurea* root) on cytochrome P450 activity in vivo, *Clinical Pharmacology and Therapeutics* 75:89, 2004.

Halbert SC, French B, Gordon RY, et al: Tolerability of red yeast rice (2,400 mg twice daily) versus pravastatin (20 mg twice daily) in patients with previous statin intolerance, *American Journal of Cardiology* 105:1504, 2010.

Hong B, Ji YH, Hong JH, et al: A double-blind crossover study evaluating the efficacy of Korean red ginseng in patients with erectile dysfunction: a preliminary report, *Journal of Urology* 168:2070, 2002.

Huxley R, Lee CMY, Barzi F, et al: Decaffeinated coffee and tea consumption in relation to incident type 2 diabetes mellitus: a systematic review with meta-analysis. *Archives of Internal Medicine* 169:2053, 2009.

Inoue M, Sasazuki S, Wakai K, et al: Green tea consumption and gastric cancer in Japanese: a pooled analysis of six cohort studies, *Gut* 58:1323, 2009.

Islami F, Pourshams A, Nasrollahzadeh D, et al: Tea drinking habits and oesophageal cancer in a high risk area in northern Iran: population based case–control study, *BMJ* 338:b929, 2009.

Israel D, Youngkin E: Herbal therapies for common health problems. In Youngkin E, Sawin KJ, Kissinger JF, et al., editors: *Pharmacotherapeutics: a primary care guide*, ed 2, Upper Saddle River, NJ, 2005, Pearson Prentice Hall.

Izzo AA, Ernst E: Interactions between herbal medicines and prescribed drugs: an updated systematic review, *Drugs* 69:1777, 2009.

Jellin J, editor: Camomile. Natural Medicines Comprehensive Database. 1995-2011a. Available at www.naturaldatabase.com. Accessed January 2011.

Jellin J, editor: Echinacea. Natural Medicines Comprehensive Database. 1995-2011b. Available at www.naturaldatabase.com. Accessed January 2011.

Jellin J, editor: Garlic. Natural Medicines Comprehensive Database. 1995-2011c. Available at www.naturaldatabase.com. Accessed January 2011.

Jellin J, editor: Ginko biloba. Natural Medicines Comprehensive Database. 1995-2011d. Available at www.naturaldatabase.com. Accessed January 2011.

Jellin J, editor: Ginseng. Natural Medicines Comprehensive Database. 1995-2011e. Available at www.naturaldatabase.com. Accessed January 2011.

Jellin J, editor: Glucosamine sulfate. Natural Medicines Comprehensive Database. 1995-2011f. Available at www.naturaldatabase.com. Accessed January 2011.

Jellin J, editor: Hawthorn. Natural Medicines Comprehensive Database. 1995-2011g. Available at www.naturaldatabase.com. Accessed January 2011.

Jellin J, editor: St John's Wort. Natural Medicines Comprehensive Database. 1995-2011h. Available at www.naturaldatabase.com. Accessed January 2011.

Jellin J, editor: Saw Palmetto. Natural Medicines Comprehensive Database. 1995-2011i. Available at www.naturaldatabase.com. Accessed January 2011.

Jellin J, editor: Milk thistle. Natural Medicines Comprehensive Database. 1995-2011j. Available at www.naturaldatabase.com. Accessed January 2011.

Jellin J, editor: natural products / Drug interaction checker. Natural Medicines Comprehensive Database. 1995-2011k. Available at www.naturaldatabase.com. Accessed January 2011.

Jellin J, editor: Fenugreek. Natural Medicines Comprehensive Database. 1995-2011L. Available at www.naturaldatabase.com. Accessed January 2011.

Jellin J, editor: Cinnamon. Natural Medicines Comprehensive Database. 1995-2011m. Available at www.naturaldatabase.com. Accessed January 2011.

Jellin J, editor: Natural medicines in the management of diabetes. Natural Medicines Comprehensive Database. 1995-2011n. Available at www.naturaldatabase.com. Accessed January 2011.

Kales HC, Blow FC, Welsh DE, et al: Herbal products and other supplements: use by elderly veterans with depression and dementia and their caregivers, *Journal of Geriatric Psychiatry and Neurology* 17:25, 2004.

Kaye AD, Kucera I, Sabar R: Perioperative anesthesia clinical considerations of alternative medicines, *Anesthesiology Clinics of North America* 22:125, 2004.

Kerr M: *Echinacea cuts cold incidence (big pharma eats their shorts)*. (2006). Boston, 2006, Reuters Health. Available at http://www.freerepublic.com/focus/f-news/1705280/posts. Accessed December 2010.

Kirkham S, Akilen R, Sharma S, et al: The potential of cinnamon to reduce blood glucose levels in patients with type 2 diabetes and insulin resistance, *Diabetes, Obesity, & Metabolism* 11:1100, 2009.

Kuhn M: Herbal remedies: drug–herb interactions, *Critical Care Nurse* 22:22, 2002.

Kuriyama S, Shimazu T, Ohmori K, et al: Green tea consumption and mortality due to cardiovascular disease, cancer, and all causes in Japan: the Ohsaki Study, *JAMA* 296:1255, 2006.

Ladenheim D, Horn O, Werneke U, et al: Potential health risks of complementary alternative medicines in HIV patients, *HIV Medicine* 9:653, 2008.

Lam A, Bradley G: Use of self-prescribed nonprescription medications and dietary supplements among assisted living facility residents, *Journal of the American Pharmacists Association* 46:547, 2006.

Lawvere S, Mahoney MC: St. John's wort, *American Family Physician* 72:2249, 2005.

Lee SH, Ahn YM, Ahn SY, et al: Interaction between warfarin and *Panax ginseng* in ischemic stroke patients, *Journal of Alternative Complementary Medicine* 14:715, 2008.

Libster M: *Delmar's integrative herb guide for nurses*, Albany, NY, 2002, Delmar Thompson.

Linde K, Berner MM, Kriston L: St. John's wort for major depression, *Cochran Database of Systematic Reviews* 4:CD000448, 2008.

Liu J et al: Herbal medicines for treatment of irritable bowel syndrome, 2006. Cochran Database of System Reviews, Jan 25(1): CD004116.

Loya AM, Gonzalez-Stuart A, Rivera JO: Prevalence of polypharmacy, polyherbacy, nutritional supplement use and potential interactions among older adults living on the United States–Mexico border: a descriptive, questionnaire-based study, *Drugs & Aging* 26:423, 2009.

Marcus MB: Coffee's endless health debate is grounded in fact, *USA Today*. Available at http://www.usatoday.com/news/health/2010-06-14-coffee14_ST_N.htm. Accessed December 2010.

Marcus MB: Exercise, tea and vitamin D to ward off dementia, *USA Today*. Available at http://www.usatoday.com/news/health/2010-07-12-alzheimerslifestyle12_ST_N.htm. Accessed December 2010.

Messina BA: Herbal supplements: facts and myths—talking to your patients about herbal supplements, *Journal of Perianesthesia Nursing* 21:268, 2006.

Moquin B, Blackman MR, Mitty E, et al: Complementary and alternative medicine (CAM), *Geriatric Nursing* 30:196, 2009.

Nahin R, Pecha M, Welmerink DB, et al; Ginkgo Evaluation of Memory Study Investigators: Concomitant use of prescription drugs and dietary supplements in elderly people, *Journal of the American Geriatrics Society* 57:1197, 2009.

Nahin RL, Barnes PM, Stussman BA, et al: Costs of complementary and alternative medicine (CAM) and frequency of visits to CAM practitioners: United States, 2007, *CDC National Health Statistics Report* 18:1, 2009.

NATIONAL CENTER FOR COMPLEMENTARY AND ALTERNATIVE MEDICINE (NCCAM):

Ginkgo biloba does not slow cognitive decline in large cohort study of older adults. Available at http://nccam.nih.gov/research/results/spotlight/20091229.htm. Accessed December 2010

Ginkgo ineffective against high blood pressure in large study of older adults. Available at http://nccam.nih.gov/research/results/

spotlight/031810.htm. Accessed December 2010.

Ginkgo does not shield seniors' hearts, but it may protect their leg arteries. Available at http://nccam.nih.gov/research/results/spotlight/052110.htm. Accessed December 2010.

A review of St. John's wort extracts for major depression. Available at http://nccam.nih.gov/research/results/spotlight/120908.htm. Accessed December 2010.

NATURAL STANDARD: THE AUTHORITY ON INTEGRATIVE MEDICINE

The following articles are available at http://www.naturalstandard.com. Accessed December 2010:

Chamomile
Echinacea
Garlic
Ginkgo
Ginseng
Glucosamine
Hawthorn
Red yeast rice
St. John's wort
Saw palmetto
Hypertension
HIV/AIDS
Gastrointestinal disorders
Cancer (in chronic diseases)
Alzheimer's disease
Diabetes mellitus type 2

NATURAL STANDARD: NEWS

The following articles are available at http://naturalstandard.com/newsAlerts.asp. Accessed December 2010:

Echinacea update, July 2007
Review: echinacea for the common cold, September 2007
Glucosamine may not slow osteoarthritis progress, October 2009
Prescription chondroitin for knee arthritis, February 2009
Glucosamine for hip osteoarthritis, February 2008

Niu K, Hozawa A, Kurlyama S, et al: Green tea consumption associated with depressive symptoms in the elderly, *American Journal of Clinical Nutrition* 90:1615, 2009.

Oba S, Nagata C, Nakamura K, et al: Consumption of coffee, green tea, oolong tea, black tea, chocolate snacks and the caffeine content in relation to risk of diabetes in Japanese men and women, *British Journal of Nutrition* 103:453, 2010.

O'Hara EM, Zhan L: Cultural and pharmacologic considerations when caring for Chinese elders, *Journal of Gerontological Nursing* 20:11, 1994.

Pham AQ, Kourlas H, Pham DQ: Cinnamon supplementation in patients with type 2 diabetes mellitus, *Pharmacotherapy* 27:595, 2007.

Pittler MH, Guo R, Ernst E: Hawthorn extract for treating chronic heart failure, *Cochrane Database of Systematic Reviews* 1:CD005312, 2008.

Radimer K, Bindewald B, Hughes J, et al: Dietary supplement use by U.S. adults: data from the National Health and Nutrition Examination

Survey, 1999-2000, *American Journal of Epidemiology* 160:339, 2004.

Ravindran AV, Lam RW, Filteau, MJ, Lesperance F, Kennedy SH, Parikh SV, Patten SB; Canadian Network for Mood and Anxiety Treatments (CANMAT): Canadian network for Mood and Anxiety Treatments (CANMAT) clinical guidelines for the management of major depressive disorder in adults. V. Complementary and alternative medicine treatments, *Journal of Affective Disorders* 117(Suppl 1):S54, 2009.

Reinhart KM, Coleman CI, Teevan C, et al: Effects of garlic on blood pressure in patients with and without systolic hypertension: a meta-analysis, *Annals of Pharmacotherapy* 42:1766, 2008.

Ried K, Frank OR, Stocks NP, et al: Effect of garlic on blood pressure: a systematic review and meta-analysis. *BMC Cardiovascular Disorders* 8:13, 2008.

Rouanet JM, Decorde K, Del Rio D, et al: Berry juices, tea, antioxidants and the prevention of atherosclerosis in hamsters, *Food Chemistry* 118:266, 2009.

Rowe DJ, Baker AC: Perioperative risks and benefits of herbal supplements in aesthetic surgery, *Aesthetic Surgery Journal* 29:150, 2009.

Ryder PT, Wolpert B, Orwig D, et al: Complementary and alternative medicine use among older urban African Americans: individual and neighborhood associations, *Journal of the National Medical Association* 100:1186, 2008.

Scorza E: *Use of herbal and nutritional supplements.* Paper presented at the National Conference of Gerontological Nurse Practitioners, September 18-21, Chicago, 2002.

Sego S: Alternative meds update: St. John's wort, *Clinical Advisor* July:134, 2006.

Shah, SA, Sander S, White CM, et al: Evaluation of *Echinacea* for the prevention and treatment of the common cold: a meta-analysis, *Lancet Infect Diseases* 7:473, 2007.

Shahrokh LE, Lukaszuk JM, Prawitz AD: Elderly herbal supplement users less satisfied with medical care than nonusers, *Journal of the American Dietetic Association* 105:1138, 2005.

Shelton RC: St. John's wort (*Hypericum perforatum*) in major depression, *Journal of Clinical Psychiatry* 70(Suppl 5):23, 2009.

Shrubsole MJ, Lu W, Chen Z, et al: Drinking green tea modestly reduces breast cancer risk, *Journal of Nutrition* 139:310, 2009.

Singh DK, Banerjee S, Porter TD: Green and black tea extracts inhibit HMG-CoA reductase and activate AMP kinase to decrease cholesterol synthesis in hepatoma cells, *Journal of Nutritional Biochemistry* 20:616, 2009.

Skidmore-Roth L: *Mosby's handbook of herbs and natural supplements*, St. Louis, MO, 2005, Mosby.

Spector RE: *Cultural diversity in health & illness*, ed 5, Upper Saddle River, NJ, 2000, Prentice Hall.

Snyder FJ, Dundas ML, Kirkpatrick C, et al: Use and safety perceptions regarding herbal supplements: a study of older persons in southeast Idaho, *Journal of Nutrition for the Elderly* 28:81, 2009.

Srivastava JK, Pandey M, Gupta S: Chamomile, a novel and selective COX-2 inhibitor with anti-inflammatory activity, *Life Sciences* 85:663, 2009.

St. Hill PF, Lipson JG, Meleis AI: *Caring for women cross-culturally*, Philadelphia, 2003, Davis.

Stupay S, Sivertsen L: Herbal and nutritional supplement use in the elderly, *Nurse Practitioner* 25:56, 2000.

Sugimoto N, Ichikawa M, Siriliang B, et al: Herbal medicine use and quality of life among people living with HIV/AIDS in northeastern Thailand, *AIDS Care* 17:252, 2005.

Swanson B: Beware bitter orange, *ADVANCE for Nurses* (September 4):43, 2006.

Tachjian A, Maria V, Jahangir A: Use of herbal products and potential interactions in patients with cardiovascular diseases, *Journal of the American College of Cardiology* 55:515, 2010.

Tacklind J, MacDonald R, Rutks I, et al: *Serenoa repens* for benign prostatic hyperplasia, *Cochrane Database of Systematic Reviews* 2:CD001423, 2009.

Tang N, Wu Y, Zhou B, et al: Green tea, black tea consumption and risk of lung cancer: a meta-analysis, *Lung Cancer* 65:274, 2009.

Tang N, Wu Y, Ma J, et al: Coffee consumption and risk of lung cancer: a meta-analysis, *Lung Cancer* 67:17, 2010.

Tillisch K: Complementary and alternative medicine for functional gastrointestinal disorders, *Gut* 55:593, 2006.

Tshibangu K, Worku ZB, de Jongh MA, et al: Assessment of effectiveness of traditional herbal medicine in managing HIV/AIDS

patients in South Africa, *East African Medical Journal* 81:499, 2004.

U.S. Food and Drug Administration: FDA warns consumers to avoid red yeast rice products promoted on Internet as treatments for high cholesterol; products found to contain unauthorized drug (2007). Available at http://www.fda.gov/NewsEvents/Newsroom/PressAnnouncements/2007/ucm108962.htm. Accessed December 2010.

van der Watt G, Laughame J, Janca A: Complementary and alternative medicine in the treatment of anxiety and depression, *Current Opinion in Psychiatry* 21:37, 2008.

Venero CV, Venero JV, Wortham DC, et al: Lipid-lowering efficacy of red yeast rice in a population intolerant to statins, *American Journal of Cardiology* 105:664, 2010.

Waddell DL, Hummell ME, Sumners AD: Three herbs you should get to know, *American Journal of Nursing* 101:48, 2001; quiz 54.

Walker AF, Marakis G, Simpson E, et al: Hypotensive effects of hawthorn for patients with diabetes taking prescription drugs: a randomized controlled trial, *British Journal of General Practice* 56:437, 2006.

Walubo A: The role of cytochrome P450 in antiretroviral drug interactions, *Expert Opinions on Drug Metabolism & Toxicology* 3:583, 2007.

Weng YL, Raab C, Georgiou C, et al: Herbal and vitamin/mineral supplement use by retirement community residents: preliminary findings, *Journal of Nutrition for the Elderly* 23:1, 2004.

Williams P, Piamjariyakul U, Ducey K, et al: Cancer treatment, symptom monitoring, and self-care in adults: pilot study, *Cancer Nursing* 29:347, 2006.

Wold RS, Lopez ST, Yau CL, et al: Increasing trends in elderly persons' use of nonvitamin, nonmineral dietary supplements and concurrent use of medications, *Journal of the American Dietetic Association* 105:54, 2005.

Yeh G, Davis RB, Phillips RS: Use of complementary therapies in patients with cardiovascular disease, *American Journal of Cardiology* 98:673, 2006.

Yoon SL: Racial/ethnic differences in self-reported health problems and herbal use among older women, *Journal of the National Medical Association* 98:918, 2006.

Yoon SL, Horne CH: Herbal products and conventional medicines used by community-residing older women, *Journal of Advanced Nursing* 33:51, 2001.

Yoon SL, Schaffer SD: Herbal, prescribed, and over-the-counter drug use in older women: prevalence of drug interactions, *Geriatric Nursing* 27:118, 2006.

Yoon SL, Horne CH, Adams C: Herbal product use by African American older women, *Clinical Nursing Research* 13:271, 2004.

Youngkin EQ, Israel DS: A review and critique of common herbal alternative therapies, *Nurse Practitioner* 21:39, 1996.

Zeilmann C, Dole EJ, Skipper BJ, et al: Use of herbal medicine by elderly Hispanic and non-Hispanic white patients, *Pharmacotherapy* 23:526, 2003.

Zhou SF, Lai X: An update on clinical drug interactions with the herbal antidepressant St. John's wort, *Current Drug Metabolism* 9:394, 2008.

Elimination, Sleep, Skin, and Foot Care

Theris A. Touhy

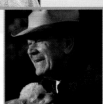

e·volve *http://evolve.elsevier.com/Ebersole/TwdHlthAging*

A STUDENT SPEAKS

I am so stressed and tired all the time in this nursing program. The workload is so intense, there is never enough time to sleep. When I have any time, I would go to bed at 7 pm and sleep until 11 in the morning if I could. When will I ever feel rested and not tired?
Marybeth, 22 years old

AN ELDER SPEAKS

The years have changed the sleep patterns. Bedtime rituals take longer. Nature wakens me two or three times a night for trips to the bathroom. Sleep returns at once unless my mind turns on and it gets launched on a needless project. The earlier remedies are called on to slow down the activities, or the next day is a disaster. My 90-year-old aunt, who slept very little and lightly and lay awake many nights, said she went to the bathroom several times just for something to do instead of just lying there.
Ricarda, 90 years old

LEARNING OBJECTIVES

On completion of this chapter, the reader will be able to:

1. Identify age-related changes that affect sleep, elimination, skin and foot care.
2. Use evidence-based protocols in assessment and development of interventions for sleep and promotion of bowel and bladder health.
3. Identify common foot and skin problems of older adults.
4. Identify preventive, maintenance, and restorative measures for skin and foot health.
5. Identify risk factors for pressure ulcers and design interventions for prevention and evidence-based treatment.

This chapter addresses sleep, bowel and bladder elimination, promotion of healthy skin and feet, and prevention of pressure ulcers. The maintenance of adequate sleep patterns, normal elimination, and healthy skin and feet can be compromised in older adults as a result of aging changes and disease processes. These areas of function may often be overlooked when the focus is on management of disease or acute problems. However, insomnia, incontinence, and skin and foot problems, can be some of the most complex and challenging concerns faced by older adults, affecting health and compromising quality of life. Thorough assessment and intervention based on age-related, evidence-based protocols, is important to healthy aging and best practice gerontological nursing. Chapter 4 provides a framework for understanding changes in body systems with age.

BLADDER ELIMINATION

The body must remove waste products of metabolism to sustain healthy function, but bladder and bowel activity are fraught with social implications. Bladder and bowel function in later life, although normally only slightly altered by the physiological changes of age, can contribute to problems severe enough to interfere with the ability to continue independent living and can seriously threaten the body's capacity to function and to survive. The effects of uncontrolled bladder and bowel action are a threat to the person's independence and well-being.

Elimination is a private matter, not publicized socially. As children, correct behavior in dealing with our own body waste is taught early. Deviations from this are socially unacceptable and can lead to chastisement, ostracism, and social withdrawal.

Bladder Function

Normal bladder function requires an intact brain and spinal cord, competent lower urinary tract function, the motivation to maintain continence, the functional ability to use a toilet, and an environment that facilitates the process (Dowling-Castronovo and Bradway, 2008). A full bladder increases pressure and signals the spinal cord and the brainstem center of the desire to micturate. Social training then dictates whether micturition should be attended to or should be postponed until there is an appropriate opportunity to seek out toilet facilities. However, when the bladder contents reach 500 mL or more, the pressure is such that it becomes more difficult to control the urge to void. As volume increases, emptying the bladder becomes an uncontrollable act.

Age-Related Changes

Bladder changes with aging include decreased capacity, increased irritability, contractions during filling, and incomplete emptying. In about 10% to 20% of well older adults, aging of the urinary tract is associated with an increased frequency of involuntary bladder contractions (Ham et al., 2007). These changes may lead to frequency, nocturia, urgency, and vulnerability to infection. The warning period between the desire to void and actual micturition is shortened. Postvoid residual urine volume increases to 75 to 100 mL in some cases. The first urge to void occurs at a lower bladder volume (150 to 300 mL) and total bladder capacity decreases to 300 to 600 mL (Ham et al., 2007). In combination with age-related changes, illness, cognitive impairments, difficulty in walking to the toilet or in handling a bedpan or urinal, and problems in manipulating clothing can affect an older person's ability to maintain continence. Drugs that increase urinary output and sedatives, tranquilizers, and hypnotics, which produce drowsiness, confusion, or limited mobility, promote incontinence by dulling the transmission of the desire to urinate.

Urinary Incontinence

Urinary incontinence (UI) is the involuntary loss of urine sufficient to be a problem (Dowling-Castronovo and Bradway, 2007, 2008). UI is a stigmatized, underreported, underdiagnosed, undertreated condition that is erroneously thought to be part of normal aging. About half of persons with UI have never discussed the concern with their primary care provider, and only one in eight who have experienced bladder control problems has been diagnosed. On average, women wait 6.5 years from the first time they experience symptoms until they obtain a diagnosis for their bladder control problems (Muller, 2005).

Individuals may not seek treatment for UI because they are embarrassed to talk about the problem or think that it is a normal part of aging. They may be unaware that successful treatments are available. Men may be unlikely to report UI to their primary care provider because they feel it is a woman's disease. Further research is necessary to explore the prevalence and experience of UI in men. A guideline for UI in men can be found in Box 11-1. Older people want more information about bladder control, and nurses must take the lead in implementing approaches to continence promotion and public health education about UI (Palmer and Newman, 2006).

Without an adequate knowledge base of continence care and use of evidence-based practice guidelines, nursing care will continue to consist of containment strategies, such as the use of pads and briefs, to manage UI (Dowling-Castronovo and Bradway, 2008). UI tends to be viewed as an inconvenience rather than a condition requiring assessment and treatment (MacDonald and Butler, 2007). Nurses in all practice settings with older adults should be prepared to assess data that relate to urine control and implement nursing interventions that promote continence (Dowling-Castronovo and Bradway, 2008). There is a growing role for nurses in continence care and advanced training and certification are available through specialty organizations such as the Society of Urologic Nurses and Associates (www.suna.org) and the Wound, Ostomy, and Continence Nurses Society (www.wocncb.org). See Evolvefor additional resources and Box 11-1 for evidence-based protocols for continence care.

Prevalence of UI

UI affects millions of adults worldwide. Of those who experience UI, 75% to 80% are female; the prevalence of UI increases with age and functional dependency. Estimates are that 39% of community-living older women and more than 50% of nursing home residents are incontinent. More than half of nursing home residents are incontinent on admission (Shamliyan et al., 2007; Zarowitz and Ouslander, 2007). Some evidence suggests that European American women have higher rates of moderate and severe UI compared with African American and Asian women (Dowling-Castronovo and Bradway, 2007, Townsend, et al., 2011).

UI is more prevalent than diabetes, Alzheimer's disease, and many other chronic conditions that have prompted more attention and treatment. Incontinence is also costly; the indirect costs are estimated at more than $16 billion annually. UI costs exceed those of coronary artery bypass surgery and renal dialysis combined (Weiss, 2005; Dowling-Castronovo and Bradway, 2008; Landefeld et al., 2008).

UI is an important yet neglected geriatric syndrome (Lawhorne et al., 2008). A study on UI in nursing facilities (Lawhorne et al., 2008) reported that physicians, geriatric nurse practitioners, and directors of nursing evaluated and managed UI significantly less often than five other geriatric syndromes (falls, dementia, unintended weight loss, pain, and delirium). Nursing assistants were more likely to be involved in care provision for UI than any other syndrome and rated UI second only to pain with respect to its effect on quality of life. Reasons for less then optimal care for UI are multifactorial and include inadequate knowledge and skills about UI, inability to implement specific guidelines for UI care in nursing facilities, insufficient staffing, and poor communication among professionals and nursing assistants. Because of the high prevalence and chronic but preventable nature of UI, it is most appropriately considered a public health problem.

Risk Factors for UI

Cognitive impairment, limitations in daily activities, and institutionalization are associated with higher risks of UI. Stroke, diabetes, obesity, poor general health, and comorbidities are

BOX 11-1   EVIDENCE-BASED RESOURCES FOR URINARY CONTINENCE, SLEEP, PRESSURE ULCERS

BLADDER CONTINENCE/UTI

- Guideline for UI in men:
  www.guideline.gov/content.aspx?id=14817
- Urinary incontinence tool kit:
  http://www.gericareonline.net/tools/eng/urinary/index.html
- Nursing Standard of Practice Protocol: Urinary incontinence (UI) in older adults admitted to acute care (Dowling-Castronovo and Bradway, 2008)
- Comprehensive toolkit for management of urinary incontinence in older adults in primary care:
  http://www.gericareonline.net/tools/eng/urinary/index.html
- Incontinence management useful to nurses in the long-term care setting:
  www.geronet.ucla.edu/centers/borun/modules/Incontinence_management/default.htm
- Urinary incontinence assessment in older adults: Part I: Transient urinary incontinence (Dowling-Castronovo, 2007) (http://consultgerirn.org/uploads/File/trythis/try_this_11_1.pdf) and Part II: Established urinary incontinence (Dowling-Castronovo, 2008) (http://consultgerirn.org/uploads/File/trythis/try_this_11_2.pdf).
- Video depicting a nurse assessing transient UI:
  http://consultgerirn.org/resources/media/?vid_id=5003886#player_container
- Prevention of catheter-associated UTIs in acute care:
  http://www.guideline.gov/content.aspx?id=13394&search=urinary+tract+infections+acute+care+hospitals

BOWEL CONTINENCE

- Prevention of urinary and fecal incontinence in adults (AHRQ):
  www.ahrq.gov/downloads/pub/evidence/pdf/fuiad/fuiad.pdf
- Prevention of catheter-associated UTIs in acute care:
  http://www.guideline.gov/content.aspx?id=13394&search=urinary+tract+infections+acute+care+hospitals

- Assessment and management of older adults with urinary incontinence: State of the Science papers:
  http://hartfordign.org/uploads/File/gnec_state_of_science_papers/gnec_incontinence.pdf

PRESSURE ULCERS

- Nursing Standard of Practice Protocol: Pressure ulcer prevention and skin tear prevention:
  http://consultgerirn.org/topics/pressure_ulcers_and_skin_tears/want_to_know_more
- Video demonstrating use of the Braden Scale:
  http://consultgerirn.org/resources/media/?vid_id=4200956#player_container
- National Pressure Ulcer Advisory Panel:
  http://www.npuap.org/
- American Medical Directors Association Clinical Practice Guideline: Pressure ulcers:
  http://www.amda.com/tools/cpg/pressureulcer.cfm
- Skin safety protocol: risk assessment and prevention of pressure ulcers. Health care protocol:
  http://www.guideline.gov/content.aspx?id=16004&search=pressure+ulcers

SLEEP

- Nursing Standard of Practice Protocol: Excessive sleepiness (Epworth Sleepiness Scale):
  http://consultgerirn.org/topics/sleep/want_to_know_more
- Practice parameters for the clinical evaluation and treatment of circadian rhythm sleep disorders:
  http://www.guideline.gov/content.aspx?id=12112&search=sleep
- Clinical guideline for the evaluation, management and long-term care of obstructive sleep apnea in adults:
  http://www.guideline.gov/content.aspx?id=15298&search=sleep

AHRQ, Agency for Healthcare Research and Quality; UI, urinary incontinence; UTI, urinary tract infection.

---

also associated with UI (Shamliyan et al., 2007). Older people with dementia are at high risk for UI. For individuals with dementia, UI prevalence rates range from 11% to 90% with higher prevalence rates reflecting institutionalized patients (Dowling-Castronovo and Bradway, 2007). Hospital patients with dementia are more likely than other older people to develop new incontinence. One study reported that those with dementia are five times more likely to develop new urinary incontinence when hospitalized (Mecocci et al., 2005).

Dementia does not cause urinary incontinence but affects the ability of the person to find a bathroom and recognize the urge to void. Mobility problems and dependency in transfers are better predictors of continence status than dementia, suggesting that persons with dementia may have the potential to remain continent as long as they are mobile. Making toilets easily visible, providing assistance to the bathroom at regular intervals, and implementing prompted voiding protocols can assist in continence promotion for people with dementia. Box 11-2 presents risk factors for UI.

Consequences of UI

UI affects quality of life and has physical, psychosocial, and economic consequences. UI is identified as a marker of frailty in community-dwelling older adults (Dowling-Castronovo and Bradway, 2007). UI is associated with falls, skin irritations and infections, urinary tract infections (UTIs), and pressure ulcers, and sleep disturbance. UI affects self-esteem and increases the

risk for depression, anxiety, social isolation, and avoidance of sexual activity. Older adults with UI experience a loss of dignity, independence, and self-confidence, as well as feelings of shame and embarrassment (MacDonald and Butler, 2007; Dowling-Castronovo and Bradway, 2008). The psychosocial impact of UI affects the individual as well as the family caregivers.

Types of UI

Incontinence is classified as either transient (acute) or established (chronic). Transient incontinence has a sudden onset, is present for 6 months or less, and is usually caused by treatable factors such as UTIs, delirium, constipation and stool impaction, and increased urine production caused by metabolic conditions such as hyperglycemia and hypercalcemia. Iatrogenic (or treatment-induced) incontinence is a type of transient UI that results from the use of restraints, limited fluid intake, bed rest, or intravenous fluid administration. Use of medications such as diuretics, anticholinergic agents, antidepressants, sedatives, hypnotics, calcium channel blockers, and α-adrenergic agonists and blockers can also lead to transient UI (Dowling-Castronovo and Bradway, 2007, 2008).

Established UI may have either a sudden or gradual onset and is categorized into the following types: 1)urge; 2) stress; 3) urge, mixed, or stress UI with high postvoid residual (originally termed overflow UI 4) functional UI; and mixed UI.

Urge incontinence (overactive bladder) is defined as involuntary urine loss that occurs soon after feeling an urgent need to

BOX 11-2   **RISK FACTORS FOR URINARY INCONTINENCE**

- Age
- Immobility, functional limitations
- Diminished cognitive capacity (dementia, delirium)
- Medications (those with anticholinergic properties, sedatives, diuretics)
- Smoking
- High caffeine intake
- Obesity
- Constipation, fecal impaction
- Pregnancy, vaginal delivery, episiotomy
- Low fluid intake
- Environmental barriers
- High-impact physical exercise
- Diabetes
- Stroke
- Parkinson's disease
- Hysterectomy
- Pelvic muscle weakness
- Childhood nocturnal enuresis
- Prostate surgery
- Estrogen deficiency
- Arthritis
- Hearing and vision impairments

Adapted from DeMaagd G: Urinary incontinence: treatment update with a focus on pharmacological management, *U.S. Pharmacist* 32:34, 2007. Available from: http://www.uspharmacist.com/content/d/featured_articles/c/10310/; Dowling-Castronovo A, Bradway C: Urinary incontinence (UI) in older adults admitted to acute care. In: Capezuti E, Zwicker D, Mezey M, et al., editors: *Evidence-based geriatric nursing protocols for best practice,* ed 3, New York, 2008, Springer.

void. Overactive bladder is a syndrome that overlaps with urge UI. With overactive bladder syndrome, individuals have urinary frequency (more than eight voids in 24 hours), nocturia, urgency, with or without incontinence (Zarowitz and Ouslander, 2007). The bladder muscles are overactive and cause a sudden urge to void—the "Gotta Go Right Now" syndrome (Bucci, 2007). Defining characteristics of urge UI include loss of urine in moderate to large amounts before getting to the toilet and an inability to suppress the need to urinate. Frequency and nocturia may also be present. Postvoid residual urine reveals a low volume. Urge UI is the most common type of urinary incontinence in older adults (Dowling-Castronovo and Bradway, 2007, 2008).

Stress incontinence (outlet incompetence) is defined as an involuntary loss of less than 50 mL of urine associated with activities that increase intraabdominal pressure (e.g., coughing, sneezing, exercise, lifting, bending). Stress UI is more common in women because of short urethras and poor pelvic muscle tone. Stress UI occurs in men who have experienced prostatectomy and radiation. Postvoid residual urine is low (Dowling-Castronovo and Bradway, 2007, 2008).

Urge, mixed, or stress UI with high postvoid residual incontinence (formerly called overflow UI) occurs when the bladder does not empty normally and becomes overdistended with frequent and nearly constant urine loss (dribbling). Other symptoms include hesitancy in starting urination, slow urine stream, passage of infrequent or small volumes of urine, a feeling of incomplete bladder emptying, and large postvoid residuals.

Persons with diabetes and men with enlarged prostates are at risk for this type of UI. Calcium channel blockers, anticholinergics, and adrenergics also contribute to symptoms.

Functional incontinence refers to a situation in which the lower urinary tract is intact but the individual is unable to reach the toilet because of environmental barriers, physical limitations, or severe cognitive impairment. Individuals may be dependent on others for assistance to the toilet but have no genitourinary problems other than incontinence. Older adults who are institutionalized have higher rates of functional incontinence (Dowling-Castronovo and Bradway, 2007, 2008). Functional UI may also occur in the presence of other types of UI.

Mixed incontinence is a combination of more than one urinary incontinence problem, usually stress and urge. Mixed UI is the most prevalent type of UI in women (Shamliyam et al., 2007). With increasing age, older women with stress UI begin to experience urge UI.

PROMOTING HEALTHY AGING: IMPLICATIONS FOR GERONTOLOGICAL NURSING

Assessment

Continence must be routinely addressed in the initial assessment of every older person, yet many older people do not bring up their concerns about incontinence, and many health professionals do not ask. Health care personnel must begin to change their thinking about incontinence and acknowledge that incontinence can be cured. If it cannot be cured, it can be treated to minimize its detrimental effects. Nurses are often the ones to identify urinary incontinence, but neither nurses nor physicians have been particularly aggressive in its management. "Nurses have long been the providers of personal hygiene information for those entrusted to their care. Therefore, it is essential that nurses play a leading role in assessing and managing UI. . . ." (Dowling-Castronovo and Bradway, 2007, p. 7).

To begin assessment, screening questions such as "Have you ever leaked urine? If yes, how much does it bother you?" are suggested (Dowling-Castronovo and Bradway, 2007). Assessment is multidimensional. It includes a health history, targeted physical examination (abdominal, rectal, genital), urinalysis, and determination of postvoid residual urine. For women, evaluation of the reproductive system and gynecological history and examination is recommended since gynecological factors may contribute to the urological problem. More extensive examinations are considered after the initial findings are assessed. Individuals who do not fit a simple pattern on UI should be referred promptly for urodynamic assessment (Ham et al., 2007).

A thorough health history should focus on the medical, neurological, gynecological, and genitourinary history. It should should include functional assessment, cognitive assessment, psychosocial effects; strategies currently used to control UI; a medication review of both prescribed and over-the-counter drugs; a detailed exploration of the symptoms of the urinary incontinence; and associated symptoms and other factors. In care facilities, an environmental assessment including the accessibility of bathrooms, room lighting, and the use of aids such as raised toilet seats or commodes is also important. A link to a video of a nurse performing an assessment to evaluate transient incontinence can be found in Box 11-1.

In the nursing home, continence is assessed with the Minimum Data Set (MDS), and the MDS 3.0 provides a comprehensive overview of the assessment, treatment, and evaluation of bladder and bowel continence based on the new Center for Medicare & Medicaid Services (CMS) guidelines (Johnson and Ouslander, 2006). All newly admitted nursing home residents should have a thorough assessment of continence status as well as ongoing evaluations during their length of stay. The CHAMMP (Continence, History, Assessment, Medications, Mobility, Plan) tool (Bucci, 2007) was developed by a certified wound, ostomy, and continence nurse to guide comprehensive continence assessment and implementation of individualized plans of care in nursing homes (Figure 11-1). Figure 11-2

CHAMP TOOL

(<u>C</u>ontinence, <u>H</u>istory, <u>A</u>ssessment, <u>M</u>edications, <u>M</u>obility, <u>P</u>lan)

C Resident is continent? Yes ___ No ___

H Medical / Surgical History:
    a. Diagnosis often associated with continence? Yes ___ No ___
        ___ BPH (prostate) ___ Diabetes ___ MS
        ___ CHF ___ Fracture ___ Osteoporosis
        ___ Constipation ___ Heart Disease ___ Pain
        ___ Contractures ___ HTN ___ Parkinson's
        ___ CVA ___ Immobility ___ Spinal Cord Injury
        ___ Dementia ___ Kidney Stones ___ UTI (last 90 days)
        ___ Depression
    b. Recent Acute Medical Condition (last 30 days)? Yes ___ No ___
        If yes, date and type:
    c. Recent Surgery (last 30 days)? Yes ___ No ___
        If yes, date and type:
    d. Surgical History: Hysterectomy ___ Bladder Repair ___ Prostate (TURP) ___ Other ___
    e. Lab Data ___ Urodynamic Studies ___ Imaging Studies ___
        Date and type:

A Assessment of Urinary Incontinence:
    Trigger Event (surgery, accident, other)? Yes ___ No ___
    Leak urine when cough, sneeze, laugh, stand up, change position? Yes ___ No ___
    Urge to go (Need to be there NOW)? Yes ___ No ___
    Wet without feeling the need to go? Yes ___ No ___
    Number of night time voids? ___
    Leak only at night? Yes ___ No ___
    Difficult to start or stop stream? Yes ___ No ___
    Weak stream? Yes ___ No ___
    Dribbling? Yes ___ No ___
    Products used? _____

M1 Medications.
    a. Current Medication:

___ Anticholinergic	___ Diuretic	___ Narcotic
___ Antidepressant	___ Hypnotic	___ OTC Cold Remedies
___ Antihypertensive	___ Laxative	___ Sedative
___ Other:		

    b. Medications to treat Incontinence:

___ Antibiotic	___ Estrogen	___ Proscar
___ Detrol	___ Flomax	___ Sanctura
___ Ditropan	___ Imipramine	___ VESIcare
___ Enablex	___ Other:	

M2 Mobility Status: I Independent, A Assist, D Dependent

___ Ambulation	___ Dressing	___ Toileting
___ Transfer		

    Can access bedpan, BSC, urinal, toilet independently (Circle): ___ Yes ___ No

P Plan of care:
    a. Resident is motivated to toilet: ___ Yes ___ No ___ not oriented
    b. Resident is candidate for treatment program? Yes ___ No ___
    If no, reason:
    c. Care Plan interventions: (Circle Suggestions)
        ○ Incontinence, functional–prompted voiding, behavioral modification (i.e., timed voiding), restorative toileting, physical and/or occupational therapy, environmental modifications
        ○ Incontinence, overflow–clean intermittent catheterization
        ○ Incontinence, stress–pelvic muscle exercises, behavior modification, medications
        ○ Incontinence, urge–pelvic muscle exercises, behavior modification, medication Incontinence, mixed (stress and urge)–pelvic muscle exercises, behavior modification, medications
        ○ Incontinence, total–check and change
    d. Bladder treatment initiated (date):
    Nurse Signature: _____ Date: _____

FIGURE 11-1 CHAMMP Tool. BPH, BSC, bedside commode; benign prostatic hyperplasia; CHF, congestive heart failure; CVA, cardiovascular accident; HTN, hypertension; MS, multiple sclerosis; OTC, over the counter; TURP, transurethral resection of the prostate; UTI, urinary tract infection. (From Bucci A: Be a continence champion: use the CHAMMP tool to individualize the plan of care, *Geriatric Nursing* 28:123, 2007.)

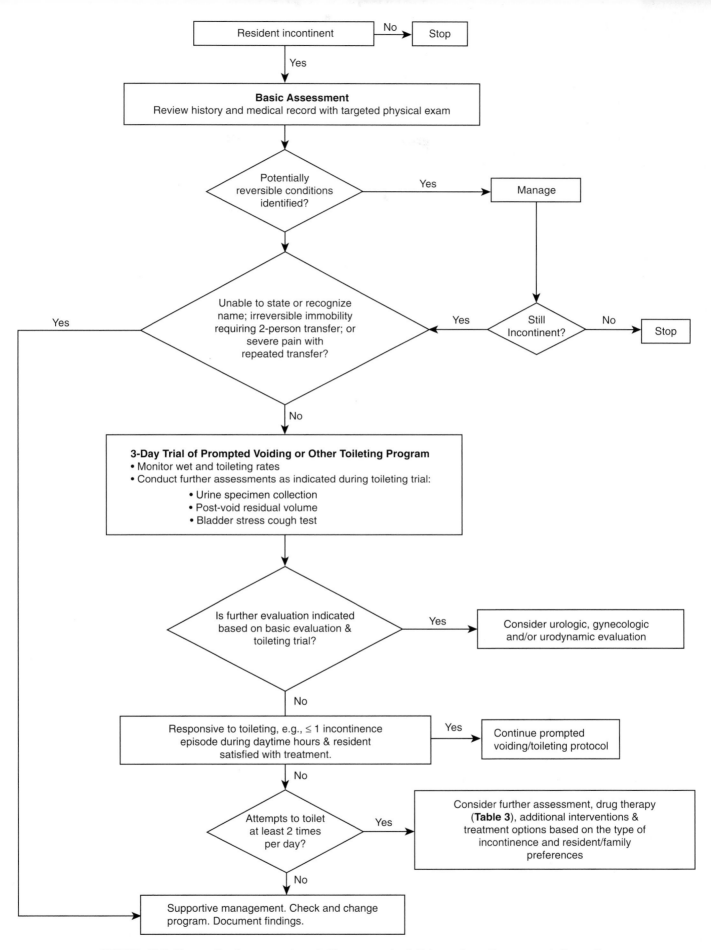

FIGURE 11-2 Diagnostic Assessment and Management of Urinary Incontinence and Overactive Bladder in the Nursing Home. (From Zarowitz B, Ouslander J: The application of evidence-based practice principles of care in older persons (issue 6): urinary incontinence, *Journal of the American Medical Directors Association* 8:35, 2007.)

	Time Interval	Urinated in Toilet	Incontinent Episode[1]	Reason for Episode[1]	Liquid Intake[3]	Bowel Movement	Product Use[3]
A.M. HOURS	12:00–01:00 AM						
	01:00–02:00 AM						
	02:00–03:00 AM						
	03:00–04:00 AM						
	04:00–05:00 AM						
	05:00–06:00 AM						
	06:00–07:00 AM						
	07:00–08:00 AM						
	08:00–09:00 AM						
	09:00–10:00 AM						
	10:00–11:00 AM						
	11:00–12:00 PM						
P.M. HOURS	12:00–01:00 PM						
	01:00–02:00 PM						
	02:00–03:00 PM						
	03:00–04:00 PM						
	04:00–05:00 PM						
	05:00–06:00 PM						
	06:00–07:00 PM						
	07:00–08:00 PM						
	08:00–09:00 PM						
	09:00–10:00 PM						
	10:00–11:00 PM						
	11:00–12:00 AM						

[1] **Incontinent episodes:** (++) = SMALL: did not have to change pad/ clothing; (+++) = LARGE: needed to change pad/clothing
[2] **Examples of reasons for incontinent episodes:** leaked while sneezing; leaked while running to the bathroom
[3] **Examples of type and amount of liquid intake:** 12 oz can of cola, 2 cups regular coffee
[4] **Examples of product use:** pad, undergarment; track times you changed

FIGURE 11-3 Sample Voiding or Bladder Diary. (Adapted from Fantl C, Newman, DK, Colling J, et al: *Urinary incontinence in adults: acute and chronic management.* Clinical Practice Guideline No. 2. AHCPR Publication No. 96-0682. Rockville, MD, 1996, Agency for Health Care Policy and Research, U.S. Department of Health and Human Services.)

presents a guide for diagnostic assessment and management of UI in the nursing home setting.

One of the best ways to establish the presence of and describe incontinence problems is with a voiding diary. This is considered the "gold standard" for obtaining objective information about the person's voiding patterns and the UI episodes and their severity (Dowling-Castronovo and Bradway, 2008, p. 314) (Figure 11-3). The voiding diary can be used by both community-dwelling and institutionalized elders. Older adults in the community can usually keep a bladder diary without much difficulty. Bladder diaries for those in long-term care are usually maintained by the staff and are used in conjunction with a trial of individualized, resident-centered toileting programs. The character of the urine (color, odor, sediment, or clear) and difficulty starting or stopping the urinary stream should be recorded. Activities of daily living (ADLs), such as ability to reach a toilet and use it and finger dexterity for clothing manipulation, should be documented.

Interventions

Behavioral   Urinary incontinence can be improved when appropriate care is provided. A number of behavioral interventions have a good basis in research and can be implemented by nurses without extensive and expensive evaluation. These treatments are viewed as healthy bladder behavior skills (HBBSs) (Dowling-Castronovo and Bradway, 2007, 2008).

These interventions will do no harm and if there is no improvement, further evaluation can be sought. Before instituting HBBSs, the nurse should assess the motivation of the patient, informal caregiver, and/or nursing staff because behavior management is the premise of HBBSs. Behavioral techniques, such as scheduled voiding, prompted voiding, bladder training, biofeedback, and pelvic floor muscle exercises (PFMEs), are recommended as first-line treatment of UI.

Selection of a modality and interventions will depend on a comprehensive assessment, the type of incontinence and its underlying cause, and whether the outcome is to cure or to minimize the extent of the incontinence. Interventions for UI should be multidisciplinary, and everyone involved with the person's care should be involved in the treatment plan. If the person has mobility impairments, physical and occupational therapy and/or restorative nursing programs should be implemented as part of the treatment plan for UI. Box 11-3 lists the numerous modalities available in the treatment of incontinence. Nursing interventions focus primarily on the appropriate assessment of continence and implementation and evaluation of supportive and therapeutic modalities to promote and restore continence and to prevent incontinence-related complications, such as skin breakdown.

Scheduled (timed) voiding is used to treat urge and functional UI in both cognitively intact and cognitively impaired older adults. The schedule or timing of voiding is based on the

---

BOX 11-3 THERAPEUTIC MODALITIES IN THE TREATMENT OF INCONTINENCE

SUPPORT MEASURES
- Appropriate attitude
- Accessible toilet substitutes (bedpan, urinal, commode)
- Avoidance of iatrogenic conditions (urinary tract infections, constipation/impaction, excessive sedation, inaccessible toilets, drugs adversely affecting the bladder or urethral function)
- Protective undergarments
- Absorbent bed pads
- Behavioral techniques: bladder training, scheduled (timed) voiding, prompted voiding, biofeedback, pelvic floor muscle exercises (PFMEs)
- Good skin care

DRUGS
- Bladder relaxants
- Bladder outlet stimulants

SURGERY
- Suspension of bladder neck
- Prostatectomy
- Prosthetic sphincter implants
- Urethral sling
- Bladder augmentation

MECHANICAL AND ELECTRICAL DEVICES: CATHETERS
- External (condom or "Texas" catheter)
- Intermittent
- Suprapubic
- Indwelling

---

person's bladder diary patterns or common voiding patterns (voiding on arising, before and after meals, midmorning, midafternoon, and bedtime). In general, toileting is scheduled at 2- to 4-hour intervals. People can be taught to do this routinely or they can be assisted to the bathroom according to the scheduled intervals.

Prompted voiding (PV) combines scheduled voiding with monitoring, prompting, and verbal reinforcement. The objective of PV is to increase self-initiated voiding and decrease the number of episodes of UI. The person is assisted to the toilet during waking hours if he or she requests it and receives positive feedback if he or she voids successfully. Between 25% and 40% of incontinent nursing home residents respond well to prompted voiding (Zarowitz and Ouslander, 2007). In a systematic review of randomized trials of interventions in nursing home residents with UI, Fink and colleagues (2010) concluded that prompted voiding is associated with modest short-term improvement in daytime UI in nursing home residents.

Newly admitted nursing home residents should receive a thorough assessment of continence, and those who are incontinent (and able to use the toilet) should receive a 3- to 5-day trial of prompted voiding. The trial can be helpful in demonstrating responsiveness to toileting and determining patterns of and symptoms associated with the incontinence. Residents who do not respond to prompted voiding but consistently attempt to toilet should receive further evaluation and may be appropriate candidates for drug therapy in addition to a PV program. Residents who are unresponsive to toileting programs or unable or unwilling to attempt toileting can be provided supportive

management including absorbent pads and briefs, and attention to skin breakdown prevention (Zarowitz and Ouslander, 2007; Lawhorne et al., 2008).

Continence programs in nursing homes are both needed and required by CMS regulations (Johnson and Ouslander, 2006). Monitoring and documentation of continence status in relation to implemented continence care is a quality of care indicator for nursing homes (Shamliyan et al., 2007). Despite a growing body of evidence suggesting that toileting programs can be successful in long-term care, they are difficult to sustain. Barriers to implementation and continuation of toileting programs include inadequate staffing, lack of knowledge about UI and existing evidence-based protocols, and insufficient professional staff. A major advantage of PV programs is that they target residents who are likely to be successful and direct scarce staff resources to residents most likely to benefit.

Johnson and Ouslander (2006, p. 599) remind us that "cure of incontinence in nursing home residents is unusual and not a realistic goal for most." However, every resident who is incontinent deserves appropriate medical and nursing assessment and interventions that restore continence, if possible, or provide supportive care and prevention of complications related to incontinence. Successful implementation of continence programs requires a systems-based approach with consideration of individual, group, organizational, and environmental level factors (Holroyd-Leduc and Straus, 2004).

Bladder training aims to increase the time interval between the urge to void and voiding. This method is appropriate for people with urge UI who are cognitively intact and independent in toileting or after removal of an indwelling catheter. The person follows an established voiding schedule until UI episodes cease. Once this is achieved, the interval between voidings is extended and techniques for overcoming the urge and postponing urination are taught (pelvic floor muscle exercises).

Pelvic floor muscle exercises (PFMEs), also called Kegel exercises, involve repeated voluntary pelvic floor muscle contraction. The targeted muscle is the pubococcygeal muscle, which forms the support for the pelvis and surrounds the vagina, the urethra, and the rectum. The goal of the repetitive contractions is to strengthen the muscle and decrease UI episodes. PFMEs are recommended for stress, urge, and mixed UI in older women.

Although there are some nursing home residents who may benefit from PFMEs and are capable of learning and practicing, the numbers may be insufficient to justify emphasis on this approach in this setting (Johnson and Ouslander, 2006). PFMEs have also been shown to be helpful for men who have undergone prostatectomy. Contractions should be repeated 30 to 100 times a day; the contraction is held for 10 seconds and followed by 10 seconds of relaxation.

Correct identification of the pelvic floor muscles and adherence to the exercise regimen are key to success. Improvement may not be noted until two to four weeks of exercises have been successfully completed. To help identify the correct muscle groups, it may be helpful to tell the person to try to tighten the anal sphincter (as if to control the passage of flatus or feces) and then tighten the urethral and/or vaginal muscles (as if to stop the flow of urine). Muscles of the stomach, thigh, and buttocks should not be contracted because this increases intraabdominal pressure. PFMEs may be taught during a vaginal or rectal examination when the clinician manually assists the person to identify the pelvic muscles by instructing the patient to squeeze around a gloved examination finger (Dowling-Castronovo and Bradway, 2008). Biofeedback may be helpful in identifying the correct muscle and visualizing the strength and time of the contraction.

Vaginal weight training was introduced in Europe as an alternative for women who have difficulty identifying the pelvic floor muscles. Graded-weight vaginal balls or cones are worn during two 15-minute periods each day or are used in addition to PFMEs. When the weighted cone is placed in the vagina, the pelvic floor muscle contractions keep it from slipping out. Although this technique involves less time and is more easily taught than PFMEs, difficulty inserting the cones and discomfort have been noted as deterrents to use.

Lifestyle Modifications   Several lifestyle factors are associated with either the development or exacerbation of UI. These include dietary factors (increased fluid, avoidance of caffeine), weight reduction, smoking cessation, bowel management, and physical activity. Recent research findings suggest that coffee and tea consumption has limited or no effects on incontinence (Tettamanti et al., 2011). This calls into question the common practice of advising women with UI to stop drinking coffee and tea. Box 11-4 presents other interventions helpful to noninstitutionalized elders to control or eliminate incontinence.

Urinary Catheters   Intermittent catheterization may be used in people with urinary retention related to a weak detrusor muscle (e.g., diabetic neuropathy), those with a blockage of the urethra (e.g., benign prostatic hypertrophy), or those with reflux incontinence related to a spinal cord injury. The goal is to maintain 300 mL or less of urine in the bladder. Most of the research on intermittent catheterization has been conducted with children or young adults with spinal cord injuries, but it may be useful for older adults who are able to self-catheterize. It provides an important alternative to indwelling catheterization.

Indwelling catheter use is not appropriate for long-term management (more than 30 days) except in certain clinical conditions. Continuous indwelling catheter use is indicated for urethral obstruction or urinary retention or in patients with the following conditions:

- When surgical or pharmacological interventions are inappropriate or unsuccessful
- If contraindications are present to intermittent catheterization to treat retention
- When changes of bedding, clothing, and absorbent products may be painful or disruptive for a patient with an irreversible medical condition, such as metastatic terminal disease, coma, or end-stage congestive heart failure
- For patients with severely impaired skin integrity
- For patients who live alone without a caregiver or with a caregiver who is unable to routinely change the person (Newman and Palmer, 2003; Johnson and Ouslander, 2006)

Regulatory standards in nursing homes follow these same guidelines, and the use of indwelling catheters must be justified on the basis of medical conditions and failure of other efforts to maintain continence. In hospitals, the use of indwelling catheters is often unjustified, and they are used inappropriately (convenience of staff) or left in place too long. Misuse of catheterization should be considered a medical error. About one in four indwelling catheters in hospitalized patients aged 70 years and older and one in three in patients aged 85 years and older turn out to be unnecessary (Inelmen et al., 2007). Cognitive impairment and the presence of pressure ulcers almost double the risk of receiving a catheter and severe functional decline is associated with a fourfold risk of catheter placement (Inelmen et al., 2007).

BOX 11-4   HELPFUL INTERVENTIONS FOR NONINSTITUTIONALIZED ELDERS TO CONTROL OR ELIMINATE INCONTINENCE

- Empty bladder completely before and after meals and at bedtime.
- Urinate whenever the urge arises; never ignore it.
- A schedule of urinating every two hours during the day and every four hours at night is often helpful in retraining the bladder. Use of an alarm clock may be necessary.
- Drink 1.5 to 2 quarts of fluid a day before 8 PM. This helps the kidneys to function properly. Limit fluids after supper to 0.5 to 1 cup (except in very hot weather).
- Eliminate or reduce the use of coffee, tea, brown cola, and alcohol, because they have a diuretic effect.
- Take prescription diuretics in the morning on rising.
- Limit the use of sleeping pills, sedatives, and alcohol because they decrease sensation to urinate and can increase incontinence, especially at night.
- If overweight, lose weight.
- Exercises to strengthen pelvic muscles that help support the bladder (PFMEs) are often helpful for women with stress, urge, and mixed UI. The may also be helpful for men after prostatectomy.
- Make sure the toilet is nearby, with a clear path to it and good lighting, especially at night. Grab bars or a raised toilet seat may be needed.
- Dress protectively with cotton underwear and protective pants or incontinence pads if necessary.

⚠ SAFETY ALERT

Long-term catheter use increases the risk of recurrent urinary tract infections leading to urosepsis, urethral damage in men, urethritis, or fistula formation. Catheter-associated urinary tract infection is the most frequent health care–associated infection in the United States and Medicare no longer reimburses hospitals for this infection. Indwelling catheters should be inserted only for appropriate conditions, must be removed as soon as possible, and alternatives should be investigated (e.g., condom catheters, intermittent catheterization, toileting programs).

External catheters (condom catheters) are used in male patients who are incontinent and cannot be toileted. Long-term use of external catheters can lead to fungal skin infections, penile skin maceration, edema, fissures, contact burns from urea, phimosis, UTIs, and septicemia. The catheter should be removed and replaced daily and the penis cleaned, dried, and aired to prevent irritation, maceration, and the development of pressure ulcers and skin breakdown. If the catheter is not sized appropriately and applied and monitored correctly, strangulation of the penile shaft can occur.

Prevention of catheter-associated UTIs includes the following: (1) Using as small a catheter as possible that is consistent with proper drainage, to minimize urethral trauma; (2) maintaining unobstructed urine flow to a bag below the level of the bladder; (3) properly securing the catheter to prevent movement and urethral traction; and (4) removing catheters when no longer needed. Interventions such as topical meatal antimicrobials, antimicrobial coatings for catheters, and antimicrobial irrigations have not been shown to decrease the incidence of infection. (Dowling-Castronovo and Bradway, 2007). Catheter care should consist of washing the meatal area with soap and water daily. A protocol to prevent catheter-associated urinary tract infections in acute care hospitals can be found in Box 11-1.

Urinary Tract Infections
Urinary tract infections (UTIs) are the most common cause of bacterial sepsis in older adults and are 10 times more common in women than in men. The majority of UTIs in older adults are asymptomatic. Assessment and appropriate treatment of UTIs in older people, particularly nursing home residents, is complex. Cognitively impaired residents may not recall or report symptoms, older people frequently do not present with classic symptoms (fever, dysuria, flank pain), and other illnesses (e.g., pneumonia) may present with nonspecific symptoms similar to UTI. Changes in mental status, character of urine, decreased appetite, abdominal pain, chills, low back pain, urethral discharge in men, new onset of incontinence, or even respiratory distress may signal a possible UTI in older people (Juthani-Mehta et al., 2009).

Bacteremia plus pyuria alone are not sufficient to make a diagnosis of UTI in nursing home residents (Juthani-Mehta et al., 2009; Mouton et al., 2010). Asymptomatic bacteria in the urine is considered benign in older people and should not be treated with antibiotics. Screening urine cultures should also not be performed in patients who are asymptomatic. Symptomatic UTIs necessitate antibiotic treatment, but it is important to pay attention to the range of symptoms older patients may present. An assessment and treatment algorithm for UTI is presented in Figure 11-4.

Absorbent Products
A variety of protective undergarments or adult briefs are available for the older adult who is incontinent. Disposable types come in several sizes, determined by hip and waist measurements, or as one size made to fit all. Many of these undergarments look like regular underwear and contribute more to dignity than the standard "diaper." Referring to protective undergarments as diapers is demeaning and infantilizing to older people and should be avoided. Some individuals may prefer to use absorbent products in addition to toileting interventions to maintain "social continence," and a wide variety of products is available.

Pharmacological
Pharmacological treatment may be indicated for urge UI and overactive bladder (OAB). OAB symptoms include urgency, frequency, and nocturia. Drugs for urge UI and OAB include anticholinergic (antimuscarinic) agents. Commonly prescribed medications include oxybutynin (Ditropan), tolterodine (Detrol), and trospium chloride, darifenacin, and solifenacin, as well as a transdermal formulation of oxybutynin. Toviaz (fesoterodine fumarate) is another approved drug for the treatment of OAB and UI. The extended-release forms of oxybutynin and tolterodine seem to have fewer adverse effects compared with immediate-release formulations (Zarowitz and Ouslander, 2007).

In a randomized placebo-controlled trial, short-term treatment with extended-release oxybutynin was shown to be safe and well tolerated in a group of female nursing home residents with severe dementia and urge UI (Lackner et al., 2008). More research is needed to determine the effectiveness of pharmacological treatment of UI among nursing home residents.

Dosages should be started low in older adults and titrated slowly with careful attention to side effects and drug interactions. A trial of four to eight weeks is adequate and recommended; there is no clear advantage in terms of efficacy between the various medications (DeMaagd, 2007; DuBeau, 2009). Undesirable side effects of anticholinergic medications such as dry mouth and eyes, constipation, confusion, or the precipitation of glaucoma are problematic in older people. These medications can be especially problematic for older adults with cognitive impairment (Barton et al., 2008). Medications are not considered first-line treatment but can be considered in combination with behavioral therapies in some cases.

Medications for the treatment of benign prostatic hypertrophy include α-adrenergic blockers and 5-α-reductase inhibitors. α-Adrenergic blockers are usually the therapy of choice in early, mild disease. Careful monitoring of side effects and drug interactions is necessary. The herbal saw palmetto, reported to have 5-α-reductase inhibitor activity, may also be used, but reports about its effectiveness are mixed (DeMaagd, 2007)(Chapter 10).

Surgical
Surgical intervention is appropriate for some conditions of incontinence. Surgical suspension of the bladder neck (sling procedure) in women has proved effective in 80% to 95% of persons electing to have this surgical corrective procedure. Outflow obstruction incontinence secondary to prostatic hypertrophy is generally corrected by prostatectomy. Sphincter dysfunction resulting from nerve damage following surgical trauma or radical perineal procedures is 70% to 90% repairable through sphincter implantation. Periurethral bulking has been added to the number of surgical procedures that address urinary incontinence. Collagen or polytetrafluoroethylene (PTFE) is injected into the periurethral area to increase pressure on the urethra. This adds bulk to the internal sphincter and closes the gap that allowed leakage to occur.

Nonsurgical Devices
Stress UI can be treated with intravaginal support devices, pessaries, and urethral plugs. The pessary, used primarily to prevent uterine prolapse, is a device that is fitted into the vagina and exerts pressure to elevate the urethrovesical junction of the pelvic floor. The patient is taught to insert and remove the pessary, much like inserting and removing a diaphragm used for contraception. The pessary is removed weekly or monthly for cleaning with soap and water and then reinserted. Adverse effects include vaginal infection, low back pain, and vaginal mucosal erosion. Another concern is the danger of forgetting to remove the pessary.

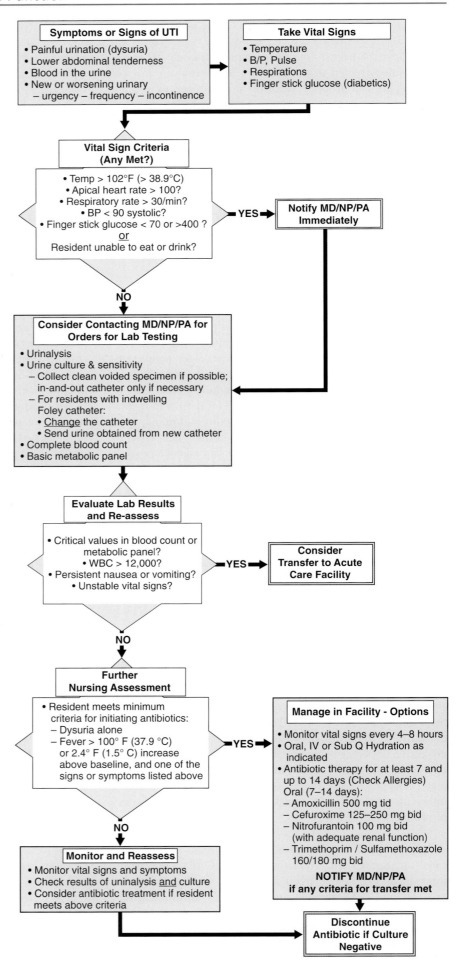

FIGURE 11-4 CARE PATH: Symptoms of Urinary Tract Infection (UTI). bid, twice daily; BP, blood pressure; IV, intravenous; MD/NP/PA, doctor/nurse practitioner/physician's assistant; sub Q, subcutaneous; tid, three times daily; WBC, white blood cell count. (Developed by Joe Ouslander. Copyright © 2010 Florida Atlantic University.)

BOWEL ELIMINATION

Bowel function of the older adult, although normally only slightly altered by the physiological changes of age, can be a source of concern and a potentially serious problem, especially for the older person who is functionally impaired. Normal elimination should be an easy passage of feces, without undue straining or a feeling of incomplete evacuation or defecation. The urge to defecate occurs when the distended walls of the sigmoid and the rectum, which are filled with feces, stimulate pressure receptors to relax the sphincters for the expulsion of feces through the anus. Evacuation of feces is accomplished by relaxation of the sphincters and contraction of the diaphragm and abdominal muscles, which raises the intraabdominal pressure.

Constipation is the most common gastrointestinal (GI) complaint made to the health care provider. The annual estimated expenditure for laxatives in the general population of the United States is $800 million annually. This figure is probably low because many people use over-the-counter medications before they seek out prescription medications. The extensive use of laxatives among older adults in the United States can be considered a cultural habit. During earlier times, weekly doses of rhubarb, cascara, castor oil, and other types of laxatives were consumed and believed by many to promote health. The belief that cleaning out the colon and having a daily bowel movement is paramount to maintaining good health still persists in some groups.

Constipation is a symptom. It is a reflection of poor habits, postponed passage of stool, and many chronic illnesses—both physical and psychological—as well as a common side effect of medication. Diet and activity level play a significant role in constipation. Constipation and other changes in bowel habits can also signal more serious underlying problems, such as colonic dysmotility or colon cancer. Thorough assessment is important, and these complaints should not be blamed on age alone. Numerous precipitating factors or condition can cause or worsen constipation (Box 11-5).

Fecal Impaction

Fecal impaction is a major complication of constipation. It is especially common in incapacitated and institutionalized older people and is reported to occur in more than 40% of older adults admitted to the hospital (Roach and Christie, 2008). Symptoms of fecal impaction include malaise, urinary retention, elevated temperature, incontinence of bladder or bowel, alterations in cognitive status, fissures, hemorrhoids, and intestinal obstruction. Unrecognized, unattended, or neglected

---

BOX 11-5   PRECIPITATING FACTORS FOR CONSTIPATION

PHYSIOLOGICAL
- Dehydration
- Insufficient fiber intake
- Poor dietary habits

FUNCTIONAL
- Decreased physical activity
- Inadequate toileting
- Irregular defecation habits
- Irritable bowel disease
- Weakness

MECHANICAL
- Abscess or ulcer
- Fissures
- Hemorrhoids
- Megacolon
- Pelvic floor dysfunction
- Postsurgical obstruction
- Prostate enlargement
- Rectal prolapse
- Rectocele
- Spinal cord injury
- Strictures
- Tumors

OTHER
- Lack of abdominal muscle tone
- Obesity
- Recent environmental changes
- Poor dentition

PSYCHOLOGICAL
- Avoidance of urge to defecate
- Confusion
- Depression
- Emotional stress

SYSTEMIC
- Diabetic neuropathy
- Hypercalcemia
- Hyperparathyroidism
- Hypothyroidism
- Hypokalemia
- Porphyria
- Uremia
- Parkinson's disease
- Cerebrovascular disease
- Defective electrolyte transfer

PHARMACOLOGICAL
- ACE inhibitors
- Antacids: calcium carbonate, aluminum hydroxide
- Antiarrhythmics
- Anticholinergics
- Anticonvulsants
- Antidepressants
- Anti-Parkinson's medications
- Calcium channel blockers
- Calcium supplements
- Diuretics
- Iron supplements
- Laxative overuse
- Nonsteroidal antiinflammatories
- Opiates
- Phenothiazines
- Sedatives
- Sympathomimetics

ACE, angiotensin-converting enzyme.

Adapted from Allison OC, Porter ME, Briggs GC: Chronic constipation: assessment and management in the elderly, *Journal of the American Academy of Nurse Practitioners* 6:311, 1994; Tabloski PA: *Gerontological nursing*, Upper Saddle River, NJ, 2006, Pearson/Prentice Hall.

constipation eventually leads to fecal impaction. Paradoxical diarrhea, caused by leakage of fecal material around the impacted mass, may occur. Reports of diarrhea in older adults must be thoroughly assessed before the use of antidiarrheal medications, which further complicate the problem of fecal impaction. Digital rectal examination for impacted stool and abdominal x-rays will confirm the presence of impacted stool. Stool analysis for *Clostridium difficile* toxin should be ordered in patients who develop new-onset diarrhea. Continued obstruction by a fecal mass may eventually impair sensation, leading to the need for larger stool volume to stimulate the urge to defecate, which contributes to megacolon.

Removal of a fecal impaction is at times worse than the misery of the condition. Management of fecal impaction requires the digital removal of the hard, compacted stool from the rectum with use of lubrication containing lidocaine jelly. In general, this is preceded by an oil-retention enema to soften the feces in preparation for manual removal. Use of suppositories is not effective, because their action is blocked by the amount and size of the stool in the rectum. Suppositories do not facilitate the removal of stool in the sigmoid, which may continue to ooze once the rectum is emptied.

Several sessions or days may be necessary to totally cleanse the sigmoid colon and rectum of impacted feces. Once this is achieved, attention should be directed to planning a regimen that includes adequate fluid intake, increased dietary fiber, administration of stool softeners if needed, and many of the suggestions presented for prevention of constipation. For patients who are hospitalized or residing in long-term care settings, accurate bowel records are essential; unfortunately, they are often overlooked or inaccurately completed. Education about the importance of bowel function, and the accurate reporting of size, consistency, and frequency of bowel movements, should be provided to all direct care providers. This is especially important for frail or cognitively impaired elders to prevent fecal impaction, a serious and often dangerous condition for older people.

PROMOTING HEALTHY AGING: IMPLICATIONS FOR GERONTOLOGICAL NURSING

Assessment

The precipitants and causes of constipation must be included in the evaluation of the patient. A review of these factors will also determine whether the patient is at risk for altered bowel function. Older people at high risk for constipation and subsequent fecal impaction are those who have hypotonic colon function, who are immobilized and debilitated, or who have central nervous system lesions. It is important to note that alterations in cognitive status, incontinence, increased temperature, poor appetite, or unexplained falls may be the only clinical symptoms of constipation in the cognitively impaired or frail older person.

Recognizing constipation can be a challenge because there may be a significant disconnect between patient definitions of constipation and those of clinicians. Constipation has different

BOX 11-6   ROME III CRITERIA FOR DEFINING CHRONIC FUNCTIONAL CONSTIPATION IN ADULTS

Chronic constipation is defined by symptoms that have persisted for the last three months with an onset at least six months before diagnosis. All three of the following criteria must be met:
- At least two of the following:
  - Hard or lumpy stool in ≥25% of defecations
  - Straining during ≥25% of defecations
  - Sensation of incomplete evacuation in ≥25% of defecations
  - Sensation of anorectal obstruction or blockage for ≥25% of defecations
  - Manual maneuvers (e.g., digital evacuation or pelvic floor support) to facilitate ≥25% of defecations
  - Fewer than three defecations per week
- Loose stools rarely present without the use of laxatives. However, it is important to check for impaction if loose stools are present
- Insufficient criteria for irritable bowel syndrome (IBS)

Adapted from Cash B: Chronic constipation—defining the problem and clinical impact, *Medscape Gastroenterology* 7:2005. Available at www.medscape.com/viewarticle/501467. Accessed December 2010. Longstreth GF, Thompson WG, Chey WD, et al: Functional bowel disorders, *Gastroenterology* 130:1480, 2006.

meanings to different people. Assessment begins with clarification of what the patient means by constipation. It is important to obtain a bowel history including usual patterns, frequency of bowel movements, size, consistency, and any changes. Many clinicians think of constipation as bowel movement infrequency but according to several large epidemiological studies, patients with chronic constipation are more likely to report straining, a sense of incomplete or ineffective defecation, and hard or lumpy stools as the most bothersome symptoms of constipation (Cash, 2005).

The Rome III criteria for defining chronic functional constipation in adults can be used to guide the evaluation and treatment of constipation (Box 11-6). The Bristol Stool Form Scale can also be used to provide a visual depiction of stool appearance (Lewis and Heaton, 1997).

A physical examination is needed to rule out systemic causes of constipation such as neurological, endocrine, or metabolic disorders. Symptoms that may suggest the presence of an underlying GI disorder are abdominal pain, nausea, cramping, vomiting, weight loss, melena, rectal bleeding, rectal pain, and fever. A review of food and fluid intake may be necessary to determine the amount of fiber and fluid ingested. Questions should be asked about the level of physical activity and the use of medications, including over-the-counter products, herbs, and supplements. A psychosocial history with attention to depression, anxiety, and stress management is also indicated.

The abdomen is examined for masses, distention, tenderness, and high-pitched or absent bowel sounds. A rectal examination is important to reveal painful anal disorders, such as hemorrhoids or fissures, that will impede the evacuation of stool and to evaluate sphincter tone, rectal prolapse, stool presence in the vault, strictures, masses, anal reflex, and enlarged prostate. Biochemical tests should include a complete blood count, fasting glucose, chemistry panel, and thyroid studies. Other diagnostic studies such as flexible sigmoidoscopy, colonoscopy, computed tomography (CT) scan of the abdomen, or abdominal x-ray study may also be indicated.

Interventions

The first intervention is to examine the medications the person is taking and eliminate those that are constipation-producing, preferably changing to medications that do not carry that side effect. Medications are the leading cause of constipation, and almost any drug can cause it. Drugs that affect the central nervous system, nerve conduction, and smooth muscle function are associated with the highest frequency of constipation. Anticholinergics, pain opiates, and many psychoactive medications can be especially problematic.

Nonpharmacological interventions for constipation that have been implemented and evaluated can be grouped into four areas: (1) fluid- and fiber-related, (2) exercise, (3) environmental manipulation, and (4) a combination of these. Adequate hydration is the cornerstone of constipation therapy, with fluids coming mainly from water. A low-fiber diet and insufficient fluid intake contribute to constipation, and the importance of dietary fiber to adequate nutrition and bowel function is discussed in Chapter 14.

Exercise   Exercise is important as an intervention to stimulate colon motility and bowel evacuation. Daily walking for 20 to 30 minutes is helpful, especially after a meal. Pelvic tilt exercises, and range of motion (passive or active) exercises are beneficial for those who are less mobile or who are bedridden. Exercise and physical activity is discussed in Chapters 2 and 12.

Positioning   The squatting or sitting position, if the patient is able to assume it, facilitates bowel function. A similar position may be obtained by leaning forward and applying firm pressure to the lower abdomen or by placing the feet on a stool. Massaging the abdomen may help stimulate the bowel.

Regularity   Establishing a routine for toileting promotes or normalizes bowel function (bowel retraining). The gastrocolic reflex occurs after breakfast or supper and may be enhanced by a warm drink. Given privacy and ample time (a minimum of 10 minutes), many will have a daily bowel movement. However, any urge to defecate should be followed by a trip to the bathroom. Older people dependent on others to meet toileting needs should be assisted to maintain normal routines and provided opportunities for routine toilet use. Box 11-8 presents a bowel-training program.

Laxatives   When changes in diet and lifestyle are not effective, the use of laxatives is considered. Older persons receiving opiates need to have a constipation prevention program in place, because these drugs delay gastric emptying and decrease peristalsis. Correction of constipation associated with opiate use calls for a senna or osmotic laxative to overcome the strong opioid effect. Stool softeners and bulking agents alone are inadequate.

Laxatives commonly used in chronic constipation include the following:
- Bulking agents (e.g., psyllium, methylcellulose)
- Stool softeners (surfactants) (e.g., docusate sodium)
- Osmotic laxatives (e.g., lactulose, sorbitol)
- Stimulant laxatives (e.g., senna, bisacodyl)
- Saline laxatives (e.g., magnesium hydroxide [Milk of Magnesia])

Bulk laxatives are often the first prescribed because of their safety. Bulk laxatives absorb water from the intestinal lumen and increase stool mass. Adequate fluid intake is essential, and use of these laxatives is contraindicated in the presence of obstruction or compromised peristaltic activity. A saline or osmotic laxative can be added if the bulk laxative is not effective. Use of saline laxatives should be avoided in patients with poor renal function or congestive heart failure because they may cause electrolyte imbalances.

Stimulant laxatives should be used when other laxatives are ineffective. The emollient laxative, mineral oil, should be avoided because of the risk of lipoid aspiration pneumonia. Stool softeners (surfactants) are frequently used as laxatives. They are poorly absorbed and have a detergent-like effect of reducing the water–oil interface in the stool. Studies of surfactants, such as docusate, have reported minimal effectiveness, particularly in older adults with limited mobility. Use should be limited to patients in whom excessive straining or painful defecation occurs, or for individuals at high risk for developing constipation in combination with other types of laxatives and bowel programs (Hall et al., 2007; Ham et al., 2007).

Combinations of natural fiber, fruit juices, and natural laxative mixtures are often recommended in clinical practice, and some studies have found an increase in bowel frequency and a decrease in laxative use when these mixtures are used. One study (Hale et al., 2007) showed that older long-term care residents receiving the Beverley–Travis natural laxative mixture (Beverley and Travis, 1992) at a dosage of two tablespoons twice per day had a significant increase in number of bowel movements compared with residents receiving daily prescribed laxatives. The Beverley–Travis natural laxative recipe and an additional recipe for an alternative natural laxative mixture are presented in Box 11-7.

Enemas   Enemas of any type should be reserved for situations in which other methods produce no response or when it is known that there is an impaction. Enemas should not be used on a regular basis. A normal saline or tap water enema (500 to 1000 mL) at a temperature of 105° F is the best choice. Soapsuds and phosphate enemas irritate the rectal mucosa and should not be used. Oil retention enemas are used for refractory constipation and in the treatment of fecal impaction.

A program to prevent as well as treat constipation that incorporates a high-fiber diet, liberal fluid intake, daily exercise, and environmental modifications that promote a regular pattern of bowel elimination must be developed for each client. Interventions in any setting are based on a thorough assessment. Assessment and management of bowel function are an important nursing responsibility.

Fecal Incontinence

Fecal incontinence (FI) is defined as "continuous or recurrent uncontrolled passage of fecal material for at least one month in a mature person" (Stevens and Palmer, 2007). Estimates are that more than 6.5 million Americans have fecal incontinence.

BOX 11-7   BOWEL-TRAINING PROGRAM

1. Obtain bowel history, and establish a schedule for the bowel-training program that is normal and comfortable for the patient and conforms to his or her lifestyle.
2. Ensure adequate fiber and fluid intake (normalize stool consistency).
    a. Fiber
        i. Add high-fiber foods to diet (dried fruit, dried beans, vegetables, and wheat products).
        ii. Suggest adding one to three tablespoons (tbsp) of bran or Metamucil to the diet once or twice each day. (Titrate dosage on the basis of response.)
    b. Fluid
        i. Two to three liters daily (unless contraindicated).
        ii. Four ounces of prune, fig, or pear juice (or a warm fluid) may be given daily as a stimulus (e.g., 30-60 min before the established time for defecation).
3. Encourage an exercise program.
    a. Pelvic tilt, modified sit-ups for abdominal strength
    b. Walking for general muscle tone and cardiovascular system
    c. More vigorous program if appropriate
4. Establish a regular time for the bowel movement.
    a. Established time depends on patient's schedule.
    b. Best times are 20 to 40 minutes after regularly scheduled meals, when the gastrocolic reflex is active.
    c. Attempts at evacuation should be made daily within 15 minutes of the established time and whenever the patient senses rectal distention.
    d. Instruct patient in normal posture for defecation. (The patient normally sits on the toilet or bedside commode; for the patient who is unable to get out of bed, the left side–lying position is best.)
    e. Instruct the patient to contract the abdominal muscles and "bear down."
    f. Have the patient lean forward to increase the intraabdominal pressure by use of compression against the thighs.
    g. Stimulate the anorectal reflex and rectal emptying if necessary.
5. (1) Insert a rectal suppository or minienema into the rectum 15 to 30 minutes before the scheduled bowel movement, placing the suppository against the bowel wall, or (2) insert a gloved, lubricated finger into the anal canal and gently dilate the anal sphincter.

BOX 11-8   NATURAL LAXATIVE RECIPES

1. BEVERLEY–TRAVIS NATURAL LAXATIVE MIXTURE
Ingredients
1. 1 cup raisins
2. 1 cup pitted prunes
3. 1 cup figs
4. 1 cup dates
5. 1 cup currants
6. 1 cup prune concentrate

Directions
Combine contents in a grinder or blender and blend to a thickened consistency. Store in refrigerator between uses.

Dosage
Administer two tablespoons (tbsp) twice per day (once in the morning and once in the evening). May increase or decrease according to the frequency of bowel movements.

Nutritional Composition
Each 2-tbsp dose contains the following:
- 61 calories
- 137 mg potassium
- 8 mg sodium
- 11.9 g sugar
- 0.5 g protein
- 1.4 g fiber

2. POWER PUDDING
Ingredients
- 1 cup wheat bran
- 1 cup applesauce
- 1 cup prune juice

Directions
Mix and store in refrigerator. Start with administration of one tbsp/day. Increase *slowly* until the desired effect is achieved and no disagreeable symptoms occur.

Beverley–Travis natural laxative mixture from Hale E, Smith E, St. James J, et al: Pilot study of the feasibility and effectiveness of a natural laxative mixture, *Geriatric Nursing* 28:104, 2007.

Accurate estimates are difficult to obtain because many people are reluctant to discuss this disorder and many primary care providers do not ask about it. Prevalence varies with the study population: 2% to 17% in community-dwelling older people, 50% to 65% in older adults in nursing homes, and 33% in hospitalized older adults. Fecal incontinence is a significant risk factor for nursing home placement. Higher prevalence rates are found among patients with diabetes, irritable bowel syndrome, stroke (new onset, 30%; 15% at three years poststroke), multiple sclerosis, and spinal cord injury (Roach and Christie, 2008; Grover et al., 2010).

Often FI is associated with urinary incontinence and as many as 50% to 70% of patients with UI also carry the diagnosis of FI. FI can be transient (episodes of diarrhea, acute illness, fecal impaction) or persistent. Fecal incontinence, like urinary incontinence, has devastating social ramifications for the individuals and families who experience it. UI and FI share similar contributing factors, including damage to the pelvic floor as a result of surgery or trauma, neurological disorders, functional impairment, immobility, and dementia. Bowel continence and defecation depend on coordination of sensory and motor innervation of the rectum and anal sphincters. Impairment of the anorectal unit, such as weakness from prolonged straining secondary to constipation or overt anal tears seen after vaginal delivery in women (35%) are common causes of FI. Injury from obstetric trauma is often delayed in onset, and many women do not manifest symptoms until after the age of 50 years (Roach and Christie, 2008).

PROMOTING HEALTHY AGING: IMPLICATIONS FOR GERONTOLOGICAL NURSING

Assessment

Assessment should include a complete client history as in urinary incontinence (described earlier in this chapter) and investigation into stool consistency and frequency, use of laxatives or enemas, surgical and obstetrical history, medications, effect of FI on quality of life, focused physical examination with attention to the gastrointestinal system, and a bowel record. A digital rectal examination should be performed to identify any presence of a mass, impaction, or occult blood.

Interventions

Nursing interventions are aimed at managing and/or restoring bowel continence. Therapies similar to those used to treat urinary incontinence such as environmental manipulation (access to toilet), diet alterations, habit-training schedules, improving transfer and ambulation ability, sphincter-training exercises, biofeedback, medications, and/or surgery to correct underlying defects are effective.

Keeping accurate bowel records and identifying triggers that influence incontinence are important. For example, eating a meal stimulates defecation 30 minutes after completion of the meal, or defecation occurs after the morning cup of coffee. If the fecal incontinence occurs only once or twice each day, it can be controlled by being prepared. Placing the individual on the toilet, commode, or bedpan at a given time after the trigger event facilitates defecation in the appropriate place at the appropriate time (Box 11-7). The judicious use of nonirritant laxatives can help to maintain bowel function and prevent constipation.

The effectiveness of interventions in fecal incontinence will be self-evident but will take time. As in the treatment of urinary incontinence, goals must be realistic. It cannot be stated too often or too strongly that the nurse must always provide immaculate skin care to persons with incontinence, because self-esteem and skin integrity depend on it.

SLEEP

The human organism needs rest and sleep to conserve energy, prevent fatigue, provide organ respite, and relieve tension. Sleep occupies a third of our lives and is a vital function that affects cognition and performance. Attention to sleep health is one of the foci on Healthy People 2020 and includes the goal of increasing public knowledge of how adequate sleep and treatment of sleep disorders improve health, productivity, wellness, quality of life, and safety on roads and in the workplace (United States Department of Health and Human Services, 2010).

In older adults, sleep is a barometer of health. Sleep assessment and interventions for sleep concerns should receive as much attention as other vital signs. As many as 57% of older adults complain of significant sleep disruption (Bloom et al., 2009). Aging is associated with changes in the amount of sleep, sleep quality, and specific sleep pathologies and disorders such as insomnia, sleep apnea, restless legs syndrome, and circadian rhythm disturbances (Subramanian and Surani, 2007; Mitty and Flores, 2009).

Biorhythm and Sleep

Our lives proceed in a series of rhythms that influence and regulate physiological function, chemical concentrations, performance, behavioral responses, moods, and the ability to adapt. Biorhythms vary between individuals. Gerontologists are beginning to seriously study the relevance of age-related changes in biorhythms (circadian rhythms) to health and the process of aging. It is clear that body temperature, pulse, blood pressure, and hormonal levels change significantly and predictably in a circadian rhythm. Circadian rhythms are linked to the 24-hour day by time cues (zeitgebers), the most important of which is the light–dark cycle (Ham et al., 2007). These rhythms tend to be a bit longer than 24 hours and vary between individuals. With aging, there is a reduction in the amplitude of all of these circadian endogenous responses.

The most important and obvious biorhythm is the circadian sleep–wake rhythm. As people age, the natural circadian rhythm may become less responsive to external stimuli, such as changes in light during the course of the day.

Sleep and Aging

The predictable pattern of normal sleep is called sleep architecture (Subramanian and Surani, 2007). The body progresses through the five stages of the normal sleep pattern, consisting of rapid eye movement (REM) sleep and non–rapid eye movement (NREM) sleep. Sleep structure is shown in Box 11-9.

Most of the changes in sleep architecture in healthy adults begin between the ages of 40 and 60 years. Healthy aging per se does not result in insomnia (Simonson et al., 2007). Less time is spent in stages 3 and 4 sleep and more time is spent awake or in stage 1 sleep. Declines in stages 3 and 4 sleep begin between 20 and 30 years of age and are nearly complete by the age of 50 to 60 years. The amount of deep sleep in stages 3 and 4 contributes to how rested and refreshed a person feels the next day. Time spent in REM sleep also declines with age, and transitions between stages 1 and 2 are more common.

Older adults need as much sleep as younger adults, but with age sleep is lighter, more fragmented, and characterized by frequent awakenings. Older people report more time in bed, reduced total sleep time, prolonged sleep latency (time it takes to fall asleep), more frequent awakenings, increased wakefulness after sleep onset, and increased daytime somnolence (excessive

---

BOX 11-9   THE FIVE STAGES OF SLEEP

NON–RAPID EYE MOVEMENT (NREM) SLEEP

Stage 1
- Lightest level
- Easy to awaken
- Comprises 5% of sleep in young

Stage 2
- Decreases with age
- Low-voltage activity on electroencephalogram (EEG)
- May cease in old age

Stage 3
- Decreases with age
- High-voltage activity on EEG
- May cease in old age

Stage 4
- Decreases with age
- High-voltage activity on EEG
- Comprises 15% of sleep in elders

RAPID EYE MOVEMENT (REM) SLEEP
- Alternates with NREM sleep throughout the night
- Rapid eye movements are the key feature
- Breathing increases in rate and depth
- Muscle tone relaxed
- 85% of dreaming occurs in REM sleep

Adapted from Beers MH, Berkow R: *The Merck manual of geriatrics,* ed 3, Whitehouse Station, NJ, 2000, Merck Research Laboratories.

sleepiness) and daytime napping (Mitty and Flores, 2009). Sleep deprivation and fragmentation of sleep in older adults may adversely affect cognitive, emotional, and physical functioning as well as quality of life (Martin et al., 2010; Teodorescu and Husain, 2010). The changes that occur in sleep with aging are summarized in Box 11-10.

Older adults with good general health, positive moods, and engagement in more active lifestyles and meaningful activities report better sleep and fewer sleep complaints. Poor sleep is not an inevitable consequence of aging but rather an indicator of health status and calls for investigation.

SLEEP DISORDERS

Insomnia

Insomnia is defined as "a complaint of disturbed sleep in the presence of an adequate opportunity and circumstance for sleep" (Bloom et al., 2009, p. 6). The diagnosis of insomnia requires that the person have difficulty falling asleep for at least one month and that impairment in daytime functioning results from difficulty sleeping. Insomnia is classified as either primary or comorbid. Primary insomnia implies that no other cause of sleep disturbance has been identified. Comorbid insomnia is more common and is associated with psychiatric and medical disorders, medications, and primary sleep disorders, such as obstructive sleep apnea or restless legs syndrome. Comorbid insomnia does not suggest that these conditions cause insomnia but that insomnia and the other conditions co-occur and each may require attention and treatment (Bloom et al., 2009). Insomnia has a higher prevalence in older adults and, there are many influencing factors, both physiological and behavioral (Box 11-11).

Prescription and nonprescription medications also create sleep disturbances. Drugs and alcohol use are thought to account for 10% to 15% of cases of insomnia (Ham et al., 2007). Problematic drugs include serotonin reuptake inhibitors (SSRIs), antihypertensives (clonidine, β-blockers, reserpine, methyldopa), anticholinergics, sympathomimetic amines, diuretics, opiates, cough and cold medications, thyroid preparations, phenytoin, cortisone, and levodopa. The times of day that medications are given can also contribute to sleep problems—

for example, a diuretic given before bedtime or sedating medication given in the morning (Rose and Lorenz, 2010).

Sleep Apnea

Sleep apnea is a condition in which people stop breathing while asleep. Apneas (complete cessation of respiration) and hypopneas (partial decrease in respiration) result in hypoxemia and changes in autonomic nervous system activity. The result is increases in systemic and pulmonary arterial pressure and changes in cerebral blood flow. The episodes are generally terminated by an arousal (brief awakening), which results in fragmented sleep and excessive daytime sleepiness (Bloom et al., 2009). Other symptoms of sleep apnea include loud periodic snoring, gasping and choking on awakenings, unusual nighttime activity such as sitting upright or falling out of bed, morning headache, poor memory and intellectual functioning, and irritability and personality change. If the person has a sleeping partner, it is often the person who reports the nighttime symptoms.

The two types of sleep apnea are obstructive sleep apnea (OSA) and central sleep apnea (CSA). OSA, caused by obstruction of the upper airway, is the most common; CSA is due to central nervous system or cardiac dysfunction. OSA occurs in about 70% of men and 56% of women over the age of 65 years (Bloom et al., 2009). OSA is more common in Asians compared with Caucasians (Bloom et al., 2009). In long-term care facilities, the prevalence of OSA has been estimated to be as high as 70% to 80% (Rose and Lorenz, 2010). The age-related decline in the activity of the upper airway muscles, which results in compromised pharyngeal patency, predisposes older adults to OSA.

BOX 11-12   RISK FACTORS FOR SLEEP APNEA

- Increasing age
- Increased neck circumference
- Male sex
- Anatomical abnormalities of the upper airway
- Upper airway resistance and/or obstruction
- Family history
- Excess weight
- Use of alcohol, sedatives, or tranquilizers
- Smoking
- Hypertension

Data from McCance KL, Huether SE: *Pathophysiology: the biologic basis for disease in adults and children,* ed 5, St. Louis, MO, 2006, Mosby; Phillips B: Sleep apnea, periodic leg movement, restless legs syndrome and cardiovascular complications. In Sleep disorders in the geriatric population: implications for health, *Clinical Geriatrics* 12:1, 2005 (December 2005 supplement).

Older adults with sleep apnea demonstrate significant cognitive decline compared with younger people with the same disease severity. The diagnosis of sleep apnea is often delayed in older adults and symptoms are blamed on age (Subramanian and Surani, 2007). Risk factors for sleep apnea are listed in Box 11-12.

PROMOTING HEALTHY AGING: IMPLICATIONS FOR GERONTOLOGICAL NURSING

Assessment

Assessment includes information from the sleeping partner, and a sleep study is usually considered. A sleep study or polysomnogram (PSG) is a multiple-component test which electronically transmits and records specific physical activities during sleep. The data obtained is analyzed by a qualified physician to determine whether or not the person has a sleep disorder. In most cases, sleep studies take place in a sleep lab specially set up for the test and are monitored by a technician, but can also be conducted at home (http://www.talkaboutsleep.com/sleep-basics/viewasleepstudy.htm). Recognition of OSA in older adults may be more difficult because many are widowed and may not have a sleeping partner to report symptoms (Subramanian and Surani, 2007). If there is a sleeping partner, he or she may move to another room to sleep because of the disturbance to his or her own rest.

Although obesity is often associated with OSA in younger people, older adults with OSA may not necessarily be obese (Bloom et al., 2009). The neck is often short and thick. The upper airway, including the nasal and pharyngeal airways, should be examined for anatomic obstruction, tumors, or cysts. A medication review is always indicated when investigating sleep complaints.

Interventions

Therapy will depend on the severity and type of sleep apnea, as well as the presence of comorbid illnesses. Specific treatment of sleep apnea may involve weight loss, avoidance of alcohol and sedatives, cessation of smoking, and avoidance of supine sleep positions. There should be risk counseling about impaired judgment from sleeplessness and the possibility of accidents when driving. Continuous positive airway pressure (CPAP) is the most effective treatment and the treatment of choice for older adults. The CPAP device delivers pressurized air through tubing to a nasal mask or nasal pillows, which are fitted around the head. The pressurized air acts as an airway splint and gently opens the patient's throat and breathing passages, allowing them to breathe normally, but only through their nose. CPAP has been shown to be well tolerated and effective for OSA in older adults with dementia (Rose and Lorenz, 2010).

Restless Legs Syndrome

Restless legs syndrome (RLS) is a sensorimotor neurological disorder characterized by unpleasant leg sensations that disrupt sleep. RLS is categorized as primary or secondary. Primary (idiopathic) develops at a younger age with no predisposing factors and probably has a genetic basis. Secondary RLS can result from a variety of medical conditions that have iron deficiency in common, the most common being iron deficiency anemia, end-stage renal disease, and pregnancy.

Individuals with RLS have an uncontrollable need to move the legs, often accompanied by discomfort in the legs. Other symptoms include paresthesias; creeping sensations; crawling sensations; tingling, cramping, and burning sensations; pain; or even indescribable sensations. RLS has a circadian rhythm, with the intensity of the symptoms becoming worse at night and improving toward the morning. It may be temporarily relieved by movement. Impairment in dopamine transport in the substantia nigra due to reduced intracellular iron seems to play a critical role in the disease.

The estimated prevalence of RLS among people over 65 years of age is 10% to 20%, and it affects women more than men (Bloom et al., 2009). Another sleep disorder, periodic limb movements of sleep (PLMS), and periodic limb movement disorder (PLMD) are often associated with RLS. These movement disorders of sleep are sometimes called nocturnal myoclonus or periodic leg movements and involve repeated rhythmical extensions of the big toe and dorsiflexion of the ankle. Disrupted sleep is the reason people with these disorders seek help.

Antidepressants and neuroleptic medications can aggravate RLS symptoms. Increased body mass index, caffeine use, tobacco, and sedentary lifestyle are also contributing factors. Diagnosis of RLS includes ruling out and/or treating as indicated any medical condition. Oral iron supplements should be prescribed for patients with serum iron levels lower than 45 μg/L (Winkelman et al., 2007). Dopamine receptor agonists (pramipexole, ropinirole) are the drugs of choice for RLS. Gabapentin may also be effective for individuals with comorbid RLS and peripheral neuropathy (Winkelman et al., 2007; Bloom et al., 2009). Nonpharmacological therapy includes mild to moderate physical activity, hot baths, and engrossing mental activity before bedtime, avoidance of alcohol, and antidepressants and dopamine antagonist medications.

Rapid Eye Movement Sleep Behavior Disorder

Rapid eye movement sleep behavior disorder (RBSD) is a sleep disorder common in older adults. The mean age at emergence is 60 years, and RBSD is more common in males. Characteristics of RBSD are loss of normal voluntary muscle atonia during REM sleep associated with complex behavior while dreaming (Subramanian and Surani, 2007). Patients report elaborate enactment of their dreams, often with violent content, during sleep. This may include violent behaviors, such as punching and kicking, with the potential for injury of both the patient and the bed partner.

RBSD may be primary or secondary to neurodegenerative diseases such as Parkinson's disease, diffuse Lewy body disease, Alzheimer's disease, and progressive supranuclear palsy. It may also be idiopathic (Bloom et al., 2009). RBSD may be an early sign of Parkinson's disease. Within five to eight years of being diagnosed with RBSD, 60% to 80% of individuals develop Parkinson's disease (Brooks and Peever, 2008). Caffeine and some medications (SSRIs, tricyclic antidepressants) may also contribute to RBSD. Interventions include neurological examination, removal of aggravating medications, and counseling related to safety measures in the sleep environment. Clonazepam and/or melatonin may be effective in treating RBSD.

Circadian Rhythm Sleep Disorders

In circadian rhythm sleep disorders (CRSDs) relatively normal sleep occurs at abnormal times. Two clinical presentations are seen: advanced sleep phase disorder (ASPD) and irregular sleep–wake disorder (ISWD). In ASPD, the individual begins and ends sleep at unusually early times (e.g., going to bed as early as 6 or 7 PM and waking up between 2 and 5 AM). Not all individuals with an advanced sleep phase have ASPD. If the person is not bothered by their sleep phase and has no functional impairment, we may just consider them "morning" people. In irregular sleep–wake disorder, sleep is dispersed across the 24-hour day in bouts of irregular length. Factors contributing to these disorders are age-related changes in sleep and circadian rhythm regulation combined with decreased levels of light exposure and activity.

A combination of good sleep hygiene practices and methods to delay the timing of sleep and wake times are recommended as treatment for ASPD. Bright light therapy (2500 to 10,000 lux) for one to two hours at about 7 to 8 PM can help normalize or delay circadian rhythm patterns (Bloom et al., 2009).

In ISWD, the individual may obtain enough sleep over the 24-hour period, but time asleep is broken into at least three different periods of variable length. Erratic napping occurs during the day, and nighttime sleep is severely fragmented and shortened. Chronic insomnia and/or daytime sleepiness are present. ISWD is most commonly encountered in individuals with dementia, particularly those who are institutionalized. In individuals with dementia who are up at night, serious consequences such as falls and unattended home exits can occur. "Approximately 40% of individuals with dementia who died after becoming lost in the community exited the home during the night" (Rowe et al., 2010, p. 339). Sleep disturbances of individuals with dementia are often among the reasons for nursing home placement. Other central nervous system disorders can also lead to this condition. Treatment consists of increasing the duration and intensity of light exposure during the daytime and avoiding exposure to bright light in the evening. Structured activity during the day and a quiet sleeping environment may also improve ISWD (Bloom et al., 2009).

PROMOTING HEALTHY AGING: IMPLICATIONS FOR GERONTOLOGICAL NURSING

Assessment

Sleep habits should be reviewed with older adults in all settings. Many people do not seek treatment for insomnia and may blame poor sleep on the aging process. Nurses are in an excellent position to assess sleep and suggest interventions to improve the quality of the older person's sleep. Assessment for sleep disorders and contributing factors to poor sleep (pain, chronic illness, medications, alcohol use, depression, anxiety) are important.

The nurse should learn how well the person sleeps at home, how many times the person is awakened at night, what time the person retires, and what rituals occur at bedtime. Rituals include bedtime snacks, watching television, listening to music, or reading—activities whose execution is crucial to the individual's ability to fall asleep. Other assessment data should include the amount and type of daily exercise; favorite position when in bed; room environment, including temperature, ventilation, and illumination; activities engaged in several hours before bedtime; medications taken for sleep as well as information about all medications taken. Additional assessment data include information about the individual's involvement in hobbies, life satisfaction, perception of health status, and assessment for depression. The patient's bed partner, caregivers, and/or family members can also provide valuable information about the person's sleep habits and lifestyle.

In institutions, there is often limited communication between night and day staff, as well as a lack of emphasis on the importance of sleep patterns. Night shift nursing staff have the opportunity to assess sleep patterns and implement appropriate interventions to enhance sleep. Kerr and Wilkinson (2010) offer comprehensive suggestions for night staff, including the development of overnight care plans. The sleep diary or log is also an important part of assessment (Box 11-13). This information will provide an accurate account of the person's sleep problem

---

BOX 11-13   SLEEP DIARY

Instructions: Record the following for two to four weeks. To be completed by the person or caregiver if the person is unable.

- The number of times a call for assistance to the bathroom or for pain medication or subjective symptoms of inability to sleep (e.g., anxiety) occur
- Whether the person appears to be asleep or awake when checked during the night
- If sleep medication was given and if repeated
- The time the person awakens in the morning
- Where the person falls asleep in the evening
- Daytime naps
- Daytime activity/exercise

and help identify the sleep disturbance. Usually a family member, or the caregiver if the older person is institutionalized, records the person's behavior 24 hours per day for five days. In addition to sleep behaviors at night, the sleep log also provides information about daytime sleepiness or changes in behavior during the day. A period of two to four weeks is needed to obtain a clear picture of the sleep problem.

Subjective and objective measures included in sleep assessment that are available to nurses include visual analog scales, subjective rating scales (e.g., 0 to 10 or 0 to 100), questionnaires that determine whether one's sleep is disturbed, interviews, and daily sleep charts. A self-rating scale, the Pittsburgh Sleep Quality Index (PSQI), can be used to measure the quality and patterns of sleep in the older adult, and daytime sleepiness can be assessed with the Epworth Sleepiness Scale (see Box 11-1). Objective measures include polysomnography conducted in sleep laboratories, including electroencephalograms (EEGs), electromyograms (EMGs), wrist actigraphy, and direct observations.

Interventions

Nonpharmacological Treatment   Interventions begin after a thorough sleep history has been recorded and, if possible, a sleep log obtained. Management is directed at identifiable causes. Pharmacological treatment should be considered an adjuvant treatment to nonpharmacological interventions. Attention to sleep hygiene principles is important to promote good sleep habits (Box 11-14). Cognitive behavioral therapy using stimulus control, sleep restriction therapy, relaxation

therapy, and exercise is effective and produces sustained positive effects. These administered behaviour treatments have been reported to be an effective and practical treatment for chronic insomnia in older adults (Buysse et al., 2011). Tai Chi Chih can be considered a useful nonpharmacological approach for sleep complaints (Irwin et al., 2008) (see Chapter 12).

Results of the Nighttime Insomnia Treatment and Education in Alzheimer's Disease study (NITE-AD) (McCurry et al., 2005), a treatment program using behavioral strategies with persons with dementia and their caregivers living in the community, suggest the following behavioral techniques to enhance sleep for individuals with AD: sleep hygiene education, daily walking, and increased light exposure. A sleep education program, designed for adult family homes, derived from this research, is provided by McCurry and colleagues (2009). Caregivers of individuals with dementia also experience poor sleep quality, and this influences caregiver stress as well as health problems (Rowe et al., 2010).

In hospital and institutional settings, promotion of a good sleep environment is important. A sleep improvement protocol, including do-not-disturb periods; provision of usual bedtime routines; and use of soft music, relaxation techniques, massage, and aromatherapy might improve sleep in hospital and nursing home settings. A multidisciplinary approach to identify sources of noise and light, such as equipment and staff interactions, could result in modification without compromising safety and quality of patient care. "Because a full sleep cycle of 90 minutes can have a positive influence on sleep effectiveness," efforts to allow sufficient time for a full sleep cycle are important (Missildine, 2008; Missildine et al., 2010).

Further research is needed on the sleep problems of older adults in both community and institutional settings. "Correcting a complex phenomenon like sleep–wake pattern disturbance will require bundled interventions" (Richards et al., 2005, p. 1516). Suggested interventions to reduce daytime sleepiness and enhance nighttime sleep among residents of long-term care facilities are presented in Box 11-15.

Pharmacological Treatment   Medications may be used in combination with behavioral interventions but must be chosen carefully, started at the lowest possible dosage, and monitored closely to avoid untoward effects in older adults. Patients should be educated on the proper use of medications and their side effects. Sedatives and hypnotics, including benzodiazepines and barbiturates, should be avoided. In long-term care settings, there are specific regulatory guidelines on the use of hypnotics, including appropriate prescribing and tapering and discontinuation of use. Over-the-counter (OTC) drugs such as diphenhydramine, often thought to be relatively harmless, should be avoided because of antihistaminic and anticholinergic side effects.

Benzodiazepine receptor agonists, such as zolpidem, eszopiclone, and zaleplon, have shorter half-lives and more favorable safety profiles for older adults. Because of the rapid action of these drugs, they should be taken immediately before bedtime. Ramelteon, a melatonin receptor agonist that promotes sleep via action on the circadian system, may cause less psychomotor and cognitive impairment in older people (Zee and Bloom, 2006; Subramanian and Surani, 2007).

BOX 11-14   SLEEP HYGIENE RULES

- Make sure the bedroom is restful and comfortable.
- Use the bedroom only for sleep and sex; do not watch television from bed or work in bed.
- Have a regular bedtime and wake-up time even on weekends.
- Avoid naps. If you must nap, sleep no longer than 30 minutes in the early afternoon (before 3 PM).
- Get regular exercise, but avoid exercising within four hours of bedtime.
- Get regular exposure to natural light.
- Wind down during the evening; have a bedtime routine, such as brush teeth, set alarm clock, and read.
- Limit caffeine (tea, cola, coffee, chocolate), nicotine, and diuretics, especially late in the day.
- Avoid alcohol for at least two hours before bedtime, and don't use alcohol to promote sleep.
- If you have reflux, eat the evening meal at least three to four hours before bedtime; have a light snack if needed before bedtime. Avoid being too hungry or too full at bedtime.
- Give attention to the bed environment (comfortable bed, pillows between the knees, quiet, darkness, comfortable temperature).
- Do not watch the clock, which increases anxiety and pressure to sleep; if anxious, take a warm bath.
- Avoid working on the computer before bedtime.
- If you cannot fall asleep, get up and go to another room. Stay up as long as needed to feel sleepy. Return to bed when sleepy. If unable to sleep again after 10 minutes, repeat and get up as long as needed.

Adapted from Beers MH, Berkow R: *The Merck manual of geriatrics*, ed 3, Whitehouse Station, NJ, 2000, Merck Research Laboratories; Zee P, Bloom H: Understanding and resolving insomnia in the elderly, *Geriatrics* (Suppl May):1-12, 2006.

- Encouraging residents to stay out of bed between 8:00 AM and 8:00 PM
- Providing 30 minutes or more of sunlight exposure in a comfortable outdoor location
- Providing low-level physical activity three times a day
- Keeping noise down, reducing light in hallways and resident rooms, quiet music, and performing necessary care (e.g., turning, changing) when the individual is awake rather than waking the individual up between the hours of 10:00 PM and 6:00 AM
- Limit intake of caffeine and other fluids in excess before bedtime.
- Provide a light snack or warm beverage before bedtime.
- Maintain a quiet environment: soft lights, quiet music, and limited noise and staff intrusions when possible.
- Discontinue invasive treatments when possible (Foley catheters, percutaneous gastrostomy tubes, intravenous lines).
- Encourage and assist to the bathroom before bed and as needed.
- Give pain medication before bedtime for patients with pain.
- Allow resident to stay out of bed and out of the room for as long as possible before bed.
- Institute the same time for resident to arise and get out of bed every morning.
- Maintain comfortable temperature in room; provide blankets as needed.
- Provide meaningful activities (individualized and group) during the daytime.

Adapted from Cefalu C: Evaluation and management of insomnia in the institutionalized elderly, *Annals of Long-term Care* 12:25, 2004; and Richards K, Beck C, O'Sullivan P, et al: Effect of individualized social activity on sleep in nursing home residents with dementia, *Journal of the American Geriatrics Society* 53:1510, 2005.

| BOX 11-16 | PHYSIOLOGICAL FUNCTIONS OF THE SKIN |

- Protects underlying structures
- Regulates body temperature
- Serves as a vehicle for sensation
- Stores fat
- Is a component of the metabolism of salt and water
- Is a site for two-way gas exchange
- Is a site for the production of vitamin D when exposed to sunlight

| BOX 11-17 | TIPS FOR HEALTHY SKIN |

- Watch for any break in the skin, and initiate treatment as soon as possible.
- For those with diabetes or peripheral vascular disease (PVD), consult a health care provider promptly if a skin break occurs.
- Use a humidifier if necessary to keep the room humid.
- When bathing, use tepid water only; and limit time in the water, which dehydrates skin.
- Use only mild skin cleaners without perfume or lanolin. Apply to damp skin after bathing or washing.
- Pat dry; do not rub.
- Do not add bath oil to water to minimize the risk of slipping.
- Apply moisturizers as often as necessary to maintain continuous coverage.
- Choose clothing made of soft cotton or other nonabrasive materials.
- Drink several glasses of water every day to maintain systemic hydration.
- Protect the skin from exposure to cold temperatures.

SKIN

The skin is the largest organ of the body and has at least seven physiological functions (Box 11-16). Exposure to heat, cold, water, trauma, friction, and pressure notwithstanding, the skin's function is to maintain a homeostatic environment. Healthy skin is durable, pliable, and strong enough to protect the body by absorbing, reflecting, cushioning, and restricting various substances and forces that might enter and alter its function; yet it is sensitive enough to relay subtle messages to the brain. When the integument malfunctions or is overwhelmed, discomfort, disfigurement, or death may ensue. However, the nurse can both promptly recognize and help to prevent many of the sources of danger to a person's skin in the promotion of the best possible health. Tips for maintaining healthy skin can be found in Box 11-17.

Many skin problems are seen with aging, both in health and when compromised by illness or mobility limitations. The skin problems seen in older adults are influenced by the environment and age-related changes. The most common skin problems of aging are xerosis (dry skin), pruritus, seborrheic keratosis, herpes zoster, and cancer. Those who are immobilized or medically fragile, such as residents of nursing facilities, are at risk for fungal infections and pressure ulcers, both major threats to wellness.

Common Skin Problems
Xerosis

Xerosis is extremely dry, cracked, and itchy skin. Xerosis is the most common skin problem experienced by older people and may be linked to a dramatic age-associated decrease in

epidermal filaggrin, a protein required for binding keratin filaments into macrofibrils. This leads to separation of dermal and epidermal surfaces, which compromises the nutrient transfer between the two layers of the skin. Xerosis occurs primarily in the extremities, especially the legs, but can affect the face and the trunk as well. The thinner epidermis of older skin makes it less efficient, allowing more moisture to escape. Inadequate fluid intake worsens xerosis as the body will pull moisture from the skin in an attempt to combat systemic dehydration.

Exposure to environmental elements such as artificial heat, decreased humidity, use of harsh soaps, and frequent hot baths or hot tubs contributes to skin dryness (called a "winter itch"). Nutritional deficiencies and smoking lead to dehydration of the outer layer of the epidermis. Hospitals and nursing homes accelerate the development of xerosis through routine bathing, use of drying soap, prolonged bed rest, and the action of bed linen on the patient's skin. For persons with incontinence, the skin must be protected from both the burning of urine or feces and from excess dryness that arises from the frequent washing and drying that is necessary. Dry skin may be just dry skin, but it may also be a symptom of more serious systemic disease (e.g., diabetes mellitus, hypothyroidism, renal disease) or dehydration.

Pruritus

One of the consequences of xerosis is *pruritus,* that is, itchy skin. It is a symptom, not a diagnosis or disease, and is a threat to skin integrity because of the attempts to relieve it by scratching. It is aggravated by perfumed detergents, fabric softeners, heat, sudden temperature changes, pressure, vibration, electrical stimuli, sweating, restrictive clothing, fatigue, exercise, and anxiety. Pruritus also may accompany systemic disorders such as chronic renal failure, biliary or hepatic disease, and iron deficiency anemia. The gerontological nurse should always listen carefully to the patient's ideas of why the pruritus is occurring and what relieves it and what aggravates it.

Scabies

Scabies is a skin condition that causes intense itching, particularly at night. Scabies is caused by a tiny burrowing mite called *Sarcoptes scabiei*. Scabies is contagious and can spread quickly though close physical contact in a family, child care group, school class, or other close communal living facilities such as nursing homes. To diagnose scabies, a close skin examination is conducted to look for signs of mites, including their characteristic burrows. A scraping may be taken from an area of skin for microscopic examination to determine the presence of mites or their eggs.

Scabies treatment involves eliminating the infestation with prescribed lotions and creams (Elimite, Lindane). Treatment is usually provided to family members and other close contacts even if they show no signs of scabies infestation. Medication kills the mites but itching may not stop for several weeks. The oral medication ivermectin (Stromectol) may be prescribed for individuals with altered immune systems, for those with crusted scabies, or for those who do not respond to prescription lotions and creams. All clothes and linen used at least three times before treatment should be washed in hot, soapy water and dried with high heat.

Purpura

Thinning of the dermis leads to increased fragility of the dermal capillaries and to blood vessels rupturing easily with minimal trauma. Extravasation of the blood into the surrounding tissue, commonly seen on the dorsal forearm and hands, is called *purpura*. These are not related to a bleeding disorder, and individuals who are prone to purpura should be advised to protect the skin against trauma and friction. Health care personnel must be advised to be gentle when handling the skin of older patients because even minor trauma can cause purpura. Long-sleeved shirts reduce shear and friction, and protect the skin against trauma. If a skin tear occurs, use non-adherent dressings secured with tubular retention bandages (Ham et al., 2007).

Keratoses

There are two types of keratosis: seborrheic and actinic. *Actinic keratosis* is a precancerous lesion and is discussed later in the chapter. *Seborrheic keratosis* is a benign growth that appears mainly on the trunk, the face, the neck, and the scalp as single or multiple lesions. One or more lesions are present on nearly all adults older than 65 years and are more common in men. An individual may have dozens of these benign lesions. Seborrheic keratosis is a waxy, raised, verrucous lesion, flesh-colored or pigmented in various sizes. The lesions have a "stuck on" appearance, as if they could be scraped off. Seborrheic keratoses may be removed by a dermatologist for cosmetic reasons. A variant seen in darkly pigmented persons occurs mostly on the face and appears as numerous small, dark, possibly taglike lesions (see www.dermatlas.com).

Herpes Zoster

Herpes zoster (HZ), or shingles, is a viral infection frequently seen in older adults. HZ is caused by reactivation of latent varicella-zoster virus (VZV) within the sensory neurons of the dorsal root ganglion decades after initial VZV infection is established. Approximately one in three persons will develop zoster during their lifetime, resulting in an estimated one million episodes in the United States annually. HZ occurs most commonly in adults over the age of 50 years, those who have medical conditions that compromise the immune system, or people who receive immunosuppressive drugs.

HZ always occurs along a nerve pathway, or *dermatome*. The more dermatomes involved, the more serious the infection, especially if it involves the head. When the eye is affected it is always a medical emergency. Most HZ occurs in the thoracic region but it can also occur in the trigeminal area and cervical, lumbar, and sacral areas. HZ vesicles never cross the midline. In most cases, the severity of the infection increases with age.

The onset may be preceded by itching, tingling, or pain in the affected dermatome several days before the outbreak of the rash. It is important to differentiate HZ from herpes simplex. Herpes simplex does not occur in a dermatome pattern and is recurrent. During the healing process, clusters of papulovesicles develop along a nerve pathway. The lesions themselves eventually rupture, crust over, and resolve. Scarring may result, especially if scratching or poor hygiene leads to a secondary bacterial infection. HZ is infectious until it becomes crusty. HZ may be very painful and pruritic.

Prompt treatment with the oral antiviral agents acyclovir, valacyclovir, and famciclovir decreases the severity and duration of acute pain from zoster. Zoster vaccine is recommended for all persons aged 60 years and over who have no contraindications, including persons who report a previous episode of zoster or who have chronic medical conditions. Before administration of the vaccine, patients do not need to be asked about their history of varicella or have serologic testing to determine varicella immunity (Centers for Disease Control and Prevention, 2008).

A common complication of HZ is postherpetic neuralgia (PHN), a chronic, often debilitating pain condition that can last months or even years. The risk of PHN in patients with HV is 10% to 18%. Another complication of HZ is eye involvement, which occurs in 10% to 25% of zoster episodes and can result in prolonged or permanent pain, facial scarring, and loss of vision. The pain of PHN has been difficult to control and can significantly affect one's quality of life. The American Academy of Neurology (2004) treatment guidelines for PHN include the use of tricyclic antidepressants, anticonvulsants, lidocaine skin patches, and opioids, as well as nonpharmacological treatments such as stress reduction techniques and behavioral cognitive therapy. Assessment and management of pain are discussed in Chapter 17.

Photo Damage of the Skin

Although exposure to sunlight is necessary for the production of vitamin D, the sun is also the most common cause of skin damage and skin cancer. "Photo-damage, not the aging process, has been estimated to account for 90% of age-associated cosmetic problems" (Ham et al., 2007, p. 616). With the accumulated years of sun exposure, the risk is significantly increased for older adults. The damage (photo or solar damage) comes from prolonged exposure to ultraviolet (UV) light from the environment or in tanning booths. Although the amount of sun-induced damage varies with skin type and genetics, much of the associated damage is preventable. Ideally, preventive measures begin in childhood, but clinical evidence has shown that some improvement can be achieved at any time by limiting sun exposure and using sunscreens regularly.

Skin Cancers

Cancer of the skin (including melanoma and nonmelanoma skin cancer) is the most common of all cancers. The exact number of basal and squamous cell cancers is not known for certain because they are not reported to cancer registries, but it is estimated that there are more than two million basal and squamous cell skin cancers found each year. Most of these (about 800,000 to 900,000) are basal cell cancers. Squamous cell cancer is less common. Most of these are curable; the type with the greatest potential to cause death is melanoma.

The American Cancer Society estimates that about 68,130 new melanomas will be diagnosed in the United States during 2010 (about 38,870 in men; 29,260 in women). Incidence rates for melanoma have been increasing for at least 30 years. In recent years, the increases have been most pronounced in young white women and in older white men. Melanoma is more than 10 times more common in white Americans than in African Americans. It is slightly more common in men than in women (American Cancer Society, 2010).

Persons with a history of sunburns, use of tanning beds, skin cancer, or exposure to carcinogenic materials, or with sun sensitivity or a depressed immune system, are at particular risk. Increasing age along with a history of sun exposure increases one's risk even further.

Actinic Keratosis

Actinic keratosis is a precancerous lesion that may become a squamous cell carcinoma. It is directly related to years of overexposure to UV light. Risk factors are older age and fair complexion. It is found on the face, the lips, and the hands and forearms, areas of chronic sun exposure in everyday life. Actinic keratosis is characterized by rough, scaly, sandpaper-like patches, pink to reddish-brown on an erythematous base (Figure 11-5). Lesions may be single or multiple; they may be painless or mildly tender. The person with actinic keratoses should be monitored by a dermatologist every 6 to 12 months for any change in appearance of the lesions. Early recognition, treatment, and removal of these lesion is easy and important. Removal is aimed at preventing the possible conversion to a malignant lesion.

Basal Cell Carcinoma

Basal cell carcinoma is the most common malignant skin cancer. It occurs mainly in older age groups but is occurring more and more in younger persons. It is slow-growing, and metastasis is rare. A basal cell lesion can be triggered by extensive sun

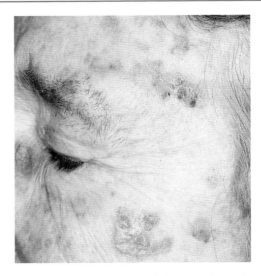

FIGURE 11-5 Actinic Keratosis in an Older Adult in an Area of Sun Exposure. (From Habif TP: *Clinical dermatology: a color guide to diagnosis and therapy,* ed 3, St. Louis, MO, 1996, Mosby.)

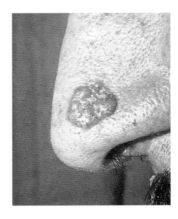

FIGURE 11-6 Basal Cell Carcinoma, the Most Commonly Occurring Skin Cancer. (Courtesy Gary Monheit, MD, University of Alabama at Birmingham School of Medicine.)

exposure, especially burns, chronic irritation, and chronic ulceration of the skin. It is more prevalent in light-skinned persons. It usually begins as a pearly papule with prominent telangiectasias (blood vessels) or as a scarlike area with no history of trauma (Figure 11-6). Basal cell carcinoma is also known to ulcerate. It may be indistinguishable from squamous cell carcinoma and is diagnosed by biopsy. Early detection and treatment are necessary to minimize disfigurement.

Squamous Cell Carcinoma

Squamous cell carcinoma is the second most common skin cancer. However, it is aggressive and has a high incidence of metastasis if not identified and treated promptly. Squamous cell cancer is more prevalent in fair-skinned, elderly men who live in sunny climates and is usually found on the head, the neck, or the hands. Individuals in their mid-60s who have been or are chronically exposed to the sun (e.g., persons who work out of doors, are athletes, etc.) are prime candidates for this type of cancer. Less common causes include chronic stasis ulcers, scars from injury, and exposure to chemical carcinogens, such as topical hydrocarbons, arsenic, and radiation. The lesion begins

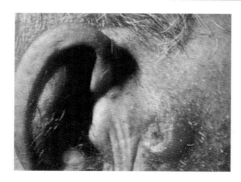

FIGURE 11-7 Squamous Cell Carcinoma. (Courtesy Gary Monheit, MD, University of Alabama at Birmingham School of Medicine.)

BOX 11-18 ABCD RULES FOR MELANOMA

*A*symmetry: One half does not match the other half.
*B*order irregularity: The edges are ragged, notched, or blurred.
*C*olor: The pigment is not uniform in color, having shades of tan, brown, or black, or a mottled appearance with red, white, or blue areas.
*D*iameter: The diameter is greater than the size of a pencil eraser or increasing in size.

---

as a firm, irregular, fleshy, pink-colored nodule that becomes reddened and scaly, much like actinic keratosis, but it may increase rapidly in size. It may also be hard and wartlike with a gray top and horny texture, or it may be ulcerated and indurated with raised, defined borders (Figure 11-7). Because it can appear so differently, it is often overlooked or thought to be insignificant. The best advice to give older patients, especially those who live in sunny climates, is that they should be regularly screened by a dermatologist.

Melanoma

Melanoma, a neoplasm of the melanocytes, accounts for less than 5% of skin cancer cases, but it causes most skin cancer deaths. The number of new cases of melanoma in the United States has been increasing for at least 30 years. Overall, the lifetime risk of getting melanoma is about 1 in 50 for the white population, 1 in 1,000 for black individuals, and 1 in 200 for the Hispanic population. Men have a higher rate of melanoma than women and a person who has already had a melanoma has a higher risk of developing another one. The risk of melanoma is more than 10 times higher for white Americans than for African Americans. White individuals with fair skin, freckles, and red or blond hair have a higher risk for melanoma. Red-haired people have the highest risk. The legs and backs of women, and the backs of men, are the most common sites of melanoma. Although melanoma occurs more often in older people, it is one of the most common cancers in people under the age of 30 years. Melanoma has a high mortality rate because of its ability to metastasize quickly (American Cancer Society, 2010).

The primary risk factor for melanoma is too much exposure to UV radiation. Many studies have linked melanoma on the trunk, legs, and arms to frequent sunburns, especially in childhood. Blistering sunburns before the age of 18 years are thought to damage Langerhans cells, which affect the immune response of the skin and increase the risk for a later melanoma. Two thirds of melanomas develop from preexisting moles; only one third arise alone. Melanoma has a classical multicolor, raised appearance with an asymmetrical, irregular border. It may appear to be of any size, but the surface diameter is not necessarily reflective of the size beneath the surface, similar in concept to an iceberg. It is treatable if caught early, before it has a chance to invade surrounding tissue. If the nurse finds any questionable lesions, the individual should be referred to a dermatologist immediately. The "ABCD" approach to assessing such potential lesions is used (Box 11-18).

PROMOTING HEALTHY AGING: IMPLICATIONS FOR GERONTOLOGICAL NURSING

The nurse caring for older adults is in an ideal position to promote healthy skin in older adults and provide health education to prevent skin problems. In doing so, quality of life and comfort can be significantly improved.

Xerosis

Because one of the major causes of xerosis is age-related changes, the nurse attends to environmental prevention and treatment and provides expert skin care. Maintaining an environment of about 60% humidity is a start. The challenge is to find ways to rehydrate the epidermis, especially the outer layer, called the *stratum corneum.*

The skin can only be hydrated with water. Topical skin products can help retain natural moisture in the skin. Most lubricants such as creams, lotions, and emollients work by trapping moisture and are most effective when applied to towel-patted, damp skin immediately after a bath. Bath oils and other hydrophobic preparations may also be used to hold in moisture. Light mineral oil is as effective and more economical than commercial brands of lotions and oils. However, oils poured directly into a tub or shower increase the risk for falls. It is safer and more effective to apply the oil directly to the moist skin. Water-laden emulsions without perfumes or alcohol are best.

To prevent excessive loss of moisture and natural oil during bathing, only tepid water temperatures and super-fatted soaps or skin cleansers without hexachlorophene or alcohol should be used. Older people may not need daily baths or showers. "Sponge" bathing armpits, groin, perineal areas, and any other parts of the body that need care can be recommended. The need for "squeaky clean" skin is an American cultural oddity. Products such as Cetaphil, Basis, Dove, Tone, and Caress soaps or Jergens, Neutrogena, and Oil of Olay bath washes are effective in helping to prevent the loss of the protective lipid film from the skin surface. Deodorant soaps and detergents contain alcohol as drying agents and should be avoided, except in places such as the axilla and the groin.

In cases of extreme dryness, petroleum jelly can be applied to the affected areas before bed, and the skin will be smoother and moister in the morning. Oils and ointments with zinc oxide are designed to coat the skin and replace the skin's natural oil barrier. This approach is often used to prevent excoriations from feces or urine. However, these can only be used on clean skin.

Pruritus

When xerosis leads to pruritus, the goal is to reduce and hopefully alleviate the itching. If rehydration of the stratum corneum is not sufficient to control itching, cool compresses, or oatmeal or Epsom salt baths, may be helpful. Failure to control the itching increases the risk for eczema, excoriations, cracks in the skin, inflammation, and infection arising from the usually linear excoriations from scratching. The nurse should be alert to signs of infection; rough, scaly, or flaky skin; and accompanying pruritus anywhere on the body.

Cancer

The nurse also has an active role in the prevention and early recognition of skin cancers. This role may include working with community awareness and education programs, screening clinics, and direct care. In promoting skin health, the nurse is vigilant in observing skin for the changes that require further evaluation.

Age-related skin changes, such as thinning and diminished melanocytes, significantly increase the risk for solar damage and subsequent skin cancer. By far the most important preventive nursing intervention is to provide education regarding the risks of photo and smoke damage. Preventive strategies include the use of sunscreens and protective clothing and limiting sun exposure (Box 11-19).

Secondary prevention is in the form of early diagnosis. After a thorough clinical screening, the elder and his or her intimate partner can be taught to perform regular "checks" of each other's skin, watching for signs of change and the need to contact a primary care provider or dermatologist promptly. For the person with keratosis and multiple freckles (nevi), photographing the body parts may be a useful reference. The adage "when it doubt, get it checked" is an important one and regular screenings should be a part of the health care of all older adults.

BOX 11-19   SUN PROTECTION RECOMMENDATIONS

- Avoid the midday sun (10 AM to 3 PM), when the ultraviolet radiation is most intense.
- Use sunscreen daily (if going outside) regardless of the weather in sunny or potentially sunny regions.
- For partial protection, wear clothing that covers the exposed areas of the skin and a broad-brimmed hat to protect the face and the top of head, especially if working outside in sunny regions.
- Select and use a sunscreen with a sun protection factor (SPF) of 15 or higher. Apply before sun exposure, and reapply periodically after perspiring heavily or swimming.
- Avoid getting sunburned, and limit sun exposure at all times.
- Be aware of reflection from sand, snow, and water, which will intensify the radiation.
- Avoid sun if taking photosensitizing drugs such as the tetracyclines.
- Avoid sunscreens with para-aminobenzoic acid (PABA) if allergic to procaine, sulfonamides, or hair dyes, because of cross-sensitization.
- Avoid tanning beds and sun lamps.

Other Skin Conditions

Combined with the skin changes discussed previously, older people who are more frail or physically ill and in hospitals or nursing homes are at more risk for the development of pressure ulcers as well as fungal skin infections.

Candidiasis (Candida albicans)

The fungus *Candida albicans* (referred to as "yeast") is present on the skin of healthy persons of any age. However, under certain circumstances and in the right environment, a fungal infection can develop. Persons who are obese, malnourished, receiving antibiotic or steroid therapy, or have diabetes are at increased risk. *Candida* grows especially well in areas that are moist, warm, and dark, such as in skinfolds, in the axilla and the groin, and under pendulous breasts. It can also be found in the corners of the mouth associated with the chronic moisture of angular cheilitis. In the vagina it is also called a "yeast infection." If this is found in an older woman, it may mean that her diabetes either has not yet been diagnosed or is in poor control.

Inside the mouth a *Candida* infection is referred to as "thrush" and is associated with poor hygiene and immunocompromise, such as those with long-term steroid use (e.g., because of chronic obstructive pulmonary disease), who are receiving chemotherapy, or who test positive for or are infected with human immunodeficiency virus (HIV) or have acquired immunodeficiency syndrome (AIDS). In the mouth, candidiasis appears as irregular, white, flat to slightly raised patches on an erythematous base that cannot be scraped off. The infection can extend down into the throat and cause swallowing to be painful. In severely immunocompromised persons the infection can extend down the entire gastrointestinal tract.

On the skin, *Candida* is usually maculopapular, glazed, and dark pink in persons with less pigmentation and grayish in persons with more pigmentation. If it is advanced, the central area may be completely red and/or dark, and weeping with characteristic bright red and/or dark satellite lesions (distinct lesions a short distance from the center). At this point the skin may be edematous, itching, and burning.

The best approach to managing fungal infections is to prevent them, and the key to prevention is limiting the conditions that encourage fungal growth. Prevention is prioritized for persons who are obese, bedridden, incontinent, or diaphoretic. In contrast to the treatment of dry skin, attention is given to the adequate drying of bodily target areas after bathing, the prompt management of incontinent episodes, the use of loose-fitting cotton clothing and underwear, the changing of clothing when damp, and the avoidance of incontinence products that are tight or have plastic that touches the skin.

One of the best ways to dry hard-to-reach, vulnerable areas is with a hair dryer set on low. A folded, dry washcloth or cotton sanitary pad can be placed under the breasts or between skinfolds to promote exposure to air and light. Cornstarch should never be used because it promotes the growth of *Candida* organisms. Optimizing nutrition and glycemic control is also important.

The goal of treatment is to eradicate the infection. This includes not only the use of prescribed antifungal medication, but also the active involvement of the nurse to reduce or eliminate the conditions that created the problem. The affected area of the skin must be cleansed carefully and dried thoroughly before antifungal preparations are applied. A mild soap or cleansing agent, such as Cetaphil, should be used. Antifungal preparations come as powders, creams, and lotions. Because the latter two trap moisture, the powder is recommended. They are usually needed for 7 to 14 days or until the infection is completely cleared. Antifungal medications include miconazole (Micatin), clotrimazole (Lotrimin), nystatin (Mycostatin), and econazole (Spectazole). Treatment of oral *Candida* infection includes mouth swishing and swallowing with an antifungal suspension and/or sucking on antifungal troches. Angular cheilitis is treated by application of a topical antifungal ointment to the corners of the mouth. If the *Candida* cannot be eliminated in the usual course of therapy, it may be necessary to use ketoconazole or fluconazole systemically for a prescribed period.

Pressure Ulcers
Definition
The European Pressure Ulcer Advisory Panel (EPUAP) and the National Pressure Ulcer Advisory Panel (NPUAP) constitute an international collaboration convened to develop evidence-based recommendations to be used throughout the world to prevent and treat pressure-related wounds. According to this group, a pressure ulcer is "an injury to the skin and/or underlying tissue resulting from pressure or in combination with shear, usually over a bony prominence" (EPUAP and NPUAP, 2009). As tissue is compressed, blood is diverted and blood vessels are forcibly constricted by the persistent pressure on the skin and underlying structures; thus cellular respiration is impaired and cells die from ischemia and anoxia. Intervention at any point in this development can stop the advancement of the pressure ulcer.

Just how much pressure can be endured by tissue (tissue tolerance) is highly variable from body location to location and person to person. Tissue tolerance is inversely affected by moisture, amount of pressure, friction, shearing, and age and is directly related to malnutrition, anemia, and low arterial pressure.

Prevalence
There are few good nationwide studies of pressure ulcers but estimates are that they affect 1.3 to 3 million people in the United States. Older people account for 70% of all pressure ulcers (Jamshed and Schneider, 2010). Several studies have reported a higher prevalence and incidence of pressure ulcers among African Americans in nursing homes than other race groups, and these differences remain after adjustment for clinical risk factors and sociodemographic and facility characteristics (Baumgarten et al., 2004; Lapane et al., 2005; Howard and Taylor, 2009).

Pressure ulcers occur in all settings across the continuum, with the highest incidence reported in hospitalized vulnerable older people undergoing orthopedic procedures (9% to 19%) and individuals with quadriplegia (33% to 60%). Baumgarten and colleagues (2009) reported that approximately one third of hip fracture patients develop at least one new pressure ulcer, at stage 2 or higher, within 32 days of hospital admission.

The NPUAP reported that the prevalence of pressure ulcers in acute care settings ranged from 10% to 18%, with 2.3% to 28% in long-term care and 0% to 29% in home care. There is wide variability among institutions. Differences in sample characteristics and study methodologies affect these statistics, but it is clear that pressure ulcers are a significant problem in all settings (Jamshed and Schneider, 2010; Plawecki et al., 2010).

Cost and Regulatory Requirements
Prevention of pressure ulcers is seen as a "key quality indicator of nursing care and pressure ulcers are widely supported as a nursing sensitive outcome" (Jull and Griffiths, 2010, p. 531). In gerontological nursing, pressure ulcers are recognized as a geriatric syndrome and efforts at prevention have always been considered an essential nursing intervention, particularly in long-term care (Armstrong et al., 2008). "Though nursing homes have been grappling with increasingly tight regulatory standards regarding wound care for two decades, there have been no similar regulatory incentives for hospitals" (Levine, 2008).

In 2008, the Centers for Medicare & Medicaid (CMS) included hospital-acquired pressure ulcers as one of the eight preventable adverse events. Hospitals will no longer receive additional reimbursement to care for a patient who has acquired pressure ulcers under the hospital's care (https://www.cms.gov/HospitalAcqCond/06_Hospital-Acquired_Conditions.asp?). With estimated annual costs for pressure ulcer treatment in hospitals in excess of $5 billion (average cost per case estimated at $43,180 per hospital stay), this has the potential to greatly increase the financial strain for facilities that fail to rise to this challenge (Armstrong et al., 2008; Levine, 2008).

Characteristics
Pressure ulcers can develop anywhere on the body but are seen most frequently on the posterior aspects, especially the sacrum, the heels, and the greater trochanters. Secondary areas of breakdown include the lateral condyles of the knees and the ankles. The pinna of the ears is another area subject to breakdown, as are the elbows and the scapulae. If one is lying prone, the knees, the shins, and the pelvis sustain undue pressure.

Heels are particularly prone to the development of pressure ulcers because they are small surfaces that receive a high degree of pressure. In many cases, heel ulcers are inevitable in the presence of peripheral vascular insufficiency combined with immobility. In the acute care setting, patients who are supine for prolonged periods, such as during surgical procedures, may exit the operating room with newly acquired pressure ulcers.

Classification
The EPUAP and NPUAP recommend a four-category classification of pressure ulcers. The NPUAP also describes two additional categories for the United States that do not fall into one of the established or classifiable categories: suspected deep tissue injury and unstageable or unclassified wound (Box 11-20). Suspected deep tissue injury is defined by a localized area of intact skin or blood-filled blister, maroon or purple in color, caused by damage of the underlying soft tissue from shear and/or pressure (Plawecki et al., 2010). Wounds that are covered

BOX 11-20   PRESSURE ULCER STAGES

SUSPECTED DEEP TISSUE INJURY

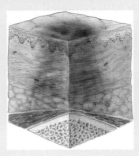

Purple or maroon localized area of discolored intact skin or blood-filled blister due to damage of underlying soft tissue from pressure and/or shear. Visible damage in the area may be preceded by tissue that is painful, firm, mushy, boggy, warmer, or cooler as compared with adjacent tissue.

Further description—Deep tissue injury may be difficult to detect in individuals with dark skin tones. Evolution may include a thin blister over a dark wound bed. The wound may further evolve and become covered by thin eschar. Evolution may be rapid, exposing additional layers of tissue even with optimal treatment.

STAGE I

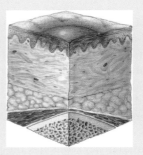

Intact skin with nonblanchable redness of a localized area, usually over a bony prominence. Darkly pigmented skin may not have visible blanching; its color may differ from the surrounding area.

Further description—The area may be painful, firm, soft, warmer, or cooler as compared with adjacent tissue. Stage I may be difficult to detect in individuals with dark skin tones. May indicate "at risk" persons (a heralding sign of risk).

STAGE II

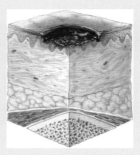

Partial thickness loss of dermis presenting as a shallow open ulcer with a reddish pink wound bed, without slough. May also present as an intact or open/ruptured serum-filled blister.

Further description—Presents as a shiny or dry shallow ulcer without slough or bruising.*

This stage should not be used to describe skin tears, tape burns, perineal dermatitis, maceration, or excoriation.

STAGE III

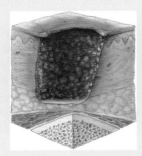

Full-thickness tissue loss. Subcutaneous fat may be visible but bone, tendon, and muscle are not exposed. Slough may be present but does not obscure the depth of tissue loss. May include undermining and tunneling.

Further description—The depth of a stage III pressure ulcer varies by anatomical location. The bridge of the nose, ear, occiput, and malleolus do not have subcutaneous tissue, and stage III ulcers can be shallow. In contrast, areas of significant adiposity can develop extremely deep stage III pressure ulcers. Bone or tendon is not visible or directly palpable.

STAGE IV

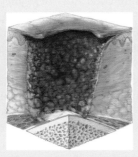

Full-thickness tissue loss with exposed bone, tendon, or muscle. Slough or eschar may be present on some parts of the wound bed. Often includes undermining and tunneling.

Further description—The depth of a stage IV pressure ulcer varies by anatomical location. The bridge of the nose, ear, occiput, and malleolus do not have subcutaneous tissue, and these ulcers can be shallow. Stage IV ulcers can extend into muscle and/or supporting structures (e.g., fascia, tendon, or joint capsule), making osteomyelitis possible. Exposed bone or tendon is visible or directly palpable.

UNSTAGEABLE

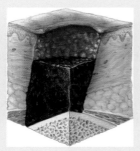

Full-thickness tissue loss in which the base of the ulcer is covered by slough (yellow, tan, gray, green, or brown) and/or eschar (tan, brown, or black) in the wound bed.

Further description—Until enough slough and/or eschar is removed to expose the base of the wound, the true depth, and therefore stage, cannot be determined. Stable (dry, adherent, intact without erythema or fluctuance) eschar on the heels serves as "the body's natural (biological) cover" and should not be removed.

*Bruising indicates suspected deep tissue injury.

with black (eschar) or yellow fibrous (slough) necrosis cannot be staged because it is not possible to determine the condition of the underlying wound bed. These wounds are documented as unstageable or unclassified. Once the dead tissue has been removed (debrided), the wound can be staged.

The ulcer is always classified by the highest stage "achieved," and reverse staging is never used. This means that the wound is documented as the stage representing the maximal damage and depth that has occurred. As the wound heals, it fills with granulation tissue composed of endothelial cells, fibroblasts, collagen, and an extracellular matrix. Muscle, subcutaneous fat, and dermis are not replaced. A stage IV pressure sore that is healing does not revert to stage III and then stage II. It remains defined as a healing stage IV pressure ulcer.

Risk Factors

Many factors increase the risk of pressure ulcers in older adults including changes in the skin, comorbid illnesses, nutritional status, cognitive deficits, and reduced mobility. "The primary risk factors for pressure ulcer development are immobility and limited activity with positioning that exerts unrelieved pressure on tissue confined between nonpliable surfaces" (Ham et al., 2007, p. 374). Individuals confined to bed or chair, who are unable to shift weight or reposition themselves at regular intervals, are at greatest risk. Tissue tolerance, in addition to unrelieved pressure, contributes to the risk of a pressure ulcer. Tissue tolerance is related to the ability of the tissue to distribute and compensate for pressure exerted over bony prominences. Factors that affect tissue tolerance include moisture, friction, shear force, nutritional status, age, sensory perception, and arterial pressure (de Souza et al., 2010).

Prevention

Although often repeated, prevention is the key to pressure ulcer treatment. Systematic prevention programs have been shown to decrease hospital-acquired pressure ulcers by 34% to 50% (Ham et al., 2007; Armstrong et al., 2008). However, "despite a number of national prevention initiatives and existing evidence-based protocols, pressure ulcer frequency has not declined in recent years and pressure ulcers continue to have a negative impact on patient outcomes and health care costs in a variety of care settings" (Baumgarten et al., 2009, p. 253). Several studies have reported that compliance with evidence-based protocol recommendations is a concern (Spillsbury et al., 2007; Baumgarten et al., 2009) (Box 11-21).

Early identification of risk status is critical so that timely interventions can be designed to address specific risk factors. The Braden Scale for Predicting Pressure Sore Risk, developed by Barbara Braden and Nancy Bergstrom, is widely used and clinically validated. This scale assesses the risk of pressure ulcers on the basis of a numerical scoring system of six risk factors: sensory perception, moisture, activity, mobility, nutrition, and friction/shear. For a video on the use of the Braden Scale see Box 11-1. Because the Braden Scale does not include all of the risk factors for pressure ulcers, it is recommended that it be used as an adjunct rather than in place of clinical judgment. A thorough patient history to assess other risk factors such as age, medications, comorbidities (diabetes, peripheral vascular disease [PVD]), history of pressure ulcers,

BOX 11-21 RESEARCH HIGHLIGHTS

Use of Pressure-redistributing Support Services among Patients with Hip Fractures

The purpose of the study was to estimate the frequency of pressure-redistributing support surfaces (PRSS) among patients with hip fractures and to determine whether higher pressure ulcer risk is associated with greater PRSS use. The sample included 658 individuals over the age of 65 years (Mean, 83.2) who had surgery for hip fracture. Participants were examined by research nurses at baseline and on alternating days for 21 days. Information was obtained on PRSS use and pressure ulcer risk factors.

The odds of PRSS use were lower in the rehabilitation setting, in the nursing home, and during readmissions to acute care than in the initial acute setting. The relationships between PRSS use and pressure ulcer risk factors were not strong. Adherence to guidelines for PRSS use was low, with only 57% of the participants in the acute care setting using PRSS. Hip fracture is a significant risk factor for pressure ulcers and PRSS is a recommendation in evidence-based practice guidelines. Adherence to guidelines for PRSS use was low and not guided by the evidence or adequate assessment of patient risk. There is an urgent need for improvement of care to prevent pressure ulcers in high-risk patients.

Baumgarten M, Margolis D, Orwig D, et al: Use of pressure-redistributing support services among elderly hip fracture patients across the continuum of care: adherence to pressure ulcer prevention guidelines, *The Gerontologist* 50:253, 2009.

and other factors is important to fully address the risk of pressure ulcer development so that appropriate preventive interventions can be developed (Armstrong et al., 2008; Jull and Griffiths, 2010).

A consensus paper from the International Expert Wound Care Advisory Panel (Armstrong et al., 2008) provides recommendations for prevention of pressure ulcers that include patient education, clinician training for all members of the health care team, strategies in developing communication and terminology materials, implementation of toolkits and protocols (prevention bundles), documentation checklists, outcome evaluation, quality improvement efforts, evidence-based treatment protocols, and appropriate products. It is important to note that not all pressure ulcers may be avoidable. Gravely ill patients facing multiple organ failure, reduced tissue perfusion, and no mobility (e.g., at the end of life) are especially at high risk Armstrong and colleagues (2008) note: "the skin, like any other organ in the body, can fail."

Consequences

Pressure ulcers are costly to treat and prolong recovery and extend rehabilitation. Complications include the need for grafting or amputation, sepsis, or even death, and may lead to legal action by the individual or his or her representative against the caregiver. The personal impact of a pressure ulcer on health and quality of life is also significant and not well understood or researched. Findings from a study exploring patients' perceptions of the impact of a pressure ulcer and its treatment on health and quality of life suggest that pressure ulcers cause suffering, pain, discomfort, and distress that is not always recognized or adequately treated by nursing staff. Pressure ulcers had a profound impact on the patients' lives, physically, socially, emotionally, and mentally (Spillsbury et al., 2007).

PROMOTING HEALTHY AGING: IMPLICATIONS FOR GERONTOLOGICAL NURSING

The treatment and prevention of pressure ulcers is complex and does not belong to any one specialty; a team approach that involves primary care providers, nursing staff, physical therapists, nutritionists, and other clinicians is the most effective approach (Armstrong et al., 2008). Nursing staff, as direct caregivers, are key team members who perform skin assessment, identify risk factors, and implement numerous preventive interventions. The nurse alerts the health care provider of the need for prescribed treatments, recommends treatments, and administers and evaluates the changing status of the wound(s) and adequacy of treatments.

Assessment

Assessments are performed on admission and whenever there is a change in the status of the patient. Assessment begins with a history, detailed head-to-toe skin examination, nutritional evaluation, and analysis of laboratory findings. Laboratory values that have been correlated with risk for the development and the poor healing of pressure ulcers include those that reflect anemia and poor nutritional status. Visual and tactile inspection of the entire skin surface with special attention to bony prominences is essential. Inspection is best accomplished in nonglare daylight or, if that is not possible, with focused lighting. Special attention should be directed to affected areas when an individual uses orthotic devices such as corsets, braces, prostheses, postural supports, splints, slings, or casts.

The nurse looks for any interruption of skin integrity or other changes, including redness or hyperemia. If pressure is present, it should be relieved and the area reassessed in one hour. In darker-pigmented persons, redness and blanching may not be observed. The wound may appear like a bruise. Observe for induration, darkening, change in color from surrounding skin, or a shadowed appearance of the skin. The affected skin area, when compared with adjacent tissues, may be firm, warmer, cooler, or painful (Plawecki et al., 2010).

It is necessary to look for induration, darkening, or a shadowed appearance of the skin and to feel for warmth or a boggy texture to the affected tissue compared with the surrounding tissue. Pressure areas and surrounding tissue should be palpated for changes in temperature and tissue resilience. Blisters or pimples with or without hyperemia and scabs over weight-bearing areas in the absence of trauma should be considered suspect.

Ulcers are assessed with each dressing change for worsening, with a detailed assessment repeated on a weekly, biweekly, and as-needed basis (see Box 11-22). The purpose is to specifically and carefully evaluate the effectiveness of treatment. If there are no signs of healing from week to week or worsening of the wound is seen, then either the treatment is insufficient or the wound has become infected; in both cases, treatment must be changed.

Lastly, careful and detailed documentation of the condition of the skin is required. The PUSH tool (Pressure Ulcer Scale for

---

BOX 11-22   KEY ASPECTS OF ASSESSMENT OF A PRESSURE ULCER

- Location and exact size (width, depth, length)
- Condition of the surrounding tissue
- Condition of the wound edges: for example, smooth and white or irregular and pink
- Wound bed: warmth, moisture, color, odor, amount, and color of exudates

---

Healing) provides a detailed form that covers all aspects of assessment, but contains only three items and takes only a short time to complete (Gardner et al., 2005). Most institutions have special forms or screens on their computer software for recording skin assessments. The Agency for Healthcare Research and Quality (AHRQ) provides the On-Time Pressure Ulcer Healing Project (http://www.ahrq.gov/research/pressureulcerhealing/). The focus of this project is on prevention and timely treatment of pressure ulcers in long-term care. Tools to document pressure ulcer healing and treatments and reports to monitor the healing process are available. For those persons with ulcers, photographic documentation is highly recommended both at the onset of the problem and at intervals during its treatment (Ahn and Salicido, 2008). The reader is referred to the NPUAP website (www.npuap.org) for more information.

Interventions

The goal of nurses is to help maintain skin integrity against the various environmental, mechanical, and chemical assaults that are potential causes of breakdown. In promoting healthy aging of all persons, nurses focus on prevention, taking action to eliminate friction and irritation to the skin, such as from shearing; to reduce moisture so that tissues do not macerate; and to displace body weight from prominent areas to facilitate circulation to the skin. The nurse should be familiar with the types of supportive surfaces and types of dressings so that the most effective products are used. The nurse should assess the frequency of position change, adding pillows so that skin surfaces do not touch, and establish a turning schedule if needed.

Nutritional intake should be monitored, as well as the serum albumin, hematocrit, and hemoglobin levels (Chapters 8 and 14). Caloric, protein, vitamin, and/or mineral supplementation can be considered if there is evidence of deficiencies of these nutrients. Routine use of higher than the recommended daily allowance of vitamin C and zinc for the prevention and/or treatment of pressure ulcers is not supported by evidence (Jamshed and Schneider, 2010). The nurse promotes nutritional health by ensuring that the person receives adequate assistance with eating and that dining time is a pleasant experience for the person (see Chapter 14).

Although a full discussion of the treatment options and indications for their use in the nursing care and treatment of pressure ulcers is beyond the scope of this text, key points in the promotion of healing can be found in Box 11-23. The type of dressing selected is based on the condition of the ulcer; the presence of granulation, necrotic tissue, and slough; the amount of drainage; microbial status; and the quality of the surrounding skin. "Too frequently, aggressive and expensive interventions are implemented without attention to basic care practices

BOX 11-23   PROMOTING WOUND HEALING

- Keep wound warm at all times.
- Keep wound clean and moist at all times.
- Protect wound from further injury.
- Promptly absorb exudate and fill dead space with a biofriendly material (e.g., alginate).
- Use normal saline for cleansing; do not subject tissue to caustic products (e.g., povidone-iodine [Betadine]).

such as provision of adequate nutrition, good hygiene, and proper positioning" (Ham et al., 2007, p. 375).

Provision of education to patients, families, and professional staff must also be included in any skin care program. Consultation with a wound care specialist is advisable for wounds that are extensive or nonhealing. Specialized nurses such as enterostomal therapists or nurse practitioners who may work with wound centers or surgeons provide consultation in nursing homes, offices, or clinics.

HEALTHY FEET

Feet influence one's physical, psychological, and social well-being. Feet carry one's body weight, hold the body erect, coordinate and maintain balance in walking, and must be rigid yet loose and adaptable enough to conform to changing walking surfaces. Little attention is given to one's feet until they interfere with walking and moving and ultimately the ability to remain independent.

Nurses and people in general have a fairly strong negative reaction to having contact with others' feet. It is aesthetically unpleasant to many. Foot problems in older people often are unrecognized and untreated, leading to considerable dysfunction (Anderson et al., 2010). Yet, promoting healthy feet and good care of the feet can alleviate disability and pain, and decrease the risk for falling. It is for these reasons that this text emphasizes the importance of feet to the well-being of the older adult.

Common Foot Problems

The human foot is a complex structure with many bones, joints, tendons, muscles, and ligaments. Some foot irregularities and problems are genetically inherited; however, many problems occur because of the shoes we wear, wear and tear, and misuse of feet. Shoe styles affect the foot, the hip, and the leg.

Older feet, subjected to a lifetime of stress, may not be able to continue to adapt, and inflammatory changes in bone and soft tissue can occur. Many older adults are limited by foot problems; approximately 90% of adults 65 and older have some form of altered foot integrity such as nail fungus, dry skin, and corns and calluses (Anderson et al., 2010). Foot health and function may reflect systemic disease or give early clues to physical illness. Sudden or gradual changes in the condition of the nails or the skin of the feet or the appearance of recurring infections may be precursors of more serious health problems. Rheumatological disorders such as the various forms of arthritis usually affect other joints but can also affect the feet.

Gout occurs most often in the joint of the great toe but is a systemic disease. Both diabetes and PVD commonly cause problems in the lower extremities that can quickly become life-threatening.

Major abnormalities occur gradually. Without proper care and treatment, these conditions become disabling and threatening to the person's mobility and independence. Care of the foot takes a team approach, including the person, the nurse, the podiatrist, and the person's primary health care provider. Nurses have the opportunity to promote healthy aging by applying their knowledge of the common problems of the feet and their skills in foot care.

Corns, Calluses, and Bunions

Corns and *calluses* are both growths of compacted skin that occur as a result of prolonged pressure, usually from ill-fitting, tight shoes. Corns are cone-shaped and develop on the top of the toe joints from the rubbing of the shoe on the joint. Soft corns form between opposing surfaces of the toes from prolonged squeezing. Both can interfere with the ability to walk and wear shoes comfortably. Once formed, continued pressure on the corn will cause pain. Unless the friction and pressure are relieved, they will continue to enlarge and cause increasing pain.

Many elders self-treat corns and calluses by following what they or their parents have done for years. Over-the-counter preparations may remove the corn temporarily but may also burn the surrounding healthy tissue. Chemical burns and ulcerations from these products can result in the loss of toes or a leg for the person with diabetes, with neurological impairment, or with poor circulation in the lower extremity. Some people use razor blades and scissors to removed the affected tissue; this is dangerous and is never recommended. Padding and protecting the affected area is the best practice. Oval corn pads, moleskin, or lamb's wool, with a hole cut in the center for the corn, can be used for more proper treatment. This can be placed around the corn, protecting it from pressure without restricting circulation to healthy tissue.

Moleskin is a skin-protective product available in the foot care section of pharmacies and hiking supply stores. Moleskin adheres for several days or longer but should be removed when it becomes wet or excessively soiled. Removing moleskin from the feet should be done slowly to prevent tearing of skin. For persons prone to calluses, daily lubrication of the feet is important. For persons with PVD and diabetes, foot care should be performed only by a trained nurse, doctor, or podiatrist.

Irritation from soft corns between the toes can be eased by loosely wrapping small amounts of lamb's wool around the involved toe, or cotton balls can be placed between the toes. Newer pads of a gel type are also useful to protect against friction and pressure. Mild corns may resolve themselves when pressure is removed and the offending shoes are replaced by others with a better fit. Larger or resistant corns may need surgical removal by a podiatrist. Corns are not usually removed from high-risk persons, such as those with diabetes or PVD, because of the risk of poor wound healing at the surgical site.

Bunions are bony deformities that also develop from longstanding squeezing together of the first (great) and second toes. Bony prominences develop over the medial aspect of the joint of the great toe and, at times, at the lateral aspect of the fifth metatarsal head (the joint of the little toe). In this last area, the bunion is called a *tailor's bunion* or a *bunionette*. There may be a hereditary factor in their development. Walking can be markedly compromised with any of these. Bunions may be treated with corticosteroid injections or antiinflammatory pain medications. A custom-made shoe should be considered. Shoes that provide forefront space (e.g., running shoes) work well. Surgery is an option as well.

Hammer Toes

A *hammer toe* is permanently flexed with a clawlike appearance; the condition is a result of muscle imbalance and pressure from the big toe slanting toward the second toe. The toe then contracts, leaving a bulge on top of the joint. It is aggravated, again, by poor-fitting shoes and is often seen in conjunction with bunions. This condition limits the ability to walk and restricts balance and comfort. As with bunions, treatment includes professional orthotics or specially designed protective devices; properly fitting, nonconstricting shoes; and/or surgical intervention.

Fungal Infections

Fungal infections are common on the aging foot, and the incidence increases with age. A fungal infection may affect the skin of the foot as well as the nails. Nail fungus, or *onychomycosis*, the most common nail disorder, is characterized by degeneration of the nail plate with color changes to yellow or brown and opaque, brittleness, and thickening of the nail (Figure 11-8). A fine powdery collection of fungus forms under the center of the nail, separating the layers and pushing it up, causing the sides of the nail to dig into the skin like an ingrown toenail. Culturing is the only definitive way to diagnose onychomycosis. Hands should be washed each time feet with a fungal infection are handled.

When nails are involved, cure is difficult to impossible because of the limited circulation to the nails. Several oral medications are available, but all are expensive and of limited effectiveness, are taken for long periods of time (3 to 12 months), and are potentially toxic to the liver and heart. A promising treatment is photodynamic therapy (PDT). In PDF, near infrared, dual wave length optical energy is pulsed on the skin using special equipment. While further study is necessary to support the use of PDT for superficial fungal infections of the skin and nails, the technology is well established for other dermatological conditions with good outcomes (Anderson et al., 2010).

Fungal infection of the foot *(tinea pedis)* is due to many of the same causes as *Candida* infections elsewhere on the body. *Tinea pedis* is treated similarly to any other fungal infections. Feet, especially the areas between the toes, should be kept dry and clean and regularly exposed to sun and air. Topical application of antifungal powders, in addition to the hygiene measures already noted, is the usual treatment. If exacerbated by diabetes, glycemic control is an additional goal.

PROMOTING HEALTHY AGING: IMPLICATIONS FOR GERONTOLOGICAL NURSING

Assessment

The gerontological nurse is an advocate for promoting the best foot health possible. Foot care is a prime factor in the maintenance of mobility and independence. Nursing care of the person with foot problems should be directed toward optimal comfort and function, removing possible mechanical irritants, and decreasing the likelihood of infection. The nurse has the important function of assessing the feet for clues of functional ability and their owner's well-being—not just bathing and applying lotion to the feet (Box 11-24). Nurses can identify potential and actual problems and make referral to or seek assistance as needed from the primary care provider or podiatrist for any changes in the feet.

Assessment also includes observation of gait, postural deformities, physical limitations, position of the foot with the heel strike, and the type of shoe worn and its condition, including sole wear. Inspect feet for irritation, abrasions, and other lesions; check for hazards to the maintenance of adequate circulation to the lower extremities and the existing circulatory status; and observe the individual's general mobility. Routine assessment of the feet is especially important for persons with diabetes, heart disease, PVD, and thyroid or renal conditions as well as any neurological impairment, such as reduced or absent sensation resulting from a stroke.

Interventions

Care of the Toenails

Care of the feet and nails of persons in the long-term care setting falls to the nurse. Poor close vision, difficulty bending, obesity, or increased nail thickness makes self-care difficult. Normal nails that become too long will begin to interfere with stockings, hose, or shoes. Ideally, toenails should be trimmed after the bath or shower when they are softened, but if this is not possible, soaking the feet for 20 to 30 minutes before care is sufficient. They should be clipped straight across and even with the top of the toe, with the edges filed slightly to remove the sharpness but not to the point of rounding (Figure 11-9).

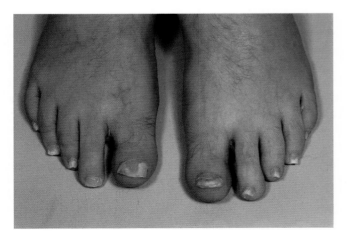

FIGURE 11-8 Onycholysis, Yellowing, Crumbling, and Thickening of the Toenails. (From Bolognia J, Jorizzo JL, Rapini RP: *Dermatology*, ed 2, St. Louis, MO, 2007, Mosby.)

BOX 11-24   ESSENTIAL ASPECTS OF FOOT ASSESSMENT

OBSERVATION OF MOBILITY
- Gait
- Use of assistive devices
- Footwear type and pattern of wear

PAST MEDICAL HISTORY
- Neuropathies
- Musculoskeletal limitations
- PVD
- Vision problems
- History of falls
- Pain affecting movement

BILATERAL ASSESSMENT
- Color
- Circulation and warmth
- Pulses
- Structural deformities
- Skin lesions
- LE edema
- Evidence of scratching
- Rash or excessive dryness
- Condition and color of toenails

LE, lower extremity; *PVD*, peripheral vascular disease.

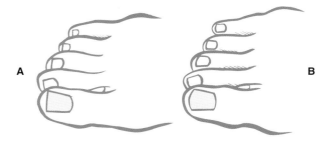

FIGURE 11-9 Cutting Toenails. A, Correct method. **B,** Incorrect method.

Diabetic foot care should be done only by a podiatrist or registered nurse (RN) with some experience, with special care to prevent accidental damage or trauma to the skin. Diabetic nail care can never be delegated to the licensed practical nurse (LPN) or certified nurse assistant (CNA). Persons with diabetes or peripheral neuropathy should never have pedicures from commercial establishments.

Nails that are neglected will become long and curved. This type of nail is known as *ram's horn* because of its appearance.

Hard, thickened nails indicate inadequate nutrition to the nail matrix because of trauma or poor circulation. Once the nail becomes thickened, it will remain so. Nails that are thick and hard split easily, causing trauma to the matrix, pain, and possibly infection. Any attempt by the nurse or other caregiver to cut these nails may result in further damage to the matrix or precipitate an infection. These conditions should be brought to the attention of a podiatrist.

An ingrown toenail is a fragment of nail that pierces the skin at the edge of the nail. Often this problem is a consequence of the hypertrophy of the nail with onychomycosis, of improper cutting of the nail, or of pressure exerted on the toes by tight hosiery or shoes. Ingrown toenails should be referred to the podiatrist because of the risk of infection. Temporary relief can be provided by inserting a small piece of cotton under the affected nail corner.

Nursing interventions include assisting the older person to understand the necessity of appropriate footwear and how to obtain it. Shoes should be new enough to provide support and should not have excessive sole wear, especially in any one area. For persons with diabetes or other neurological impairments, the shoes should cover and protect the foot entirely without pressure areas. For persons with arthritis, firm soles are more comfortable than soft soles and may decrease pain associated with walking.

Shoes should be functional, that is, they should cover, protect, and stabilize the foot and provide maximal toe space. They must also be the right size. One foot is usually larger than the other, and feet lengthen slightly with age and are largest in the afternoons. Shoes should be fitted to the largest foot, and afternoon purchases are advised. There should be about a half inch of space (a "thumb's width") from the longest toe to the tip of the shoe while the person is standing. Shoes should provide enough forefoot space laterally and dorsally with a wide toe box and comfortable fit, such as that found in ultralight walking shoes and running shoes. Fabric shoes are not recommended for persons with diabetes or PVD. Low-heeled shoes place less stress on the legs and back than completely flat shoes and are ideal for comfort.

Slip-on shoes are helpful for those who are unable to bend or lace shoes, but care must be taken that the person will not accidentally "slip out" of the shoe, which can lead to a fall. Velcro closures are useful for those who have limited finger dexterity. Custom-made shoes, although expensive, may be necessary for persons with bunions or any other deformity. These come in a broad range of prices. As the time of this writing, Medicare will cover the cost of one pair of orthotic shoes per year for persons with diabetes when purchased from an approved vendor.

KEY CONCEPTS

- Use of evidence-based protocols and best practice gerontological nursing care is essential to promote normal elimination, sleep, and healthy skin and feet. Alterations in these basic needs can significantly affect health, well-being, and quality of life as one ages.
- UI is a symptom of an underlying problem and needs thorough assessment. Many therapeutic modalities are available for treatment of UI.
- In addition to age-related changes in sleep architecture, many chronic conditions interfere with quality and quantity of sleep in older adults. Complaints of sleep difficulties should be thoroughly investigated and not attributed to age. Nonpharmacological interventions should always be included in any plan of care to improve sleep.
- The skin is the largest and most visible organ of the body; it has multiple roles in maintaining one's health.
- With aging, maintaining adequate hydration and skin lubrication will reduce the incidence of xerosis and other skin problems.
- The best way to minimize the risk of skin cancer is to avoid prolonged sun and smoke exposure.

- The primary risk factors for pressure ulcer development are immobility and reduced activity. Changes in the skin with age, comorbid illnesses, nutritional status, low body mass, shear, and friction also increase pressure ulcer risk. Individuals at greatest risk include those who are confined to bed or chair and unable to shift weight or reposition themselves.
- Structured protocols and prevention bundles (toolkits) should be present in all facilities and have been shown to reduce pressure ulcer development.
- A pressure ulcer is documented by stage, which reflects the greatest degree of tissue damage; as a pressure ulcer heals, reverse staging is not appropriate.
- A pressure ulcer that is covered with dead tissue (eschar or slough) cannot be staged until it has been debrided.
- Darkly pigmented persons will not display the "typical" erythema of a stage I pressure ulcer. Deep tissue injury may be difficult to detect in individuals with dark skin tones. Evolution may include a thin blister over a dark wound bed.
- Mobility is fundamental to independence; therefore care of the feet and toenails is an important area for the gerontological nurse.

CASE STUDY   REST AND SLEEP

Gerald, 80 years old, had a sleeping disorder and was tired most of the day and lonely at night. His wife of 45 years had recently moved into her sewing room on the couch at night because she could no longer cope with his loud snoring. He sometimes even seemed to stop breathing, which kept her awake watching his abdomen rise and fall, or not. Sometimes he would awaken suddenly, gasping for air. However, he had tolerated it because he thought nothing could be done for it. Because it had become a threat to his marriage, he became motivated to investigate possible solutions. Gerald said to his nurse clinician, "This isn't anything, but it upsets my wife." Although he did not admit it, he was also worried because he was beginning to feel rather weak and listless during the day. When he had consulted the clinic nurse, Gerald was diagnosed with obstructive sleep apnea. He found that some very practical means of dealing with this problem of sleep apnea were available, and if these were not effective, she had reassured him that additional medical interventions could be helpful.

On the basis of the case study, develop a nursing care plan using the following procedure*:
- List Gerald's comments that provide subjective data.
- List information that provides objective data.
- From these data, identify and state, using accepted format, two nursing diagnoses you determine are most significant to Gerald at this time. List two of Gerald's strengths that you have identified from the data.

- Determine and state outcome criteria for each diagnosis. These must reflect some alleviation of the problem identified in the nursing diagnosis and must be stated in concrete and measurable terms.
- Plan and state one or more interventions for each diagnosed problem. Provide specific documentation of the source used to determine the appropriate intervention. Plan at least one intervention that incorporates Gerald's existing strengths.
- Evaluate the success of the intervention. Interventions must correlate directly with the stated outcome criteria to measure the outcome success.

CRITICAL THINKING QUESTIONS
1. What lifestyle factors may be increasing Gerald's episodes of sleep apnea?
2. In what circumstances is sleep apnea particularly dangerous to health?
3. Compose a list of 10 questions you would ask Gerald to obtain a clear picture of factors contributing to his sleep apnea. Discuss the rationale behind each.
4. List some of the common methods for dealing with this problem that Gerald's nurse may have given to him.

*Students are advised to refer to their nursing diagnosis text and identify possible or potential problems.

CASE STUDY   ELIMINATION

Stella, at 78 years old, had never had problems with her bowel movements. They had been regular—each morning about an hour after breakfast. In fact, she hardly thought about them because they had been so regular. While hospitalized for podiatric surgery last year, she never regained her usual pattern of bowel function. She was greatly distressed by this because it had been a symbol to her of her good health. Admittedly, she did not move about as much now or as well and had begun using a cane. And she had heard that pain medications sometimes made one constipated, so she tried to use them very sparingly despite

the pain. She tried to reestablish her pattern of having a bowel movement every morning after breakfast but with little success. She now began to worry about constipation and to use laxatives. She thought, "This constipation really upsets me. I just don't feel like myself if I don't have a bowel movement every day."

On the basis of the case study, develop a nursing care plan using the following procedure*:
- List Stella's comments that provide subjective data.
- List information that provides objective data.

Continued

- From these data, identify and state, using accepted format, two nursing diagnoses you determine are most significant to Stella at this time. List two of Stella's strengths that you have identified from the data.
- Determine and state outcome criteria for each diagnosis. These must reflect some alleviation of the problem identified in the nursing diagnosis and must be stated in concrete and measurable terms.
- Plan and state one or more interventions for each diagnosed problem. Provide specific documentation of the source used to determine the appropriate intervention. Plan at least one intervention that incorporates Stella's existing strengths.
- Evaluate the success of the intervention. Interventions must correlate directly with the stated outcome criteria to measure the outcome success.

CRITICAL THINKING QUESTIONS

1. What information will you need to obtain from Stella to help her determine the causes of her constipation?
2. What advice will you give Stella regarding the use of laxatives?
3. What dietary changes will you suggest to her, and how will you do this to encourage modifications?
4. What information regarding the relationship of medications to constipation will be useful to Stella?
5. When you are constipated, how do you feel?
6. Do you know any elders who focus a lot of their conversation on elimination? How do you handle that? How should you handle that?

*Students are advised to refer to their nursing diagnosis text and identify possible or potential problems.

RESEARCH QUESTIONS

Elimination

1. What strategies can enhance the use of nonpharmacological interventions to promote normal bowel function?
2. What are the specific concerns of older people related to constipation?
3. Do childhood training experiences affect one's eliminatory functions in late life?
4. What is the knowledge level of graduating nursing students and practicing nurses in UI care?
5. What factors are associated with effective implementation and maintenance of PV programs in long-term care?

Rest and Sleep

6. How do sleep patterns correlate with various disease states?
7. What is the average time of the total sleep cycle as experienced by a healthy individual older than 70 years?

8. How much does exercise contribute to a good night's sleep?
9. What is the effect of nonpharmacological interventions on sleep?
10. What are the concerns of caregivers of persons with dementia as they relate to sleep?

Skin and Foot Care/Pressure Ulcers

11. What is the knowledge level of older adults about pressure ulcer risk?
12. What are the major barriers identified by nursing staff to implementation of preventive interventions for pressure ulcers?
13. How effective are current patient education materials in enhancing knowledge of pressure ulcer risk among racially and culturally diverse older people?

REFERENCES

Ahn C, Salicido RS: Advances in would photography and assessment methods, *Advances in Skin & Wound Care* 21:94, 2008

Anderson J, White K, Kelechi T: Managing common foot problems in older adults, *Jour Gerontol Nurs* 36(10):9-14, 2010.

American Academy of Neurology: AAN evidence-based guideline summary for clinicians: treatment of postherpetic neuralgia (2004). Available at http://www.aan.com/professionals/practice/pdfs/pn_guideline_physicians.pdf. Accessed December 2010.

American Cancer Society: Learn about cancer (2010). Available at http://www.cancer.org/Cancer/index. Accessed December 2010.

Armstrong D, Ayello E, Capitulo K, et al: Opportunities to improve pressure ulcer prevention and treatment: implementation of the CMS inpatient hospital care present on admission (POA) indicators/hospital acquired conditions (HCA) policy, *Wounds* 20:A14, 2008. Available at http://www.medscape.com/viewarticle/581767. Accessed December 2010.

Barton C, Sklenicka J, Sayegh P, et al: Contraindicated medication use among patients in a memory disorders clinic,

American Journal of Geriatric Pharmacotherapy 6:147, 2008.

Baumgarten M, Margolis D, van Doorn C, et al: Black/white differences in pressure ulcer incidence in nursing home residents, *Journal of the American Geriatrics Society* 52:1293, 2004.

Baumgarten M, Margolis D, Orwig D, et al: Use of pressure-redistributing support surfaces among elderly hip fracture patients across the continuum of care: adherence to pressure ulcer prevention guidelines, *The Gerontologist* 50:253, 2009.

Beverley L, Travis I: Constipation: proposed natural laxative mixtures, *Journal of Gerontological Nursing* 18:5, 1992.

Bloom H, Ahmed I, Alessi C, et al: Evidence-based recommendations for the assessment and management of sleep disorders in older persons, *Journal of the American Geriatrics Society* 57:761, 2009.

Brooks P, Peever J: Glycinergic and GABAA–mediated inhibition of somatic motor neurons does not mediate rapid eye movement sleep motor atonia, *Journal of Neuroscience* 28:3535, 2008.

Bucci A: Be a continence champion: use the CHAMMP tool to individualize the plan of care, *Geriatric Nursing* 28:120, 2007.

Buysse D, Germain A, Moul D, Franzen P, Brar L, et al: Efficacy of brief behavioral treatment for chronic insomnia in older adults, Archives of Internal Medicine. Published online January 24, 2011. doi: 10.1001/*Arch Intermed*, 535: E1-E8, 2010.

Cash B: Chronic constipation—defining the problem and clinical impact, *Medscape Gastroenterology* 7:2005. Available at www.medscape.com/viewarticle/501467. Accessed December 2010.

Centers for Disease Control and Prevention (CDC): Prevention of herpes zoster: recommendations of the Advisory Committee on Immunization Practices (ACIP) (2008). Available at http://www.cdc.gov/mmwr/preview/mmwrhtml/rr57e0515a1.htm?s_cid=rr57e0515_e. Accessed December 2010.

DeMaagd G: Urinary incontinence: treatment update with a focus on pharmacological management, *U.S. Pharmacist* 32:34, 2007.

de Souza DM, Santos V, Iri H, et al: Predictive validity of the Braden Scale for pressure ulcer risk in elderly residents of long-term care facilities, *Geriatric Nursing* 31:95, 2010.

Dowling-Castronovo A, Bradway C: Assessment and management of older adults with urinary incontinence (2007). Available at http://hartfordign.org/uploads/File/gnec_state_of_science_papers/gnec_incontinence.pdf. Accessed December 2010.

Dowling-Castronovo A, Bradway C: Urinary incontinence (UI) in older adults admitted to acute care. In: Capezuti E, Zwicker D, Mezey M, et al, editors: *Evidence-based geriatric nursing protocols for best practice*, ed 3, New York, 2008, Springer.

DuBeau CE: Therapeutic/pharmacologic approaches to urinary incontinence in older adults, *Clinical Pharmacology* 85:98, 2009.

European Pressure Ulcer Advisory Panel and National Pressure Ulcer Advisory Panel: Pressure ulcer treatment: quick reference guide (2009). Available at http://www.npuap.org/Final_Quick_Treatment_for_web.pdf. Accessed December 2010.

Fink H, Taylor B, Tacklind J, et al: Treatment interventions in nursing home residents with urinary incontinence: a systematic review of randomized trials (2010). Available at http://www.mayoclinicproceedings.com/content/83/12/1332.full. Accessed December 2010.

Gardner SE, Frantz RA, Bergquist S, et al: A prospective study of the pressure ulcer scale for healing (PUSH), *Journals of Gerontology Series A, Biological Sciences and Medical Sciences* 60:93, 2005.

Grover M, Busby-Whitehead J, Palmer MH, et al: Survey of geriatricians on the effect of fecal incontinence on nursing home referral, *Journal of the American Geriatrics Society* 58:1058, 2010.

Hale E, Smith E, St. James J, et al: Pilot study of the feasibility and effectiveness of a natural laxative mixture, *Geriatric Nursing* 28:104, 2007.

Hall K, Karstens M, Rakel B, et al: Managing constipation in the elderly, *Geriatrics* A CME-Accredited Supplement, August: 2007.

Ham R, Sloane P, Warshaw G, et al: *Primary care geriatrics: a case-based approach*, ed 4, St. Louis, MO, 2007, Mosby/Elsevier.

Holroyd-Leduc JM, Straus SE: Management of urinary incontinence in women: clinical applications, *JAMA* 291:996, 2004.

Howard D, Taylor Y: Racial and gender differences in pressure ulcer development among nursing home residents in the southeastern United States, *Journal of Women & Aging* 21:266, 2009.

Inelmen E, Giuseppe S, Giuliano E: When are indwelling catheters appropriate in elderly patients? *Geriatrics* 62:18, 2007.

Irwin MR, Olmstead R, Motivala SJ: Improving sleep quality in older adults with moderate sleep complaints: a randomized controlled trial of tai chi chih, *Sleep* 31:1001, 2008.

Jamshed N, Schneider E: Is the use of supplemental vitamin C and zinc for the prevention and treatment of pressure ulcers evidence-based? *Annals of Long-term Care* 18:28, 2010.

Johnson T, Ouslander J: The newly revised F-Tag 315 and surveyor guidance for urinary incontinence in long-term care, *Journal of the American Medical Directors Association* 7:594, 2006.

Jull A, Griffiths P: Is pressure sore prevention a sensitive indicator of the quality of nursing care? A cautionary note. *International Journal of Nursing Studies* 47:531, 2010.

Juthani-Mehta M, Quagliarello V, Perrelli E, et al: Clinical features to identify urinary tract infection in nursing home residents: a cohort study, *Journal of the American Geriatrics Society* 57:963, 2009.

Kerr D, Wilkinson H: *Providing good care at night for older people*, London, 2010, Jessica Kingsley Publishers.

Lackner T, Wyman J, McCarthy T, et al: Randomized placebo-controlled trial of the cognitive effect, safety, and tolerability of oral extended release oxybutynin in cognitively impaired nursing home residents with urge urinary incontinence, *Journal of the American Geriatrics Society* 56:862, 2008.

Landefeld C, Bowers B, Feld A, et al: National Institutes of Health State-of-the-Science Conference Statement: prevention of fecal and urinary incontinence in adults, *Annals of Internal Medicine* 148:449, 2008.

Lapane K, Jesdale W, Zierler S: Racial differences in pressure ulcer prevalence in nursing homes, *Journal of the American Geriatrics Society* 55:1663, 2005.

Lawhorne L, Ouslander J, Parmelee P, et al: Urinary incontinence: a neglected geriatric syndrome in nursing facilities, *Journal of the American Medical Directors Association* 9:9, 2008.

Levine J: What hospitals can learn about pressure ulcers form long-term care clinicians, *Caring for the Ages* September:6, 2008.

Lewis SJ, Heaton KW: Stool Form Scale as a useful guide to intestinal transit time, *Scandinavian Journal of Gastroenterology* 32:920, 1997.

MacDonald DG, Butler L: Silent no more: elderly women's stories of living with urinary incontinence in long-term care, *Journal of Gerontological Nursing* 33:14, 2007.

Martin J, Fiorentino L, Jouldjian S, et al: Sleep quality in residents of assisted living facilities: effect on quality of life, functional status, and depression, *Journal of the American Geriatrics Society* 58:829, 2010.

McCurry S, Gibbons L, Logsdon R, et al: Nighttime insomnia treatment and education for Alzheimer's disease: a randomized, controlled trial, *Journal of the American Geriatrics Society* 53:793, 2005.

McCurry S, LaFazia D, Pike K, et al: Managing sleep disturbances in adult family homes: recruitment and implementation of a behavioral treatment program, *Geriatric Nursing* 30:36, 2009.

Mecocci P, von Strauss E, Cherubini A, et al: Cognitive impairment is the major risk factor for development of geriatric syndromes during hospitalization: results from the GIFA Study, *Dementia and Geriatric Cognitive Disorders* 20:262, 2005.

Missildine K: Sleep and the sleep environment of older adults in acute care settings, *Journal of Geriatric Nursing* 34:15, 2008.

Missildine K, Bergstrom N, Meininger J, et al: Sleep in hospitalized elders: a pilot study, *Geriatric Nursing* 31:263, 2010.

Mitty E, Flores S: Sleepiness or excessive daytime somnolence, *Geriatric Nursing* 30:53, 2009.

Mouton C, Adenuga B, Vijayan J: Urinary tract infections in long-term care, *Annals of Long-term Care* 18:35, 2010.

Muller N: What Americans understand and how they are affected by bladder control problems: highlights of recent nationwide consumer research, *Urologic Nursing* 25:109, 2005.

Newman DK, Palmer MH, editors: The state of the science on urinary incontinence, *American Journal of Nursing* 3(suppl):1, 2003.

Palmer M, Newman D: Bladder control: educational needs of older adults, *Journal of Gerontological Nursing* 32:28, 2006.

Plawecki L, Amrhein D, Zortman T: Under pressure: nursing liability and skin breakdown in older patients, *Journal of Gerontological Nursing* 36:23, 2010.

Richards K, Beck C, O'Sullivan P, et al: Effect of individualized social activity on sleep in nursing home residents with dementia, *Journal of the American Geriatrics Society* 53:1510, 2005.

Roach M, Christie J: Fecal incontinence in the elderly, *Geriatrics* 63:13, 2008.

Rose K, Lorenz R: Sleep disturbances in dementia: what they are and what to do, *Journal of Gerontological Nursing* 36:9, 2010.

Rowe M, Kairalla J, McCrae C: Sleep in dementia caregivers and the effects of a nighttime monitoring system, *Journal of Nursing Scholarship* 42:338, 2010.

Shamliyan T, Wyman J, Bliss DZ, et al: *Prevention of fecal and urinary incontinence in adults*. Evidence Report/Technology Assessment No. 161 (Prepared by the Minnesota Evidence-based Practice Center under Contract No. 290-02-0009) AHRQ Publication No 08-E003. Rockville, MD, 2007, Agency for Healthcare Research and Quality.

Simonson W, Bergeron C, Crecelius C, et al: Improving sleep management in the elderly, *Supplement to the Annals of Long-term Care: Clinical Care and Aging* 15(12 Suppl 1):1, 2007.

Spillsbury K, Nelson A, Cullum N, et al: Pressure ulcers and their treatment and effects on quality of life: hospital inpatient perspectives, *Journal of Advanced Nursing* 57:494, 2007.

Stevens T, Palmer R: Fecal incontinence in LTC patients, *Long-term Care Interface* 8:35, 2007.

Subramanian S, Surani S: Sleep disorders in the elderly, *Geriatrics* 62:10, 2007.

Teodorescu M, Husain N: Nonpharmacological approaches to insomnia in older adults, *Annals of Long-term Care* 18:36, 2010.

Townsend M, Curhan G, Resnik N, Grodstein F: Rates of remission improvement, and progression of urinary incontinence in Asian

Black, and white women, *American Journal of Nursing* 111(4):26–33, 2011.

Tettamanti G, Altman D, Pedersen NL, Bellocco R, Milsom I, Iliadou AN: Effects of coffee and tea consumption on urinary incontinence in female twins, BJOG An international journal of obstetrics and gynaecology, 2011. Article published online March 15 2011. DOI: 10: 1111/J. 1471–0528.2011.02930.x, 1–7.

U.S. Department of Health and Human Service, Office of Disease Prevention and Health Promotion: *Healthy People 2020 Framework. s: Phase 1 report: recommendations for the framework and format of Healthy People 2020* (2010). Available at http://www.healthypeople.gov. Accessed December 2010.

Weiss B: Selecting medications for the treatment of urinary incontinence, *American Family Physician* 71:315, 2005.

Winkelman J, Allen R, Tenzer P, et al: Restless legs syndrome: nonpharmacologic and pharmacologic treatments, *Geriatrics* 62:13, 2007.

Zarowitz B, Ouslander J: The applications of evidence-based principles of care in older persons (issue 6): urinary incontinence, *Journal of the American Medical Directors Association* 8:35, 2007.

Zee P, Bloom H: Understanding and resolving insomnia in the elderly, *Geriatrics* (Suppl May):1, 2006.

Theris A. Touhy

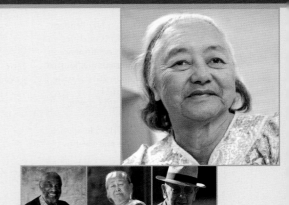

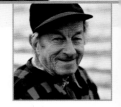

evolve *http://evolve.elsevier.com/Ebersole/TwdHlthAging*

A STUDENT SPEAKS

The thought of needing someone to help me shower and dress and transfer me from a chair to bed requires more acceptance than I have ever had to muster. I'm very good at making the best out of a bad situation, but somehow adapting to something like never walking again cannot be equated with a "bad situation." It is permanent, and it is the sacrifice of my precious independence. I was born on Independence Day! Thinking about these things overwhelms me with sadness.

Holiday, age 22

AN ELDER SPEAKS

I hate to have the family see me like this. You know, I was a military man. I took pride in the way I marched ... or just stood at attention. I never imagined a time when I wouldn't be able to walk without assistance.

Jerry, age 78

LEARNING OBJECTIVES

On completion of this chapter, the reader will be able to:

- Discuss the effects of impaired mobility on general function and quality of life.
- Describe age-related changes in bones, joints, and muscles that may predispose older adults to limitations in mobility.
- Discuss risk factors for impaired mobility.
- Describe the beneficial effects of exercise and appropriate exercise regimens for older adults.

- Discuss factors that increase vulnerability to falls.
- Describe assessment measures to determine gait and walking stability.
- Describe the effects of restraints, and identify alternative safety interventions.
- List several measures to reduce fall risks, and identify those at high risk.
- Develop a plan of care for an older adult at risk for falls.

Mobility is the capacity one has for movement within the personally available microcosm and macrocosm. This includes abilities such as moving oneself by turning over in bed, transferring from lying to sitting and sitting to standing, walking, using assistive devices, or transportation within the community environment. In infancy, moving about is the major mode of learning and interacting with the environment. In old age, one moves more slowly and purposefully, sometimes with more forethought and caution. Throughout life, movement remains a significant means of personal contact, sensation, exploration, pleasure, and control. Pride, maintaining dignity, self-care, independence, social contacts, and activity are all needs identified as important to elders, and all are facilitated by mobility. "Mobility is fundamental to active aging and is intimately linked to health status and quality of life" (Webber et al., 2010, p. 443). Impairment of mobility is an early predictor of physical

disability and associated with poor outcomes such as falling, loss of independence, decreased quality of life, institutionalization, and death (Webber et al., 2010). Maintenance of mobility and functional ability for older adults is one of the most important aspects of gerontological nursing.

This chapter focuses on maintaining maximal mobility and physical activity; assessing gait, mobility, and fall risk factors; fall risk-reduction interventions; restraints and restraint-free care; and interventions that are useful when mobility is impaired.

MOBILITY AND AGING

Mobility and comparative degrees of agility are based on muscle strength, flexibility, postural stability, vibratory sensation, cognition, and perceptions of stability. Aging produces changes in muscles and joints, particularly of the back and legs. Strength and flexibility of muscles decrease and movements and range of motion (ROM) become more limited. Normal wear and tear reduce the smooth cartilage of joints. Movement is less fluid as one ages, and joints change as regeneration of tissue slows and muscle wasting occurs. Gait changes in late life include a narrower standing base, wider side-to-side swaying when walking, slowed responses, a greater reliance on proprioception, diminished arm swing, and increased care in gait. Steps are shorter, and there is a decrease in step height (lifting of the foot when taking a step). One third to one half of individuals 65 years of age or older report difficulties related to walking or climbing stairs (Webber et al., 2010).

Sarcopenia (age-related loss of muscle mass, strength and function), a condition prevalent in older people and a marker of frailty, contributes to mobility impairments and disability (Janssen, 2006). Limitations in mobility are approximately three times greater in older women and two times greater in older men with sarcopenia (Yeom et al., 2008). Findings from studies in the United Kingdom suggest that pre- and postnatal development of muscle fibers and muscle growth during puberty may have critical effects on musculoskeletal aging, development of sarcopenia, and risk of frailty (Kuh, 2007).

Mobility impairments are caused by diseases and impairments across many organ systems. For some older people, osteoporosis, gait disorders, Parkinson's disease, strokes, and arthritic conditions markedly affect movement and functional capacities. Mobility may be limited by paresthesias; hemiplegia; neuromotor disturbances; fractures; foot, knee, and hip problems; respiratory diseases, and illnesses that deplete one's energy. All these conditions are likely to occur more frequently and have more devastating effects as one ages. Many older adults have some of these impairments, with women significantly outnumbering men in this respect (see Chapter 15).

Regular physical activity throughout life is likely to enhance health and functional status as people age while also decreasing the number of chronic illnesses and functional limitations often assumed to be a part of growing older. The frail health and loss of function we associate with aging is in large part due to physical inactivity. A sedentary lifestyle, excess weight, and smoking are associated with mobility problems (Yeom et al., 2008). Few factors contribute as much to health in aging as being physically active. The old adage "Use it or lose it" certainly applies to our muscles and physical fitness (Agency for Healthcare Research and Quality, 2002.

PROMOTING HEALTHY AGING: IMPLICATIONS FOR GERONTOLOGICAL NURSING

Assessment

Assessment of functional abilities and screening should be included as part of the health assessment of all older adults. The purpose of screening is to (1) identify medical problems while allowing the individual to achieve the maximal benefit from physical activity; (2) identify functional limitations that will be addressed in the exercise program; and (3) minimize injury or other serious adverse effect. Exercise stress tests are no longer recommended by either the U.S. Preventive Services Task Force or the American College of Cardiology and the American Heart Association for the screening of low-risk, asymptomatic individuals before starting a physical activity program. The consensus is that there is minimal cardiovascular risk to engaging in physical activity and a much greater risk in maintaining a sedentary lifestyle (Resnick et al., 2006).

The Exercise and Screening for You (EASY) tool (www. easyforyou.info) is a screening tool that can be used to determine a safe exercise program for older adults on the basis of underlying physical problems. The programs recommended have all been reviewed and endorsed by national organizations such as the National Institute on Aging (Bethesda, MD) and can be printed and given to the person (Resnick, 2009). There are many resources available on the Internet that provide excellent information on physical activity in a useable format (see Evolve Resources). The Senior Fitness Test (SFT) is another instrument that has been used to assess physical fitness levels before and after an exercise intervention (Purath et al., 2009).

The Get-Up-and Go Test (Mathias et al., 1986) (Figure 12-2) can also be used to assess mobility, gait, and gait speed. This tool is a practical assessment tool for older people that can be adapted to any setting. The client is asked to rise from a straight-backed chair, stand briefly, walk forward about 10 feet, turn, walk back to the chair, turn around and sit down. The test can be timed as well and gait speed has been found to be a predictor of mobility. On the basis of the results of initial screening, older adults may need further evaluation.

Frail older adults will need more comprehensive assessment and close monitoring to ensure benefit without compromising safety. Exercise goals for the frail older adult are different from those for younger adults. Exercise in younger adults helps prevent disease and increases life expectancy. For frail older people, exercise is important to minimize the effects of aging, reverse the effects of disuse, and maximize psychological health. Absolute contraindications to exercise testing and training include recent electrocardiogram changes or myocardial infarction; unstable angina; and uncontrolled arrhythmias, third degree heart block, and acute heart failure. Poorly controlled diabetes, severe hypertension, respiratory disease, acute musculoskeletal pain, and arthritis are other conditions that warrant careful assessment before exercise programs are begun exercise programs may need to be adapted depending on the condition of the individual (e.g., pool exercise programs rather than resistance activities, such as lifting weights or using stretchy bands, if the elder has arthritis). Extremely frail individuals may not be able to engage in aerobic activities and should begin with strength and balance training before engaging in as little as five minutes of aerobic training.

INTERVENTIONS

Physical Fitness

Despite a large body of evidence about the benefits of physical activity to maintain and improve function, only about one third of men and 25% of women aged 65 to 74 years engage in leisure-time activity. With advancing age participation is even lower, with 16% of men and 11% of women 75 years and older engaged in leisure-time strengthening activities (lifting weights, calisthenics) (Purath et al., 2009; Centers for Disease Control and Prevention [CDC], 2010c). Older African-American women are the least physically active race-sex subgroup in the United States (Duru et al., 2010). Older people are also less likely to receive exercise counseling from their primary care providers than younger individuals. Research has noted that health care providers value the benefits of physical activity but have inadequate knowledge of specific recommendations (Tompkins et al., 2009; CDC, 2010c). The levels of physical activity among older adults have not improved over the past decade in the United States. Many older people mistakenly believe that they are too old to begin a fitness program. Physical activity is important for all older people, not just active healthy elders. Even a small amount of time (at least 30 minutes of moderate activity several days a week) can improve health.

Physical activity is also associated with better cognitive functioning in old age. For women, physical activity at any time during the life course, especially as teenagers, is associated with a lower likelihood of cognitive impairment in later life (Middleton et al., 2010). Erickson and colleagues reported that people 65 years of age and over who walked at least six miles a week had greater gray matter volume and halved their risk of developing memory problems (Erickson et al., 2010). Once weekly progressive strength training exercise programs have also been shown to improve cognitive abilities in women aged 65 to 75 years of age (Davis et al., 2010).

Studies have found that increasing physical activity improves health outcomes in persons with chronic illnesses (regardless of severity) and in those with functional impairment (Sherrington et al., 2008; Yeom et al., 2009). The benefit of exercise (improvement in walking speed, strength, functional ability) of frail nursing home residents with diagnoses ranging from arthritis to lung disease and dementia has also been shown (Heyn et al., 2008). Physical activity can also improve emotional health and quality of life. Regardless of age or situation, the older person can find some activity suitable for his or her condition. It is important to keep older people moving any way possible for as long as possible. Following are examples of myriad ways in which older people keep fit:

Em, an 84-year-old nursing home resident, jogged every morning in place for about five minutes and then briskly walked around outside the facility. Although she had occasional lapses of memory, she was vital, erect, and interested in life around her.

Nellie, 83 years old, began swimming to ease the discomfort of a short left arm, the residual effect of poliomyelitis, and for a frozen left shoulder. She became an award-winning synchronized swimmer with 20 gold medals, 12 blue ribbons, and 13 trophies to her credit. Nellie continued to exercise this way despite the need to wear cataract goggles.

Guidelines for Physical Activity

Recommendations for all adults are participation in 30 minutes of moderate-intensity physical activity for five or more days of the week. People do not have to be active for 30 minutes at a time but can accumulate 30 minutes over 24 hours. As little as 10 minutes of exercise has health benefits and three 10-minute bouts of activity have the same fitness effects as one 30-minute bout. Health care practitioners should counsel all patients on how to incorporate exercise into their daily routines (CDC, 2010c).

Guidelines for physical activity for adults 65 years of age or older who are generally fit and have no limiting health conditions are as follows:

- Two hours and 30 minutes (150 minutes) of moderate-intensity aerobic activity (e.g., brisk walking, swimming, bicycling) every week AND muscle-strengthening activi-

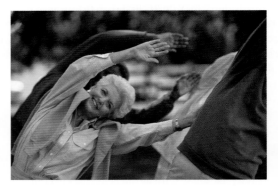

Stretching. (© 2010 Photos.com, a division of Getty Images. All rights reserved.)

BOX 12-1   RESEARCH HIGHLIGHTS

Influence of Intense Tai Chi Training on Physical Performance and Hemodynamic Outcomes in Transitionally Frail Older Adults

This study explored the extent and time course over which tai chi (TC) impacts measures of physical performance and cardiovascular function in older adults who are becoming frail. Participants ranged in age from 70 to 97 years (mean, 80.9 yr) and were living in 20 independent congregate living facilities in the greater Atlanta area.

A 48-week randomized trial was provided to 291 women and 20 men who were transitionally frail (older than 70 years and had fallen at least once in the past year). Participants were randomized to either TC exercise or wellness education (control) interventions. Physical performance (gait speed, reach, chair rises, 360-degree turn, picking up an object from the floor, and single limb support) and hemodynamic outcomes (heart rate and blood pressure) were obtained at baseline and after 4, 8, and 12 months.

The TC training had a positive impact on body mass index, systolic blood pressure, and heart rate as well as on chair rises. Fall occurrences were also reduced. Positive outcomes became apparent after four or eight months of training and persisted through completion of the intervention. TC exercise programs have positive benefits for frail older adults, including improved cardiovascular performance, decreased falls, and increased functional ability, and these benefits are demonstrated after at least four months of training.

Data from Wolf S, O'Grady M, Easley KA, et al: The influence of intense tai chi training on physical performance and hemodynamic outcomes in transitionally frail older adults, *Journals of Gerontology Series A, Biological Sciences and Medical Sciences* 61:184, 2006.

ties on two or more days that work all major muscle groups (legs, hips, abdomen, chest, shoulders, and arms) (CDC, 2010c). See www.cdc.gov/physicalactivity/everyone/guidelines/olderadults.html for video presentations of exercise as well as an explanation of guidelines and tips for physical activity.

- Stretching (flexibility) and balance exercises (particularly for older people at risk of falls) are also recommended. Yoga and tai chi exercises have been shown to be of benefit to older people in terms of improving flexibility and balance as well as pain reduction and improved psychological well-being (Rogers et al., 2010). Tai chi can be adapted for level of function and mobility status (Wolf et al., 2006; Yeom et al., 2009) (Box 12-1). Home-based balance-training exercise programs are also available.

One does not have to invest in expensive equipment or gym memberships or follow a structured exercise regimen to benefit from increased activity. The older person may be able to integrate activity into daily life rather than doing a specific exercise. Examples include walking to the store instead of driving, golfing, raking leaves, gardening, washing windows or floors, washing and waxing the car, and swimming. The Wii game system offers other possibilities for exercise at all levels and is increasingly being used in nursing homes and assisted living facilities to encourage physical activity and enjoyable entertainment. One study reported significant improvement in the ADL (activities of daily living) ability of frail community-dwelling older people following a program of twice-weekly water exercises. Benefits from the water exercise program were evident during the exercise period and for one year afterward (Sato et al., 2009). Water-based exercises are particularly beneficial for older people with arthritis or other mobility limitations.

Special Considerations

Nonambulatory older people can also engage in physical activity and may benefit most from an exercise program in terms of function and quality of life. "Muscle weakness and atrophy are probably the most functionally relevant and reversible aspects to exercise in nonambulatory older adults" (Resnick et al., 2006, p. 174). Suggested exercises might include upper extremity cycling, marching in place, stretching, range of motion, use of resistive bands, and chair yoga. At the Louis and Anne Green Memory and Wellness Center at Florida Atlantic University (Boca Raton, FL), 90-year-old Vera Paley leads groups of cognitively impaired elders as well as caregivers in chair yoga sessions. See Evolve resources for a DVD by Vera describing gentle chair yoga.

The benefits of physical activity extend to the more physically frail older adult, those with cognitive impairment, and those residing in assisted living facilities (ALFs) or skilled nursing facilities (SNFs) (Rolland et al., 2007; Heyn et al., 2008; Sato et al., 2009). Nurse researcher Barbara Resnick has written extensively on exercise and health promotion for older people and conducted numerous studies evaluating interventions to improve function and physical activity in older adults. The Res-Care intervention (Resnick et al., 2006), a self-efficacy–based approach to restore and/or maintain the residents' physical function, can be used as a model for restorative care in ALFs and SNFs. The focus of restorative care is on "the restoration and/or maintenance of physical function and helping older adults to compensate for functional impairments so that the highest level of function is obtained and secondary complications of physical dependence are minimized" (Galik et al., 2009, p. 48). Restorative care programs should be integral activities in all facilities for older people.

Following a recent study, the Res-Care intervention has been revised to be appropriate for individuals with moderate to severe cognitive impairment (Res-Care-CI) (Galik et al., 2009). This intervention holds promise to enhance therapeutic care of older adults with cognitive impairment and to focus interventions on quality of life rather than only on safety and behavior. Results of research suggest that older adults with cognitive impairment who participate in exercise rehabilitation programs have similar outcomes in strength and endurance as those who are not cognitively impaired (Heyn et al., 2008). However, those with cognitive impairment are often not included in physical

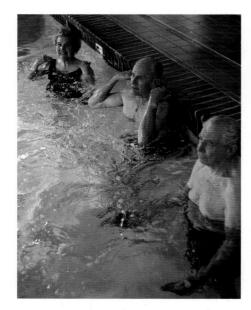

Aquatic Exercise. Aquatic exercise programs are beneficial for elders with mobility problems; they improve circulation, muscle strength, and endurance; and provide socialization and relaxation. (Copyright © Getty Images.)

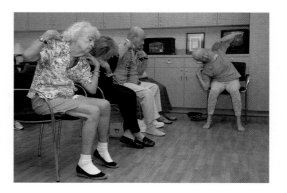

Yoga. Vera Paley leads Yoga class. (Courtesy of Louis and Anne Green Memory & Wellness Center, Boca Raton, FL.)

activity programs or physical rehabilitation. Physical activity may also have a beneficial effect on mood in cognitively impaired older people. Nursing home residents who participated in a comprehensive 16-week exercise program with whole body movement (targeting balance, endurance, and upper and lower extremity strength), rather than walking alone, exhibited higher positive and lower negative affect and mood (Williams and Tappen, 2007a,b).

Physical activity can be adapted in creative and enjoyable ways for people with cognitive impairment and may include activities such as ball toss, chair yoga, parachute toss, marching in place, shaking tambourines, dancing, Wii games, as well as ADL self-care activities and endurance and strength-training programs. Galik and colleagues (2009, p. 53) offer further suggestions for enhancing restorative nursing care programs for cognitively impaired nursing home residents, including "knowing what makes them tick, verbal encouragement, cueing, role modeling, humor and persistence."

Exercise Prescription

Prescribing an exercise plan that includes the specific exercises the individual should do as well as the reasonable short- and long-term goals and safety tips is suggested. As suggested by the CDC, the program should include endurance, strength, balance, and flexibility (Table 12-1). Examples of strength-training exercises that can be done at home are presented in Figure 12-1. Varied activities that involve interaction with peers and fit the person's lifestyle and culture will encourage participation (Yeom et al., 2009). The individual should be informed of resources in their community, and communities should be encouraged to provide accessible and affordable options for physical activity. Motivational interventions are important when encouraging older adults to begin and sustain a physical activity program. Collaborate with the individual on the goals they hope to achieve. Most older people are interested in how physical activity will improve the quality of

---

TABLE 12-1   GUIDELINES FOR TEACHING ABOUT EXERCISE

EXERCISE	DESCRIPTION	BENEFITS	INTENSITY	FREQUENCY	EXAMPLES
Moderate-intensity aerobic activity	Continuous movement involving large muscle groups that is sustained for a minimum of 10 min	Improves cardiovascular functioning, strengthens heart muscle, decreases blood glucose and triglycerides, increases HDL, improves mood	On a 10-point scale, where sitting is 0 and working as hard as you can is 10, moderate-intensity aerobic activity is a 5 or 6. You will be able to talk but not sing the words to your favorite song	30 min, 5 d/wk. Perform for at least 10 min at a time	Biking, swimming, dancing, brisk walking, lifestyle activities that incorporate large muscle groups (pushing a lawn mower, climbing stairs)
Muscle-strengthening activities that involve moving or lifting some type of resistance and work all major muscle groups (legs, hip, back, abdomen, chest, shoulders, arms)	Activities that involve moving or lifting some type of resistance and work all major muscle groups (legs, hip, back, abdomen, chest, shoulders, arms)	Increases muscle strength, prevents sarcopenia, reduces fall risk, improves balance, modifies risk factors for cardiovascular disease and type 2 diabetes	To gain health benefits, muscle-strengthening activities need to be done to the point at which it is difficult to do another repetition without help. A repetition is one complete movement of an activity such as lifting a weight. An effort should be made to do 8-12 repetitions per activity, which counts as one set. At least one set should be done	2 d/wk, but not consecutive days to allow muscles to recover between sessions	Lifting weights, working with resistance bands, exercises that use the body's own weight for resistance (push-ups, sit-ups), heavy gardening (digging, shoveling), yoga
Stretching (flexibility)	A therapeutic maneuver designed to elongate shortened soft tissue structures and increase flexibility	Facilitates ROM around joints, prevents injury	Stretch muscle groups but not past the point of resistance or pain	At least 2 d/wk	Yoga, range-of-motion exercises
Balance exercises	Movements that improve the ability to maintain control of the body over the base of support to avoid falling	Improves lower body strength, improves balance, helps prevent falls	Safety precautions are essential (holding onto a chair, working with another person)	Can be incorporated into regularly scheduled strength exercises. More formal balance programs may be appropriate for those at high risk for falls	Tai chi Exercises such as standing on one leg, walking heel to toe, leg raises, hip extensions (can be done holding onto a chair) (see http://www.nia.nih.gov/HealthInformation/Publications/ExerciseGuide/04d_balance.htm for pictorial description)

HDL, high-density lipoprotein; ROM, range of motion.
Data from Centers for Disease Control and Prevention: *How much physical activity do older adults need?* (2010c). Available at http://www.cdc.gov/physicalactivity/everyone/guidelines/olderadults.html. Accessed December 2010; Resnick B, Ory M, Rogers M, et al: Screening and prescribing exercise for older adults, *Geriatrics and Aging* 9:174, 2006.

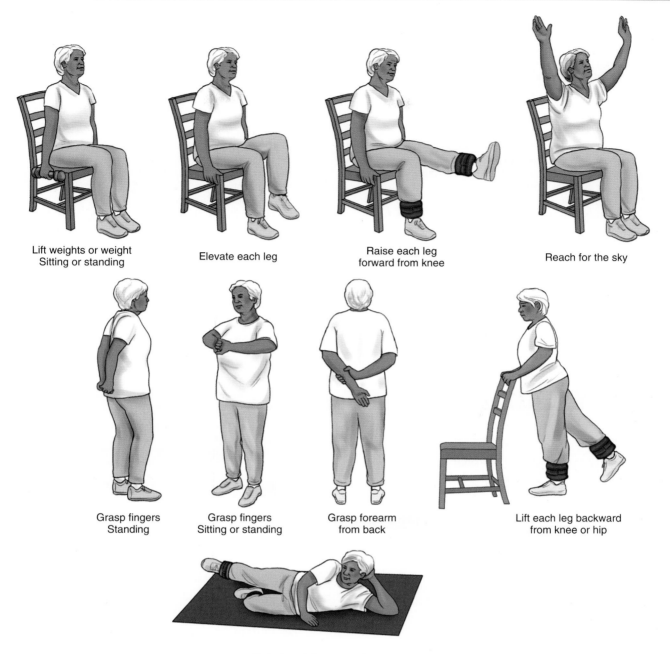

Lift weights or weight
Sitting or standing

Elevate each leg

Raise each leg
forward from knee

Reach for the sky

Grasp fingers
Standing

Grasp fingers
Sitting or standing

Grasp forearm
from back

Lift each leg backward
from knee or hip

Abduct each leg upward

FIGURE 12-1 Examples of Strength-training Exercises. [Modified from Centers for Disease Control and Prevention: *Growing stronger: strength training for older adults: exercises: stage 1*. Available at www.cdc.gov/nccdphp/dnpa/physical/growing_stronger/exercises/index.htm. Accessed December 2010.]

their life and enhance their functional ability. The immediate benefits that can be expected should be emphasized—for example, improving walking ability or decreasing risk of falls. Specific types of exercises that are to be done daily as well as daily and long-term goals can be written down. Individuals can keep a journal or diary reflecting their experience and progress.

Follow up with the older individual so that they can share their progress. Support from experts such as nurse practitioners and family and peers is a significant factor in encouraging continued physical activity programs (Resnick et al., 2009, 2010). Group exercise programs with a lay trainer or nurse, and teaching a peer within the group to take on the leadership for

long-term sustainability have been shown to be effective for older adults (Dorgo et al., 2009; Resnick, 2009). Duru and colleagues (2010) reported that a faith-based physical activity program (Sisters in Motion) led to an increase in walking and a decrease in systolic blood pressure among sedentary African-American women. Suggestions for exercise programs are presented in Box 12-2. Sharing stories of older people's experience with physical fitness can be motivating. To hear the stories of older people (65 to 85 years) who maintain exercise regimens, see www.cdc.gov/physicalactivity/everyone/getactive/olderadults.html.

Similar to prescriptions for medication, a prescription for exercise should include potential exercise side effects, tips for

BOX 12-2 SUGGESTIONS FOR EXERCISE PROGRAMS FOR OLDER ADULTS

- Provide appropriate screening before beginning an exercise program.
- Provide information about the benefits of exercise, emphasizing short-term benefits such as sleeping better.
- Clarify the misconceptions associated with exercise (fatigue, injury).
- Assess for functional abilities and discuss how exercise can enhance function.
- Assess barriers to exercise and how to overcome.
- Provide an "exercise prescription" that specifies what exercises and how often the person should exercise. Include daily and long-term goals.
- Collaborate with the person to set short- and long-term goals that are specific, achievable, and match the older person's perceived need, health, cognitive abilities, culture, gender, as well as their interests.
- Provide choices as to types of exercises, and design the program so that the person can do it at home or elsewhere when formal training ends.
- Refer to community resources for physical fitness (e.g., YMCA, mall walking).
- Provide self-monitoring methods to assist in visualizing progress.

- Group-based programs and exercising with a buddy may be more successful.
- Try to make the program fun and entertaining (walking with favorite music, socializing with friends).
- Discuss potential exercise side effects and any symptoms that should be reported.
- Provide safety tips.
- Share stories about your own personal exercise program and those of older people and the benefits.
- Follow up frequently on progress, and provide reinforcement.
- Begin with low-intensity physical activity for sedentary older adults.
- Initiate low-intensity activities in short sessions (less than 10 minutes), and include warm-up and cool-down components with active stretching.
- Progression from low to moderate intensity is important to obtain maximal benefits, but activity level changes should be instituted gradually.
- Lifestyle activities (e.g., raking, gardening) can build endurance when performed for at least 10 minutes.

Data from Cress ME, Buchner DM, Prohaska T, et al: Best practices for physical activity programs and behavior counseling in older adult populations, *Journal of Aging and Physical Activity* 13:61, 2005; Jitrarnontree N: *Evidence-based protocol: exercise promotion: walking in elders.* Iowa City, IA, 2001, University of Iowa Gerontological Nursing Interventions Research Center, Research Dissemination Core; Schneider JK, Eveker A, Bronder DR, et al: Exercise training program for older adults: incentives and disincentives for participation, *Journal of Gerontological Nursing* 29:21, 2006; Struck B, Ross K: Health promotion in older adults: prescribing exercise for the frail and home bound, *Geriatrics* 61:22, 2006; Resnick B, Ory M, Rogers M, et al: Screening for and prescribing exercise for older adults, *Geriatrics and Aging* 9:174, 2006.

BOX 12-3 SAFETY TIPS

Follow these EASY safety tips for when to start and stop exercise. Use the recommendations below for exercising safely with your condition.

Exercise Safety Tips to Always Consider Before Starting Exercise

- Always wear comfortable, loose-fitting clothing and appropriate shoes for your activity.
- Warm up: Perform a low to moderate intensity warm-up for 5-10 minutes.
- Drink water before, during and after your exercise session.
- When exercising outdoors, evaluate your surroundings for safety: traffic, pavement, weather, and strangers.
- Wear clothes made of fabrics that absorb sweat and remove it from your skin.
- Never wear rubber or plastic suits. These could hold the sweat on your skin and make your body overheat.
- Wear sunscreen when you exercise outdoors.

Exercise Safety Tips for When to STOP Exercising

Stop exercising right away if you:
- Have pain or pressure in your chest, neck, shoulder, or arm.
- Feel dizzy or sick.
- Break out in a cold sweat.
- Have muscle cramps.
- Feel acute (not just achy) pain in your joints, feet, ankles, or legs.
- Slow down if you have trouble breathing. You should be able to talk while exercising without gasping for breath.

Exercise Safety Tips to Recognize Days/Times When Exercise Should NOT be Initiated:

- Avoid hard exercise for two hours after a big meal. (A leisurely walk around the block would be fine).
- Do not exercise when you have a fever and/or viral infection accompanied by muscle aches.
- Do not exercise if your systolic blood pressure is greater than 200 and your diastolic is greater than 100.
- Do not exercise if your resting heart rate is greater than 120.
- Do not exercise if you have a joint that you are using to exercise (such as a knee or an ankle) that is red and warm and painful.
- If you have osteoporosis, always avoid stretches that flex your spine or cause you to bend at the waist, and avoid making jerky, rapid movements.
- Stop exercising if you experience severe pain or swelling in a joint. Discomfort that persists should always be evaluated.
- Do not exercise if you have a new symptom that has not been evaluated by your health care provider such as pain in your chest, abdomen or a joint; swelling in an arm, leg or joint; difficulty catching your breath at rest; or a fluttering feeling in your chest.

Additional Safety Information is provided at the National Institute of Health Web page www.nlm.nih.gov/medlineplus/safety.html

From Program on Healthy Aging, School of Rural Public Health, Texas A&M Health Science Center: Easy exercise and screening for you, 2007, available at http://www.easyforyou.info/downloads/EASYSafetyTipsFINAL111507.pdf

prevention and management, and safety precautions (Box 12-3). Exercise side effects may include sensations associated with activity (shortness of breath) or things that might occur the day after exercise (muscle soreness) or more untoward things that require medical attention. Any exercise intervention should begin slowly and gradually progress with careful evaluation and monitoring of response. Proper instruction in technique and performance is important as well as the importance of warming up and cooling down. An extended cool-down period should be encouraged to diminish the risk of postexercise hypotension, syncopal episodes, or arrhythmias during recovery. Adequate hydration is important because total body water declines with age, and perspiration from exercise can increase the risk of dehydration. Proper footwear is also essential because of potential circulatory limitations, muscle sarcopenia, or degenerative changes in bones or joints.

Increasing physical activity and improving function and mobility are possible even for the most frail older person and are essential to health and quality of life. Nurses must be well prepared to support older adults in enhancing physical activity and mobility. Many older people have misconceptions about exercise, and the nurse can assess beliefs and understanding and provide education. Screening and assessment of function before beginning a physical activity program and exercise counseling should be a routine part of assessment of older adults. Nurses can also design and lead exercise and restorative programs in many settings as well as teach others best practices in physical activity for older adults. Maintenance of mobility and function is an essential component of best practice in gerontological nursing and is effective in preventing falls, unnecessary decline, and loss of independence.

FALLS

Falls are one of the most important geriatric syndromes and the leading cause of morbidity and mortality for people older than 65 years (Gray-Micelli, 2008). One in three people aged 65 years and older falls each year (Rantz et al., 2008). Nursing home residents, who are more frail, fall frequently and repeatedly (Quigley et al., 2010). Falls among nursing home residents are estimated at 2.6 per year (Gray-Micelli, 2010).

It is important to use a consistent definition of falls in practice and research because the word *fall* is interpreted in many different ways (Zecevic et al., 2006). A fall has been defined in the literature as unintentionally coming to rest on a lower area such as the ground or floor (Buchner et al., 1993). Often, the terms *slips, trips,* and *falls* are used interchangeably, and *near falls, mishaps,* or *missteps,* not usually reported, may be important in assessing fall risk. Exactly what constitutes a fall for reporting procedures in institutions is also problematic and can lead to inconsistencies in data (Zecevic et al., 2006). Therefore it is important to define a fall in words that seniors understand and to use an operational definition of falls in all research and fall-reporting data.

Falls are a significant public health problem, and the rate of fall-related deaths among older persons has risen significantly over the past decade (Stevens et al., 2006) (Box 12-4). In the hospital, falls with resultant fractures, dislocations, and crushing injuries are considered one of the 10 hospital-acquired conditions (HCAs) that are not covered under Medicare. HCAs are conditions that (1) are high-cost or high-volume or both; (2) result in the assignment of a case to a DRG (diagnosis-related group) that has a higher payment when present as a secondary diagnosis; and (3) could reasonably have been prevented through the application of evidence-based guidelines (www.cms.gov/HospitalAcqCond/06_Hospital-Acquired_Conditions.asp).

Falls are considered a nursing-sensitive quality indicator. Patient falls have been reported to account for at least 40% of all hospital adverse occurrences (Ireland et al., 2010). All falls in the nursing home setting are considered sentinel events and must be reported to the Centers for Medicare & Medicaid Services (CMS). The Joint Commission (JC) has established

BOX 12-4   STATISTICS ON FALLS AND FALL-RELATED CONCERNS

- One third of people older than 65 years fall at least one time each year, and about half of those fall repeatedly.
- Of those who fall, 20% to 30% suffer moderate to serious injuries, such as hip fractures or head traumas.
- Falls account for 40% of nursing home admissions annually.
- Older adults (75 years of age and older) have the highest rates of traumatic brain injury (TBI)-related hospitalization and death. TBIs account for 46% of fatal falls among older adults.
- More than half of deaths related to falls occur within the home.
- Up to 20% of hospitalized patients and 45% of those in long-term care facilities will fall. In these settings, injury rates are considerably higher, with 10% to 25% of institutional falls resulting in fracture, laceration, or the need for hospital care.
- Men are more likely to die from a fall.
- Rates of fall-related fractures among older adults are more than twice as high for women as for men. White women have significantly higher rates of fall-related hip fractures than black women.
- More than 95% of hip fractures among older adults are caused by falls.
- Between 18% and 33% of older patients with hip fractures die within one year of their fracture.
- Up to 25% of adults who lived independently before their hip fracture have to stay in a nursing home for at least one year after their injury.
- In 2000, more than $19 billion were spent on fall injuries in older people and costs are estimated to rise to nearly 44 billion by 2030 (Lach, 2010).

Centers for Disease Control and Prevention: *Falls among older adults: an overview* (2010). Available at www.cdc.gov/homeandrecreationalsafety/falls/adultfalls.html. Accessed December 2010; Lach H: The costs and outcomes of falls: what's a nursing administrator to do? *Nursing Administration Quarterly* 34:147, 2010.

national patient safety goals (NPSG) for fall reduction in all JC-approved institutions across the health care continuum (Capezuti et al., 2008).

The Quality and Safety Education for Nurses (QSEN) project has developed quality and safety measures for nursing and proposed targets for the knowledge, skills, and attitudes to be developed in nursing prelicensure and graduate programs. Education on falls and fall risk reduction is an important consideration in the QSEN safety competency, which addresses the need to minimize risk of harm to patients and providers through both system effectiveness and individual performance (http://www.qsen.org/competencies.php).

Falls are a symptom of a problem and are rarely benign in older people. The etiology of falls is multifactorial; falls may indicate neurological, sensory, cardiac, cognitive, medication, and musculoskeletal problems or impending illness. Episodes of acute illness or exacerbations of chronic illness are times of high fall risk. The presence of dementia increases risk for falls twofold, and individuals with dementia are also at increased risk of major injuries (fracture) related to falls (Oliver et al., 2007).

In institutional settings, iatrogenic factors such as limited staffing, lack of toileting programs, and restraints and side rails also increase fall risk. A JC review of falls between 1995 and 2004 reported that the root causes of fatal falls included the following: (1) inadequate staff communication and training, (2) incomplete patient assessments and reassessments, (3) environmental issues, (4) incomplete care planning or delayed care provision, and (5) inadequate organizational culture of safety (Tzeng and Yin, 2008).

Consequences of Falls

Among older adults, falls are the leading cause of injury deaths and the most common cause of nonfatal injuries and hospital admissions for trauma (CDC, 2010a). Falls and their subsequent injuries result in physical and psychosocial consequences. Twenty percent to 30% of people who fall suffer moderate to severe injuries (bruises, hip fractures, TBI). Estimates are that up to two thirds of falls may be preventable (Lach, 2010).

Hip Fractures

More than 95% of hip fractures among older adults are caused by falls. Hip fracture is the second leading cause of hospitalization for older people, occurring predominantly in older adults with underlying osteoporosis (Andersen et al., 2010). Hip fractures are associated with considerable morbidity and mortality. Negative outcomes include mortality; limitations in mobility; decline in bone mineral density, lean body mass, and strength; and quality of life issues such as persistent pain and depression. Only 50% to 60% of patients with hip fractures will recover their prefracture ambulation abilities in the first year postfracture. Older adults who fracture a hip have a five to eight times increased risk of mortality during the first three months after hip fracture. This excess mortality persists for 10 years after the fracture and is higher in men. Existing research also suggests that mortality and morbidity limitations are higher in nonwhite people as compared with white people. Most research on hip fractures has been conducted with older women, and further studies of both men and racially and culturally diverse older adults are necessary (Thompson et al., 2006; Andersen et al., 2010; CDC, 2010a; Haentjens et al., 2010).

Traumatic Brain Injury

Older adults (75 years of age and older) have the highest rates of TBI-related hospitalization and death. TBI has been called the "silent epidemic" and older adults with TBI are an even more silent population within this epidemic. Falls are the leading cause of TBI for older adults (51%), and motor vehicle crashes are second (9%). In 2006, more than $2.8 billion was spent on treating TBI in individuals over the age of 65 years. Advancing age negatively affects the outcome after TBI, even with relatively minor head injuries (Timmons and Menaker, 2010). Yet, there is scant research on TBI and its management in older adults. Some authors question whether current protocols, based on work with younger adults, are appropriate for older people who may present differently with TBI (Thompson et al., 2006). A new CDC initiative, *Help Seniors Live Better Longer: Prevent Brain Injury*, provides educational resource materials on TBI for older adults, caregivers, and health care professionals in both Spanish and English (http://www.cdc.gov/traumaticbraininjury/seniors.html

Factors that place the older adult at greater risk for TBI include the presence of comorbid conditions, use of aspirin and anticoagulants, and changes in the brain with age (Thompson et al., 2006). Brain changes with age, although clinically insignificant, do increase the risk of TBIs and especially subdural hematomas, which are much more common in older adults. There is a decreased adherence of the dura matter to the skull,

increased fragility of bridging cerebral veins, an increase in the subarachnoid space, and atrophy of the brain, which creates more space within the cranial vault for blood to accumulate before symptoms appear (Karnath, 2004; Timmons and Menaker, 2010). Falls are the leading cause of TBI, but older people may experience TBI with seemingly more minor incidents (e.g., sharp turns or jarring movement of the head). Some patients may not even remember the incident.

In cases of moderate to severe TBI, there will be cognitive and physical sequelae obvious at the time of injury or shortly afterward that will require emergency treatment. However, older adults who experience a minor incident with seemingly lesser trauma to the head often present with more insidious and delayed symptom onset. Because of changes in the aging brain, there is an increased risk for slowly expanding subdural hematomas. TBIs are often missed or misdiagnosed among older adults (CDC, 2010b). Health professionals should have a high suspicion of TBI in an older adult who falls and strikes the head or experiences even a more minor event, such as sudden twisting of the head. Further, symptoms of cognitive or physical decline occurring over a period of weeks or months should be investigated to rule out subdural hematomas. Manifestations of TBI are often misinterpreted as signs of dementia, which can lead to inaccurate prognoses and limit implementation of appropriate treatment (Flanagan et al., 2006). Table 12-2 presents signs and symptoms of TBI.

Fallophobia

Even if a fall does not result in injury, falls contribute to a loss of confidence that leads to reduced physical activity, increased dependency, and social withdrawal (Rubenstein et al., 2003; Hill et al., 2010). Fear of falling (fallophobia) may restrict an individual's life space (area in which an individual carries on activities). Fear of falling is an important predictor of general functional decline and a risk factor for future falls. Hill and colleagues (2010) reported that 60% of older individuals presenting to an emergency room after a fall had fear of falling as measured by the Modified Falls Efficacy Scale. Assessing the presence of fallophobia and referring for further assessment and management are important in all settings.

Resnick (2002) suggests that nursing staff may also contribute to fear of falling in their patients by telling them not to get up by themselves or by using restrictive devices to keep them from independently moving about. More appropriate nursing responses include assessing fall risk and designing individual interventions and safety plans that will enhance mobility and independence, as well as reduce fall risk.

Factors Contributing to Falls

Individual risk factors can be categorized as either intrinsic or extrinsic. Intrinsic risk factors are unique to each patient and are associated with factors such as reduced vision, unsteady gait, cognitive impairment, acute and chronic illnesses, and effect of medications. Extrinsic risk factors are external to the patient and related to the physical environment and include lack of support equipment by bathtubs and toilets, height of beds, condition of floors, poor lighting, inappropriate footwear, improper use of assistive devices, or inadequate assistive devices (Tzeng and Yin, 2008). Factors such as limited staffing, lack of toileting

TABLE 12-2 SIGNS AND SYMPTOMS TRAUMATIC BRAIN INJURY IN OLDER ADULTS

SYMPTOMS OF MILD TBI	SYMPTOMS OF MODERATE TO SEVERE TBI
Low-grade headache that won't go away	Severe headache that gets worse or does not go away
Having more trouble than usual remembering things, paying attention or concentrating, organizing daily tasks, or making decisions and solving problems	Repeated vomiting or nausea
Slowness in thinking, speaking, acting, or reading	Seizures
Getting lost or easily confused	Inability to wake from sleep
Feeling tired all of the time, lack of energy or motivation	Dilation of one or both pupils
Change in sleep pattern (sleeping much longer than usual, having trouble sleeping)	Slurred speech
Loss of balance, feeling light-headed or dizzy	Weakness or numbness in the arms or legs
Increased sensitivity to sounds, lights, distractions	Loss of coordination
Blurred vision or eyes that tire easily	Increased confusion, restlessness, or agitation
Loss of sense of taste or smell	
Ringing in the ears	
Change in sexual drive	
Mood changes (feeling sad, anxious, listless or becoming easily irritated or angry for little or no reason)	

Note: Older adults taking blood thinners should be seen immediately by a health care provider if they have a bump or blow to the head, even if they do not have any of the symptoms listed here.
From Centers for Disease Control and Prevention: *Preventing Traumatic Brain Injury in Older Adults* (2010). Available at http://www.cdc.gov/traumaticbraininjury/pdf/PreventingBrainInjury_Factsheet_508_080227.pdf. Accessed January 2011.

TABLE 12-3 FALL RISK FACTORS FOR ELDERS

CONDITIONS	SITUATIONS
Sedative and alcohol use, psychoactive medications, opiods, diuretics, anticholinergics, antidepressants, cardiovascular agents, anticoagulants, bowel preparations	Urinary incontinence, urgency, nocturia
Four or more medications	Environmental hazards
Unrelieved pain	Recent relocation, unfamiliarity with new environment
Previous falls and fractures	Inadequate response to transfer and toileting needs
Female, 80 years of age or older	Assistive devices used for walking
Acute and recent illness	Inadequate or missing safety rails, particularly in bathroom
Cognitive impairment (delirium, dementia)	Poorly designed or unstable furniture
Diabetes	High chairs and beds
Chronic pain	Uneven floor surfaces
Dehydration	Glossy, highly waxed floors
Weakness of lower extremities	Wet, greasy, icy surfaces
Abnormalities of gait and balance	Inadequate visual support (glare, low wattage bulbs, lack of nightlights)
Unsteadiness, dizziness, syncope	
Foot problems	
Depression, anxiety	General clutter
Decreased vision or hearing	Inappropriate footwear/clothing
Fear of falling	Pets that inadvertently trip an individual
Orthostatic hypotension	
Postprandial drop in blood pressure	Electrical cords
Decreased weight	Loose or uneven stair treads
Sleep disorders	Throw rugs
Skeletal and neuromuscular changes that predispose to weakness and postural imbalance	Reaching for a high shelf
Functional limitations in self-care activities	Inability to reach personal items, lack of access to call bell or inability to use it
Inability to rise from a chair without using the arms	Side rails, restraints
Slow walking speed	Lack of staff training in fall risk–reduction techniques
Wheelchair-bound	

Data from: National Institute on Aging, National Institutes of Health: *Senior health: falls and older adults* (2008). Available at http://nihseniorhealth.gov/falls/causesandriskfactors/01.html. Accessed December 2010. Feinsod F, Capezutti EA, Felix V: Reducing fall risk in long-term care residents through the interdisciplinary approach, *Annals of Long-term Care* 13:25, 2005; Rubinstein T, Alexander N, Hausdoff J: Evaluating fall risks in older adults: steps and missteps, *Clinical Geriatrics* 11:52, 2003; Tinetti ME, Speechley J, Ginter SF: Risk factors for falls among elderly persons living in the community, *New England Journal of Medicine* 319:1701, 1988; Tinetti ME, Baker DI, King M, et al: Effect of dissemination of evidence in reducing injuries from falls, *New England Journal of Medicine* 359:252, 2008.

programs, and restraints and side rails also interact to increase fall risk.

Falls in the young-old and the more healthy old occur more frequently because of external reasons; however, with increasing age and comorbid conditions, internal and locomotor reasons become increasingly prevalent as factors contributing to falls. The risk of falling increases with the number of risk factors. A community-dwelling older adult with four or more risk factors has an overall 80% risk of suffering a serious fall in the next year (Tinetti et al., 2008; Lach, 2010). Most falls occur from a combination of intrinsic and extrinsic factors that come together at a certain point in time (Table 12-3). Some of the fall risk factors that increase proportionally as one ages include the following:

- Disturbances in visual acuity
- Cognitive impairment
- Chronic pain
- Orthostatic (postural) hypotension
- Cardiac arrhythmias
- Uncontrolled diabetes
- Depressive symptoms
- Lower extremity weakness
- Gait disturbances
- Use of four or more prescription medications

Gait Disturbances

Gait disturbances are frequently seen in older people, especially those 85 years of age and older. Marked gait disorders are not normally a consequence of aging alone but are more likely indicative of an underlying pathological condition. Arthritis of the knee may result in ligamentous weakness and instability, causing the legs to give way or collapse. Muscle weakness is often experienced in hyperthyroidism and hypothyroidism, hypokalemia, hyperparathyroidism, osteomalacia, and hypophosphatemia, and in some cases, it is brought on by various medications. Diabetes, dementia, Parkinson's disease, stroke, alcoholism, and vitamin B deficiencies, may cause neurological damage and resultant gait problems.

Foot Deformities

Foot deformities and ill-fitting footwear also contribute to gait problems. Care of the feet is an important aspect of mobility, comfort, and a stable gait, and is often neglected (Chapter 11). Some older persons are unable to walk comfortably, or at all, because of neglect of corns, bunions, and overgrown nails. Other causes of problems may be traced to loss of fat cushioning and resilience with aging, diabetes, ill-fitting shoes, poor arch support, excessively repetitive weight-bearing activities, obesity, or uneven distribution of weight on the feet. As many as 35% of persons living at home may have significant foot disability that goes untended. Feet and footwear should be inspected as a part of assessment and proper foot care taught to older people and their caregivers. Podiatric referral should be available to older people in both home and institutional settings. Well-fitting walking shoes with low heels and a relatively thin, firm sole (leather) and interior are recommended. Rubber-soled shoes such as sneakers, often recommended for older people, may increase the risk of stumbling while walking, particularly if the person is not accustomed to this type of shoe. This type of shoe may provide too much "sway" and may not promote good balance (American Geriatrics Society, 2010). Orthotic and orthopedic shoes may be indicated for certain foot problems and can greatly enhance mobility and comfort.

Postural and Postprandial Hypotension

Declines in depth perception, proprioception, vibratory sense, and normotensive response to postural changes are important factors that contribute to falls, although the majority of falls occur in individuals with multiple medical problems. Appropriate assessment of postural changes in pulse and blood pressure is important. Clinically significant postural hypotension (orthostasis) is detected in up to 30% of older people (Tinetti, 2003). Postural hypotension is considered a decrease of 20 mm Hg (or more) in systolic pressure or a decrease of 10 mm Hg (or more) in diastolic pressure.

Assessment of postural hypotension in everyday nursing practice is often overlooked or assessed inaccurately. Postural hypotension is more common in the morning, and therefore assessment should occur then (Morley, 2002). All older persons should be cautioned against sudden rising from sitting or supine positions, particularly after eating. Postprandial hypotension (PPH) occurs after ingestion of a carbohydrate meal and may be related to the release of a vasodilatory peptide. PPH is more common in people with diabetes and Parkinson's disease but has been found in approximately 25% of persons who fall (Morley, 2002).

Cognitive Impairment

Older adults with cognitive impairment, such as dementia and delirium, are at increased risk for falls. Fall risk assessments may need to include more specific cognitive risk factors, and cognitive assessment measures may need to be more frequently scheduled for at-risk individuals. One study (Harrison et al., 2010) reported that use of the Confusion Assessment Method

(CAM) to screen for delirium, and the symptom of inattention, has the potential to improve early detection of fall risk in cognitively impaired hospitalized individuals.

PROMOTING HEALTHY AGING: IMPLICATIONS FOR GERONTOLOGICAL NURSING

Screening and Assessment

The American Geriatrics Society/British Geriatrics Society *Clinical Practice Guideline: Prevention of Falls in Older Persons* (2010) recommends that all older individuals should be asked whether they have fallen in the past year and whether they experience difficulties with walking or balance. In addition, ask about falls that did not result in an injury and the circumstances of a near fall, mishap, or misstep because this may provide important information for prevention of future falls (Zecevic et al., 2006). Older people may be reluctant to share information about falls for fear of losing independence, so the nurse must use judgment and empathy in eliciting information about falls, assuring the person that there are many modifiable factors to increase safety and help maintain independence.

If the person reports a fall, they should be asked about the frequency and circumstances of the fall(s) and should be evaluated for gait and balance. Multifactorial fall risk assessments should be performed if the individual cannot perform or performs poorly on a standardized gait and balance test (see Appendix 12-A) or presents for medical attention because of a fall, reports recurrent falls in the past year, or reports difficulty in walking or balance.

Patients who fall present a complex diagnostic challenge and require multifactorial assessment (Table 12-4). In the acute and long-term care settings, an integrated multidisciplinary team (physician, nurse, health care provider, risk manager, physical and occupational therapist, and other designated staff) should be involved in planning care on the basis of findings from an individualized assessment (Gray-Micelli, 2008). Attention to modifying risk factors through appropriate medical management is essential, and this may include medication reduction, treatment of cardiac irregularities, cataract surgery, and management of pain.

Assessment is an ongoing process that includes "multiple and continual types of assessment, reassessment, and evaluation following a fall or intervention to reduce the risk of a fall. Assessment includes: 1) assessment of the older adult at risk; 2) nursing assessment of the patient following a fall; 3) assessment of the environment and other situational circumstances upon admission and during institutional stays; 4) assessment of the older adult's knowledge of falls and their prevention, including willingness to change behavior, if necessary, to prevent falls" (Gray-Micelli, 2008, p. 164).

Fall Risk Assessment Instruments

Various fall risk assessment instruments are available and can be used to identify people who are at risk for falls in community and institutional settings. Instruments that have been evaluated for reliability and validity should be used rather than creating

TABLE 12-4 RECOMMENDED COMPONENTS OF CLINICAL ASSESSMENT AND MANAGEMENT FOR OLDER PERSONS LIVING IN THE COMMUNITY AND WHO ARE AT RISK FOR FALLING

ASSESSMENT AND RISK FACTOR	MANAGEMENT
Circumstances of previous falls*	Changes in environment and activity to reduce the likelihood of recurrent falls
Medication use	Review and reduction of medications
High-risk medications (e.g., benzodiazepines, other sleeping medications, neuroleptics, antidepressants, anticonvulsants, or class IA antiarrhythmic)*,†,‡	
Four or more medications‡	
Vision*	Ample lighting without glare; avoidance of multifocal glasses while walking; referral to an ophthalmologist
Acuity <20/60	
Decreased depth perception	
Decreased contrast sensitivity	
Cataracts	
Postural blood pressure (after ≥5 min in a supine position, immediately after standing, and 2 min after standing)‡	Diagnosis and treatment of underlying cause, if possible; review and reduction of medications; modification of salt restriction; adequate hydration; compensatory strategies (e.g., elevation of head of bed, rising slowly, or dorsiflexion exercises); pressure stockings; pharmacological therapy if the previous strategies fail
≥20 mm Hg (or ≥20%) drop in systolic pressure, with or without symptoms, either immediately or after 2 min of standing	
Balance and gait†,‡	Diagnosis and treatment of underlying cause, if possible; reduction of medications that impair balance; environmental interventions; referral to physical therapist for assistive devices and for gait and progressive balance training
Patient's report or observation of unsteadiness	
Impairment on brief assessment (e.g., the Get Up and Go Test or performance-oriented assessment of mobility)	
Targeted neurological examination	Diagnosis and treatment of underlying cause, if possible; increase in proprioceptive input (with an assistive device or appropriate footwear that encases the foot and has a low heel and thin sole); reduction of medications that impede cognition; awareness on the part of caregivers of cognitive deficits; reduction of environmental risk factors; referral to physical therapist for gait, balance, and strength training
Impaired proprioception*	
Impaired cognition*	
Decreased muscle strength†,‡	
Targeted musculoskeletal examination: examination of legs (joints and range of motion) and examination of feet*	Diagnosis and treatment of the underlying cause, if possible; referral to physical therapist for strength, range-of-motion, and gait and balance training and for assistive devices; use of appropriate footwear; referral to podiatrist
Targeted cardiovascular examination†	Referral to cardiologist; carotid-sinus massage (in the case of syncope)
Syncope	
Arrhythmia (if there is known cardiac disease, an abnormal electrocardiogram, and syncope)	
Home hazard evaluation after hospital discharge†,‡	Removal of loose rugs and the use of nightlights, nonslip bathmats, and stair rails; other interventions as necessary

From Tinetti M: Preventing falls in elderly persons, *New England Journal of Medicine* 348:42, 2003.
*Recommendation of this assessment is based on observational data that the finding is associated with an increased risk of falling.
†Recommendation of this assessment is based on one or more randomized controlled trials of a single intervention.
‡Recommendation of this assessment is based on one or more randomized controlled trials of a multifactorial intervention strategy that included this component.

new instruments (Gray-Micelli, 2008). Fall risk assessments provide general information about a person's risk factors but must be used in combination with additional individual assessment so that appropriate fall risk-reduction interventions can be developed and modifiable risk factors identified and managed.

The following concerns have been identified related to fall risk assessment instruments:

- In institutions, nurses often complete these assessments every shift in a routine manner and risk factors identified may not be addressed. In addition, risk factors may not be known due to lack of assessment and knowledge of patient's history.
- The scores used to identify patients at high risk may not be based on research.
- So many patients are considered at high risk that nurses may become desensitized to fall risks and have difficulty prioritizing interventions.
- Nurses' clinical judgment is not considered and may be as effective at identifying high-risk patients as use of fall-risk screening tools (Harrison et al., 2010; Lach, 2010).

Lach (2010) reported that "the problems with fall risk assessment tools caused one author to wonder whether these tools should be 'put to bed'" (p. 152). Additional research is needed to develop valid, reliable instruments to differentiate levels of fall risk in various settings.

The Hendrich II Fall Risk Model (Hendrich et al., 2003) (Figure 12-2), recommended by the Hartford Foundation for Geriatric Nursing (New York, NY), is an example of an instrument that has been validated with skilled nursing and rehabilitation populations. A *Nursing Standard of Practice Protocol: Fall Prevention* and a video demonstrating the Hendrich II Fall Risk Model are available at http://consultgerirn.org/topics/falls/want_to_know_more). The Morse Fall Scale (Morse et al., 1989) is also widely used in hospitals and other inpatient settings. In the skilled nursing facility, the Minimum Data Set (MDS 3.0) includes information about history of falls and hip fractures as well as an assessment of balance during transitions and walking (moving from seated to standing, walking, turning around, moving on and off toilet, and transfers between bed and chair or wheelchair) (Chapter 7).

Hendrich II Fall Risk Model™

Confusion Disorientation Impulsivity		4	
Symptomatic Depression		2	
Altered Elimination		1	
Dizziness Vertigo		1	
Male Gender		1	
Any Administered Antiepileptics		2	
Any Administered Benzodiazepines		1	
Get Up & Go Test			
Able to rise in a single movement – No loss of balance with steps		0	
Pushes up, successful in one attempt		1	
Multiple attempts, but successful		3	
Unable to rise without assistance during test (OR if a medical order states the same and/or complete bed rest is ordered) * If unable to assess, document this on the patient chart with the date and time		4	
A Score of 5 or Greater = High Risk		**Total Score**	

FIGURE 12-2 The Hendrich II Fall Risk Model. The Hendrich II fall risk model is a fall risk assessment tool recommended by the Hartford Institute for Geriatric Nursing. (© 2007 AHI of Indiana Inc. All rights reserved. U.S. patent (US20050182305) has been allowed. Reproduction and use prohibited except by written permission from AHI of Indiana Inc.)

Postfall Assessment

Incomplete analysis of the reasons for a fall can result in repeated incidents. "When important details are overlooked, missing information leads to an inappropriate plan of care" (Gray-Micelli, 2008, p. 33). Postfall assessments (PFAs) are essential to prevention of future falls and implementation of risk-reduction programs, particularly in institutional settings. The initial post-fall assessment includes assessment of the patient for any obvious injuries and the provision of appropriate treatment. If the older adult cannot tell you about the circumstances of the fall, information should be obtained from staff or witnesses. The purpose of the PFA is to identify the underlying cause(s) of the fall and assist in implementing appropriate individualized risk-reduction interventions. Because complications of falls may not occur immediately, all patients should be observed for 48 hours after a fall. Standard "incident report" forms do not provide adequate postfall assessment information. The Department of Veterans Affairs National Center for Patient safety (http://www.patientsafety.gov/SafetyTopics/fallstoolkit/

index.html) provides a guide for a PSA as well as comprehensive information about fall assessment, fall risk reduction, and policies and procedures. Box 12-5 presents information for a PFA that can be used in health care institutions.

Results of a qualitative study describing the intentions of older homebound women to prevent a fall (Porter et al., 2010) suggest that postfall assessments should include the person's explanation of the fall, description of any changes the individual has made as a result of the fall, and what interventions they are taking to prevent further falls. Information such as this would contribute to individualizing fall prevention interventions.

Interventions

Randomized controlled trials support the effectiveness of multicomponent fall prevention strategies in reducing fall risks (Tinetti et al., 2008; Cameron et al., 2010). However, Frick and colleagues (2010) suggest that multifactorial approaches aimed at all older people, or high-risk elders, are not necessarily more cost-effective or better than focused intervention approaches

BOX 12-5   POSTFALL ASSESSMENT SUGGESTIONS

HISTORY

- Description of the fall from the individual or witness
- Individual's opinion of the cause of the fall
- Circumstances of the fall (trip or slip)
- Person's activity at the time of the fall
- Presence of comorbid conditions, such as a previous stroke, Parkinson's disease, osteoporosis, seizure disorder, sensory deficit, joint abnormalities, depression, cardiac disease
- Medication review
- Associated symptoms, such as chest pain, palpitations, light-headedness, vertigo, fainting, weakness, confusion, incontinence, or dyspnea
- Time of day and location of the fall
- Presence of acute illness

PHYSICAL EXAMINATION

- Vital signs: postural blood pressure changes, fever, or hypothermia
- Head and neck: visual impairment, hearing impairment, nystagmus, bruit
- Heart: arrhythmia or valvular dysfunction
- Neurological signs: altered mental status, focal deficits, peripheral neuropathy, muscle weakness, rigidity or tremor, impaired balance
- Musculoskeletal signs: arthritic changes, range of motion (ROM), podiatric deformities or problems, swelling, redness or bruises, abrasions, pain on movement, shortening and external rotation of lower extremities

FUNCTIONAL ASSESSMENT

Observe and inquire about the following:

- Functional gait and balance: observe resident rising from chair, walking, turning, and sitting down
- Balance test, mobility, use of assistive devices or personal assistance, extent of ambulation, restraint use, prosthetic equipment
- Activities of daily living: bathing, dressing, transferring, toileting

ENVIRONMENTAL ASSESSMENT

- Staffing patterns, unsafe practice in transferring, delay in response to call light
- Faulty equipment
- Use of bed, chair alarm
- Call light within reach
- Wheelchair, bed locked
- Adequate supervision
- Clutter, walking paths not clear
- Dim lighting
- Glare
- Uneven flooring
- Wet, slippery floors
- Poorly-fitted seating devices
- Inappropriate footwear
- Inappropriate eyewear

---

and that further research is needed. An important consideration is individual assessment and tailoring interventions to identified risk factors. Interventions should include an education component complementing and addressing issues specific to the intervention being provided and tailored to individual cognitive function and language (American Geriatrics Society, 2010).

As part of a randomized study of fall prevention in an acute care hospital, Dykes and colleagues (2010), developed a fall prevention tool kit utilizing a health information technology program. The tool kit included a fall risk assessment, patient-specific prevention plan, a patient/family educational handout (at a consumer level of literacy), and a poster for over the bed. Results suggested that the use of the tool kit significantly reduced the rate of falls, particularly among older patients. While most hospitals routinely screen all patients for fall risk, tailoring interventions based on individual risks is done less frequently. Additionally, the individualized fall prevention plan was communicated in an effective manner to patients, families, and staff through the use of the poster and the handout. Further research is needed to determine if a similar program evaluated over a longer period of time can significantly reduce falls.

Lach (2010) reminds us that "while there is much that the nurse can do to manage falls, it may be unrealistic to think that they can be eliminated" (p. 151). Fall risk-reduction programs are a shared responsibility of all health care providers caring for older adults. Choosing the most appropriate interventions to reduce the risk of falls depends on appropriate assessment at various intervals depending on the person's changing condition. A one-size-fits-all approach is not effective and further research is needed to determine the type, frequency, and timing of interventions best suited for specific populations (community-living, hospital and institutionalized, and racially and culturally diverse older adults).

In a comprehensive review of fall prevention and injury protection for nursing home residents, Quigley and colleagues (2010) suggest that the "dose, intensity, duration, and components of an effective fall and injury prevention program are not clear . . . and there is little firm evidence demonstrating the cost benefit or return on investment of fall prevention and injury protection in the nursing home" (p. 284). Ireland and colleagues (2010) also suggest that each institution needs to design strategies to meet organizational needs and to match patient population needs and clinical realities of the staff.

Box 12-6 presents an innovative fall risk-reduction program, designed by a nurse in an acute care facility, that has been adopted around the country and included in fall risk-reduction guidelines. Other innovative programs in nursing homes include the Visiting Angels and neighborhood watch teams. In the Visiting Angels program, alert residents visit and converse with cognitively impaired residents in the late afternoon and evening when fall risk starts to rise. Neighborhood watch teams involve the evening and night staff in morning reviews of any fall or incident that happened during the night (Kilgore, 2010). The components most commonly included in efficacious interventions are shown in Box 12-7.

Exercise

The relationship between exercise and fall risk reduction is strong, particularly when combined with balance training, for elders in the community (Sherrington et al., 2008). Although the best type, duration, and intensity of exercise have not been determined, exercise programs must be at least 10 weeks in duration, must be individualized, and must target strength, gait, and balance for maximal benefit. In institutional settings, depending on the condition of the patient, early mobilization and measures to increase mobility are important. Group exercises may also be of benefit. Further research is needed to

BOX 12-6   THE RUBY SLIPPER FALL INTERVENTION PROGRAM

Nurse Ginny Goldner of St. Joseph's Hospital in Tucson, Arizona, started the "Ruby Slipper" program to identify patients at risk for falling and to help prevent falls in elderly patients. Patients at risk for falls wear red socks with nonslip treads so that anyone from a housekeeper to a head nurse who sees them walking around or trying to get out of bed will know to stay with them until they are safely back in bed. Education on fall risk reduction, identification of patients at high risk, and Ruby Slipper rounds on high-risk patients to see whether they need anything, such as to go to the bathroom, are included in the program as well. The program has reduced patient falls by nearly 75%. Ginny was awarded the March of Dimes Arizona Innovation and Creativity Nurse of the Year Award for the program. The ruby slipper program has been adopted by many hospitals across the country and is also included in the evidence-based guideline for fall prevention from the Institute for Clinical Systems Improvement: *Health Care Protocol: Prevention of Falls (Acute Care)* (http://www.icsi.org/falls__acute_care___prevention_of__protocol_/falls__acute_care___prevention_of__protocol__24255.html).

Data from Arizona Hospital and Healthcare Association, *www.azhha.org.* For information, contact Ginny Goldner RN, MS at (520) 873-3722 or email vgoldner@carondelet.org.

BOX 12-7   SELECTED COMPONENTS OF FALL RISK-REDUCTION INTERVENTIONS

- Adaptation or modification of home environment
- Withdrawal or minimization of psychoactive medications
- Withdrawal or minimization of other medications
- Management of postural hypotension
- Continence programs such as prompted voiding
- Management of foot problems and footwear
- Exercise, particularly balance, strength, and gait training
- Staff and patient education

Source: American Geriatrics Society: *AGS clinical practice guideline: prevention of falls in older persons* (2010). Available at http://www.americangeriatrics.org/health_care_professionals/clinical_practice/clinical_guidelines_recommendations/2010. Accessed December 2010; *Nursing standard of practice protocol: fall prevention.* Available at www.consultgerirn.org/topics/falls/want_to_know_more. Accessed December 2010.

evaluate the effect of exercise on fall risk reduction in long-term care settings.

Medication Review

Reduction of medications is an important component of effective fall risk-reduction programs. Medications, including over-the-counter (OTC) and herbals, should be reviewed and limited to those that are absolutely essential. Risk of falls increases with the use of four or more medications, particularly neuroleptics and benzodiazepines. Frick and colleagues (2010), in a study of the cost-effectiveness of fall prevention programs that reduce hip fracture in older adults, reported that management of psychotropics was the most effective and least expensive falls management option of those considered. Home modifications, group tai chi, and vitamin D supplementation were also reported to be effective and cost-efficient interventions.

A recent study (Buckeridge et al, 2010) reports that the use of low-potency opiods for chronic pain, particularly codeine

combinations, are increasing among older adults. Higher doses of these medications result in twice the risk of injury from falls. Short acting episode may be especially problematic in increasing fall risk when compared to longer acting episode medication (American Public Health Association, 2010). Further research is needed but if these medications are being used, patient teaching should be provided related to fall risk, appropriate dosing and use of other medications, such as benzodiazepines, as well as alcohol use.

Environmental Modifications

Environmental modifications alone have not been shown to reduce falls, but when included as part of a multifactorial program, they may be of benefit in risk reduction. However, a home environmental assessment including mitigation of hazards and interventions to promote the safe performance of daily activities is recommended (see Chapter 13, Table 13-1). Another valuable resource for older adults is the Check for Safety available at www.cdc.gov/ncipc/pub-res/toolkit/Falls_Tool/DesktopPDF/English/booklet_Eng_desktop.pdf. Assistive technologies, such as fall sensors and devices that monitor gait and stability, are discussed in Chapter 13. In institutional settings, the patient care environment should be assessed routinely for extrinsic factors that may contribute to falls and corrective action taken. Patients should be able to access the bathroom or be provided with a bedside commode, routine assistance to toilet, and programs such as prompted voiding (Chapter 11). The majority of falls in acute care occur in patient rooms (79.5%) followed by bathrooms (11%) and hallways (9.5%) (Tzeng and Yin, 2008).

The following is a list of important areas to check for safety:

- Outdoor grounds and indoor floor surfaces for spills, wet areas, and unevenness
- Proper illumination and functioning of lights, including night lights
- Tabletops, furniture, and beds are sturdy and in good repair
- Grab rails and grab bars are in place in the bathroom
- Adaptive aids work properly and are in good repair
- Bed rails do not collapse when used for transitioning or support
- Patient gowns/clothing do not cause tripping; proper footwear is provided
- IV poles are sturdy if used during ambulation and tubing does not cause tripping

Behavior and Education Programs

As a single strategy, behavior and education programs do not reduce falls but are recommended as part of multifactorial intervention programs. Information should be provided to the older person, to health care professionals, and to caregivers on fall risk factors and fall risk-reduction strategies. There are many excellent sources of information for both consumers and health care professionals on interventions to reduce fall risk (see Box 12-10 and Resources on Evolve).

Assistive Devices

Research on multifactorial interventions including the use of assistive devices has demonstrated benefits in fall risk reduction. It is important to provide instruction and supervision on the

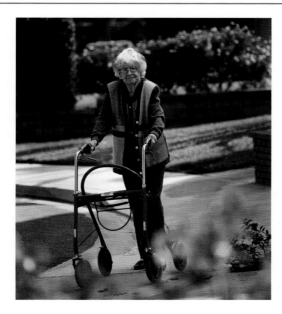

Maintaining Ambulation and Safety with Appropriate Assistive Devices. (Courtesy Corbis Images.)

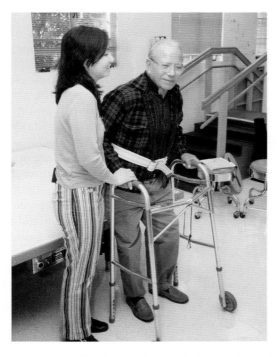

A Physical Therapist Helping a Client to Ambulate. (From Ignatavicius DD, Workman ML: *Medical-surgical nursing: patient-centered collaborative care*, ed 6, St. Louis, MO, 2010, WB Saunders.)

correct use of assistive devices. Assist the person in obtaining a written prescription for the assistive device because Medicare may cover up to 80% of the cost of the device; other insurance coverage varies.

Many devices are available that are designed for specific conditions and limitations. Physical therapists provide training on use of assistive devices, and nurses can supervise correct use. New technologies such as canes that "talk" and provide feedback to the user, sensors that detect when falls have occurred or when risk of falling is increasing, and other developing assistive

technologies hold the potential to significantly improve functional ability, safety, and independence for older people (Rantz et al., 2008) (Chapter 13).

When an assistive device is obtained, the individual will need assistance in learning to use it correctly. Following are some general principles for walker and cane use:

- Place your cane firmly on the ground before you take a step, and do not place it too far ahead of you. Put all of your weight on your unaffected leg, and then move the cane and your affected leg at a comfortable distance forward. With your weight supported on both your cane and your affected leg, step through with your unaffected leg.
- Always wear low-heeled, nonskid shoes.
- When using a cane on stairs, step up with the unaffected leg and down with the affected leg. Use the cane as support when lifting the affected leg. Bring the cane up to the step just reached before climbing another step. When descending, place the cane on the next step down, move the affected leg down, and then move the unaffected leg down.
- When using a walker, stand upright and lift or roll the walker with both hands a step's length ahead of you. Lean slightly forward, and hold the arms of the walker for support. Step toward it with the weaker leg, and then bring the stronger leg forward. Do not climb stairs with a walker.
- Every assistive device must be adjusted to individual height; the top of the cane should align with the crease of the wrist.
- Choose a size and shape of cane handle that fits comfortably in the palm; like a tight shoe, it will be a constant irritant if it is not properly fitted.
- Cane tips are most secure when they are flat at the bottom and have a series of rings. Replace tips frequently because they wear out, and a worn tip is insecure.

Wheelchairs are a necessary adjunct at some level of immobility and for some individuals, but are overused in nursing homes, with up to 80% of residents spending time sitting in a wheelchair every day. Often, the individual is not assessed for therapeutic treatment and restorative ambulation programs to improve mobility and function. Improperly maintained or ill-fitting wheelchairs can cause pressure ulcers, skin tears, bruises and abrasions, nerve impingement, and account for 16% of nursing home falls (Gavin-Dreschnack et al., 2010). There are many new assistive devices that could replace wheelchairs, such as small walkers with wheels and seats and automative brakes.

All nursing homes need to implement programs that promote ambulation and improve function. Brief walks and repeated chair stands four times a day improved walking and endurance in frail, deconditioned, cognitively impaired nursing home residents. Tappen and colleagues (2000) reported that a combination of assisted walking with conversation reduced decline in functional ability and improved mood in nursing home residents with Alzheimer's. If the person is unable to ambulate without assistance, they should be seated in comfortable chairs with frequent repositioning and wheelchairs should be used for transport only. Electric scooters and wheelchairs may be appropriate for some residents as well, but instruction on safe use is necessary. At one Veterans Affairs medical center, the physical therapists held driving classes to teach safety with these devices. It is important that a professional evaluate the wheelchair for proper fit and provide training on proper use as well as evaluate the resident for more appropriate mobility and seating devices and ambulation programs.

The GROW initiative (Getting Residents Out of Wheelchairs) (www.growcoalition.org) was conceived by a group of health professionals to lobby against the overuse of wheelchairs in nursing homes and advocates for increased ambulation whenever possible and decreasing the use of wheelchairs when regular chairs could be used for stationary seating. Their mission is to support the Advancing Excellence in America's Nursing Homes campaign (http://www.nhqualitycampaign.org/), which is discussed further in Chapter 16 (Gavin-Dreschnack et al., 2010).

Other Interventions

Other potential interventions include assessment and treatment of osteoporosis to reduce fracture rates (Chapter 15). Older people with osteoporosis are more likely to experience serious injury from a fall. Vitamin D supplementation is recommended for nursing home residents. The use of hip protectors for prevention of hip fractures in high-risk individuals may be considered, and there is some evidence that they may have an overall effect on rates of hip fracture (Oliver et al., 2007; Hayes et al., 2008; Quigley et al., 2010), but further research is needed to determine their effectiveness (Kiel et al., 2007). Compliance has been a concern related to the ease of application and getting them off quickly enough for toileting.

Formal vision assessment is also an important intervention to identify remediable visual problems. Although a significant relationship exists between visual problems and falls and fractures, little research has been conducted on interventions for visual problems as part of fall risk-reduction programs. Poor visual acuity, reduced contrast sensitivity, decreased visual field, cataracts, and use of nonmiotic glaucoma medications have all been associated with falls.

RESTRAINTS AND SIDE RAILS

Definition and History

A physical restraint is defined as any manual method, physical or mechanical device, material, or equipment that immobilizes or reduces the ability of a patient to move his or her arms, legs, body, or head freely. A chemical restraint is when a drug or medication is used as a restriction to manage the patient's behavior or restrict the patient's freedom of movement and is not a standard treatment or dosage for the patient's condition. Historically, restraints and side rails have been used for the "protection" of the patient and for the security of the patient and staff. Originally, restraints were used to control the behavior of individuals with mental illness considered to be dangerous to themselves or others (Evans and Strumpf, 1989).

The problem of restraint use was first brought to the forefront of nursing attention by a request from Doris Schwartz, one of the gerontological nursing pioneers, for information from practicing nurses regarding their observations and concerns about restraint usage. Research over the last 20 years by nurses such as Lois Evans, Neville Strumpf, and Elizabeth Capezuti has shown that the practice of physical restraint is ineffective and hazardous. Through research, increased knowledge about restraint alternatives, advocacy groups' efforts, and changed standards and regulations concerning restraints there has been a significant reduction in restraint use, particularly in long-term care settings. According to the Agency for Healthcare Research and Quality (AHRQ) 2009 National Health Disparities Report, the number of residents in nursing homes who were physically restrained dropped by more than half from 1999 to 2007 in long-term care (www.ahrq.gov/qual/qrdr09.htm).

Consequences of Restraints

Physical restraints, intended to prevent injury, do not protect patients from falling, wandering, or removing tubes and other medical devices. Physical restraints may actually exacerbate many of the problems for which they are used and can cause serious injury and death as well as emotional and physical problems. "The most common mechanism of restraint-related death is by asphyxiation—that is, the person is suspended by a restraint from a bed or chair and the ability to inhale is inhibited by gravitational chest compression" (Wagner et al., 2008, p. 168). Physical restraints are associated with higher mortality rates, injurious falls, nosocomial infections, incontinence, contractures, pressure ulcers, agitation, and depression. Although prevention of falls is most frequently cited as the primary reason for using restraints, restraints do not prevent serious injury and may even increase the risk of injury and death. Injuries occur as a result of the patient attempting to remove the restraint or attempting to get out of bed while restrained.

The use of restraints is a great source of physical and psychological distress to older adults and may intensify agitation and contribute to depression. Side rails may be seen as a barrier rather than a reminder of the need to request assistance with transfers. And, for some older people, especially those with a history of trauma (such as that induced by war, rape, or domestic violence), side rails may cause fear and agitation and a feeling of being jailed or caged (Sullivan-Marx, 1995; Talerico and Capezuti, 2001). The following quotes from a qualitative study on restraints by Strumpf and colleagues (1992, p. 126) illustrate the reactions of two patients:

> "I felt like a dog and cried all night. It hurt me to have to be tied up. I felt like I was nobody, that I was dirt. It makes me cry to talk about it. The hospital is worse than a jail."

> "I don't remember misbehaving, but I may have been deranged from all the pills they gave me. Normally, I am spirited, but I am also good and obedient. Nevertheless, the nurse tied me down, like Jesus on the cross, by bandaging both wrists and ankles. . . . It felt awful, I hurt and I worried. Callers, including men friends, saw me like that and thought I lost something. I lost a little personal prestige. I was embarrassed, like a child placed in a corner for being bad. I had been important . . . and to be tied down in bed took a big toll . . . I haven't forgotten the pain and the indignity of being tied."

Side Rails

Side rails are no longer viewed as simply attachments to a patient's bed but are considered restraints with all the accompanying concerns just discussed. Side rails are now defined as restraints or restrictive devices when used to impede a person's ability to voluntarily get out of bed and the person cannot lower them by themselves. Restrictive side rail use is defined as two full-length or four half-length raised side rails. If the patient uses a half- or quarter-length upper side rail to assist in getting in and out of bed, it is not considered a restraint (Talerico and Capezuti, 2001). "Because the use of body restraints, such as vest and wrist restraints, has been drastically reduced in nursing homes, restrictive siderails have become the most frequently used restraint to prevent older adults from bed-related falls" (Wagner et al., 2007, p. 132).

There is no evidence to date that side rail use decreases the risk or rate of fall occurrence. There are numerous reports and studies documenting the negative effects of side rail use, including entrapment deaths and injuries that occur when the person slips through the side rail bars or between split side rails, the side rail and the mattress, or between the head or footboard, side rail, the mattress; or between the head or footboard, side rail, and mattress (Talerico and Capezuti, 2001; Wagner et al., 2007). The U.S. Food and Drug Administration (2006) issued a hospital bed design guidance to reduce side rail entrapment (http://www.fda.gov/NewsEvents/Newsroom/PressAnnouncements/2006/ucm108612.htm).

The Centers for Medicare & Medicaid Services (CMS) require nursing homes to conduct individualized assessments of residents, provide alternatives, or clearly document the need for restrictive side rails (Sollins, 2009). Capezuti and colleagues (1998) describe an individualized assessment tool for side rail use. A side rail utilization assessment, adapted from the work of Capezuti and colleagues (1999), can be found at the TMF Health Quality Institute (Austin, TX) website (http://nursinghomes.tmf.org/Portals/16/Documents/NH/Toolkits/Restraints/SideRailUtilizationAssessment.pdf).

Restraint-Free Care

Restraint-free care is now the standard of practice and an indicator of quality care in all health care settings, although transition to that standard is still in progress, particularly in acute care settings. The Hartford Geriatric Nursing Institute provides an evidence-based protocol on physical restraints (Box 12-10) and a guideline for restraint use in acute care has been developed by Park and Hsiao-Chen Tang (2007) (Figure 12-3).

Flaherty (2004) remarked that a "restraint-free environment should be held as the standard of care and anything less is substandard. The fact that it is done in some European hospitals (de Vries et al., 2004) and in some U.S. hospitals, even among delirious patients, and in skilled nursing facilities should be evidence enough that it can be done everywhere" (p. 919). Implementing best practice nursing in fall risk reduction and restraint-free care is a complex clinical decision-making process and calls for recognition, assessment, and intervention for physical and psychosocial concerns contributing to patient safety, knowledge of restraint alternatives, interdisciplinary teamwork, and institutional commitment. Antonelli (2008) described a comprehensive restraint management program in an acute care that was successful in improving care practices and reducing restraint use. Included in the program were the development of a restraint prevention cart to increase the

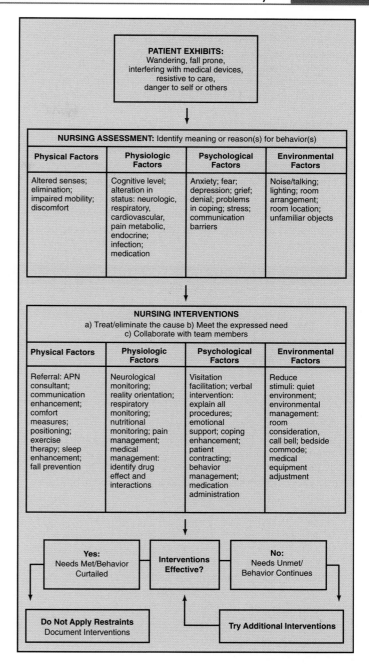

FIGURE 12-3 Decision Algorithm: Behavior Management and Restraint-free Care. *APN,* advanced practice nurse. (From Park M, Hsiao-Chen Tang J: Evidence-based guidelines: changing the practice of physical restraint use in acute care, *Journal of Gerontological Nursing* 33:9, 2007.)

accessibility of alternatives to restraints, rounds and consultation led by a geriatric nurse practitioner, the use of college and high school students as activity assistants, and staff education.

Removing restraints without careful attention to underlying fall-risk factors and effective alternative strategies can jeopardize safety. The use of advanced practice nurse consultation in implementing alternatives to restraints has been most effective (Bourbonniere and Evans, 2002; Capezuti, 2004; Wagner et al., 2007). Important areas of focus derived from research on advanced practice nurse consultations include compensating for memory loss (e.g., improving behavior, anticipating needs, providing visual and physical cues; improving impaired mobility; reducing injury potential); evaluating nocturia/incontinence; and reducing sleep disturbances. The key to successful implementation of restraint-free fall prevention interventions is conducting careful individualized assessments. What works for one resident may not necessarily be effective for another (Wagner et al., 2007, pp. 134, 138).

Staff education is also important and one study reported increased knowledge, attitude change, and reduction of the use of physical restraints without any change in the incidence of falls or use of psychoactive medications after a six-month education program (Pellfolk et al., 2010). Many of the suggestions on safety and fall risk reduction in this chapter can be used

to promote a safe and restraint-free environment. Fall risk reduction and alternative strategies to restraints are presented in Boxes 12-8 and 12-9. A list of resources can be found in Box 12-10 and on the Evolve website.

PROMOTION OF HEALTHY AGING: IMPLICATIONS FOR GERONTOLOGICAL NURSING

Gerontological nurses need to be knowledgeable about fall risk factors and fall risk-reduction interventions in all settings. Health promotion interventions to maintain fitness and mobility; appropriate assessment of fall risk; teaching older adults, their caregivers, and staff about fall risk factors; fall

---

BOX 12-8   SUGGESTIONS FOR FALL RISK REDUCTION AND RESTRAINT ALTERNATIVES

ASSESSMENT
- Work with the interdisciplinary team; nurses cannot manage these complicated challenges alone.
- Perform fall risk screening; gait, balance, and mobility assessment. Multifactorial assessment as indicated.
- Individualize the patient's plan of care based on risk factors and condition.
- Assess ambulation ability; refer to physical therapy for walking and/or strengthening.
- Check for postural hypotension (orthostasis).
- Use a behavior log to track when the person is trying to get up, and/or when he or she seems agitated.
- Assess mental status (delirium/dementia).
- Assess vision and hearing. If the person wears glasses, hearing aid, or dentures, see that they are worn.
- Assess continence status.
- Assess for pain and ensure that pain is well managed.
- Involve family and all staff in fall risk-reduction education and activities.
- Inform all staff of fall risk, and put fall risk and fall risk-reduction interventions on care plan.
- Use identification bracelet or door sign to indicate patients at risk for falling. Use red socks with treads to identify patient at risk.

PATIENT ROOM
- Lower the bed to the lowest level, or use a bed that is especially designed to be low to the floor.
- Use a concave mattress.
- Use bed boundary markers to mark the edges of the bed, such as mattress bumpers, rolled blanket, or "swimming noodles" under sheets.
- If the person is (or has been married), line the spouse's side of the bed with pillows or bolsters.
- Place a soft floor mat or a mattress by the bed to cushion any falls.
- Use a water mattress to reduce movement to the edge of the bed.
- Have the person at risk sleep on a mattress on the floor.
- Remove wheels from the bed.
- Clear the floor of debris, excessive furniture; make sure it is not wet or slippery.
- Place nonskid strips on the floor next to the bed; ensure that floors are nonskid.
- Use night lights in the bedroom and bathroom.
- Place a call bell within reach, and make sure the patient can use it—attach the call bell to the patient's garment or obtain an adapted call device.
- Provide visual reminders to encourage the patient to use the call bell.
- Have a purse (empty or without harmful items or important papers or money) in the bed with the person, if a woman.
- Ensure all personal items are within reach.
- Have ambulation devices within reach, and make sure the patient knows how to use them properly.

- Use bed, chair, or wrist alarms (the best alarm tells you only that there is an emergency; still need frequent checks, supervised areas). Apply a patient-worn sensor (lightweight alarm worn above the knee that is position-sensitive).
- Provide a trapeze or patient assist handles (transfer bars) to enhance mobility in bed.
- If the person is able, he or she should walk at every opportunity possible. If the patient walked in or could walk before hospitalization, make every effort to keep the patient walking during hospitalization.
- Do frequent bed checks, especially during the evening and at night.
- Be especially alert at change-of-shift times.
- Understand that very few people spend all day in bed; activity is necessary.
- Provide diversional activities (catalogues, puzzles, therapeutic activity kit) (http://consultgerirn.org/uploads/File/trythis/try_this_d4.pdf).
- Know sleeping patterns—if the person is usually up during the night, get him or her up in a chair and keep at nursing station or involve in activities.

BATHROOM
- Establish toileting plan, and take the person to the bathroom frequently.
- Have the person use a bedside commode.
- Make sure the person knows the location of the bathroom—leave the door open so he or she can see the toilet, or put a picture of a toilet on the door; clear the path to the bathroom.
- Provide grab bars in the bathroom and shower; provide a shower chair with suction bottom.
- Provide an elevated toilet seat.
- Have the person wear clothing that is easy to pull down for toileting.

ON THE UNIT
- Assess for environmental hazards.
- Keep the person in a supervised area or room within view of the nursing station.
- Have the person sit in a reclining chair, chair with a deep seat, bean bag chair, rocker—keep close to nurses' station in the chair.
- Consider occupational therapy evaluation for seating devices.
- Provide a supervised area and meaningful activities.
- If the person is wandering or trying to exit, create a grid with masking tape on the floor in front of the doorway, use a black half-rug, and camouflage exit doors with wallpaper, window treatments, and so on.
- Provide hip protectors, helmets, and arm pads for high-risk individuals
- Investigate the Hospital Elder Life Program (HELP) and consider implementing (http://www.hospitalelderlifeprogram.org/public/public-main.php).
- Provide a restraint management cart with alternative restraint products arranged in order of least restrictive measures as described by Antonelli (2008).

BOX 12-9 TIPS FOR DEALING WITH TUBES, LINES, AND OTHER MEDICAL DEVICES

- Assessment: First question: "Is the device really necessary?" Remove as soon as possible.
- Preoperative teaching about the device allowing the person to see and the tubes may be effective in decreasing anxiety about devices.
- Use guided exploration and a mirror to help the patient understand what devices are in place and why.
- Provide comfort care to the site—oral and nasal care, anchoring of tubing, topical anesthetic on site.
- Foley catheters should be used only if the patient needs intensive output monitoring or has an obstruction.
- Weigh risks and benefits of restraint versus therapy: Are alternatives available, e.g., replace intravenous (IV) tubing with heparin lock, deliver medications intramuscularly (IM), consider intermittent IV administration or hypodermoclysis.
- Use camouflage: clothing or elastic sleeves, temporary air splint (occupational therapy can be helpful), skin sleeves to prevent IV tube dislodgement.
- Use mitts instead of wrist restraints; roll belts instead of vest restraints.
- Use diversional activity aprons (zipping–unzipping, threading exercises, dials and knobs), busy box, or therapeutic activity kit.
- Hide lines by placing them in an unobtrusive place; place tubing behind the patient, out of his or her view; have patient wear long sleeves or double surgical gowns with cuffs to prevent access.
- Hang IV bags behind the patient's field of vision.
- Nasogastric (NG) tubes—replace with percutaneous endoscopic gastrostomy (PEG) tube if necessary but obtain comprehensive speech therapy swallowing evaluation. If NG tube is used, use as small a lumen as possible to minimize irritation; consider taping with occlusive dressings.
- Cover the PEG tube or abdominal incisions and other tubes with an abdominal binder, sweat pants.
- For men with Foley catheters—shave area just above pubis, and tape catheter to pubis. *Never* secure catheter to leg (causes discomfort and can cause a fistula). Run tubing around back and down leg to a leg bag. Patient should wear underpants and pajama pants.
- Take restraints off while working with the patient.
- Use a modified soft collar for tracheostomy protection.

BOX 12-10 GUIDELINES AND PROTOCOLS FOR EXERCISE, FALL PREVENTION AND RESTRAINT ALTERNATIVES

- American Geriatrics Society/British Geriatrics Society Clinical Practice Guideline for Prevention of Falls in Older Persons: http://www.americangeriatrics.org/health_care_professionals/clinical_practice/clinical_guidelines_recommendations/2010/
- Dementia Series: Tools and strategies in the assessment of older adults with dementia (includes avoiding restraints in older adults with dementia in print and video): http://consultgerirn.org/resources/#issues_on_dementia
- Exercise Promotion: Walking in Older Adults: http://www.guideline.gov/content.aspx?id=10948&search=exercise+promotion+walking+in+older+adults
- National Center for Patient Safety: http://www.patientsafety.gov/SafetyTopics/fallstoolkit/index.html
- National Guideline Clearing House: Fall Management Guideline: http://www.guideline.gov/summary/summary.aspx?doc_id=13484
- Physical activity and public health in older adults: recommendation from the American College of Sports Medicine and the American Heart Association: http://www.guideline.gov/content.aspx?id=11691&search=exercise+promotion+walking+in+older+adults
- The Nursing Standard of Practice: Fall Prevention: www.consultgerirn.org/topics/falls/want_to_know_more
- Side rail utilization assessment: http://nursinghomes.tmf.org/Portals/16/Documents/NH/Toolkits/Restraints/SideRailUtilizationAssessment.pdf
- Use of physical restraints with elderly patients: http://consultgerirn.org/topics/physical_restraints/want_to_know_more/

---

risk reduction interventions; and restraint-free care are important nursing responses. For community-dwelling older adults, nurses need to have knowledge of home, community, and environmental safety factors, as well as assistive devices and technology, environmental modifications, and resources to aid in maintaining independence and functional abilities. In institutions, working as members of the interdisciplinary team, nurses bring expert knowledge of patient activities, abilities, and needs from a 24 hr/day, 7 day/week perspective to help the team implement the most appropriate interventions and evaluate outcomes. Accidents and injuries among older adults in all settings are significant in terms of morbidity and mortality, and using evidence-based practice can ensure improvement of many modifiable and preventable injuries, as well as mobility limitations and functional decline.

In summary, the capacity to move about, on two legs, horses, and wheeled vehicles, has been portrayed from the earliest recorded time. The nurse can be significant in facilitating this most fundamental human need, to assist our patients to maintain independence, preserve autonomy, and move as far as their reach extends and as far as the imagination will allow.

ℯvolve To access your student resources, go to *http://evolve.elsevier.com/Ebersole/TwdHlthAging*

KEY CONCEPTS

- Mobility provides opportunities for exercise, exploration, and pleasure and is the crux of maintaining independence.
- Changes in bones, muscles, and ligaments affect one's balance and gait as one ages and increase instability.
- Ease of mobility is thought to be the most visible measure of one's overall health and survival capacity.
- Muscle weakness must be investigated because it is often a result of reversible problems, such as endocrine imbalances (particularly hypothyroidism) or medication reactions.
- Gait disorders are often the obvious indexes of systemic problems and should be investigated thoroughly.
- A thorough nursing assessment must include descriptions of gait and mobility patterns, as well as fall risk factors.
- Restraint-appropriate care is the standard of practice in all settings, and knowledge of restraint alternatives and safety measures is essential for nurses.
- Many illnesses that may accompany aging affect mobility and safety. Nursing interventions to enhance functional ability, prevent excess disability, and promote safety are essential.

CASE STUDY   EXERCISE AND ACTIVITY

Tom, 75 years old, had lost his wife Ella a year ago and had been feeling down and tired much of each day. He had retired at age 70 from his job as a housing contractor and had spent much of his time with Ella. They had been married for 50 years. He now sometimes seemed to sit in front of the television most of the day without actually remembering what it was that he had seen. Many of the couple's friends had moved away or to retirement settings, and other than his daughter who lived about 45 minutes from his house, he rarely saw anyone any more. He had lived like this for nearly a year, and it had become his daily pattern of life. Tom took the initiative after a suggestion from his daughter to go to the local senior citizen center. He went and had lunch there nearly every day. At one point he was asked if he would allow a nursing student to spend time with him during her semester in a gerontology course. He agreed. In the course of her assessment, she (and he) found that his activity level was nearly completely sedentary. She gave Tom information about the ramifications of such a sedentary life. She pointed out that the center had an exercise class every day between 10 AM and 12 noon. Because he came every day (except Saturday and Sunday) for lunch, it seemed a good thing to do. Tom said to his nursing student, "This isn't anything I am really interested in doing, but I will give it a try." Though he did not admit it, he was also worried because he usually felt weak and listless during the day after his lunch. When he did attend the first class, he found that there were basic exercises and more advanced ones for elders who had participated regularly for six months. He found after a few weeks that he was enjoying the social aspect of the exercise, if not the exercise itself. After nearly a year of fairly regular participation, Tom began playing golf with some of the men from the center. Once he attended a dance.

On the basis of the case study, develop a nursing care plan for the nursing student using the following procedure*:

- List Tom's comments that provide subjective data.
- List information that provides objective data.
- From these data identify and state, using accepted format, two nursing diagnoses you determine are most significant to Tom at this time. List two of Tom's strengths that you have identified from these data.
- Determine and state outcome criteria for each diagnosis. These must reflect some alleviation of the problem identified in the nursing diagnosis and must be stated in concrete and measurable terms.
- Plan and state one or more interventions for each diagnosed problem. Provide specific documentation of the source used to determine the appropriate intervention. Plan at least one intervention that incorporates Tom's existing strengths.
- Evaluate the success of the intervention. Interventions must correlate directly with the stated outcome criteria to measure the outcome success.

CRITICAL THINKING QUESTIONS

1. What lifestyle factors that Tom had developed after his wife Ella's death became dangerous to his health?
2. Compose a list of 10 questions you would ask Tom to obtain a clear picture of factors contributing to his activity level. Discuss the rationale behind each.
3. List some of the common methods for motivating Tom that his nursing student may have used.
4. Describe the level of activity that Tom should begin with and what symptoms he might expect as he increases his activity.

*Students are advised to refer to their nursing diagnosis text and identify possible or potential problems.

RESEARCH QUESTIONS

1. What types of gait disorders trigger falls and in what situations?
2. How does cognitive impairment influence risk of falls?
3. What activities and exercises are most useful in maintaining mobility in elders?
4. What are the psychological reactions of elders to the use of assistive devices for ambulation?
5. What factors in the institutional environment induce immobility?
6. What factors outside home and institution (in the community) are most hazardous for the mobility of elders? Where do most falls occur?
7. How does a new environment affect mobility? Is the incidence of falls higher in the first few weeks of adaptation to a new environment as compared with later?
8. How does obesity affect agility mobility, and risk for falls?
9. How often and in what circumstances are falls precipitated by the distractions or actions of another individual?
10. What interventions would increase adherence to use of hip protectors?

REFERENCES

Agency for Healthcare Research and Quality: *Physical activity and older Americans: benefits and strategies* (2002). Available at http://www.ahrq.gov/ppip/activity.htm. Accessed December 2010.

American Geriatrics Society/British Geriatrics Society: *Clinical practice guideline: prevention of falls in older persons* (2010). Available at http://www.americangeriatrics.org/health_care_professionals/clinical_practice/clinical_guidelines_recommendations/2010/. Accessed January 2011.

American Public Health Association, 138th Annual Meeting Abstract 42840 Presented November 9, 2010.

Andersen D, Osei-Boamah E, Gambert S: Impact of trauma-related hip fractures on the older adult, *Clinical Geriatrics* 18:18, 2010.

Antonelli M: Restraint management: moving from process to outcome, *Journal of Nursing Care Quality* 23:227, 2008.

Bourbonniere M, Evans LK: Advanced practice nursing in the care of frail older adults, *Journal of the American Geriatrics Society* 50:2062, 2002.

Buchner DM, Hornbrook MC, Kutner NG, et al: Development of the common data base for the FICSIT trials, *Journal of the American Geriatrics Society* 41:297, 1993.

Buckeridge D, Huang A, Hanley J, Kelome A, et al: Risk of injury associated with opiod use in older adults, *JAGS* 58(9):1664-1670, 2010.

Cameron I, Murray G, Gillespie L, et al: Interventions for preventing falls in older people in nursing facilities and hospitals,

Cochrane Database of Systematic Reviews 1:CD005465, 2010.

Capezuti E: Building the science of falls-prevention research, *Journal of the American Geriatrics Society* 52:461, 2004.

Capezuti E, Talerico KA, Strumpf N, et al: Individualized assessment and intervention in bilateral siderail use, *Geriatric Nursing* 19:322, 1998.

Capezuti E, Talerico K, Cochran I, et al: Individualized intervention to prevent bed-related falls and reduced siderail use, *Journal of Gerontological Nursing* 25:26, 1999.

Capezuti E, Zwicker D, Mezey M, et al: *Evidence-based geriatric nursing protocols for best practice*, ed 3, New York, 2008, Springer.

Centers for Disease Control and Prevention: *Hip fractures among older adults* (2010a).

Available at http://www.cdc.gov/HomeandRecreationalSafety/Falls/adulthipfx.html. Accessed December 2010.

Centers for Disease Control and Prevention: *Preventing traumatic brain injury in older adults* (2010b). Available at http://cdc.gov/BrainInjuryinSeniors. Accessed December 2010.

Centers for Disease Control and Prevention: *How much physical activity do older adults need?* (2010c). Available at http://www.cdc.gov/physicalactivity/everyone/guidelines/olderadults.html. Accessed December 2010.

Davis J, Marra C, Beattie L, Robertson M et al: Sustained cognitive and economic benefits of resistance training among community-dwelling senior women: a 1-year follow-up study of the brain power study, *Arch Intern Med* 170(22):2036-2038, 2010.

de Vries OJ, Ligthart GJ, Nikolaus T; on behalf of the participants of the European Academy of Medicine of Ageing—Course III: Differences in period prevalence of the use of physical restraints in elderly inpatients of European hospitals and nursing homes [letter], *Journals of Gerontology Series A, Biological Sciences and Medical Sciences* 59:922, 2004.

Dorgo S, Robinson K, Bader J: The effectiveness of a peer-mentored older adult fitness program on perceived physical, mental and social function, *Journal of the American Academy of Nurse Practitioners* 21:116, 2009.

Dykes P, Carroll D, Hurley A, Lipsitz S et al: Fall prevention in acute care hospitals: a randomized trial, *JAMA* 304(17):1912-1918, 2010.

Duru O, Sarkisian C, Leng M, Mangione C: Sisters in motion: a randomized controlled trial of a faith-based physical activity intervention, *JAGS* 58:1863-1869, 2010.

Erickson KI, Raji CA, Lopez OL, Becker JT et al: Physical activity predicts gray matter volume in late adulthood, *Neurology* 75:1415-1422, 2010.

Evans L, Strumpf N: Tying down the elderly: a review of literature on physical restraint, *Journal of the American Geriatrics Society* 37:65, 1989.

Flaherty J: Zero tolerance for physical restraints: difficult but not impossible, *Journals of Gerontology Series A, Biological Sciences and Medical Sciences* 59:M919, 2004.

Flanagan S, Hibbard M Riordan B, et al: Traumatic brain injury in the elderly: diagnostic and treatment challenges, *Clinics in Geriatric Medicine* 22:449, 2006.

Frick K, Kung J, Parrish J, et al: Evaluating the cost-effectiveness of fall prevention programs that reduce fall-related hip fractures in older adults, *Journal of the American Geriatrics Society* 58:136, 2010.

Galik E, Resnick B, Pretzer-Aboff I: "Knowing what makes them tick": motivating cognitively impaired older adults to participate in restorative care, *International Journal of Nursing Practice* 15:48, 2009.

Gavin-Dreschnack D, Volicer L, Morris C: Prevention of overuse of wheelchairs in nursing homes, *Annals of Long-term Care* 18:34, 2010.

Gray-Micelli D: Preventing falls in acute care. In Capezuti E, Zwicker D, Mezey M, et al, editors: *Evidence-based geriatric nursing protocols for best practice*, New York, 2008, Springer.

Gray-Micelli D: Falls in the environment. 1. Faulty footwear or footing? An interdisciplinary case-based perspective, *Annals of Long-term Care* 18:32, 2010.

Haentjens P, Magaziner J, Colon-Emeric C, et al: Meta-analysis: excess mortality after hip fracture among older men and women, *Annals of Internal Medicine* 152:380, 2010.

Harrison B, Ferrari M, Campbell C, et al: Evaluating the relationship between inattention and impulsivity-related falls in hospitalized older adults, *Geriatric Nursing* 31:8, 2010.

Hayes N, Witchard S, Awan-Bux R, et al: What predicts compliance rates with hip protectors in older hospital in-patients? *Age and Ageing* 37:225, 2008.

Hendrich AL, Bender PS, Nyhuis A: Validation of the Hendrich II fall risk model: a large concurrent case/control study of hospitalized patients, *Applied Nursing Research* 16:9, 2003.

Heyn PC, Johnson KE, Kramer AF: Endurance and strength training outcomes on cognitively impaired and cognitively intact older adults: a meta-analysis, *The Journal of Nutrition, Health & Aging* 12:401, 2008.

Hill K, Womer M, Russell M, et al: Fear of falling in older fallers presenting at emergency departments, *Journal of Advanced Nursing* 66:1769, 2010.

Ireland S, Lazar T, Mavrak C, et al: Designing a falls prevention strategy that works, *Journal of Nursing Care Quality* 25:198, 2010.

Janssen I: Influence of sarcopenia on the development of physical disability: the cardiovascular health study, *Journal of the American Geriatrics Society* 54:56, 2006.

Karnath B: Subdural hematoma: presentation and management in older adults, *Geriatrics* 59:18, 2004.

Kiel D, Magaziner J, Zimmerman S: Efficacy of a hip protector to prevent hip fracture in nursing home residents: the HIP PRO randomized controlled trial, *JAMA* 298:413, 2007.

Kilgore C: Fall-prevention efforts must be multifaceted, *Caring for the Ages* 11:26, 2010.

Kuh D: A life course approach to healthy aging, frailty, and capability, *Journals of Gerontology Series A, Biological Sciences and Medical Sciences* 62:717, 2007.

Lach H: The costs and outcomes of falls: what's a nursing administrator to do? *Nursing Administration Quarterly* 34:147, 2010.

Leveille S, Jones R, Keily D, et al: Chronic musculoskeletal pain and occurrence of falls in an older population, *JAMA* 302:2214, 2009.

Mathias S, Nayak US, Isaacs B: Balance in elderly patients: the "get up and go test", *Arch Phys Med Rehabil* 67(6): 387-389, 1986.

Middleton L, Barnes D, Lui L, Yaffe K: Physical activity over the life course and its association with cognitive performance and impairment in old age, *Journal of the American Geriatrics Society* 58(7):1322-1326, 2010.

Morley J: A fall is a major event in the life of an older person, *Journal of Gerontology* 57A:M492, 2002.

Morse J, Morse R, Tylko S: Development of a scale to identify the fall-prone patient, *Canadian Journal of Aging* 8:366, 1989.

Oliver D, Connelly J, Victor C, et al: Strategies to prevent falls and fractures in hospitals and care homes and effect of cognitive impairment: systematic review and meta-analyses, *BMJ* 334:82, 2007. Available at https://www.ncbi.nlm.nih.gov/pmc/articles/PMC1767306/. Accessed December 2010.

Park M, Hsiao-Chen Tang J: Evidence-based guideline: changing the practice of physical restraint use in acute care, *Journal of Gerontological Nursing* 33:9, 2007.

Pellfolk T, Gustafson Y, Bucht G, et al: Effects of a restraint minimization program on staff knowledge, attitudes, and practice: a cluster randomized trial, *Journal of the American Geriatrics Society* 58:62, 2010.

Porter E, Matsuda S, Lindbloom E: Intentions of older homebound women to reduce the risk of falling again, *Journal of Nursing Scholarship* 42:101, 2010.

Purath J, Bucholz S, Kark D: Physical fitness assessment of older adults in the primary care setting, *Journal of the American Academy of Nurse Practitioners* 21:101, 2009.

Quigley P, Bulat T, Kurtzman E, et al: Fall prevention and injury protection for nursing home residents, *Journal of the American Medical Directors Association* 11:284, 2010.

Rantz M, Aud M, Alexander G, et al: Falls, technology, and stunt actors: new approaches to fall detection and fall risk assessment, *Journal of Nursing Care Quality* 23:195, 2008.

Resnick B: In Henkel G: Beyond the MDS: team approach to falls assessment, prevention and management, *Caring for the Ages* 3:15, 2002.

Resnick B: Promoting exercise for older adults, *Journal of the American Academy of Nurse Practitioners* 21:77, 2009.

Resnick B, Ory M, Rogers M, et al: Screening for and prescribing exercise for older adults, *Geriatrics & Aging* 9:174, 2006.

Resnick B, Galik E, Gruber-Baldini A, et al: Implementing a restorative care philosophy of care in assisted living: pilot testing of Res-Care-AL, *Journal of the American Academy of Nurse Practitioners* 21:123, 2009.

Resnick B, Galik E, Gruber-Baldini AL, Zimmerman S. *Geriatr Nurs* 2010 May-Jun;31(3):197-205.

Rogers C, Keller C, Larkey L: Perceived benefits of meditative movement in older adults, *Geriatric Nursing* 31:37, 2010.

Rolland Y, Pillard F, Klapouszczak A, et al: Exercise program for nursing home residents with Alzheimer's disease: a 1-year randomized controlled trial, *Journal of the American Geriatrics Society* 55:158, 2007.

Rubenstein T, Alexander NB, Hausdorff JM: Evaluating fall risk in older adults: steps and missteps, *Clinical Geriatrics* 11:52, 2003.

Sato D, Kaneda K, Wakabayashi H, et al: Comparison of 2-year effects of once and twice weekly water exercise on activities of daily living of community dwelling frail elderly, *Archives of Gerontology and Geriatrics* 49:123, 2009.

Sherrington C, Whitney J, Lord S, et al: Effective exercise for the prevention of falls: a systematic review and meta-analysis, *Journal of the American Geriatrics Society* 56:2234, 2008.

Sollins H: Bed rails—be vigilant, but know the rules and guidelines, *Geriatric Nursing* 30:414, 2009.

Stevens J, Ryan G, Krenow M: Fatalities and injuries from falls among older adults—United States, 1993-2003 and 2001-2005, *MMWR Morbidity and Mortality Weekly Report* 50:1221, 2006.

Strumpf N, Wagner L, Evans L: *Reducing restraints: individualized approaches to behavior*, Huntington Valley, PA, 1992, The Whitman Group.

Sullivan-Marx E: Psychological responses to physical restraint use in older adults, *Journal of Psychosocial Nursing and Mental Health Services* 33:20, 1995.

Talerico K, Capezuti E: Myths and facts about side rails, *American Journal of Nursing* 101:43, 2001.

Tappen R, Roach K, Applegate E, et al: Effect of a combined walking and conversation intervention on functional mobility of nursing home residents with Alzheimer's disease, *Alzheimer Disease and Associated Disorders* 14:196-201, 2000.

Thompson H, McCormick W, Kagan S: Traumatic brain injury in older adults: epidemiology,

outcomes, and future implications, *Journal of the American Geriatrics Society* 54:1590, 2006.

Timmons T, Menaker J: Traumatic brain injury in the elderly, *Clinical Geriatrics* 18:20, 2010.

Tinetti M: Preventing falls in elderly persons, *New England Journal of Medicine* 348:42, 2003.

Tinetti M, Baker D, King M, et al: Effect of dissemination of evidence in reducing injuries from falls, *New England Journal of Medicine* 359:252, 2008.

Tompkins T, Belza B, Brown M: Nurse practitioner practice patterns for exercise counseling, *Journal of the American Academy of Nurse Practitioners* 21:79, 2009.

Tzeng H, Yin C: The extrinsic risk factors for inpatient falls in hospital patient rooms, *Journal of Nursing Care Quality* 23:233, 2008.

U.S. Food and Drug Administration: *FDA news release: FDA issues guidance on hospital bed design to reduce patient entrapment* (2006). Available at http://www.fda.gov/NewsEvents/Newsroom/PressAnnouncements/2006/ucm108612.htm. Accessed December 2010.

Wagner L, Capezuti E, Brush B, et al: Description of an advanced practice nursing consultative model to reduce restrictive siderail use in nursing homes, *Research in Nursing and Health* 30:131, 2007.

Wagner LM, Capezuti E, Brush BL, et al: Contractures in frail nursing home residents, *Geriatric Nursing* 29:259, 2008.

Webber S, Porter M, Menec V: Mobility in older adults: a comprehensive framework, *The Gerontologist* 50:443, 2010.

Williams C, Tappen R: Exercise training for depressed older adults with Alzheimer's disease, *Aging & Mental Health* 12:72, 2007a.

Williams C, Tappen R: Effect of exercise on mood in nursing home residents with Alzheimer's disease, *American Journal of Alzheimer's Disease and Other Dementias* 22:389, 2007b.

Wolf S, O'Grady M, Easley KA, et al: The influence of intense tai chi training on physical performance and hemodynamic outcomes in transitionally frail elders, *Journals of Gerontology Series A, Biological Sciences and Medical Sciences* 61:184, 2006.

Yeom HA, Fleury J, Keller C: Risk factors for mobility limitation in community-dwelling older adults: a social ecological perspective, *Geriatric Nursing* 29:133, 2008.

Yeom H, Keller C, Fleury J: Interventions for promoting mobility in community-dwelling older adults, *Journal of the American Academy of Nurse Practitioners* 21:95, 2009.

Zecevic A, Salmoni AW, Speechley M, et al: Defining a fall and reasons for falling: comparisons among the views of seniors, health care providers, and the research literature, *The Gerontologist* 46:367, 2006.

Tinetti Balance and Gait Evaluation

Scoring: Scoring of the Tinetti Assessment Tool is done on a three-point ordinal scale with a range of 0 to 2. A score of 0 represents the most impairment and a score of 2 would represent independence of the patient. The individual scores are then combined to form three measures: an overall gait assessment score, an overall balance score, and a gait and balance score.

Interpretation: The maximal score for the gait component is 12 points. The maximal score for the balance component is 16 points. The maximal score is 28 points. In general, patients who score below 19 are at high risk for falls. Patients who score in the range of 19 to 24 are considered at risk for falls.

BALANCE

Instructions: Subject is seated in a hard, armless chair. The following maneuvers are tested.

1. Sitting balance
   0 = Leans or slides in chair
   1 = Steady, safe
2. Arise
   0 = Unable without help
   1 = Able but uses arms to help
   2 = Able without use of arms
3. Attempts to arise
   0 = Unable without help
   1 = Able but requires more than one attempt
   2 = Able to arise with one attempt
4. Immediate standing balance (first five seconds)
   0 = Unsteady (staggers, moves feet, marked trunk sway)
   1 = Steady but uses walker/cane or grabs other object for support
   2 = Steady without walker or cane or other support
5. Standing balance
   0 = Unsteady
   1 = Steady but wide stance (medial heels >4 inches apart) or uses cane/walker or other support
   2 = Narrow stance without support
6. Nudge (subject at maximal position with feet as close together as possible. Examiner pushes lightly on subject's sternum with palm of hand three times)
   0 = Begins to fall
   1 = Staggers, grabs but catches self
   2 = Steady
7. Eyes closed (at maximal position #6)
   0 = Unsteady
   1 = Steady
8. Turn 360°
   0 = Discontinuous steps
   1 = Continuous steps
   0 = Unsteady (grabs, staggers)
   1 = Steady

9. Sit down
   0 = Unsafe (misjudged distance, falls into chair)
   1 = Uses arms or not a smooth motion
   2 = Safe, smooth motion
BALANCE SCORE: _____

GAIT

Instructions: Subject stands with examiner. Walks down hallway or across room, first at his/her usual pace, then back at a "rapid but safe" pace (using usual walking aid such as cane/walker).

10. Initiation of gait (immediately after told "go")
    0 = Any hesitancy or multiple attempts to start
    1 = No hesitancy
11. Step length and height (right foot swing)
    0 = Does not pass L. stance foot with step
    1 = Passes L. stance foot
    0 = R. foot does not clear floor completely with step
    1 = R. foot completely clears floor
12. Step length and height (left foot swing)
    0 = Does not pass R. stance foot with step
    1 = Passes R. stance foot
    0 = L. foot does not clear floor completely with step
    1 = L. foot completely clears floor
13. Step symmetry
    0 = R. and L. step length not equal (estimate)
    1 = R. and L. step length appear equal
14. Step continuity
    0 = Stopping or discontinuity between steps
    1 = Steps appear continuous
15. Path (estimated in relation to floor tiles, 12 inches wide. Observe excursion of one foot over about 10 feet of course)
    0 = Marked deviation
    1 = Mild/moderate deviation or uses a walking aid
    2 = Straight without walking aid
16. Trunk
    0 = Marked sway or uses walking aid
    1 = No sway but flexion of knees or back or spreads arms out while walking
    2 = No sway, no flexion, no use of arms, and no walking aid
17. Walk stance
    0 = Heels apart
    1 = Heels almost touching while walking
GAIT SCORE: _____
TOTAL MOBILITY SCORE (BALANCE AND GAIT): _____

From Brady R, Chester FR, Pierce LL, et al: Geriatric falls: prevention strategies for the staff, *Journal of Gerontological Nursing* 19:26, 1993. (Reprinted with permission, Mary Tinetti, MD.)

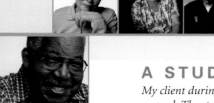

Environmental Safety and Security

Theris A. Touhy

evolve *http://evolve.elsevier.com/Ebersole/TwdHlthAging*

A STUDENT LEARNS

My client during the community nursing experience decided to stay in her own home in spite of being barely able to shuffle around. The state gave a homemaker a small sum each month to provide a few hours of assistance on a daily basis. She had to rely on the goodwill of neighbors when the budget for those services was discontinued. She wants so much to remain in her own home. I worry about her but don't know what I should do.   **Jennifer, age 24**

AN ELDER SPEAKS

I have been in my home for 50 years and widowed for 25 of those 50. The upkeep on my home is expensive and my resources are limited. I'm hoping I can manage to remain here, but I need some modifications to make it safe and I really don't know how to go about getting assistance to make the necessary changes.   **Esther, age 79**

LEARNING OBJECTIVES

On completion of this chapter, the reader will be able to:

1. Identify interactions of intrapersonal, interpersonal, geographical, economic, and health factors that influence environmental safety and security for older adults.
2. Discuss the effects of declining health, reduced mobility, isolation, and unpredictable life situations on the older adult's perception of security.
3. Explain the underlying vulnerability of older adults to effects of extreme temperatures, and identify actions to prevent and treat hypothermia and hyperthermia.
4. Define strategies and programs designed to prevent, detect, or alleviate crimes against older adults.
5. Consider the impact of available transportation and driving in relation to independence.
6. Discuss the use of assistive technologies to promote self-care, safety, and independence.

INFLUENCES OF CHANGING HEALTH AND DISABILITY ON SAFETY AND SECURITY

Physical Vulnerability

Vulnerability to environmental risks and mistreatment by others increases as people become less physically or cognitively able to recognize or cope with real or potential hazards. Aging itself does not necessarily bring about failing health or disease, yet some physical changes can be anticipated in all body systems. Older adults and their caregivers need to be knowledgeable about risks and interventions to avoid unsafe behaviors and situations. A safe environment is one in which the older person is capable, with reasonable caution, of carrying out activities of daily living (ADLs) and instrumental activities of daily living (IADLs), as well as the activities that enrich one's life without fear of attack, accident, or imposed interference.

Helping the older person to be vigilant about hazardous surroundings includes offering suggestions for adequate lighting, placement of furniture and rugs, and markings on sidewalks and steps, and providing information on crime prevention. Sensory deficits, whether visual, auditory, or olfactory, reduce the individual's ability to detect dangerous conditions or imminent threats. Tactile or neurosensory impairment raises the risk of tissue injury from burns, pressure, or beginning inflammation that escapes the person's awareness.

225

This chapter discusses the influences of changing health and disability on the safety and security of older adults. Included is vulnerability to temperature extremes, natural disasters, crime against older people, fire safety, driving safety, and the role of assistive technology in enhancing independence and the ability to live safely at home. Elder-friendly communities that foster aging in place and promote safety and security are also discussed.

Home Safety

Home safety assessments must be multifaceted and individualized to the areas of identified risks. They are particularly important for the older adult with fall risk and are recommended in evidence-based protocols for fall-risk reduction. An evidence-based home safety assessment tool, developed by Tanner (2003), includes fall and injury risk, as well as fire and crime risk assessment (Table 13-1). Home safety assessments targeted at fall-risk reduction are available from www.cdc.gov.injury in formats easy for older adults to access and use. Hurley and colleagues (2004) describe a home safety injury model for persons with Alzheimer's disease and their caregivers that addresses the physical environment and caregiver competence. Special home modifications for persons with Alzheimer's disease have also been described (Warner, 2000). Chapter 19 discusses safety and dementia as well.

Vulnerability to Environmental Temperatures

Given the nation's growing problems with supply and costs of energy, many older adults are exposed to temperature extremes in their own dwellings. Environmental temperature extremes impose a serious risk to older persons with declining physical health. Preventive measures require attentiveness to impending climate changes, as well as protective alternatives. Early intervention in extreme temperature exposure is crucial because excessively high or low body temperatures further impair thermoregulatory function and can be lethal.

Thermoregulation

To be vigilant or aware of older adults at risk, it is important to understand the basis of thermal vulnerability. Neurosensory changes in thermoregulation delay or diminish the older person's awareness of temperature changes and may impair behavioral and thermoregulatory response to dangerously high or low environmental temperatures (Chapter 4). Decline in thermoregulatory responsiveness to temperature extremes as one ages is well documented, yet these changes vary widely among individuals and are related more to general health than to age. The delicate equilibrium required to maintain thermal balance at any age involves the generation or replacement of body heat at about the same rate as heat is lost to the environment.

A number of physiological changes associated with aging affect heat generation, distribution, and conservation. The aging of the skin, with the loss of subcutaneous fat, is a factor in temperature regulation. Heat conservation is especially affected by changes in body density, water content, and insulation that accompany aging. Circulatory impairment and changes in vascular responsiveness affect the distribution of heat carried by blood. As a result, thermoregulatory sensitivity declines with age, and both cooling and warming responses appear to be blunted. Many of the drugs taken by older people affect thermoregulation by affecting the ability to vasoconstrict or vasodilate, both of which are thermoregulatory mechanisms. Other drugs inhibit neuromuscular activity (a significant source of kinetic heat production), suppress metabolic heat generation, or dull awareness (tranquilizers, pain medications). Alcohol is notorious for inhibiting thermoregulatory function by affecting vasomotor responses in either hot or cold weather.

Economic, behavioral, and environmental factors may combine to create a dangerous thermal environment in which older persons are subjected to temperature extremes from which they cannot escape or that they cannot change. Caretakers and family members should be aware that persons are vulnerable to environmental temperature extremes if they are unable to shiver, sweat, control blood supply to the skin, take in sufficient liquids, move about, add or remove clothing, adjust bedcovers, or adjust the room temperature. Economic conditions often play a role in this vulnerability, such as when an older person cannot afford air conditioning or adequate heating. During winter months, the older person may try using little or no room heat to either reduce or eliminate the high cost of fuel. Fear of unsafe neighborhoods in some urban areas prompts many elders to keep doors and windows bolted throughout the year. Although most of these problems occur in the home setting, older adults with multiple physical problems who reside in institutions may be especially vulnerable to temperature changes.

Temperature Monitoring in Older Adults. Diminished thermoregulatory responses and abnormalities in both the production and response to endogenous pyrogens may contribute to differences in fever responses between older and younger patients in response to an infection. Up to one-third of older people with acute infections may present without a robust febrile response, leading to delays in diagnosis and appropriate treatment, as well as increased morbidity and mortality (Outzen, 2009). Careful attention to temperature monitoring in older adults is very important, and often this technical task is not given adequate attention by professional nurses.

Frail older adults have lower baseline temperatures than healthy younger persons. In one study, the mean oral baseline temperature of randomly selected nursing home residents was 36.3° C (97.34° F). Therefore, a temperature of 98.34° F can represent one degree of elevation and may be significant in indicating infection. It is important to remember that acute infection in older adults frequently presents with a change in functional status, regardless of whether or not there is a temperature elevation. Fever in older adults can be defined as a persistent oral or TM temperature ≥37.2° C (98.96° F) or a

---

! SAFETY ALERT

A temperature of 98.6° F may indicate fever in frail older people. Because of thermoregulatory changes, up to one-third of older people with acute infections may present without a febrile response. Additionally, baseline temperatures in frail older people may be lower than the expected 98.6° F. If the baseline temperature is 97° F, a temperature of 98° F is a one-degree elevation and may be significant. Temperatures reaching or exceeding 100.94° F are very serious in older people and are more likely to be associated with serious bacterial or viral infections. Careful attention to temperature monitoring in older adults is very important and can prevent morbidity and mortality. Accurate measurement and reporting of body temperature requires professional nursing supervision.

TABLE 13-1	ASSESSMENT AND INTERVENTIONS OF THE HOME ENVIRONMENT FOR OLDER PERSONS

PROBLEM	INTERVENTION
Bathroom	
Getting on and off toilet	Raised seat; side bars; grab bars
Getting in and out of tub	Bath bench; transfer bench; hand-held shower nozzle; rubber mat; hydraulic lift bath seat
Slippery or wet floors	Nonskid rugs or mats
Hot water burns	Check water temperature before bath; set hot water thermostat to 120° F or less
	Use bath thermometer
Doorway too narrow	Remove door and use curtain; leave wheelchair at door and use walker
Bedroom	
Rolling beds	Remove wheels; block against wall
Bed too low	Leg extensions; blocks; second mattress; adjustable-height hospital bed
Lighting	Bedside light; night-light; flashlight attached to walker or cane
Sliding rugs	Remove; tack down; rubber back; two-sided tape
Slippery floor	Nonskid wax; no wax; rubber-sole footwear; indoor-outdoor carpet
Thick rug edge/doorsill	Metal strip at edge; remove doorsill; tape down edge
Nighttime calls	Bedside phone; cordless phone; intercom; buzzer; lifeline
Kitchen	
Open flames and burners	Substitute microwave; electrical toaster oven
Access items	Place commonly used items in easy-to-reach areas; adjustable-height counters, cupboards, and drawers
Hard-to-open refrigerator	Foot lever
Difficulty seeing	Adequate lighting; utensils with brightly colored handles
Living Room	
Soft, low chair	Board under cushion; pillow or folded blanket to raise seat; blocks or platform under legs; good armrests to push up on; back and seat cushions
Swivel and rocking chairs	Block motion
Obstructing furniture	Relocate or remove to clear paths
Extension cords	Run along walls; eliminate unnecessary cords; place under sturdy furniture; use power strips with breakers
Telephone	
Difficult to reach	Cordless phone; inform friends to let phone ring 10 times; clear path; answering machine and call back
Difficult to hear ring	Headset; speaker phone
Difficult to dial numbers	Preset numbers; large button and numbers; voice-activated dialing
Steps	
Cannot handle	Stair glide; lift; elevator; ramp (permanent, portable, or removable)
No handrails	Install at least on one side
Loose rugs	Remove or nail down to wooden steps
Difficult to see	Adequate lighting; mark edge of steps with bright-colored tape
Unable to use walker on stairs	Keep second walker or wheelchair at top or bottom of stairs
Home Management	
Laundry	Easy to access; sit on stool to access clothes in dryer; good lighting; fold laundry sitting at table; carry laundry in bag on stairs; use cart; use laundry service
Mail	Easy-to-access mailbox; mail basket on door
Housekeeping	Assess safety and manageability; no-bend dust pan; lightweight all-surface sweeper; provide with resources for assistance if needed
Controlling thermostat	Mount in accessible location; large-print numbers; remote-controlled thermostat
Safety	
Difficulty locking doors	Remote-controlled door lock; door wedge; hook-and-chain locks
Difficulty opening door and knowing who is there	Automatic door openers; level doorknob handles; intercom at door
Opening and closing windows	Lever and crank handles
Cannot hear alarms	Blinking lights; vibrating surfaces
Lighting	Illumination 1 to 2 feet from object being viewed; change bulbs when dim; adequate lighting in stairways and hallways; night-lights
Leisure	
Cannot hear television	Personal listening device with amplifier; closed captioning
Complicated remote	Simple remote with large buttons; universal remote control; voice control–activated remote control; clapper
Cannot read small print	Magnifying glass; large-print books
Book too heavy	Read at table; sit with book resting on lap pillow
Glare when reading	Place light source to right or left; avoid glossy paper for reading material; black ink instead of blue ink or pencil
Computer keys too small	Replace keyboard with one with larger keys

Modified from Rehabilitation Engineering Research Center on Aging (RERC-Aging), Center for Assistive Technology, University at Buffalo.

TABLE 13-2	HEAT SYNDROMES	
ILLNESS	**SYMPTOMS**	**TREATMENT**
Heat fatigue/heat syncope	Pale, sweaty skin that is still cool and moist to the touch Elevated heart rate and patient feels exhausted and weak Body temperature remains normal Some loss of vascular volume and electrolytes from sweating Sudden syncopal spell or dizziness after exercising in the heat	Oral hydration with electrolyte replacement Cooler, less humid environment Rest
Heat cramps and heat exhaustion	Muscle cramping of legs, arms, or abdominal wall. Skin remains moist or cool and clammy, tachycardia, decreased pulse pressure, and thirst usually present. Altered mental status (giddy, confused, weak), nausea. Core temperature normal or mildly elevated.	Cool environment, hydration, IV normal saline, rest
Heat stroke	Mechanisms to control heat are lost, core temperature rises quickly (>104° F) and causes cellular and end organ damage, skin flushed and hot and dry. Mental status changes, tachycardia, hypotension, hyperventilation.	Complex medical emergency; if untreated will cause death. Cool person as rapidly as possible, IV infusions. Complications during treatment include hypoglycemia, shivering, seizures, renal failure, and hypotension.

Modified from: Ham R, et al: *Primary care geriatrics: A case-based approach*, ed 5, St. Louis, 2007, Mosby; Ebersole P, et al: *Toward Healthy Aging: Human needs and nursing response*, ed 7, St. Louis, 2008, Mosby.

persistent rectal temperature ≥37.5° C (99.5° F). Temperatures reaching or exceeding 38.3° C (100.94° F) are very serious in older people and are more likely to be associated with serious bacterial or viral infections (Norman, 2000).

Hyperthermia

More older people die from excessive heat than from hurricanes, lightening, tornadoes, floods, and earthquakes combined (Centers for Disease Control and Prevention, 2006). When body temperature increases above normal ranges because of environmental or metabolic heat loads, a clinical condition called heat illness, or *hyperthermia*, develops. Heat illnesses tend to follow a continuum (Table 13-2), beginning with mild heat fatigue and ending with the potentially fatal heat stroke, so it is imperative to assess hyperthermia quickly and appropriately. Heat fatigue is usually caused by exposure to high outside temperatures or overexertion in a hot environment. It is characterized by pale or sweaty skin that is still moist and cool to touch, elevated heart rate, and feelings of exhaustion and weakness. Core body temperature remains normal (Ham et al., 2007). Diuretics and low intake of fluids exacerbate fluid loss and can precipitate the onset of hyperthermia in hot weather.

Heat stroke, the most serious form of heat illness, is a medical emergency that usually arises from failure of normal body-cooling mechanisms to cope with extremely high environmental heat or humidity. Heat stroke affects the hypothalamic thermoregulatory center and impairs the ability to sweat or lose heat by vasodilation. This condition can quickly lead to death unless treated, and rising core temperatures above 40° C (104° F) increase the likelihood of irreversible brain damage. Hyperthermia requires active cooling and fluid replacement. Because hyperthermia induces loss of thermoregulatory control, temperature must be closely monitored to avoid inducing hypothermia.

Box 13-1 presents interventions to prevent hyperthermia when the ambient temperature exceeds 90° F (32.2° C). Local governments and communities must coordinate response strategies to protect the older person when environmental temperatures rise. Strategies may include providing fans, opportunities to spend part of the day in air-conditioned buildings, and identification of high-risk older people.

Hypothermia

Nearly 50% of all deaths from hypothermia occur in older adults (Ham et al., 2007). Hypothermia is produced by exposure to cold environmental temperatures and is defined as a core temperature of less than 35° C (95° F). Hypothermia is categorized into mild, moderate, and severe, depending on the core temperature taken with a rectal probe thermometer. Hypothermia is a medical emergency requiring comprehensive assessment of neurological activity, oxygenation, renal function, and fluid and electrolyte balance.

During cold weather, two situations tend to produce hypothermia: (1) exposure involving a healthy individual in severely cold environmental conditions for a prolonged period; or (2) exposure involving a person with impaired thermoregulatory ability in room temperature without protection. The more severe the impairment or prolonged the exposure, the less able are thermoregulatory responses to defend against heat loss. Older adults are particularly predisposed to hypothermia because the opportunity for heat loss frequently coexists with the decline in heat generation and conservation responses. Such coexistence occurs frequently among persons who are homeless or cognitively impaired; persons who are injured in falls or from trauma; and persons with cardiovascular, adrenal, or thyroid dysfunction, and diabetes. Other risk factors include excessive alcohol use, exhaustion, poor nutrition, inadequate housing, as well as the use of sedatives, anxiolytics, phenothiazines, and tricyclic antidepressants.

Unfortunately, a dulling of awareness accompanies hypothermia, and persons experiencing the condition rarely recognize the problem or seek assistance. For the very old and frail, environmental temperatures below 65° F (18° C) may cause a serious drop in core body temperature to 95° F (35° C). Factors that increase the risk of hypothermia are numerous, as shown in Box 13-2.

Under normal temperature conditions, heat is produced in sufficient quantities by cellular metabolism of food, friction produced by contracting muscles, and the flow of blood.

BOX 13-1 INTERVENTIONS TO PREVENT HYPERTHERMIA

- Drink 2 to 3 L of cool fluid daily.
- Minimize exertion, especially during the heat of the day.
- Stay in air-conditioned places, or use fans when possible.
- Wear hats and loose clothing of natural fibers when outside; remove most clothing when indoors.
- Take tepid baths or showers.
- Apply cold wet compresses, or immerse the hands and feet in cool water.
- Evaluate medications for risk of hyperthermia.
- Avoid alcohol.

BOX 13-2 FACTORS THAT INCREASE THE RISK OF HYPOTHERMIA IN OLDER ADULTS

THERMOREGULATORY IMPAIRMENT
Failure to vasoconstrict promptly or strongly on exposure to cold
Failure to sense cold
Failure to respond behaviorally to protect oneself against cold
Diminished or absent shivering to generate heat
Failure of metabolic rate to rise in response to cold

CONDITIONS THAT DECREASE HEAT PRODUCTION
Hypothyroidism, hypopituitarism, hypoglycemia, anemia, malnutrition, starvation
Immobility or decreased activity (e.g., stroke, paralysis, parkinsonism, dementia, arthritis, fractured hip, coma)
Diabetic ketoacidosis

CONDITIONS THAT INCREASE HEAT LOSS
Open wounds, generalized inflammatory skin conditions, burns

CONDITIONS THAT IMPAIR CENTRAL OR PERIPHERAL CONTROL OF THERMOREGULATION
Stroke, brain tumor, Wernicke's encephalopathy, subarachnoid hemorrhage
Uremia, neuropathy (e.g., diabetes, alcoholism)
Acute illnesses (e.g., pneumonia, sepsis, myocardial infarction, congestive heart failure, pulmonary embolism, pancreatitis)

DRUGS THAT INTERFERE WITH THERMOREGULATION
Tranquilizers (e.g., phenothiazines)
Sedative-hypnotics (e.g., barbiturates, benzodiazepines)
Antidepressants (e.g., tricyclics)
Vasoactive drugs (e.g., vasodilators)
Alcohol (causes superficial vasodilation; may interfere with carbohydrate metabolism and judgment)
Others: methyldopa, lithium, morphine

BOX 13-3 FACTORS ASSOCIATED WITH LOW BODY TEMPERATURE IN OLDER ADULTS

AGE-RELATED CHANGES
Increases risk of thermoregulatory dysfunction.
Increases risk of acute and chronic conditions that predispose one to hypothermia.

LOW ENVIRONMENTAL TEMPERATURE
Risk of hypothermia increases below 65° F.

THINNESS AND MALNUTRITION
Very thin people have less thermal insulation and higher surface area/volume ratios.
Prolonged malnutrition can decrease the metabolic rate by 20% to 30%.

POVERTY
Increases risk of thinness and malnutrition, inadequate clothing, and low environmental temperature secondary to poor housing conditions and inadequate heat.

LIVING ALONE
Associated with poverty, delayed detection of hypothermia, and delayed rescue if person falls.

NOCTURIA/NIGHT RISING
Associated with falls; if rescue delayed and person lies immobilized for a long time, hypothermia may develop as heat is conducted away from the body to the cold floor.

ORTHOSTATIC HYPOTENSION
An indicator of autonomic nervous system impairment; dizziness and postural instability are associated with falls.

Paralyzed or immobile persons lack the ability to generate significant heat by muscle activity and become cold even in normal room temperatures. Persons who are emaciated and have poor nutrition lack insulation, as well as fuel for metabolic heat-generating processes, so they may be chronically mildly hypothermic. Box 13-3 lists factors that may induce low basal body temperatures in elders.

When exposed to cold temperatures, healthy persons conserve heat by vasoconstriction of superficial vessels, shunting circulation away from the skin where most heat is lost. Heat is generated by shivering and increased muscle activity, and a rise in oxygen consumption occurs to meet aerobic muscle requirements. Circulatory, cardiac, respiratory, or musculoskeletal impairments affect either the response to or function of thermoregulatory mechanisms. Older persons with some degree of thermoregulatory impairment, when exposed to cold temperatures, are at high risk for hypothermia if they undergo surgery, are injured in a fall or accident, or are lost or left unattended in a cool place.

All body systems are affected by hypothermia, although the most deadly consequences involve cardiac arrhythmias and suppression of respiratory function. Correctly conducted rewarming is the key to good management, and the guiding principle is to warm the core before the periphery and raise the core temperature 0.5° C to 2° C per hour. Heating blankets and specially designed heating vests are used in addition to warm humidified air by mask, warm IV boluses, and other measures depending on the severity of the hypothermia (Ham et al., 2007).

Recognition of clinical signs and severity of hypothermia is an important nursing responsibility. Nurses are responsible for keeping frail elders warm for comfort and prevention of problems. It is important to closely monitor body temperature in older people and pay particular attention to lower-than-normal readings compared with the person's baseline. The potential risk of hypothermia and its associated cardiorespiratory and metabolic exertion makes prevention important and early recognition vital.

Detecting hypothermia among community-dwelling older adults is sometimes difficult, because unlike in the clinical setting, no one is measuring body temperature. For persons exposed to low temperatures in the home or the environment, confusion and disorientation may be the first overt signs. As judgment becomes clouded, a person may remove clothing or

BOX 13-4	NURSING INTERVENTIONS TO PREVENT COLD DISCOMFORT AND THE DEVELOPMENT OF ACCIDENTAL HYPOTHERMIA IN FRAIL ELDERS

DESIRED OUTCOMES
- Hands and limbs warm
- Body relaxed, not curled
- Body temperature >97° F
- No shivering
- No complaints of cold

INTERVENTIONS
- Maintain a comfortably warm ambient temperature no lower than 65° F. Many frail elders will require much higher temperatures.
- Provide generous quantities of clothing and bedcovers. Layer clothing and bedcovers for best insulation. Be careful not to judge your patient's needs by how you feel working in a warm environment.
- Limit time patients sit by cold windows or air conditioners to short periods in which they are adequately dressed and covered.
- Provide a head covering whenever possible—in bed, out of bed, and particularly out-of-doors.
- Cover patients well when in bed, bathing. The standard—a light bath blanket over a naked body—is not enough protection for frail elders.
- Cover patients with heavy blankets for transfer to and from showers; dry quickly and thoroughly before leaving shower room; cover head with a dry towel or hood while wet. Shower rooms and bathrooms should have warming lights.
- Dry wet hair quickly with warm air from an electric dryer. Never allow the hair of frail elders to air-dry.
- Use absorbent pads for incontinent patients rather than allowing urine to wet large areas of clothing, sheets, and bedcovers. Avoid skin problems by changing pads frequently, washing the skin well, and applying a protective cream.
- Provide as much exercise as possible to generate heat from muscle activity.
- Provide hot, high-protein meals and bedtime snacks to add heat and sustain heat production throughout the day and as far into the night as possible.

fail to seek shelter, and hypothermia can progress to profound levels. For this reason, regular contact with home-dwelling elders during cold weather is crucial. For those with preexisting alterations in thermoregulatory ability, this surveillance should include even mildly cool weather. Because heating costs are high in the United States, the Department of Health and Human Services provides funds to help low-income families pay their heating bills. Specific interventions to prevent hypothermia are shown in Box 13-4. Additional resources can be found on the Evolve website.

Vulnerability to Natural Disasters

Natural disasters such as hurricanes, tornadoes, floods, and earthquakes claim the lives of many people worldwide each year. In addition, human-made or human-generated disasters include chemical, biological, radiological, and nuclear terrorism and food and water contamination. The events of September 11, 2001, have prompted much thought and planning related to human-generated disasters. Older people are at great risk during and after disasters, and the older population had the highest casualty rate during disaster events when compared to all other age groups (Burnett et al., 2008).

The tragedies that occurred during Hurricane Katrina in 2005 highlighted the serious consequences of disasters on older people living both in the community and in institutions. Before Hurricane Katrina, older people composed 15% of the population in New Orleans, but after the event they accounted for 70% of the dead (Campbell, 2008). Fifty-six percent of the evacuees at the Astrodome following Katrina were 65 years of age or older.

Older adults at most risk include, but are not limited to, those who depend on others for daily functioning; those with limited mobility; and those who are socially isolated, cognitively impaired, or institutionalized (Brown, 2008). Older people may be less likely to seek formal or informal help during disasters and may not get as much assistance as younger individuals. Nursing home residents compose a particularly vulnerable group due to their frailty. Many nursing homes in Louisiana were not prepared for Katrina, and of the 60 nursing homes in Louisiana affected by Katrina, only 21 evacuated before the storm. Many were not prepared for the storm or for evacuation of residents, and 56 nursing home residents died. Better preparation of nursing homes for disasters is essential. Rhoads and Clayman (2008) provide a guide to preparing long-term care facilities for disasters.

Gerontological nurses must be knowledgeable about disaster preparedness and assist in the development of plans to address the unique needs of older adults, as well as educate fellow professionals, older adult clients, and community agencies about disaster preparedness. Comprehensive planning is necessary to respond to the needs of the aging population in emergency situations around the world. Lach and colleagues (2005) provide excellent information for nurses considering disaster planning for older people. Adelman and Legg (2010) discuss the impact of a disaster on older adults with dementia. Ready America (http://www.ready.gov/america/getakit/seniors.html) provides a disaster-planning tool kit for older adults as well as other resources for weather related emergencies.

CRIMES AGAINST OLDER ADULTS

Risks and Vulnerability

Older individuals share many of the same fears about violent crime held by the rest of the population, but they may feel more vulnerable because of frailness or disability. Living alone, memory impairments, and loneliness may make elders more susceptible to crime. Property crime is the most common crime against persons age 65 years and older. Older people are more likely to be victims of consumer fraud and scams that include telemarketing fraud, e-mail scams, and undelivered services. Older people also experience rising problems with identity theft.

Several crime-prevention programs for older adults have been established through combined efforts of agencies and provide information about crime prevention for seniors (National Association of Triads [website]: www. nationaltriad. org). The National Crime Prevention Council also offers information on prevention of crime for older people.

Community-centered projects have demonstrated the effectiveness of neighborhood crime prevention networks, public education in self-protective measures, avoidance of fraudulent schemes, community safety inspection programs, security advice in homes, and civic and organizational assistance in obtaining security devices and escort services. In some instances, older volunteer peer counselors provide support and counseling to victims of crime and violence. Strategies for promoting security-conscious behaviors among elders are aimed at decreasing vulnerability to criminal victimization and teaching self-protection skills. Nurses can be instrumental in reducing fear of crime and assisting elders in exploring ways they may protect themselves and feel more secure. Box 13-5 offers crime-reduction suggestions.

Fraudulent Schemes Against Elders

Fraud against elders ranges from solicitations from seemingly worthwhile charities to requests for a cash deposit to win a nonexistent prize. Trusting elderly persons may be duped into giving money to pen pals, Internet acquaintances, phony religious causes, or new acquaintances who "need help."

Attractive prices of fraudulent door-to-door contractors, who offer services the older adult cannot perform, may entice a substantial cash outlay. According to the Internal Revenue Service (IRS), every year impersonators swindle vulnerable taxpayers out of thousands of dollars by posing as IRS agents. Older people are often targets of these frauds. Scams may involve announcements that they have won a large cash sweepstakes that requires payment of taxes before the prize is delivered. Other IRS impersonators have called on widows or widowers to pay the "back taxes" owed by their deceased spouse. These abuses often go unpunished because the older person waits too long to report the fraud or feels embarrassment at having been taken in. Several key precautions should be shared with those at risk for fraud from IRS impersonators:

- All IRS employees carry identification and are required to show it to taxpayers when visiting a home or office.
- All citizens can obtain an IRS office address in their local telephone directory or call the national IRS directory number at 1-800-829-1040 to find its location.
- No check should ever be made payable to an IRS employee. Checks for federal taxes should be made payable to the Internal Revenue Service, not IRS; spelling out the full name makes it more difficult for criminals to alter the check.

Medical fraud is another serious type of fraud that affects older citizens on a national scale. Medical supplies and equipment delivered to homes by various suppliers have either been grossly overpriced or charged for but never received by the client. Scams to defraud Medicare beneficiaries for the new Medicare Part D benefit have also been reported. Callers ask for bank information and use the account numbers to electronically withdraw money for a Medicare card and drug plan that is not legitimate.

The Centers for Medicare and Medicaid Services (CMS) has offices to inform Medicare and Medicaid beneficiaries of ways to avoid fraud and also provides toll-free numbers to report suspected fraud. National agencies have combined forces to bring about reform. CMS offers the following advice for seniors:

- No one should come to your house uninvited.
- No one can ask for personal information during his or her marketing activities.
- Keep personal information safe, including your Medicare number, and do not give out any information about bank accounts or credit cards to marketers.
- Legitimate Medicare drug plans will not ask for payment over the telephone or Internet and must send a bill to the beneficiary for the monthly premium (Centers for Medicare and Medicaid Services, 2006.)
- Most states offer the volunteer program Seniors Health Information Needs of Elders (SHINE), which offers assistance on Medicare and health insurance–related concerns, and local area agencies on aging often offer assistance to older people on completion of tax returns.

FIRE SAFETY FOR ELDERS

Risk Factors for Elders

According to the U.S. Fire Administration, people older than 65 years are one of the groups at highest risk of dying in a fire.

BOX 13-6   REDUCING FIRE RISKS IN THE HOME

1. When you smell smoke, see flames, or hear the sound of fire, evacuate everyone in the house before doing anything else.
2. Use normal exits unless blocked by smoke or flame. Never use elevators during fire evacuation.
3. Stay near the floor because gases and smoke collect near the ceiling.
4. In a high-rise apartment, remain in the room with doors and hall vents closed unless smoke is in your apartment. Open or break a window to obtain fresh air.
5. Home fire alarm systems and smoke detectors should have a label indicating Underwriters' Laboratories (UL) approval. Smoke detectors should be installed outside each sleeping area, at the top of the basement stairs, in the bedrooms of smokers, and in all levels of the house. Do not install a smoke detector too near a window, door, or forced-air register, where drafts could interfere with the detector's operation. Do not install a smoke detector within six inches of where walls and ceilings meet, because air is less likely to circulate smoke to the alarm.
6. Rehearse what to do: If clothing catches fire, do not run; lie down, and then roll over and over ("stop, drop, and roll"). If someone else's clothing is burning, smother the flames with the handiest item, such as a rug, a coat, a blanket, or drapes.

BOX 13-7   MEASURES TO PREVENT FIRES AND BURNS

- Do not smoke in bed or when sleepy.
- When cooking, do not wear loose-fitting clothing (e.g., bathrobes, nightgowns, pajamas).
- Set thermostats for water heater or faucets so that the water does not become too hot.
- Install a portable hand fire extinguisher in the kitchen.
- Keep access to outside door(s) unobstructed.
- Identify emergency exits in public buildings.
- If you consider entering a boarding or foster home, check to see that it has smoke detectors, a sprinkler system, and fire extinguishers.
- Wear clothing that is nonflammable or treated with a permanent fire-retardant finish. Fabrics of animal hair, wool, and silk are less flammable.
- Use several electrical outlets rather than overloading one outlet.

Fire-related mortality rates are three times higher in people older than 80 years than in the rest of the population. The risk of injury during a fire is greater if medication or illness slows response time or decision making, and if help is not available to contain the fire and help the person escape.

A number of factors predispose the older person to fire injuries. In home-dwelling elders, economic or climatic conditions may promote the use of ill-kept heating devices. Attempts to cook over an open flame while wearing loose-fitting clothing or inability to manage spattering grease from a frying pan can often start a fire from which the elder cannot escape. Those living in apartment dwellings are often at the mercy of inadequate repair and safety measures and the careless behaviors of others. Many older people living in their own homes cannot afford home repairs, placing them at risk for fire. Failing vision can contribute to an elderly person's setting a cook-top burner, heating pad, or hot plate at too high a temperature, resulting in fire or thermal injury.

Most fires occur at home during the night, and deaths are attributed to smoke injury more often than burns. Smoking materials are the most common sources of residential fires. Fire-related deaths are more common among men than women, which may be related to higher incidence of smoking and alcohol consumption. Plastic articles and other synthetics can produce noxious fumes that are deadly, particularly to persons with preexisting respiratory disorders. Even flame-retardant garments have been linked to noxious fume release when burned, and therefore they are a possible hazard to elders. Specific fire prevention guidelines for elders appear in Box 13-6, and Box 13-7 presents information about preventing fires and burns and reducing fire risks in the home. The National Fire Protection Association offers a fire prevention program for older adults. Additional resources can be found on the Evolve website.

Reducing Fire Risks in Group Residential Settings

Residents of institutional settings, such as nursing homes or assisted living facilities, are particularly vulnerable to fire because of the high numbers of frail or immobilized elderly. Activities to promote a fire-safe institutional environment include use of noncombustible building materials, sprinkler systems, smoke detectors, closed air spaces, written fire procedures, orientation of personnel, and assessment of environment by fire prevention officials. Nurses are in a position to ensure familiarity of personnel with fire safety procedures and evacuation protocol and also to report or remove any potential fire hazards.

TRANSPORTATION SAFETY

Available transportation is a critical link in the ability of the elderly to remain independent and functional. The lack of accessible transportation may contribute to other problems, such as social withdrawal, poor nutrition, or neglect of health care. Even when municipal transportation service is available, elders may not use it. Urban buses and subways not only are physically hazardous but also are often dangerous. A "crisis in mobility" exists for many older people because of the lack of an automobile, an inability to drive, limited access to public transportation, health factors, geographical location, and economic considerations. Culturally and ethnically diverse older people may experience more difficulty getting around than older whites, and rural residents may experience more difficulty than urban residents.

Older people may desire increased contact with other people, particularly relatives. However, even more crucial is the need to reach medical services, shopping areas, and service agencies. If mobility is hampered, both security and the sense of belonging to the mainstream of society may be blocked. The emphasis on a "barrier-free" (structurally revised) transportation system and reduced fares has been helpful to many older people, but some cannot avail themselves of public transportation because of physical disability or residence in a high-crime area.

County, state, or federally subsidized transportation is being provided in certain areas to assist older people in reaching social services, nutrition sites, health services, emergency care, recreational centers, day care programs, physical and vocational rehabilitation, continuing education, grocery, and library services. Although transportation can often be found for special needs, it is virtually impossible to locate transportation for pleasure or recreation. Senior centers offer a wide range of activities for older people, as well as transportation services. Nurses can refer older people to local social service and aging organizations, such as area agencies on aging, for information on transportation resources and financial assistance for services.

Driving

Driving is one of the instrumental activities of daily living (IADLs) for most elders because it is essential to obtaining necessary resources. Driving is a highly complex activity that requires a variety of visual, motor, and cognitive skills (Mathias and Lucas, 2009). Assessments of functional capacities often neglect this important activity. We should evaluate whether an individual can drive, feels safe driving, and has a driver's license. Giving up mobility and independence afforded by driving one's own car has many psychological ramifications and inconveniences. Giving up driving is a major loss for an older person both in terms of independence and pleasure, as well as feelings of competence and self-worth. Driving cessation has been associated with decreased social integration, decreased out-of-home activities, increased depressive and anxiety symptoms, decreased quality of life, and increased risk of nursing home placement (Carr and Ott, 2010; Siren and Hakamies-Blomqvist, 2009).

For many older people, alternate transportation is not available, and consequently, they may continue driving beyond the time when it is safe. Almost 90% of people age 65 years and older continue to drive, and these numbers are expected to grow as "baby boomers" age and more people live into their 80s and 90s. Women are more likely than men to give up driving for less pressing reasons than health, and at a younger age (Oxley and Charlton, 2009). Older men seem to place more value on the ability to drive, as well as owning a car, than older women. Therefore, one can expect more stress involved with the decision not to drive for older men.

Driving Safety

Older drivers typically drive fewer miles than younger drivers and tend to drive less at night, during adverse weather conditions, or in congested areas. Generally, they choose familiar routes and drive fewer miles per year than younger drivers. Fewer older drivers speed or drive after drinking alcohol than drivers of other ages. However, when compared with younger age-groups, older people have more accidents per mile driven, and older drivers and passengers are three times more likely to die than younger people following an auto crash. The leading cause of injury-related deaths among drivers age 65 to 74 years is a motor vehicle accident; for those older than 75 years, motor vehicle accidents are the second leading cause of death after falls (Hooyman and Kiyak, 2011). Age-related changes in driving skills, including vision changes, cognitive impairment, and various medical illnesses and functional impairments, are all factors related to driving safety for older adults. Box 13-8 presents information that can be used by older adults and their caregivers to identify driving concerns.

BOX 13-8	DRIVING SKILLS AND SAFETY FACTORS

DIRECTIONS:

If you answer "yes" to one or more of the following questions, you may want to limit your driving or take steps to improve a problem.

If you answer "yes" to most of the questions, it may be time to consider letting someone else do your driving.

- Does driving make you feel nervous or physically exhausted?
- Do you have difficulty seeing pedestrians, signs, and vehicles?
- Do cars frequently seem to appear from nowhere?
- At night, does the glare from oncoming headlights temporarily "blind" you?
- Do you find intersections confusing?
- Are you finding it harder to judge the distance between cars?
- Do you have difficulty coordinating your hand and foot movements?
- Do you have difficulty staying in a lane?
- Are you slower than you used to be in reacting to dangerous situations?
- Do you sometimes get lost in familiar neighborhoods?
- Do other drivers often honk at you?
- Have you had any tickets?
- Have you been pulled over by the police?
- Have you had an increased number of traffic violations, accidents, or near-accidents in the past year?
- Do you have any vision problems?
- Do you have any hearing problems?
- Do you take any of the following medications: antihistamines, antipsychotics, tricyclic antidepressants, benzodiazepines, barbiturates, sleeping medications, muscle relaxants?
- Do you have any memory impairment?
- Do you have any muscle stiffness or weakness?

Adapted From Carr D, Ott B: The older adult driver with cognitive impairment: "It's a very frustrating life," *JAMA* 303:1632-1641, 2010.

Driving and Dementia

Driving has been identified as one of the top 10 tough ethical issues associated with dementia (Dobbs et al., 2009). Dementia, even in the early stages, can impair cognitive and functional skills required for safe driving. Evidence from some studies of motor vehicle crashes suggests that drivers with dementia have at least a two-fold risk of crashes compared to those without cognitive impairment. The risk of a crash for the driver with cognitive impairment appears to increase with the duration of driving after disease onset. In driving simulation studies, older drivers with dementia consistently perform more poorly than drivers without dementia and are more likely to drive off the road, drive more slowly than the speed limit, apply less brake pressure when trying to stop, and make slower turns. Inattention and slow or inappropriate responses are the major factors leading to crashes, but this has not been studied well in actual performance situations (Carr and Ott, 2010; Gray-Vickrey, 2010a).

Older individuals with frontotemporal lobe dementia and Lewy body dementia may be particularly at risk as a result of disinhibition, agitation, and visuoperceptual and attention deficits associated with these types of dementia. As many as 30% of older individuals with dementia continue to drive (Carr and Ott, 2010; Gray-Vickrey, 2010b). Many individuals early in the course of dementia are still able to pass a driving performance test, so a diagnosis of dementia should not be the sole justification for revocation of a driver's license (Carr and Ott, 2010).

BOX 13-9 ACTION STRATEGIES USED TO BRING ABOUT DRIVING CESSATION

IMPOSED TYPE	INVOLVED TYPE
Report person to division of motor vehicles for possible license suspension	All family members and individual meet, discuss the situation, and come to a mutual agreement of the problem
Use of deception or threats such as false keys, disabling the car, saying car was stolen	Dialog is ongoing from the earliest signs of cognitive impairment about the eventuality of the need to stop driving
Attempts to order or control, such as provider writing a prescription, commands from children to stop driving	Arrangements are made for alternative transportation plans that are available when needed and acceptable to the individual

From Jett K, et al: Imposed versus involved: different strategies to effect driving cessation in cognitively impaired older adults, *Geriatric Nursing* 26:111-116, 2005.

BOX 13-10 ADAPTATIONS FOR SAFER DRIVING

- Wider rear-view mirrors
- Pedal extensions
- Less complicated, larger, and legible instrument panels
- Electronic detectors in front and back that signal when the car is too close to other cars
- Better protection on doors
- Booster cushions for shorter-stature drivers
- "Smart" driving assistants (under development) that automatically plan a safe driving route based on the person's driving habits
- GPS devices

Modified from: Hooyman N, Kiyak H: *Social Gerontology: A multidisciplinary perspective*, Boston, 2011, Allyn & Bacon.

However, discussions should begin about the inevitability of driving cessation. Additionally, driving evaluations should be conducted every six months or as needed as the disease progresses.

The legal regulations regarding driver's license renewal in older drivers and the responsibility of medical practitioners to identify unsafe drivers vary from state to state and country to country (Mathias and Lucas, 2009). Driver's license renewal procedures vary from state to state and may include accelerated renewal cycles, renewal in person rather than electronically or by mail, and vision and road tests. Additional information can be found at www.iihs.org/laws/state_laws/older_drivers.html. The issues of driving in the older adult population are the subject of a great deal of public discussion. Many older drivers and their families struggle with issues related to continued safety in driving, and families struggle with when and how to tell older people they are no longer safe to drive.

Driving Cessation

Planning for driving cessation should occur for all older adults before their mobility situations become urgent (Carr & Ott, 2010). Health care providers should encourage open discussion of issues related to driving with the older person and his or her family and should identify impairments that affect safe driving, correct them when possible, and offer alternatives for transportation. It is generally agreed that voluntarily giving up a driver's license, rather than having it revoked, is associated with more positive outcomes (Oxley & Charlton, 2009). Jett and colleagues (2005) provide useful strategies for driving counseling for people with dementia from a qualitative study involving guided interviews with participants (Box 13-9).

Suggestions for easing the transition from driving to not driving are to encourage the individual to modify driving habits such as not driving on unfamiliar roads, during rush hour, at dusk or at night, in inclement weather, or in heavy traffic. Other strategies to decrease the need to drive include

home-delivered groceries, prescriptions, and meals; personal services provided in the home; asking a caregiver to obtain needed supplies or act as a copilot; and exploring community resources for transportation (Gray-Vickrey, 2010b). Additional suggestions include asking the provider to "prescribe" driving cessation, use medical conditions other than dementia (impaired vision, slowed reaction time) as the reason to stop driving, and request the family lawyer to discuss financial and legal implications of crash or injury (Carr & Ott, 2010). Disabling the care in some way, such as replacing keys with ones that will not start the vehicle, disabling the ignition, and removing the car, are other suggestions, but often the older person can circumvent these strategies by hiring a mechanic to repair the car or buying a new vehicle.

Vehicle adaptations (Box 13-10), sensory aids, elder driving training, and driving assessment programs are helpful in promoting safe driving (Gillian & Schwartzberg, 2005; Perkinson et al., 2005). There is no gold standard for determining driving competency, but driving evaluations are offered by driver rehabilitation specialists through local hospitals and rehabilitation centers and private or university-based driving assessment programs. State Departments of Motor Vehicles (DMVs) also conduct performance-based road tests. Specialized driving cessation support groups (Box 13-11) aimed at the transition from driver to non-driver may also be beneficial in decreasing the negative outcomes associated with this decision (Dobbs et al., 2009).

A mnemonic, SAFE DRIVE, addresses key components to screen for in older drivers (McGregor, 2002). The components include the following:

S Safety record
A Attention skills
F Family report
E Ethanol use
D Drugs
R Reaction time
I Intellectual impairment
V Vision and visuospatial function
E Executive functions

The American Medical Association, in partnership with the National Highway Traffic Safety Administration, provides the Guide to Assessing and Counseling Older Drivers with

Transition from Driving to Driving Cessation: The Role of Specialized Driving Cessation Support Groups for Individuals with Dementia

The loss of driving privileges due to a dementing illness is an issue that is likely to impact a sizeable number of individuals now and in the next several decades. For many individuals with dementia, the loss of driving privileges is a major occurrence in the course of their illness. Yet, few, if any, interventions have been available to assist individuals in coping with the loss.

In this study, individuals with dementia (47) who had experienced a loss of driving privileges and their caregivers participated in an experimental-control design study in which they participated either in a driving cessation support group (DCSG) or a support group offered by the Alzheimer's Society. The mean age of the participants was 77 years of age, and 57% of them were males. 50% of the participants had failed a formal driving assessment, and the remainder had stopped driving based on advice of physicians, their family, or of their own accord.

Before stopping driving, 25% of the participants reported having had a crash (14% had one crash; 11% had two or more); 13% reported receiving a citation (11% received two or more) in the six months before driving cessation.

Participants attending the DCSGss had an improvement in depression scores, were less angry, and were happier. All participants reported that attending the DCSG had made a difference in their lives and had helped them cope with the illness and with not driving. Support groups designed specifically to deal with loss of driving privileges among individuals with dementia may be important in alleviating depressive symptoms and other negative outcomes associated with cessation of driving. DCSG interventions may represent an important step in the management of a very difficult aspect of dementia.

From Dobbs B, et al: Transitioning from driving to driving cessation: The role of specialized driving cessation support groups for individuals with dementia, *Topics in Geriatric Rehabilitation* 25:73-86, 2009.

step-by-step plans for assessing older driver safety. Many states have implemented the Silver Alert system. Similar to Amber Alerts for missing children, the Silver Alert is designed to create a widespread lookout for older adults who wander from their surroundings. Silver Alert features a public notification system to broadcast information about missing persons, especially older adults with Alzheimer's disease or other mental disabilities, in order to aid in their return. Silver Alert uses a wide array of media outlets, such as commercial radio stations, television use stations, and cable TV, to broadcast information about missing persons. Silver Alert also uses message signs on roadways to alert motorists to be on the lookout for missing elders and provides the car make, model, and the license information. In cases in which a missing person is believed to have gone missing on foot, Silver Alert uses reverse 911 or other emergency notification systems to notify nearby residents of the neighborhood surrounding the missing person's last known location.

EMERGING TECHNOLOGIES TO ENHANCE SAFETY OF OLDER ADULTS

Advancements in all types of technology hold promise for improving quality of life, decreasing the need for personal care, and enhancing independence and the ability to live safely at home and age-in-place (Daniel et al., 2009). Assistive technology is any device or system that allows a person to perform a task independently or that makes the task easier and safer to perform. Assistive technology is decreasing the number of older people who depend on others for personal care in ADLs and presents cost-effective alternatives to human services and institutionalization (Daniel et al., 2009). Delaying the need to send people from their homes to assisted living or nursing facilities by even one month can save $1.12 billion annually (Bezaitis, 2009). Gerotechnology is the term used to describe assistive technologies for older people and is expected to significantly influence how we live in the future. Health care technologies, telemedicine, mobility and activities-of-daily-living (ADL) aids,

and environmental control systems (smart houses/intelligent homes) are some examples of assistive technology.

Telemedicine offers exciting possibilities for managing medical problems in the home or other setting, reducing health care costs, and promoting self-management of illness. The number of telemedicine programs is increasing, and these programs offer exciting possibilities for nurses, particularly advanced practice nurses. Smart medical homes (www.futurehealth.rochester.edu) are being studied as a way to aid in the prevention and early detection of disease through the use of sensors and monitors. These devices keep data on vital signs and other measures such as gait, behavior, and sleep and provide an interactive medical-advising system. Devices to monitor gait and detect balance problems, such as the iShoe and the "smart carpet" (a sensor system embedded in carpet that detects gait abnormalities that may predispose to falls, and also as detects falls and summons assistance), are being developed (Aud et al., 2010; Rantz et al., 2008).

Remote-controlled houses are becoming more popular and allow the individual to control the house from anywhere (e.g., devices that turn lights on and off, automatically water plants, or feed pets; motion detectors; and leak detectors). The first of a series of smart houses is already on the market to enable older people to live safely in their own homes. An example is the Quiet Care 24-hour monitoring service. This system uses an ordinary home security infrastructure to keep a close eye on what happens in the house and transfers information about the occupant's daily living activities, triggering when a normal routine is broken. Caregivers and family can perform virtual check-ins with their older relative over the Internet (Bezaitis, 2009).

The MedCottage (http://www.medcottage.com) is a 12-by-24 foot portable and modular medical home equipped with technology and amenities for the health, safety, and comfort of older adults recovering from illness or injury. The MedCottage provides a family communication center that provides telemetry, environmental control, and dynamic interaction to offsite caregivers through smart and robotic technology. Technology inside includes monitoring of vital signs and safety, medication reminders, and adaptive devices. The MedCottage can be purchased or leased and temporarily placed on the caregiver's family property. It is similar to an RV and connects to a single–family home's electrical and water supplies.

Motion and pressure sensors may be useful in the homes of older adults with cognitive impairment. These sensors can detect movement as well as its absence. If there has been no movement for a period of time, a monitoring system is activated and a plan of action initiated depending on the person's response or lack of response. Pressure sensors can be used under the mattress and can turn on bedside lights when the individual gets out of bed and activate an alarm if he or she does not return to bed in a specified period of time. Sensors placed in entry doors can detect if a person leaves the home and can send messages to caregivers that the individual has left the house (Daniel et al., 2009). See http://www.agingtech.org/imagine_video.aspx for a video depicting home technology for older adults.

On the horizon are technology developments such as household robots that can help lift things, check a person's vital signs, and assist with baths and meals. A child-size therapist robot on wheels with a humanlike torso is being developed for use in homes and long-term care facilities to assist with the high level of attention individuals with dementia require for safety and function. Wheelchair technology that enables the user to go down stairs, move to an upright position, be reminded to change positions to alleviate pressure, or use mechanical arms to change a light bulb or get things out of the refrigerator are other developing technologies.

Robotic technology for health care is more advanced in Europe and Japan than in the United States at this time. Since 2001, Japan has spent $210 million on research to deploy robots to support its aging workforce (Robinson & Reinhard, 2009). A novel type of animal-assisted therapy being researched in Japan is the use of mental commit robots, which have the appearance of real animals. Paro, a seal-like robot, was developed with tactile, vision, audition, and posture sensors and a behavior-generation system that simulates the behaviors of a real animal. A seal was chosen since it is a nonfamiliar animal, and it is thought that people may accept it more easily without preconception. Early research has shown decreased stress levels, enhanced communication, and improvement of mood among nursing home elders who were exposed to Paro. Paro is amazingly lifelike and is even able to respond and turn its head in response to voices and touch. More information can be found at http://paro.jp/english.

Other futuristic developments include first-person vision in which a camera located on the shirt lapel or within eyeglasses would enable a computer to familiarize itself with all the elements in an older person's environment. First-person vision would be equipped with facial recognition software to remind the user of people's names and even help with driving by taking over control of the care for short preprogrammed stints. The Mem Exerciser has been developed for older adults with mild memory loss and is a camera worn around the neck that captures what the individual sees through a series of frequent photographs recorded throughout the day. It then automatically extracts the images and sounds that represent pleasant actions or events and plays them back for the individual so he or she can recollect the event (Bezaitis, 2009).

In hospitals and long-term care facilities, devices such as wireless pendants that track people's movements, load cells built into beds that create an alert when residents get out of bed as well as monitor patients' weights and sleep patterns, and bed lifts that allow persons to go from lying down to standing up with the push of a button are being used.

As the baby boomers and future generations age, comfort with technology will be increased, and people will seek options for better, safer, and more independent ways not yet imagined. At this time, many of the assistive technologies can be cost-prohibitive for older people, but with more development they may be more accessible and affordable for more people. Research is needed on assistive technologies and their acceptance among older people. It is important for nurses to be aware of available technology to improve safety. See the Evolve website for more information.

ELDER-FRIENDLY COMMUNITIES

Efforts to create communities for older adults that enhance safety, security, and quality of life go beyond simply providing a safe physical environment and freedom from violence and crime. Physical, social, and personal environmental spaces and their relationship to stress and health are beginning increased attention. The physical components of environmental sensitivity (air, water, and land mass) and the social components (government, economics, and culture) are avenues through which the individual's health and wellness can be enhanced or limited. Older people are often confronted with social and economic issues that force environmental changes against their wishes.

Developing elder-friendly communities and increasing opportunities to age in place can enhance the health and well-being of older people. Enabling the community to become the good neighbor to older citizens provides mutual benefits to all who are involved. Many state and local governments are assessing the community and designing interventions to enhance the ability of older people to remain in their homes and familiar environments. These interventions range from adequate transportation systems to home modifications and universal design standards for barrier-free housing. Home design features such as 36-inch-wide doors and hallways, a bathroom on the first floor, an entry with no steps, outlets at wheelchair level, and reinforced walls in bathrooms to support a grab bar will become standard nationwide in the next 50 years (Robinson & Reinhard, 2009).

Naturally Occurring Retirement Communities (NORCs) are neighborhoods or buildings in which a large segment of the residents are older adults. They are not purpose-built senior housing or retirement communities but are places where community residents have aged in place within the same housing constructs or neighborhoods and where they intend to spend the rest of their lives. NORCs provide a range of health and social services for the residents as well as individual assessments of risk, coordination of non-professional services, and referrals and follow-up. The prototypical NORC is Beacon Hill Village in Boston. The U.S. Administration on Aging (AoA) administers the Older Americans Act programs, including the National

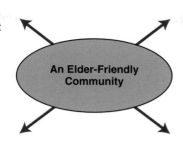

Addresses Basic Needs

• Provides appropriate and
  affordable housing
• Promotes safety at home and
  in the neighborhood
• Ensures no one goes hungry
• Provides useful information about
  available services

Promotes Social and Civic Engagement

• Fosters meaningful connections
  with family, neighbors, and friends
• Promotes active engagement
  in community life
• Provides opportunities for meaningful
  paid and voluntary work
• Makes aging issues a community-wide priority

**Optimizes Physical and Mental
Health and Well-Being**

• Promotes healthy behaviors
• Supports community activities
  that enhance well-being
• Provides ready access to
  preventive health services
• Provides access to medical,
  social, and palliative services

**An Elder-Friendly
Community**

**Maximizes Independence for
Frail and Disabled**

• Mobilizes resources to
  facilitate "living at home"
• Provides accessible transportation
• Supports family and other caregivers

FIGURE 13-1 Essential elements of an elder-friendly community. (From AdvantAge Initiative, Center for Home Care Policy and Research, Visiting Nurse Service of New York, www.vnsny.org/advantage).

NORCs Initiative. Since 2002, more than $22 million in federal funds and matching funds exceeding $7 million has been used to fund these types of programs (www.norcs.com; http://www.aoa.gov/AoARoot/AoA_Programs/HCLTC/NORC/index.aspx#resources).

Components of an elder-friendly community include the following: 1) addresses basic needs; 2) optimizes physical health and well-being; 3) maximizes independence for the frail and disabled; and 4) provides social and civic engagement. Figure 13-1 presents elements of an elder-friendly community.

evolve To access your student resources, go to *http://evolve.elsevier.com/Ebersole/TwdHlthAging*

KEY CONCEPTS

• With increasing age and dependency, the environment becomes a larger factor in maintaining a sense of security.
• Anxiety and insecurity increase when situations and conditions become unpredictable.
• Sensory deficits increase feelings of insecurity and uncertainty in the environment.
• Because of declining thermoregulatory mechanisms in older adults, extremes of heat and cold must be avoided.
• Severe hypothermia and hyperthermia are medical emergencies and may result in death if not properly attended.
• Neighborhoods change over the years, and long-term dwellers may find themselves in dangerous or crime-ridden areas as they age.

• Elders are often targets of fraud and deception.
• Reducing fire hazards is essential to feelings of security.
• Transportation for older adults is critical to their physical, psychological, and social health.
• Driving safety for older people is an important issue, and health care professionals must be knowledgeable about assessment, safety interventions, and transportation resources.
• A familiar and comfortable environment allows an elder to function at his or her highest capacity.

RESEARCH QUESTIONS

1. What criminal activities are of most concern to older people?
2. What percentage of major cities or states provide crime victimization programs?
3. What environmental safety factors are most frequently neglected by older people?
4. What home safety factors most frequently cause trouble for older people?

5. What is the geographical distribution and incidence of hypothermia and hyperthermia in the United States?
6. What are the most frequent causes of fires among elders?
7. What do older people fear most in their environment?
8. What are the barriers to the use of assistive technology in institutions and personal homes?

CASE STUDY   CHANGING LIFE SITUATIONS AND ENVIRONMENTAL VULNERABILITY

Ethel had lived in one home for all her married life, but when her husband died her children worried about her safety being alone in a big home. She could fall and lie undiscovered to die of hypothermia, the deteriorating neighborhood was no longer considered safe, and she could no longer drive so was limited in her ability to get around. They convinced her to move to a community in Phoenix near them.

They were able to find a suitable apartment that she could afford. For a while they visited her each week, but each visit became more depressing for them as she continually talked about her old home, old friends, old furniture, old priest—everything old. Their visits became less frequent. She called them faithfully each morning but detected their urge to get off the phone and on with their lives. One morning she called her daughter Gladys and said, "I'm so sick! Yesterday I walked outside and I swear I saw my friend Rose from the old neighborhood getting on the bus, but she didn't see me. I was so disappointed but managed to make it home, then couldn't find the key to my apartment so finally had to call 911 for help. They were really irritated with me when I said I had lost my key. I want to go back to Detroit. I know how things work there." After a family conclave, they found a nice place in assisted living for her and were much relieved. Ethel said, "I don't know where I am anymore. Seems I bounce around like a rubber ball." She seldom left her room except for meals, and soon she needed meals brought to her. Last week she wandered out and, when found, had suffered a serious case of heat stroke.

Based on the case study, develop a nursing care plan using the following procedure*:

- List Ethel's comments that provide subjective data.
- List information that provides objective data.
- From these data, identify and state, using accepted format, two nursing diagnoses you determine are most significant to Ethel at this time. List two of Ethel's strengths that you have identified from data.
- Determine and state outcome criteria for each diagnosis. These must reflect some alleviation of the problem identified in the nursing diagnosis and must be stated in concrete and measurable terms.

- Plan and state one or more interventions for each diagnosed problem. Provide specific documentation of the source used to determine the appropriate intervention. Plan at least one intervention that incorporates Ethel's existing strengths.
- Evaluate the success of the intervention. Interventions must correlate directly with the stated outcome criteria to measure the outcome success.

CRITICAL THINKING QUESTIONS

1. Locate low-cost housing in your area, and assess for convenience and safety.
2. Are purse snatching and mugging of elders commonplace in your city?
3. What resources are available to prevent or assist those who may be vulnerable to attack?
4. Discuss how you would assist your parents in making a decision regarding a change in living situations as they become increasingly disabled and unable to care for themselves.
5. List several aspects of your environment that are important to you, and discuss their significance.
6. Discuss housing options that would be most suitable and feasible for you if you were unable to get around without the assistance of a walker.
7. Discuss the meanings and the thoughts triggered by the student's and elder's viewpoints expressed at the beginning of the chapter. How do these vary from your own experience?
8. Make a plan for assistance to your older parents when they are no longer able to fully care for themselves. Discuss the signals that will let you know they are insecure in their environment.
9. What are your city's and state's plans for disaster preparedness for disabled and older people living in the community and in institutions?
10. Compare your community to the characteristics of an elder-friendly community.
11. Survey the homes of elders you are serving in your clinical practice for the presence or absence of safety features.

*Students are advised to refer to their nursing diagnosis text and identify possible or potential problems.

REFERENCES

Adelman D, Legg T: Caring for older adults with dementia when disaster strikes. *Journal of Gerontological Nursing* 36:13-17, 2010.

Aud M, et al: Smart carpet: developing a sensor system to detect falls and summon assistance, *Journal of Gerontological Nursing* 36:8-12, 2010.

Bezaitis A: Robot technologies: exciting new frontier, *Aging Well* 2:10, 2009.

Brown L: Issues in mental health care for older adults after disasters, *Generations* 31:21-26, 2008.

Burnett J, et al: Rapid needs assessment for older adults in disasters, *Generations* 31:10-15, 2008.

Campbell J: Applying the "disaster lens" to older adults, *Generations* 31:5-7, 2008.

Carr D, Ott B: The older adult driver with cognitive impairment: "It's a very frustrating life," *Journal of the American Medical Association* 303:1632-1641, 2010.

Centers for Disease Control and Prevention: Heat-related deaths—United States, 1999-2003, *Morbidity and Mortality Weekly Report* 55:796-798, 2006.

Centers for Medicare and Medicaid Services (CMS): *Medicare fights against new schemes to defraud beneficiaries.* Available at: www.cms.

hhs.gov/apps/media/press/release.asp? Counter=1882.Accessed June 16, 2006.

Daniel K, et al: Emerging technologies to enhance the safety of older people in their homes, *Geriatric Nursing* 30:384-389, 2009.

Dobbs B, et al: Transitioning from driving to driving cessation: The role of specialized driving cessation support groups for individuals with dementia, *Topics in Geriatric Rehabilitation* 25:73-86, 2009.

Gillian C, Schwartzberg J: Addressing the at-risk older driver, *Clinics in Geriatric Medicine* 13:27-34, 2005.

Gray-Vickrey P: Enhancing driver safety in dementia, *Alzheimer's Care Today* 11:147-148, 2010a.

Gray-Vickrey P: Research updates: driving and dementia, *Alzheimer's Care Today* 11:149-150, 2010b.

Ham R, et al: *Primary care geriatrics: A case-based approach*, ed 5, St Louis, 2007, Elsevier.

Hooyman N, Kiyak H: *Social Gerontology: A multidisciplinary perspective*, Boston, 2011, Allyn & Bacon.

Hurley A, et al: Promoting safer home environments for persons with Alzheimer's disease: the home safety/injury model, *Journal of Gerontological Nursing* 30:43-51, 2004.

Jett K, et al: Imposed versus involved: different strategies to effect driving cessation in cognitively impaired older adults, *Geriatric Nursing* 26:111-116, 2005.

Lach H, Langan J, James D: Disaster planning: Are gerontological nurses prepared? *Journal of Gerontological Nursing* 31:21-28, 2005.

Mathias J, Lucas L: Cognitive predictors of unsafe driving in older drivers: A meta-analysis, *Inter Psychogeriatrics* 21:637-653, 2009.

McGregor D: Driving over 65: proceed with caution, *Journal of Gerontological Nursing* 28:221-226, 2002.

National Association of Triads, Inc. *NATI resources*: Frauds, scams, and the senior citizen Available at: www.nationaltriad.org/tools/ NATI_Resource_Frauds_and_Scams.pdf. Accessed July 10, 2006.

Norman D: Fever in the elderly, *Clinical Infectious Diseases* 31:148-151, 2000.

Outzen M: Management of fever in older adults, *Journal of Gerontological Nursing* 35:17-23, 2009.

Oxley J, Charlton J: Attitudes to and mobility impacts of driving cessation, *Topics in Geriatric Rehabilitation* 25:43-54, 2009.

Perkinson M, et al: Driving and dementia of the Alzheimer type: beliefs and cessation strategies, *Gerontologist* 45:676-685, 2005.

Rantz M, et al: Falls, technology, and stunt actors, *Journal of Nursing Care Quality* 23:195-201, 2008.

Rhoads J, Clayman A: Learning from Katrina: preparing long-term care facilities for disasters, *Geriatric Nursing* 29:253-258, 2008.

Robinson K, Reinhard S: Looking ahead in long-term care: the next 50 years, *Nursing Clinics of North America* 44:253-262, 2009.

Siren A, Hakamies-Blomqvist L: Mobility and well-being in old age, *Topics in Geriatric Rehabilitation* 25:3-11, 2009.

Tanner E: Assessing home safety in homebound older adults, *Geriatric Nursing* 24:250-255, 2003.

Warner M: *The complete guide to Alzheimer's proofing your home*, Lafayette, Ind, 2000, Purdue University Press.

CHAPTER

14

Nutrition and Hydration

Theris A. Touhy

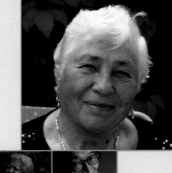

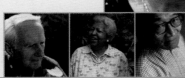

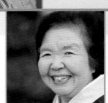

evolve http://evolve.elsevier.com/Ebersole/TwdHlthAging

A STUDENT SPEAKS

I work as a certified nursing assistant in a skilled nursing facility and I am responsible for feeding 10 residents at the dinner meal. I try to get them to eat but they are very slow and we only have a limited amount of time. Sometimes, I end up just mixing the food and getting them to take a few spoonfuls. The people with dementia need even more time and I know that they are not getting enough to eat. It makes me feel terrible and we need so much more help to do a good job.

Marcia, age 21

AN ELDER SPEAKS

If I do reach the point where I can no longer feed myself, I hope that the hands holding my fork belong to someone who has a feeling for who I am. I hope my helper will remember what she learns about me and that her awareness of me will grow from one encounter to another. Why should this make a difference? Yet I am certain that my experience of needing to be fed will be altered if it occurs in the context of my being truly known . . . I will want to know about the lives of the people I rely on, especially the one who holds my fork for me. If she would talk to me, if we could laugh together, I might even forget the chagrin of my useless hands. We would have a conversation, rather than a feeding. **From Lustbader W: Thoughts on the meaning of frailty, Generations 13:21-22, 1999.**

LEARNING OBJECTIVES

On completion of this chapter, the reader will be able to:

1. Discuss nutritional requirements and factors affecting nutrition for older adults.
2. Describe a nutritional screening and assessment.
3. Identify strategies to assist in ensuring adequate nutrition for older adults experiencing hospitalization, institutionalization, and physical and cognitive impairments.
4. Delineate risk factors for poor nutrition and malnutrition, and identify strategies for management.

5. Discuss assessment and interventions for older adults with dysphagia.
6. Discuss interventions that promote good oral hygiene for older people.
7. Develop a plan of care to assist an older person in developing and maintaining good nutritional status.

Adequate nutrition is critical to preserving the health of older people. The quality and quantity of diet are important factors in preventing, delaying onset, and managing chronic illnesses associated with aging (American Dietetic Association, American Society for Nutrition, Society for Nutrition Education, 2010). Results of studies provide growing evidence that diet can affect longevity and, when combined with lifestyle changes, reduce disease risk. "While diet is only one component in the development and exacerbation of illness (heredity, environment, medical care, social circumstances, and other lifestyle risk factors play a part), eating and drinking habits have been

implicated in 6 of the 10 leading causes of death in this country (heart disease, cancer, stroke, diabetes, atherosclerosis, liver disease) as well as in several debilitating disorders such as osteoporosis and diverticulosis" (Haber, 2007). About 87% of older adults have diabetes, hypertension, dyslipidemia, or a combination of these diseases that may have dietary implications. (American Dietetic Association, American Society for Nutrition, Society for Nutrition Education, 2010).

Proper nutrition means that all of the essential nutrients (i.e., carbohydrates, fat, protein, vitamins, minerals, and water) are adequately supplied and used to maintain optimal health and well-being. Although some age-related changes in the gastrointestinal system do occur, these changes are rarely the primary factors in inadequate nutrition. Fulfillment of an older person's nutritional needs is more often affected by numerous other factors, including chronic disease, life-long eating habits, ethnicity, socialization, income, transportation, housing, food knowledge, functional impairments, health, and dentition. Data from the National Health and Nutrition Examination Survey (NHANES) showed that only about 17% of older adults consumed a "good" quality diet, with non-Hispanic white persons having the highest scores on the Healthy Eating Index (HEI) and non-Hispanic black persons having the lowest scores (Ervin, 2008).

This chapter discusses the dietary needs of older adults, age-related changes affecting nutrition, risk factors contributing to inadequate nutrition and hydration, obesity, and the effect of diseases and functional and cognitive impairments on nutrition. Dysphagia and oral care are included as additional concerns related to adequate nutrition in older adults. Readers are referred to a nutrition text for more comprehensive information on nutrition and aging and disease.

AGE-RELATED REQUIREMENTS

Modified MyPyramid

The Modified MyPyramid for Older Adults (over 70 years) has been adapted from the United States Department of Agriculture's (USDA) MyPyramid. The Modified MyPyramid provides the types and amounts of food that should be eaten to optimize nutrient intake (Figure 14-1). Modifications for older adults include the addition of eight 8-ounce glasses of water to the foundation of the pyramid. Older adults have reduced thirst mechanism and may not consume adequate fluids. Fluid intake is important for older adults to prevent cardiovascular and kidney complications as well as constipation. Additionally, a flag was added at the top to remind older adults that they may not be getting adequate calcium, vitamin D, and vitamin B_{12}, and may need supplements.

The foundation of MyPyramid depicts physical activities characteristic of older adults and emphasizes the importance of regular physical activity. The food guide emphasizes whole grains, fiber, nutrient-dense food, monounsaturated fats, reducing sodium, and fruits and vegetables. Generally, older adults need fewer calories because they may not be as active and metabolic rates slow down. However, they still require the same or higher levels of nutrients for optimal health outcomes. The recommendations may need modification for the older adult with illness.

With proper instruction, the Modified MyPyramid is an easy and systematic way for a person to evaluate his or her own nutritional intake and independently make corrective adjustments. Pictures can be used to transcend cultural and educational barriers. The USDA also provides ethnic-cultural and vegetarian food pyramids (www.fda.gov). The Dietary Approaches to Stop Hypertension (DASH) eating plan is another highly recommended eating plan for older people that assists older adults with maintenance of optimal weight and management of hypertension. This plan consists of fruits, vegetables, whole grains, low-fat dairy products, poultry, and fish, and restriction of salt intake (http://www.nhlbi.nih.gov/health/public/heart/hbp/dash/new_dash.pdf).

Other Dietary Recommendations
Fats

Similar to other age groups, older adults should limit intake of saturated fat and trans fatty acids. High fat diets cause obesity and increase the risk of heart disease and cancer. Recommendations are that 20% to 35% of total calories should be from fat, 45% to 65% from carbohydrates, and 10% to 35% from proteins. Monounsaturated fats, such as olive oil, are the best type of fat since they lower low-density lipoprotein (LDL) but leave the high density lipoprotein (HDL) intact or even slightly raise it. A simple technique to determine how much fat a person should consume is to divide the ideal weight in half and allowing that number of grams of fat (Haber, 2007).

Protein

Presently, the Institute of Medicine's Recommended Dietary Allowance (RDA) for protein of 0.8 g/kg per day, based primarily on studies in younger men, may be inadequate for older adults. Results of a recent study (Beasley et al., 2010) suggest that higher protein consumption, as a fraction of total caloric intake, is associated with a decline in risk of frailty in older adults. Protein intake of 1.5 g/kg per day, or 20% to 25% of total calorie intake, may be more appropriate for older adults at risk of becoming frail.

Older people who are ill are the most likely segment of society to experience protein deficiency. Those with limitations affecting their ability to shop, cook, and consume food are at risk for protein deficiency and malnutrition.

Fiber

Fiber is an important dietary component that some older people do not consume in sufficient quantities. Older adults should increase dietary fiber intake to 14 g per 1000 calories consumed (Ham et al., 2007). Insufficient amounts of fiber in the diet, as well as insufficient fluids, contribute to constipation. Fiber is the indigestible material that gives plants their structure. It is abundant in raw fruits and vegetables and in unrefined grains and cereals. The benefits of fiber include the following: facilitates the absorption of water; helps control weight by delaying gastric emptying and providing a feeling of fullness; improves glucose tolerance by delaying movement of carbohydrate into the small intestine; prevents or reduces constipation by increasing the weight of the stool and shortening the transit time; helps prevent hemorrhoids and diverticulosis by decreasing pressure in the colon, shortening transit time, and increasing stool weight; reduces the risk of heart disease by binding with bile (which contains cholesterol) and causes its excretion; and protects against cancer.

Individuals who can chew well could benefit from eating increased amounts of fresh fruits and vegetables daily or combining unsweetened bran with other types of food. It is better to get fiber from food than from fiber supplements such as Metamucil, since they do not contain the essential nutrients found in high-fiber foods and their anticancer benefits are

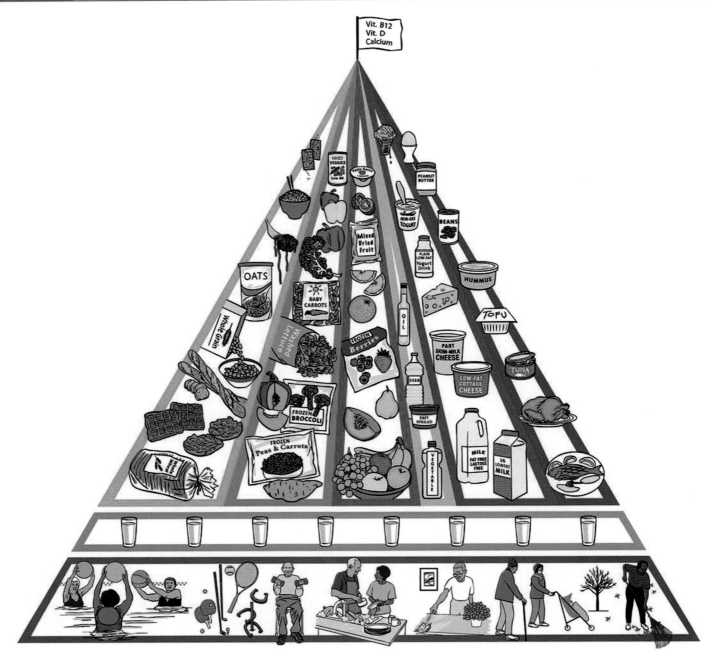

FIGURE 14-1 Modified MyPyramid for Older Adults. (Copyright 2007 Tufts University. Reprinted with permission from Lictenstein AH, Rasmussen H, Yu WW, et al. Modified MyPyramid for Older Adults, *Journal of Nutrition* 138: 78-82, 2008.)

questionable. Ways to increase fiber intake include eating cooked dry beans, peas, and lentils; leaving skins on fruits and vegetables; eating whole fruit rather than drinking fruit juice; and eating whole-grain breads and cereals (National Institute on Aging, 2010). Those who have difficulty chewing could sprinkle oat bran on cereals or in soups, meat loaf, or casseroles.

The quantity of bran depends on the individual, but generally, one to two tablespoons daily is sufficient. Individuals who have not used bran should begin with one teaspoon and progressively increase the quantity until the fiber intake is enough to accomplish its purpose. If bran is used in larger amounts to start, bloating, gas, diarrhea, and other colon discomforts will initially occur and discourage further use of this important

dietary ingredient. Fluid intake of 64 ounces daily is essential as well.

Vitamins and Minerals

Older people who consume five servings of fruits and vegetables daily will obtain adequate intake of vitamins A, C, and E, and potassium. Americans of all ages eat less than half of the recommended amounts of fruits and vegetables (Haber, 2007).

After age 50, the stomach produces less gastric acid, which makes vitamin B_{12} absorption less efficient. Vitamin B_{12} deficiency in a common and underrecognized condition that is estimated to occur in 12% to 14% of community-dwelling older adults and up to 25% of those residing in institutional settings (Ahmed & Haboubi, 2010).

Atrophic gastritis and pernicious anemia are the most common causes of vitamin B_{12} deficiency. Less common causes are a strict vegetarian diet over a long period of time or inadequate absorption after gastrectomy or ileostomy. While intake of this vitamin is generally adequate, older adults should increase their intake of the crystalline form of vitamin B_{12} from fortified foods such as whole-grain breakfast cereals. Use of proton pump inhibitors for more than one year, as well as histamine H2 receptor blockers can lead to lower serum vitamin B_{12} levels by impairing absorption of the vitamin from food. Metformin, colchicine, and antibiotic and anticonvulsant agents may also increase the risk of vitamin B_{12} deficiency (Cadogan, 2010).

Calcium and vitamin D are essential for bone health and may prevent osteoporosis and decrease the risk of fracture. Chapter 15 discusses recommendations for calcium and vitamin D supplementation. Calcium is a difficult mineral to absorb, and some foods inhibit calcium absorption (e.g., green beans, peanuts, and summer squash) (Table 14-1). High levels of protein, sodium, or caffeine also cause more calcium to be excreted in the urine and should be avoided. For older adults with inadequate calcium intake from diet, supplemental calcium can be used.

OBESITY (OVERNUTRITION)

While most of the research on nutrition and older adults has centered on underweight and frailty, the increase in the prevalence of obesity in the general population, and in older adults, is getting increased attention. More than two-thirds of all adults in the United States are overweight (BMI = 25 to 29.9) or obese (BMI ≥30), and the proportion of older adults who are obese has doubled in the past 30 years (Bales & Buhr, 2008; Flicker et al., 2010; Newman, 2009). "The obesity epidemic is occurring in parallel with the aging of the baby boomer generation. Current estimates in the United States indicate that nearly 70% of those aged 65 and older are overweight or obese and 29% are obese" (Jarosz and Bellar, 2009).

TABLE 14-1	CALCIUM CONTENT OF SEVERAL COMMON FOODS	
FOOD ITEM	**SERVING SIZE**	**CALCIUM (MG)**
Plain yogurt, fat-free	8 oz	452
American cheese	2 oz	312
Yogurt with fruit (low fat or fat-free)	8 oz	345
Milk	8 oz	300
Orange juice, calcium-fortified	8 oz	350
Dried figs	10 figs	269
Cheese pizza	1 slice	240
Ricotta cheese, part skim	½ cup	334
Ice cream, soft serve	4 oz	103
Spinach	4 oz	139
Cooked soybeans	1 cup	298

Source: National Institutes of Health: Sources of calcium, Washington, D.C. Available at: www.nichd.nih.gov/milk. Accessed November 1, 2008.

Similar trends are observed in other developed and developing countries. Overweight and obesity are growing global public health concerns and are associated with increased health care costs, functional impairments, disability, chronic disease, and nursing home admission (Felix, 2008; Newman, 2009). Socioeconomic deprivation and lower levels of education have been linked to obesity. African Americans have a 51% higher prevalence of obesity compared with whites, and Hispanics have a 21% higher prevalence (CDC, 2010).

While there is strong evidence that obesity in younger people lessens life expectancy and has a negative effect on functionality and morbidity, it remains unclear whether overweight and obesity are predictors of mortality in older adults. Concerns have been raised about encouraging apparently overweight older people to lose weight (Bales and Buhr, 2008; Flicker et al., 2010). In what has been termed the *obesity paradox*, for people who have survived to age 70, mortality risk is lowest in those with a BMI classified as overweight (Felix, 2008, p. 36). Flicker and colleagues (2010) conclude that "BMI thresholds for overweight and obese are overly restrictive for older people. Overweight older people are not at greater mortality risk, and there is little evidence that dieting in this age group confers any benefit; these findings are consistent with the hypothesis that weight loss is harmful" (p. 239). For nursing home residents with severely decreased functional status, obesity may be regarded as a protective factor with regard to functionality and mortality (Kaiser et al., 2010).

However, as Jarosz and Bellar (2009) point out, the reduction in muscle mass that occurs with aging (sarcopenia) is increasingly being paired with an increased fat mass in obese older adults (sarcopenic obesity). This may make it more difficult to recognize frailty and/or malnutrition in obese older people. The growing prevalence of obesity in middle and late life could further exacerbate a number of age-related health concerns, depending on body weight gain patterns and the health history of the individual. Felix (2008) also notes the effect on nursing homes expenditures and staff workload in light of the increasing number of obese individuals being admitted for care.

At this time, maintaining weight in older persons seems to be a clinical recommendation, and any weight loss interventions in older persons must be "carefully considered on an individualized basis with special attention to the weight history and the medical conditions of each individual" (Bales and Buhr, 2008, p. 311). Maintaining a healthy weight throughout life is one of the most important goals for people of all ages.

MALNUTRITION

Malnutrition is defined as a state in which a deficiency, excess or imbalance of energy, protein and other nutrients causes adverse effects on body form, function, and clinical outcome" (Ahmed and Haboubi, 2010, p. 207). The rising incidence of malnutrition among older adults has been documented in acute care, long-term care, and the community. Between 16% and 30% of older adults are malnourished or at high risk, and about half of this population has protein levels consistent with malnutrition when they are admitted to hospitals (Duffy, 2010). Older adults in skilled nursing facilities and long-term nursing home residents also have a higher incidence of malnutrition.

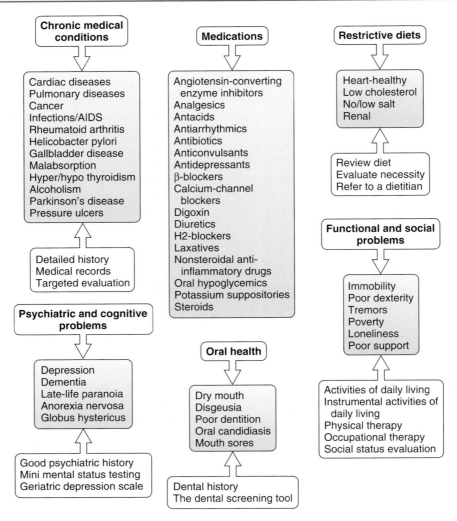

FIGURE 14-2 Risk factors for undernutrition illustrated by clinical approach. (From Omran M, Salem P: *Clinics in Geriatric Medicine* 18:719-36, 2002).

An estimated 15% of community-dwelling older people experience malnutrition, and a recent study links malnutrition in this population to socioeconomic status, functional limitations, and social isolation (Lee & Berthelot, 2010). The diseases and functional impairments that prompt admission to a skilled nursing facility make older people extremely vulnerable to malnutrition. These figures are projected to rise dramatically in the next 30 years (Ahmed & Haboubi, 2010). Malnutrition among older people is clearly a serious challenge for health professionals in all settings.

Malnutrition has serious consequences, including infections, pressure ulcers, anemia, hypotension, impaired cognition, hip fractures, and increased mortality and morbidity. "Malnourished older adults take 40% longer to recover from illness, have 2-3 times as many complications, and have hospital stays that are 90% longer" (Haber, 2007, p. 211). Many factors contribute to the occurrence of malnutrition in older adults (Figure 14-2).

Protein-energy malnutrition (PEM) is the most common form of malnutrition in older adults. PEM is characterized by the presence of clinical signs (muscle wasting, low BMI) and biochemical indicators (albumin, cholesterol, or other protein changes) indicative of insufficient intake. Two clinical patterns

of PEM are marasmus and kwashiorkor (hypoalbuminemic malnutrition). Marasmus develops gradually over months or years when energy intake is insufficient. Skeletal muscle, rather than plasma or visceral protein, is metabolized. In this condition, serum albumin level is generally normal.

Kwashiorkor is more acute or subacute but may frequently be superimposed on marasmus. It is precipitated by the stress of an acute illness and develops over weeks. Serum proteins are depleted with consequent edema, and there may be no weight loss. This PEM syndrome has a high mortality rate. Signs and symptoms of PEM are nonspecific, and it is important that other conditions such as malignancy, hyperthyroidism, peptic ulcer, and liver disease are ruled out (Ham et al., 2007). Comprehensive nutritional screening and assessment are essential in identifying older adults at risk for nutrition problems or who are malnourished.

FACTORS AFFECTING FULFILLMENT OF NUTRITIONAL NEEDS

Fulfillment of the older person's nutritional needs is affected by numerous factors including change associated with aging, lifelong eating habits, chronic disease, medication regimens, ethnicity and culture, socialization, socioeconomic deprivation, transportation, housing, and food knowledge.

Age-Associated Changes

Some age-related changes in the senses of taste and smell (chemosenses) and the digestive tract do occur as the individual ages and may affect nutrition. For most older people, these changes do not seriously interfere with eating, digestion, and the enjoyment of food. However, combined with other factors, they may contribute to inadequate nutrition and decreased eating pleasure (Chapter 4).

Taste

The sense of taste has many components and primarily depends on receptor cells in the taste buds. Taste buds are scattered on the surface of the tongue, the cheek, the soft palate, the upper tip of the esophagus, and other parts of the mouth. Components in food stimulate taste buds during chewing and swallowing, and tongue movements enhance flavor sensation. Fine, subtle taste to discriminate between flavors is an olfactory function, whereas crude taste (e.g. sweet and sour) depends on the taste buds. Individuals have varied levels of taste sensitivity that seem predetermined by genetics and constitution, as well as age variations. Early studies suggested that a decline in the number of taste cells occurs with aging, but more recent studies suggest that "taste cells can regenerate but that the lag time of this turnover may account for the diminished taste response in older adults" (Miller, 2008, p. 363).

Age-related changes do not affect all taste sensations equally. With age, the inability to detect sweet taste seems to remain intact, whereas the ability to detect sour, salty, and bitter taste declines. Many denture wearers say they lose some of their satisfaction with food taste, possibly because dentures cover the palate and because texture is a very important element in food enjoyment. Difficulty in flavor appreciation comes from individual variables such as smoking, olfactory sensitivity, attitude toward food and eating, and the presence of moistening secretions. There are also aberrations in flavor sensation caused by certain medications and medical conditions. The addition of flavor enhancers (bouillon cubes) and concentrated flavors (jellies or sauces) can amplify both taste and smell. Fresh herbs and spices also give an extra boost to flavor and may increase enjoyment and interest in eating. The bland diets often found in hospitals and institutions contribute to decreased appetite.

Smell

Age-related changes in the sense of smell and the consequent effect on nutrition is in need of further research. In the past, studies have shown a decline in the sense of smell as the individual ages. Recent research (Markovic et al., 2007) disputes this belief. Results of this study suggested that for perceived odors, olfactory pleasure increases at later stages in the life span, and the perceived intensity of odors remains stable. Decrease in the sense of smell may be related to many factors, including the following: nasal sinus disease, repeated injury to olfactory receptors through viral infections, age-related changes in central nervous system functioning, smoking, medications, and

periodontal disease and other dentition problems. Changes in the sense of smell are also associated with Parkinson's disease and Alzheimer's disease (Cacchione, 2008).

Smell occurs when nerve receptors in the nose send messages to the brain. The oral and nasal senses interact to give us the impression of a certain food, combining to heighten the sensory perceptions we receive. Smells also create emotional responses (positive or negative) to food because emotions and smell sensations overlap in the brain. Think how the smell of freshly baked chocolate chip cookies makes you feel compared with the smell of burned popcorn. Many older people, particularly those in institutions, no longer cook and never have the experience of smelling food as it is cooking, an important appetite stimulant. Many long-term care institutions have adapted kitchens and dining rooms so that the residents can smell the food cooking and even participate in the preparation of food as a way of increasing interest and enjoyment in food.

Digestive System

Age-related changes in the oral cavity, the esophagus, the stomach, the liver, the pancreas, the gallbladder, and the small and large intestines may influence nutritional status in concert with other factors. However, these changes do not significantly affect function, and the digestive system remains adequate throughout life. *Presbyesophagus*, a decrease in the intensity of propulsive waves, may be an age-related change in the esophagus. Some of these changes may be more attributable to pathological conditions rather than to age alone. The functional impact of presbyesophagus seems to be minimal, but combined with other conditions, may contribute to dysphagia.

Buccal Cavity

Age-related changes in the buccal cavity also predispose older people to orodental problems that can significantly affect nutrition (Box 14-1). Aging teeth become worn and darker in color and tend to develop longitudinal cracks. The dentin, or the layer beneath the enamel, becomes brittle and thickens so that pulp space decreases. In addition to years of exposure of the teeth and related structures to microbial assault, the oral cavity shows evidence of wear and tear as a result of normal use (chewing and talking) and destructive oral habits such as bruxism (habitual grinding of the teeth). People who are edentulous and are using complete dentures, continue to have oral health care needs. Ill-fitting dentures affect chewing and hence nutritional intake. People without teeth remain susceptible to oral cancer and other oral diseases.

Another common oral problem among older adults is dry mouth (xerostomia). Approximately 25% to 40% of older adults experience xerostomia. More than 500 medications have the side effect of reducing salivary flow. A reduction in saliva and a dry mouth make eating, swallowing, and speaking difficult. It can also lead to significant problems of the teeth and their supporting structure (Jablonski, 2010). Artificial saliva preparations are available (avoid those containing sorbitol), and adequate fluid intake is also important when xerostomia occurs. Chewing on xylitol-flavored fluoride tablets, sugar-free candies, or sugar-free gum with xylitol 15 minutes after meals may

BOX 14-1   AGE-RELATED CHANGES OF THE BUCCAL CAVITY

- Decrease in the cellular compartment
- Loss of submucosal elastin in oral mucosa
- Loss of connective tissue (collagen)
- Increase in thickness of collagen fibers
- Decrease in function of minor salivary glands
- Decrease in number and quality of blood vessels and nerves
- Attrition on occlusive contact surfaces
- Enamel less permeable and teeth more brittle
- Tooth color change
- Excessive secondary dentin formation
- Decrease in rate of cementin deposition
- Decrease in size of pulp chamber and root canals
- Decrease in size and volume of the tooth pulp
- Increase in pulp stones and dystrophic mineralization

stimulate saliva flow and promote oral hygiene (Miller, 2008). Medication review is also indicated to eliminate, if possible, medications contributing to xerostomia.

Regulation of Appetite

Appetite in persons of all ages is influenced by factors such as physical activity, functional limitations, smell, taste, mood, socialization, and comfort. With age, appetite and food consumption decline. Healthy older people are less hungry and are fuller before meals, consume smaller meals, eat more slowly, have fewer snacks between meals, and become satiated after meals more rapidly than younger people (Ahmed and Haboubi, 2010). Appetite is regulated by a combination of a peripheral satiation system and a central feeding drive. There is some evidence that alterations in the endogenous opioid feeding and drinking drive may decline in aging and contribute to decreased appetite and risk for dehydration. Nearly 20% of old-old individuals have anorexia. Individuals with anorexia are likely to be frailer and more disabled, and are likely to have an increased rate of mortality (Morley, 2010).

Older men have a greater degree of anorexia than do women. This is thought to be related to testosterone level decline in men and associated increase in leptin levels. Gastrointestinal hormones, such as cholecystokinin (CCK), also regulate satiety to varying degrees. CCK is increased both basally and following a meal in older persons and also has a more potent satiating effect in older persons. Disease states also increase cytokine levels as a result of its release by diseased tissues. An increase in cholecystokinin levels also occurs in malnourished individuals, which may further decrease appetite.

Decreased stomach fundal compliance, decreased testosterone, and increased leptin and amylin also contribute to decreases in appetite among older people. "Much of the anorexia of aging seems to be related to changes in gastrointestinal activities that occur with aging, with less antral distention, and thus earlier satiety" (Ham et al., 2007, p. 282). Other factors that contribute to decreases in appetite include depression, polypharmacy, oral and dental problems, dementia, and other chronic illnesses, as well as feeding techniques and mealtime ambience in institutions (Morley 2003; Morley, 2010).

Lifelong Eating Habits

The nutritional state of a person reflects the individual's dietary history and present food practices. Lifelong eating habits are also developed out of tradition, ethnicity, and religion, all of which collectively can be called culture. Food habits established since childhood may influence the intake of older adults.

Eating habits do not always coincide with fulfillment of nutritional needs. Rigidity of food habits may increase with age as familiar food patterns are sought. Ethnicity determines if traditional foods are preserved, whereas religion affects the choice of foods possible. Throughout life, then, preferences for particular foods bring deep satisfaction and possess emotional significance. Such foods are called *soul food* or comfort food. Preferences for soul food influence food choices and affect nutrient intake. Foods prepared or served in a special way provide "soul" and are not unique to any one group but, rather, are found all over the world. Rice with every meal and homemade chicken soup given to the individual when ill are examples of what people consider their soul food.

Members of a particular ethnic or religious group will have unique eating patterns, so individual assessment is important. Cultural preferences affect nutrition and culturally and religiously appropriate diets should be available in any institution or congregate dining program.

Lifelong habits of dieting or eating fad foods also echo through the later years. Older people may fall prey to advertisements that claim specific foods maintain youth and vitality or rid one of chronic conditions. Everyone can benefit from improved eating habits, and it's never too late to change dietary habits to improve health. Following the Modified MyPyramid for Older Adults (Figure 14-1) is best for an ideal diet, with changes based on particular problems, such as hypercholesteremia. Older adults should be counseled to base their dietary decisions on valid research and consultation with their primary care provider. For the healthy older adult, essential nutrients should be obtained from food sources rather than relying on dietary supplements.

Socialization

The fundamentally social aspect of eating has to do with sharing and the feeling of belonging that it provides. All of us use food as a means of giving and receiving love, friendship, or belonging. Often, older adults may be isolated from the mainstream of life because of chronic illness, depression, and other functional limitations. When one eats alone, the outcome is often either overindulgence or disinterest in food. The presence of others during meals is a significant predictor of caloric intake (Locher et al., 2008).

Disinterest in food may also result from the effects of medication or disease processes. Misuse and abuse of alcohol are prevalent among older adults and are growing public health concerns. Excessive drinking interferes with nutrition. Drinking alcohol depletes the body of necessary nutrients and often replaces meals, thus making an individual susceptible to malnutrition (Chapter 18).

The elderly nutrition program, authorized under Title III of the Older Americans Act (OAA), is the largest national food and nutrition program specifically for older adults.

Programs and services include congregate nutrition programs, home-delivered nutrition services (Meals-on-Wheels), and nutrition screening and education. The program is not means-tested, and participants may make voluntary confidential contributions for meals. However, the OAA Nutrition Program reaches less than one-third of older adults in need of its program and services, and those served receive only three meals a week. With the emphasis on community-based care rather than institutional care, expansion of nutrition services should be a priority. These programs enable older adults to avoid or delay costly institutionalization and allow them to stay in their homes and communities. The American Dietetic Association estimates that the cost of one day in a hospital equals the cost of one year of OAA Nutrition Program meals, while the cost of one month in a nursing home equals that of providing midday meals five days a week in the community for about seven years (American Dietetic Association, 2010).

Chronic Diseases and Conditions

Many chronic diseases and their sequela pose nutritional challenges for older adults. Functional impairments associated with chronic disease interfere with the person's ability to shop, cook, and eat independently. For example, heart failure and chronic obstructive pulmonary disease (COPD) are associated with fatigue, increased energy expenditure, and decreased appetite. Dietary interventions for diabetes are essential but may also affect customary eating patterns and require lifestyle changes.

The side effects of medications prescribed for these conditions may further impair nutritional status. A number of prevalent disorders of the gastrointestinal (GI) tract are associated with nutritional concerns including gastroesophageal reflux disease (GERD), ulcers, constipation, diverticulosis, and colon cancer. Dysphagia, often a result of stroke or dementia, significantly affects nutrition. Diseases affecting function, such as arthritis and Parkinson's disease, may impair eating ability. Cancers and subsequent treatment impair appetite and ability to consume adequate nutrition. More detailed information on chronic illness can be found in Chapter 15.

Many medications affect appetite and nutrition. These include digoxin, theophylline, nonsteroidal anti-inflammatory drugs (NSAIDs), iron supplements, antidepressants, and psychotropics. There are clinically significant drug-nutrient interactions that result in nutrient loss, and evidence is accumulating that shows the use of nutritional supplements may counteract these possible drug-induced nutrient depletions. A thorough medication review is an essential component of nutritional assessment and individuals should receive education about the effects of prescription medications, as well as herbals and supplements, on nutritional status (Chapters 9, 10).

Socioeconomic Deprivation

There is a strong relationship between poor nutrition and socioeconomic deprivation. According to the federal government, fewer than 1 in 10 adults age 65 and older is living in poverty. However, poverty rates among older African Americans are nearly triple those of whites, and rates among Hispanics are more than double those of whites (Butrica, 2008). Older single women are also at high risk for poverty. Older adults with low incomes may need to choose among fulfilling needs such as food, heat, telephone bills, medications, and health care visits. Some older people eat only once per day in an attempt to make their income last through the month.

Programs such as the food stamp program have the potential for increasing the purchasing power of older adults who qualify, but older adults are less likely than any other age group to use the food stamp program. Of all older Americans living in poverty, approximately one in five receives food stamps (Fuller-Thomson & Redmond, 2008). Many older people may find that the amount of money required to purchase the food stamps is greater than they think they can afford, or they do not see the benefit to them. Transportation may be limited and the distance may be too great for an older person to travel to grocery stores or to acquire food stamps, which are obtained only at designated locations in cities. In addition, many older people, especially those who lived through the Great Depression, are very reluctant to accept "welfare."

Fuller-Thomson and Redmond (2008) suggest the use of focused outreach programs and public education to destigmatize the food stamp program and encourage greater use by older adults in need. Suggestions to improve the use of the food stamp program include creating mobile and satellite food stamp offices separate from welfare offices; increasing the availability of on-line application forms; creating more user-friendly applications; providing home visits by food stamp workers; providing more extensive multilingual services; and targeting information to older adults who receive Supplemental Security Income (SSI) or Medicaid, those who live in public housing, and those whose Social Security payments are below the poverty line.

Free food programs, such as donated commodities, are also available at distribution centers (food banks) for those with limited incomes. Although this is another valuable option for older people, use of such programs is not always feasible. One takes a chance on the types of food available on any particular day or week; quantities distributed are frequently too large for the single older person or the older couple to use or even carry from the distribution site; the site may be too far away or difficult to reach; and the time of food distribution may be inconvenient.

Cafeterias and restaurants that provide special meal prices for older people have had to increase their prices as food costs have risen. Thus the previous advantages of eating out have diminished. Yet, many single elders eat out for most meals. More and more are eating at fast food restaurants that typically do not offer low fat/low salt menu items. Older adults should be educated about nutritional content of fast food and other convenient ways to enhance healthy nutritional intake.

Transportation

Available and easily accessible transportation may be limited for older people. Many small, long-standing neighborhood food stores have been closed in the wake of the expansion of larger supermarkets, which are located in areas that serve a greater segment of the population. It may become difficult to walk to the market, to reach it by public transportation, or to carry a bag of groceries while using a cane or walker. Fear is apparent in elders' consideration of transportation. They may fear walking in the street and being mugged, not being able to cross the street in the time it takes the traffic light to change, or being knocked down or falling as they walk in crowded streets. Despite reduced senior citizen bus fares, many older people remain very fearful of attack when using public transportation. Functional impairments also make the use of public transportation difficult for some older people.

Transportation by taxicab for an individual on a limited income is unrealistic, but sharing a taxicab with others who also need to shop may enable the older person to go where food prices are cheaper and to take advantage of sale items. Senior citizen organizations in many parts of the United States have been helpful in providing older adults with van service to shopping areas. In housing complexes, it may be possible to schedule group trips to the supermarket. Many urban communities have multiple sources of transportation available, but the older adult may be unaware of them. Resources in rural areas are more limited. It is important for nurses to be knowledgeable about resources in the community that are available to older people.

In addition, many older adults, particularly widowed men, may have never learned to shop and prepare food. Often, older adults have to rely on others to shop for them, and this may be a cause of concern depending on availability of support and the reluctance to be dependent on someone else, particularly family. For older adults who own a computer, shopping over the Internet and having groceries delivered offers advantages, although prices may be higher than in the stores. Fresh From the Kitchen is a service that prepares and delivers meals that do not contain additives or preservatives and can be used immediately or stored for future use (www.freshfromthekitchen.net).

Hospitalization and Long-Term Care Residence

Older adults in hospitals and long-term care settings are more likely to experience a number of the problems that contribute to inadequate nutrition. In the United States, 40% to 60% of hospitalized older adults are malnourished or at risk for malnutrition (DiMaria-Ghalili, 2008). In addition to the risk factors mentioned earlier in the chapter, severely restricted diets, long periods of nothing-by-mouth (NPO) status, and insufficient time and staff for feeding assistance contribute to inadequate nutrition. Malnutrition is related to prolonged hospital stay, increased risk for poor health status, institutionalization, and mortality (DiMaria-Ghalili, 2008). Assessment of nutritional status to identify malnutrition and the risk factors for malnutrition is important and required by the Joint Commission. Sufficient time, care, and attention should be given to feeding dependent older people.

The incidence of eating disability in long-term care is high with estimates that 50% of all residents cannot eat independently (Burger et al., 2000). Inadequate staffing in long-term care facilities is associated with poor nutrition and hydration, and as Kayser-Jones (1997, p. 19) states: "Certified nursing assistants (CNAs) have an impossible task trying to feed the number of people who need assistance." Having one staff person for every two or three residents who need feeding assistance would allow the resident 20 to 30 minutes with the CNA (Burger et al., 2000). In a study by Simmons and colleagues (2001), 50% of residents significantly increased their oral food and fluid intake during mealtime when they received one-on-one feeding assistance. The time required to implement the feeding assistance (38 minutes) greatly exceeded the time nursing staff spent assisting residents in usual mealtime conditions (9 minutes).

In response to concerns about the lack of adequate assistance during mealtime in long-term care facilities, the Centers for Medicare and Medicaid Services (CMS) implemented a rule that allows feeding assistants with eight hours of approved training to help residents with eating. Feeding assistants must be supervised by a registered nurse (RN) or licensed practical–vocational nurse (LPN-LVN). Family members may also be willing and able to assist at mealtimes and also provide a familiar social context for the patient. Nurses need to provide guidance and support on feeding techniques, supervise eating, and evaluate outcomes.

The use of restrictive therapeutic diets for frail elders in long-term care (low cholesterol, low salt, no concentrated sweets) often reduces food intake without significantly helping the clinical status of the resident (Morley, 2003). If caloric supplements are used, they should be administered at least one hour before meals or they interfere with meal intake. These products are widely used and can be costly. Often, they are not dispensed or consumed as ordered. Powdered breakfast drinks added to milk are an adequate substitute (Duffy, 2010).

Dispensing a small amount of calorically dense oral nutritional supplement (2 calories/ml) during the routine medication pass may have a greater effect on weight gain than a traditional supplement (1.06 calories/ml) with or between meals. Small volumes of nutrient-dense supplement may have less of an effect on appetite and will enhance food intake during meals and snacks. This delivery method allows nurses to observe and document consumption. Further studies and randomized clinical trials are needed to evaluate the effectiveness of nutritional supplementation (Doll-Shankaruk et al., 2008).

Attention to the environment in which meals are served is important. It is not uncommon to hear over the public address system at mealtimes: "Feeder trays are ready." This reference to the need to feed those unable to feed themselves is, in itself, degrading and erases any trace of dignity the older person is trying to maintain in a controlled environment. It is not malicious intent by nurses or other caregivers but rather a habit of convenience. Feeding older people who have difficulty eating can become mechanical and devoid of feeling. The feeding

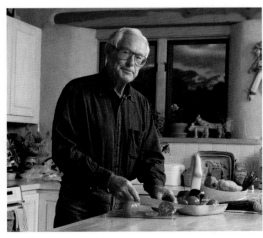

An older man preparing a meal. (Courtesy Corbis Images.)

BOX 14-2 SUGGESTIONS TO IMPROVE INTAKE IN INSTITUTIONAL SETTINGS

- Serve meals with the person in a chair rather than in bed when possible.
- Provide analgesics and antiemetics on a schedule that provides comfort at mealtime.
- Determine food preferences; provide for choices in food; include culturally appropriate food.
- Make food available 24 hours/day—provide snacks between meals and at night.
- Avoid prolonged periods of NPO status, and restore regular eating as soon as possible.
- Do not interrupt meals to administer medication if possible.
- Limit staff breaks to before and after mealtimes to ensure adequate staff are available to assist with meals.
- Walk around the dining area or the rooms at mealtime to determine if food is being eaten or if assistance is needed.
- Encourage family members to share the mealtimes for a heightened social situation.
- If caloric supplements are used, offer them between meals or with the medication pass.

- Recommend an exercise program that may increase appetite.
- Ensure proper fit of dentures and denture use.
- Provide oral hygiene, and allow the person to wash his or her hands before meals.
- Have the person wear his or her glasses during meals.
- Sit while feeding the person who needs assistance, use touch, and carry on a social conversation.
- Provide soft music during the meal.
- Use small, round tables seating six to eight people. Consider using tablecloths and centerpieces.
- Seat people with like interests and abilities together, and encourage socialization.
- Involve in restorative dining programs if in a nursing home.
- Make diets as liberal as possible depending on health status, especially for frail elders who are not consuming adequate amounts of food.
- Consider a referral to a speech-language pathologist for persons experiencing difficulties with eating and/or an occupational therapist for adaptive equipment.

process becomes rapid, and if it bogs down and becomes too slow, the meal may be ended abruptly, depending on the time the caregiver has allotted for feeding the person. Any pleasure derived through socialization and eating and any dignity that could be maintained is often absent (see "An Elder Speaks" at the beginning of this chapter). Older adults accustomed to certain table manners may feel ashamed at their inability to behave in what they feel is an appropriate manner.

In addition to adequate staff, many innovative and evidence-based ideas can improve nutritional intake in institutions. Many suggestions are found in the literature including the following: restorative dining programs; homelike dining rooms; individualized menu choices, including ethnic foods; cafeteria style service; refreshment stations with easy access to juices, water, and healthy snacks; kitchens on the nursing units; availability of food around the clock; choice of mealtimes; liberal diets; finger foods; visually appealing pureed foods with texture and shape; music; touch; verbal cueing; hand-over-hand feeding; and sitting while assisting the person to eat. Other suggestions can be found in Box 14-2.

Dementia

Older adults with dementia are particularly at risk for weight loss and inadequate nutrition. Weight loss often becomes a considerable concern in late-stage dementia. Significant weight loss affects 40% of individuals with dementia (Dunne et al., 2004). Some of the factors predisposing older people with dementia to nutritional inadequacy include lack of awareness of the need to eat, depression, loss of independence in self-feeding, agnosia, apraxia, vision impairments (deficient contrast sensitivity), and behavior disturbances. Modification of feeding techniques can assist in improving intake.

One of the best strategies for managing poor intake is establishing a routine so the older person does not have to remember time and places for eating. Caregivers should continue to serve foods and fluids that the person likes and has always eaten. Nutrient-dense foods are preferred. Attention to mealtime ambience is important, and the person should be able to take

BOX 14-3 SUGGESTIONS TO IMPROVE INTAKE FOR INDIVIDUALS WITH DEMENTIA

- Serve only one dish at a time.
- Provide only one utensil at a time.
- Consider using a "spork" (combination spoon-fork).
- Serve finger foods such as fried chicken, chicken strips, pizza in bite-size pieces, fish sticks, sandwiches.
- Serve soup in a mug.
- Remove any hot items or items that should not be eaten.
- Cut up foods before serving.
- Sit next to the person at their level.
- Demonstrate eating motions that the person can imitate.
- Use hand-over-hand feeding technique to guide self-feeding.
- Use verbal cueing and prompting (e.g., take a bite, chew, swallow).
- Use gentle tone of voice, and avoid scolding or demeaning remarks.
- Provide verbal encouragement to participate in eating by talking about food taste and smell.
- Offer small amounts of fluid between bites.
- Help person focus on the meal at hand; turn off background noise, remove clutter from the table.
- Avoid patterned dishes or table coverings.
- Use red plates/glasses/cups. Dunne et al., 2004 reported increased food intake when food was served using high contrast tableware.
- Use unbreakable dishes that won't slide around.
- Serve smaller more frequent meals rather than expecting the person to complete a big meal.

Data from Dunne T, Neargarder S, Cipolloni P, Cronin-Golomb A: Visual contrast enhances food and liquid intake in advanced Alzheimer's disease, *Clinical Nutrition* 23(4):533-538, 2004, Spencer P: How to solve eating problems common to people with Alzheimer's and other dementias. Retrieved August 30, 2010 from www.caring.com/articles/Alzheimer's-eating-problems.

as much time as needed to eat the food. Food should be available 24 hours a day, and the person should be allowed to follow his or her accustomed eating schedule (e.g., late breakfast, early dinner). Other suggestions to enhance food intake for individuals with dementia are presented in Box 14-3. Amella and Lawrence (2007) provide a protocol: *Eating and Feeding Issues in Older Adults with Dementia* (Box 14-4). Chapter 19 provides more discussion of dementia.

PROMOTING HEALTHY AGING: IMPLICATIONS FOR GERONTOLOGICAL NURSING

Nutritional Screening and Assessment

Older people are less likely than younger people to show signs of malnutrition and nutrient malabsorption. Evaluation of nutritional health can be difficult in the absence of severe malnutrition, but a comprehensive assessment can reveal deficits. A nutritional assessment that provides the most conclusive data about a person's actual nutritional state consists of the following steps: interview, physical examination, anthropometrical measurements, and biochemical analysis. The collective results provide the data needed to identify the immediate and the potential nutritional problems of the client so that plans for supervision, assistance, and education in the attainment of adequate nutrition for the older person can be implemented. Multidisciplinary approaches are key to appropriate assessment and intervention and should involve medicine; nursing; dietary, physical, occupational, and speech therapy; and social work.

A Nutrition Screening Initiative checklist (Figure 14-3) can be used by older people or staff in any setting to identify risk factors for poor nutrition and determine the need for a more comprehensive assessment and nutritional interventions. The Mini Nutritional Assessment (MNA), developed by Nestle of Geneva, Switzerland, is intended for use by professionals to screen for malnutrition (www.consultgerirn.org) (Figure 14-4). A video demonstration of the MNA can be found at http://www.nursingcenter.com/prodev/ce_article.asp?tid=771233.

In intensive care units, the APACHE II score (Acute Physiology and Chronic Health Evaluation II), is used to measure the severity of disease for adult patients. The APACHE II score can help identify those patients with severe degrees of critical illness who are at high risk for rapid deterioration in nutritional status, low likelihood for early advancement to oral diet, and in greatest need for aggressive enteral nutritional support (Box 14-4).

The Minimum Data Set (MDS), used in long-term care facilities, includes assessment information that can be used to identify potential nutritional problems, risk factors, and the potential for improved function. Triggers for more thorough investigation of problems include weight loss, alterations in taste, medical therapies, prescription medications, hunger, parenteral or intravenous feedings, mechanically altered or therapeutic diets, percentage of food left uneaten, pressure ulcers, and edema. Other protocols and guidelines for nutritional assessment of older adults can be found in Box 14-4.

BOX 14-4	PROTOCOLS AND GUIDELINES: NUTRITION, ORAL CARE, HYDRATION

Unintentional weight loss in the elderly *(www.guideline.gov)*

Mealtime difficulties for older persons: assessment and management *(www.guideline.gov)*

Preventing aspiration in older adults with dysphagia *(www.consultgerirn.org)*

Assessing nutrition in older adults *(www.consultgerirn.org)*

Eating and feeding issues in older adults with dementia. Part I: Assessment *(www.consultgerirn.org)*

Eating and feeding issues in older adults with dementia. Part II: Interventions *(www.consultgerirn.org)*

Nutrition in the elderly: Nursing Standard of Practice Protocol: Nutrition in Aging *(www.consultgerirn.org)*

Nursing Standard of Practice Protocol: Providing Oral Health Care to Older Adults *(www.consultgerirn.org)*

Nursing Standard of Practice Protocol: Oral Hydration Management *(www.consultgerirn.org)*

APACHE II *(https://apachefoundations.cernerworks.com/apachefoundations/resources/APACHE%20IV%20White%20Paper%20Version%201.0.pdf)*

Read the statements below. Circle the number in the Yes column for those that apply to you or someone you know. For each "yes" answer, score the number listed. Total your nutritional score.

	YES
I have an illness or condition that made me change the kind or amount of food I eat.	2
I eat fewer than two meals per day.	3
I eat few fruits, vegetables or milk products.	2
I have three or more drinks of beer, liquor, or wine almost every day.	2
I have tooth or mouth problems that make it hard for me to eat.	2
I don't always have enough money to buy the food I need.	4
I eat alone most of the time.	1
I take three or more different prescriptions or over-the-counter drugs each day.	1
Without wanting to, I have lost or gained 10 pounds in the past 6 months.	2
I am not always physically able to shop, cook, and/or feed myself.	2

Total Nutritional Score _____

0-2 indicates good nutrition
3-5 moderate risk
6+ high nutritional risk

FIGURE 14-3 Nutritional assessment and approaches. (Courtesy The Nutrition Screening Initiative, Washington, DC.)

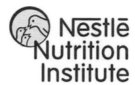

Mini Nutritional Assessment
MNA®

Last name:			First name:		
Sex:	Age:	Weight, kg:	Height, cm:	Date:	

Complete the screen by filling in the boxes with the appropriate numbers. Total the numbers for the final screening score.

Screening

A Has food intake declined over the past 3 months due to loss of appetite, digestive problems, chewing or swallowing difficulties?
0 = severe decrease in food intake
1 = moderate decrease in food intake
2 = no decrease in food intake ☐

B Weight loss during the last 3 months
0 = weight loss greater than 3 kg (6.6 lbs)
1 = does not know
2 = weight loss between 1 and 3 kg (2.2 and 6.6 lbs)
3 = no weight loss ☐

C Mobility
0 = bed or chair bound
1 = able to get out of bed / chair but does not go out
2 = goes out ☐

D Has suffered psychological stress or acute disease in the past 3 months?
0 = yes   2 = no ☐

E Neuropsychological problems
0 = severe dementia or depression
1 = mild dementia
2 = no psychological problems ☐

F1 Body Mass Index (BMI) (weight in kg) / (height in m^2)
0 = BMI less than 19
1 = BMI 19 to less than 21
2 = BMI 21 to less than 23
3 = BMI 23 or greater ☐

IF BMI IS NOT AVAILABLE, REPLACE QUESTION F1 WITH QUESTION F2.
DO NOT ANSWER QUESTION F2 IF QUESTION F1 IS ALREADY COMPLETED.

F2 Calf circumference (CC) in cm
0 = CC less than 31
3 = CC 31 or greater ☐

Screening score ☐☐
(max. 14 points)

12-14 points: Normal nutritional status
8-11 points: At risk of malnutrition
0-7 points: Malnourished

Ref.   Vellas B, Villars H, Abellan G, et al. Overview of the MNA® - Its History and Challenges. *J Nutr Health Aging* 2006;10:456-465.

Rubenstein LZ, Harker JO, Salva A, Guigoz Y, Vellas B. Screening for Undernutrition in Geriatric Practice: Developing the Short-Form Mini Nutritional Assessment (MNA-SF). *J. Geront* 2001;56A: M366-377.

Guigoz Y. The Mini-Nutritional Assessment (MNA®) Review of the Literature - What does it tell us? *J Nutr Health Aging* 2006; 10:466-487.

For more information: www.mna-elderly.com

FIGURE 14-4 Mini Nutritional Assessment. (Copyright Nestle, 1994, Revision 2009, Glendale, California.)

Interview The interview provides background information and clues to the nutritional state and actual and potential problems of the older adult. Questions about the individual's state of health, social activities, normal patterns, and changes that have occurred should be asked. The nurse must explore the individual's needs, the manner in which food is obtained, and the client's ability to prepare food.

Information concerning the relationship of food to daily events will provide clues to the meaning and significance of food to that person. The older person who eats alone is considered a candidate for malnutrition. Information about occupation and daily activities will suggest the degree of energy expenditure and caloric intake most appropriate for the overall activity. One's economic status will have a direct bearing on nutrition. It is therefore important to explore the client's financial resources to establish the income available for food.

Medications being taken should be included in the nutrition history. Additional medical information should include the presence or absence of mouth pain or discomfort, visual difficulty, bowel and bladder function, and history of illness. As noted earlier, depression is a major cause of weight loss, so an evaluation for depression should be obtained (Chapter 18).

Diet Histories Frequently a 24-hour diet recall compared with the Modified MyPyramid can provide an estimate of nutritional adequacy. When the older person cannot supply all of the information requested, it may be possible to obtain data from a family member or another source. There will be times, however, when information will not be as complete as one would like, or the older person, too proud to admit that he or she is not eating, will furnish erroneous information. Even so, the nurse will be able to obtain additional data from the other three areas of the nutritional assessment.

Keeping a dietary record for three days is another assessment tool. What one ate, when food was eaten, and the amounts eaten must be carefully recorded. Computer analysis of the dietary records provides information on energy and vitamin and mineral intake. Printouts can provide the older person and the health care provider with a visual graph of the intake. Accurate completion of 3-day dietary records in hospitals and nursing homes can be problematic, and intake may be either underestimated or overestimated. Standardized observational protocols should be developed to ensure accuracy of oral intake documentation as well as the adequacy and quality of feeding assistance during mealtimes. Nurses should ensure that direct caregivers are educated on the proper observation and documentation of intake and should closely monitor performance in this area.

Physical Examination The physical examination furnishes clinically observable evidence of the existing state of nutrition. Data such as height and weight; vital signs; condition of the tongue, lips, and gums; skin turgor, texture, and color; and functional ability are assessed, and the overall general appearance is scrutinized for evidence of wasting. Height should always be measured and never estimated or given by self-report. If the person cannot stand, an alternative way of measuring standing height is knee-height using knee-height calipers. BMI should be

calculated to determine if weight for height is within the normal range of 22 to 27. A BMI below 22 is a sign of undernutrition (DiMaria-Ghalili, 2008).

A detailed weight history should be obtained along with current weight. Weight loss is a key indicator of malnutrition, even in overweight older adults. History should include a history of weight loss, whether the weight loss was intentional or unintentional, and during what period it occurred. A history of anorexia is also important, and many older people, especially women, have limited their weight throughout life. Debate continues in the quest to determine the appropriate weight charts for an older adult. Although weight alone does not indicate the adequacy of diet, unplanned fluctuations in weight are significant and should be evaluated.

Accurate weight patterns are sometimes difficult to obtain. Procedures for weighing people should be established and followed consistently to obtain an accurate picture of weight changes. Weighing procedure should be supervised by licensed personnel, and changes should be reported immediately to the provider. One might meet correct weight values for height, but weight changes may be the result of fluid retention, edema, or ascites and merit investigation. An unintentional weight loss of more than 5% of body weight in one month, more than 7.5% in three months, or more than 10% in six months is considered a significant indicator of poor nutrition, as well as an MDS trigger.

Anthropometrical Measurements Anthropometrical measurements include height, weight, midarm circumference, and triceps skinfold thickness. These are obtained by simple body measurement procedures, which take less than five minutes to perform. These measurements offer information about the status of the older person's muscle mass and body fat in relation to height and weight. Muscle mass measurements are obtained by measuring the arm circumference of the nondominant upper arm. The arm hangs freely at the side, and a measuring tape is placed around the midpoint of the upper arm, between the acromion of the scapula and the olecranon of the ulna. The centimeter circumference is recorded and compared with standard values.

Body fat and lean muscle mass are assessed by measuring specific skinfolds with Lange or Harpenden calipers. Two areas are accessible for measurement. One area is the midpoint of the upper arm, the triceps area, which is also used to obtain arm circumference. The nondominant arm is again used. The nurse lifts the skin with the thumb and forefinger so that it parallels the humerus. The calipers are placed around the skinfold, 1 cm below where the fingers are grasping the skin. Two readings are averaged to the nearest half centimeter. If there is a neuropathological condition or hemiplegia following a stroke, the unaffected arm should be used for obtaining measurements.

Biochemical Examination The final step in a nutritional assessment is the biochemical examination (Chapter 8). A complete blood count, total lymphocyte count, thyroid level, comprehensive metabolic panel, and liver function tests help assess the presence of diseases known to affect weight loss or cause loss of appetite. Urinalysis to rule out infection, as well as a stool sample for fecal occult blood, should be included. Suggested biochemical parameters include serum albumin, cholesterol, hemoglobin, and serum transferrin. Although these parameters may also be abnormal in several conditions unassociated with malnutrition, they are useful as guides to interventions (Thomas, 2000). Serum proteins also decrease in an inflammatory reaction, infection, or liver disorder. In acute illness, hypoalbuminemia may occur but not be indicative of malnutrition, however, low serum protein levels need further investigation (Duffy, 2010). Serum albumin of more than 4 g/dl is desired; less than 3.5 g/dl is an indicator of poor nutritional state. Prealbumin level may be a better indicator of protein loss because it changes rapidly in the presence of malnutrition.

Transferrin, an iron transport protein, is diminished in protein malnutrition. However, it increases in iron deficiency anemia, which is common in older adults, so it is not a sensitive indicator of PEM. Laboratory test results, although not definitive for malnutrition, provide important clues to nutritional status but should be evaluated in relation to the person's overall health status. There is no single biochemical marker of malnutrition as a screening test, and unintentional weight loss remains the most important indicator of a potential nutritional deficit (Ahmed and Haboubi, 2010).

Interventions

Interventions are formulated around the identified nutritional problem or problems. Nursing interventions are centered on techniques to increase food intake and enhance and manage the environment to promote increased food intake (DiMaria-Ghalili, 2008). Collaboration with the interdisciplinary team (e.g., dietitian, pharmacist, social worker, occupational or speech therapist) is important in planning interventions. For the community-dwelling elder, nutrition education and problem solving with the elder and family members on how to best resolve the potential or actual nutritional deficit is important. Causes of poor nutrition are complex, and all of the factors emphasized in this chapter are important to assess when planning individualized interventions to ensure adequate nutrition for older people.

Pharmacological Therapy   Drugs that stimulate appetite (orexigenic drugs) can be considered to reverse resistant anorexia but only after all other interventions have been tried. They must be monitored closely for side effects and have had little evaluation in frail older people. Benefits are restricted to small weight gains without indication of decreased morbidity or mortality or improved quality of life or functional ability (Vitale et al., 2009).

Megestrol (Megace) can improve appetite, although studies of its effectiveness have produced contradictory results. The onset of action is several weeks, and it should be discontinued if no response occurs after eight weeks of therapy. Patients should be monitored closely for adrenocortical insufficiency. Megestrol should not be used with bedridden patients because of the risk for deep venous thrombosis. Dronabinol (Marinol), although not adequately tested in older people, may be an appropriate drug for end-of-life and palliative care and dementia-induced anorexia. It stimulates appetite, has

antinausea properties, decreases pain, and enhances general well-being. Weight gain from the use of these two drugs is primarily adipose tissue as opposed to lean body mass (Duffy, 2010; Vitale et al., 2009; University of Texas, 2006). Oxandrolone (Osandrin), an exogenous anabolic hormone, is used to increase net protein synthesis but there is little research on use of this medication in older people. If the older person is depressed and with poor appetite and weight loss, mirtazapine (Remeron), an antidepressant, has been shown to increase appetite and weight gain as well as improve depressed mood (University of Texas, 2006).

Patient Education   Education should be provided to older adults on nutritional requirements for health, special diet modifications for chronic illness management, the effect of age-associated changes and medication on nutrition, and community resources to assist in maintaining adequate nutrition. Medicare covers nutrition therapy for select diseases, such as diabetes and kidney disease, which creates unprecedented opportunities for older Americans to access information.

SPECIAL CONSIDERATIONS IN NUTRITION FOR OLDER PEOPLE: HYDRATION, DYSPHAGIA, ORAL CARE

Several conditions warrant further discussion because they are frequently encountered in care of older adults and are related to adequate diet and nutritional status. These include dehydration, dysphagia, oral health, and bowel function.

Hydration Management

Hydration management is the promotion of an adequate fluid balance, which prevents complications resulting from abnormal or undesirable fluid levels. Water, an accessible and available commodity to almost all people, is often overlooked as an essential part of nutritional requirements. Water's function in the body includes thermoregulation, dilution of water-soluble medications, facilitation of renal and bowel function, and creation of requisite conditions for and maintenance of metabolic processes.

Daily needs for water can usually be met by functionally independent older adults through intake of fluids with meals and social drinks. However, a significant number of older adults (up to 85% of those 85 years of age and over) drink less than 1 liter of fluid per day. Older adults, with the exception of those requiring fluid restrictions, should consume at least 1500 ml of fluid per day (Mentes, 2006).

Maintenance of fluid balance (fluid intake equals fluid output) is essential to health, regardless of a person's age (Mentes, 2006). Age-related changes, medication use, functional impairments, and comorbid medical and emotional illnesses place some older adults at risk for changes in fluid balance, especially dehydration (Mentes, 2008). See Box 14-4 for a hydration management guideline.

Dehydration

Dehydration is defined clinically as "a complex condition resulting in a reduction in total body water. In older people, dehydration most often develops as a result of disease, age-related changes, and/or the effects of medication and NOT primarily due to lack of access to water" (Thomas et al., 2008, p. 293). Dehydration is considered a geriatric syndrome that is frequently associated with common diseases (e.g., diabetes, respiratory illness, heart failure) and declining stages of the frail elderly (Crecelius, 2008). It is often an unappreciated comorbid condition that exacerbates an underlying condition such as a urinary tract infection, respiratory infection, or worsening depression (Thomas et al., 2008).

Dehydration is a problem prevalent among older adults in all settings. If not treated adequately, mortality from dehydration can be as high as 50% (Faes et al., 2007). Dehydration is a significant risk factor for delirium, thromboembolic complications, infections, kidney stones, constipation and obstipation, falls, medication toxicity, renal failure, seizure, electrolyte imbalance, hyperthermia, and delayed wound healing (Mentes, 2006; Faes et al., 2007).

Thomas and colleagues (2008) comment that there are few diagnoses that generate as much concern about causes and consequences as does dehydration. Due to a lack of understanding of the pathogenesis and consequences of dehydration in older adults, the condition is often attributed to poor care by nursing home staff and/or physicians. However, the majority of older people develop dehydration as a result of increased fluid losses combined with decreased fluid intake, related to decreased thirst. The condition is rarely due to neglect (Thomas et al., 2008).

Risk Factors for Dehydration

Most healthy older adults maintain adequate hydration, but the presence of physical or emotional illness, surgery, trauma, or conditions of higher physiological demands increase the risk of dehydration. When the fluid balance of older adults is at risk, the limited capacity of homeostatic mechanisms becomes significant (Faes et al., 2007).

Age-related changes in the thirst mechanism, decrease in total body water (TBW), and decreased kidney function increase the risk for dehydration. TBW decreases with age. In young adults, TBW is about 60% of body weight in men and 52% in women. In older people, TBW decreases to about 52% of body weight in men and 46% in women. The loss of muscle mass with age increases the proportion of fat cells. This loss is greater in women because they have a higher percentage of body fat and less muscle mass than men. Because fat cells contain less water than muscle cells, older people have a decreased intracellular fluid volume (Mentes, 2006).

Thirst sensation diminishes, resulting in the loss of an important defense against dehydration. In a mechanism that is not well understood, thirst in older adults is not "proportional to metabolic needs in response to dehydrating conditions" (Mentes, 2008, p. 371). Creatinine clearance also declines with age, and the kidneys are less able to concentrate urine. These changes are more pronounced in older people with illnesses affecting kidney function.

Other risk factors for dehydration include medications, particularly those that directly affect renal function and fluid balance (diuretics, laxatives, angiotensin-converting enzyme [ACE] inhibitors) and psychotropic medications that have anticholinergic effects (dry mouth, urinary retention, constipation). The use of four or more medications is also a risk factor (Mentes, 2006; Faes et al., 2007).

Functional deficits, communication and comprehension problems, oral problems, dysphagia, delirium, depression, dementia, hospitalization, low body weight, diagnostic procedures necessitating fasting, inadequate assistance with fluid intake, diarrhea, fever, vomiting, infections, bleeding, draining wounds, artificial ventilation, fluid restrictions, high environmental temperature, and multiple comorbidities have all been noted as risk factors for dehydration in older people (Mentes, 2006; Faes et al., 2007). NPO requirements for diagnostic tests and surgical procedures should be as short as possible for older adults, and adequate fluids should be given once tests and procedures are completed. A 2-hour suspension of fluid intake is recommended for many procedures (www.asahq.org/publicationsAndServices/NPO.pdf).

PROMOTING HEALTHY AGING: IMPLICATIONS FOR GERONTOLOGICAL NURSING

Assessment

Prevention of dehydration is essential, but assessment is complex in older people. Clinical signs may not appear until dehydration is advanced. Attention to risk factors for dehydration in older adults using a screen (Box 14-5) is very important. In addition, the MDS has triggers for dehydration/fluid maintenance. Education should be provided to older people and their caregivers on the need for fluids and the signs and symptoms of dehydration. Acute situations such as vomiting, diarrhea, or febrile episodes should be identified quickly and treated. Older adults over age 85 years who have experienced volume deficits, weight loss, malnutrition, or infections, and those with dementia, delirium, and functional impairments are at high risk for dehydration.

Typical signs of dehydration may not always be present in older people, and most clinical signs and symptoms are not very sensitive or specific. "The large variability in the way different organs are affected by dehydration will cause symptoms to remain atypical in older adults" (Faes et al., 2007, p. 3). Skin turgor, assessed at the sternum and commonly included in the assessment of dehydration, is an unreliable marker in older adults because of the loss of subcutaneous tissue with aging. Dry mucous membranes in the mouth and nose, longitudinal furrows on the tongue, orthostasis, speech incoherence, extremity weakness, dry axilla, and sunken eye may indicate dehydration. However, the diagnosis of dehydration is biochemical (Thomas et al., 2008).

If dehydration is suspected, laboratory tests include blood urea nitrogen (BUN), sodium, creatinine, glucose, and bicarbonate. Osmolarity should be either directly measured or calculated. While most cases of dehydration have an elevated BUN, there are many other causes of an elevated BUN/creatinine ratio, so this test cannot be used alone to diagnose dehydration in older adults (Thomas et al., 2008). Mentes (2006) notes that "as is true with other standard tests, serum markers confirm a diagnosis of dehydration once it is too late to prevent it from

BOX 14-5	SIMPLE SCREEN FOR DEHYDRATION

Drugs, e.g., diuretics
End of life
High fever
Yellow urine turns dark
Dizziness (orthostasis)
Reduced oral intake
Axilla dry
Tachycardia
Incontinence (fear of)
Oral problems/sippers
Neurological impairment (confusion)
Sunken eyes

From Thomas D, Cote T, Lawhorne L, et al: Journal of the American Medical Directors Association 9:292-301, 2008.

BOX 14-6	ONGOING MANAGEMENT OF ORAL INTAKE

1. Calculate a daily fluid goal.
   - All older adults should have an individualized fluid goal determined by a documented standard for daily fluid intake. At least 1500 ml of fluid/day should be provided.
2. Compare current intake to fluid goal to evaluate hydration status.
3. Provide fluids consistently throughout the day.
   - Provide 75% to 80% of fluids at mealtimes and the remainder during non-mealtimes such as medication times.
   - Offer a variety of fluids and fluids that the person prefers.
   - Standardize the amount of fluid that is offered with medication administration—for example, at least 6 oz.
4. Plan for at-risk individuals.
   - Fluid rounds midmorning and midafternoon.
   - Provide two 8-oz glasses of fluid in the morning and evening.
   - "Happy hour" or "tea time," when residents can gather for additional fluids and socialization.
   - Provide modified fluid containers based on resident's abilities—for example, lighter cups and glasses, weighted cups and glasses, plastic water bottles with straws (attach to wheelchairs, deliver with meals).
   - Make fluids accessible at all times and be sure residents can access them—for example, filled water pitchers, fluid stations, or beverage carts in congregate areas.
   - Allow adequate time and staff for eating or feeding. Meals can provide two thirds of daily fluids.
   - Encourage family members to participate in feeding and offering fluids.
5. Perform fluid regulation and documentation.
   - Teach individuals, if they are able, to use a urine color chart to monitor hydration status.
   - Document complete intake including hydration habits.
   - Know volumes of fluid containers to accurately calculate fluid consumption.
   - Frequency of documentation of fluid intake will vary among settings and is dependent on the individual's condition. In most settings, at least one accurate intake and output recording should be documented, including amount of fluid consumed, difficulties with consumption, and urine specific gravity and color. For individuals who are not continent, teach caregivers to observe incontinent pads or briefs for amount and frequency of urine, color changes, and odor, and report variations from individual's normal pattern.

Adapted from: Mentes JC: Managing oral hydration. In Capezuti E, Zwicker D, Mezey M, et al., editors: Evidence-based geriatric nursing protocols for best practice, ed 3, New York, 2008, Springer; www.consultgerirn.org.

occurring" (p. 5). Attention to risk factors is important to identify possible dehydration and to intervene early. Body weight changes should also be assessed as indicators of changes in hydration (Faes et al., 2007).

Urine color, which is measured using a urine color chart, has been suggested as helpful in assessing hydration status (not dehydration) in older individuals in nursing homes with adequate renal function (Mentes, 2008). The urine color chart has eight standardized colors, ranging from pale straw (number 1) to greenish brown (number 8) approximating urine specific gravities of 1.003 to 1.029 (Mentes, 2006, 2008). Urine color should be assessed and charted over several days. Pale straw–colored urine usually indicates normal hydration status, and as urine darkens, poor hydration may be indicated (after taking into account discoloration by food or medications). For older adults, a reading of 4 or less is preferred (Mentes, 2006). If a person's urine becomes darker than his or her usual color, fluid intake assessment is indicated, and fluids can be increased before dehydration occurs (Mentes, 2008).

Interventions

Interventions are derived from a comprehensive assessment and consist of risk identification and hydration management (Mentes, 2008) (Box 14-6). Hydration management involves both acute and ongoing management of oral intake. Oral hydration is the first treatment approach for dehydration. Individuals with mild to moderate dehydration who can drink and do not have significant mental or physical compromise due to fluid loss may be able to replenish fluids orally (Thomas et al., 2008). Water is considered the best fluid to offer, but other clear fluids may also be useful depending on the person's preference. One study found a significant reduction in lab values indicative of dehydration among nursing home residents who received verbal prompting and were given the type of beverage they requested (Simmons et al., 2001).

Rehydration methods depend on the severity and the type of dehydration and may include intravenous or hypodermoclysis (HDC). A general rule is to replace 50% of the loss within the first 12 hours (or 1 L/day in afebrile elders) or sufficient quantity to relieve tachycardia and hypotension. Further fluid replacement can be administered more slowly over a longer period of time.

HDC is an infusion of isotonic fluids into the subcutaneous space. HDC is safe, easy to administer, and a useful alternative to intravenous administration for persons with mild to moderate dehydration, particularly those patients with altered mental status. HDC cannot be used in severe dehydration or for any situation requiring more than 3 L over 24 hours. Common sites of infusion are the lateral abdominal wall; the anterior or lateral aspects of the thighs; the infraclavicular region; and the back, usually the interscapular or subscapular regions with a fat fold of at least 1 inch thick (Mei and Auerhahn, 2009). Normal saline (0.9%), half-normal saline (0.45%), 5% glucose in water infusion (D_5W), or Ringer's solution can be used (Thomas et al., 2008). Hypodermoclysis can be administered in almost any

- Cerebrovascular accident
- Parkinson's disease
- Neuromuscular disorders (ALS, MS, myasthenia gravis)
- Dementia
- Head and neck cancer
- Traumatic brain injury
- Aspiration pneumonia
- Inadequate feeding technique
- Poor dentition

| BOX 14-8 | SYMPTOMS OF DYSPHAGIA OR POSSIBLE ASPIRATION |

- Difficult, labored swallowing
- Drooling
- Copious oral secretions
- Coughing, choking at meals
- Holding or pocketing of food/medications in the mouth
- Difficulty moving food or liquid from mouth to throat
- Difficulty chewing
- Nasal voice or hoarseness
- Wet or gurgling voice
- Excessive throat clearing
- Food or liquid leaking from the nose
- Prolonged eating time
- Pain with swallowing
- Unusual head or neck posturing while swallowing
- Sensation of something stuck in the throat during swallowing; sensation of a lump in the throat
- Heartburn
- Chest pain
- Hiccups
- Weight loss
- Frequent respiratory infections, pneumonia

setting, so hospital admissions may be avoided. Hypodermoclysis is "an evidence-based low-cost therapy in geriatrics" (Faes et al., 2007).

Ongoing management of oral intake includes the following five components: (1) calculate a daily fluid goal; (2) compare the individual's current intake to the amount calculated from applying the standard, to evaluate the individual's hydration status; (3) provide fluids consistently throughout the day; (4) plan for at-risk individuals; and (5) perform fluid regulation and documentation (Mentes, 2008).

Dysphagia

Dysphagia, or difficulty swallowing, is a common problem in older adults. The prevalence of swallowing disorders is 16% to 22% in adults over age 50 years, and up to 60% of nursing home residents have clinical evidence of dysphagia (Tanner, 2010). Dysphagia can be the result of behavioral, sensory, or motor problems and is common in individuals with neurologic disease and dementia, as well as in people at the end of life. Changes in esophageal sphincter function and peristalsis with age can result in dysphagia, but changes associated with stroke, neuromuscular disorders such as Parkinson's disease, and central nervous system disorders are more frequent causes of dysphagia. Other factors such as poor dentition, inadequate feeding techniques, and reduced salivation may also predispose the older adult to dysphagia. Box 14-7 presents risk factors for dysphagia.

Dysphagia is a serious problem and has negative consequences, including weight loss, malnutrition, dehydration, aspiration pneumonia, and even death. Aspiration pneumonia is the leading cause of death and the second most common cause for hospitalization among nursing home residents (Sarin et al., 2008). Dysphagia can be categorized as transfer or oropharyngeal dysphagia (difficulty moving the food from the mouth to the esophagus), transport dysphagia (difficulty passing the ingested food down the esophagus), or delivery dysphagia (the propulsion of a bolus of food to the stomach is difficult).

PROMOTION OF HEALTHY AGING: IMPLICATIONS FOR GERONTOLOGICAL NURSING

Assessment

It is important to obtain a careful history of the older adult's response to dysphagia and to observe the person during mealtime. Symptoms that alert the nurse to possible swallowing problems are presented in Box 14-8. Silent aspiration (lack of protective cough reflex at the vocal folds) is common. A recent study found that 55% of the patients who aspirated on video flouroscopic examination had no protective cough reflex (Garon et al., 2009). Among the highest risk groups were those with brain cancer, brainstem stroke, head-neck cancer, pneumonia, dementia, chronic obstructive lung disease, seizures, myocardial infarcts, neurodegenerative pathologies, right and left hemisphere stroke, and closed head injury. These "red flag" patients require close observation by nursing staff for clinical symptoms associated with silent aspiration and early referral for dysphagia evaluation.

Patients referred for a dysphagia evaluation ("swallowing study") must be assumed to be dysphagic and at risk for aspiration. NPO status should be maintained until the swallowing evaluation is completed. During this period, if necessary, nutrition and hydration needs can be met by intravenous, nasogastric, or gastric tubes (Tanner, 2010). A comprehensive evaluation by a speech-language pathologist, usually including a video fluoroscopic recording of a modified barium swallow, should be considered when dysphagia is suspected.

Interventions

After the swallowing evaluation, a decision must be made about the person's potential for functional improvement of the swallowing disorder and their safety in swallowing liquid and solid food. The goal is safe oral intake to maintain optimal nutrition and caloric needs. Compensatory interventions include postural changes, such as chin tucks or head turns while swallowing, and modification of bolus volume, consistency, temperature, and rate of presentation (Easterling and Robbins, 2008). Neuromuscular electric stimulation has received clearance by the U.S. Food and Drug Administration for treatment of dysphagia. This therapy

BOX 14-9   INTERVENTIONS TO PREVENT ASPIRATION IN PATIENTS WITH DYSPHAGIA: HAND FEEDING

- Provide a 30-minute rest period before meal consumption; a rested person will likely have less difficulty swallowing.
- The person should sit at 90 degrees during all oral (PO) intake.
- Maintain 90-degree positioning for at least 1 hour after PO intake.
- Adjust rate of feeding and size of bites to the person's tolerance; avoid rushed or forced feeding.
- Alternate solid and liquid boluses.
- Follow speech therapist's recommendation for safe swallowing techniques and modified food consistency (may need thickened liquids, pureed foods).
- If facial weakness is present, place food on the nonimpaired side of the mouth.
- Avoid sedatives and hypnotics that may impair cough reflex and swallowing ability.
- Keep suction equipment ready at all times.
- Supervise all meals.
- Monitor temperature.
- Observe color of phlegm.
- Visually check the mouth for pocketing of food in cheeks.
- Provide mouth care every four hours.

Adapted from: Metheny N, Boltz M, Greenberg S: *American Journal of Nursing* 108:45-46, 2008.

BOX 14-10   MYTHS AND FACTS ABOUT PEG TUBES

MYTHS

- PEGs prevent death from inadequate intake.
- PEGs reduce aspiration pneumonia.
- Not feeding people is a form of euthanasia, and we can't let people starve to death.
- PEGs improve albumin levels and nutritional status.
- PEGs assist in healing pressure ulcers.
- PEGs provide enhanced comfort for people at the end-of-life.

FACTS

- PEGs do not improve quality of life.
- PEGs do not reduce risk of aspiration and increase the rate of pneumonia development and death rate.
- PEGs do not prolong survival in dementia.
- Nearly 50% of patients die within 6 months following PEG tube insertion.
- PEGs cause increased discomfort from both the tube presence and use of restraints.
- PEGs are associated with infections, gastrointestinal symptoms, and abscesses.
- PEG tube feeding deprives people of the taste of food and contact with caregivers during feeding.
- PEGs are popular because they are convenient and labor beneficial.

Data from Aparanji K, Dharmarajan T: Pause before a Peg: A feeding tube may not be necessary in every candidate, *JAMDA* 11:453-456, 2010; Vitale C, Monteleoni C, Burke L, Frazier-Rios D, Volicer L: Strategies for improving care for patients with advanced dementia and eating problems: optimizing care through physician and speech pathologist collaboration, *Annals of Long-Term Care* 32-39, 2009.

involves the administration of small electrical impulses to the swallowing muscles in the throat and is used in combination with traditional swallowing exercises.

Aspiration is the most profound and dangerous problem for older adults experiencing dysphagia. It is important to have a suction machine available at the bedside or in the dining room in the institutional setting. Suggested interventions helpful in preventing aspiration during hand feeding are presented in Box 14-9. The gerontological nurse must work closely with other members of the interdisciplinary team, such as dietitians and speech-language pathologists, in implementing suggested interventions to prevent aspiration. Research on the appropriate management of swallowing disorders in older people, particularly during acute illness and in long-term care facilities, is very limited, and additional study is essential. A comprehensive protocol for preventing aspiration in older adults with dysphagia and other resources, including a video presentation of assessment of dysphagia, can be found in Box 14-4.

Feeding Tubes   Comprehensive assessment of swallowing problems and other factors that influence intake must be conducted before initiating severely restricted diet modifications or considering the use of feeding tubes, particularly in older people with dementia or those at the end of life. Feeding tube placement "does not reduce the risk of aspiration, and is not indicated to lower the likelihood of recurrent aspiration, irrespective of the presence or absence of dysphagia" (Aparanji and Dharmarajan, 2010, p. 455). Patients who aspirate oral feedings are just as likely to aspirate tube feedings, either via nasogastric tubes or gastrostomy tubes (Metheny et al., 2008).

However, the use of percutaneous endoscopic gastrostomy (PEG) feeding tubes has increased at an astonishing rate in older adults over recent years. It is estimated that 8.1% of all nursing home residents were receiving tube feedings in 2006. State-to-state rates varied widely, with Nebraska having the lowest rate of 3.8% and the District of Columbia having the highest rate of 44.8% (Gavi et al., 2008). Higher rates of feeding tube insertion for nursing home residents with advanced cognitive impairment are associated with for-profit ownership versus hospitals owned by state or local governments, hospitals with a higher number of beds, and those with more intensive care unit use for chronically ill patients in the last six months of life (Teno et al., 2010).

No scientific study demonstrates improved survival, reduced incidence of pneumonia or other infections, improved function, or fewer pressure ulcers with the use of feeding tubes (Teno et al., 2010). Few complications occur with insertion of a PEG tube. However, numerous complications occur from having a PEG tube, including aspiration pneumonia, diarrhea, metabolic problems, and cellulitis. "Nearly 50% of patients die within 6 months following PEG insertion; the procedure is often overused and its value has been questioned" (Aparanji and Dharmarajan, 2010, p. 453). Box 14-10 presents myths and facts about PEG tube placement.

As discussed earlier in the chapter, food and eating are closely tied to socialization, comfort, pleasure, love, and the meeting of basic biological needs. Decisions about feeding tube placement are challenging and require thoughtful discussion with patients and caregivers, who should be free to make decisions without duress and with careful consideration of the patient's advance directives, if available. Aparanji and

Dharmarajan (2010) suggest that decisions to place a feeding tube are often taken without completely exhausting means to maintain a normal oral intake and that physician discussions before insertion are often inadequate with room for improvement. Discussion about advance directives and feeding support should begin early in the course of the illness rather than waiting until a crisis develops. The best advice for individuals is to state preferences for the use of a feeding tube in a written advance directive. Surrogate decision makers should use advance directives and previously expressed wishes to decide what the patient with advanced dementia who is not eating would want under the present circumstances.

Individuals have the right to use or not use a feeding tube but should be given information about the risks and benefits of enteral feeding, particularly in late-stage dementia. In difficult situations, an ethics committee may be consulted to help make decisions. Nursing homes should have policies to ensure that patients with remediable causes of weight loss are appropriately evaluated and treated and that enteral feeding is not regarded as the only treatment. It is important that everyone involved in the care of the patient be informed of the risks and benefits of tube feeding and the uncertainty of whether enteral feeding provides any benefit for the patient. The decision should never be understood as a question of tube feeding versus no feeding. No family member should be made to feel that they are starving their loved one to death if a decision is made not to institute enteral feeding. Efforts to provide nutrition should continue, and patients should be able to take any type of nutrition they desire any time they desire.

Strict dietary restrictions, such as low salt or no concentrated sweets, should be replaced with liberalized diet choices. Attention to all factors contributing to inadequate intake should be investigated, including attention to mealtime ambience, feeding techniques, food preferences, medication side effects, and treatment of depression if present. Excellent information for patients and families about enteral feeding can be found at http://www.chcr.brown.edu/dying/consumerfeedingtube.htm. The Northern California chapter of GAPNA has produced a brochure about nutrition and hydration for caregivers and families of persons with dementia and health care professionals (http://ecom.gapna.org/cgi-bin/WebObjects/GAPNA.woa/1/wa/viewSection?wosid=iOvYhk7vfJs82mV8zap66b7Hsrj&tName=chapterNorthernCalifornia&s_id=1073744814&ss_id=536873909).

Short-term enteral feeding may be indicated for some conditions. When tube feeding is indicated, formulas for feedings should vary based on certain diseases such as glucose intolerance, which would entail finding a formula with low carbohydrate content, high fiber to reduce glucose response, and high monounsaturated fatty acids to reduce the risk of heart disease. Most commercial products are lactose free because of intolerance in many older adults and those with malabsorption syndromes. Most of the formulas given through tube feedings are concentrated, and the hydration status of the patient must be closely monitored. To improve safety in medication administration via feeding tubes, the "Be A.W.A.R.E." campaign sponsored by the Nestle HealthCare Nutrition and the American Society for Parenteral and Enteral Nutrition has been launched (see Safety Alert).

! SAFETY ALERT

Be A.W.A.R.E.: Medication administration and feeding tubes
- Do not add medication directly into an enteral feeding formula.
- Administer each medication separately.
- Flush the tube before and after each medication is administered.
- Dilute solid or liquid medication as appropriate.
- Administer each medication using a clean oral or enteral syringe.

From: http://www.nestle-nutrition.com/Media_Room/News_Article_Detail.aspx?ArticleId=03166266-87f0-45f2-8348-c7470a9a0c59. Accessed August 30, 2010.

Oral Care

Dental health of older adults is a basic need that is increasingly neglected with advanced age, debilitation, and limited mobility. Orodental health is integral to general health. Poor oral health is recognized as a risk factor for dehydration and malnutrition, as well as a number of systemic diseases, including pneumonia, joint infections, cardiovascular disease, and poor glycemic control in type 1 and type 2 diabetes (Jablonski, 2010; O'Connor, 2008; Sarin et al., 2008). Poor oral health, which leads to difficulty chewing, missing teeth, teeth in ill repair, and oral pain, contributes to chewing and swallowing problems that affect adequate nutritional intake (Locher et al., 2008).

The percentage of older people without natural teeth is more than 30%, primarily as a result of periodontitis, which occurs in about 95% of those older than 65 years (American Geriatrics Society, 2006a). Prevalence of this disease is decreasing as knowledge increases and more people use fluorides, improve nutrition, engage in new oral hygiene practices, and take advantage of improved dental health care. However, older people may not have had the advantages of new preventive treatment, and those with functional and cognitive limitations may be unable to perform oral hygiene. Oral care is often lacking in institutions, and the "oral health status of nursing home residents has been described as deplorable" (Jablonski, 2010, p. 21). Decades ago, dental care was extremely painful, and fear of the dentist still exists. Access to dental care for older people may be limited as well as cost-prohibitive.

In the existing health care system, dental care is a low priority, reflected by the absence or inadequacy of third-party reimbursement for the type of dental care needed by older adults. Medicare does not provide any coverage for oral health care services, and few Americans age 75 years or older have private dental insurance. Elders have fewer dentist visits than any other age group. Older Americans with the poorest oral health are those who are economically disadvantaged, lack insurance, and are members of racial and ethnic minorities. Being disabled, homebound, or institutionalized increases the risk of poor oral health (Centers for Disease Control and Prevention, 2006).

Oral cancers occur more frequently in late life; men are affected twice as often as women. Oral cancers occur more frequently in black men, and the incidence of oral cancer varies in different countries. It is much more common in Hungary and France than in the United States and much less common in Mexico and Japan (American Geriatrics Society, 2006b). For all stages combined, the 5-year survival rate is 59%, and the 10-year survival rate is 48%. This has not changed significantly in the past 20 years. Oral examinations are important and can assist in early detection and treatment of oral cancers and other orodental problems. Box 14-11 presents common signs and symptoms of oral cancer.

Risk factors for oral cancer are tobacco use, alcohol use, and exposure to ultraviolet light, especially for cancer of the lips.

Pipe, cigar, and cigarette smoking are all implicated. Other risk factors are age, sex, local irritation of the tissues, poor nutrition, mouthwash with high alcohol content, human papillomavirus (HPV) infection, and immune suppression from immunosuppressant drugs. Therapy options are based on diagnosis and staging and include surgery, radiation, and chemotherapy. If detected early, these cancers can almost always be treated successfully.

BOX 14-11　SIGNS AND SYMPTOMS OF ORAL AND THROAT CANCER

- Swelling or thickening, lumps or bumps, or rough spots or eroded areas on the lips, gums, or other areas inside the mouth
- Velvety white, red, or speckled patches in the mouth
- Persistent sores on the face, neck, or mouth that bleed easily
- Unexplained bleeding in the mouth
- Unexplained numbness or pain or tenderness in any area of the face, mouth, neck, or tongue
- Soreness in the back of the throat; a persistent feeling that something is caught in the throat
- Difficulty chewing or swallowing, speaking, or moving the jaw or tongue
- Hoarseness, chronic sore throat, or changes in the voice
- Dramatic weight loss
- Lump or swelling in the neck
- Severe pain in one ear—with a normal eardrum
- Pain around the teeth; loosening of the teeth
- Swelling or pain in the jaw; difficulty moving the jaw

PROMOTING HEALTHY AGING: IMPLICATIONS FOR GERONTOLOGICAL NURSING

Assessment

Good oral hygiene and assessment of oral health are essentials of nursing care. In addition to identifying oral health problems, examination of the mouth can serve as an early warning system for some diseases and lead to early diagnosis and treatment. All persons, especially those over age 50 years, with or without dentures, should have oral examinations on a regular basis. Federal regulations mandate an annual examination for residents of long-term care facilities. Although the oral examination

KAYSER-JONES BRIEF ORAL HEALTH STATUS EXAMINATION

Resident's Name _____　　Date _____
Examiner's Name _____　　TOTAL SCORE _____

CATEGORY	MEASUREMENT	0	1	2
LYMPH NODES	Observe and feel nodes	No enlargement	Enlarged, not tender	Enlarged and tender*
LIPS	Observe, feel tissue, and ask resident, family or staff (e.g., primary caregiver)	Smooth, pink, moist	Dry, chapped, or red at corners*	White or red patch, bleeding or ulcer for 2 weeks*
TONGUE	Observe, feel tissue, and ask resident, family, or staff (e.g., primary caregiver)	Normal roughness, pink and moist	Coated, smooth, patchy, severely fissured or some redness	Red, smooth, white or red patch; ulcer for 2 weeks*
TISSUE INSIDE CHEEK, FLOOR, AND ROOF OF MOUTH	Observe, feel tissue, and ask resident, family, or staff (e.g., primary caregiver)	Pink and moist	Dry, shiny, rough, red, or swollen*	White or red patch, bleeding, hardness; ulcer for 2 weeks*
GUMS BETWEEN TEETH AND/OR UNDER ARTIFICIAL TEETH	Gently press gums with tip of tongue blade	Pink, small indentations; firm, smooth, and pink under artificial teeth	Redness at border around 1-6 teeth; one red area or sore spot under artificial teeth*	Swollen or bleeding gums, redness at border around 7 or more teeth, loose teeth; generalized redness or sores under artificial teeth*
SALIVA (EFFECT ON TISSUE)	Touch tongue blade to center of tongue and floor of mouth	Tissues moist, saliva free flowing and watery	Tissues dry and sticky	Tissues parched and red, no saliva*
CONDITION OF NATURAL TEETH	Observe and count number of decayed or broken teeth	No decayed or broken teeth/roots	1-3 decayed or broken teeth/roots*	4 or more decayed or broken teeth/roots; fewer than 4 teeth in either jaw*
CONDITION OF ARTIFICIAL TEETH	Observe and ask patient, family, or staff (e.g., primary caregiver)	Unbroken teeth, worn most of the time	1 broken/missing tooth, or worn for eating or cosmetics only	More than 1 broken or missing tooth, or either denture missing or never worn*
PAIRS OF TEETH IN CHEWING POSITION (NATURAL OR ARTIFICIAL)	Observe and count pairs of teeth in chewing position	12 or more pairs of teeth in chewing position	8-11 pairs of teeth in chewing position	0-7 pairs of teeth in chewing position*
ORAL CLEANLINESS	Observe appearance of teeth or dentures	Clean, no food particles/tartar in the mouth or on artificial teeth	Food particles/tartar in one or two places in the mouth or on artificial teeth	Food particles/tartar in most places in the mouth or on artificial teeth

Upper dentures labeled: Yes_____ No _____ None _____　Lower dentures labeled: Yes_____ No _____ None _____　Italic*—refer to dentist immediately
Is your mouth comfortable? Yes_____ No _____ If no, explain: _____
Additional comments:_____

FIGURE 14-5 Kayser-Jones Brief Oral Health Status Examination. (With permission of Jeanie Kayser-Jones, RN, PhD, School of Nursing, University of California, San Francisco.)

is best performed by a dentist, nurses can provide basic screening examinations to persons using an instrument such as The Kayser-Jones Brief Oral Health Status Examination (BOHSE) (Figure 14-5). Gil-Montoya and colleagues (2006) developed an oral clinical history appropriate for residents of long-term care institutions (Figure 14-6).

Interventions

Prescribed oral hygiene for the individual with some or all teeth is to brush, floss, and use a fluoride dentifrice and mouthwash daily. It is best if individuals can brush their teeth after each meal. There is evidence that cleaning the person's teeth with a toothbrush after meals lowers the risk of developing aspiration pneumonia (Metheny, 2007). Impaired manual dexterity may make it difficult for elders to adequately maintain their dental routine and remove plaque adequately. The hand grip of manual toothbrushes is too small to grasp and manipulate easily. Using a child's toothbrush or enlarging the handle of an adult-sized toothbrush by adding a foam grip or wrapping it with gauze to increase handle size has been effective in facilitating grasp. Caregivers may also bend a toothbrush handle back approximately 45 degrees to improve access in dependent older people or those who are resistant (Stein & Henry, 2009).

The ultrasonic toothbrush is an effective tool for elders or for those who must brush the teeth of elders. The base is large enough for easy grasp, and the ultrasonic movement of the bristles in concert with the usual brushing movement is very effective in plaque removal. The Collis Curve toothbrush, with curved bristles of differing lengths, may also be useful (Stein & Henry, 2009). Use of a commercial floss handle may provide the leverage and ease necessary for the person to continue flossing. Occupational therapists can be helpful in assessment of functional impairments and provision of adaptive equipment for oral care.

Foam swabs are available to provide oral hygiene but do not remove plaque as well as toothbrushes. Foam swabs may be used to clean the oral mucosa of an edentulous older adult. Lemon glycerin swabs should never be used for older people.

Oral Clinical History	
Date of examination:	
Name:	
Room No:	
1. Does he/she have any natural teeth? ( ) No ( ) Yes, Upper ( ) Yes, Lower	
2. Does he/she use removable dental prosthesis? ( ) No ( ) Yes, Upper ( ) Yes, Lower	
3. Are his/her gums inflamed (reddened or bleeding)? ( ) No ( ) Yes	
4. Does he/she have bacterial plaque or tartar on teeth or prosthesis? ( ) No ( ) Medium amount ( ) A lot	
5. Does his/her mouth slow signs of dryness? ( ) No ( ) Yes	
6. He/she carries out hygiene ( ) on his/her own ( ) with some help ( ) someone has to do it for him/her	
7. ( ) Immediate dental care by the dental service is required.	Reason
Recommendations for care of teeth and prostheses	

	Encourage/supervise tooth and/or prosthesis brushing
	Remove prostheses at bedtime
	Clean teeth with electric toothbrush
	Clean prostheses with electric toothbrush
	Clean oral mucosa with gauze - 0.12% CLX
	Rinse with 0.12% Chlorhexidine solution
	Moisten/coat lips with vaseline or lip balm
	Transfer for immediate dental care

Dates	Incidences

FIGURE 14-6 Oral clinical history appropriate for residents of long-term care institutions. (From Gil-Montoya JA, de Mello AL, Cardenas CB, et al: *Geriatric Nursing* 27:98, 2006.)

In combination with decreased salivary flow and xerostomia, they dry the oral mucosa and erode the tooth enamel (O'Connor, 2008).

Therapeutic rinses contain an agent that is beneficial to the surface of the teeth and the oral environment. Some therapeutic rinses require a prescription, such as Peridex (chlorhexidine), which contains alcohol but is also a broad-spectrum antimicrobial agent that helps control plaque. The commercial product, Listerine, is an over-the-counter product that carries the American Dental Association approval, but it should not be used by persons taking Antabuse, or who have severe oral mucositis, because it contains a high quantity by volume of alcohol (26.9%). Listerine and generic equivalents that contain alcohol may be mixed with water but should always be used in conjunction with, not instead of brushing.

Infected teeth and poor oral hygiene are associated with pneumonia following aspiration of contaminated oral secretions. Research results indicate that tube feeding in older adults is associated with significant pathologic colonization of the mouth, greater than that observed in people who received oral feeding. Oral care should be provided every four hours for patients with gastrostomy tubes, and teeth should be brushed with a toothbrush after each meal to decrease the risk of aspiration pneumonia (Metheny et al., 2008; O'Connor, 2008). The oral mucosa of unconscious or severely cognitively impaired patients should be hydrated using gauze soaked in physiological saline, and lips should be coated with petroleum jelly or lip balm (Gil-Montoya et al., 2006).

When the person is unable to carry out his or her dental/oral regimen, it is the responsibility of the caregiver to provide oral care (Box 14-12). Oral care is an often neglected part of daily nursing care and should receive the same priority as other kinds of care (Stein, 2009). Poor oral health and lack of attention to oral hygiene are major concerns in institutional settings and contribute significantly to poor nutrition and other negative outcomes such as aspiration pneumonia. Many reasons exist for this deficit, including inadequate knowledge of how to assess and provide care, difficulty providing oral care to dependent and cognitively impaired elders, inadequate training and staffing, and lack of appropriate supplies.

Older people with cognitive impairment may be resistive to mouth care, and this is one of the reasons caregivers may neglect oral care. Placing yourself at eye level and explaining all actions in step-by-step instructions with cues and gestures may decrease mouth care–resistive behavior. Even with individuals who need help, caregivers should encourage as much self-care as possible. Caregivers can have the person hold the toothbrush but place their hand over the person's hand (hand-over-hand technique (Jablonski, 2010; Jablonski et al., 2009; Stein & Henry, 2009).

Jablonski and colleagues (2009) describe an educational program using interventions derived from the Need-Driven Dementia-Compromised Behavior Model (see Chapter 19) that addresses oral care techniques that minimize care-resistive behaviors often encountered during oral care to residents with dementia. The Southern Association of Institutional Dentists also provides specific guidelines on oral hygiene in residents with mental and developmental disabilities (Stein & Henry, 2009) (www.saiddent.org/modules.asp).

Many long-term care institutions have implemented programs, such as special training of aides for dental care teams, providing visits from mobile dentistry units on a routine basis, or using dental students to perform oral screening and cleaning of teeth. "Implementation of evidence-based protocols combined with educational training sessions have been shown to have a positive impact on oral care being provided and on the oral health status of older adults" (O'Connor, 2008, p. 394).

Many elders believe that there is no longer a need for oral care once they have dentures. Older adults with dentures should be taught the proper home care of their dentures and oral tissue to prevent odor, stain, plaque buildup, and oral infections. Care should include removal of debris under dentures to prevent pressure on and shrinkage of underlying support structures. Dentures and other dental appliances, such as bridges, should be rinsed after each meal and brushed thoroughly once a day, preferably at night (Box 14-13). Dentures should be worn constantly except at night (to allow relief of compression on the gums) and replaced in the mouth in the morning.

Dentures are very personal and expensive possessions. In communal living situations of nursing homes, hospitals, and other care centers, dentures have often been misplaced or mixed up with those of others. The utmost care should be taken when handling, cleaning, and storing dentures. Dentures should be marked, and many states require all newly made dentures to contain the client's identification. A commercial denture marking system called Identure, produced by the 3M Company, provides a simple, efficient, and permanent means of marking dentures.

BOX 14-12 DENTAL CARE: INSTRUCTIONS FOR CAREGIVERS

1. Explain all actions to the person; use gestures and demonstration as needed; cue and prompt to encourage as much self-care performance as possible.
2. If the patient is in bed, elevate his or her head by raising the bed or propping it with pillows, and have the patient turn his or her head to face you. Place a clean towel across the chest and under the chin, and place a basin under the chin.
3. If the patient is sitting in a stationary chair or wheelchair, stand behind the patient and stabilize his or her head by placing one hand under the chin and resting the head against your body. Place a towel across the chest and over the shoulders. (It may be helpful to secure it with a safety pin.) The basin can be kept handy in the patient's lap or on a table placed in front of or at the side of the patient. A wheelchair may be positioned in front of the sink.
4. If the patient's lips are dry or cracked, apply a light coating of petroleum jelly or use lip balm.
5. Brush and floss the patient's teeth as you have been instructed (use an electric toothbrush if possible, with sulcular brushing). It may be helpful to retract the patient's lips and cheek with a tongue blade or fingers in order to see the area that is being cleaned. Use a mouth prop as needed if the patient cannot hold his or her mouth open. If manual flossing is too difficult, use a floss holder or interproximal brush to clean the proximal surfaces between the teeth. Use a dentifrice-containing fluoride.
6. Provide the conscious patient with fluoride rinses or other rinses as indicated by the dentist or hygienist.

BOX 14-13   INSTRUCTIONS FOR DENTURE CLEANING

1. Rinse your denture or dentures after each meal to remove soft debris. Do not use toothpaste on dentures since it abrades denture surfaces.
2. Once each day, preferably before retiring, remove your denture and brush it thoroughly.
   a. Although an ordinary soft toothbrush is adequate, a specially designed denture brush may clean more effectively. (Caution: Acrylic denture material is softer than natural teeth and may be damaged by being brushed with very firm bristles.)
   b. Brush your denture over a sink lined with a facecloth and half-filled with water. This will prevent breakage if the denture is dropped.
   c. Hold the denture securely in one hand, but do not squeeze. Hold the brush in the other hand. It is not essential to use a denture paste, particularly if dentures are soaked before being brushed to soften debris. Never use a commercial tooth powder, because it is abrasive and may damage the denture materials. Plain water, mild soap, or sodium bicarbonate may be used.
   d. When cleaning a removable partial denture, great care must be taken to remove plaque from the curved metal clasps that hook around the teeth. This can be done with a regular toothbrush or with a specially designed clasp brush.
3. After brushing, rinse your denture thoroughly; then place it in a denture-cleaning solution and allow it to soak overnight or for at least a few hours. (Note: Acrylic denture material must be kept wet at all times to prevent cracking or warping.) In the morning, remove your denture from the cleaning solution, rinse it thoroughly, and then insert it into your mouth. Use denture paste if necessary to secure dentures.

Broken or damaged dentures and dentures that no longer fit because of weight loss are a common problem for older adults. Rebasing of dentures is a technique to improve the fit of dentures. Ill-fitting dentures or dentures that are not cleaned contribute to oral problems as well as to poor nutrition and reduced enjoyment of food. Daily removal and cleaning of dentures and brushing of teeth should be a part of the care routines in institutions.

Both nursing students and nursing staff need to be knowledgeable about oral hygiene and techniques to care for teeth and dentures. Oral hygiene protocols and appropriate oral care equipment should be available in institutions. Patients and families also need education on the importance of good oral health in older adults and techniques for providing adequate oral care.

Maintenance of adequate nutritional health as a person ages is extremely complex. Knowledge of nutritional needs in later years and of the many factors contributing to inadequate nutrition is essential for the gerontological nurse and should be a part of every assessment of an older person. Working with members of the interdisciplinary team in appropriate assessment and development of therapeutic interventions is a major role in community, hospital, and long-term care settings. Use of evidence-based practice protocols is important in determining nursing interventions to support and enhance nutritional and hydration status and promote adequate bowel function.

Prevention of undernutrition and malnutrition and the maintenance of dietary needs and food enjoyment until the end of life are also ethical responsibilities. No older person should be hungry or thirsty because he or she cannot shop, cook, buy and prepare food, or eat independently. Nor should any older person have to suffer because of a lack of assistance with these activities in whatever setting in which they may reside.

evolve To access your student resources, go to *http://evolve.elsevier.com/Ebersole/TwdHlthAging*

KEY CONCEPTS

- Many factors affect adequate nutrition in later life, including lifelong eating habits, income, age-associated changes, chronic illness, dentition, mood disorders, capacity for food preparation, and functional limitations.
- Protein-energy malnutrition (PEM) is the most common form of malnutrition in older adults and occurs among older adults in all settings. Malnutrition has serious consequences, including infections, pressure ulcers, anemia, hypotension, impaired cognition, hip fractures, and increased mortality and morbidity.
- A comprehensive nutritional assessment is an essential component of the assessment of older adults.
- Medications may interfere with adequate food intake, absorption, digestion, and elimination. A comprehensive medication review must be included in a nutritional assessment.
- Making mealtimes pleasant and attractive for the older person who is unable to eat unassisted is a nursing challenge; mealtimes must be made enjoyable, and adequate assistance must be provided.
- Age-related changes in the thirst mechanism, decrease in TBW, and decreased kidney function increase the risk for dehydration in older adults.
- Dysphagia is a serious problem and has negative consequences, including weight loss, malnutrition, dehydration, aspiration pneumonia, and even death. Aspiration pneumonia is the leading cause of death and the second most common cause for hospitalization among nursing home residents. Nurses must carefully assess risk factors for dysphagia, observe for signs and symptoms, refer for evaluation, and collaborate with speech-language pathologists on interventions to prevent aspiration.
- Dental health of older adults is a basic need that is often neglected. Poor oral health is a risk factor for dehydration, malnutrition, and aspiration pneumonia.

CASE STUDY   NUTRITION

Helen, 77 years old, had dieted all her life—or so it seemed. She often chided herself about it. "After all, at my age who cares if I'm too fat? I do. It depresses me when I gain weight and then I gain even more when I'm depressed." At 5 feet, 4 inches tall and 148 pounds, her weight was ideal for her height and age, but Helen, like so many women of her generation, had incorporated Donna Reed's weight of 105 pounds as ideal. She had achieved that weight for only a few weeks three or four times in her adult life. She had tried high-protein diets, celery and cottage cheese diets, fasting, commercially prepared diet foods, and numerous fad diets. She always discontinued the diets when she perceived any negative effects. She was invested in maintaining her general good health. Her most recent attempt at losing 30 pounds on an all-liquid diet had been unsuccessful and left her feeling constipated, weak, irritable, and mildly nauseated and experiencing heart palpitations. This really frightened her. Her physician criticized her regarding the liquid diet but seemed rather amused while reinforcing that her weight was "just perfect" for her age. In the discussion, the physician pointed out how fortunate she was that she was able to drive to the market, had sufficient money for food, and was able to eat anything with no dietary restrictions. Helen left his office feeling silly. She was an independent, intelligent woman; she had been a successful manager of a large financial office. Before her retirement seven years ago, her work had consumed most of her energies. There had been no time for family, romance, or hobbies. Lately, she had immersed herself in reading the Harvard Classics as she had promised herself she would when she retired. Unfortunately, now that she had the time to read them, she was losing interest. She knew that she must begin to "pull herself together" and "be grateful for her blessings" just as the physician had said.

Based on the case study, develop a nursing care plan using the following procedure*:

- List Helen's comments that provide subjective data.
- List information that provides objective data.
- From these data, identify and state, using accepted format, two nursing diagnoses you determine are most significant to Helen at this time. List two of Helen's strengths that you have identified from the data.
- Determine and state outcome criteria for each diagnosis. These must reflect some alleviation of the problem identified in the nursing diagnosis and must be stated in concrete and measurable terms.
- Plan and state one or more interventions for each diagnosed problem. Provide specific documentation of the source used to determine the appropriate intervention. Plan at least one intervention that incorporates Helen's existing strengths.
- Evaluate the success of the intervention. Interventions must correlate directly with the stated outcome criteria to measure the outcome success.

CRITICAL THINKING QUESTIONS

1. Discuss how you would counsel Helen regarding her weight.
2. If Helen insists on dieting, what diet would you recommend, considering her age and activity level?
3. What lifestyle changes should Helen make?
4. What lifestyle changes would you suggest to Helen?
5. What are the specific health concerns that require attention in Helen's case?
6. What factors may be involved in Helen's preoccupation with her weight?
7. What are some of the reasons that fad diets are dangerous?

*Students are advised to refer to their nursing diagnosis text and identify possible or potential problems.

RESEARCH QUESTIONS

1. What are the dietary patterns of older women living alone?
2. What percentage of women over age 60 are satisfied with their weight? What is the percentage for men?
3. What factors influence older people to implement dietary changes suggested by nurses, dietitians, or primary care providers?
4. What nursing interventions can enhance nutritional intake of frail older adults in nursing facilities?
5. What is the level of knowledge of acute care and long-term care nurses about dysphagia?
6. What strategies are most helpful in enhancing fluid intake of older adults in long-term care facilities?
7. What are the barriers to adequate oral care for older people in hospitals and long-term care facilities?

REFERENCES

Ahmed T, Haboubi N: Assessment and management of nutrition in older people and its importance to health, *Clinical Interventions in Aging* 5:207, 2010.

Amella E, Lawrence J: Eating and feeding issues in older adults with dementia, 2007. Available at www.hartfordign.org. Accessed June 30, 2008.

American Dietetic Association, the American Society for Nutrition, and the Society for Nutrition Education: Position of the American Dietetic Association, American Society for Nutrition and Society for Nutrition Education: Food and nutrition programs for community-residing older adults. *Journal of the American Dietetic Association* 110:463, 2010.

American Geriatrics Society: *Geriatrics at your fingertips*, New York, 2006a, The Society.

American Geriatrics Society: *Geriatric review syllabus*, New York, 2006b, The Society.

Aparanji K, Dharmarajan T: Pause before a PEG: A feeding tube may not be necessary in every candidate, *Journal of the American Medical Directors Association* 11:453, 2010.

Bales C, Buhr G: Is obesity bad for older persons? A systematic review of the pros and cons of weight reduction in later life, *Journal of the American Medical Directors Association* 9:302, 2008.

Beasley J, LaCroix A, Neuhouser M, et al: Protein intake and incident frailty in the Women's Health Initiative Observational Study, *Journal of the American Geriatrics Society* 58:1063, 2010.

Burger S, et al: Malnutrition and dehydration in nursing homes: key issues in prevention and treatment, 2000. Available at www.cmwf.org/programs/elders/burger_mal_386.asp. Accessed July 23, 2004.

Butrica B: Do assets change the racial profile of poverty among older adults? February 9, 2008, Urban Institute. Available at http://www.urban.org/publications/411620.html. Accessed August 30, 2010.

Cadogan M: Clinical concepts: functional consequences of vitamin B12 deficiency, *Journal of Gerontological Nursing* 36:18, 2010.

Cacchione PZ: Sensory changes. In Capezuti E, Zwicker D, Mezey M, et al, editors: *Evidence-based geriatric nursing protocols for best practice*, ed 3, New York, 2008, Springer.

Centers for Disease Control and Prevention: Oral health for older Americans, 2006. Available at www.cdc.gov/Oralhealth/publications/factsheets/adult_older.htm. Accessed August 31, 2010.

Centers for Disease Control and Prevention: U.S. Obesity Trends. Available at http://www.cdc.gov/obesity/data/trends.html. Accessed August 31, 2010.

Crecelius C: Dehydration: myth and reality, *Journal of the American Medical Directors Association* 9:287, 2008.

DiMaria-Ghalili R: Nutrition. In Capezuti E, Zwicker D, Mezey M, et al, editors:

Evidence-based geriatric nursing protocols for best practice, ed 3, New York, 2008, Springer.

Doll-Shankaruk M, Yau E. Oekle C: Implementation and effects of a medication pass nutritional supplement program in a long-term care facility, *Journal of Gerontological Nursing* 34:45, 2008.

Duffy E: Malnutrition in older adults, Advance for NPs and PAs, 2010. Available at *http://nursepractitioners-and-physician-assistants.advanceweb.com/Editorial/Content/PrintFriendly.aspx?C.* Accessed August 31, 2010.

Dunne T, Neargarder S, Cipolloni P, et al: Visual contrast enhances food and liquid intake in advanced Alzheimer's disease, *Clinical Nutrition* 23:533, 2004.

Easterling C, Robbins E: Dementia and dysphagia, *Geriatric Nursing* 29:275, 2008.

Ervin B: *Healthy eating index scores among adults 60 years of age and over, by sociodemographic and health characteristics: United States, 1999-2002.* Advance data from vital and health statistics; no. 395. Hyattsville, MD: National Center for Health Statistics, 2008. Available at www.cdc.gov/nchs/data/ad/ad395.pdf. Accessed August 27, 2010.

Faes MC, Spift MG, Olde et al: Dehydration in geriatrics, *Geriatric Aging* 10:590, 2007.

Felix H: Obesity, disability and nursing home admission, *Annals of Long-Term Care* 16:33, 2008.

Flicker L, McCaul K, Hankey G, et al: Body mass index and survival in men and women aged 70 to 75, *Journal of the American Geriatrics Society* 58:234-241, 2010.

Fuller-Thomson E, Redmond M: Falling through the social safety net: food stamp use and nonuse among older impoverished Americans, *Gerontologist* 48:235-244, 2008.

Garon B, Sierzant T, Ormiston C, et al: Silent aspiration: results of 2,000 video fluoroscopic evaluations, *Journal of Neuroscience Nursing* 41:178-185, 2009.

Gavi S, Hensley J, Cervo F, et al: Management of feeding tube complications in the long-term care resident, *Annals of Long-Term Care* 16:28, 2008. Available at http://www.annalsoflongtermcare.com/article/8614. Accessed August 31, 2010.

Gil-Montoya JA, Ferreira A, Lopez I: Oral health protocol for the dependent institutionalized elderly, *Geriatric Nursing* 27:95, 2006.

Haber D: *Health promotion and aging*, ed 4, New York, 2007, Springer.

Ham R, Sloane P, Warshaw G, et al: *Primary care geriatrics: A case-based approach*, ed 5, St Louis, 2007, Mosby.

Jablonski R: Examining oral health in nursing home residents and overcoming mouth-care resistive behaviors, *Annals of Long-Term Care* 18:21, 2010.

Jablonski R, Munro C, Grap M, et al: Mouth care in nursing homes: knowledge, beliefs, and practices of nursing assistants, *Geriatric Nursing* 30:99, 2009.

Jarosz P, Bellar A: Sarcopenic obesity: An emerging cause of frailty in older adults, *Geriatric Nursing* 30:64, 2009.

Kaiser R, Winning K, Uter W, et al: Functionality and mortality in obese nursing home residents: An example of "risk factor paradox?" *Journal of the American Medical Directors Association* 11:428, 2010.

Kayser-Jones J: Inadequate staffing at mealtime: implications for nursing and health policy, *Journal of Gerontological Nursing* 23:14, 1997.

Lee M, Berthelot E: Community covariates of malnutrition based mortality among older adults, *Annals of Epidemiology* 20:371, 2010.

Locher J, Ritchie C, Robinson C, et al: A multidimensional approach to understanding under-eating in homebound older adults: the importance of social factors, *Gerontologist*, 48:223, 2008.

Lustbader W: Thoughts on the meaning of frailty, *Generations* 13:21, 1999.

Markovic K, Reulbach U, Vassiliadu A, et al: Good news for elderly persons: olfactory pleasure increases at later stages of the life span, *The Journals of Gerontology. Series A, Biological Sciences and Medical Sciences* 62:1287, 2007.

Mei A, Auerhahn C: Hypodermoclysis: maintaining hydration in the frail older adult, *Annals of Long-Term Care* 17:28, 2009.

Mentes JC: Oral hydration in older adults: greater awareness is needed in preventing, recognizing and treating dehydration, *American Journal of Nursing* 106:40, 2006.

Mentes JC: Managing oral hydration. In Capezuti E, et al, editors: *Evidence-based geriatric nursing protocols for best practice*, ed 3, New York, 2008, Springer.

Metheny M: Preventing aspiration in older adults with dysphagia, 2007, Available at http://consultgerirn.org/uploads/File/trythis/try_this_20.pdf. Accessed January 2011.

Metheny M, Boltz M, Greenberg S: Preventing aspiration in older adults with dysphagia, *American Journal of Nursing* 108:45, 2008.

Miller C: *Nursing for wellness in older adults*, ed 5, Philadelphia, 2008, Wolters Kluwer Lippincott Williams & Wilkins.

Morley JE: Anorexia and weight loss in older persons, *The Journals of Gerontology. Series A, Biological Sciences and Medical Sciences* 58:131, 2003.

Morley J: Anorexia, weight loss, and frailty, *Journal of the American Medical Directors Association* 11:225, 2010.

National Institute on Aging: Healthy Eating after 50, 2010. Available at www.nia.nih.gov/healthinformation/publications/healthyeating.htm. Accessed August 31, 2010.

Newman A: Obesity in older adults, *The Online Journal of Issues in Nursing* 14, Manuscript 3, 2009. (website): *http://www.nursingworld.org/MainMenuCategories/ANAMarketplace/ANAPeriodicals/OJIN/TableofConte.* Accessed August 31, 2010.

O'Connor L: Oral health care. In Capezuti E, et al, editors: *Evidence-based geriatric nursing protocols for best practice*, ed 3, New York, 2008, Springer.

Sarin J, Balasubramaniam R, Corcoran A, et al: Reducing the risk to aspiration pneumonia among elderly patients in long-term care facilities through oral health interventions, *Journal of the American Medical Directors Association* 9:128, 2008.

Simmons S, Osterweil D, Schnelle J: Improving food intake in nursing home residents with feeding assistance, *The Journals of Gerontology. Series A, Biological Sciences and Medical Sciences* 12:M790, 2001.

Stein P, Henry R: Poor oral hygiene in long-term care, *American Journal of Nursing* 109:44, 2009.

Tanner D: Lessons from nursing home dysphagia malpractice litigation, *Journal of Gerontological Nursing* 36:41, 2010.

Teno J, Mitchell S, Gozalo P, et al: Hospital characteristics associated with feeding tube placement in nursing home residents with advanced cognitive impairment, *Journal of the American Medical Association* 303:544, 2010.

Thomas D, Cote T, Lawhorne L, et al: Understanding clinical dehydration and its treatment, *Journal of the American Medical Directors Association* 9:292, 2008.

Thomas DR, Ashmen W, Morley JE, et al: Nutritional management in long-term care: development of a clinical guideline, *The Journals of Gerontology. Series A, Biological Sciences and Medical Sciences* 55:M725, 2000.

University of Texas: *Unintentional weight loss in the elderly.* Austin, University of Texas School of Nursing, 2006. Available at www.guideline.gov. Accessed November 3, 2010.

Vitale C, Monteleoni C, Burke L, et al: Strategies for improving care for patients with advanced dementia and eating problems: optimizing care through physician and speech pathologist collaboration, *Annals of Long-Term Care* 17:32, 2009.

Chronic Conditions

Kathleen Jett

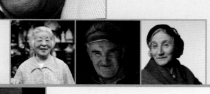

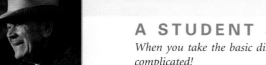

evolve *http://evolve.elsevier.com/Ebersole/TwdHlthAging*

A STUDENT SPEAKS

When you take the basic disease and add it to the normal changes with aging things get pretty complicated!

Nursing Student, age 20

AN ELDER SPEAKS

If I'd known I was going to live this long, I'd have taken better care of myself.

Eubie Blake, on his 100th birthday

LEARNING OBJECTIVES

On completion of this chapter, the reader will be able to:

1. Identify the most common chronic disorders of late life and their sequela.
2. Develop strategies that have been used successfully to maintain maximum function and comfort in the person with a chronic disorder.
3. Suggest nursing interventions appropriate to the care of an individual with a chronic disorder.
4. Construct nursing interventions that are consistent with a theoretical framework of maximizing wellness in the presence of chronic disease.

The relationship between chronic disease and aging is complex. Chronic disease, such as heart failure, was once viewed intrinsic to aging. This belief was challenged as the science of preventive medicine advanced. How is it that some persons develop many of the "chronic diseases of old age" and others do not? Now, with increasing understanding of the most basic cellular process in aging cells (e.g., oxidation) and advances in the genomic sciences, the line between aging and chronic conditions is blurred. We now know that most lung disease in late life can be avoided by not smoking earlier in life; yet as one ages one is more susceptible to pneumonia. A diagnosis of an HIV infection no longer means imminent death. With the introduction of antiretroviral therapy in the 1990s, persons are living longer than they ever had before. A large number of persons with stabilized and therefore chronic HIV are now in middle age and soon to be entering late life (see Chapter 21). The worldwide incidence of stroke has fallen as people are able to better control their blood pressure, exercise, and eat healthier, yet heart disease remains the primary cause of death for persons across the globe.

A chronic health problem is one that is managed rather than cured. It is always present although not always visible. The onset may be insidious and identified only during a health screening or while being treated for another problem that is actually a complication or late-stage effect. For example, a person sees an ophthalmologist for problems with deteriorating vision, only to be found to have diabetic retinopathy; diabetes is diagnosed already in a later stage.

Persons with new chronic conditions often continue to work and perform their usual routine. Later, and with increasing age, the effects of the limitations caused by the condition become noticeable (Figure 15-1). The person may receive assistance and rehabilitation in the home or in a designated rehabilitation center when the disabilities are first significant or during exacerbations in the limitations. As the limitations increase further, the person at home may move to the home of another and receive informal help or into an institutional setting where formal help is available.

The most common chronic condition in persons over 65 is hypertension, followed by arthritis (Figure 15-2). Yet for the

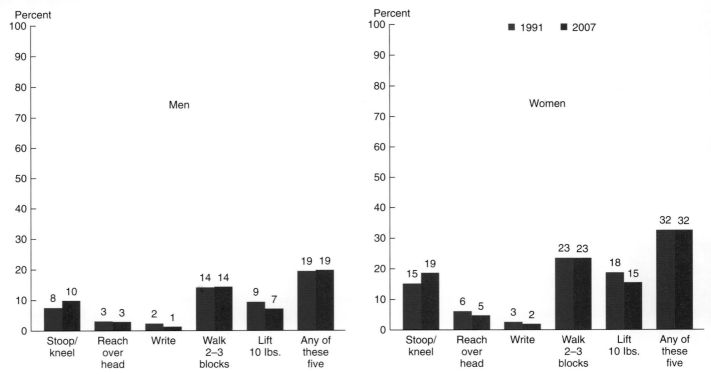

NOTE: Rates for 1991 are age adjusted to the 2007 population.
Reference population: These data refer to Medicare enrollees.
SOURCE: Centers for Medicare and Medicaid Services, Medicare Current Beneficiary Survey.

FIGURE 15-1 Percentage of Medicare enrollees age 65 and over who are unable to perform certain physical functions, by sex, 1991 and 2007. (Redrawn from Federal Interagency Forum on Aging-Related Statistics: *Older Americans 2010: Key indicators of well-being*, Washington DC, 2010, U.S. Government Printing Office.)

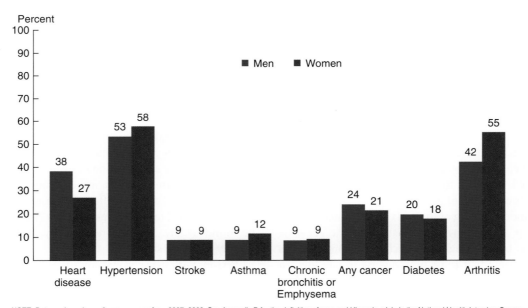

NOTE: Data are based on a 2-year average from 2007–2008. See Appendix B for the definition of race and Hispanic origin in the National Health Interview Survey.
Reference population: These data refer to the civilian noninstitutionalized population.
SOURCE: Centers for Disease Control and Prevention, National Center for Health Statistics, National Health Interview Survey.

FIGURE 15-2 Chronic health conditions among the population age 65 and over, by sex, 2007-2008. (Redrawn from Federal Interagency Forum on Aging-Related Statistics: *Older Americans 2010: Key indicators of well-being*, Washington DC, 2010, U.S. Government Printing Office.)

older adult, the presence or absence of a condition is not as important as its affect on function. The effect may be as little as an inconvenience or as great as an impairment of one's ability to live independently (Figure 15-3).

Working with those with chronic health conditions means that the gerontological nurse has the opportunity to decrease mortality of older adults and minimize the potentially disabling effects of chronic disease, that is, to be instrumental in decreasing morbidity. This chapter provides a snapshot of the most common chronic conditions the nurse will see in persons who depend on him or her for care and proposes strategies to promote healthy living regardless of the limitations with which one lives. We neither cover all possible conditions nor do we provide comprehensive medical management of these disorders. However, certain disorders are encountered frequently enough in late life to merit special attention. These include specific medical diagnoses and conditions in body systems. Other conditions such as those of the eyes and skin are addressed in Chapters 6 and 11.

It is anticipated that this chapter will enable the nurse to develop and implement strategies to promote healthy aging in the presence of the chronic disease.

THEORETICAL FRAMEWORKS FOR CHRONIC DISEASE

Chronic Illness Trajectory

While there are many conceptual models from which chronic illness can be viewed, the trajectory model originally conceptualized by Anselm Strauss and Barney Glaser (1975) and later Corbin and Strauss (1992) has long aided health care providers to understand the realities of chronic illness and its effect on individuals. According to this theoretical approach, chronic illness can be viewed from a life course perspective or along a trajectory trace. In this way, the course of a person's illness can be viewed as an integral part of their lives rather than an isolated event. The nurse's response is then holistic rather than isolated. Woog (1992) divided Glaser and Strauss' model into eight phases for the purpose of identifying goals and developing interventions. The trajectory may include a preventive phase (pretrajectory), a definitive phase (trajectory onset), a crisis phase, an acute phase, a stable phase, an unstable phase, a downward phase, and dying phase (Table 15-1). The shape and stability of the trajectory is influenced by the combined efforts, attitudes, and beliefs held by the elder, family members and significant others, and the involved health care providers. Key points of the model are based on the theoretical assumptions listed in Box 15-1.

TABLE 15-1	THE CHRONIC ILLNESS TRAJECTORY
PHASE	**DEFINITION**
1. Pre-trajectory	Before the illness course begins, the preventive phase, no signs or symptoms present
2. Trajectory onset	Signs and symptoms are present, includes diagnostic period
3. Crisis	Life-threatening situation; acute threat to self-identity
4. Acute	Active illness or complications that require hospitalization for management
5. Stable	Controlled illness course/symptoms
6. Unstable	Illness course/symptoms not controlled by regimen but not requiring or desiring hospitalization
7. Downward	Progressive decline in physical/mental status characterized by increasing disability/symptoms
8. Dying	Immediate weeks, days, hours preceding death

Examples of goals that nurses might establish include the following:
1. To assist a client in overcoming a plateau by increasing adherence to a regimen so that he or she might reach the highest level of functional ability possible within limits of the disability.
2. To assist a client in making the attitudinal and lifestyle changes that are needed to promote health and prevent disease.
3. To assist a client who is in a downward trajectory to be able to maintain sense of self and receive expert palliative care.
4. To assist with advance care planning to assure wishes are met.
5. To assist the client who is in an unstable phase to gain greater control over symptoms that are interfering with his or her ability to carry out everyday activities.

See Woog P: *The chronic illness trajectory framework: the Corbin and Strauss nursing model*, New York, 1992, Springer.

BOX 15-1	KEY POINTS IN THE CHRONIC ILLNESS TRAJECTORY FRAMEWORK

- The majority of health problems in late life are chronic.
- Chronic illnesses may entail lifetime adaptations.
- Chronic illness and its management often profoundly affect the lives and identities of both the individual and the family members or significant others.
- The acute phase of management is designed to stabilize physiological processes and promote recovery.
- Other phases of management are designed primarily to maximize and extend the period of stability in the home with the help of family and by visits to and from health care providers and other members of the rehabilitation and restoration team as appropriate.
- A primary care nurse is often in the role of coordinator of the multiple resources that may be needed to promote quality of life along the trajectory.
- The nurse has multiple opportunities to promote the health of persons during the chronic phase.

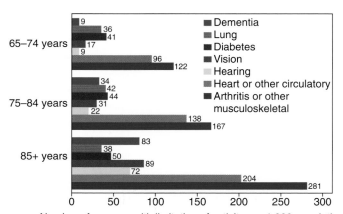

SOURCE: CDC/NCHS, *Health, United States, 2009*, Figure 15. Data from the National Health Interview Survey.

FIGURE 15-3 Activity limitation caused by chronic conditions among older adults, 2006-2007. (National Center for Health Statistics: Health, United States, 2009: with special feature on medical technology, Hyattsville, MD, 2010.)

The person's perceptions of both needs met and functional limitations are paramount to predicting movement along the illness trajectory (Corbin & Strauss, 1992). By using this approach, the gerontological nurse may have the biggest impact on promoting the health of the person with a chronic condition.

CARDIOVASCULAR DISEASE

In 2009 the National Heart, Lung and Blood Institute reported that as of 2006 17.6 million persons in the United States had some form of cardiovascular disease (CVD). It is the leading cause of death for all persons over 65 and living in the United States with the exception of Asian Americans, for whom it is second (National Heart, Lung and Blood Institute [NHLBI], 2010). It is also the primary diagnosis of persons admitted to long-term care facilities and acute care hospitals (Auerhahn, et al., 2007). The high rate of CVD in later life is caused from a combination of genetics, normal changes with aging, risk factors such as smoking, and environmental factors such as pollution and stress, and in some cases, discrimination and racism (Box 15-2). Treatment approaches, mortality, and morbidity are highly variable by ethnicity, gender, and socioeconomic group.

Cardiovascular diseases derive from damage to the blood vessels or to the heart wall or from prolonged effects on either. Hypertension, coronary heart disease (CHD), and heart failure (HF) are reviewed in this section with an emphasis on health promotion. For a more detailed examination of these conditions, the reader is referred to gerontological nursing and geriatric medicine texts that are disease-based.

Hypertension

Hypertension (HTN) is the most common chronic cardiovascular disease encountered by the gerontological nurse. Both the definition of and the guidelines for treatment of HTN are provided by the Joint National Committee of the Detection, Evaluation, and Treatment of High Blood Pressure (JNC)*. According to JNC, HTN is diagnosed any time the diastolic blood pressure reading is 90 or higher or the systolic reading is 140 or higher on two separate occasions (JNC 7, 2003) (Table 15-2). However, the average of three readings is recommended for older adults due to age-related variability. Blood pressure, especially systolic blood pressure, increases with age, and an elevation of 140 mm Hg or more is a much more important risk indicator than a diastolic elevation in persons over age 50. Contrary to prior knowledge, it was found that the parameters for the diagnosis of HTN did not change with age (Box 15-3). The current blood pressure goal of all persons is less than 140/90 and equal to or less than 130/80 for persons with diabetes (JNC 7, 2003). The U.S. Prevention Task Force has recommend that persons with blood pressure readings of <120/80 be screened every two years and once a year for those with SBP of 120-139 or DBP 80-90 (U.S. Preventive Services Task Force [USPSTF], 2007a).

---

*Publication date for JNC 8 is expected in Spring 2011 at which time the definition may change.

BOX 15-2   RISK FACTORS FOR CARDIOVASCULAR DISEASE

- Age (>55 years for men; >65 years for women)
- Family history of premature CHD (<55 years for men; <65 years for women)
- Microalbuminuria or estimated GFR <60 mL/min
- Hypertension*
- Cigarette smoking
- Central obesity (BMI ≥30)*
- Physical inactivity
- Dyslipidemia*
- Diabetes, IGT, or IFG*

*Components of metabolic syndrome.
CHD, Coronary heart disease; *GFR,* glomerular filtration rate; *BMI,* body mass index; *IGT,* impaired glucose tolerance; *IFG,* impaired fasting glucose.

TABLE 15-2   BLOOD PRESSURE CLASSIFICATION

CLASSIFICATION	BLOOD PRESSURE
Normal	<120 systolic and <80 diastolic
Prehypertension	120-139 systolic or 80-89 diastolic
Stage 1 HTN	140-159 systolic or 90-99 diastolic
Stage 2 HTN	>160 systolic or >100 diastolic

HTN, Hypertension.

BOX 15-3   KEY POINTS OF THE JNC 7

- For persons older than age 50, SBP is more important than DBP as a CVD risk factor.
- Starting at 115/75 mm Hg, CVD risk doubles with each increment of 20/10 mm Hg throughout the BP range.
- Persons who are normotensive at age 55 still have a 90% lifetime risk for developing HTN.
- Those with SBP 120-139 mm Hg or DBP 80-89 mm Hg should be considered prehypertensive and require health-promoting lifestyle modifications to prevent CVD.
- Thiazide-type diuretics should be the initial drug therapy either alone or combined with other drug classes unless compelling reasons are present.
- Certain high-risk conditions are compelling indications for other drug classes, e.g., diabetes.
- Most patients will require two or more antihypertensive drugs to achieve goal BP.
- If BP is >20/10 mm Hg above goal, initiate therapy with two agents; one usually should be a thiazide-type diuretic.

Adapted from JNC 7: USHHS Pub No 03-5233, 2003. Available at www.nhlbi.nih.gov. JNC 8 is expected to be published in Fall 2011. *SBP,* Systolic blood pressure; *DBP,* diastolic blood pressure; *CVD,* cardiovascular disease; *BP,* blood pressure; *HTN,* hypertension.

All persons with hypertension should be screened for diabetes.

As of 2007, over 74 million Americans were thought to have HTN. The prevalence is highest among African Americans at all ages and lowest among Mexican Americans (NHLBI, 2010). Although the genetic predisposition cannot be controlled, many risk factors for both the disease and complications are modifiable (Box 15-4).

A common problem related to the measurement blood pressure disorders in the older adult is "white coat syndrome," wherein the blood pressure readings in the office are higher than they would otherwise be. Management is also difficult due to the frequency of postural or orthostatic hypotension, and postprandial hypotension. As a result, it may be necessary to include ambulatory blood pressure monitoring and positional measurement in the diagnostic evaluation. The subsequent evaluation includes the determination of contributing factors and end-organ damage. Only when all of the information is available can a holistic plan of care be developed.

Etiology

Hypertension is a multigenic disease with strong familial clustering, however the effect of the environment and other endogenous factors are so significant that research is ongoing in an attempt to both understand and control the disease. Arterial stiffness and reduced vascular compliance, both normal changes with aging, are the factors most likely to account for the increased incidence of HTN among older adults. Decreased baroreceptor sensitivity may explain the variability of the blood pressure. Both changes in renal function and the neurohumoral system may explain the fact that approximately two thirds of older adults have sodium-sensitive hypertension, especially in the black population (Auerhahn, et al., 2007). Secondary causes are relatively rare in older adults and include pheochromocytoma, Cushing's syndrome, obstructive sleep apnea, thyroid/parathyroid disease, and chronic kidney disease (NHLBI, 2008).

Signs and Symptoms

Many persons are found to have HTN during health screening. The person may be completely asymptomatic until suffering an acute cardiovascular event or found to have already progressed from simple HTN to heart disease. Some persons complain of a headache, lightheadedness, "swimmy head" or a "full head" when the BP is elevated. On the contrary, the lightheadedness and "swimmy head" or other cultural expressions of dizziness may also suggest periods of hypotension.

Complications

As with other CVDs, it may not be diagnosed until some degree of end-organ damage has occurred. Uncontrolled hypertension is a remarkable harbinger for complex and life-threatening end-organ damage, especially heart disease. Older persons with HTN have an absolute higher risk for cardiac disease (e.g., coronary heart disease, atrial fibrillation, and heart failure), as well as acute cardiovascular and cerebrovascular events (e.g., myocardial infarction, stroke, and sudden death). Poorly controlled HTN is also implicated in chronic renal insufficiency, end-stage renal disease, and peripheral vascular disease.

BOX 15-4	MODIFIABLE FACTORS THAT INCREASE THE RISK FOR ESSENTIAL HYPERTENSION

- Cigarette smoking, tobacco use or exposure
- Excessive alcohol intake
- Sedentary lifestyle
- Inadequate stress/anger management
- High-sodium diet
- High-fat diet

PROMOTING HEALTHY AGING; IMPLICATIONS FOR GERONTOLOGICAL NURSING: HYPERTENSION

Both pharmacological and non-pharmacological interventions that promote a healthy lifestyle have been found to be effective in controlling HTN and minimizing the complications that can significantly interfere with quality of life. The universal use of thiazide-type diuretics (e.g. chlorothiazide) was recommended when the evidence was conclusive that this would improve both mortality and morbidity of persons with HTN. It is expected that in most cases more that one type of antihypertensive medications will be needed based on concurrent co-conditions, such as diabetes and race. Pharmacological guidelines, including adjustments by race, can be found in the JNC 7 report supported by the National Heart, Lung and Blood Institute (www.nhlbi.nih.gov).

By reducing or eliminating modifiable risk factors, hypertension can be controlled or prevented leading to healthier aging (Table 15-3). With few exceptions (e.g., late-stage dementia), maintaining blood pressure control is recommended regardless of the overall disease state. This means reducing the pulse pressure and keeping the blood pressure less than 140/90 mm Hg for otherwise healthy adults and less than 130/80 mm Hg for persons with diabetes.

There is considerable evidence regarding the importance of diet. Healthy eating habits and weight loss have been found to irrefutably lower blood pressure (Table 15-4). Even modest reductions in sodium intake and weight may make a significant difference. A healthy diet includes control of cholesterol, sodium, and calories. It is now recommended that all persons limit their daily sodium intake to less than 2400 mg/day. Teaching people how to read food labels can be a first step. An evidence-based DASH diet is available from the National

TABLE 15-3	BENEFITS OF CONTROLLING BLOOD PRESSURE
	AVERAGE PERCENT REDUCTION IN RISK FOR NEW EVENTS
Stroke decreased	30%-40%
Myocardial infarction decreased	20%-25%
Heart failure decreased	50%

TABLE 15-4	RELATIONSHIP BETWEEN LIFESTYLE CHANGE AND REDUCTION IN SYSTOLIC BLOOD PRESSURE
LIFESTYLE CHANGE	**APPROXIMATE REDUCTION IN SBP**
Weight reduction	Decrease of 5-20 mm Hg per 10-lb loss
Adopt the DASH diet	Decrease of 8-14 mm Hg
Lower sodium intake	Decrease of 2-8 mm Hg
Increase physical activity	Decrease of 4-9 mm Hg
ETOH in moderation	Decrease of 2-4 mm Hg

SBP, Systolic blood pressure; DASH, Dietary Approaches to Stop Hypertension; ETOH, alcohol.

Heart, Lung and Blood Institute at www.nhlbi.nih.gov (*see* Chapter 14*).* When combined with the appropriate medications, the long-term complication of heart disease can be reduced (Box 15-5).

Unfortunately, less is known about the appropriate management of hypertension for persons over age 85 or those who are medically fragile, such as many residing in long-term care settings or those with advanced dementia. A careful risk-benefit analysis should be done related to treatment effects, side effects, and both short-and-long term outcomes in such situations. For someone with a limited life expectancy, the significant side effects of some medications and limitations in food choices may result in an unnecessary decrease in quality of life.

Coronary Heart Disease

The beating heart, like other muscles, needs oxygen and nutrients to survive. Despite all the blood that passes through it, the muscle depends on the coronary arteries for oxygenation. While not an expected change of aging, the incidence of CHD rises significantly with age, most often as a result of prolonged hypertension. CHD includes both atherosclerotic *coronary artery disease* (CAD) and ischemic heart disease, conditions that either completely or partially obstruct the flow of oxygenated blood to the heart.

While 425,000 deaths in 2006 were attributed to CHD, the death rate has declined dramatically in the past 20 years. While

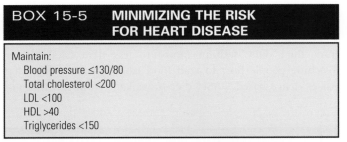

BOX 15-5   MINIMIZING THE RISK FOR HEART DISEASE

Maintain:
  Blood pressure ≤130/80
  Total cholesterol <200
  LDL <100
  HDL >40
  Triglycerides <150

LDL, Low-density lipoprotein; *HDL,* high-density lipoprotein.

this rate has declined for persons of all races, it remains highest among African Americans and lowest among Asian Americans (NHLBI, 2010) (Figure 15-4). The incidence in men exceeds the incidence in women until after menopause, at which time the rate in women accelerates. It has been found that 70% of persons over age 70 had ≥50% atherosclerotic obstruction in at least one coronary artery on autopsy (Auerhahn, et al., 2007).

Etiology

Narrowed or blocked arterial lumina probably result from a complicated interaction of processes that may begin before birth. The walls of the normally pliable artery thicken and stiffen with age as a result of cross-linking. There are changes in lipid, cholesterol, and phospholipid metabolism. Although many of these changes are associated with normal aging, the sequela can be life threatening when coupled with pathophysiological conditions, such as hypertension.

Blockage may be from atherosclerosis, referred to as hardening of the arteries caused by the accumulation of lipid-laden macrophages within the arterial wall and the formation of plaques (Figure 15-5). The plaques reduce the capacity for oxygenation of the surrounding tissue. With complete obstruction, ischemic pain and tissue necrosis occur, and death may follow. With only partial blockage, the pain may be intermittent and experienced as angina. In severe cases of complete blockage, the result is acute myocardial infarction (AMI) and tissue necrosis. Risk factors for an AMI are both intrinsic and extrinsic and therefore somewhat modifiable (Figure 15-6).

Signs and Symptoms

The pain of ischemic cardiac origin is classically described as a pressing or squeezing, usually in the chest under the breastbone, but sometimes in the shoulders, arms, neck, jaws, or back. While these are the classic signs and symptoms earlier in life (especially for men), this varies greatly with age and varies by gender. In later life, only 19% to 66% of persons complain of chest pain, 20% to 59% complain first of dyspnea, 15% to 33% have neurological manifestations, and up to 19% may have

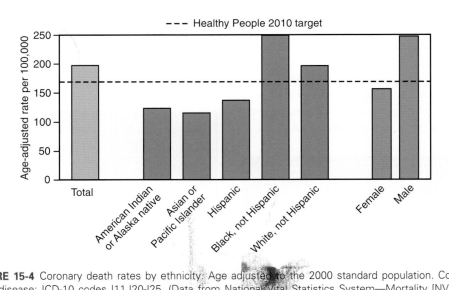

FIGURE 15-4 Coronary death rates by ethnicity. Age adjusted to the 2000 standard population. Coronary heart disease: ICD-10 codes I11,I20-I25. (Data from National Vital Statistics System—Mortality [NVSS-M], NCHS, CDC. Redrawn from www.cdc.gov/nchs/hphome.htm. Focus area No. 12.)

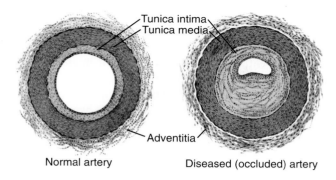

FIGURE 15-5 Arteriosclerosis. (From McCance K, Huether S, editors: *Pathophysiology: the biological basis for disease in adults and children*, ed 5, St Louis, 2006, Mosby, p. 1082.)

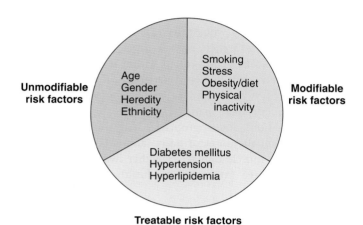

FIGURE 15-6 Risk factors for cardiovascular (CV) events. (From www.nhlbi.gov; Grundy SM. *J Am Coll Cardiol* 34:1348-1359, 1999.)

gastrointestinal symptoms (e.g., nausea and vomiting) associated with an AMI (Auerhahn, et al., 2007). This array of nonspecific and atypical symptoms often leads to misdiagnosis, which delays the prompt medical intervention needed for optimal outcomes.

Both non-invasive (e.g., ECG, stress test) and invasive (e.g., coronary angiography, thallium perfusion scintigraphy) tests may be necessary to make a definitive diagnosis of CAD or estimate the extent of damage. A definitive diagnosis of an AMI (MI) requires the documentation of changes in biochemical markers within 24 to 72 hours of the event (see Chapter 8). In late life, many, but not all, diagnoses of CAD and cardiac events are made at the time of a screening electrocardiogram (ECG). However, because of the high numbers of false-negative ECGs, delayed recognition leads to increases in the rate of complications.

Complications

The potential problems and complications from CAD are the result of either acute or long-term reduced oxygenation of the heart muscle, i.e. angina. In stable angina, all reversible factors are addressed (e.g., smoking, exercise), and most persons are prescribed a combination of aspirin, clopidogrel (Plavix), nitrates, and beta blockers (e.g., metroprolol, atenolol). Unstable angina is characterized by ischemic symptoms

that increase in frequency, intensity, or duration and occur with less and less provocation. It is associated with arrhythmias, tachycardia, and ventricular fibrillation. During more acute events, additional treatment is needed, usually sublingual or aerosol nitroglycerine.

An AMI can cause a small or extensive amount of damage to the heart muscle. The acute event may be triggered by a sudden increase in myocardial oxygen demand, such as from an infection or bleeding and the arteries' inability to respond adequately, or from a sudden occlusion of an artery from a blood clot or plaque passing through a narrowed vessel. Tissue death occurs quickly, and with extensive damage death may follow if the damage is not reversed in the first several hours after the event.

In chronic CHD, the body attempts to compensate for the damage through a process called remodeling in which the heart enlarges and changes shape. This remodeling eventually leads to a decrease in cardiac pumping efficiency, and it can lead to a more gradual onset of heart failure, months or years after the AMI (see below).

PROMOTING HEALTHY AGING; IMPLICATIONS FOR GERONTOLOGICAL NURSING: CORONARY ARTERY DISEASE

As with most chronic conditions, optimizing health for persons with CHD requires a multimodal team approach. After diagnosis, pharmacological management is always required. Lipid-lowering medications, such as the statins, are always recommended regardless of laboratory values. Nonpharmacologic approaches are directed at reducing risk factors and compensating for damage that has already occurred. After an acute event, the person may experience depression and anxiety because of the changes in functional ability, self-image, and fear of another event.

The rehabilitation team includes physical therapists, occupational therapists, counselors, indigenous healers, and nutritionists working alongside the nurse, nurse practitioner, and physician and the patient and significant others. Cardiac exercise rehabilitation programs often are the cornerstone of the plan to return the person to maximum functioning after an acute event. They are designed to build endurance and self-reliance to facilitate self-care and improve quality of life. Typical programs begin with light activity and progress to moderate levels under the supervision of a nurse or physical therapist or both. For more impaired persons, it is necessary to help them identify energy conservation measures applicable to their daily tasks.

Promoting the health of the person with CAD differs from those with other chronic problems in that most exacerbations of CAD require hospitalization and intensive treatment, whereas many of the other chronic disorders can be managed at home. Onset of illness or exacerbation of chronic disorders may be quite different in older clients. For those with cardiac problems, subtle cues of potential alterations in health must be attended to in order to minimize the likelihood of an outcome that is unnecessarily adverse. The nurse can work with the persons and significant others to conduct advanced planning prior to a cardiac crisis.

Heart Failure

Heart failure (HF) is a general term used to describe the end result of the combination of normal changes with aging and other cardiac disorders. As more persons live longer with heart disease, more failure is seen in both men and women, affecting about five million persons in the United States. Seventy-five percent of the 500,000 new cases each year occur to persons over 65 (Bashore et al., 2010). It is the most common cause for hospitalization, re-hospitalization, and disability among persons over age 65 (Figure 15-7). Clinical heart failure is categorized as systolic failure, diastolic failure, or both. End-stage and acute heart failure is known as congestive heart failure (CHF) and is quite common (Auerhahn et al., 2007).

When left ventricular (LV) *systolic* remains within normal limits in the presence of LV *diastolic* dysfunction it is referred to as left-sided failure. The ejection fraction remains ≥50%, but persons are unable to increase their stroke volume with exertion. There is pulmonary and systemic venous congestion with resultant inadequate perfusion.

In contrast, right-sided heart failure is associated with LV systolic dysfunction; the ejection fraction is ≤50%, and the person is symptomatic and may be very ill. Long-standing left-sided failure will eventually cause right-sided failure as well. While the overall prevalence of CHF in African Americans is higher than in whites, persons from the latter group have a 30% to 50% higher rate of hospitalization (Jones-Burton & Saunders, 2006).

Diagnosis is often made empirically, that is, based on presenting symptoms and examination. A definitive diagnosis requires the finding of enlargement of the heart's chambers, especially the ventricles. A determination of ejection fraction (per ECG) is then essential in the determination of the appropriate pharmacological management and advance planning. A serum BNP is useful in differentiating dyspnea due to heart failure with that caused by other conditions. Both the BNP and the N-terminal pro-BNP are excellent biomarkers with similar accuracy (see Chapter 8) (Bashore, et al., 2010).

Etiology

Most heart failure is the result of end-organ damage from pre-existing conditions such as hypertension and coronary heart disease. To compensate for the damage, the heart, especially the ventricles, enlarge and dilate. In most cases, this enlargement decreases heart muscle function as the walls are remodeled but weakened. Eventually, the heart cannot compensate for the lost stroke volume, and evidence of failure appears.

Secondary causes of heart failure include alcohol abuse, cocaine or amphetamine abuse, and chronic hyperthyroidism. Another common cause of the dilated cardiomyopathy of heart failure is inflammation of the heart muscle, a condition termed myocarditis. Myocarditis is usually caused by viral infections but also can be caused by bacterial infections and by non-infectious causes, such as lupus and other inflammatory diseases. Valvular heart disease, especially aortic regurgitation and mitral regurgitation, is increasingly seen as a cause of heart failure, especially as people live longer with these underlying disorders.

Persons with CAD who suffer extensive ischemic damage with necrosis have a high risk of developing heart failure, and its onset can be acute—often within the first few hours or days after an AMI. But even patients with only a moderate amount of muscle damage can eventually advance to heart failure. For these patients, lifestyle adjustments (e.g., smoking cessation) and appropriate drug therapy can often delay or prevent the onset of heart failure. For patients with only moderate muscle damage, whether heart failure ensues depends to a large extent on the health of the remaining heart muscle.

Signs and Symptoms

Failure can appear quickly in persons who suffer simultaneous multivessel myocardial infarctions or more slowly in persons with long-standing and uncontrolled hypertension. If the failure develops slowly, symptoms may not appear until it is quite advanced. It is common for the person to find ways to compensate for declining cardiac function without realizing they are doing so. For example, a person slowly reduces their activity level saying they are "not so fit" (which they attribute to advancing age), when it is a pathological condition that requires treatment. Others may complain of "just not feeling right" or having "a case of the dwindles," complaints that indicate an evaluation for failure or other signs of decline (Box 15-6).

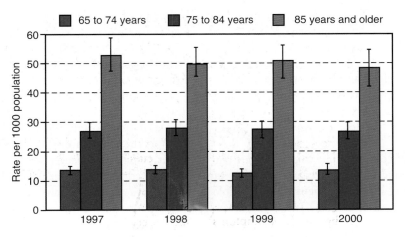

FIGURE 15-7 Hospitalization rate for heart failure. Age adjusted to the 2000 standard population; 95% confidence interval. Heart failure: ICD-9-CM code 428.0. (Data from National Hospital Discharge Survey, NCHS, CDC. Redrawn from www.cdc.gov/nchs/hphome.htm. Focus area No. 12.)

BOX 15-6 SIGNS OF POTENTIAL EXACERBATION OF ILLNESS IN AN OLDER ADULT WITH CORONARY HEART DISEASE

- Lightheadedness or dizziness
- Disturbances in gait and balance
- Loss of appetite or unexplained loss of weight
- Inability to concentrate or shortened attention span
- Changes in personality or mood
- Changes in grooming habits
- Unusual patterns in urination or defecation
- Vague discomfort, frequent bouts of anxiety
- Excessive fatigue, vague pain
- Withdrawal from usual sources of pleasure

BOX 15-7 CLASSIFICATION OF HEART FAILURE BY THE AMERICAN COLLEGE OF CARDIOLOGISTS

STAGE A
High risk but no symptoms or structural disorder (e.g., CAD, HTN)

STAGE B
No symptoms but with structural disorder (e.g., LVH, hx MI)

STAGE C
Current or past symptoms and structural disorder
  Especially dyspnea from LVSD

STAGE D
End-stage disease
  Symptomatic at rest despite optimal treatment

Data from Jessup M, Brozema S: *New England Journal of Medicine* 348:2003, 2007-2018.
CAD, Coronary artery disease; *HTN,* hypertension; *LVH,* left ventricular hypertrophy; *hx,* history; *MI,* myocardial infarction; *LVSD,* left ventricular systolic dysfunction.

BOX 15-8 CLASSIFICATION OF HEART FAILURE BY THE NEW YORK HEART ASSOCIATION

CLASS 1 MILD
No evidence of symptoms at rest or during activity

CLASS 2 MILD
Ordinary activities result in fatigue, palpitation, or dyspnea

CLASS 3 MODERATE
Less than ordinary activities cause symptoms

CLASS 4 SEVERE
Symptoms at rest, any activity increases discomfort

Data from Heart Failure Society of America: The states of heart failure—NYHA classification, 2002. Last modified 9/28/2006. Available at http://www.abouthf.org/questions_stages.htm. Accessed January 15, 2010.

BOX 15-9 ATYPICAL SYMPTOMS OF HEART FAILURE IN OLDER ADULTS

NON-CEREBRAL
- Chronic cough
- Insomnia
- Weight loss
- Nocturia
- Syncope

CEREBRAL
- Delirium
- Falls
- Anorexia
- Decreased functional capacity

Early in left-sided failure, symptoms are present only with exertion, but eventually progress to orthopnea, paroxysmal nocturnal dyspnea, and rest dyspnea. The predominate sign of right-sided failure is edema and hepatic congestion. The typical clinical pattern of a person with heart failure is periods of "baseline" symptomatology, then periods of exacerbation leading to hospitalization for stabilization and a return to baseline. Heart failure symptoms are ranked by their affect on function and activity (Boxes 15-7 and 15-8). As with other disorders, older adults often have atypical manifestations of the disease (Box 15-9).

Complications

Because heart failure is the end-stage of heart disease, the complications are "limited" to exacerbations of symptoms and decline in physical functioning. Common signs of exacerbations of heart failure are often noticeable. They include tachycardia, tachypnea, S3 or S4 gallop, pulmonary crackles, and dependent edema depending on the type of failure. As the severity increases, the pulse pressure narrows and signs of impaired tissue perfusion may develop, such as cool skin and central or peripheral cyanosis. Diminished cognition, perhaps to the point of delirium, is common. Recurrent hospitalization is usually required until the point is reached when only palliative care is possible. Sudden death is always a possibility, especially associated with ventricular tachycardia or fibrillation. In these patients, an episode of syncope should be regarded as a harbinger of sudden death.

PROMOTING HEALTHY AGING; IMPLICATIONS FOR GERONTOLOGICAL NURSING: HEART FAILURE

It is still possible to promote healthy aging in a person with a life-limiting illness such as heart failure. The emphasis is not on a cure, but on alleviating symptoms, improving functioning, minimizing or preventing exacerbations of symptoms, and maximizing both functioning and comfort. In doing so, quality of life may be optimized and hospitalizations delayed or prevented.

Careful pharmacological management is of utmost importance in the control of the disease to prevent ventricular remodeling. Common medications include angiotensin-converting enzyme (ACE) inhibitors, beta-blockers, diuretics, digitalis,

<table>
<tr></tr>
</table>

BOX 15-10	TOPICS OF EDUCATION RELATED TO LIVING WITH HEART FAILURE

1. Activities: pacing and tolerance
2. Exercise: strategizing adherence to prescribed program
3. Medications: timing, side effects, evaluation of effectiveness, obstacles to adherence
4. Disease self-management: signs and symptoms of exacerbation, intake, output and weight, when to call for help or questions, interpreting laboratory values, diet
5. Diet: low cholesterol, fat, and sodium
6. Fluid restriction if necessary

aldosterone antagonists (spironolactone), and, in some cases, isosorbide dinitrate with hydralazine. All of these have been found to improve mortality and quality of life. Calcium channel blockers may worsen the failure and are usually contraindicated.

Non-pharmacological interventions focus on adaptation and function, anticipatory teaching, and advanced care planning. The nurse works with the individual and family to understand all aspects of the disease and its management, as well as strategies to prevent exacerbations and maximize function (Box 15-10). Nurses also work with persons with CHF through specialized heart failure clinics and hospice or palliative care units (Ducharme et al., 2005). The nurse negotiates with the elder for the best way to adhere to drug regimens and lifestyle changes. This includes consistent sodium restriction, in some cases fluid restriction and often supplemental oxygen. The nurse helps the elder determine the best way to perform activities of daily living while not overtaxing the heart. The nurse teaches about the early signs of exacerbations, such as weight changes, and then works to discover the most effective interventions while aggressively pursuing comfort measures.

In some cases, when in otherwise good health, the elder may elect an aggressive approach. If in otherwise relatively good health, some of the options may be resynchronization, a heart transplant, or an implantable cardioverter defibrillator. The nurse helps the patient navigate the considerable ethical and technological challenges of such choices.

In the long-term care setting, the nurse is the key health care provider to promote healthy aging and to advocate and secure appropriate interventions for the elder who is dependent on others. The nurse is responsible for the accurate assessment of the resident's heart sounds, pulses, respiratory status, and oxygenation, as well as the atypical signs and symptoms. Jugular venous distention, unless extreme, is not a reliable indicator in late life due to the loss of adipose tissue in the neck. The nurse is often the first to identify progressive heart failure or sudden decompensation and alerts the resident's nurse practitioner or physician about the changes. The nurse practitioner is then responsible for the prescriptive interventions that are consistent with the latest evidence-based practice and the patient and family wishes and advanced directives.

Peripheral Vascular Disease

Occlusive peripheral vascular disease (PVD) is a cluster of disorders, all of which are the result of vascular insufficiency and damage to the surrounding dependent tissue. The prevalence of PVD increases with age and is ameliorated to some extent when risk factors are addressed, such as smoking cessation. Arterial PVD is known as peripheral artery disease (PAD) (also called *lower extremity arterial disease* [LEAD]). Diagnosis is made through review of symptoms and systems, a physical examination, and ankle-brachial index or Doppler studies. Chronic venous insufficiency (CVI) is the most common PVD seen in older adults.

PAD affects an estimated 12 million persons in the United States and 1 in 20 persons over age 50 (Bashore, et al., 2010). CVI is most common in persons over age 65 and is often associated with DVTs (Rapp et al., 2010). Risk factors, all of which are modifiable, include poor glycemic control and tobacco use; risk persists for >5 years after smoking cessation. (Auerhahn et al., 2007).

Etiology

Atherosclerotic vascular disease is the common cause of PAD. As arterial circulation is compromised, the capacity for oxygenation of the surrounding tissue lessens, pain occurs, and there is a risk for ulceration and gangrene. With complete obstruction, severe ischemic pain and tissue necrosis occur, and amputation may be necessary. Pain from intermittent blockage is referred to as claudication (in the calf or buttock, depending on the vessels involved). Diagnosis is made through review of symptoms and systems, a physical examination, and ankle-brachial index calculation.

Venous insufficiency is the result of reduced circulation back to the heart due to damaged or incompetent venous walls and valves. This occlusion is often the result of a chronic DVT (deep vein thrombosis). Insufficiency affects the deep or superficial veins, resulting in reverse flow and elevated pressure in the veins during ambulation. The vein becomes engorged and the surrounding tissue becomes edematous as a result of increased hydrostatic pressure pushing plasma through the stretched wall. When movement of the extremity is reduced, the circulatory problems are exacerbated. Standing or being immobile for long periods, constricting garments, crossing the legs at the knees, and obesity all significantly increase the chance of the development of venous insufficiency. Early insufficiency is seen as varicose veins, which can progress to CVI. When the ischemia is persistent long enough, the surrounding tissue breaks down, with or without trauma and may produce venous stasis ulcers.

Signs and Symptoms

Up to 50% of those with PVD are symptomatic. Symptoms include pain with use (arterial) and pain at rest (venous). In early PVD, persons are often asymptomatic, with complaints noted only when the disease has progressed. Early complaints may include numbness or tingling in the affected extremity or mild edema with standing. Although both arterial and venous diseases cause tissue necrosis in the end, their signs and symptoms (other than pain) are different, as is the disease management. Persons may also first present with a nonhealing wound. However, the characteristics of discomfort, shape, texture, and location of the wounds help differentiate the cause. In persons with known or suspected PVD, a careful history and ankle brachial index (ABI) measurement is essential to differentiate between PAD and CVI and to determine appropriate treatment.

Venous insufficiency is characterized by progressive edema and pain with dependency; in lighter pigmented persons, the limb is a bluish or purple color from the pooling of the blood. In darker pigmented persons there is a dull gray appearance. Over time, long-standing stasis of blood leads to the deposition of hemosiderin, giving the skin a dark, speckled appearance, especially in the lower calf. Varicosities of the superficial veins may be obvious. Dependent edema, dermatitis, and firm induration are common signs in CVI.

As arterial disease stops the blood from flowing into a limb, the symptoms of arterial insufficiency include resting pain that is classically described as an ache, numbness, or squeezing sensation, often in the arch of the foot and toes but also in the calf, thigh, or buttock. Classically, the pain occurs when the leg is elevated and may awaken the person. It may be instantly relieved when the limb is moved to a dependent position, when gravity helps pull the blood into the ischemic limb. Pain is increased with exertion as the tissue demands more oxygen, and relieved by rest. When elevated, the extremity may be pale and cool, consistent with ischemia; and it may be red or purple with dependency. The skin is shiny, without hair and with thickening of nails. Buerger's sign is the presence of rubor with dependency and rapid blanching with elevation (Begelman, 2004). See Table 15-3 for a comparison of CVI and PAD.

Complications

The most common complications of CVI are pain, the development of skin ulcers, and the risk for amputation. Wounds that result from PVD may never heal, and the extremity may require surgery to save the limb or a portion of it.

Arterial wounds are the result of tissue necrosis. They appear distally, at the ends of the toes, between the toes, over pressure points, on the heels, and over the lateral malleolus. They are round with well-defined edges, dry, necrotic, pale at the base, and without signs of vascularity. A dense, fibrinous exudate (slough) may be present in the ulcer. Intense pain is a hallmark of ischemic ulcers.

Wounds that develop with CVI have irregular borders, are painless, and are located most often at the medial malleolus or on the adjacent tissue. Edema and the continuing increase in hemosiderin deposits make healing difficult.

PROMOTING HEALTHY AGING; IMPLICATIONS FOR GERONTOLOGICAL NURSING: PERIPHERAL VASCULAR DISEASE

The primary management of PVD is addressing the modifiable risk factors that led to the disease itself, skin care, and pharmacological intervention for pain as needed. Optimal control of concurrent problems is essential (e.g., HTN, diabetes, CHD). The day-to-day management of health in the person with PVD falls largely within the scope of practice of the nurse.

Careful assessment of early signs of PVD in persons with CHD includes regular palpation of the peripheral pulses and examination of the color, temperature, and integrity of the extremities. It also means paying careful attention to the patient's report of pain or discomfort, especially related to activities such as walking (Box 15-11). The nurse should suspect arterial insufficiency in patients with coronary artery disease, carotid stenosis, stroke, or dystrophic toenail disease.

The sooner potential or new problems are identified, the less the risk for complications. In persons with PVD, promoting healthy aging means carefully assessing and teaching about skin,

TABLE 15-5	COMPARISON OF ARTERIAL AND VENOUS INSUFFICIENCY OF THE LOWER EXTREMITIES	
CHARACTERISTICS	**ARTERIAL**	**VENOUS**
Pain	Sudden onset with acute; gradual onset with chronic	Deep muscle pain with acute deep vein thrombosis
	Exceedingly painful	Relieved by elevation
	Claudication relieved by rest	
	Rest pain relieved by dependency (with total occlusion, no position will give complete relief)	
Pulses	Absent or weak	Normal (unless arterial disease is also present)
Associated changes in leg and foot	Thin, shiny, dry skin	Firm ("brawny") edema
	Thickened toenails	Reddish brown discoloration with postphlebitic syndrome
	Absence of hair growth	Evidence of healed ulcers
	Temperature variations (cooler if no cellulitis is present)	Dilated and tortuous superficial veins
	Elevational pallor	Swollen limb
	Dependent rubor	Increased warmth and erythema with acute deep vein thrombosis
	Atrophy or no change in limb size	
Ulcer location	Between toes or at tips of toes	Primarily the medial malleolus and the lower leg
	Over phalangeal heads	
	On heels	
	Over lateral malleolus or pretibial area over metatarsal heads, on side or sole of foot	
Ulcer characteristics	Well-defined edges	Uneven edges
	Black or necrotic tissue	Ruddy granulation tissue
	Deep, pale base	Superficial
	Non-bleeding	Bleeding

BOX 15-11   GUIDELINES FOR PERSONS LIVING WITH VENOUS INSUFFICIENCY

GIVE LEGS A REST
Elevate the feet above heart level while sleeping, while sitting and several times a day.

CHANGE POSITIONS FREQUENTLY
Avoid activities that require standing or sitting with feet dangling for long periods.

GIVE LEGS SUPPORT
As directed, wear professionally made compression stockings that apply even pressure from ankles to knees or ankles to hip.
Replace hose as needed to maintain usefulness.
Put hose on early in the morning; wear all day; remove at bedtime.
If a compression pump has been prescribed, follow the instructions.

TAKE CARE OF THE SKIN
Examine feet daily, including the soles, sides and between the toes.
Wash lower legs and feet regularly with mild soap and water.
Use moisturizing cream and emollients after washing.
Do NOT use lanolin or petroleum-based creams when wearing support hose made with latex.
Avoid activities that can injure the legs or feet.
Monitor legs for skin changes:
- Persistent edema
- Discoloration
- Dryness and/or itching
- Any bruises or wounds that do not go away in one week

APPLY DRESSINGS
Follow ulcer care directions as prescribed.

sensation, and circulation. Persons with diabetes will need more specific instruction (see the section on diabetes mellitus later in the chapter).

For persons with arterial insufficiency, exercise rehabilitation and protection of the skin are paramount. Daily skin inspection and protection against the effects of pressure, friction, shear, and maceration are essential for the early detection and prevention of wounds. Nothing should be done that limits circulation in the affected limb. Wearing restrictive clothing and compression stockings are specifically contraindicated. Exercise rehabilitation usually includes establishing a walking program to slowly and steadily increase the pain-free walking distance. The person is asked to walk until maximum tolerable pain occurs, rest, and then continue.

Although the person with chronic vascular insufficiency will need intermittent courses of diuretics for severe edema, the mainstay of management is the use of customized compression stockings. Compression facilitates wound healing, reduces venous dermatitis, improves sclerotic changes, and counteracts venous hypertension. In addition to compression stockings, other devices that have been found useful to improve venous return include Unna boots (or equivalent), pneumatic compression pumps, and orthotic devices. Elevation of the legs above the heart for 30 minutes three to four times a day can reduce edema and improve skin microcirculation.

Although the principles of the management of PVD-related ulcers are similar to those of pressure ulcers, special care must be taken to ensure that venous stasis ulcers and arterial ulcers are differentiated and treated appropriately. Because of the chronic and potentially limb-threatening nature of these ulcers, it is recommended that the nurse consult with colleagues who are wound care specialists to develop the most appropriate treatment plans.

Polymyalgia Rheumatica and Giant Cell (Temporal) Arteritis

Polymyalgia rheumatica (PMR) and Giant Cell Arteritis (GCA), which are different aspects of the same inflammatory vascular disease, co-exist in about 50% of those affected and have similar signs and symptoms, including similar patterns of cytokines. Both are associated with fever, malaise, and weight loss. Fevers occur in absence of an elevation in the white blood count. The differences are singularly important, that is, only GCA can cause blindness if not treated promptly and requires high doses of steroids compared to the lower doses used with PMR. GCA symptoms occur "above the neck," and those of PMR occur below the neck.

Polymyalgia Rheumatica

Polymyalgia rheumatica is characterized and diagnosed by pain and stiffness in the shoulder and pelvic girdle areas, muscles of the neck, shoulders, lower back, buttocks, and thighs. Nocturnal pain, especially in the shoulder, interferes with sleep, and there may be difficulty when trying to stand after sitting for awhile or when getting out of a car or bathtub (gelling phenomenon). Pain is usually greatest at night and in the early morning, but usually no joint inflammation is present. If swelling and joint inflammation are present, rheumatoid arthritis is more likely. A sharply elevated ESR (>50 mm/hr) is common, as well as mild normocytic or normochromic anemia. Diagnosis can be difficult because infection, fibromyalgia, and other diffuse connective tissue diseases may share similar symptoms, and similar pain may occur with statin medication use.

Giant Cell Arteritis

GCA is a granulomatous inflammation of the proximal branches of the aorta and its branches and the cranial arteries—the most common form of vasculitis for this age group. The typical person with GCA is white, female, and older than 70 years (Blumenthal, 2004). It is rare in African Americans or in those of Hispanic descent (O'Rourke, 2003). Initial diagnosis is made empirically and confirmed with a biopsy of the temporal artery.

Due to the affected location being the aorta, the signs and symptoms are associated with ischemia and inflammation of primarily the head. Occasionally symptoms are localized as erythema and swelling of the temporal artery. More often, a temporal headache, jaw or tongue claudication, or sudden vision loss is seen. Overt signs may be preceded by systemic symptoms such as fatigue, muscle weakness, malaise, weight loss, and fever, which is indistinguishable from polymyalgia rheumatic (PMR). Diagnosis is made on the basis of a careful analysis of the signs and symptoms combined with unexplained elevations in ESR (≥40 mm/hr) or C-reactive protein (C-RP) (Hellmann & Imboden, 2010).

The most important complication of GCA is sudden blindness, which can be prevented with prompt treatment. But once it occurs, it is permanent. Persons who have had GCA are 17 times more likely to have a thoracic aneurysm, which develops several years later (Hellmann & Imboden, 2010).

PROMOTING HEALTHY AGING: IMPLICATIONS FOR GERONTOLOGICAL NURSING

For the best outcomes, persons with either PMR or GCA need prompt treatment but especially with GCA. Persons with signs and symptoms of PMR receive low doses (10 to 20 mg) of prednisone. If there is no significant improvement in 72 hours, the diagnosis needs to be reconsidered. If accurate, the ESR and C-RP will return to normal within 14 days (Kreiner, Langberg, Galbo, 2010). However, treatment may continue for up to one year with a slow taper. If tapered too rapidly, a flair will occur. Those with GCA may require an immediate infusion of methlyprednisone, but they will always require a high dose (approximately 60 mg/day). The high dose is continued for about one month, and then a very slow taper is titrated to changes in the ESR of C-RP.

A major complication for both conditions is related to the potentially long-term use of steroids. Efforts should be made to lower the dose to the optimal level to suppress symptoms. Side effects are common and potentially life-threatening, including the development of osteoporosis, myopathy, increased blood glucose levels, and elevated total cholesterol. Nurses monitor glucose levels, blood pressure, and fluid retention. If the elder has diabetes, careful monitoring is particularly important. Relapse is common if the steroids are lowered too quickly.

NEUROLOGICAL DISORDERS

Multiple neurological disorders are seen in older adults. Their effects range from fleeting symptoms to marked cognitive compromise to significant functional decline to death. The three major neurological disorders addressed in this text are the dementia disorders (Chapter 19), the cerebrovascular disorders, and the movement disorder Parkinson's disease. There are many others that are beyond what is possible in this text.

Cerebrovascular Disorders

Cerebrovascular disorders include the Stroke syndromes of transient ischemic attack (TIA) and cerebrovascular accidents (CVA, stroke). Ischemic strokes usually result from a thrombosis or embolism and hemorrhagic strokes from vascular ruptures. Both cause neurological deficits (some transient, others permanent). Because the immediate effects of the events are similar, diagnosis is geared toward identifying the specific cause of the symptoms and location of injury to the brain. *Only when the cause is known can appropriate therapy be implemented.*

TIAs are by their nature highly transient; the associated neurological deficits usually last less than 24 hours, often only 1 or 2 hours. They most often resolve before the person is even seen by a health care provider. Instead, the person reports, "I think I had a small stroke last week." Onset is usually abrupt.

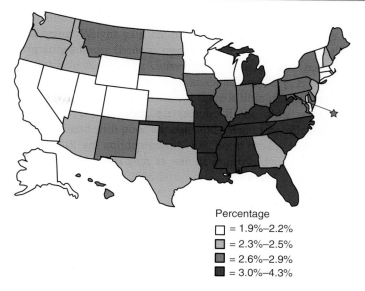

Percentage
- □ = 1.9%–2.2%
- ▨ = 2.3%–2.5%
- ▨ = 2.6%–2.9%
- ■ = 3.0%–4.3%

FIGURE 15-8 Percentage of people who were ever told they had a stroke, 2008. Age adjusted to the 2000 U.S. standard population. (Redrawn from Behavioral Risk Factor Surveillance System (BRFSS): Stroke fact sheet, Atlanta, Georgia, January 2010, Centers for Disease Control and Prevention.)

The signs and symptoms are dependent on the location of the ischemia. While not all persons with TIAs have strokes, about 30% of those who have had strokes also have had TIAs. The greatest risk for a stroke is the first 48 hours following the TIA and declines thereafter (Aminoff, 2010).

About 795,000 people have a stroke in the United States each year, most of which are first-time events; 50% occur to persons over 70. Women have strokes more often (6 out of 10). African Americans have double the number of strokes than white Euro-Americans, and both African Americans and Hispanics are more likely to die (Sugarman, 2010). Stroke is the third most common cause of death behind heart disease and cancer, and it accounts for about 1 in 17 deaths in the United States. The death rates are highest in the eleven "stroke belt" states of the Southeastern United States and lowest in the Northeast and Midwest (Figure 15-8) (CDC, 2010).

Etiology: Ischemic Events

The four main types and causes of ischemic strokes are arterial disease, cardioembolism, hematological disorders, and systemic hypoperfusion; 30% of all ischemic strokes are embolic in nature (Sugarman, 2010). Arterial disease in the form of arteriosclerosis is probably most common. Cardioembolism is caused by an arrhythmia such as atrial fibrillation, frequently seen in coronary heart disease. The use of antithrombotics (e.g., aspirin, warfarin) in persons with heart disease is an attempt to reduce the risk for ischemic events. Hematological disorders include coagulation disorders and hyperviscosity syndromes. Hypoperfusion can occur from dehydration, hypotension (including over-treatment of HTN), cardiac arrest, or syncope.

Etiology: Hemorrhagic Events

Hemorrhagic strokes account for 15% to 20% of all strokes, and 80% of these affect persons between age 40 and 70 (Auerhahn et al., 2007). The primary cause is hypertension and, less often, malformations of the blood vessels (e.g., aneurysms) or cerebral amyloid angiography. A secondary cause is excessive alcohol consumption. Although the exact mechanism is not fully understood, it appears that the chronic hypertension causes thickening of the vessel wall, microaneurysms, and necrosis. When enough damage to the vessel accumulates, it is at risk for rupture. The rupture may be large and acute or small with a slow leaking of blood into the adjacent brain tissue. In many cases, there is a rupture or seepage of blood into the ventricular system of the brain with damage to the affected tissue through necrosis (Boss, 2010a). Resolution of the event can occur only with the resorption of excess blood and damaged tissue. Hemorrhagic strokes are more significantly life threatening but much less frequent than thrombotic strokes.

Signs and Symptoms

Both strokes and TIAs present with acute neurological deficits that are reflective of the part of the brain affected. They are often heralded by a severe headache. In subarachnoid hemorrhages, the headache is not only sudden but is explosive and very severe, but without other neurological manifestations. As treatment varies significantly, it is essential that a differential diagnosis is made with a careful exam and a CAT scan to determine if there is cerebral bleeding.

Some of the clinical signs and symptoms are suggestive of either ischemia or hemorrhage (Box 15-12). Persons with hemorrhage have more focal neurological changes, a more depressed level of consciousness, and a potential for seizures. Focal neurological deficits include alternations in motor, sensory, and visual function; coordination; cognition; and language. The deficits are specific to the area of damage. Nausea and vomiting are suggestions of increased cerebral edema in response to the event. For persons with an ischemic stroke, hypertension and dehydration are common. Care must be taken to avoid both fluid overload and hypoperfusion.

Complications

Early complications of a simple TIA or stroke include extension of the amount of damage and reoccurrence. Brain edema is a problem, especially after a large infarction, and could result in obstructive hydrocephalus (Aminoff, 2010). The long-term effects of a stroke include depression, paralysis and hemiparesis, dysarthrias, dysphagias, and aphasias, depending on type, extent, and area affected. Whenever paralysis results, the development of spasticity in the affected limb(s) is a risk. Spasticity

can lead to contractures if it is not managed. Iatrogenic-type complications include DVT in a flaccid lower limb, aspiration pneumonia, and urinary tract infections. Morbidity following strokes involves neurological and functional deficits and depends on the affected area extent of the brain damage. The person with a period of non-responsiveness is unlikely to survive (Boss, 2010a).

PROMOTING HEALTHY AGING; IMPLICATIONS FOR GERONTOLOGICAL NURSING: TRANSIENT ISCHEMIC ATTACK

Promoting neurological health means working with individuals and the community to prevent TIAs and strokes and helping those affected by the disorders to achieve the highest quality of life possible. The nurse teaches and encourages the family to be alert to the signs and symptoms of stroke and to call the emergency response system quickly for the best outcomes.

Identifying high-risk or stroke-prone elders is something nurses can do in the elders' homes, in the community, or at the health facilities where the nurses work. The Stroke Scale of the National Institute of Health (http://stroke.nih.gov/resources) can be used for this identification. Once identified, persons can be guided and supported in the reduction of modifiable risk factors.

Smoking cessation may be the most important strategy in reducing risk for an initial or recurrent event. Additional primary prevention includes a healthful diet, limiting salt and alcohol, and aspirin therapy unless contraindicated. Tight control of lipids, diabetes, and fibrillation has been found to be helpful, as well as regular exercise and weight-management programs.

Acute medical management of the stroke requires careful attention to the accuracy of the diagnosis. The prompt administration of recombinant tissue-type plasminogen activator [rt-PA] can double the chance of improved outcomes after three months (Auerhahn, et al., 2007). However, it must be given within three hours of the event and *only* for occlusive, ischemic strokes and for persons with an SBP of less than 180 mm Hg and a DBP of less than 110 mm Hg (Aminoff, 2010). If a person with a hemorrhagic stroke were to receive rt-PA, bleeding will be rapidly accelerated by the rt-PA, and the person will die. Therefore, it can only be used if a CT scan confirms the absence of hemorrhage. The initial response to the hemorrhagic stroke is to find a means to stop the bleeding rather than dissolve an occlusion.

Promoting healthy aging post–ischemic stroke begins immediately with anticoagulants or antiplatelets. For those who are aspirin-sensitive, clopidogrel may be used (Box 15-13). Warfarin therapy is recommended for those with atrial fibrillation. Aspiration and sepsis precautions, pneumatic stocking devices, attention to bowel function, physical therapy, and early mobilization are necessary. A period of intense rehabilitation often takes place in a rehabilitation or skilled nursing facility setting and continues long after the person returns home or to an assisted living setting. An important role for the nurse is documenting clearly and in detail the functional capacities that are retained and those that are impaired. The assessment must be

---

BOX 15-12   SYMPTOMS OF TIA OR STROKE

- Sudden weakness or numbness on one side of the body (face, arm, or leg)
- Dimness or loss of vision in one eye
- Slurred speech, loss of speech, difficulty comprehending speech
- Dizziness, difficulty walking, loss of coordination, loss of balance, a fall
- Sudden severe headache
- Difficulty swallowing
- Sudden confusion
- Nausea and vomiting

TIA, Transient ischemic attack.

BOX 15-13 FOCUS ON GENETICS

CLOPIDOGREL (PLAVIX®)

Persons at risk for a heart attack or stroke often take the drug clopidogrel either on-going or following procedures such as stint placements. Its anti-platelet effects have been found to be highly effective in preventing strokes, but not for everyone. Recent studies have found that it is less effective in persons who have variants of the CYP2C19 gene. According to NIH these "reduced-function" variants make it difficult or impossible to convert clopido-grel to its active form. At least one third of all people may carry at least one of the variants of this gene.

Conti V: Gene variants tied to poor outcomes with heart drug. Available at http://www.nih.gov/researchmatters/november2010/11012010heart.htm.

redone routinely to carefully evaluate and document areas of progress, areas of need, and signs of depression, a common sequela.

Support services are available at community or regional stroke centers. The major elements of a stroke center are patient care areas, acute stroke teams, written care protocols, emergency medical services, stroke unit, neurology service, support services, a stroke center director with support from the medical organization, neuroimaging services, laboratory services, outcome and quality improvement activities, and continuing education.

All actual or potential cerebrovascular events are considered emergencies. Management to prevent recurrences and reduce modifiable risk is preventive and geared toward health promotion. Of significant importance is control of diabetes; it appears that persons with diabetes have a two to three times greater chance of stroke (Auerhahn, et al., 2007).

Parkinson's Disease

Parkinson's disease (PD) is a progressive disease of the basal ganglia (corpus striatum) and involves the dopaminergic nigrostriatal pathway. Considered a movement disorder, PD affects approximately 1.5 million people in the United States or 1% to 2% of the population. It appears to be slightly more common in men than in women, and the average age of onset is about 60 years. All races and ethnicities throughout the world appear to be affected; however, a number of studies have found a higher incidence in developed countries. It is speculated that this might be related to the use of pesticides or other toxins. PD is the second most common neurodegenerative disease after stroke.

PD is considered a terminal diagnosis. However, progression of the disease may take many years. Older age at onset and the presence of rigidity/hypokinesia as an initial symptom may predict a more rapid rate of motor progression and increase the urgency for advance care planning.

PD has such an insidious onset that it may be very difficult to diagnose, particularly in the early stages. By the time a person becomes overtly symptomatic, 80% to 90% of the dopamine-producing cells are lost (Boss, 2010b). Symptoms vary, and the intensity of symptoms also varies from person to person; some become severely disabled, and others experience only minor motor disturbances. Diagnosis is one of exclusion and may include a "challenge test" in which levodopa is administered. If symptoms improve, then a diagnosis of PD is made. Early falls, poor response to levodopa, symmetry of motor symptoms, lack of tremor, and early autonomic dysfunction are characteristic of other neurological disturbances.

Etiology

About 10% of persons with Parkinson's disease have a familial form; the majority of cases are sporadic or idiopathic. Several genes have been identified as associated with PD, but the trigger that activates them to evidence of disease is not known (Boss, 2010b).

If onset is early, it is more often of genetic origin; some cases have been linked to specific gene mutations. PD is the result of a deficiency of the neurotransmitter dopamine in the substantia nigra. The severity is associated with the degree of neuron loss and the reduction of dopamine receptors in the basal ganglia.

In *primary* parkinsonism, either the cause is known or it is a secondary effect of another disorder causing loss or interference with the action of dopamine in the basal ganglia (e.g., head trauma, postencephalitic parkinsonism, stroke, tumors, and toxin- and drug-induced parkinsonian syndrome). Epidemiological data suggest genetic, viral, and toxic (pesticide exposure) causes. *Idiopathic* parkinsonism is a term describing a disorder for which a cause has not yet been found.

Signs and Symptoms

While resting tremors are thought of as the key sign of PD, the most common early sign is actually akinesia or an absence or poverty of movement. All the striated muscles in the extremities, trunk, and ocular area, are affected, including the muscles of mastication (chewing), deglutition (swallowing), and articulation. The face is also affected; there is little animation (called *masked facies*) and infrequent blinking. Other signs are micrographia, bradykinesia (slow movement); rigidity; and abnormalities of posture, balance, and gait. Resting tremors are also classic signs but do not always occur.

Muscle rigidity impedes both passive and active movement. On exam of the upper extremities, there is notable "cogwheel" movement, that is, if nurses were to conduct a test of passive ROM, the extremity movement alternates with resistance. Severe muscle cramps may occur in the toes or hands. Postural reflexes are lost. The elder will have involuntary flexion of the head and neck, a stooped posture, and a tendency to fall backward.

The characteristic gait consists of very short steps and minimal arm movements and is called festination. Initiating movement is difficult, but once it starts the person moves forward with small steps and a forward lean. "Freezing" occurs. That is, if movement is stopped for any reason, the person has the appearance of being frozen in movement and restarting is difficult once again. Turning is difficult and may require many steps. If off balance, correction is very slow, so falls are common.

When present, tremors are asymmetrical and rhythmic, of low-amplitude, and disappear briefly during voluntary movement. The arm and hand are most commonly affected, but so might the leg, foot, and head. They are not present during sleep. All tremors increase with stress and anxiety.

While they may appear at different times, bradykinesia, tremor at rest, rigidity, and akinesia all will appear to some degree. Other clinical signs include sleep/wake reversals, constipation, fatigue, excessive salivation, pain, loss of smell, depression, visual disturbances, psychosis, seborrhea, sweating, and hypotension.

Complications

In late stages of the disease, complications such as pressure ulcers, pneumonia, aspiration, and falls can lead to death. Depression and the development of dementia are very common (See Chapter 19). While functional disabilities are inevitable, the greatest cause is rigidity, slowed movements, and postural instability.

PROMOTING HEALTHY AGING; IMPLICATIONS FOR GERONTOLOGICAL NURSING: PARKINSON'S DISEASE

Drug therapy focuses on replacing, mimicking, or slowing dopamine breakdown. The first-line drug approach to symptom management is most often the combination of carbidopa and levodopa in the form of Sinemet, a dopamine precursor. It must be taken one hour before or two hours after a meal to minimize GI side effects and given routinely and on time to prevent fluctuations in symptoms. While Sinemet can be highly and rapidly effective, its efficacy decreases with long-term use. Dopamine agonists such as pramipexole and ropinirole are sometimes used early in the disease or concurrently with Sinemet. These and other drugs used for movement disorders have the potential for serious side effects, including hallucinations, sleep disorders, hypotension, dyskinesias, and dystonia (see Chapter 9).

Surgical procedures include ablation (pallidotomy/thalamotomy), deep brain stimulation (DBS), and transplantation. DBS is the most commonly performed and is used in patients who have not responded to drug therapy or have intractable motor fluctuations, dyskinesias, or tremor. Transplantation is in the experimental stage. Research is ongoing and has shown promising results for both DBS and transplantation (American Academy of Neurology, 2006).

PROMOTING HEALTHY AGING: IMPLICATIONS FOR GERONTOLOGICAL NURSING

Nursing interventions can contribute greatly to quality of life and functional ability of the person with neurological disorders and reduce the burden load for their significant others (Box 15-14). These include comprehensive functional assessments with detailed fall assessments and risk reduction interventions. The goal of treatment is to preserve self-care abilities and prevent complications. There are many nonpharmacological interventions that contribute to the attainment of these goals.

Training in relaxation, stress management, and self-care management may be beneficial in helping people cope. Support groups may help the family and the person to cope with the losses associated with PD. Exercise, walking, ROM, and balance work begin early in the course of the disease, and physical therapy evaluation and treatment are important. Occupational therapy can assist with adaptive equipment, such as weighted utensils, nonslip dinnerware, and other self-care aids. Speech therapy is beneficial for dysarthria and dysphagia, and patients can be taught facial exercises and swallowing techniques.

In caring for persons with neurological disorders, regular pain assessments and appropriate management are also essential (see Chapter 17). In PD, the rigidity, contractures, and dystonias may cause a considerable amount of pain. There is also a recognized but not well understood central-pain syndromes associated with the disease itself. In stroke syndromes, the focus is primarily on neuralgias and pain associated with complications, such as pressure ulcers (see Chapter 11).

Persons with PD experience a change in roles, activities, and social participation due to the disability that accompanies movement disorders. Tremors may produce embarrassing movements. The expressionless face, slowed movement, and soft, monotone speech or aphasias may give the impression of apathy, depression, and disinterest and discourage others who might otherwise be socially active. Others, observing these symptoms, may feel that the person is unable to participate in activities and relationships and may even think the person is cognitively impaired. A sensitive nurse is aware that the visible

---

BOX 15-14   HAVING PARKINSON'S DISEASE

Parkinson is the name of the disease we got
It can strike anyone when it's cold or when it's hot
You might get tremors that cause you to shake
But living with them is a piece of cake
Stiffness of the body occurs in some
And you shuffle your feet like some old bum
Slurring of your speech makes others think you're drunk
But faith keeps you going and you gotta have spunk
Sometimes when you're walking you freeze and cannot move
And people who are watching think you've missed the groove
Penmanship is a thing of the past
In a handwriting contest you'd come in last
Simple little movements like getting in a car
Turn into big projects like draining a reservoir
You get going walking and fell like you're falling
If you weren't so stubborn you'd feel like bawling
Frequent naps are a plus if you like to sleep
But along comes your caregiver and your sleep isn't deep
Your instant response to an act that calls for action
Is harder to do than figuring out a fraction
Sharing your problems with others like you
For yourself is the best thing you can do
You meet with your cohorts in a support group
And you're with people that also have your droop
You're all in the same boat you are all afflicted
You take so many pills you think you're addicted
It's not all bad no matter what you say
You make new friends most every day
And you'll still live to a ripe old age
And no one will put you away in a cage
So don't you worry that I'm not going to fret
I'm still on this earth fighting for all I can get
For all your tribulation and what you gotta do
Chin up comrades learn to laugh at "YOU"

Author: Ken Weber, Sheboygan Wisconsin, 1987. Poem appeared in a Parkinson's Foundation newsletter.

symptoms produce an undesired façade that may hide an alert and responsive individual who wishes to interact but is trapped in a body that no longer cooperates.

Treatment focuses on relieving symptoms with medication, increasing functional ability, preventing excess disability, and decreasing risk of injury. The promotion of healthy aging for the persons with neurological disorders requires a skilled and caring interdisciplinary team to work with both the person and his or her significant others. This includes nurses; neurologists; physical, occupational and speech therapists; and support persons to work with the family as the disease progresses. When PD is in the early stages and symptoms are well maintained by first-line drugs, care is usually provided in the primary care setting by nurse practitioners and internists/geriatricians. Pharmacological interventions are also used for both the prevention and treatment of stroke syndromes. As the disease progresses or for those at risk for complications, a neurologist becomes the leader of the health care team.

The nurse also has an active role in tertiary prevention. The nurse works to prevent skin breakdown and falls, identifies confusion, monitors the lungs for pneumonia, and ensures and maximizes the capacity for self-care, especially related to mobility and activity, eating, maintaining adequate fluid intake, and continence. The nurse is alert for problems with sleep, constipation, and depression. The nurse acts as an advocate in the recommendation to or participation in support groups for both the persons and their significant others or caregivers.

Nowhere in the care of elders is the multidisciplinary team more essential than in the care of persons with a neurological disorder. The assessment of needs after stroke is extremely complex; it requires evaluation by a team coordinated by a nurse and includes a neurologist; a physiatrist; speech, occupational, and physical therapists; an ophthalmologist; a rehabilitation specialist; and a psychologist. It also may include a spiritual advisor. It always includes the person's significant other, who may be involved with the day-to-day life and needs of the elder after a stroke. The gerontological nurse is challenged to take an active role in improving the quality of life of all elders, especially those with functional limitations.

ENDOCRINE DISORDERS

As with most other systems, the signs and symptoms of endocrine disorders may be subtle and nonspecific. Their presence may only become known during a routine laboratory exam or in the work-up for vague symptoms, such as confusion or falling. The two endocrine disorders addressed in this chapter are diabetes mellitus and thyroid disturbances.

Diabetes Mellitus

Diabetes mellitus (DM) is a syndrome of disorders of glucose metabolism resulting in hyperglycemia. The two main forms are type 1 (T1DM) and type 2 (T2DM). Age alone is a major risk factor (Figure 15-9). Ninety percent of older adults with DM have Type 2. A third category of DM is related to a number of unique conditions, such as following a course of steroids or infection of the pancreas. Other metabolic disorders include impaired fasting glucose (IFG) and impaired glucose tolerance (IGT). Persons with IFG or IGT are at high risk for a

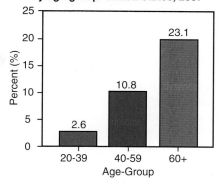

Estimated total prevalence of diabetes in people ages 20 years or older by age-group. United States, 2007

FIGURE 15-9 Prevalence of diabetes among older adults. (Data from 2003-2006 National Health and Nutrition Examination Survey estimates of total prevalence (both diagnosed and undiagnosed) projected to year 2007.)

BOX 15-15	RISK FACTORS FOR DIABETES MELLITUS

Hispanic men*
African-American men and women*
Increasing age
Blood pressure ≥140/90 mm Hg
First-degree relative (parent, sibling, child) with diabetes mellitus (DM)
History of impaired glucose tolerance or impaired fasting plasma glucose
Abnormal lipid levels
Signs of insulin resistance, e.g., acanthosis nigricans or polycystic ovarian syndrome
Obesity: ≥120% of desirable weight or body mass index (BMI) ≥30 kg/m²
History of vascular disease
Previous gestational DM or having had a child with a birth weight of ≥9 pounds
Undesirable lipid levels: high-density lipoproteins (HDLs) ≤35 mg/dL or triglycerides ≥250 mg/dL

*data regarding other groups is less accurate

progression to DM (Box 15-15). Those with problems in glucose metabolism often have problems with metabolism of lipids and proteins as well. When suspicions of DM are suggested by clinical signs and symptoms, the diagnosis requires specific laboratory testing (Box 15-16).

In 2007, 12.2 million persons or 23.1% of all persons at least age 60 in the United States were known to have diabetes (National Institute of Diabetes and Digestive and Kidney Diseases [NIDDK], 2010a). The overall death rate for persons with diabetes is double that of those without. It is the leading cause of end-stage renal disease and blindness and is strongly associated with heart disease.

The prevalence of diabetes varies considerably by ethnicity and gender (Figure 15-10). The rate is highest among Hispanic men and women and black women. Data from other groups are less accurate.

Etiology

T1DM is the result of absolute insulin deficiency due to autoimmune destruction of the β cells in the pancreas. T2DM is most

BOX 15-16   DIAGNOSIS OF DISORDERS OF GLUCOSE METABOLISM

DIAGNOSIS OF DIABETES MELLITUS REQUIRES EITHER:

ONE fasting hemoglobin A1C value of ≥6.5% tested by a certified laboratory*
OR
ONE random plasma glucose ≥200 mg/dL when exhibiting symptoms
OR
TWO of any combination of positive tests on different days:
- Fasting plasma glucose (FPG) ≥126 mg/dL on separate occasions (Note: This is not blood glucose levels that are obtained with a fingerstick.)
- Oral glucose tolerance test (OGTT) ≥200 mg/dL 2 hours after glucose
- Random plasma glucose ≥200 mg/dL without symptoms

DIAGNOSIS OF IMPAIRED FASTING GLUCOSE (IFG) REQUIRES:

Fasting blood glucose between 110 and 125 mg/dL

DIAGNOSIS OF IMPAIRED GLUCOSE TOLERANCE REQUIRES:

Glucose between 141 and 199 mg/dL 2 hours after a glucose challenge

*There remains controversy as to the exact cut off to use.

BOX 15-17   SIGNS AND SYMPTOMS SUGGESTIVE OF DIABETES

1. General symptoms such as polyphagia, polyuria, polydipsia, and occasional weight loss
2. Recurrent infections, particularly of bacterial or fungal origin, that involve the skin, intertriginous areas, or urinary tract and sores or wounds that tend to heal slowly
3. Neurological dysfunction, including paresthesia, dysesthesia, or hyperesthesia; muscle weakness and pain (amyotrophy); cranial nerve palsies; and autonomic dysfunction of the gastrointestinal tract (diarrhea); cardiovascular system (orthostatic hypotension, arrhythmias); reproductive system (impotence); and bladder (atony, overflow incontinence)
4. Arterial disease (macroangiopathy) involving the cardiovascular, cerebrovascular, or peripheral vasculature structures
5. Small-vessel disease (microangiopathy) involving the kidneys (proteinuria, glomerulopathy, uremia) and eyes (macular disease, exudates, hemorrhages)
6. Lesions of the skin, such as Dupuytren's contractures, facial rubeosis, and diabetic dermopathy
7. Endocrine-metabolic complications, including hyperlipidemia, obesity, hypertension

Data from Beers MH (ed.): Disorders of Carbohydrate Metabolism (chapter 64, updated February 2006). In *Merck manual of geriatrics*, ed 3. Available at http://www.merck.com/mkgr/mmg/home.jsp.

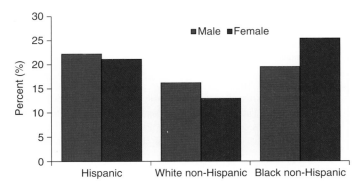

FIGURE 15-10 Percent of persons age 65 and over (age-adjusted) reporting diabetes mellitus, by sex and race/ethnicity, 2004-2005. (Redrawn from Trends in Health and Aging. Available at www.cdc.gov/nchs/agingact.htm. Accessed November 11, 2010.)

commonly due to combination of relative insulin deficiency and insulin resistance. Genetics, lifestyle, and aging are all of significant influence (NIDDK, 2007).

Signs and Symptoms

Although the classic symptoms (i.e., polyuria, polyphagia, and polydipsia) may be seen with plasma glucoses of more than 200 mg/dL, these may not be present with lesser elevations or in older adults. The presentation in elders is more often one of dehydration, confusion, delirium, and decreased visual acuity. In severe cases, the person may be found obtunded in a nonketotic hyperglycemic-hyperosmolar coma (Box 15-17) (Beers, 2006a). Instead of urinary frequency, glycosuria often causes incontinence. Women may present with recurrent candidiasis as the first sign. The catabolic state caused by lack of insulin causes polyphagia in younger persons but causes weight loss and anorexia in elders. Other vague signs and symptoms include fatigue, nausea, delayed wound healing, and paresthesias (Jones et al., 2010). Ketosis is more common among African-American elders.

Complications

Both the onset and development of complications are insidious; fatigue, weight loss, and muscle weakness may be expected. The long-term complications of DM are microvascular, macrovascular, or both and are related to prolonged periods of hyperglycemia leading to glycosylation of proteins and the production of by-products, which, in turn, cause tissue damage. Diabetes is associated with a high rate of depression, and those who are depressed have a higher mortality rate.

Complications are many, including heart disease, stroke, painless neuropathy and periodontal disease. Adults with diabetes have two to four times the rate of heart disease and stroke accounting for 82% of deaths. Nerve damage occurs in 60% to 70% of persons ranging from peripheral neuropathy to gastroporesis (NIDDK, 2010a). Wound healing is delayed, which may lead to amputation when combined with peripheral neuropathy. Older adults with DM are at higher risk for geriatric syndromes such as falls, incontinence, and confusion. Both amputations and orchidectomy occur more often in black men than in any other group. This appears related to disparities in care rather than biology (Smedley, 2003).

Combined macrovascular and microvascular damages lead to sexual dysfunction. Impotence in men is a result of reduction in vascular flow, peripheral neuropathy, and uncontrolled circulating blood glucose. Sexual dysfunction is two to five times greater in this group than in the general population.

Persons with DM commonly have problems with their lower extremities, which can have a considerable impact on functional status. Warning signs of foot problems include cold feet and intermittent claudication, neuropathic burning, tingling, hypersensitivity, and numbness of the extremities. Infections are common and difficult to treat. Both infections and many antibiotics may result in unstable glucose control.

Hypoglycemia (blood glucose <60 mg/dL) can occur from many causes, such as unusually intense exercise, alcohol intake, or medication mismanagement (Jones et al., 2010). Signs in the older adult include tachycardia, palpitations, diaphoresis, tremors, pallor, and anxiety. Later symptoms may include headache, dizziness, fatigue, irritability, confusion, hunger, visual changes, seizures, and coma. Immediate care involves giving the patient glucose either by mouth or intravenously.

Hyperglycemia appears to be well tolerated in later life. It is not unusual to find persons with fasting glucose levels of 300 mg/dL or higher. Because of this ability to tolerate high levels of circulating glucose, there is a higher risk for hyperosmolar hyperglycemic non-ketonic coma. This is especially important in persons who are otherwise medically frail and should be considered in any older adult with diabetes who is difficult to arouse. This is always considered an emergency.

PROMOTING HEALTHY AGING: IMPLICATIONS FOR GERONTOLOGICAL NURSING

The goals of nursing care of persons with diabetes are to maintain the older adult with the best health that is realistically possible and ensure that the person obtains at least the established minimum standards of care (Box 15-18). Caring for the elder with diabetes centers on prevention, early identification, and delay of complications as long as possible (Box 15-19). For persons at higher risk for DM, especially those with IFG or IGT, attention should be directed toward reducing the risk for the progression to DM. This means education and interventions to lower glucose, control blood pressure and blood lipids, and reduce to or maintain one's ideal body weight (see Table 15-5).

While glycemic control is important, more emphasis is now on the prevention of cardiovascular diseases. With benefits of better control of blood pressure and lipids seen at two to three years, promoting health in this area has the potential to be the most efficacious in the minimization of complications (Auerhahn et al., 2007). Research has indicated that it may take eight years of glycemic control before benefits are seen. At all times, interventions must be considered in the context of the life expectancy and cost:benefit ratio for the person. They are geared toward supporting self-efficacy of the patient and significant others.

Screening for DM by fasting plasma and random blood glucose testing is important for early identification of potential or actual disease. Nurses participate in screenings at community health fairs and in clinical settings. Nurses also participate in community education about the need for early diagnosis, glycemic control, and the prompt treatment of complications (Table 15-6). Some nurses make caring for persons with diabetes their professional focus and obtain additional preparation to become certified diabetes educators and clinicians.

Promoting healthy aging in the person with diabetes requires an array of interventions and an interdisciplinary team working together with the patient and his or her family/significant others in culturally appropriate ways (e.g., the persons who prepares meals). This includes ancillary nursing staff and licensed nurses, nutritionists, pharmacists, podiatrists, ophthalmologists, physicians, nurse practitioners, certified diabetic educators, and counselors. The nurse serves as team leader, educator, care provider, advocate, supporter, and guide. If the person's

---

BOX 15-18   EVIDENCED-BASED CARE: MINIMUM STANDARDS OF CARE FOR THE PERSON WITH DIABETES

- At each visit:
  - Monitor weight and BP
  - Inspect feet
  - Review self-monitoring glucose record
  - Review/adjust medications as needed
  - Review self-management skills/goals
  - Assess mood
- Quarterly visits:
  - Obtain Hemoglobin A1C (biannually if stable)
- Annual visits:
  - Obtain fasting lipid profile and serum creatinine
  - Obtain albumin to creatinine ratio
  - Refer for dilated eye exam
  - Perform comprehensive foot exam
  - Refer to dentist for comprehensive exam and cleaning
  - Administer influenza vaccination
- Once in lifetime:
  - Administer pneumococcal vaccination (consider repeat if over 5-10 years)

Modified from: National Diabetes Education Program: *Guiding principles for diabetes care: For health care professionals*, revised April 2009. Available at http://ndep.nih.gov/publications/PublicationDetail.aspx?PubId=108. Accessed January 17, 2011.

BOX 15-19   MINIMIZING CARDIOVASCULAR RISK IN PERSONS WITH DIABETES

- Eat a healthy diet (lower carbohydrate, lower sodium)
- Attain and maintain a healthy weight
- Get regular exercise
- Keep the BP <130/80
- Stop smoking
- Attain and maintain acceptable lipid levels
  - Cholesterol <200
  - LDL <100
  - HDL <40
  - Triglycerides <150

BP, Blood pressure; LDL, low-density lipoprotein; HDL, high-density lipoprotein.

TABLE 15-6   MAINTAINING GLYCEMIC CONTROL

	PREPRANDIAL	PEAK POST-PRANDIAL	3 AM
Capillary plasma glucose (mg/dL)	70-130	<180	>65

Data from National Diabetes Education Program. Modified from: National Diabetes Education Program: Guiding principles for diabetes care: For health care professionals, revised April 2009. Available at http://ndep.nih.gov/publications/PublicationDetail.aspx?PubId=108. Accessed January 18, 2011.

disease is hard to control, endocrinologists are involved, and as complications develop, more specialists are called in, such as nephrologists, cardiologists, and wound care specialists. Nurses are expected to advocate for elders and encourage them to expect and receive quality care to prevent the devastating end results of poor management.

Assessment

Health promotion for older adults with DM begins with a comprehensive geriatric assessment, especially for those with significant co-morbidities or functional limitations. Due to the high prevalence of heart disease, the initial standard assessment includes examination of pulses, lipid and thyroid panels, ECG, and other tests as indicated. This includes identifying risk to end-organs and their current status (Box 15-20). Laboratory testing includes urinalysis for protein and microalbumin; blood studies of blood urea nitrogen (BUN), albumin, and creatinine level; and the calculations of creatinine clearance and the albumin-creatinine ratio. The measurement of a glyconated hemoglobin A 1 C is the best measure of ongoing glycemic control and can now be used as a diagnostic indicator as well ($\geq 6.5\%$) (see Chapter 8) (Figure 15-11). A dilated funduscopic assessment by an ophthalmologist determines the presence of microvascular retinal changes. Assessment of painless neuropathy requires a careful neurological examination with an emphasis on sensation and history of functioning. Clinical guidelines suggest that the best means of testing neurological and sensory intactness is the use of the Semmes-Weinstein–type monofilament (Feng, et al., 2009) (Figure 15-12). The measurement of height, weight, and waist circumference may be used to calculate the BMI, however for the very old, BMI is less useful because of the replacement of muscle mass with adipose tissue. More importantly, assessment includes a careful inspection of the feet, skin, and mouth for signs of injury or the presence of lesions.

Assessing economic resources helps establish the ability to purchase medication, equipment, materials, and special foods that may be needed. Medication history of over-the-counter and prescription drugs and the use of alcohol and tobacco are all components of the assessment of someone with diabetes. All have a direct or indirect effect on renal, circulatory,

neurological, and nutritional function. The nurse uses a complete assessment to work with the elder and significant others to develop the plan of care related to both pharmacological and nonpharmacological approaches to everyday life. Finally, assessment of mood and coping is an essential component so that timely and effective interventions can be initiatied.

Medications

Promoting healthy aging with DM requires the elder and the nurse to develop expertise in the use of pharmacological interventions. These include the antiglycemics and preventive adjuvant therapy, such as ACE inhibitors and aspirin. Both have been demonstrated to improve outcomes in persons with diabetes. Medications are prescribed according to the insulin deficit identified: no secretion of insulin, insulin resistance, or inadequate secretion of insulin. Each class of drugs used has its own set of advantages and potential dangers. For example, metformin (Glucophage) is commonly prescribed for persons with T2DM. However, it is contraindicated in persons with

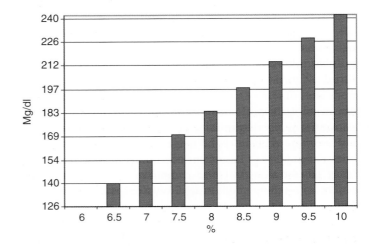

FIGURE 15-11 Comparison of HgbA1C(%) and estimated Average Glucose conversion (eAG)
Formula: $28.7 \times A1C - 46.7 = eAG$.
(Data from National Diabetes Education Program: Guiding principles for diabetes care: for health care professionals, NIH Publication No. 09-4343 NDEP-16, revised April 2009.)

BOX 15-20	FACTORS INCREASING RISK FOR DIABETES-RELATED COMPLICATIONS

- Diabetes for longer than 10 years
- Male
- Poor glucose control
- Cardiovascular, retinal, or renal complications

INCREASED RISK FOR AMPUTATION WITH THE FOLLOWING:
- Peripheral neuropathy with loss of sensation
- Evidence of increased pressure (redness, bony deformity)
- Peripheral vascular disease (diminished or absent pedal pulses)
- History of ulcers
- History of amputation
- Severe nail pathology

Data from American Diabetes Association. *Diabetes Care* 25:S69, 2002.

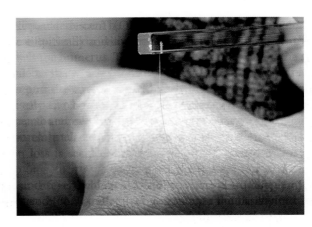

FIGURE 15-12 Semmes-Weinstein-type monofilament. (Courtesy of AliMed, Dedham, Massachusetts.)

renal insufficiency (serum creatinine ≥1.5 mg/dL in men and ≥1.4 mg/dL in women) often seen in later life. Insulin and sulfonylureas are inexpensive but also significantly increase the risk for hypoglycemia, which is particularly dangerous for older adults. If insulin is needed on a regular basis, the use of the implantable pump that monitors blood sugars and administers insulin as needed has revolutionized diabetes management for those who are candidates for this intervention.

If other medications are prescribed, they are carefully reviewed. The effects of drugs on blood glucose must be seriously considered because a number of medications commonly used for elders adversely affect blood glucose levels. Therefore, older adults should be advised to ask if the particular drug prescribed affects their therapy and should check with their primary care provider or endocrinologist before taking any over-the-counter medications.

Nutrition

Adequate and appropriate nutrition is a key factor in healthy living with DM. An initial nutrition assessment with a 24-hour recall will provide some clues to the patient's dietary habits, intake, and style of eating (see Chapter 14). If a recall is not possible, have the person bring in his or her grocery list or receipt for the past week. If the elder is from an ethnic group different from the nurse, the nurse will need to learn more about the usual ingredients and methods of food preparation to be able to give reasonable instructions. Ideally, all persons with diabetes should have culturally appropriate medical nutrition therapy by a registered dietitian annually. At the time of this writing, this service was covered by Medicare.

It is part of the nurse's responsibility to learn if access to food is difficult (including food preparation and shopping for food) and if adequate funds are available for the purchase of fresh fruits, vegetables, and other ingredients for healthful eating. Working with elders' dietary habits that have been formed over a lifetime may be difficult but not impossible. If the person is overweight or obese, a weight-loss plan is important. Control of diet (especially of portions) and weight loss may also prevent the person with impaired fasting glucose or impaired glucose tolerance from developing DM. Reductions of as little as 10% in weight will improve glycemic control and may reduce the need for oral antihyperglycemic agents or insulin or enable the DM to be controlled by diet and exercise alone.

Exercise

Exercise is also an important avenue toward healthy living with DM, because exercise increases insulin production and may increase tissue sensitivity. Walking is an inexpensive and beneficial way to exercise, however it needs to be done in a safe location, which cannot be assumed to be one's neighborhood. Exercise in conjunction with an appropriate diet may be sufficient to maintain blood glucose levels within normal levels in some cases. A more intensive exercise program should not be started until the older adult has consulted with his or her health care provider. Those who have limited mobility can still do chair exercises or, if possible, use exercise machines that enable sitting and holding on for support.

If the person is using insulin, exercise needs to be done on a regular rather than an erratic basis, and blood glucose must be checked before and after exercise to avoid or respond promptly to hypoglycemia. A large number of resources are available about exercise and diabetes are available at through the National Institute of Diabetes and Digestive Disgestive Disorders (http://diabetes.niddk.nih.gov/index.htm).

Self-Care

Because of the chronicity and complexity of DM in late life, maximum wellness is difficult to achieve without considerable self-care skills (Box 15-21). The nurse is often the professional who is responsible for working with the elder in developing such skills. In addition to diet, exercise, and medication use already discussed, self-care skills include self-monitoring of blood glucose, optimal care of the feet, "sick-day" adjustments, and knowledge about the disease and the care expected. Knowing the signs of hypoglycemia and hyperglycemia and what to do about these are diabetes self-management essentials. An identification bracelet is recommended as confusion or delirium may be a manifestation of low blood sugar and misinterpreted as dementia, which delays treatment. Self-care also includes preventive care practices for the eyes, kidneys, and feet. Nurses support patients in obtaining the needed services. Annual diabetes self-management training is covered by Medicare.

Implications for the Long-Term Care Setting

Many residents of long-term care facilities have DM. In this setting, the nurse is responsible for many of the activities that would otherwise fall on the patient or a home caregiver in addition to those as a professional. Meals, nutritional status, intake and output, and exercise/activity are monitored. The nurse assesses the person for signs of hypoglycemia and

---

BOX 15-21 SELF-CARE SKILLS NEEDED FOR THE PERSON WITH DIABETES

GLUCOSE SELF-MONITORING
Obtaining a blood sample correctly
Using the glucose monitoring equipment correctly
Troubleshooting when results indicate an error
Recording the values from the machine
Understanding the timing and frequency of the self-monitoring
Understanding what to do with the results

MEDICATION SELF-ADMINISTRATION
Where Appropriate, Insulin Use
Selecting appropriate injection site
Using correct technique for injections
Disposing of used needles and syringes correctly
Storing and transporting insulin correctly

Oral Medication Use
Knowing drug, dose, timing, and side effects.
Knowing drug-drug and drug-food interactions
Recognizing side effects and knowing when to report

FOOT CARE AND EXAMINATION
Selecting and using appropriate and safe footwear

HANDLING SICK DAYS
Recognizing the signs and symptoms of both hyperglycemia and hypoglycemia

hyperglycemia and evidence of complications. The nurse ensures that the standards of care for the person with DM are met. The nurse monitors the effect and side effects of diet, exercise, and medication use. The nurse administers or supervises the administration of medications. If the person requires what is called sliding scale insulin, wherein the dosage depends on the current glucose reading, it is the nurse who must make the determination of the dosage under "sliding scale" guidelines.

Thyroid Disease

Estimates of the prevalence of thyroid disease vary from 0.5% to 5% for overt hypothyroidism and 0.5% to 2.3% hyperthyroidism. Between 5% and 10% of older adults may have subclinical hypothyroidism. While easy to diagnose, many of the signs and symptoms in an older population are unfortunately non-specific, atypical, or absent. Signs such as a decline in cognitive function or functional status may be incorrectly attributed to normal aging, another disorder, or to side effects of medications. If abnormal the TSH is followed by the measurement of the thyroid hormone thyroxine (T4) and T3. When a patient presents with multiple symptoms without a marked change in laboratory findings, a diagnosis of subclinical disease may be made. The TSH is elevated in hypothyroidism as the pituitary gland tries to stimulate the underfunctioning thyroid; the TSH is decreased in hyperthyroidism as the pituitary gland responds to the elevated blood levels of T4 (see Chapter 8). The most common thyroid disturbance in older adults is hypothyroidism.

Etiology

Hypothyroidism, insidious in onset, is thought to be caused most frequently by chronic autoimmune thyroiditis. It may be iatrogenic, resulting from radioiodine treatment, subtotal thyroidectomy, or a number of medications. It can also be caused by a pituitary or hypothalamic abnormality (Jones et al., 2010).

Grave's disease is the most common cause of hyperthyroidism in elders. Thyroid disease from multinodular toxic goiter and adenomas are more common among older than younger adults. It can also result from ingestion of iodine or iodine-containing substances, such as seafood, radio-contrast agents, and the medication amiodarone, a commonly prescribed antiarrhythmic agent. The onset of hyperthyroidism may be abrupt.

Signs and Symptoms

As noted, when present, the signs and symptoms of thyroid disease, especially hypothyroidism, are vague or non-specific in older adults. The person may complain of slowed mentation, gait disturbances, fatigue, weakness, or heat intolerance. These and other symptoms and signs are often evaluated for other causes with consideration of possible hypothyroidism as a "rule out." The onset of symptoms is usually insidious and subtle.

The signs and symptoms of hyperthyroidism in the older adult include unexplained atrial fibrillation, heart failure, constipation, anorexia, or muscle weakness and other vague complaints. Symptoms of heart failure or angina may cloud the clinical presentation and prevent the correct diagnosis. Dementia is often suspected. On examination, the person is likely to have tachycardia, tremors, and weight loss. However, in elders a condition known as apathetic thyrotoxicosis, rarely seen in younger persons, may occur in which usual hyperkinetic activity is replaced with slowed movement and depressed affect.

Complications

Complications occur both as the result of treatment and in the failure to diagnose and therefore failure to treat in a timely manner. Myxedema coma is a serious complication of untreated hypothyroidism in the older patient. Rapid replacement of the missing thyroxin is not possible due to risk of drug toxicity. Even with the best treatment, death may ensue. Because thyroid replacement is necessary to maintain life, the person has to learn to minimize the side effects, especially increased bone loss. Over-replacement can cause the complications of hyperthyroidism.

Thyroxin increases myocardial oxygen consumption; therefore the elevations found in hyperthyroidism produce a significant risk for atrial fibrillation and exacerbation of angina in persons with pre-existing CHD, and may precipitate congestive heart failure. The most common complication is atrial fibrillation, which is present in 27% of elderly patients with hyperthyroidism.

PROMOTING HEALTHY AGING: IMPLICATIONS FOR GERONTOLOGICAL NURSING

The management of thyroid disturbances is largely one of careful pharmacological intervention and, in the case of hyperthyroidism, one of surgical or chemical ablation. As advocates, nurses can assure that a thyroid screening test be done anytime there is a possibility of concern. The nurse caring for frail elders can be attentive to the possibility that the person who is diagnosed with anxiety, dementia, or depression may instead have a thyroid disturbance.

Although the nurse may see little that can be done to prevent thyroid disturbances in late life, organizations such as the Monterey Bay Aquarium have launched campaigns to inform consumers of the iodine and mercury found in seafood (www.seafoodwatch.org) because of their association with thyroid disease.

The nurse may be instrumental in working with the person and family to understand both the seriousness of the problem and the need for very careful adherence to the prescribed regimen. If the elder is hospitalized for acute management, the life-threatening nature of both the disorder and the treatment can be made clear so that advanced planning can be done that will account for all possible outcomes.

For the person in ongoing maintenance treatment, the nurse works with the person and significant others in the correct self-administration of medications and in the appropriate timing of monitoring blood levels and signs or symptoms indicating an exacerbation.

GASTROINTESTINAL DISORDERS

While there are several physiological and functional changes in the gut, the majority of the problems are the result of extrinsic factors. Polypharmacy, co-morbid conditions, inactivity, and high-fat, high-volume meals are all aggravating factors. Gastro-esophageal reflux disease (GERD), and diverticular disease are discussed here. Constipation and dysphagia are discussed in Chapter 11.

Gastroesophageal Reflux Disease

Gastroesophageal Reflux Disease (GERD) is a syndrome defined as mucosal damage from the movement of gastric contents backwards from the stomach into the esophagus. It is the most common GI disorder affecting older adults. Once any symptoms have appeared, at least 50% of those persons will either have persistent symptoms or require intervention. If GERD is left untreated, complications can develop. It is diagnosed empirically based on history and response to treatment. When the symptoms do not resolve with standard treatment, an endoscopy is indicated.

Etiology

The majority of GERD is caused by abnormalities of the lower esophageal sphincter (LES). In 80% of persons, the LES relaxes inappropriately, and in others a sliding hiatal hernia or poor esophageal peristalsis is to blame.

Signs and Symptoms

While complaints of simple "heartburn" are often from dyspepsia, when other signs and symptoms are added it is a greater concern. The classic complaints indicative of GERD are heartburn plus regurgitation—a sensation of burning in the throat as partial digested food and stomach acid inappropriately return to the posterior oropharynx. Older adults more commonly have more atypical symptoms of persistent cough, exacerbations of asthma, laryngitis, and intermittent chest pain. Abdominal pain may occur within one hour of eating, and symptoms are worse when lying down with the added pressure of gravity on the LES. Consumption of alcohol prior to or during eating exacerbates the reflux.

Complications

Persistent symptoms may lead to esophagitis, peptic strictures, esophageal ulcers (with bleeding), and most importantly, Barrett's esophagus, a precursor to cancer (Ali & Lacy, 2004, Longstreth, 2009). The most serious complication is the development of pneumonia from the aspiration of stomach contents. Dental caries may be caused from chronic exposure to gastric acids.

Diverticular Disease

Diverticula are small herniations or saclike out-pouchings of mucosa that extend through the muscle layers of the colon wall, almost exclusive of the sigmoid colon (Huether, 2010a). They form at weak points in the colon wall, usually where arteries penetrate and provide nutrients to the mucosal layer. Usually less than 1 cm, diverticula have thin, compressible walls if empty or firm walls if full of fecal matter. Diverticular disease is primarily a "hot" illness by those persons who subscribe to the hot/cold theory of disease causation and treatment (Giger & Davidhizar, 2003). The prevalence is 5% for persons under age 40, and it increases to 30% for age 60 and to 50% for those over age 80 (McQuaid, 2010). The risk factors for diverticular

---

BOX 15-22	RISK FACTORS FOR DIVERTICULAR DISEASE

- Family history
- Personal history of gallbladder disease
- Low dietary intake of fiber
- Use of medications that slow fecal transit time
- Chronic constipation
- Obesity

---

disease can be found in Box 15-22. Diverticulitis is an acute inflammatory complication of diverticulosis. Occasionally the fecal matter in a diverticulum will become quite desiccated, even calcified.

Etiology

Although the exact etiology of diverticular disease is unknown, it is thought to be the result of a low-fiber diet, especially one accompanied by increased intraabdominal pressure and chronic constipation. There is also an association with lack of exercise, but the exact relationship is unknown (NIDDK, 2008).

Sign and Symptoms

The majority of persons with diverticulosis are completely asymptomatic, and the condition is found only when a barium enema, colonoscopy, or CT scan is performed for some other reason. Persons with uncomplicated diverticulitis complain of abdominal pain, especially in the left-lower quadrant, and may have a fever and elevated white blood cell count, although the latter symptoms may be delayed or absent in the older adult. The physical assessment may be completely negative. Rectal bleeding is typically acute in onset, is painless, and stops spontaneously.

Complications

The complications of diverticulitis are rupture, abscess, stricture, or fistula. With any perforation, peritonitis is likely. Persons with these complications may have an elevated pulse or are hypotensive; however, in the older adult, unexplained lethargy or confusion may be seen as well or instead. A lower-left quadrant mass may be palpated (Ali & Lacy, 2004). Complicated diverticulitis is always considered an emergency and requires hospitalization for treatment and possible surgical repair.

PROMOTING HEALTHY AGING: IMPLICATIONS FOR GERONTOLOGICAL NURSING

Although neither can be prevented, it may be possible to exert considerable control over exacerbation of the symptoms of GERD and diverticular disease, and to have some effect on preventing complications or, at a minimum, developing awareness of the early signs of potential complications.

The management of GERD combines lifestyle changes with pharmacological preparations, used in a stepwise fashion. Lifestyle modifications include eating smaller meals; not eating three to four hours before bed; avoiding high-fat foods, alcohol, caffeine and nicotine; and sleeping with the head of the bed elevated. Weight reduction and smoking cessation are helpful (Huether, 2010b). These strategies alone may control the majority of symptoms when complications are not present. Pharmacological preparation begins with over-the-counter antacids, such as Tums and Rolaids, and progresses to H2 blockers, such as ranitidine (Zantac), and then proton pump inhibitors, such as lansoprazole (Prevacid). In severe cases of GERD, surgical tightening of the lower esophageal sphincter may be necessary. The nurse may work with the elder to identify situations that aggravate his or her GERD (e.g., overeating, alcohol at mealtime) and come up with strategies to best deal with them. The nurse also teaches persons with GERD the alarm signs—the signs that should receive prompt evaluation by a physician or nurse practitioner (Box 15-23).

For persons with diverticulosis, the goal is prevention of diverticulitis. High-fiber diets (25 to 30 g/day) have been cited in American, European, and Asian studies as protective against diverticulosis (Rubio, 2002). In addition, persons should strive for intake of six to eight glasses of fluid per day, preferably with little caffeine.

Acute diverticulitis can be quite painful. The nurse works with the individual to find effective and safe comfort strategies that include pain medication and creative non-pharmacological approaches such as massage, hot or cold packs, stretching exercises, relaxation, music, or meditation techniques. Uncomplicated diverticulitis is treated with antibiotics and a clear liquid diet and is usually managed in the outpatient setting.

In the promotion of healthy aging, the nurse works with the elder to analyze diet, fluid intake, and activity level to ensure adequate motility and minimal pressure within the GI tract. If the person is overweight or obese, weight loss will decrease intraabdominal pressure and decrease the risk for the development of new diverticula and exacerbations of GERD. In all cases, the nurse is responsible for patient education regarding the appropriate use of medications, the warning signs of potential problems, and the best response to the signs or symptoms. When working with an elder in a cross-cultural setting, it is especially important for the nurse to communicate effectively and incorporate cultural expectations and habits (e.g., diet) into the plan of nursing care. The nurse works with the elder to achieve lifestyle modifications.

RESPIRATORY DISORDERS

Normal age-related changes increase the risk for respiratory problems, and when they occur, the mortality rate is higher in older adults than in younger adults. Diseases of the respiratory system are identified as acute or chronic and as involving the upper or lower respiratory tract. They are further defined as either obstructive—preventing airflow out as a result of obstruction or narrowing of the respiratory structures (e.g., chronic obstructive pulmonary disease)—or as restrictive—causing a decrease in total lung capacity as a result of limited expansion (e.g., asthma). While rare, tuberculosis in older adults is usually seen as a reactivation of a long-dormant infection.

Chronic Obstructive Pulmonary Disease

Chronic obstructive pulmonary disease (COPD) affects approximately 15 million people (Auerhahn et al., 2007). It encompasses conditions that limit airflow and include emphysema and chronic bronchitis. Chronic bronchitis is diagnosed clinically by a productive cough for three months in two consecutive years or six months in one year. It can be either obstructive or non-obstructive. Emphysema is a pathological process characterized by dilated air spaces distal to the terminal bronchiole and is associated with destruction of the alveolar wall (Rissmiller & Adair, 2004).

COPD is the fourth leading cause of death for both older men and women in most ethnic groups; however, it is expected to be the third leading cause of death by 2020. Both the incidence of and mortality from COPD has risen dramatically since 1980, but this increase has occurred primarily in women. For example, between 1980 and 2000 the death rate for women in the United States rose from 20.1 to 56.7 per 100,000 (CDC, 2009). COPD occurs most frequently in whites and the least often in Asians (NHLBI, 2009).

COPD contributes to activity limitations. For all persons older than 45 years, the activity limitation rate was 2.5% in 2002. This varies by ethnicity, with Hispanics with the lowest rate of activity limitation (1.4%) and the highest rate of limitation among non-Hispanic whites (2.6%) (Figure 15-13). However, poverty causes more disparity than race or ethnicity in COPD, with 5.7% of the poor with limitations compared with only 1.5% of the middle class (Beato, 2004).

Spirometry is the gold standard for diagnosis; it is a standardized and reproducible test that objectively confirms the presence of airflow obstruction. Measurement of the diffusing capacity for carbon monoxide may help differentiate between emphysema and chronic bronchitis.

Etiology

The airway obstruction of COPD is caused from airway and lung injury but usually from the inhalation of toxins and pollutants earlier in life, such as dust, chemicals, and especially tobacco smoke—either directly or from secondhand smoke. Associated tobacco use accounts for 80% to 90% of all COPD. The smoker becomes symptomatic after 35 to 40 pack-years of exposure (Rissmiller & Adair, 2004). The airflow obstruction in chronic bronchitis is caused by a combination of thickened and inflamed bronchial walls, hypertrophy of mucus glands, smooth muscle constriction, and excess mucus production, all of which cause lumen compromise stimulated by the inhalation of toxins. In rare cases, COPD may be caused by a genetic condition that causes a deficiency in alpha-1 antitrypsin, a protein made in the liver (NHLBI, n.d.)

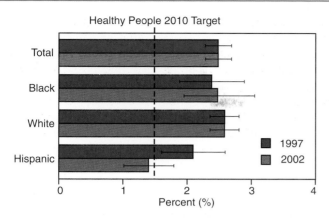

FIGURE 15-13 Activity limitation because of chronic respiratory problems. (NOTE: Data are for ages 45 years and older and age adjusted to the 2000 standard population. Black and white exclude persons of Hispanic origin. Persons of Hispanic origin may be any race. Persons reported one or more races. Data by single race category are for persons who reported only one racial group. Data from National Health Interview Survey, NCHS, CDC. Redrawn from www.cdc.gov/nchs/hphome.htm. Focus area No. 24.)

Signs and Symptoms

The most common symptoms of COPD are wheezing, cough, dyspnea on exertion, and increased phlegm production (Chesnutt et al., 2010). However, COPD has a long asymptomatic stage. Symptoms may not appear until 50% of lung function has been irretrievably lost (Stoller, 2002). Common later signs include prolonged expiration with pursed-lip breathing, barrel chest, air trapping, hyperresonance, pale lips or nail beds, fingernail clubbing, and use of accessory breathing muscles. Cough is the primary symptom of chronic bronchitis, affecting the majority of smokers. Unfortunately, the cough is often dismissed by smokers as insignificant because early in the disease there is no measurable airflow obstruction. In advanced disease, cyanosis, evidence of right-sided heart failure, and peripheral edema are present. In older adults, a high level of fatigue was found, and this in turn significantly decreased functional status (Mollaogu et al., 2010).

Complications

COPD is a progressively debilitating condition characterized by exacerbations and remissions in symptoms. Exacerbations of COPD result in the acute worsening of the baseline signs and symptoms, generally characterized by significantly worsened dyspnea and increased volume and purulence of sputum (Chesnutt et al., 2010). In addition, pulsus paradoxus, which is marked by a decrease in blood pressure of 10 mm Hg or more during inspiration compared with expiration, may occur (Estes, 2002). Spirometry of less than 150 mL, worsening orthopnea, paroxysmal nocturnal dyspnea, and respirations greater than 30 per minute signal an emergent exacerbation of COPD. Exacerbations have numerous inciting factors, including viral or bacterial infections, air pollution or other environmental exposures, and changes in the weather. Pneumonia is a frequent and serious complication.

Exacerbations frequently precipitate the need for changes in medications and may include hospitalization or respiratory support. Invasive endotracheal intubation may be needed for patients with respiratory acidosis that progresses despite therapy or for those with impaired consciousness. In the elderly, decreased alertness may indicate hypoxemia or hypercapnia. Although the acute phase of an exacerbation is usually over in 10 days to 2 weeks, lung function may take 4 to 6 weeks to return to baseline, if ever.

Asthma

Asthma is an inflammatory airway disease that is closely linked to allergic mechanisms and is seen as bronchial hyperresponsiveness and inflammation resulting in bronchorestriction. It is staged from mild to severe based on the frequency of symptoms and the need for treatment, from dyspnea only with activity to dyspnea at rest. A diagnosis is confirmed when a lung capacity increases after the administration of bronchodilators (National Heart Lung and Blood Institute [NHLBI], 2007).

While the prevalence of the disease has increased, the number of deaths is decreasing. Although the majority of asthma is diagnosed in children, the number of elders with asthma has increased, composing 45% of all asthma-related cases. The rate varies further with ethnicity, with non-Hispanic blacks having the highest rate of all other groups. Women, who have a death rate nearly double that of men, also have a hospitalization rate that is two and a half times that of men (Beato, 2004). African Americans and those from Puerto Rico bear the greatest burden (NHLBI, 2007).

Asthma is often underdiagnosed and undertreated in older adults. Instead, the symptoms are attributed to normal changes with aging or cardiovascular disease, or are simply labeled "COPD." The person with asthma may have developed a tolerance to the bronchorestriction and minimizes the reports of symptoms despite the potentially significant respiratory compromise actually present.

Etiology

The development of asthma is influenced by genetics, environment, and lifestyle. A positive family history of asthma and personal history of atopy are positive predictors. Whereas men have an increased risk in childhood, women are at increased risk in late life. After a susceptible person is exposed to an antigen, a cascade of reactions occurs with immediate, late, and recurrent effects. These reactions not only have direct effects on airway smooth muscle and mucus secretion but also recruit the participation of monocytes, lymphocytes, neutrophils, and eosinophils into the cells lining the airways. Repeated exposure potentiates the person's inflammatory response or desensitizes him or her to the antigen. Common external risk factors include exposure to tobacco smoke, air pollution, viral respiratory infections, and allergens such as pet dander, fumes, and dust.

Signs and Symptoms

Although it may be blunted, the presentation of asthma in the elderly is similar to that of younger adults. The classic presentation is one of recurrent episodes of wheezing, dyspnea on exertion, shortness of breath, non-productive cough, and chest tightness. The wheezing is characteristically limited to expiratory respirations and may increase in intensity during the night, interrupting sleep or cause paroxysmal nocturnal dyspnea.

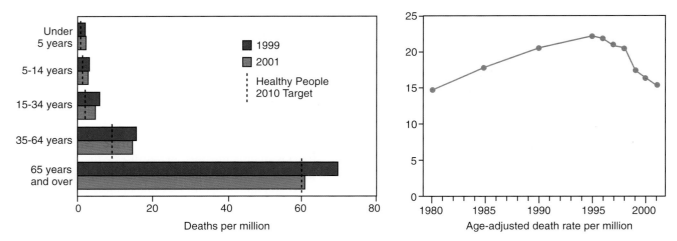

FIGURE 15-14 Asthma-related hospitalizations. NOTE: Data are age adjusted to the 2000 standard population. Black and white include persons of Hispanic or non-Hispanic origin. Persons were asked to select only one race category; selection of more than one race category was not an option in 1998. In 2001, persons reported one or more races. Data by race are shown for persons who reported one racial group. Data from National Hospital Discharge Survey, NCHS, CDC. (Redrawn from www.cdc.gov/nchs/hphome.htm. Focus area No. 24.)

Symptoms are usually worse at night or in the early morning hours but may be triggered by a variety of stimuli, including stress, cold air, pollutants, and especially infection. Asthma may be chronic and require regular doses of medications, or may be episodic, following exposure to sensitizing agents or infection. Symptoms provide a reliable measure of a person's need for and response to therapy, although differences among individuals are highly varied in regard to which symptoms are salient, how symptoms are tolerated, and how they relate to physiological alterations of lung function as measured by peak expiratory flow (PEF) meters. For those with mild to moderate disease, there are often periods of asymptomatic remission.

Complications

Asthma can interfere with the quality of one's life, and acute or severe exacerbations may require hospitalizations (Figure 15-14). When asthma is long-standing, untreated, or under-treated, structural changes to the airway can occur, such as thickening of the airway wall and peribronchial fibrosis. When a person has asthma, he or she is at higher risk for lower respiratory infections and prolonged associated debility.

Tuberculosis

Tuberculosis (TB) is a communicable and infectious disease associated with Mycobacterium bovis, Mycobacterium africanum, or especially, Mycobacterium tuberculosis. The term *tuberculosis infection* refers to a positive TB skin test with no evidence of active disease, while *tubercular disease* refers to an infection that has been documented with testing.

The number of cases of TB in the United States has steadily decreased, with the lowest overall rate recorded in 2009 (most recent data available), with infection found in only 3.9 persons per 100,000 (Figure 15-15). Persons over age 65 compose about 20% of all cases, but compose 50% when combined with those over age 45; men more than twice the number of women. While decreasing, the number of HIV/TB co-infections continues. Among those born in the United States, African Americans

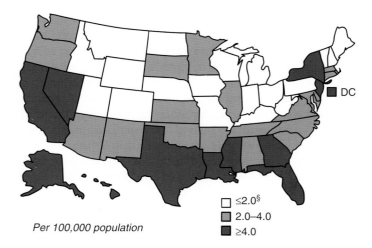

FIGURE 15-15 Rate of tuberculosis cases, by state/area—United States, 2009. (NOTE: Data are updated as of February 16, 2010, and are provisional. Redrawn from *Morbidity & Mortality Weekly Report* 59(10):289-294, 2010.)

represent 42% of all cases, followed by whites at 32%. Among persons born outside of the United States, Asians/Pacific Islanders compose 44% of cases, and Hispanics compose 36%. Since 2001, new cases of TB have been more often among those born outside of the U.S (CDC, 2010). While there are no recent statistics related to the occurrence of TB in long-term care faculties, it has been found that residents of group living settings are between two and seven times more likely to acquire the infection than those who live independently (Ferebee, 2006). Gerontological nurses working in states with a higher incidence or with high-risk populations need to be particularly knowledgeable about this potentially infectious and life-threatening disease.

Etiology

Many of today's elders contracted the disease in childhood or during wartime. The tuberculin bacilli in a person who has become infected may remain dormant for years, only to be activated should the person become immunocompromised as a result of the reduced immunity of aging, chemotherapy, or when concomitantly infected by the human immunodeficiency virus (HIV) infection. Although HIV is the greatest single risk factor for reactivation of the bacilli, other risk factors include cancer, renal failure, diabetes, long-term steroid therapy, and poor nutritional status (Brashers, 2010).

Signs and Symptoms

Symptoms include unexplained weight loss or fever and a cough lasting more than three weeks, regardless of age-group. Night sweats and generalized anxiety may be present. In more advanced stages, the person will also have dyspnea, chest pain, and hemoptysis. Because these signs and symptoms are associated with many disorders common in older adults, diagnosis often is during a health screening or when treatment of the presumed diagnosis is ineffective. Laboratory results in the elderly may show an increased sedimentation rate and lymphocytopenia. For persons with positive skin tests, it is necessary to confirm a diagnosis, traditionally with a chest film and sputum culture. However, a significant increase in the number of false-positive skin tests may necessitate use of one of the newer tools, such as deoxyribonucleic acid (DNA) probes, polymerase chain reaction (PCR) assays, and liquid media, which have been found to be more rapid and accurate biomarkers (Talat et al., 2009). In 2010 a new DNA based test the Xpert MTB/RIF successfully identified 98% of persons in less than two hours. This is expected to pave the way to lead to more rapid diagnosis and effective treatment (Jassal et al., 2010, NIH, 2010).

PROMOTING HEALTHY AGING: IMPLICATIONS FOR GERONTOLOGICAL NURSING

As for most chronic conditions, a team approach is the most useful for maximizing the quality of life and functional capacity for persons with respiratory disorders. The core team may include the nurse, a pulmonologist, a respiratory therapist, and a pharmacist. It may also include an occupational therapist to help the person adapt to declines in functional capacity as appropriate. Management of respiratory disorders in older adults is often complicated by the presence of other chronic disorders and side effects from the medications themselves. Caring for persons with respiratory disorders requires complex nursing skills (Box 15-24). For chronic conditions with repeated exacerbations or deterioration, advance care planning is especially recommended, and includes a discussion of how long rehospitalizations or intubation are desired.

The goals of COPD and asthma management include optimizing pulmonary function, controlling cough and nocturnal symptoms, maximizing functional status, preventing exacerbations, promoting prompt recognition and treatment of exacerbations, reducing the need for emergency department visits, avoiding aggravating other medical conditions, and minimizing medication adverse effects. Each of these may be more difficult to attain for older adults. The cornerstone to the management of asthma is control of triggers to prevent

---

BOX 15-24   SUGGESTIONS IN CARING FOR THE PERSON WITH COPD

EMOTIONAL SUPPORT
Accept/encourage expression of emotions.
Be an active listener.
Be cognizant of conversational dyspnea; do not interrupt or cut off conversations.

EDUCATION
Teach breathing techniques:
- Pursed-lip breathing
- Diaphragmatic breathing
- Cascade coughing (series)

Teach postural drainage.
Teach about medications: what, why, frequency, amount, side effects, and what to do if side effects occur.
Teach use and care of inhalers and spacers and equipment.
Teach signs and symptoms of respiratory infection.
Teach about sexual activity:
- Sexual function improves with rest.
- Schedule sex around best breathing time of day.
- Use prescribed bronchodilators 20 to 30 minutes before sex.
- Use positions that do not require pressure on the chest or support of the arms.

COPD, Chronic obstructive pulmonary disease.

---

symptoms and maintain as near to normal lung function as possible.

Pharmacological intervention is based on the treatment of acute and chronic manifestations of the illness. Medications for COPD and asthma include fast-acting bronchodilators administered on an as-needed basis and long-term agents that maintain bronchodilation and control inflammation. Inhaled medications may be taken a number of ways, including metered-dose inhalers (MDIs), electric nebulizers, and dry-powder inhalers. Several devices are available to facilitate effective drug administration, including spacers when coordination is limited or special devices for helping persons with hand limitations to manage medication cylinders. The nurse advances self-care when teaching the person how to use at-home peak flow meters to monitor disease and adjust medications accordingly.

In COPD, the routine use of antibiotics is controversial because the causal role of bacterial infection is often difficult to document. Antibiotics are generally indicated for patients with new pulmonary infiltrates on chest x-ray film, fever, and perhaps purulent sputum and a sudden increase in the volume of the expectorant or dyspnea. Although the use of pharmacological interventions may increase comfort and functional status, they do not affect mortality (Rissmiller & Adair, 2004). However, the use of long-term oxygen therapy in hypoxemic patients has been shown to improve survival, and smoking cessation slows the rate of decline in lung capacity.

The management of tuberculosis in older adults is one of ensuring prompt and accurate diagnosis and the completion of a specific drug regimen. Unfortunately, the emergence of multidrug-resistant tuberculosis (MDR-TB) is growing, and a new group is also erupting, one of extensively drug-resistant TB (XDR-TB) (Dheda et al., 2010). The successful completion of a treatment plan is more important than ever. When

---

BOX 15-25   CLINICAL NOTE: COMMUNITY NURSING AND PERSONS WITH TUBERCULOSIS, FIRST PERSON

As a young public health nurse, it was my responsibility to periodically check on all persons in my assigned district who were undergoing treatment for tuberculosis (TB). A new person had moved into one of the many boarding houses of this inner-city neighborhood. Mr. Jones was a pleasant, robust 60-year-old who expressed pleasure in the visit and reported that he was doing well, had plenty of medications and that they were not causing him any problems. He dashed out of the room, returned with a small suitcase, and opened it for me to assure me of his supply, and there before me were dozens of unopened bottles of isoniazid (INH), one of the staples of TB treatment at the time. I called the medical director, who recommended that Mr. Jones be sent to the local hospital and, to make sure he got there, to deliver him forthwith. So I loaded him and his suitcase into my car and away we went; thinking of what Florence Nightingale would say, I left the windows open wide. When I returned to the health department, my first stop was for a TB test for myself and the plans for a follow-up after the incubation period. All for the sake of community well-being!

Kathleen Jett

BOX 15-26   SURVEILLANCE GUIDELINES FOR TUBERCULOSIS IN THE LONG-TERM CARE SETTING*†

- Each facility should have an individual responsible for TB infection control and an infection prevention and control plan.
- Each facility should conduct a TB risk assessment on a regularly scheduled basis that considers both patients/residents and health care workers (low, moderate, and high risk).
- Determine the need for TB screening based on the results of the risk assessments.
- For low-risk settings:
  - Screen all new residents on admission and employees on hire for symptoms, and consider using the two-step TST (tuberculin skin test) or BAMT (blood assay for M. tuberculosis).
  - Repeat annually.
  - For those who test positive or have had a positive test in the past, one chest radiograph and annual review of symptoms rather than repeat of film.
- No persons with a diagnosis of TB should remain in a long-term care facility unless adequate administrative and environmental controls and a respiratory protection program are in place.

*For more details, see MMWR 54(RR17): 1-141, 2005; also available on the CDC website: www.cdc.gov.
†Each state public health unit provides guidelines and directions specific to the geographic area and the known risk estimates.

---

combined with the toxicity of the medications and normal changes in the older liver and kidneys, the physiological status must be carefully evaluated before the initiation of the drug regimen, as well as during and afterward. For persons with TB living in the community, many municipalities require a system of direct observation of compliance. This means that a community health worker visits the person on a daily basis during the course of treatment to personally observe ingestion of the medications. Resolution of the infection is confirmed by repeat sputum culture, although bacterium is increasingly resistant to treatment.

TB is a reportable condition, which means that all suspected and confirmed cases are reported to the local or state health authorities (Chesnutt et al., 2010). Local public health nurses usually conduct investigations to ensure that all potentially infected people have been tested and that all persons with the disease receive treatment (Box 15-25). The nurse actively participates in health screenings that may include TB testing. As a health care provider, the nurse is also at risk for acquiring the infection and needs to be screened regularly to prevent becoming a carrier.

Nurses, especially public health nurses, actively promote healthy respiratory aging through prevention. This means promoting or conducting smoking cessation programs and community intervention. It also means political activism with industry leaders and environmental agencies to push for clean air and water and careful and non-discriminatory TB surveillance. In occupational settings, the nurse can contribute to the health of the workers by promoting healthy work environments and in some cases monitoring patients, residents, and employees for exposure to tuberculosis and treatment effectiveness for asthma. In doing so, the nurse can decrease respiratory diseases and their associated morbidity and mortality.

Nurses have a role in monitoring laboratory values, assessing for adverse drug reactions, and monitoring drug compliance in persons with TB, all of which are crucial to treatment effectiveness, the patient's well-being, and controlling the growth of

MDR (Box 15-26). The gerontological nurse in the congregate living setting participates in screening, educating regarding the seriousness of the infection, and helping persons obtain the appropriate treatment as needed.

The nurse can also have a large impact on the quality of life for the elder with respiratory problems and his or her family members. The nurse helps the person learn to monitor symptoms and their effect on function and educates about the appropriate use of medications, oxygen, and exercise and the avoidance of triggers. The nurse encourages the person with COPD to remain as active as possible for as long as possible and to function as fully as possible within the limitations of the disease. When appropriate, the nurse can be instrumental in facilitating palliative care as appropriate.

Avoidance of infection for all older persons, especially those with respiratory diseases, is paramount to the prevention of complications, especially potentially life-limiting pneumonia. In the promotion of healthy aging, the nurse should encourage persons to avoid those with respiratory infections, practice good hand washing, and use preventive immunizations for influenza and pneumonia unless contraindicated. The nurse has a responsibility to both the public and the individual to minimize opportunities for infections and the proliferation of infective agents. This is especially important in the long-term care setting where residents are at very high risk secondary to communal living and the high rate of medical frailty.

MUSCULOSKELETAL DISORDERS

The most common disorders are osteoporosis, osteoarthritis (OA), rheumatoid arthritis (RA), gout, and polymyalgia rheumatica (PMR). Most, if not all, postmenopausal women have osteoporosis, and up to 90% of older adults have OA. All have the potential to negatively affect functional status (especially mobility) and quality of life and to cause a significant amount of pain. Giant cell (temporal) arteritis (GCA) tied to PMR may be chronic or acute and can cause blindness if not treated promptly and appropriately.

Approximately 52% of persons 65 are disabled. The two most common forms of disability are arthritis (8.6 million persons) and back or spine problems (7.6 million) (CDC, 2010). Pain or problems with function associated with these and other musculoskeletal problems are among the most common reasons older adults seek medical care. Arthritis affects 46.5 million people in the United States, with an estimated increase to 67 million by 2030.

Osteoporosis

Osteoporosis means "porous bone." It is the result of a gradual loss of cortical (outer shell) and trabecular bone (inner spongy meshwork). The degree of the loss is measured in terms of bone mineral density (BMD).

Low bone mineral density affects about 44 million, or 55% of people over age 50. Ten million people have OP, and another 34 million have *osteopenia*, a measurable, yet not as extensive loss of BMD. Eighty percent of the 44 million are women (NOF, 2010). Thin, white, postmenopausal women of Northern European or Asian descent are at the highest risk for reduced BMD (20% OP; 52% osteopenia). There is significant racial variation (Table 15-7).

The U.S. Prevention Task Force recommends that women over age 65 be routinely screened for osteoporosis. There is inadequate information to recommending intervals for repeated screening. The dual-energy x-ray absorptiometry (DEXA) scan of the femoral neck is the "gold standard" and best predictor of fractures at any site. The results (T-score) indicate the number of standard deviations from the score of a matched healthy man or woman. Osteopenia is diagnosed if the bone loss is between −1 and −2.5, and osteoporosis is diagnosed if the T-Score is greater than −2.5 (USPSTF, 2010). Medicare covers the cost of an initial scan and a repeat at 24-month intervals if the person is diagnosed with osteoporosis and receiving treatment.

Etiology

Primary osteoporosis is associated with the normal changes of aging. Secondary osteoporosis, accounting for 15% of cases, is caused by another disorder (e.g., cancer, alcoholism) or by medications (e.g., prolonged use of levothyroxine).

Signs and Symptoms

Osteoporosis (OP) is a silent condition, and a person may have no symptoms of any kind ever or for years. A person with osteoporosis may be without symptoms until a fracture occurs. Some of the more subtle signs suggestive of reduced BMD are a non-traumatic injury, loss of height of more than 3 cm or kyphosis, or the development of a *C* shape to the cervical vertebrae (Figure 15-16). The nurse may be the one to identify the changes to the spine or realize that the person had a fracture or unexplained back pain but has not received a medical diagnosis. Without a diagnosis, it is unlikely that the person will have access to the full treatments that are available. It is important to assess the person's risk factors and urge both formal screening and lifestyle changes to minimize risk and enhance prevention (Box 15-27). Once a fracture occurs, it can result in significant pain, loss of function, suffering, and mortality.

Complications

The most serious health consequence is the morbidity and mortality that results from an osteoporosis-related fall. The most common sites for such fractures are hips, vertebra, wrist, and pelvis. Hip fractures are of particular note; among persons at least age 50, 24% die in the year following the injury, 20% will require ongoing long-term care, and only 15% will be able to walk unassisted 6 months postfracture (NOF, 2010). Women who suffer osteoporotic fractures have an increased incidence of heart attack, breast cancer, and stroke combined (Zarowitz,

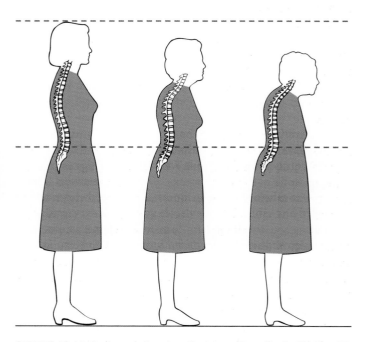

FIGURE 15-16 Osteoporosis spine alignment. (From Touhy TT, Jett KF: *Ebersole and Hess' gerontological nursing & healthy aging*, ed 3, St Louis, 2010, Mosby.)

TABLE 15-7	PREVALENCE OF OSTEOPOROSIS BY GENDER, ETHNIC, AND RACIAL GROUP	
	OSTEOPOROSIS	OSTEOPENIA
Non-Hispanic Caucasian and Asian women	20%	52%
Non-Hispanic Caucasian and Asian Men	7%	35%
Non-Hispanic black women	5%	35%
Non-Hispanic black men	4%	19%
* Hispanic women	10%	49%
* Hispanic men	3%	23%

*Hispanic may be of any race.

BOX 15-27 **RISK FACTORS FOR OSTEOPOROSIS**

NON-MODIFIABLE FACTORS
Female
Caucasian
Asian
Advanced age
Family history of osteoporosis

MODIFIABLE FACTORS
Low body weight (underweight)
Low calcium intake
Vitamin D deficiency
Low testosterone
Inadequate exercise or activity
Use of steroids or anticonvulsants
Excess coffee or alcohol intake
Cigarette smoking

2006). The FRAX Tool is now available to calculate the 10-year probability of a fracture using a combination of risk factors and T-score from the DEXA.

Vertebral fractures are often recognized by clinicians or the radiologist when an elder has back pain. Usual therapy is bedrest, with variable success and the possible complications of DVT, pneumonia, and further bone loss; fixation surgery, which has a high failure rate because of weakened bone foundation; and analgesics. Non-steroidal antiinflammatory drugs (NSAIDs) may provide the analgesia needed, but due to intensity of pain, narcotics are usually necessary. Effective pain management will allow early mobilization and prevent complications. Calcitonin may be useful in pain relief.

Newer treatments, such as vertebroplasty and kyphoplasty, may be considered in those with continued pain. Percutaneous polymethylmethacrylate vertebroplasty (PPV) is the percutaneous injection of a cement into the affected vertebral body. PPV is performed under local anesthesia with conscious sedation as an outpatient procedure. PPV is usually performed after a trial of conservative therapy. The elder is able to walk within two to four hours and usually has dramatic or complete pain relief (Syed et al., 2006).

PROMOTING HEALTHY AGING: IMPLICATIONS FOR GERONTOLOGICAL NURSING:

Osteoporosis

Promoting bone health in late life begins in the teen years, with an adequate intake of calcium and vitamin D (or light exposure). However, preventive measures are helpful at any age and include weight-bearing physical activity, and exercise, nutrition, and lifestyle changes that reduce risk factors. In addition, medications have been developed for the prevention and treatment of OP.

Weight-bearing and resistance-training exercises help maintain bone mass and muscle strength, decreasing the risk for falls. Brisk walking and working with light weights provide mechanical force and spinal and long-bone movement. Avoiding smoking and excessive alcohol intake can also help prevent OP.

Nutrition, especially the adequate intake of calcium and vitamin D, is the cornerstone to all other treatments. The recommended daily calcium intake for older adults is 1200 mg/day in divided doses. While calcium-enriched food and sunlight are the best sources, supplementation is usually needed. Calcium carbonate is the least expensive form of calcium and should be taken with meals to enhance absorption. If the person is also taking H2 blockers, then calcium citrate is the recommended formula. Patient teaching includes discussion of the factors that inhibit calcium absorption (e.g., excess alcohol, protein, or salt); excretion enhancers (e.g., caffeine, excess fiber, phosphorus in meats, sodas, and preserved foods); and the influence of the body's response to stress (decreased calcium absorption, increased excretion of calcium in the urine).

Vitamin D deficiency has been found to be very common, and the implications of this are under review. Nonetheless, it is conclusive that adequate amounts of vitamin D are necessary for bone health. The principle source of Vitamin D is ultraviolet B (UVB) through sunlight on exposed skin. How long the exposure should be and how much skin to expose is dependent on many factors, including global location, skin color, source of light, and use of sunscreens (Rhodes et al., 2010). Due to this uncertainty, supplementation of 400 to 800 I.U. is recommended.

Promoting bone health also includes education about fall prevention (see Chapter 12). Education about the sites most vulnerable to fracture through accidents, falls, back strain, and poor posture should be provided. Fall risk assessment and fall risk reduction measures should also be included in patient teaching. Hip protectors may be considered for frail older adults with OP.

For those at highest risk for OP or those with existing OP, pharmacological interventions may be used. While assuring adequate intake of vitamin D and calcium, the currently available medications include bisphosphonates, calcitonin, selective estrogen receptive modulators (SERMs), estrogen, and parathyroid hormone. While all have been found effective at reducing fracture rate in at least one location (e.g., spine), they are not without dangers. The effectiveness of pharmacological intervention is monitored through a periodic DEXA scan.

Exogenous estrogen had been the primary treatment prescribed for many years. However, the Women's Health Initiative found that while estrogen is an excellent means to prevent bone loss, it also increases the rate of breast cancer, colon cancer, and thrombotic events (Brucker & Youngkin, 2002). As a result of these findings, estrogen is not usually prescribed for osteoporosis, and if it is, it is for a limited period. The SERM raloxifene is an estrogen substitute and may have a protective effect against breast cancer, but it is contraindicated for someone with a history of deep vein thrombosis (DVT) or someone who is taking warfarin (Coumadin).

The most common treatments that are seen in older adults are the bisphosphonates alendronate (Fosamax), risedronate (Actonel), and ibandronate (Boniva); teriparatide (Forteo); or zolendronic acid (Zometa), with dosing anywhere from daily to every 6 or 12 months.

Bisphosphonates are most often prescribed for primary osteoporosis prevention and treatment. There is ample evidence that they reduce bone loss and increase bone mass at the hip, spine, and total body as early as three months into therapy, as well as reduce fractures (Zarowtiz, 2006). However, oral forms of these medications must be taken with caution and should not be administered to persons who cannot reliably follow the dosing instructions precisely. Due to the risk for esophageal erosions, ulceration, or possible rupture, bisphosphonates must be taken on an empty stomach (when first awake) with a full glass of water, and the person must remain in an upright position for at least 30 minutes and not eat or drink for at least 30 minutes.

Another medication that is quite useful is calcitonin (Miacalcin). Although the mechanism is not known, for some it not only slows bone resorption but also reduces osteoporosis-related pain and may be particularly useful in the treatment of vertebral fractures. It is given either subcutaneously or as a nasal spray.

Osteoarthritis

While persons of any age may have osteoarthritis (OA), the greatest percentage are among those who are at least age 65, with 27 million or 54% of women and 43% of men living in the community (Egan, Mentes, 2010). The most common locations for OA are the hands, knees, hips, neck (cervical spine), lower back (lumbar spine), fingers, and thumbs (Figure 15-17).

The osteoarthritic joint is one in which the normal soft and resilient cartilaginous lining becomes thin and damaged. This causes the joint space to narrow and the bones of the joint to rub together, causing destruction of the joint (Figure 15-18).

Etiology

OA results from a complex interplay of many factors, including increased age, genetic predisposition, obesity, cellular and biochemical processes, and repetitive use or trauma to the joint.

Signs and Symptoms

The diagnosis of OA is usually made clinically. In the early stages, there are no laboratory tests to confirm the diagnosis. Later stages can be confirmed with imaging of osteophytes, especially with MRI and directly with arthroscopy. In classic OA, there is stiffness with inactivity and pain with activity that is relieved by rest. The stiffness is greatest in the morning after the disuse of sleep but usually resolves within 20 to 30 minutes (Crowther-Radulewicz & McCance, 2010a). As the disease advances, pain with little activity and at rest is present as more and more joints become involved. On exam, subluxation and joint instability may be found and crepitus is common (both indicators of the deterioration of the synovial covering of the joints). Physiologically, there is bony growth of osteophytes and joint space narrowing from loss or destruction of cartilage and inflammation of the synovium lining the joint. As the joint enlarges, range of motion is lost. In the lumbar region, spinal stenosis is common.

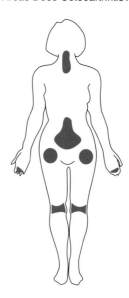

What Areas Does Osteoarthritis Affect?

FIGURE 15-17 Common locations for osteoarthritis. (Source: National Institutes of Health: Handout on health: osteoarthritis, Washington, DC. (Available at www.niams.nih.gov/hi/topics/arthritis/oahandout.htm. Accessed July 29, 2004.)

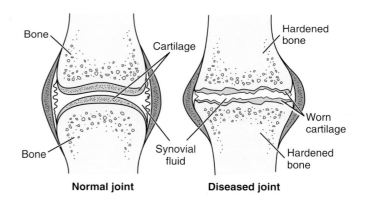

FIGURE 15-18 Normal joint and arthritic joint.

Osteophytes in the distal joints of the fingers are called Heberden's nodes, and those in the nodes in the proximal joints are called Bouchard's nodes. If present, they appear as deformities in the flexion of these joints (Figure 15-19). Heberden's nodes are thought to have a hereditary component.

Complications

As OA is a disease of the joints the complications are limited to the effect of the degenerative changes in function. Further complications may result as a result of side effects of pain medications. Fortunately, for advanced disease of the knees (the most common site) and hips, replacements are available and very successful in many cases. Persons with advanced OA of the spine often require the support of pain centers (see Chapter 17).

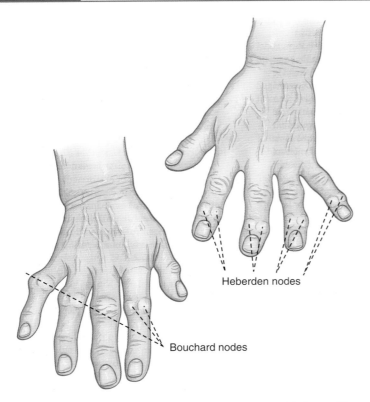

Heberden nodes

Bouchard nodes

FIGURE 15-19 Hand deformities in arthritis. (From McCance KL, Huether SE, Brashers VL, et al: *Pathophysiology: The biologic basis for disease in adults and children,* ed 6, St Louis, 2010, Mosby.)

PROMOTING HEALTHY AGING: IMPLICATIONS FOR GERONTOLOGICAL NURSING: OA

Approaches to advance healthy aging include non-pharmacological, pharmacological, and surgical interventions. The goals are controlling pain and minimizing disability (Box 15-28). As such, the nurse should be less concerned about the addictive quality of the medications and strive for adequate pain relief to allow the person to function at as high a level as possible. The recognition and management of pain in elders, particularly those with dementia or those who are non-verbal, continues to be inadequate and causes a great deal of needless suffering (see Chapter 17). To minimize disability, the joint must be used, strengthened, and protected. Exercises will not be done if they cause pain. Balancing pain relief with appropriate and safe exercise is important (NIAMS, 2006).

Pharmacological management is usually necessary, and acetaminophen (Tylenol) remains the drug of choice for the treatment of pain associated with mild arthritis (Altman, 2010). When this is not effective, the next choice is one of the NSAIDs, such as aspirin or ibuprofen; however, these are not without significant risk for GI problems such as bleeding, as well as cardiovascular side effects. Fortunately, there are formulations that combine the NSAIDs and a gastric protectant (e.g. Vimovo). Acupuncture has show to be an effective adjuvant (Miller, et al., 2009). As the disease progresses or during exacerbations, stronger medications such as narcotics may be necessary to help control pain, and the nurse may need to act as a patient advocate to ensure that the pain is satisfactorily addressed.

For persistent and disabling pain in the knees, joint injections with either steroids or intraarticular hyaluronans or surgery may be necessary for pain management (Brzusek & Petron, 2008). Surgical replacement of the joint (arthroplasty) may be highly successful and restore the person to his or her previous level of functioning. Surgical replacements are recommended for even the very old.

Non-pharmacological approaches include the use of heat and cold, joint support and protection, exercise, and diet. The use of heat and cold is well known for management of arthritic pain; patient's preference drives the selection. Devices and techniques are available that relieve some of the pressure to the hand, and in doing so may decrease pain and improve balance. A cane can relieve hip pressure by 60%. A shoe lift can improve lumbar pain. A knee brace is useful for knees, especially if there is lateral instability (the knee "gives out"). If the hands are affected, paraffin baths for the hands have been found to be very soothing. The person can also resist carrying packages by the fingers or use adaptive devices on utensils and household equipment to make a larger grip surface. A variety of adaptive equipment is available to make daily activities less problematic.

Exercise should be strongly encouraged. Working with a skilled physical therapist or rehabilitation nurse specialist will improve clinical outcomes. Regular exercise improves flexibility and increases muscle strength, which in turn support the affected joints, reduce pain, improve function, and reduce falls (Egan, Mentes, 2010). Water exercise is recommended for people with arthritis as a gentle way to exercise joints and muscles.

Attention should also be given to diet. With the decrease in activity associated with pain, it is easy for the person to gain weight. Excess weight significantly increases the pressure and wear and tear of the joints, leading to less activity and more weight gain. Weight reduction should be considered for all persons who are overweight. The dietician and nurse can work with the person to identify weight and caloric goals and develop meal plans that are culturally acceptable but still balanced and healthy. The nurse can also refer the person to a registered dietitian and then lend support and encouragement.

Rheumatoid Arthritis

Rheumatoid arthritis (RA) is a chronic, systemic, inflammatory joint disorder. It is an autoimmune disease in which the inflammation of the synovium (joint lining) causes destruction of the surrounding cartilage and eventually the bone. Prompt efforts must be made to halt or slow the significant and irreversible damage to affected joints as much as possible. The natural course of RA is highly variable, with remission and exacerbations, but it is overall a progressive condition.

Etiology

While the reason the immune system begins to confuse the host (person) with a foreign body is not known, information about causation of RA is accumulating. Three areas are the focus of research on the etiology of RA at this time. Several genes appear to be associated with a small risk for RA, however, as continues to be the case, not all persons with these genes develop RA. Instead, it appears that environmental factors may trigger the disease in those who are genetically vulnerable. These may include a viral or bacterial infection. A final area of inquiry is hormonal factors, suggested by the increased likelihood of the development of the disease or disease flare following pregnancy or breastfeeding (NIAMS, 2009).

Signs and Symptoms

As RA affects both joints and the system as a whole, fatigue, malaise, weakness, and fever may be presenting signs (NIAMS, 2009). It is characterized by symmetrical polyarticular erythema, pain and swelling of the joints, and morning stiffness lasting longer than 30 minutes, which is considerably longer than in OA. It usually affects the small joints of the wrist, knee, ankle, and hand, although it can affect large joints as well. As the disease progresses, joint deformities occur, with more than 10% of persons developing hand deformities within two years (see Figure 15-19). Older people who have had RA for many years may present with multiple deformities, especially of the hands and feet, and may have undergone joint replacement surgeries (Tabloski, 2006).

An elevated rheumatoid factor (RF) combined with an elevated erythrocyte sedimentation rate (ESR) are most suggestive but not confirmatory of RA. RA is classified as seropositive or seronegative; about 80% of people with RA are RF antibody positive, or negative with later conversion. This is associated with a more severe and progressive course and a reduced life expectancy of 10 to 15 years (Luggen, 2003). However, laboratory findings are less specific in persons with multiple chronic diseases (e.g., older adults), as there may be multiple other reasons for the elevations. RF factor is also often positive in smokers and is not necessarily indicative of rheumatism (Gornisiewicz & Moreland, 2001).

Complications

As with OA, the complications of RA are largely a consequence of orthopedic deformites and side effect of medications. The most common deformity in RA is the boutonnière deformity or hyperextension of the DIP joint with flexion of the PIP joint, followed by a "swan neck" deformity or flexion of the DIP and extension of the PIP, and a vagus deformity of the knee and volar subluxation of the MTP joints. Persons with RA also have excess cardiovascular death, but the association is unexplained (Hellmann & Imboden, 2010)

PROMOTING HEALTHY AGING: IMPLICATIONS FOR GERONTOLOGICAL NURSING: RA

In RA, a class of drugs called disease-modifying antirheumatic drugs (DMARDs), such as methotrexate, is usually the cornerstone of treatment of disease progression. Other medications may be necessary, including biological response modifiers. Protein-A immunoadsorption therapy, a blood-filtering therapy that removes antibodies and immune complexes that promote inflammation, may also be used. All DMARDs are potentially toxic, and the nurse must work closely with the patient and family to be aware of early danger signs.

For many years, it was thought that people with RA should rest their joints to protect them from damage; however, both rest and exercise are necessary. In terms of rest, this may be resting the particular affected joint, such as a hand or wrist, or total body rest. Therapeutic exercise programs are designed to help maintain or improve the ability to do ADLs. Even a warm, inflamed joint should be given ROM exercises to maintain movement in the joint. A physical or occupational therapist should be consulted for developing a program of rest and exercise. Splints and assistive devices, as well as occupational therapy consultation to enhance self-care ability, are important interventions.

Environmental modifications are often necessary for elders with RA. Zipper pulls and Velcro closures on clothing are two practical measures. Book holders, chairs to sit on while preparing foods, light switch changes, and secure stair railings are other measures.

Gout

Gout is an inflammatory arthritis that is either acute or chronic. Gout may be a one-time acute illness or become chronic with intermittent (and unpredictable) acute attacks. The joint of the great toe is the most typical site; however, it also may occur in the ankle, knee, wrist, or elbow. Men between ages 40 and 50 are most commonly affected, but the prevalence increases significantly with age. Gout may be exacerbated by medications commonly used in later life, particularly thiazide diuretics and salicylates (even in small doses).

Etiology

Gout is a cytokine-mediated inflammatory response to the accumulations of uric acid in the blood and other body fluids, such as synovial fluid of a joint or joints. Hyperuricemia is only one of the causes. Other factors include genetic predisposition (X-linked alteration in the enzyme HGPRT), excessive alcohol consumption, lead toxicity and a high purine diet (Crowther-Radulewicz & McCance, 2010a). Gout is the clinical manifestation of either an overproduction of uric acid or inadequate excretion.

Signs and Symptoms

While gout may develop insidiously, it typically starts with an acute attack. The person complains of what is called exquisite pain in the affected joint, often starting in the middle of the night awakening one from sleep. The joint is bright red, hot, and too painful to touch. They may complain that "even the sheet hurts." Fever, malaise, and chills may also be present. A laboratory test finding of elevated uric acid is likely, but it may also be within normal limits.

Complications

With prolonged elevations of uric acid, it crystallizes, forming insoluble precipitates that gather in subcutaneous tissue. They are seen as small, white tophi that may be quite painful. If they collect in the kidneys, they can form urate renal stones and cause renal failure.

PROMOTING HEALTHY AGING: IMPLICATIONS FOR GERONTOLOGICAL NURSING: GOUT

The first goal of treatment during an acute attack of gout is to stop it as promptly as possible and thereby achieve pain relief. This may include NSAIDs, colchicines, and sometimes injection of long-acting steroids into the joint. The nurse ensures that the person takes in enough fluids to help flush the uric acid through the kidneys (2 L/day if not contraindicated). During drug therapy, the person should not take salicylates, which may inhibit drug effectiveness.

After the acute attack, the goal is to prevent another attack, systemic spread of the disease, and the development of chronic gout. This may be done by avoiding drugs or foods that are high in purine and alcohol, both of which increase uric acid levels, and by taking medications to either decrease uric acid production, such as xanthine oxidase inhibitors (e.g., allopurinol or febuxostat), or increase its excretion (e.g., probenecid) (Crowther-Radulewicz & McCance, 2010). The nurse's role includes teaching the person how to decrease the likelihood of another attack by employing preventive measures. This includes avoiding high-purine foods, such as sardines in oil, organ meats, anchovies, herring, mussels, and codfish. In administering gout-related medications, the nurse pays close attention to renal function and notifies the physician or nurse practitioner of any impairment so that dosages can be adjusted.

Urologic Disorders

Incontinence and benign prostatic hyperplasia (BPH) commonly occur in late life. Incontinence is addressed in Chapter 11. BPH is addressed here. It is the most common benign condition in men, with a significant increase in prevalence with age—from 20% in men age 41 to 60 to 90% in men over age 80 (Meng et al., 2010). It affects both the epithelial and fibromuscular components of the prostate, which may be found only on autopsy or when a person becomes symptomatic due to obstruction or partial obstruction of the urethra. BPH affects 6.5 of 27 million white men (NIDDK, 2010b). However, African-American and Hispanic men have disproportionally high rates. The disparity may be related to differences in genetic factors related to androgen signaling pathways, among other factors (Hoke & McWilliams, 2008).

Etiology

The etiology of BPH remains elusive. However, in some men there appears to be a significant genetic predisposition (autosomal dominant trait), with a fourfold increased risk for men who have a first-degree relative with BPH (Meng et al., 2010).

Signs and Symptoms

The signs and symptoms of BPH are at times very close to or identical to those of prostatic cancer and prostatitis, making diagnosis difficult. Symptoms are classified as irritative (frequency, urgency, or nocturia) or obstructive (hesitancy, weak or split stream, or incomplete emptying).

The differential diagnosis is primarily through indirect measures and exclusion. These include ruling out endocrine, neurological, sexually transmitted, and medication causation. Sensitive but non-specific urological testing for postresidual void, urine flow rates, and bladder capacity will confirm evidence of obstruction. The digital rectal exam may reveal a boggy, smooth, and enlarged gland or a completely normal one. At one time, a negative PSA (prostate specific antigen) was used to differentiate BPH from prostate cancer, however, due to the very high rates of both false-negatives and false-positives with the PSA, this is no longer dependable.

Complications

Bleeding, chronic renal insufficiency, or bladder stones may all be consequences and complications of BPH. When they occur, irritative symptoms particularly affect quality of life relative to the degree of discomfort or pain. Partial obstruction may lead to overflow incontinence, chronic failure to empty increases the risk for infection and may result in renal failure due to retrograde urination. Complete obstruction is a medical emergency.

PROMOTING HEALTHY AGING: IMPLICATIONS FOR GERONTOLOGICAL NURSING

The goal of caring for the man with BPH is symptom management related to quality of life. The American Urological Association Symptom Index is used almost universally to guide a response to persons with BPH. Symptoms can be quantified by scale from absent through mild annoyance to a significant impairment. The medical management ranges from what is called "watchful waiting," during which symptoms are monitored, to surgical prostatectomy. The nurse is involved with education, specifically regarding avoidance of caffeine while maintaining adequate hydration, avoiding medications or supplements with anticholinergic effects, and appropriate response to increase in symptoms or signs of infection. Finally, the nurse and nurse practitioner work with the patient who is considering surgery or is taking α-andrenergic antagonists, 5α-reductase medications, or serenoa repens (saw palmetto) (see Chapter 10).

COPING WITH CHRONIC HEALTH PROBLEMS

Promoting healthy aging is possible at any age, from working with teenagers to get enough calcium to reach a healthy bone mass peak to leading smoking cessation campaigns. Promoting healthy aging also means being aware of special considerations that almost universally need attention and must be addressed actively by nurses and other members of the health care team. The following discussion addresses several of these, not as a comprehensive coverage of the topic but as a touchstone for further examination and discussion. Pain, which is common in some conditions, is discussed in Chapter 17.

Gender

Before the 1990s, the majority of research related to chronic conditions and their related medications was conducted on men (especially white men) and extrapolated to women and persons of color. However, significantly less work was done on understanding the health issues specific to women, such as menopause and the use of hormone replacement therapy. In the landmark study of health disparities documented in the manuscript "Unequal Treatment" (Smedley et al., 2003; www.iom.gov), women were found to experience considerable disparities in health care outcomes.

We now have good evidence that women are evaluated less intensely and diagnosed and referred less frequently than men for many problems, including those of a cardiac origin. Although CVD is the number-one cause of death for both men and women, women have been found to receive fewer "standard interventions" than men, including thrombolytic therapy, aspirin, heparin, and beta-blockers. They are also less likely to undergo cardiac catheterization and bypass graft surgery. We also know that women may have slightly different signs and symptoms of both heart disease and other common problems, especially in late life (Endoy, 2004).

In April 1991, Dr. Bernadine Healy, then-Director of the National Institutes of Health (NIH), attempted to address some of these issues when she launched the Women's Health Initiative (WHI) to examine the most common causes of death, disability, and impaired quality of life in postmenopausal women. This was the first multisite study of its size specifically designed for older women. Originally scheduled for completion in 2006, in 2001 the study was temporarily interrupted because of surprising findings in the part of the study examining hormone replacement therapy (HRT). Previous studies had used observational data to suggest that HRT protected women from a number of problems, especially heart disease. The mid-study report from the WHI refuted these observations, finding that although HRT did slightly decrease a woman's risk for colorectal cancer and hip fractures, it increased her risk for coronary heart disease, stroke, and pulmonary embolism. Almost overnight, the health care of postmenopausal women changed (Brucker and Youngkin, 2002). Only now are these findings and their implications being understood.

Fatigue

Fatigue is a common complaint of persons living on the chronic illness trajectory, especially as the number of chronic illnesses grows. It is often variable and unpredictable and is either ignored or incorrectly assumed to be a normal part of the aging process. Instead, fatigue may be a symptom of the illness, a side effect of a medication, a symptom of depression, or all of these.

In promoting healthy aging, the most important intervention of the gerontological nurse may be to validate the reality and debilitating effects of the disorder. It is also important to help the person differentiate a treatable depression that may be superimposed on the fatigue of chronic illness. Discussing patterns of fatigue and identifying the precipitants are important (Mollaoglu, Fertelli, Tuncay, 2010). If the elder can be engaged in keeping a log of the low points of energy, it may prove useful. It is also helpful to emphasize the wisdom of the body and balance rest and activity within limitations to help conserve energy for activities that are most important or necessary.

Chronic problems tax this existing energy level. Direct assistance by caregivers or families may be necessary to aid the older adult in exploring lifestyle adaptations that decrease energy expenditure and permit continued involvement in valued interests. Throughout this process, the older adult with a disability must remain involved in decision making on every level of need. He or she may have different priorities from those of the caregiver. Elderly clients may relegate their health needs to a lower priority to fulfill other needs or life demands. Based on the ethical principle of autonomy, the priorities identified by an individual are expected to be respected, regardless of their age, and established by the elder as a competent adult. Persons with chronic illnesses are the "experts" on managing their illnesses and lifestyle, with nurses as their collaborators.

Grief

Grieving the loss of appearance, function, independence, and comfort may occupy much of one's time initially when adapting to and coming to terms with a chronic illness, particularly if the onset has been abrupt and the loss interferes directly with a major source of one's pleasure (see Chapter 23). As the mother with a handicapped newborn mourns the loss of the visualized "perfect" infant, the elder may begin to memorialize the "perfect" self that no longer exists. The earlier image of the self may grow far beyond the reality that existed. The nurse's function is to encourage verbalization, talk with the elder about the lost self, recognize the grief that may be occurring, and help reframe the new self. Clearly, grief reactions will be highly individual, depending on the significance of the loss and the number of additional losses with which the individual is attempting to cope (see Chapter 23).

Iatrogenesis

While the nurse is working to reduce the complications of the chronic illness itself, a secondary risk increases—that of iatrogenesis (that which is a complication or by-product of the health care intervention itself). The majority of emphasis has been on control of the potential deleterious effects of hospitalization, yet iatrogenesis can develop in any setting (Box 15-29). The person may become incontinent with the addition of a potent diuretic, not because of a new physiological problem but from the increase in urinary frequency without an increased access to toileting facilities. A new medication may cause depression, fatigue, or erectile dysfunction while improving the control of the underlying illness. Elders with some functional disabilities may find themselves completely dependent during an acute illness. The use of warfarin to prevent stroke can cause a life-ending subdural hematoma if the person has a head injury from a fall or a game of football with a grandchild.

Whenever a negative change is likely or occurs after an intervention, the nurse can be proactive in working with the care team in identifying the potential or actual effect and facilitating

BOX 15-29   COMMON IATROGENIC PROBLEMS ASSOCIATED WITH AN INSTITUTIONAL STAY

- Loss of mobility because of insufficient ambulation
- Incontinence because of inattention when needed; sometimes becoming a permanent problem
- Confusion or delirium caused by medications, treatments, anesthesia, and translocation
- Pressure ulcers caused by immobility and reduced sensation
- Dehydration caused by limited access to fluids
- Fluid overload caused by improper use of intravenous fluids
- Nosocomial infections caused by infectious agents in surroundings
- Urinary tract infections caused by catheter usage
- Upper respiratory tract infections caused by immobility and shallow breathing and aspiration of oral secretions
- Fluid and electrolyte imbalances caused by medications and treatments
- Falls because of unfamiliar environment, weakness, and positional instability
- Impaired sleep because of treatments and environment
- Malnutrition caused by anorexia and insufficient assistance in eating

a cost-benefit discussion with the person and his or her significant other (see Chapter 16).

Fostering Self-Care

In the day-to-day life of the person with chronic illness, self-care skills are of the greatest importance. Nurse theorist Dorothy Orem has provided us with a useful language and taxonomy for both understanding and responding to calls from persons with self-care needs (1995).

According to Orem, each person has self-care needs called universal self-care requisites. Each person also develops self-care capacity or the ability to meet these requisites. However, in some circumstances, the needs exceed the individual's capacity to meet them, and a self-care deficit ensues in which an individual is unable to carry out basic functions without assistance. These deficits are primarily the result of pathophysiological disorders that impinge on neuromuscular, musculoskeletal, or sensory integrity, but they can also have a psychological or spiritual origin. They can also be the result of changes in neurological functioning or even iatrogenesis as just noted.

The appropriate nursing approach is highly individualized and may involve changing the environment, modifying the treatment, or teaching the individual strategies to compensate for the pathophysiological changes. The impact of chronic illness is also highly individual and may include identity erosion, expectation of death, dependency conflicts, and feelings of failure and fatalism.

Many of the largest health maintenance organization (HMO) providers now offer reimbursement for alternative medicine therapies, such as therapeutic massage, touch therapy, acupuncture, chiropractic, biofeedback, homeopathy, and naturopathy. This trend arises from studies showing that alternative medicine is less expensive, results in fewer hospitalizations, and tends to be used by individuals who are more concerned about managing their own health in a holistic manner. Now it is possible for more individuals to direct their own care, order their own special supplies without provider approval, and, in many cases, purchase some medications over the counter. Nursing will be called on to obtain background

information and to help to sort out options in self-care management. The nurse can also be instrumental in fostering self-care efficacy. Two strategies for fostering effective self-care that are receiving attention are the use of small groups and telephone/electronic follow-up.

Small-Group Approaches

Small-group meetings are among the most effective and economic ways of assisting clients to meet informational and psychosocial needs. They can also be designed to provide family support and counseling. Self-help groups can be seen as support systems, consumer participant systems, expressive-social influence groups, or homogeneously identified therapeutic groups. Facilitating adjustment to new roles and activities and assisting with redefinition of self and meanings constitute a large part of working with groups.

Some of the most successful groups have been those in which the members identify topics and issues on which they wish to focus. The first meeting sets the tone and expectations for the group, including ground rules. The group facilitator gathers information, brochures, and other resources that may be valuable to share based on the expressed interest of the group. In addition to information, many groups related to chronic illness address psychological issues, such as the following:

1. Fears about incapacitation, pain, abandonment, isolation, and death
2. Expressions of low self-esteem and loss of confidence
3. Feelings of helplessness and uselessness; a desire to be whole and well again
4. A desire to fit into the family system once again
5. Willingness to redefine role relationships with significant others
6. A desire to face and handle public situations without fear or embarrassment

PROMOTING HEALTHY AGING: IMPLICATIONS FOR GERONTOLOGICAL NURSING

Maximizing the quality of life and health of a person with a chronic condition is one of team work. The nurse is part of an expanded network of health professionals (e.g., nurse practitioner, physical therapist, physician or physiotherapist, occupational therapist, nutritionist) who work together with the elder and his or her support persons and loved ones. In some cultures, the nurse also works with indigenous healers, such as shamans, medicine men and women, and curanderas. In cross-cultural situations, the nurse may work with the help of an interpreter (see Chapter 5). The work always includes consideration of the psychosocial and physical needs of the person. Spiritual needs are often present as the person deals with the "Why me?" of chronic disease. Helping older adults cope with chronic diseases requires that the nurse be skilled not only in hands-on care but also skilled as a teacher, advocate, consultant, and counselor. This includes screening, patient education, advocacy, referral, and assistance with disease and symptom management. The advanced practice nurse has the added responsibility to direct medical management that is consistent with the available evidence-based guidelines. The promotion of healthy aging in relation to chronic disease revolves around reducing modifiable risk factors to prevent further damage and minimize complications. Risk-reduction programs can be instituted only with a clear understanding of the person's difficulties with changing lifelong habits. Smoking, overeating, habitual anger or irritation, and a sedentary lifestyle (all components of poor health) are often deeply embedded in the personality structure and lifestyle and are not easily eradicated by "education." The nursing role is to provide acceptance, encouragement, resources, knowledge, and affirmation of the individual and his or her right to choose.

SUMMARY

Nurses impact the quality of life for all persons with chronic diseases as they serve as resource persons, advisors, teachers, and, at times, facilitators (Box 15-30). The goals of care of persons with chronic illness are to slow decline, relieve discomfort, and support preferred lifestyle with as few restrictions as possible (Strauss and Glaser, 1975). The ability of the elder and the family to manage and cope with the problems encountered determines the need. It is necessary for those who participate in care to be reoriented and resocialized to self-care capacity in the presence of chronic illness and to recognize a different system of rewards.

The basics of the care process emphasize improving function, managing the existing illness, preventing secondary complications, delaying deterioration and disability, and facilitating death with peace, comfort, and dignity. Progress is not measured in attempts to achieve cure but, rather, in maintenance of a steady state or regression of the condition while remembering that the condition does not define the person. This thinking is essential if realistic expectations for the caregiver and the elder are to be achieved. The individual will in some manner seek to understand the meaning of the chronic disease and incorporate the old self-image with the new self-image. The nurse's involvement in this process is to ask about the meanings of the illness and to listen and learn.

BOX 15-30 NURSES' ROLE IN CARING FOR PERSONS WITH CHRONIC DISEASE

- Assessing elder and family strengths and challenges
- Teaching related to healthy lifestyle modifications, preservation of energy, and self-care strategies
- Encouraging the reduction of modifiable risk factors
- Counseling the individual in the development of reasonable expectations of self
- Providing access to resources when possible
- Referring appropriately and when needed
- Organizing and leading interdisciplinary case conferences and team meetings
- Facilitating advance care planning and palliative care when appropriate

Corbin and Strauss (1992) suggest that assisting individuals and their support persons to view chronic disorders as having a "trajectory" may help them cope with the ups and downs of the disorders, as well as the acute exacerbations. If they are able to better understand the phases of a disorder, they are likely to weather the difficult periods without undue discouragement. Often it must be seen as a lifetime situation that travels along a trajectory in which resources must be tailored accordingly. In summary, they suggest the following points that practitioners can consider:

1. Chronic illness must be seen through the eyes of the persons experiencing it.
2. The illness is often a lifelong course that passes through many phases.
3. Biographical, medical, spiritual, and everyday needs must be considered.
4. Collaborative rather than purely professional relationships may be most effective.
5. Lifelong support may be necessary, although the type, amount, and intensity of such support will vary.

evolve To access your student resources, go to http://evolve.elsevier.com/Ebersole/TwdHlthAging

KEY CONCEPTS

- The nation's goals include increasing the span of healthy life. The challenge to this is to help persons find ways to promote healthy aging in the presence of chronic disease.
- The effects of chronic illness range from mild to life-limiting, with each person responding to unique circumstances in a highly individualized manner.
- Coping with chronic illness can be a physical, psychological, and spiritual challenge.
- The Chronic Illness Trajectory is a useful framework with which to understand chronic illness and design nursing interventions.
- Cardiovascular diseases are the leading cause of death and a frequent cause of disability in the older adult.
- The careful control of hypertension and diabetes has the potential to significantly improve health and minimize complications that have significant detrimental effects on the person.
- Most disorders that become chronic diseases have atypical presentations in the older adult and may be attributed to normal aging, which delays the receipt of appropriate care and treatment.
- For most chronic diseases, optimal care includes an interdisciplinary team working closely with the elder and his or her family or significant others.
- The goals of promoting healthy aging include minimizing risk for disease, and in the presence of disease, alleviating symptoms, delaying or avoiding the development of complications including end-organ damage, and maximizing function and quality of life.
- The gerontological nurse has the potential to serve as a leader in the promotion of health and the prevention of disease.

CASE STUDY   DIABETES

Ms. P., an 82-year-old single woman, lives in a life-care community in her own apartment but has the reassurance of knowing her medical and functional needs will be taken care of, regardless of the extent of these needs. This is the primary reason she chose to sell her home and move. She is at present independent. She has been gaining weight steadily since she moved into the community and attributes that to the fact that she eats much better now that she joins others in the congregate dining room for meals. She has diabetes, which she manages with diet, exercise, and oral medications; heart failure; and mild arthritis. Although she says she feels fine, lately she has noticed some increased fatigue and that her toes are cold and somewhat numb. The great toe on her left foot seems to be discolored. Because of the lack of feeling, she often walks around her apartment barefoot because it seems to increase the sensation in her feet. She has not needed to use the health care center and goes to the clinic only to pick up her medication. Her niece stopped by last week to see her and called the clinic and spoke with the nurse. The niece reported that her aunt seemed a little confused and lethargic. The niece accompanied Ms. P. to the clinic, where the nurses checked her blood pressure and blood sugar and found them to be 170/80 and 280 mg/dL, respectively. Ms. P. said, "Oh, I don't think it is anything to worry about! I am just a little tired."

Based on the case study, develop a nursing care plan using the following procedure*:

- List Mrs. P.'s comments that provide subjective data.
- List information that provides objective data.
- From these data, identify and state, using accepted format, two nursing diagnoses you determine are most significant to Mrs. P. at this time. List two of Mrs. P.'s strengths that you have identified from the data.

- Determine and state outcome criteria for each diagnosis. These must reflect some alleviation of the problem identified in the nursing diagnosis and must be stated in concrete and measurable terms.
- Plan and state one or more interventions for each diagnosed problem. Provide specific documentation of the source used to determine the appropriate intervention. Plan at least one intervention that incorporates Mrs. P.'s existing strengths.
- Evaluate the success of the intervention. Interventions must correlate directly with the stated outcome criteria to measure the outcome success.

CRITICAL THINKING QUESTIONS

1. How would you explain that the leading cause of death worldwide is heart disease?
2. What risk factors do you have for heart disease, and what can you do to reduce them?
3. What thoughts do you have on the persistent disparities in health outcomes between white persons and persons of color?
4. What commonly held beliefs about aging would lead Ms. P. to believe that the changes in her health did not warrant seeking health care?
5. Of all of the symptoms that Ms. P. reports, which one should the nurse be most concerned about related to Ms. P.'s long-term health?
6. Of all of the symptoms that Ms. P. reports, which one should the nurse be most concerned about related to Ms. P.'s ability to live alone?

*Students are advised to refer to their nursing diagnosis text and identify possible or potential problems.

RESEARCH QUESTIONS

1. Is there any information that explains the differences in the incidence and prevalence of common chronic diseases in various ethnic groups?
2. Can the trajectory model of Glaser and Strauss be used for situations other than living with a chronic disease?
3. Discuss with an elder who has at least one chronic disease: What aspect of the disease or condition is the most difficult to manage? What strategies have he or she found to cope better?
4. What types of complementary and alternative therapies are used by persons with chronic diseases, and for what?

REFERENCES

American Academy of Neurology: AAN Summary of evidence-based guidelines for clinicians. Medical and surgical treatment of Parkinson disease with motor fluctuations and dyskinesia, 2006. Available at http://aan.com/professionals/practice/guidelines/Med_Treatment_PD_Sum.pdf.

Ali MA, Lacy BE: Abdominal complaints and gastrointestinal disorders. In Landefeld CS, et al, editors: Current geriatric diagnosis and treatment, New York, 2004, McGraw-Hill.

Altman RD: Pharmacological therapies for osteoarthritis of the hand: A review of the evidence, Drugs & Aging 27:729, 2010.

Aminoff MJ: Nervous system disorders. In McPhee SJ, Papadakis MA, editors. 2010 Current medical diagnosis and treatment. NY, 2010, McGraw-Hill Lange.

Auerhahn C, Capezuti E, Flaherty E, Resnick B, editors: Geriatric Nursing Review Syllabus: A core curriculum in advanced practice geriatric nursing, ed 2, NY, 2007, American Geriatrics Society.

Bashore TM, Granger CB, Hranitzky MR: Heart disease. In McPhee SJ, Papadakis MA, editors.

2010 Current medical diagnosis and treatment, NY, 2010, McGraw-Hill Lange.

Beato CV: Progress review: respiratory diseases, June 29, 2004, USDHHS. Available at www.healthypeople.gov/data/2010prog/-focus24/default.htm. Accessed June 22, 2006.

Beers MH, editor: Disorders of carbohydrate metabolism (Chapter 64, updated February 2006a). In Merck manual of geriatrics, ed 3. Available at http://www.merck.com/mkgr/mmg/home.jsp.

Beers MH, editor: Lower gastrointestinal tract disorders. (Chapter 107, updated February 2006). In Merck manual of geriatrics, ed 3. Updated since 2006. Available at http://www.merck.com/mkgr/mmg/sec13/ch107/ch107a.jsp.

Begelman SM: Peripheral vascular and thromboembolic disease. In Landefeld CS, et al., editors: Current geriatric diagnosis and treatment, New York, 2004, McGraw-Hill.

Blumenthal DE: Geriatric rheumatology. In Landefeld CS, et al., editors: Current geriatric diagnosis and treatment, New York, 2004, McGraw-Hill.

Boss B: Disorders of central and peripheral nervous systems and the neuromuscular junction. In McCance KL, Huether SE, Brashers VL, et al., editors: Pathophysiology: the biological basis for disease in adults and children, ed 6, St Louis, 2010a, Mosby.

Boss B: Alterations in cognitive systems, cerebral hemodynamics and motor function. In McCance KL, Huether SE, Brashers VL, et al., editors: Pathophysiology: the biological basis for disease in adults and children, ed 6, St Louis, 2010b, Mosby.

Brashers VL: Alterations of cardiovascular function. In McCance KL, Huether SE, Brashers VL, et al., editors: Pathophysiology: the biological basis for disease in adults and children, ed 6, St Louis, 2010, Mosby.

Brucker MC, Youngkin EQ: What's a woman to do: exploring HRT questions raised by the women's health initiative, AWHONN Lifelines 6:406, 2002.

Brzusek D, Petron D: Treating knee osteoarthritis with intra-articular hyaluronans, Current Medical Research and Opinion 24:3307, 2008.

Centers for Disease Control and Prevention: Stroke Facts, 2010. Available at http://www.cdc.gov/stroke/facts.htm.

Centers for Disease Control and Prevention: Tuberculosis in the United States: The national Tuberculosis Surveillance System Highlights from 2009, Updated 2010 (presentation). Available at http://www.cdc.gov/tb/statistics/surv/surv2009/default.htm.

Centers for Disease Control and Prevention: Facts about chronic obstructive pulmonary disease (COPD). 2009. Available at: http://www.cdc.gov/copd/copdfaq.htm.

Centers for Disease Control and Prevention: Osteoarthritis, 2010. Available at: http://www.cdc.gov/arthritis/basics/osteoarthritis.htm.

Chesnutt MS, Gifford AH, Prendergast TJ: Pulmonary disorders. In McPhee SJ, Papadakis MA, editors: *2010 Current medical diagnosis and treatment*, New York, 2010, McGraw-Hill.

Corbin JM, Strauss A: A nursing model for chronic illness management based upon the trajectory framework. In Woog P, editor: *The chronic illness framework: the Corbin and Strauss nursing model*, New York, 1992, Springer.

Crowther-Radulewicz CL, McCance KL: Alterations of musculoskeletal function. In McCance KL, et al., editors: *Pathophysiology: the biological basis for disease in adults and children*, ed 6, St Louis, 2010a, Mosby.

Dheda K, Warren RM, Zumla A, et al: Extensively drug-resistant tuberculosis: Epidemiology and management challenges, *Infectious Disease Clinics of North America* 24:705, 2010.

Ducharme A, Odette Doyon, Michel White, et al: Impact of care at a multidisciplinary congestive heart failure clinic: a randomized trial, *Canadian Medical Association Journal* 173:40, 2005.

Egan BA, Mentes JC: Benefits of physical activity for knee osteoarthritis: A brief review, *J Gerontol Nurs* 36(9):9-14, 2010.

Endoy MP: CVD in women: risk factors and clinical presentation, *American Journal for Nurse Practitioners* 8:33, 2004.

Estes MEZ: *Health assessment and physical examination*, Albany, NY, 2002, Delmar.

Feng Y, Schlösser FJ, Sumpio BE: The Semmes Weinstein monofilament examination as a screening tool for diabetic peripheral neuropathy, *Journal of Vascular Surgery* 50:675, 2009.

Ferebee L: Respiratory function. In Meiner SE, Luecknotte AG, editors: *Gerontologic nursing*, ed 3, St Louis, 2006, Mosby.

Giger JN, Davidhizar RE: *Transcultural nursing: assessment and intervention*, ed 4, St Louis, 2003, Mosby.

Gornisiewicz M, Moreland LW: Rheumatoid disorders. In Robbins L, editor: *Clinical care in the rheumatic diseases*, ed 2, Atlanta, 2001, Association of Rheumatology Health Professionals.

Hellmann DR, Imboden JB: Musculoskeletal and immunologic disorders. In McPhee SJ, Papadakis MA, editors: *2010 Current medical diagnosis and treatment*. NY, 2010, McGraw-Hill Lange.

Hoke GP, McWilliams GW: Epidemiology of benign prostatic hypertrophy and comorbidities in racial and ethnic populations. *American Journal of Medicine* 121(8 Suppl 2):S3, 2008.

Huether SE: Structure and function of the digestive system. In McCance KL, et al., editors: *Pathophysiology: the biological basis for disease in adults and children*, ed 6, St Louis, 2010a, Mosby.

Huether SE: Alterations of digestive function. In McCance KL, et al., editors: *Pathophysiology: the biological basis for disease in adults and children*, ed 6, St Louis, 2010b, Mosby.

Jassal MS, Nedeltchev GG, Lee SW, et al: [C]-Urea breath test as a novel point-of-care biomarker for tuberculosis treatment and diagnosis, *Public Library of Science* 5:2010 pii: e12451.

JNC 7: JNC 7 Express: the seventh report of the Joint National Commission of the Prevention, Detection, Evaluation and Treatment of High Blood Pressure, USHHS Pub No 03-5233, 2003. Available at www.nhlbi.nih.gov.

Jones RE, Brashers VL, Huether SE: Alterations in hormonal regulation. In McCance KL, Huether SE, Brashers VL, et al, editors: *Pathophysiology: the biological basis for disease in adults and children*, ed 6, St Louis, 2010, Mosby.

Jones-Burton C, Saunders E: Cardiovascular disease and hypertension. In Satcher D, Pamies RJ, editors: *Multicultural medicine and health disparities*, NY, 2006, McGrawHill.

Kreiner F, Langberg H, Galbo H: Increased muscle interstitial levels of inflammatory cytokines in polymyalgia rheumatic, *Arthritis and Rheumatism* 2010, e-pub ahead of print, PMID 20812339.

Longstreth GF: Barrett's esophagus, 2009. Available at http://www.nlm.nih.gov/medlineplus/ency/article/001143.htm.

Luggen AS: Arthritis in older adults: current therapy with self-management as a centerpiece, *Advance for Nurse Practitioners* 11:26, 2003.

Meng MV, Stoller ML, Walsh T: Urologic disorders. In McPhee SJ, Papadakis MA, editors: *2010 Current medical diagnosis and treatment*. NY, 2010, McGraw-Hill Lange.

McQuaid KR: Gastrointestinal disorders. In McPhee SJ, Papadakis MA, editors. *2010 Current medical diagnosis and treatment*. NY, 2010, McGraw-Hill Lange.

Miller E, Maimon Y, Rosenblatt Y, et al: Delayed effect of acupuncture treatment in OA of the knee: A blinded, randomized, controlled trial, *Evidence-Based Complementary and Alternative Medicine*. e-print, PMID 19124552, 2009.

Mollaoglu M, Fertelli TK, Tuncay FO: Fatigue and disability in elderly patients with chronic obstructive pulmonary disease (COPD*)*, *Arch Geronotol Geriatr* August 2010 epub ahead of print.

National Heart Lung and Blood Institute (NHLBI): *NHLBI Fact Book Fiscal Year, 2010*, Bethesda, Md, 2010, The Institute. Available at http://www.nhlbi.nih.gov/about/factbook/factbook_2010.pdf. Accessed April 27, 2011.

National Heart Lung and Blood Institute: What is High Blood Pressure? 2008, Available at http://www.nhlbi.nih.gov/health/dci/Diseases/Hbp/HBP_WhatIs.html.

National Heart Lung and Blood Institute: NAEPP Expert Panel Report 3: guidelines for the diagnosis and management of asthma, 2007. Available at http://www.nhlbi.nih.gov/guidelines/asthma/01_front.pdf.

National Heart, Lung and Blood Institute: What causes COPD? n.d. Available at http://www.nhlbi.nih.gov/health/dci/Diseases/Copd/Copd_Causes.html.

National Institute of Arthritis and Musculoskeletal and Skin Disease (NIAMS): Rheumatoid arthritis. Revised 2009. Available at http://www.niams.nih.gov/health_info/Rheumatic_Disease/default.asp#ra_5.

National Institute of Arthritis and Musculoskeletal and Skin Disease: Osteoarthritis. Revised 2006. Available at http://www.niams.nih.gov/health_info/Osteoarthritis/default.asp.

National Institute of Diabetes and Digestive and Kidney Diseases. Important information about diabetes and blood tests: For people of African, Mediterranean or Southeast Asian heritage, 2007. Available at http://diabetes.niddk.nih.gov/dm/pubs/traitA1C.

National Institute of Diabetes and Digestive and Kidney Diseases: Diverticulosis and Diverticulitis. NIH Publication no 08-1163, 2008. Available at http://digestive.niddk.nih.gov/ddiseases/pubs/diverticulosis/index.htm#cause.

National Institute of Diabetes and Digestive and Kidney Diseases. 2007 National Diabetes Fact Sheet, 2010a. Available at http://www.cdc.gov/diabetes/pubs/estimates07.htm#4.

National Institute of Diabetes and Digestive and Kidney Diseases. Kidney and Urologic Disease Statistics for the United States. Publication no. 10-3895, 2010b. Available at: http://kidney.niddk.nih.gov/kudiseases/pubs/kustats/index.htm.

National Institute of Health (NIH): NIH Research matters: New test detects TB in less than two hours, September 13, 2010. Available at: http://www.nih.gov/researchmatters/september2010/09132010tbtest.htm.

National Osteoporosis Foundation: Fast Facts on Osteoporosis, 2010. Available at http://www.nof.org/osteoporosis/diseasefacts.htm.

Orem DE: *Nursing: concepts of practice*, St Louis, 1995, Mosby.

O'Rourke KS: Myopathies, polymyalgia rheumatica and giant cell arteritis. In Hazzard WR et al., editors: *Principles of geriatric medicine and gerontology*, ed 5, New York, 2003, McGraw-Hill.

Rapp JH, Sarkar R, Owens CD: Blood vessels and lymphatic disorders, In McPhee SJ, Papadakis MA, editors. *2010 Current medical diagnosis and treatment*, New York, 2010, McGraw-Hill Lange.

Rhodes LE, Webb AR, Fraser HI, et al: Recommended summer sunlight exposure levels can produce sufficient (> or =20 ng ml (−1)) but not the proposed optimal (> or

=32 ng ml(−1)) 25(OH)D levels at UK latitudes, *Journal of Investigative Dermatology* 130:1411, 2010.

Rissmiller RW, Adair NE: Respiratory diseases. In Landefeld C, Palmer R, Johnson M, et al., editors: *Current geriatric diagnosis and treatment*, New York, 2004, McGraw-Hill.

Rubio MA: Implications of fiber in different pathologies, *Nutrición hospitalaria* 17:17, 2002.

Smedley BD, Stith AY, Nelson AR, editors: *Unequal treatment: confronting racial and ethnic disparities in health care*, Washington, DC, 2003, National Academies Press.

Syed M, Solomon J, Patel NA, et al: Vertebroplasty: The alternative treatment for osteoporotic vertebral compression fractures in the elderly, *Clinical Geriatrics* 14:20, 2006.

Stoller JK: Acute exacerbations of chronic obstructive pulmonary disease, *New England Journal of Medicine* 346:988, 2002.

Strauss A, Glaser B: *Chronic illness and the quality of life*, St Louis, 1975, Mosby.

Sugarman RA: Structure and function of the neurological system. In McCance KL, Huether SE, Brashers VL, et al., editors: *Pathophysiology: the biological basis for disease in adults and children*, ed 6, St Louis, 2010, Mosby.

Tabloski P: *Gerontological nursing*. Upper Saddle River, NJ, 2006, Pearson Prentice Hall.

Talat N, Shahid F, Dawood G, et al: Dynamic changes in biomarker profiles associated with clinical and subclinical tuberculosis in a high transmission setting: A four year follow-up study, *Scandinavian Journal of Immunology* 69:537, 2009.

U.S. Preventive Services Task Force (USPSTF): Screening for high blood pressure: USPSTF Reaffirmation Recommendation Statement, AHRQ Pub No. 08-05105-EF-2, December 2007a. Available at http://www.uspreventiveservicestaskforce.org/uspstf07/hbp/hbprs.htm.

U.S. Preventive Services Task Force: Screening for osteoporosis: Updated July 2010. Available at http://www.uspreventiveservicestaskforce.org/uspstf/uspsoste.htm.

Woog P: *The chronic illness trajectory framework: the Corbin and Strauss nursing model*, New York, 1992, Springer.

Zarowitz BJ: Management of Osteoporosis in order persons, *Geriatric Nursing* 27(1):16-18, 2006.

Care Across the Continuum

Theris A. Touhy

evolve *http://evolve.elsevier.com/Ebersole/TwdHlthAging*

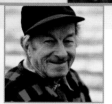

A STUDENT SPEAKS

I feel so depressed when I see all those old people in nursing homes. I don't know how families can put loved ones into a nursing home and I have promised my parents I will never do that to them. **John, age 25**

AN ELDER SPEAKS

This nursing home is my home now. We are all like a family, and I will die here. The girls that help me during the day, we treat one another like family members. We have some days when we are grumpy, some days we are happy, and we don't hold our feelings back, like you would do with your own family at home. **Helen, age 88**

LEARNING OBJECTIVES

Upon completion of this chapter, the reader will be able to:

1. Compare the major features, advantages, and disadvantages of several residential options available to the older adult.
2. Assist older adults and their families in making an informed choice when relocation to a more protected setting becomes necessary.
3. Describe factors influencing the provision of long-term care.
4. Identify interventions to improve care for older adults in acute and long-term care settings.
5. Discuss interventions to improve transitions of care and outcomes for older adults moving between health care settings.

A mobile, youth-oriented society may find it difficult to fully comprehend the insecurity that elders feel when moving from one site to another in their later years. In addition to the stress of relocation and the initial anxiety of adapting to a new setting, elders typically move to ever more restrictive environments, often in times of crisis. This chapter discusses residential care options across the continuum with related implications for nursing practice. The major issues are the choice and control elders have about relocation, assistance provided to the elder in making personally appropriate choices, strategies to improve outcomes of transition between health care settings, and creation of environments that enhance care outcomes in whatever situation the elder is encountering.

RESIDENTIAL OPTIONS IN LATER LIFE

"Home" provides basic shelter, is a place to establish security, and is the place where one "belongs." It should provide the highest possible level of independence, function, and comfort. Most older people prefer to remain in their own homes and "age-in-place," rather than relocate, particularly to institutional living. The ability to age in place depends on appropriate support for changing needs so the older person can stay where he or she wants. Developing elder-friendly communities and increasing opportunities to "age in place" can enhance the health and well-being of older people (Chapter 13).

Some older people, by choice or by need, move from one type of residence to another. A number of options exist, especially for those with the financial resources that allow them to have a choice. Residential options range along a continuum from remaining in one's own home; to senior retirement communities; to shared housing with family members, friends, or others; to residential care communities such as assisted living settings; to nursing facilities for those with the most needs, (Figure 16-1). There are many different models of senior housing, and older people may seek assistance from nurses in choosing what kind

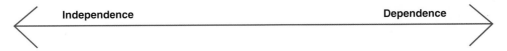

Independence

Home ownership
Single-room occupation (SRO)
Condominium ownership
Apartment dwelling
Shared housing
Congregate lifestyles

Independent to partial dependence

Retirement communities
Public housing complexes
Residence with family
Foster homes
Board and care
Residential homes
Continuing care retirement communities (CCRCs)

Partial dependence to complete dependence

Nursing facilities
Skilled nursing facilities
Acute care facilities
Inpatient hospice care facilities

Independence ←————————————————————→ Dependence

FIGURE 16-1 Continuum of residential options based on level of assistance needed. From Touhy TT, Jett KF: *Ebersole and Hess' gerontological nursing & healthy aging*, ed 3, 2010, Mosby.

of living situation will be best for them. It is important to be aware of the various options available in your local community as well as the advantages, disadvantages, cost, and services provided in each option. When discharging older people from the hospital, knowledge of where they live or the type of setting to which they are being discharged, will assist in individualizing teaching so that outcomes can be enhanced for both the older adult and his or her family.

Shared Housing

Shared housing among adult children and their older relatives has become a choice for many because of cultural preferences or need. The sharing may relieve the economic burdens of maintaining a home after widowhood or retirement on a fixed income. However, strong cultural influences predict the frequency of multigenerational residences. Among Asians, South Americans, and African Americans, it is often an expectation. A variation of multigenerational housing has long existed in what has become known as "granny flats." These may be apartments added to existing homes or the construction of small housing units on family property with privacy as well as sharing of time and resources. Such arrangements allow families to be close enough to be of assistance if needed but to remain separate. They are practical and economical, and their production has continually expanded, particularly in Australia. In the United States, use of this model is minimal, but existing "mother-in-law" cottages and apartments have served a similar purpose for many families for years.

Another model of shared housing is that of opening one's personal home to others. Older people often live in houses, which were purchased in their young adult years, and find that as they age, much of the space may be underused. Sharing a house can be easily implemented by locating, screening, and matching older people looking for houses to share with those who have them. The National Shared Housing Resource Center (NSHRC) (http://www.nationalsharedhousing.org/) has established subgroups nationally to assist individuals interested in home sharing. Those who have done so report feeling safer and less lonely. Studies on home sharing focus on the effects on well-being, finances, health, social life, and daily satisfaction.

Community Care

PACE (Program for All Inclusive Care for the Elderly) is an alternative to nursing home care for frail older people who want to live independently in the community with a high quality of life. It provides a comprehensive continuum of primary care, acute care, home care, nursing home care, and specialty care by an interdisciplinary team. PACE is a capitated system in which the team is provided with a monthly sum to provide all care to the enrollees, including medications, eyeglasses, and transportation to care as well as urgent and preventive care. Participants must meet the criteria for nursing home admission, prefer to remain in the community, and be eligible for Medicare and Medicaid. Adult day services are also provided.

PACE is now recognized as a permanent provider under Medicare and a state option under Medicaid. In 2009, there were 72 PACE programs operational in 30 states. PACE has been approved by the U.S. Department of Health and Human Services (USDHHS) Substance Abuse and Mental Health Services Administration (SAMHSA) as an evidence-based model of care. Models such as PACE are innovative care delivery models, and continued development of such models are important as the population ages. More information about PACE models and outcomes of care can be found at www.cms.hhs.gov/QualityInitiativesGenInfo/10_PACE.asp and at http://www.npaonline.org/website/article.asp?id=12.

Adult Day Services

Adult day services (ADS) are community-based group programs designed to provide social and some health services to adults who need supervised care in a safe setting during the day. They also offer caregivers respite from the responsibilities of caregiving, and most provide educational programs for caregivers and support groups. There are more than 4,600 adult day services centers across the United States—a 35% increase since 2002. Adult day centers are serving populations with higher levels of physical disability and chronic disease, and the number of older people receiving adult day services has increased 63% over the last eight years (National Adult Day Services Association, Ohio State University College of Social Work, MetLife Mature Market Institute, 2009).

Adult day services are an important part of the long-term care continuum and a cost-effective alternative or supplement to home care or institutional care. While further research is needed on patient and caregiver outcomes of ADS, findings suggest that they improve health-related quality of life for participants and improve caregiver well-being. ADS are increasingly being utilized to provide community-based care for conditions like Alzheimer's disease and for transitional care and short-term rehabilitation following hospitalization.

Historically, ADS has been divided into three models of care: social (meals, recreation, some health-related services), medical-health (social activities and more intensive health and therapeutic services), and specialized (services provided only to specific care recipients such as those with dementia or developmental disabilities). However, more and more ADS are offering a range of comprehensive services. Staff ratios in ADS are one direct care worker to six clients. Almost 80% of centers have professional nursing staff, and 50% have a social worker and physical, occupational, and speech therapists. Most also offer transportation services.

The average ADS cost/day is $66.71. Some ADS are private pay, and others are funded through Medicaid home and community-based waiver programs, state and local funding, and the Veteran's Administration. The Patient Protection and Affordable Care Act provides additional funding to states for home and community-based care. Pilot programs have been implemented through Medicare and are being evaluated. ADS hold the potential to meet the need for cost-efficient and high-quality long-term care services, and continued expansion and funding is expected. Local area agencies on aging are good sources of information about adult day services and other community-based options (National Adult Day Services Association, Ohio State University College of Social Work, MetLife Mature Market Institute, 2009).

Foster Care

Adult foster care offers a community-based living arrangement to adults who are unable to live independently because of physical or mental impairment or disabilities and are in need of supervision or personal care.

Homes providing foster care offer 24-hour supervision, protection, and personal care in addition to room and board. They may also provide additional services. Adult foster care serves a designated, small number of individuals (generally from one to six) in a homelike and family-like environment; one of the primary caregivers often resides in the home. A growing number of foster care homes are under corporate ownership, and in these situations, the home-like atmosphere tends to be lost. However, with state-regulated, outcome-oriented quality assurance strategies focused on achieving maximal function, autonomy, and social integration, adult foster care may fill a real need.

Residential Care Facilities

Residential care facility is the broad term for a range of nonmedical, community-based residential settings that house two or more unrelated adults and provide services such as meals, medication supervision or reminders, activities, transportation, or assistance with activities of daily living (ADLs). These kinds of facilities are for elders who need more care than is available in shared housing, or for whom shared housing is not an option and nursing home care is not needed. Residential care facilities are known by more than 30 different names across the country, including *adult congregate facilities, foster care homes, personal care homes, homes for the elderly, domiciliary care homes, board and care homes, rest homes, family care homes, retirement homes,* and *assisted living facilities.*

Residential care facilities are the fastest growing housing option available for older adults in the United States. This kind of facility is viewed as more cost effective than nursing homes while providing more privacy and a homelike environment. Medicare does not cover the cost of care in these types of facilities. In some states, costs may be covered by private and long-term care insurance and some other types of assistance programs. Assisted living is primarily private pay, although 41 states currently have a Medicaid Waiver/Medicaid State Plan for a limited amount of residents (AAHSA, 2011). The rates charged and what services those rates include vary considerably, as do regulations and licensing.

Assisted Living

A popular type of residential care can be found in assisted living facilities (ALFs), also called *board and care homes* or *adult congregate living facilities* (ACLFs). Assisted living is a residential long-term care choice for older adults who need more than an independent living environment but do not need the 24 hours/day skilled nursing care and the constant monitoring of a skilled nursing facility. The typical assisted living resident is an 86-year-old woman who is mobile but needs assistance with 2 ADLs (Box 16-1).

Assisted living settings may be a shared room or a single-occupancy unit with a private bath, kitchenette, and communal meals. They all provide some support services. Assisted living provides security with independence and privacy, and supports physical and social well-being with the health care supervision it provides.

Assisted living is more expensive than independent living and less costly than skilled nursing home care, but it is not

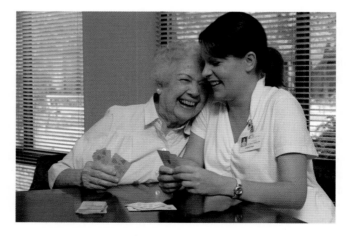

Providing nursing services in assisted living facilities promotes physical and psychosocial health. (From Potter PA: *Basic nursing: essentials for practice,* ed 7, 2010, Mosby).

inexpensive. There are 39,500 assisted living facilities in the United States. Costs vary by geographical region, size of the unit, and relative luxury. The average base rate (room and board and limited other services) in an assisted facility is $2,930 monthly, or $35,160 annually in 2010 (Prudential Life Insurance Company of America, 2011). Most ALFs offer two or three meals per day, light weekly housekeeping, and laundry services, as well as optional social activities. Each added service increases the cost of the setting but also allows for individuals with resources to remain in the setting longer, as functional abilities decline.

Many seniors and their families prefer ALFs to nursing homes because they cost less, are more homelike, and offer more opportunities for control, independence, and privacy. However, many residents of ALFs have chronic care needs and over time may require more care than the facility is able to provide. Services (e.g., home health, hospice, homemakers) can be brought into the facility, but some question whether this adequately substitutes for 24-hour supervision by registered nurses (RNs). Not every ALF has an RN or licensed practical–vocational nurse (LPN/LVN), and, in most states, any skilled nursing provided by the staff other than nurse-delegated assistance with self-administered medication is prohibited. In the ALF, there is no organized team of providers such as that found in nursing homes (i.e., nurses, social workers, rehabilitation therapists, pharmacists).

With the growing numbers of older adults with dementia residing in ALFs, many are establishing dementia-specific units. It is important to investigate services available as well as staff training when making decisions as to the most appropriate placement for older adults with dementia. Continued research is needed on best care practices as well as outcomes of care for people with dementia in both ALFs and nursing homes. The Alzheimer's Association has issued a set of dementia care practices for ALFs and nursing homes (Alzheimer's Association, 2009) (http://www.alz.org/national/documents/brochure_DCPRphases1n2.pdf) and an evidence-based guideline, *Dementia Care Practice Recommendations for Assisted Living Residences and Nursing Homes* (Tilly & Reed, 2006) (www.guideline.gov) is also avaliable.

The Joint Commission and the Commission for Accreditation of Rehabilitation Facilities have published standards for accreditation of ALFs, but many are advocating for more comprehensive federal and state standards and regulations. The nonmedical nature of ALFs is a primary factor in keeping costs more reasonable than those in nursing facilities, but costs are still high for those without adequate funds. Appropriate standards of care must be developed and care outcomes monitored to ensure that residents are receiving quality care in this setting, which is almost devoid of professional nursing. Further research is needed on care outcomes of residents in ALFs and the role of unlicensed assistive personnel, as well as RNs, in these facilities.

The American Assisted Living Nurses Association has established a certification mechanism for nurses working in these facilities and has also developed a *Scope and Standards of Assisted Living Nursing Practice for Registered Nurses* (www.alnursing.org). Advanced practice gerontological nurses are well suited to the role of primary care provider in ALFs, and many have assumed this role. Consumers are advised to inquire as to exactly what services will be provided and by whom if an ALF resident becomes more frail and needs more intensive care. The Assisted Living Federation of America (2010) provides a consumer guide for choosing an assisted living residence (http://www.alfa.org/images/alfa/PDFs/getfile.cfm_product_id=94&file=ALFAchecklist.pdf).

Continuing Care Retirement Communities

Life care communities, also known as continuing care retirement communities (CCRCs), provide the full range of residential options, from single-family homes to skilled nursing facilities all in one location. Most of these communities provide access to these levels of care for a community member's entire remaining lifetime, and for the right price, the range of services may be guaranteed. Having all levels of care in one location allows community members to make the transition between levels without life-disrupting moves. For married couples in which one spouse needs more care than the other, life care communities allow them to live nearby in a different part of the same community. This industry is maturing, and there are 1900 CCRCs in the United States, housing more than 745,000 older adults (AAHSA, 2011).

Most CCRCs are managed by not-for-profit organizations. They usually charge an entry fee ranging from $60,000 to $120,000 that covers and reflects the cost of the residence in which the member will live, the possible future care needed, and the quality and quantity of the community services. The average monthly cost of living in a not-for-profit CCRC is $2,672. Important to remember about these types of communities is that the residence purchased usually belongs to the community after the death of the owner.

Population-Specific Communities

As the number of senior communities expands, older adults will have more options of moving somewhere that they find especially welcoming. These options include communities that emphasize a particular sport, like tennis or golf. Groups of people can also come together to form intentional communities, buying a cluster of home tracts and building in such a way to support their particular lifestyles or needs or personalities. Still others provide unique additional services, such as those in communities that specialize in providing residences for persons with, for example, a mental illness, alcoholism, or developmental disabilities.

Lesbian, gay, bisexual, and transgender (LGBT) seniors face several problems in housing in their older years. They may have little family support and may face discrimination in housing options. Many LGBT seniors say they do not feel welcome at traditional residential options. Those who wish to live together are discouraged from doing so by some organizations. Residential facilities and communities designed specifically for LGBT seniors are increasing in number across the country. Nurses should be aware of this heretofore invisible group of older adults who need access to welcoming resources. Chapters 21 and 22 discusses issues specific to LGBT seniors in more depth.

Senior Retirement Communities

Communities designed for elders are proliferating. Numerous combinations of single-family homes, apartments, activities, optional services, meals in the home, cafeterias, restaurants, housekeeping, golf, tennis, and security are available. In some cases, emergency services and health clinics are adjacent. These are all designed to make independent living feasible with the least effort on the part of the elder. Some senior communities are luxurious and have a wide range of physical and cultural amenities; others are simpler, providing only the basic necessities. Prices are consistent with the level of luxury provided and the range of services available.

Although the costs of the majority of senior communities are borne by the consumers, for elders with limited incomes, federally subsidized rental options are available in some areas of the country. Older adults benefiting from this option are assisted through rental housing subsidized by the U.S. Department of Housing and Urban Development (HUD). Although not all HUD housing is designated for senior living, Section 202 of the Housing Act, U.S. Department of Housing and Urban Development, approved the construction of low-rent units especially for elders. These units may also have provisions for health care, recreation, and transportation. Under Section 8 of the Housing Act of 1983, tenants locate their own unit. Usually the tenant pays 30% of his or her adjusted gross income toward the rent, and HUD assists with supplementary vouchers to meet the fair market value of the rental (American Association of Homes and Services for the Aging [AAHSA], 2011).

ACUTE CARE FOR OLDER ADULTS

Older adults often enter the health care system with admissions to acute care settings. The admission rate for older adults is as high as three times those of younger individuals (Resnick, 2009). Exacerbations of chronic illnesses and injuries are often the cause of hospitalizations for older adults. Acutely ill older adults frequently have multiple chronic conditions and comorbidities and present many care challenges. Hospitals are dangerous places for elders: 34% experience functional decline, and iatrogenic complications occur in as many as 29% to 38%, a rate three to five times higher than in younger patients (Inouye et al, 2000; Kleinpell, 2007). Common iatrogenic complications include functional decline, pneumonia, delirium, new-onset incontinence, malnutrition, pressure ulcers, medication reactions, and falls.

Recognizing the impact of iatrogenesis, both on patient outcomes and cost of care, the Centers for Medicare and Medicaid Services (CMS) has instituted changes to the inpatient prospective payment system that will reduce payment to hospitals relative to poor care. The changes target conditions that are high cost or high volume, result in a higher payment when present as a secondary diagnosis, are not present on admission, and could have reasonably been prevented through the use of evidence-based guidelines. Targeted conditions include catheter-associated urinary tract infections, pressure ulcers, and falls.

Nursing Roles and Models of Care

Nurses caring for older adults in hospitals may function in the direct care provider role, as well as in leadership and management positions. Most nurses who work in hospitals are caring for older patients, and many have not had gerontological nursing content in their basic nursing education programs. In a survey of hospital nurses, only 37% reported participating in a hospital in-service training program on care of older adults (Mezey et al., 2007). "Few of the country's 6,000 hospitals have institutional practice guidelines, educational resources, and administrative practices that support best practices care of older adults" (Boltz et al., 2008, p. 176). As part of the Nurse Competence in Aging project, the American Association of Nurse Executives (AONE) has developed guiding principles for the elder-friendly hospital/facility (Box 16-2).

Recognizing the need for models of nursing practice to prevent iatrogenesis and improve outcomes for older hospitalized patients, the Hartford Geriatric Nursing Institute developed, in 1992, the Nurses Improving Care for Health System Elders (NICHE) program. "NICHE is built on the premise that the bedside nurse plays a pivotal role in influencing the older adult's hospital experience and outcomes, through direct nursing care, as well as coordination of interdisciplinary activities" (Resnick, 2009, p. 81). More than 300 hospitals in more than 40 states, as well as parts of Canada, are involved in NICHE projects. NICHE units of various types have been developed including the geriatric resource nurse (GRN) model and the acute care of the elderly (ACE) unit (www. nicheprogram.org).

The GRN model is the most frequently implemented NICHE model. In this model, staff nurses receive competency-based training and are mentored by advanced practice nurses in care of hospitalized older adults. GRNs then function as clinical resource experts on geriatric issues to staff on their unit. Evidence-based interdisciplinary protocols, geriatric-specific resources, management strategies, policies to meet the specialized needs of older adults, as well as an online knowledge center providing educational support, are features of the NICHE

BOX 16-2	GUIDING PRINCIPLES FOR THE ELDER-FRIENDLY HOSPITAL/FACILITY

FOR THE PATIENT
- Each patient is a unique individual and should be evaluated as such
- Measures are taken to accommodate the patient and family's special needs

FOR THE STAFF
- Nurses demonstrate clinical competence in geriatric nursing
- Nurses provide therapeutic response, patience and presence when caring for geriatric patients
- Nurses and staff who provide direct care identify and address the patient's individual needs and preferences; staff creates a positive experience for the patient and family
- Nurses coordinate care across the continuum and "Manage the Journey" of the patient and family
- Excellent communication, tailored to meet the needs of the geriatric patient, results in a "Climate of Confidence" for the patient and the nurse
- The organization provides appropriate resources and systems that support best practice in geriatric nursing care

FOR THE ENVIRONMENT
- The physical environment supports the needs of the geriatric patient and family and the staff who care for them
- An Elder-Friendly environment, as defined by the patient and family, also enhances the practice environment for the staff
- The Elder-Friendly environment is embraced hospital-wide

From American Association of Nurse Executives: *The guiding principles for creating elder-friendly hospitals.* Available at www.aone.org/resource/elderguiding.html. Accessed October 31, 2010. Copyright 2010 by the American Organization Nurse Executives (AONE) ALL Rights Reserved.

---

model (Resnick, 2009). This is an innovative role for a hospital staff nurse interested in care of older adults. Outcomes in hospitals using NICHE models include enhanced nursing knowledge and skills related to treatment of common geriatric syndromes, patient and nurse satisfaction, decreased length of stay, reductions in admission rates, and reductions in hospital costs (Fulmer et al., 2002; Mezey et al., 2004b; Boltz et al., 2008; Steele, 2010). Further research on patient outcomes, patient and staff satisfaction, and cost of implementation of NICHE models is needed.

The ACE model was originally developed at University Hospitals in Cleveland in conjunction with the Frances Payne Bolton School of Nursing at Case Western Reserve University. A 29 bed medical surgical specialty unit was renovated and dedicated as an ACE unit to prevent functional decline of targeted older adult patients. The NICHE ACE model designates a specific unit or section of a unit to deliver interventions known to improve the clinical outcomes of older adult patients. Key elements include environmental modifications for older patients and interdisciplinary staff with expertise in geriatrics and prevention of geriatric syndromes (www.nicheprogram.org/niche_models).

COMMUNITY-BASED AND HOME-BASED CARE

Nurses will care for older adults in hospitals and long-term care, but the majority of older adults live in the community. Community-based care settings include home care,

independent senior housing, retirement communities, residential care facilities, adult day health programs, primary care clinics, and public health departments. The growth in home- and community-based health care is expected to continue because older people prefer to age in place. Other factors influencing the growth of home-based care include rapidly escalating health care costs. The Independence at Home Act, part of the Affordable Care Act, supports home-based primary care teams, including physicians and nurse practitioners, to deliver primary care services to high-risk patients. This three-year demonstration project will receive mandatory appropriations of $5 million per year. After the project ends, the Department of Health and Human Services will evaluate the program and report to Congress (AARP, 2010; Landers, 2010). Advances in technology for remote monitoring of health status and safety, and point-of-care testing devices show promise in improving outcomes for elders who want to age in place. These technologies present exciting opportunities for nurses in the management and evaluation of care and call for increased education and practice experiences for nursing students in home-based care.

Nurses in the home setting provide comprehensive assessments and care management. They may provide and supervise care for elders with a variety of care needs including chronic wounds, intravenous therapy, tube feedings, unstable medical conditions, and complex medication regimens, and for those receiving rehabilitation and palliative and hospice services. Gerontological nurses will find opportunities to create practices in community-based settings with a focus not only on care for those who are ill, but also on health promotion.

NURSING HOMES

Nursing homes are the settings for the delivery of around-the-clock care for those needing specialized care that cannot be provided elsewhere. Nursing homes today have evolved into a significant location where health care is provided across the continuum of care. Nursing homes are a complex health care setting that is a mix of hospital, rehabilitation facility, hospice, and dementia-specific units, and they are a final home for many elders. When used appropriately, nursing homes fill an important need for families and elders.

Characteristics of Nursing Homes

The settings called *nursing homes or nursing facilities* most often include up to two levels of care: a *skilled nursing care* (also called *subacute care*) facility is required to have licensed professionals with a focus on the management of complex medical needs; and a *chronic care* (also called *long-term* or *custodial*) facility is required to have 24-hour personal assistance that is supervised and augmented by professional and licensed nurses. Often, both kinds of services are provided in one facility. Most nursing homes offer subacute units that function much like the general medical-surgical hospital units of the past.

Subacute care is more intensive than traditional nursing home care and several times more costly, but far less costly than care in an acute-care hospital. Skilled nursing facilities are the most frequent site of postacute care in the United States, and they treat 50% of all Medicare beneficiaries requiring postacute care following hospitalization (Alliance for Quality Nursing Home Care and the American Health Care Association, 2010). The expectation is that the patient will be discharged home or to a less intensive setting. In addition to skilled nursing care, rehabilitation services are an essential component of subacute units. Length of stay is usually less than one month and is largely reimbursed by Medicare. Patients in subacute units are usually younger and less likely to be cognitively impaired than those in traditional nursing home care. Generally, higher levels of professional staffing are found in the subacute setting than those in the traditional nursing home setting because of the acuity of the patient's condition.

Nursing homes also care for patients who may not need the intense care provided in subacute units but still need ongoing 24-hour care. This may include individuals with severe strokes, dementia, or Parkinson's disease, and those receiving hospice care. More than 50% of residents in nursing homes are cognitively impaired, and nursing homes are increasingly caring for people at the end of life. Twenty-three percent of Americans die in nursing homes, and this figure is expected to increase 40% by 2040 (Carlson, 2007). Nursing home residents represent the most frail of all older adults. Their needs for 24-hour care could not be met in the home or residential care setting, or may have exceeded what the family was able to provide.

There are approximately 16,100 certified nursing homes in the United States, and more than 1.4 million older adults reside in nursing homes. The majority of nursing homes are for-profit organizations (67%), with 31% managed by not-for-profit organizations (AAHSA, 2011). Nursing home chains own 54% of all nursing homes (Harrington et al., 2010). The number of nursing home beds is decreasing in the United States and the number of Medicaid-only beds has decreased by half since 1995 (Gleckman, 2010). This is most likely a result of the increased use of residential care facilities and more reimbursement by Medicaid programs for community-based care alternatives.

Residents of long-term facilities are predominantly women, 80 years or older, widowed, and dependent in ADLs and instrumental activities of daily living (IADLs). While the percentage of older people living in nursing homes at any given time is low (4% to 5%), those who live to age 85 will have a 1 in 2 chance of spending some time in a nursing home. This could be for subacute care, ongoing long-term care, or end-of-life care.

With the increasing number of older people, projections are that there will be a threefold increase in the number of older people needing nursing home care by 2030. People who reach age 65 will likely have a 40% chance of entering a nursing home, and about 10% who enter a nursing home will stay there 5 years or more (Medicare.gov, 2010a). Continued attention to the development of a range of appropriate, high-quality alternatives and different models of long-term care and services is needed.

Rehabilitation and Restorative Care Services

Rehabilitation is a philosophy, not a place of care, or a set of specific services. In all settings, rehabilitation and restorative care is focused on maximizing the individual's strengths and supporting limitations to assist the patient to achieve the highest practicable level of function. Rehabilitation and restorative care

"seeks to improve the individual's quality of life in any way, no matter how small, in relation to physical, emotional, or spiritual well-being; and ultimately return that individual to a residence of his choice and at minimal personal risk. This implies integration into society plus support in and by the community" (Williams, 1993, p. 361).

People who are cared for in subacute units, as well as long-term units of nursing facilities, require access to rehabilitation and restorative care services that maintain or improve their function and prevent excess disability. These services are required under federal and state regulations and are integral to quality indicators in nursing facilities. Barbara Resnick, a noted gerontological nursing researcher, has published extensively on restorative care in both nursing facilities and residential care facilities (Chapters 2 and 12). Restorative nursing programs for ADLs, toileting, range of motion, ambulation, and feeding contribute to restoration and maintenance of function for nursing facility residents who may have been discharged or who are not eligible for reimbursement for rehabilitation services by physical, occupational, or speech therapists. Both rehabilitation and restorative programs require comprehensive multidisciplinary assessment and involvement of the patient and family in development of a plan of care with short and long-term goals (Box 16-3). Rehabilitation and restorative care is increasingly important in light of shortened hospital stays that may occur before conditions are stabilized and the older adult is not ready to function independently.

Costs of Care

Costs for nursing homes vary by geographical location, ownership, and amenities, but the average annual cost for a semiprivate room is $215 per day or $78,475 annually. Nursing home rates have increased more than 10% since 2008 and nearly 50% since 2004 (Prudential Insurance Company of America, 2010). The majority of the cost of care in nursing homes is borne by Medicaid (42%), followed by Medicare (25%), out of pocket (22%), and private insurance and other sources (11%) (AAHSA, 2011). Medicare covers 100% of the costs for the first 20 days. Beginning on day 21 of the nursing home stay, there is a significant co-payment. This co-payment may be covered by a Medigap policy. After 100 days the individual is responsible for all costs.

BOX 16-3	MEMBERS OF THE REHABILITATION CARE TEAM

- Rehabilitation nurse specialist
- Physical therapist
- Occupational therapist
- Speech therapist
- Social worker
- Discharge planner
- Psychologist
- Prosthetist and orthotist
- Audiologist
- Physician, nurse practitioner
- Vocational rehabilitation specialist
- Person in rehabilitation
- Person's significant others

In order for a nursing home stay to be covered by Medicare, you must enter a Medicare-approved "skilled nursing facility" or nursing home within 30 days of a hospital stay that lasted at least 3 days (Medicare.gov, 2010). Complex medical treatments (e.g., feeding tube, tracheostomy, intravenous [IV] therapy) and rehabilitation services such as occupational therapy (OT), physical therapy (PT), or speech therapy (ST), are considered skilled care. Medicare does not cover the costs of care in chronic, custodial, and long-term units. If the older person was admitted to the nursing home because of a dementia diagnosis and the need for assistance with ADLs and maintenance of safety, Medicare would not cover the cost of care unless there was some skilled need (Chapter 20).

Concern is growing nationwide about the financing of long-term care and the ability of the states and the federal government to continue to support costs through the Medicaid programs. The reimbursement levels of both Medicare and Medicaid do not cover actual costs, and there is fear that if further cuts are made, quality of care will be more drastically compromised. The increasing burden on Medicaid is unsustainable, and assuming present growth, Medicaid costs for long-term care will double by 2025 and increase fivefold by 2045 (AAHSA, 2008).

The purchase of long-term care insurance is an option, but it is expensive and pays for less than 5% of long-term care costs (AAHSA, 2011). The Community Living Assistance Services and Support (CLASS), approved as part of the Patient Population and Affordable Care Act, is a voluntary, federally administered, consumer-directed, long-term insurance plan. The CLASS plan provides those who participate with cash to help pay for needed assistance if they become functionally limited, in a place they call home, from independent living to a nursing facility.

Health care coverage for people with long-term care needs is a major national issue that demands attention along with the growing numbers of uninsured individuals of all ages and the rising costs of care in the United States. In response to the nation's need for a long-term care financing solution, the AAHSA has made recommendations for a model for future financing for long-term care (www.thelongtermcareresolution.org/problem.aspx).

Quality of Care

Nursing homes are one of the most highly regulated industries in the United States. The Omnibus Reconciliation Act (OBRA) of 1987, and the frequent revisions and updates, are designed to improve the quality of resident care and have had a positive impact. Some of the requirements of OBRA and subsequent legislation include the following: comprehensive resident assessments (Minimum Data Set [MDS]), increased training requirements for nursing assistants, elimination of the use of medications and restraints for the purpose of discipline or convenience, higher staffing requirements for nursing and social work staff, standards for nursing home administrators, and quality assurance activities.

Both the federal and state governments describe the standards that nursing facilities must meet to comply with the law and qualify for reimbursement. Quality trends are monitored and available to the public (http://www4.cms.gov/MDSPubQIandResRep/03_qireports.asp?qtr=21&isSubmitted=qi2). Nursing homes were the first to publish on-line quality information, which is now available for hospitals and other health care organizations. Findings from the recent report on care quality in nursing and rehabilitation facilities report that a majority of key government-measured quality trends are improving, while others still require ongoing attention (Alliance for Quality Nursing Home Care and the American Health Care Association, 2010).

Although nursing homes recognize the need to ensure quality and have responded to improvement initiatives, the lack of additional funding for legislated initiatives has left many nursing homes struggling to maintain quality and meet standards with few resources. Care of the frail elderly and seriously ill persons is labor-intensive, costly, and requires specialized knowledge. Reasonable workloads, enhanced education and training, and adequate reimbursement are essential. Oversight has too often been conducted in a punitive fashion rather than a collaborative effort to enhance outcomes similar to that which is seen in other health care institutions.

The Five-Star Quality Rating system for nursing homes, established by the CMS, was created to help consumers, their families, and caregivers to compare nursing homes (www.medicare.gov/NHCompare). This rating system is based on the nursing home's most recent health inspection, staffing, and quality measures. The CMS advises consumers to use additional sources of information because the Five Star rating system should not substitute for visiting nursing homes since it is a "snap shot" of the care in individual nursing homes, (www.medicare.gov, 2010b).

The most appropriate method of choosing a nursing home is to personally visit the facility, meet with the director of nursing, observe care routines, discuss the potential resident's needs, and use a format such as the one presented in Box 16-4 to ask questions. The CMS provides a nursing home checklist on their website, and the National Citizens' Coalition for Nursing Home Reform also provides resources for choosing a nursing home (www.nccnhr.org). Nurse researchers Marilyn Rantz and Mary Zywgart-Stauffacher (2009) published a book, *How to Find the Best Eldercare*, based on their research.

Regulations have also been created to protect the rights of the residents of nursing homes. Residents in long-term care facilities have rights under both federal and state law. The staff of the facility must inform residents of these rights and protect and promote their rights. The rights to which the residents are entitled should be conspicuously posted in the facility (Box 16-5). Also, the Long-Term Care Ombudsman Program is a nationwide effort to support the rights of both the residents and the facilities. In most states, the program provides trained volunteers to investigate rights and quality complaints or conflicts. All reporting is anonymous. Each facility is required to post the name and contact information of the ombudsman assigned to the facility.

Professional Nursing in Nursing Homes

There are a wide range of opportunities for professional nursing in nursing homes. Eldercare is projected to be the fastest-growing employment sector in the health care industry, and the demand for professional nurses, other health care professionals, and direct care workers is projected to rise dramatically.

BOX 16-4 SELECTING A NURSING HOME

CENTRAL FOCUS
- Residents and families are the central focus of the facility

INTERACTION
- Staff members are attentive and caring
- Staff members listen to what residents say
- Staff members and residents smile at one another
- Prompt response to resident and family needs
- Meaningful activities provided on all shifts to meet individual preferences
- Residents engage in activities with enjoyment
- Staff members talk to cognitively impaired residents; cognitively impaired residents involved in activities designed to meet their needs
- Staff members do not talk down to residents, talk as if they are not present, ignore yelling or calling out
- Families are involved in care decisions and daily life in facility

MILIEU
- Calm, active, friendly
- Presence of community, volunteers, children, plants, animals

ENVIRONMENT
- No odor, clean and well maintained
- Rooms personalized
- Private areas
- Protected outside areas
- Equipment in good repair

INDIVIDUALIZED CARE
- Restorative programs for ambulation, ADLs
- Residents well dressed and groomed
- Resident and family councils
- Pleasant mealtimes, good food, residents have choices
- Adequate staff to serve meals and assist residents
- Flexible meal schedules, food available 24 hours per day
- Ethnic food preferences available

STAFF
- Well trained, high level of professional skill
- Professional in appearance and demeanor
- RNs involved in care decisions and care delivery
- Active staff development programs
- Physicians and advanced-practice nurses involved in care planning and staff training
- Adequate staff (more than the minimum required) on each shift
- Low staff turnover

SAFETY
- Safe walking areas indoors and outdoors
- Monitoring of residents at risk for injury
- Restraint-appropriate care, adequate safety equipment and training on its use

ADLs, Activities of daily living; *RNs,* registered nurses.
Adapted from Rantz MJ, Mehr DR, Popejoy L, et al: Nursing home care quality: a multidimensional theoretical model, *Journal of Nursing Care Quality* 12:30-46, 1998.

BOX 16-5 BILL OF RIGHTS FOR LONG-TERM CARE RESIDENTS

- The right to voice grievances and have them remedied
- The right to information about health conditions and treatments and to participate in one's own care to the greatest extent possible
- The right to choose one's own health care providers and to speak privately with one's health care providers
- The right to consent to or refuse all aspects of care and treatments
- The right to manage one's own finances if capable, or to choose one's own financial advisor
- The right to be transferred or discharged only for appropriate reasons
- The right to be free from all forms of abuse
- The right to be free from all forms of restraint to the extent compatible with safety
- The right to privacy and confidentiality concerning one's person, personal information, and medical information
- The right to be treated with dignity, consideration, and respect in keeping with one's individuality
- The right to immediate visitation and access at any time for family, health care providers, and legal advisors; the right to reasonable visitation and access for others

Note: This list of rights is a sampling of federal and several states' lists of rights of residents or participants in long-term care. Nurses should check the rules of their own state for specific rights in law for that state.

This negative image is compounded by reimbursement policies that significantly limit the ability to provide high-quality care" (p. 365).

Nursing homes are often blamed for all of the societal problems associated with the aging of our population. Daily, millions of dedicated caregivers in nursing homes are providing competent and compassionate care to very sick older people against great odds, such as a lack of support, inadequate salaries and staff, inadequate funding, and a lack of respect. It is time for their stories to be told, and it is time to recognize their needs for adequate and well-trained staff to do this very important work. Although there are continued challenges and opportunities to improve care in nursing homes (and care in all settings for older adults) and in the fabric of the long-term care system, many nursing homes provide an environment that truly represents the best of caring and quality of life.

Professional Nurse Staffing

For those of us committed to quality care for the most frail of our elders, the lack of professional nurse staffing in nursing facilities is reason for grave concern. A study by the CMS revealed that registered nurse staffing levels below 0.75 hours/resident per day can jeopardize health and safety, and yet approximately 97% of nursing homes do not meet this standard (Mezey & Harrington, 2004). In 2009, the average number of RN hours per day was 0.67 (Harrington et al, 2010). Current federal regulations require only one RN in the nursing facility for eight hours a day, a figure quite shocking considering the ratio of RNs to patients in acute care, even in the face of shortages in this setting. More RN direct-care time per resident in nursing facilities is associated with fewer pressure ulcers, fewer hospitalizations, fewer urinary tract infections, less weight loss, fewer catheterizations, and less deterioration in the ability to perform ADLs

However, there are few health care workers who are interested and prepared to care for older people (Institute of Medicine, 2008) (Chapter 1). We agree with Eliopoulos (2010) who states: "The many positive aspects of geriatric nursing in long-term care facilities are often overshadowed by an uncomplimentary image of care in this setting, influenced by a history laden with scandals and the media's readiness to highlight the abuses and substandard conditions demonstrated by a small minority.

(Horn et al., 2005). Total nursing staffing and RN staffing levels are predictors of nursing home quality and are negatively associated with total deficiencies, quality of care deficiencies, and serious deficiencies that may cause harm or jeopardy to nursing homes residents (Kim et al., 2009).

An expert panel on nursing home care convened by the John A. Hartford Institute for Geriatric Nursing (Harrington et al., 2000) provided comprehensive recommendations for improved RN staffing, increased gerontological nursing education requirements for all staff, including a bachelor of science in nursing (BSN) degree for directors of nursing, and increased staffing ratios for RNs, LPNs, and nursing assistants. Additional recommendations were that most nursing homes should have a full-time CNS or GNP on staff. Many groups dealing with issues of the aging, as well as the ANA, have supported the critical need for adequate staffing in nursing homes, but to date the federal government has not acted to mandate increases in minimum staffing requirements.

There are several new initiatives nurses can be involved with that are aimed at improving professional nursing practice and quality outcomes in long-term care, including Sigma Theta Tau's new Center for Nursing Excellence in Long Term Care, and the Advancing Excellence in America's Nursing Homes (www.nhqualitycampaign.org/). The culture change movement, discussed later in the chapter, provides many exciting opportunities for professional nurses to lead the change from institution-centered care to a person-centered culture in nursing facilities. Continued research on new models of care delivery and the appropriate mix of all levels of nursing staff in subacute and long-term units is needed to improve outcomes.

Professional Nursing Roles

Professional nurses in nursing facilities must be highly skilled in the complex care concerns of older people, ranging from subacute care to end-of-life care. Excellent assessment skills; ability to work with multidisciplinary teams in partnership with residents and families; skills in acute, rehabilitative, and palliative care; and leadership, management, supervision, and delegation skills are essential. Practice in this setting calls for independent decision making and is guided by a nursing model of care because there are fewer physicians and other professionals on site at all times. Roles for nursing may include nursing administrator, manager, supervisor, charge nurse, educator, infection control nurse, Minimum Data Set (MDS) coordinator, case manager, quality improvement coordinator, and direct care provider. Box 16-6 presents leadership resources for nurses in long-term care. The American Health Care Association (2010) predicts a 41% increase in the need for RNs in long-term care between 2000 and 2020.

Nurses accustomed to practicing in an acute care hospital will find many differences in subacute and skilled nursing facilities. Differences in focus of care and goals between acute and long-term care are presented in Boxes 16-7 and 16-8. For many, nursing in long-term care offers the opportunity to practice the full scope of nursing, establish long-term relationships with patients and families, and make a significant difference in patient outcomes. While medical management is important, the need for expert nursing care is the most essential service provided.

BOX 16-6 LEADERSHIP RESOURCES FOR NURSES IN LONG-TERM CARE

- Sullivan-Marx E, Gray-Micelli D: Leadership and Management Skills for Long-Term Care, New York, 2008, Springer.
- Long-Term Care Nursing Leadership and Management, University of Minnesota Center for Gerontological Nursing. Available at www.nursing.umn.edu/CGN/LTCNurseLeader/LeadershipResources/home.html.
- American College of Health Care Administrators: Effective Leadership in Long-Term Care: The Need and the Opportunity, 2008. Available at http://www.achca.org/content/pdf/achca_leadership_need_and_opportunity_paper_dana-olson.pdf.

BOX 16-7 FOCUS OF ACUTE AND LONG-TERM CARE

ACUTE CARE ORIENTATION
- Illness
- High technology
- Short term
- Episodic
- One-dimensional
- Professional
- Medical model
- Cure

LONG-TERM CARE ORIENTATION
- Function
- High touch
- Extended
- Interdisciplinary model
- Ongoing
- Multidimensional
- Paraprofessional and family
- Care

Adapted from Ouslander J, Osterweil D, Morley J: *Medical care in the nursing home*, New York, 1997, McGraw-Hill.

BOX 16-8 GOALS OF LONG-TERM CARE

1. Provide a safe and supportive environment for chronically ill and functionally dependent people.
2. Restore and maintain highest practicable level of functional independence.
3. Preserve individual autonomy.
4. Maximize quality of life, well-being, and satisfaction with care.
5. Provide comfort and dignity at the end of life for residents and their families.
6. Provide coordinated interdisciplinary care to subacutely ill residents who plan to return to home or a less restrictive level of care.
7. Stabilize and delay progression, when possible, of chronic medical conditions.
8. Prevent acute medical and iatrogenic illnesses, and identify and treat them rapidly when they do occur.
9. Create a homelike environment that respects the dignity of each resident.

Adapted from Ouslander J, Osterweil D, Morley J: *Medical care in the nursing home*, New York, 1997, McGraw-Hill.

Nursing Assistants. Although it is important to promote professional nursing care for all elders, nursing assistants provide the majority of direct care in nursing homes and significantly contribute to the quality of life for nursing home residents. Critical shortages of nursing assistants exist now in residential care facilities, skilled care, and home care, and these shortages will worsen in the future. "Difficulty recruiting and retaining these long-term care workers continues to plague nursing homes, as turnover rates approach 100%" (Carpenter & Thompson, 2008). Several recent studies have investigated the relationship of factors such as turnover, work satisfaction, staffing, and power relations to quality of care and positive outcomes in nursing homes. Results support the importance of developing a culture of respect in which the work of nursing assistants is understood and valued at all levels of the organization. An important nursing role in long-term care is the supervision and education of nursing assistants to enable them to competently perform in their role as an essential member of the care team.

Results of several studies confirm the deep commitment and passion that nursing assistants bring to their jobs as they "struggle to find and maintain a balance between the task-oriented needs of residents (e.g., bathing, toileting, feeding) and develope relationships and building community" (Carpenter & Thompson, 2008, p. 31). The significance and importance of close personal relationships between nursing assistants and residents, often described as "like family," is emerging as a central dimension of quality of care and positive outcomes (Bowers, Esmond et al., 2000, 2003; Carpenter & Thompson, 2008; Ersek, Kraybill and Hansberry, 2000; Fisher and Wallhagen, 2008; Sikma, 2006; Touhy, Strews and Brown, 2005). The commitment and dedication of nursing home staff must be honored and supported. They have much to teach us about aging, nursing, and caring. Box 16-9 presents a description of caring themes expressed by nursing home caregivers.

BOX 16-9 HOW WE CARE: VOICES OF NURSING HOME STAFF

RESPONDING TO WHAT MATTERS
Taking time to do the little things, competence, cleanliness, meeting basic needs, safe administration of medications, kindness and consideration

CARING AS A WAY OF EXPRESSING SPIRITUAL COMMITMENT
Spiritual beliefs led staff to long-term care and continue to motivate and guide the special care they give to residents; they reflect a spiritual commitment to caring for residents as expressed in the golden rule: "Do unto others as you would like done to you."

DEVOTION INSPIRED BY LOVE FOR OTHERS
Deep connection between staff and residents described as being like family, caring for residents as you would for your own mother or father, sharing of good and bad times, going out on a limb to be an advocate, listening and staying with residents when others had given up

COMMITMENT TO CREATING A HOME ENVIRONMENT
Nursing home is the resident's home, staff are guests in the home; the importance of cleanliness, privacy, good food, and feeling part of a family

COMING TO KNOW AND RESPECT PERSON AS PERSON
Treating residents, families, and one another with respect and dignity, being recognized for the person you are, intimate knowing of likes and dislikes, individualized care

From Touhy T, Strews W, Brown C: Expressions of caring as lived by nursing home staff, residents, and families, *International Journal for Human Caring* 9:31, 2005.

One of the most important components of the culture change movement is the creation of models of care that value and honor the important work of nursing assistants. Culture change must be equally concerned about the needs of residents and the well-being of staff (Thomas & Johnson, 2003). "An organization that learns to give love, respect, dignity, tenderness, and tolerance to all members of the staff will soon find these same virtues being practiced by the staff" (Thomas & Johnson, 2003, p. 3). Until health care professionals and our society make a real commitment to providing adequate wages, individual supports (e.g., health insurance, education, career ladders), and an appreciation of their significant contribution to quality of nursing home care, these neglected workers cannot be expected to have the energy or incentive to extend themselves to the elders in their care (Kash et al., 2007).

An important organization for nursing assistants in nursing homes is the National Association of Geriatric Nursing Assistants (NAGNA). NAGNA was established in 1995 as a professional association of nursing assistants. The purpose of NAGNA is to ensure that the highest quality of care is provided to our elders living in nursing homes, achieved by elevating the professional standing and performance of the caregivers. With a membership of more than 30,000 CNAs representing more than 500 nursing homes, the organization provides recognition for outstanding achievements, development training for CNAs, mentoring programs to reduce CNA turnover, and advocacy for issues important to long-term care and CNAs.

Another organization, the National Clearinghouse on the Direct Care Workforce, supports efforts to improve the quality of jobs for frontline workers who assist people who are elderly and/or living with disabilities. This organization provides information resources needed to effect change in industry practice, public policy, and public opinion. The clearinghouse is also working with the Paraprofessional Healthcare Institute to improve understanding for the direct care workforce crisis through research and analysis funded by the U.S. Department of Health and Human Services and the Center for Medicare and Medicaid Services.

The Culture Change Movement

Across the United States, the movement to transform nursing homes from the typical medical model into "homes" that nurture quality of life for older people and support and empower frontline caregivers is changing the face of long-term care. Begun by the Pioneer Network, a national not-for-profit organization that serves the culture change movement, many facilities are changing from a rigid institutional approach to one that is person-centered (http://www.pioneernetwork.net/). "Culture change is the process of moving from a traditional nursing home model—characterized as a system unintentionally designed to foster dependence by keeping residents, as one observer put it, 'well cared for, safe, and powerless'—to a regenerative model that increases residents' autonomy and sense of control" (Brawley, 2007, p. 9).

Older people in need of long-term care want to live in a homelike setting that does not look and function like a hospital. They want a setting that allows them to make decisions they are used to making for themselves, such as when to get up, take a bath, eat, or go to bed. They want caregivers who know them

BOX 16-10 INSTITUTION-CENTERED VERSUS PERSON-CENTERED CULTURE

INSTITUTION-CENTERED CULTURE

- Schedules and routines are designed by the institution and staff, and residents must comply.
- Focus is on tasks to be accomplished.
- Rotation of staff from unit to unit occurs.
- Decision making is centralized with little involvement of staff or residents and families.
- There is a hospital environment.
- Structured activities are provided to all residents.
- There is little opportunity for socialization.
- Organization exists for employees rather than residents.
- There is little respect for privacy or individual routines.

PERSON-CENTERED CULTURE

- Emphasis is on relationships between staff and residents.
- Individualized plans of care are based on residents' needs, usual patterns, and desires.
- Staff members have consistent assignments and know the residents' preferences and uniqueness.
- Decision making is as close to the resident as possible.
- Staff members are involved in decisions and plans of care.
- Environment is homelike.
- Meaningful activities and opportunities for socialization are available around the clock.
- There is a sense of community and belonging—"like family."
- There is involvement of the community—children, pets, plants, outings.

Adapted from The Pioneer Network. Available at www.pioneernetwork.net. Accessed August 8, 2008.

and understand and respect their individuality and their preferences. "No matter how old, how sick, how disabled, how forgetful we are, each of us deserves to have a home—not an institution" (Baker, 2007; Baker as cited by Haglund, 2008, p. 8). Box 16-10 presents some of the differences between an institution-centered culture and a person-centered culture.

While further research is needed, some results suggest that person-centered care is associated with improved organizational performance, including higher resident and staff satisfaction, better workforce performance, and higher occupancy rates (Alliance for Quality Nursing Home Care and the American Health Care Association, 2010). Examples of philosophies and programs of culture change are the Eden Alternative (www.edenalt.com) founded by Dr. Bill Thomas, the Green House Project (www.thegreenhouseproject.org), and the Wellspring Model developed by Wellspring Innovative Solutions in Seymour, Wisconsin (http://www.innovations.ahrq.gov/content.aspx?id=259).

The Eden Alternative is best known for the addition of animals, plants, and children to nursing homes. However, cats and dogs are not the heart of culture change. Truly transforming a nursing home starts at the top and requires involvement of all levels of staff and changes in values, attitudes, structures, and management practices. Some of the principles of culture change activities are as follows:

- Staff empowerment
- Resident involvement in decision making
- Individualized rather than routine task-oriented care

- Relationship building
- A sense of community and belonging
- Meaningful activities
- A homelike environment
- Increased attention to respect of staff and the value of caring

Culture change has moved from a grassroots movement to one "that is embraced and supported by policy makers, providers, national and state associations, and CMS" (The Commonwealth Fund, 2010). The CMS has endorsed culture change and has also released a self-study tool for nursing homes to assess their own progress toward culture change. The Affordable Care Act includes a national demonstration project on culture change to develop best practices and the development of resources and funding to undertake culture change.

Nurses should take a leadership role in the culture change movement. The Hartford Institute of Geriatric Nursing, in collaboration with the Coalition for Geriatric Nursing Organizations and the Pioneer Network, are working together to identify the principles and characteristics of a nursing practice model that includes role definition and culture change competencies of all members of the nursing service team (e.g., directors of nursing, nursing supervisors, RNs, LPNs, nursing assistants, and advanced practice nurses) (www.pioneernetwork.net/AboutUs/Strategic/Hartford/). Several position papers on nurses' involvement in nursing home culture change are available at www.hartfordign.org/policy/position_papers.briefs/. The culture change movement is growing rapidly, and ongoing research is needed to demonstrate costs, benefits, and outcomes (Rahman & Schnelle, 2008; White-Chu et al., 2009).

IMPROVING TRANSITIONS ACROSS THE CONTINUUM OF CARE

Care transition refers to the movement of patients from one health care practitioner or setting to another as their condition and care needs change. Older people have complex health care needs and often require care in multiple settings across the continuum. An older person may be treated by a family practitioner, hospitalized and treated by an hospitalist, discharged to a nursing home and followed by another practitioner, and then discharged home or to a less care-intensive setting (e.g., ALF) where the family practitioner may or may not continue to follow him or her. Most health care providers practice in only one setting and are not familiar with the specific requirements of other settings. "Many factors contribute to gaps in care during critical transitions including poor communication, incomplete transfer of information, inadequate education of older adults and their family members, medication errors, limited access to essential services, and the absence of a single point person to ensure continuity of care" (Naylor & Keating, 2008, p. 65). Language and health literacy issues and cultural differences exacerbate the problem (Corbett et al., 2010).

Transitions happen often, and there is increasing evidence that serious deficiencies exist for older patients undergoing transitions across sites of care. Approximately one-fifth of Medicare beneficiaries discharged from a hospital were

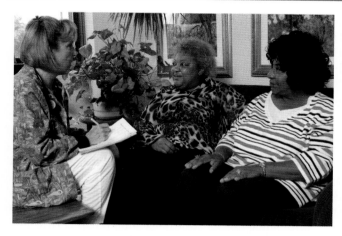

Working with the patient and the caregiver to provide education to enhance self-care abilities and to facilitate linkages to resources is important for the consideration of promoting safe discharges and transitions to home and other care settings. (From Potter PA: *Basic nursing: essentials for practice*, ed 7, 2010, Mosby).

⚠ SAFETY ALERT

Medication discrepancies are the most prevalent adverse event following hospital discharge and the most challenging component of a successful hospital-to-home transition. Nurses' attention to an accurate prehospital medication list, medication reconciliation during hospitalization and at discharge, and patient and family education about medications is required to enhance safety (see Box 16-11).

🔬 BOX 16-11 RESEARCH HIGHLIGHTS

Medication Discrepancies During Transitions

Medication discrepancies are the most prevalent adverse event following hospital discharge and the most challenging component of a successful hospital-to-home transition. The purpose of this study was to describe the most common medication discrepancies identified by nurses within 72 hours of the patient's transition from hospital to home. A medication discrepancy was defined as "any difference between the discharge medication list and the medications patients report actually taking at home" (Corbett et al., 2010, p. 188). 261 patients participated in the study. Inclusion criteria was age over 50 years and with at least one of the following diagnoses: cardiovascular condition, peripheral vascular disease, diabetes mellitus, cerebral vascular accident, chronic obstructive pulmonary disease.

94% of the participants had at least one discrepancy with a mean of 3.3 per participant. This was higher than results reported in other research, where findings range from 15% to 76%. On average, the study participants consumed 10 medications daily. Anticoagulants, insulin, aspirin, and opioids were common medications involved in a discrepancy. Suggestions to decrease medication discrepancies include clinician training to improve medication history on admission, assigning specific staff to reassess medication history and reconcile discrepancies during hospitalization for high-risk patients (e.g., older adults with 10 or more medications and those with heart failure or diabetes); improved patient and family education about medications during hospital stay as well as upon discharge (culturally and linguistically appropriate with attention to health literacy); provision of a medication table that includes the purpose, dose, and frequency of each medication, as well as correct administration and side effects to be reported; assessment of ability to pay for medications; and encouraging patients to obtain all medications from the same pharmacy.

Source: Corbett C, Setter S, Daratha K, et al: Nurse identified hospital to home medication discrepancies: implications for improving transitional care, *Geriatric Nursing* 31:188-196, 2010.

rehospitalized within 30 days, and 34% were rehospitalized within 90 days of hospital discharge. Of these rehospitalizations, about 10% were planned. Estimated costs to Medicare for unplanned hospitalizations is $17.4 billion (Jenks et al., 2009). Additionally, 1 in 4 Medicare patients admitted to skilled nursing facilities from hospitals is readmitted to the hospital within 30 days. Up to two thirds of hospital transfers are rated as potentially avoidable by expert long-term care health professionals (http://interact2.net/). These rehospitalizations are costly, potentially harmful, and often preventable.

Transitions during the course of hospitalization can also be problematic for older patients. Minimizing the number of transfers from unit to unit during a single hospitalization is associated with more consistent nursing care, fewer adverse incidents (e.g., nosocomial infections, falls, delirium, medication errors), shorter hospital stays, and lower overall costs (Kanak et al., 2008).

Individuals at high risk for transitional care problems include older people with multiple medical conditions or depression or other mental health disorders, isolated elders without family or friends, non-English speakers, recent immigrants, and low-income individuals (Graham et al., 2009). Compared to other groups of older adults, ethnically and racially diverse elders have slower rates of recovery after hospitalization and increased incidence of potentially preventable rehospitalizations (Graham et al., 2009). Heart failure is the most frequent reason for rehospitalization, and patients with heart failure experience a 27% rate of readmission within 30 days of a hospital discharge (Hines et al, 2010).

Improving Transitional Care

Transitional care "encompasses a broad range of services and environments designed to promote the safe and timely passage of patients between levels of care and across care settings (Naylor & Keating, 2008, p. 65). National attention to improving patient safety during transfers is increasing, and a growing body of evidence-based research provides data for design of care to improve transition outcomes. Nurses play a very important role in ensuring the adequacy of transitional care, and many of the successful models involve the use of advanced practice nurses and registered nurses in roles such as transition coaches and care managers (Coleman et al., 2006; Chalmers & Coleman, 2008; Naylor et al., 2009).

Nurse researchers Dorothy Brooten and Mary Naylor, and their colleagues, have significantly contributed to knowledge in the area of transitional care. The Transitional Care Model (TCM): Hospital Discharge Screening Criteria for High Risk Older Adults (Bixby and Naylor, 2009) can be found at http://consultgerirn.org/uploads/File/trythis/try_this_26.pdf. In addition to roles as care managers and transition coaches, nurses play a key role in many of the elements of successful transitional care models, such as medication management, family caregiver education, comprehensive discharge planning, and adequate and timely communication between providers and sites of service (Box 16-12).

Further research is needed to evaluate what transitional care models are most effective in various settings and for which group of patients. Particularly important is research on transitions from nursing home to hospital, racial and cultural disparities in transitional care, and ways to improve family caregiver

BOX 16-12 SUGGESTED ELEMENTS OF TRANSITIONAL CARE MODELS

- Utilize interdisciplinary teams guided by evidence-based protocols
- Performance measures and evaluation
- Utilize information systems such as electronic medical records that span traditional settings
- Target high-risk patients
- Improve communication between patients, family caregivers, and providers
- Improve communication between sending and receiving clinicians
- Well-designed and structured patient transfer records
- Simplify posthospital medication regimen
- Reconcile of patients' prehospital and posthospital medication lists
- Improve patient/family knowledge of medications prior to discharge
- Adapt educational materials for language and health literacy
- Schedule follow-up care appointments prior to discharge
- Discuss of warning signs that require reporting and medical evaluation
- Follow-up discharge with home visits/telephone calls
- Care coordination by advanced nurse practitioners
- Assess of informal support
- Involvement, education, and support of family caregivers
- Knowledge of community resources and appropriate referrals to resources and financial assistance
- Interventions to enhance discussions of palliative and end-of-life care and communication of advance directives

preparation and involvement during transitions. The Family Caregiver Alliance provides a hospital discharge planning guide for families and caregivers (www.caregiver.org). Other care transitional care resources can be found at http://interact2.net/care.html and www.ahrq.gov/qual/pips.

The CMS and The Joint Commission (TJC) have also increased efforts to promote better outcomes, patient safety, and effective care by requiring hospitals to collect data on the core measures and other quality indicators. The CMS posts 30-day, all cause, risk-adjusted readmission rates on its website for heart failure, acute myocardial infarction, and pneumonia. Participating hospitals are classified as better than U.S. national rate; no different than U.S. national rate; or worse than U.S. national rate (www.hospitalcompare.gov). Medicare is also implementing initiatives to reduce the amount of improper payments to providers as a result of medically unnecessary care (American Association of Retired Persons, 2010; Hines, Yu, Randall, 2010).

A major goal of the Patient Protection and Affordable Care Act (PPACA) is improving care coordination and outcomes for individuals with multiple comorbid conditions who require high-cost care. The health care reform law creates several programs based on promising models that include the following: the Medicare Community-Based Care Transitions Program; the Medicare Independence at Home demonstration; bonus payments for Medicare Advantage plans with care management programs; Medical (Health) Home models in Medicare and Medicaid; and Community Health Teams to support the Medical (Health) Homes (AARP, 2010). Many of these new initiatives include nurse practitioners and offer opportunities for new roles for registered nurses with preparation in care of older adults as well. The American Nurses Association (2011) has prepared a

paper on key provisions related to nursing in health care reform (http://www.nursingworld.org/MainMenuCategories/HealthcareandPolicyIssues/HealthSystemReform/Key-Provisions-Related-to-Nurses.aspx).

RELOCATION

For many older adults, relocation is a major stressor and often a crisis for the older person and his or her family. Relocation to a long-term care facility is identified as one of the most stressful and one that many older people fear. With each move, if the adaptation is to be satisfying, one must begin to claim personal space by somehow placing one's stamp of individuality on the new surroundings. Because the older adult is particularly likely to move or be moved, the subject of relocation is significant. Nurses in hospitals, the community, and long-term care institutions frequently care for elders who have experienced relocation.

The first issue to address in any move is whether it is necessary and whether it will provide the least restrictive lifestyle appropriate for the individual. Questions that must be asked to assess the impact on the individual after a move are presented in Box 16-13. Nurses' concerns are with assessing the impact of relocation and determining methods to mitigate any negative reactions.

Relocation stress syndrome is a nursing diagnosis describing the confusion resulting from a move to a new environment. Characteristics of relocation stress syndrome include anxiety, insecurity, altered mental status, depression, insecurity, loss of control, and physical problems. An abrupt and poorly prepared transfer actually increases illness and disorientation. Research suggests that individuals are better able to meet the challenges of relocation if they have a sense of control over the circumstances and the confidence to carry out the needed activities associated with a move. Self-efficacy, defined as "the beliefs in one's capability to organize and execute the courses of action

BOX 16-13 ASSESSMENT OF RELOCATION

- Are significant persons as accessible in the new location as they were before the move?
- Is the individual developing new and reciprocal relationships in the new setting?
- Is the individual functioning as well, better, or not as well in the new location? This determination cannot be made immediately, but this assessment must be done within at most six weeks of the move.
- Was the individual given options before the move?
- Was the individual given the opportunity to assess the new environment before making a decision to move?
- Has the individual been able to move important items of furniture and memorabilia to the new setting?
- Has a particular individual who is familiar with the environment been available to assist with orientation?
- Was the decision to move made hastily or with inadequate information?
- Does the new situation provide adequately for basic needs (food, shelter, physical maintenance)?
- Are individual idiosyncratic needs recognized, and is there an opportunity to actualize them?
- Does the new situation decrease the possibility of privacy and autonomy?
- Is the new living situation an improvement over the previous situation, similar in quality, or worse?

BOX 16-14   RELOCATION STRESS SYNDROME

Relocation stress syndrome is a physiological and/or psychosocial disturbance as a result of transfer from one environment to another.

DEFINING CHARACTERISTICS
Major
Change in environment or location
Anxiety
Apprehension
Increased confusion
Depression
Loneliness

Minor
Verbalization of unwillingness to relocate
Sleep disturbance
Change in eating habits
Dependency
Gastrointestinal disturbances
Increased verbalization of needs
Insecurity
Lack of trust
Restlessness
Sad affect
Unfavorable comparison of posttransfer and pretransfer staff
Verbalization of being concerned or upset about transfer
Vigilance
Weight change
Withdrawal

RELATED FACTORS
Past, concurrent, and recent losses
Losses involved with the decision to move
Feeling of powerlessness
Lack of adequate support system
Little or no preparation for the impending move
Moderate to high degree of environmental change
History and types of previous transfers
Impaired psychosocial health status
Decreased physical health status

SAMPLE DIAGNOSTIC STATEMENT
Relocation stress syndrome related to admission to long-term care setting as evidenced by anxiety, insecurity, and disorientation

EXPECTED OUTCOMES
1. The resident will socialize with family members, staff, and/or other residents.
2. Preadmission weight, appetite, and sleep patterns will remain stable. If previous patterns were dysfunctional, more appropriate health patterns will develop.
3. The resident will verbalize feelings, expectations, and disappointments openly with members of the staff and/or family.
4. Inappropriate behaviors (e.g., "acting out," refusing to take medicines) will not occur.

Expected Short-Term Goals
1. The resident will become independent in moving to and from areas within the facility during the next three months.
2. The resident will react in a positive manner to staff effort to assist in adjusting to nursing home placement in the next three months.
3. The resident will express his or her thoughts or concerns about placement when encouraged to do so during individual contacts in the next three months.
4. During the next three months, the resident will not develop physical or psychosocial disturbances indicative of translocation syndrome as a result of the change in living environment.

Expected Long-Term Goals
1. The resident will verbalize acceptance of nursing home placement within the next six months.
2. The resident will indicate acceptance of nursing home placement through positive body language within the next 6 months.

Specific Nursing Interventions
1. Identify previous coping patterns during admission assessment. Clearly document these, and share the information with other staff members.
2. Include the resident in assessing problems and developing the care plan on admission.
3. Adjust for limitations in sensory-perceptual disturbances when planning care for residents. Visual disturbances necessitate special intervention to assist residents in finding their way around.
4. Staff members will introduce themselves when entering the resident's room, indicating the nature of their relationship with the resident. Example: "Hello, Mr. S. My name is Nancy. I'll be your nurse attendant today, helping you with your meals and your bath."
5. Each staff member providing care for the resident should make it a point to spend at least five minutes each day with new admissions to "just visit."
6. Allow the resident as many opportunities to make independent choices as possible.
7. Identify previous routines for activities of daily living (ADLs). Try to maintain as much continuity with the resident's previous schedule as possible. Example: If Mr. S. has taken a bath before bed all of his life, adjust his schedule to continue that practice.
8. Familiarize the resident with unit schedules.
9. Encourage family participation through frequent visits, phone calls, and activity sessions. Be sure to let the family know schedules.
10. Establish familiar landmarks for the resident when leaving his or her room so that he or she can recognize areas more quickly.
11. Encourage family members to bring familiar belongings from home for the resident's room decorations.
12. Provide reorientation cues frequently. Example: "You are in the dining room. Your room is down the hall three doors just past the window."
13. Encourage the resident to talk about expectations, anger, and/or disappointments and the recent life changes that he or she has experienced.
14. Review the patient's medication list with the physician to verify the need for medications that might promote disorientation.
15. Provide for constructive activities. Initiate activity therapy consultation.

required to manage prospective situations" (Bandura, 1997, p. 2), may be an important variable in positive adjustment to a relocation. The Self-Efficacy Relocation Scale (SERS), developed by Rossen and Gruber (2007), can be used to assess self-efficacy in individuals who are relocating, identify potential pre-relocation adjustment issues, and guide interventions to promote positive relocation outcomes.

To avoid some of the effects of relocation stress syndrome, the individual must have some control over the environment,

preparation regarding the new situation, and maintenance of familiar situations to the greatest degree possible. Nurses must carefully assess and monitor older people for relocation stress syndrome effects. Working with families to help them plan relocations, understanding the effects of relocation, and implementing effective approaches are also necessary. It is important that some familiar and some treasured items accompany the transfer. Too often, elders arrive at long-term care institutions via ambulance stretcher from the hospital with nothing but a hospital gown. Everything familiar and necessary in their lives remains at the home they have left when they became ill. Even more distressing is when families or responsible parties sell the home to finance long-term care stays without the input of the elder. It is no wonder so many residents with dementia in nursing homes wander the hallways looking for home and for something familiar and comforting. Family members will need considerable support when an elder is moved into an institution. No matter what the circumstances, the family invariably feels that they have in some way failed the elder (Chapter 22). A summary of relocation stress syndrome and nursing actions to prevent relocation stress during transition to long-term care are presented in Box 16-14. An evidence-based practice guideline, *Management of relocation in cognitively intact older adults* (Hertz et al, 2005) is available at www.guideline.gov.

PROMOTING HEALTHY AGING: IMPLICATIONS FOR GERONTOLOGICAL NURSING

Nurses in all practice settings play a key role in improving care for older people across the continuum. New roles for nursing are emerging in the era of health care reform and heightened attention to improved patient outcomes. Most nurses work in only one setting and are not familiar with the requirements of other settings or the needs of patients in those settings. As a result, there are often significant misunderstandings and criticisms of care in the different settings across the continuum. As Barbara Resnick pointed out: "We can stop the finger pointing and start working together through the common transitions patients endure in our health care system. This will be a win-win situation for patients and providers alike" (2008, p. 154).

It is essential that educational programs prepare students for competent care of older adults in a variety of health care settings, including acute, long-term, home, and community-based care. Nurses in all settings need to increase awareness of the roles and responsibilities of nursing practice across the continuum and work collaboratively to improve care outcomes, particularly during times of transition. We can no longer work in our individual "silos" and not be concerned with what happens after the patient is out of our particular unit or institution. Nurses are well positioned "to create services and environments that embrace values that are at the core of this profession—patient/caregiver centered care, communication and collaboration, and continuity (Naylor, 2002, p. 140).

evolve   To access your student resources, go to *http://evolve.elsevier.com/Ebersole/TwdHlthAging*

KEY CONCEPTS

- A familiar and comfortable environment allows an elder to function at his or her highest capacity.
- Nurses must be knowledgeable about the range of residential options for older people so they can assist the elder and the family to make appropriate decisions.
- Nursing homes are an integral part of the long-term care system, providing both skilled (subacute) care and chronic, long-term, and palliative care. Projections are that this setting will provide increasing amounts of care to the growing numbers of older adults.
- The present long-term care system is fragmented, cost-prohibitive, difficult to access, and in need of major

transformation to meet the needs of individuals of all ages in need of this type of care.
- Culture change in nursing homes is a growing movement to develop models of person-centered care and improve care outcomes and quality of life.
- Relocation has variable effects, depending on the individual's personality, health, cognitive capacities, sense of control, opportunities for choice, self-esteem, and preferred lifestyle.
- Nurses play a key role in ensuring optimal outcomes during transitions of care.

RESEARCH QUESTIONS

1. What are the factors influencing choice of housing options for older adults, and how do these vary between young-old and old-old?
2. How do care outcomes differ between assisted living facilities with professional nursing involvement and those that provide care with only unlicensed assistive personnel?
3. How do care outcomes and perceived quality of care differ for residents in assisted living facilities compared to nursing facilities?
4. What are the primary concerns of family caregivers of older persons experiencing transitions?
5. How does the family caregiver role change when a family member is admitted to a nursing facility?
6. Do nurses and nursing assistant who work in nursing facilities embracing culture change report greater job satisfaction and less turnover?
7. What practice settings are most commonly included in nursing education programs?
8. How can we encourage collaboration of nurses across the care continuum? Does this make a difference in attitudes and knowledge about patient needs and differing nursing roles in various practice settings?

CASE STUDY   TRANSITIONS ACROSS THE CONTINUUM

Ray is 85 years old and was recently admitted to the hospital from his own home following a fall with resultant fracture of the right hip. He was brought to the hospital by paramedics after a neighbor checked on him because they had not heard any sounds from his apartment. He had laid on the floor for eight hours unable to call for help. He lives alone in a one bedroom apartment. His wife of 50 years died 4 years ago. His three adult children and their families live out of state but keep in close contact with their father and visit several times a year. The last time they saw their father was four months before his hospitalization.

Prior to the hip fracture, Ray was fairly capable of taking care of himself but since the death of his wife, his memory and mood have declined. He is hard of hearing in both ears but often refuses to wear his hearing aids, claiming that they distort all sounds and were a bother. He only occasionally left his apartment and had lost a great deal of weight. His neighbors reported that he was falling frequently and there were repeated calls to 911 for assistance. He had several "fender-benders" and had limited his driving to shopping and church. His children were becoming increasingly worried about him living alone. He refused to consider moving to live nearer or with his children or to assisted living. He did not want to be a bother to his children. His home is full of family pictures, pictures from his world-wide travels with his wife, memorabilia from his days as a police officer, and antique furniture. He has a little dog who gives him great enjoyment.

Following a surgical repair of his fractured hip, he experienced a delirium and his mental status declined. He received physical therapy but had difficulty following the orders for partial weight bearing on the affected leg. He became incontinent and required an adult brief. He also developed a necrotic pressure ulcer on his right heel. The hospital case manager recommended to the family that he be transferred to a skilled nursing facility for further rehabilitation, treatment of the pressure ulcer, and possible long-term care placement. It was felt that he could not return safely to is home related to his mental status and functional decline. His finances were limited so a home that accepted both Medicare and Medicaid was recommended.

Even though the family had promised their father that they would never put him in a nursing home and felt terrible, they agreed with the decision and felt relieved that he would not be living alone. Worried that he would be upset, they decided not to tell him that he would not be going home. They decided to sell his apartment to provide some money for his nursing home care. The children divided the furniture and memorabilia between them and sold the remaining household items. They chose not to tell him that they had done this and when he asked, they said: "When you get better, then you can go home." Ray's mental status continued to decline. He was unable to walk independently, experienced weight loss and sleep problems and became more withdrawn.

Based on the case study, develop a nursing care plan using the following procedure*:
- List Ray's and the family comments that provide subjective data.
- List information that provides objective data.
- From these data, identify and state, using accepted format, two nursing diagnoses you determine are most significant to Ray at this time. List two of Ray's strengths that you have identified from the data.
- Determine and state outcome criteria for each diagnosis. These must reflect some alleviation of the problem identified in the nursing diagnosis and must be stated in concrete and measurable terms.
- Plan and state one or more interventions for each diagnosed problem. Provide specific documentation of the source used to determine the appropriate intervention. Plan at least one intervention that incorporates Ray's strengths.
- Evaluate the success of the interventions. Interventions must correlate directly with the stated outcome criteria to measure the outcome success.

CRITICAL THINKING QUESTIONS
- If you were in the role of a hospital case manager, how might you have helped this family with the discharge decision?
- Would Ray be appropriate for an assisted living facility upon discharge from the hospital? Why or why not? What services would need to be in place for him to be discharged to an assisted living facility? How would he pay for these services?
- Would Ray be appropriate for discharge home following hospitalization? What would home health provide under Medicare? What other services might he need? How would he pay for these services?
- What type of interventions might you have implemented to enhance Ray's adjustment to the nursing home?
- What are some of the obstacles that families of older people face when their loved one needs a great deal of care? Do you think that families should provide the care rather than placing loved ones with 24-hour care needs in nursing homes? If this was your family, what challenges might present in providing 24-hour care for a loved one?
- Do you feel the system of long-term care in this country is adequate? Do you think the government (state, local, federal) has a role in improving the financing and structure of long-term care or do you think the individual is responsible for paying for this type of care?

*Students are advised to refer to their nursing diagnosis text and identify possible a potential problems.

REFERENCES

Alliance for Quality Nursing Home Care and the American Health Care Association: 2010 Annual quality report: A comprehensive report on the quality of care in America's nursing homes and rehabilitation facilities. Available at http://www.aqnhc.org/www/file/AHCA_Alliance_2010_Quality_Report_v2.pdf. Accessed October 27, 2010.

Alzheimer's Association: Dementia care practice: Recommendations for assisted living residences and nursing homes 2009. Available at http://www.alz.org/national/documents/brochure_DCPRphases1n2.pdf. Accessed November 1, 2010.

American Association of Retired Persons Public Policy Institute: Health care reform initiative to improve care coordination and transitional care for chronic conditions. Available at http://www.assets.aarp.org/rgcenter/ppi/health-care/fs191-health-reform.pdf. Accessed October 31, 2010.

American Health Care Association: U.S. long-term care workforce at a glance. Available at www.acha.org. Accessed October 28, 2010.

American Association of Homes and Services for the Aging: Aging Services: Finding the right aging services. Available at http://www2.aahsa.org/choice.aspx. Accessed January 15, 2011.

American Association of Homes and Services for the Aging: Future of Aging, June 2008. Available at http://futureofaging.aahsa.org/2008/06/. Accessed January 15, 2011.

Assisted Living Federation of America: Guide to choosing an assisted living residence. Available at http://www.alfa.org/images/alfa/PDFs/getfile.cfm_product_id=94&file=ALFAchecklist.pdf. Accessed October 22, 2010.

American Nurses Association: Health care reform: key provisions related to nursing. Available at http://www.nursingworld.org/MainMenu Categories/HealthcareandPolicyIssues/HealthSystemReform/Key-Provisions-

Related-to-Nurses.aspx. Accessed January 15, 2011.

Baker B: Old age in a new age: the promise of transformative nursing homes, Nashville, Tenn, 2007, Vanderbilt University Press.

Baker B, as cited in Haglund K: Closing keynote speaker found hope in changes benefiting residents and staff, Caring Ages 9:8, 2008.

Bandura A: Self-efficacy: the exercise of control, New York, 1997, W.H. Freeman.

Bixby M, Naylor M: The Transitional Care Model (TCM): Hospital Discharge Screening Criteria for High Risk Older Adults, Try This: Best Practices in Nursing Care to Older Adults, 26, 2009. Available at http://consultgerirn.org/uploads/File/trythis/try_this_26.pdf. Accessed November 16, 2010.

Boltz M, Capezuti E, Bower-Ferres S, et al: Changes in the geriatric care environment associated with NICHE, Geriatric Nursing 29:176, 2008.

Bowers B, Esmond S, Jacobson N: The relationship between staffing and quality in long-term care facilities: Exploring the views of nurses aides, *Journal of Nursing Care Quality* 14:55, 2000.

Bowers BJ, Esmond S, Jacobson N: Turnover reinterpreted: CNAs' talk about why they leave, *Journal of Gerontological Nursing* 29(3), 36-43:2003.

Brawley E: What culture change is and why an aging nation cares, *Aging Today* 28:9-10, 2007.

Carlson A: Death in the nursing home: resident, family and staff perspectives, *Journal of Gerontological Nursing* 33:33, 2007.

Carpenter J, Thompson SA: CNAs experience in the nursing home: "It's in my soul," *Journal of Gerontological Nursing* 34:25, 2008.

Chalmers S, Coleman E: Transitional care. In Capezuti E, Swicker D, Mezey M, et al., editors: *The encyclopedia of elder care*, ed 2, New York, 2008, Springer.

Coleman EA, Parry C, Chalmers S, et al: The Care Transitions Intervention: results of a randomized controlled trial, *Archives of Internal Medicine* 166:1822, 2006.

Corbett C, Setter S, Daratha K, et al: Nurse identified hospital to home medication discrepancies: implications for improving transitional care, *Geriatric Nursing* 31:188, 2010.

Eliopoulos C: *Gerontological nursing*, Philadelphia, 2010, Wolters Kluwer/Lippincott Williams & Wilkins.

Ersek M, Kraybill B, Hansberry J: Assessing the educational needs and concerns of nursing home staff regarding end-of-life care, *Journal of Gerontological Nursing* 26:16, 2000.

Fisher L, Wallhagen M: Day-to-day care: The interplay of CNAs' views of residents and nursing home environments, *Journal of Gerontological Nursing* 34:26, 2008.

Fulmer T, Mezey M, Bottrell M, et al: Nurses improving care for health system (NICHE): Using outcomes and benchmarks for evidence-based practice, *Geriatric Nursing* 23:121, 2002.

Gleckman H: The death of nursing homes. Available at www.kaiserhealthnews.org/Columns/2009/September092809Gleckman.aspx. Accessed October 28, 2010.

Graham C, Ivey S, Neuhauser L: From hospital to home: assessing the transitional care needs of vulnerable seniors, *The Gerontologist* 49:23, 2009.

Harrington C, Kovner C, Mezey M, et al: Experts recommend minimum staffing standards for nursing facilities in the United States, *Gerontologist* 40:5, 2000.

Harrington C, Carrillo H, Blank B, et al: Nursing facilities, staffing, residents and deficiencies by state, 2001-2007. Available at www.theconsumervoice.org/node/444. Accessed October 28, 2010.

Hertz J, Rossetti J, Koren N, et al: *Management of relocation in cognitively intact older adults*, Iowa City, IA, University of Iowa Gerontological Nursing Interventions Research Center, Research Dissemination Core, 2005. Available at www.guidelines.gov. Accessed October 31, 2010.

Hines P, Yu K, Randall M: Preventing heart failure readmissions: Is your organization prepared? *Nursing Economics* 28:74, 2010.

Horn S, Buerhas P, Bergstrom N, Smout R: RN staffing time and outcomes of long-stay nursing home residents, *Am J Nurs* 105(11):58-70, 2005.

Inouye S, Baker DI, Leo-Summmers L: The hospital elder life program: A model of care to prevent cognitive and functional decline in older hospitalized patients, *Journal of the American Geriatrics Society* 48:1657, 2000.

Institute of Medicine: Retooling for an aging America: Building the healthcare workforce, 2008. Available at http://www.iom.edu/Reports/2008/Retooling-for-an-Aging-America-Building-the-Health-Care-Workforce.aspx. Accessed June 7, 2010.

Jenks SF, Williams MV, Coleman EA: Rehospitalizations among patients in the Medicare fee-for-service program, *New England Journal of Medicine* 360:1457, 2009.

Kanak MF, Titler M, Shever L, et al: The effect of hospitalization on multiple units, *Applied Nursing Research* 21:15, 2008.

Kash B, Castle N, Phillips C: Nursing home spending, staffing and turnover, *Health Care Management Review* 43:253, 2007.

Kim H, Kovner C, Harrington C, et al: A panel data analysis of the relationships of nursing home staffing levels and standards of regulatory deficiencies, *The Journals of Gerontology. Series B, Psychological Sciences and Social Sciences* 64B:269, 2009.

Kleinpell R: Supporting independence in hospitalized elders in acute care, *Critical Care Nursing Clinics of North America* 19:242, 2007.

Landers SJ: Why health care is going home, *New England Journal of Medicine* 363:1690, 2010.

Medicare.gov: Long-Term Care. Available at www.medicare.gov/longtermcare/static/home.asp. Accessed October 28, 2010a.

Medicare.gov: Nursing home important information: Five Star Quality Rating. Available at www.medicare.gov/NHCompare/static/tabHelp.asp?activeTab=6. Accessed October 28, 2010b.

MetLife Mature Market Institute: The 2009 MetLife Market Survey of Nursing Home, Assisted Living, Adult Day Services, and Home Care Costs. Available at http://www.metlife.com/assets/cao/mmi/publications/studies/mmi-market-survey-nursing-home-assisted-living.pdf. Accessed October 22, 2010.

Mezey M, Harrington C, Kluger M: NPs in nursing homes: An issue of quality, *American Journal of Nursing* 104:71, 2004a.

Mezey M, Kobayashi M, Grossman S: Nurses improving care to health system elders (NICHE): implementation of best practice models, *Journal of Nursing Administration* 34:451, 2004b.

Mezey M, Stierle L, Huba G, et al: Ensuring competence of specialty nurses in care of older adults, *Geriatric Nursing* 28:9, 2007.

National Adult Day Services Association, Ohio State University College of Social Work, MetLife Mature Market Institute: The MetLife National Study of Adult Day Services: Providing support to individuals and their family caregivers. Available at http://www.metlife.com/assets/cao/mmi/publications/studies/2010/mmi-adult-day-services.pdf. Accessed October 21, 2010.

Naylor M: Transitional care of older adults. In Archbold P, Fitzpatrick J, Stewart B, editors: *Annual Review of Nursing Research*. New York, 2002, Springer, p. 127-147.

Naylor M, Keating S: Transitional care: moving patients from one care setting to another, *American Journal of Nursing* 108(9 Suppl):58, 2008.

Naylor M, Kurtzman E, Pauly M: Transitions of elders between long-term care and hospitals, *Policy, Politics, and Nursing Practice* 10:187, 2009.

Prudential Life Insurance Company of America: Long-term care cost study. Available at http://www.prudential.com/media/managed/LTCCostStudy.pdf. Accessed January 15, 2011.

Rahman A, Schnelle J: The nursing home culture change movement: recent past, present, and future directions for research, *Gerontologist* 48:142-148, 2008.

Rantz M, Zwygart-Stauffacher M: *How to find the best elder care*, Minneapolis, MN, 2009, Fairview Press.

Resnick G: A big welcome to our NICHE hospitals, *Geriatric Nursing* 3:81, 2009.

Rossen E, Gruber K: Development and psychometric testing of the relocation self-efficacy scale, *Nursing Research* 56:244, 2007.

Sikma S: Staff perceptions of caring: The importance of a supportive environment, *Journal of Gerontological Nursing* 32:22, 2006.

Steele J: Current evidence regarding models of acute care for hospitalized geriatric patients, *Geriatric Nursing* 31(5):331-339, 2010.

The Commonwealth Fund: States in Action: New Roles in Changing the Culture of Long-Term Care. Available at www.commonwealthfund.org/Content/Newsletters/States-in-Action/2010/Oct/September-Oct-2010/. Accessed October 28, 2010.

Tilly J, Reed P, editors: Dementia care practice recommendations for assisted living residences and nursing homes, Washington, DC, Alzheimer's Association, 2006. Available at www.guideline.gov. Accessed October 22, 2010.

Thomas WH, Johansson C: Elderhood in Eden, *Topics in Geriatric Rehabilitation* 19:282, 2003.

Touhy T, Strews W, Brown C: Expressions of caring as lived by nursing home staff, residents, and families, *International Journal for Human Caring* 9:31, 2005.

White-Chu E, Graves W, Godfrey S, et al: Beyond the medical model: The culture change revolution in long-term care, *Journal of the American Medical Directors Association* 6:370, 2009.

Williams J: Rehabilitation challenge, *Nursing Times* 18:66, 1993.

Pain and Comfort

Kathleen Jett

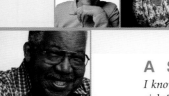

evolve http://evolve.elsevier.com/Ebersole/TwdHlthAging

A STUDENT SPEAKS

I know she has pain all of the time, but if I give her too many pills she will get addicted and that would be a bad thing, right?
Ana, age 23 regarding Molly age 89

AN ELDER SPEAKS

It seems to have crept up on me—first one joint, now the other, I wouldn't call it pain really, and just an ache that never goes away and keeps me from dancing like I used to.
Gloria, age 78

LEARNING OBJECTIVES

On completion of this chapter, the reader will be able to:
1. Define the concept of pain.
2. Identify factors that affect the elder's pain experience.
3. Identify barriers that interfere with pain assessment and treatment.
4. Describe data to include in a pain assessment.
5. Discuss pharmacological and non-pharmacological pain management therapies.
6. Develop a nursing plan of care for an elder with pain.

The International Association for the Study of Pain defines pain as "an unpleasant sensory and emotional experience associated with actual or potential tissue damage . . . always subjective . . . a sensation . . . always unpleasant" (International Association for the Study of Pain, 2010). Physical pain can be a fleeting discomfort or something so pervasive that it wears heavily on one's spirit. In young adulthood, pain is frequently the result of an acute event. The cause is clear (e.g., a fracture or infection), and treatment is based on intensity of the pain, which resolves when the underlying cause is treated. While those at midlife and beyond continue to experience acute events, the pain experience itself becomes more complex; acute pain occurs in the presence of co-morbidities including chronic, that is, persistent pain. The pain is more likely to be multidimensional with sensory, physical, psychosocial, emotional, and spiritual components. How we respond to pain is a part of who we are—part of our personalities (Box 17-1). Even the words used to describe it are many, an *ache*, a *burn*, a *pester*—with the language and the willingness to express it a manifestation of the person's culture and relationship with whom he or she is speaking to (Campbell, Andrews, Scipio et al., 2009).

In 2001, The Joint Commission on Accreditation of Healthcare Organizations, made pain management a patient right, referring to it as the fifth vital sign (Joint Commission, 2009; Schofield, 2010). It became the expectation that health care professionals recognize and treat pain effectively and efficiently and, in doing so, provide comfort and caring. Additionally, in the nursing home setting, pain is one of the quality indicators, and the nurse is required to determine the presence or absence of pain when completing the Minimum Data Set (MDS 3.0) assessment. Knowing skills were needed to meet this basic standard of human caring, the American Nurses Association, in collaboration with the American Society of Pain Management Nursing, developed Pain Management Nursing: Scope and Standards of Practice, and the American Nurses Credentialing Center (ANCC) offers a certification examination on pain management for nurses at the generalist level. Yet research continues to tell us that pain in the older adult is undertreated, especially those with cognitive impairments and most especially elders of color (Arnstein, 2010; Herr, 2010; Papaleontiou et al., 2010).

Pain is usually first classified as cancer or non-cancer related. It is either acute or persistent, and, finally, it is nociceptive,

BOX 17-1   VARIATIONS IN INDIVIDUAL RESPONSES TO PAIN

- Minimizes pain with significant others

or

- Uses pain to elicit sympathy and support from others
- Carefully controls the expression of pain (calm and unemotional)

or

- Is vocal about pain (cries and moans, complains)
- Withdraws and wants to be alone when pain is severe

or

- Seeks attention and presence of others
- Willingly accepts pain relief measures

or

- Avoids pain relief measures in the belief that they indicate weakness
- Wants and expects quick pain relief

or

- Accepts pain for long periods before requesting help

BOX 17-3   CONSEQUENCES OF UNTREATED PAIN

Falls and other accidents
Functional impairment
Slowed rehabilitation
Mood changes
Increased health care costs
Caregiver strain
Sleep disturbance
Changes in nutritional status
Impaired cognition
Increased dependency and helplessness
Depression, anxiety, fear
Decline in social and recreational activities
Increased health care utilization and costs

Data from American Geriatrics Society: *Journal of the American Geriatrics Society 57*:1331-1346, 2009.

BOX 17-2   TYPES OF PAIN SENSATIONS

- **Nociceptive pain** is associated with injury to the skin, mucosa, muscle, or bone and is usually the result of stimulation of pain receptors. This type of pain arises from tissue inflammation, trauma, burns, infection, ischemia, arthropathies (rheumatoid arthritis, osteoarthritis, gout), nonarticular inflammatory disorders, skin and mucosal ulcerations, and internal organ and visceral pain from distention, obstruction, inflammation, compression, or ischemia of organs. Pancreatitis, appendicitis, and tumor infiltration are common causes of visceral pain. Nociceptive mechanisms usually respond well to common analgesic medications and non-pharmacological interventions.
- **Neuropathic pain** involves a pathophysiological process of the peripheral or central nervous system and presents as altered sensation and discomfort. Conditions causing this type of pain include postherpetic or trigeminal neuralgia, poststroke or postamputation pain (phantom pain), diabetic neuropathy, or radiculopathies (e.g., spinal stenosis). This type of pain may be described as stabbing, tingling, burning, or shooting. Neuropathic pain is very difficult to treat and may occur at the same time as nociceptive and idiopathic pain.
- **Mixed or unspecified pain** usually has mixed or unknown causes. Examples include recurrent headaches and vasculitis. A compression fracture causing nerve root irritation, common in older people with osteoporosis, is an example of a mix of nociceptive and neuropathic pain.

See: Horgas A: Nursing standard of practice protocol: Pain management in older adults. Updated January 2008. Available at http://consultgerirn.org/topics/pain/want_to_know_more. Accessed January 22, 2011.

neuropathic, or idiopathic (Box 17-2). Acute pain is temporary and usually controllable with adequate dosages of analgesia. For example, the acute pain of a myocardial infarction is relieved temporarily with morphine and permanently when oxygen is restored to the myocardium. Everyone experiences acute physical pain at some point in their lives.

The most common type of pain in late life is chronic (i.e., persistent), and while the intensity may vary from day to day or hour to hour it is present most of the time (if not always) in the older adult. It is most likely felt in more than one location at a time, such as in both knees or both hands. Persistent pain is multifactorial in nature and can manifest as depression, eating and sleeping disturbances, impaired function, and

confusion (Jansen, 2008). If left untreated, the effects are broad ranging, regardless of the cognitive capacity of the person in pain (Box 17-3).

PAIN IN THE OLDER ADULT

Research has found that pain in late life tends to be persistent, moderate to severe, and present in about 50% of those over 65 living in the community in the United States (Schofield, 2010). For those living in long-term care settings, the number of persons with pain, largely untreated, is thought to be much higher (Robinson, 2010). The barriers to adequate pain management in older adults are many (Boxes 17-4 and 17-5).

The most common causes of non-cancer pain in late life are musculoskeletal in nature, especially from arthritis and degenerative spinal conditions, with neuralgias common as well (American Geriatrics Society [AGS], 2009). Neuralgias occur frequently as a result of long-standing diabetes, peripheral vascular disease, herpes zoster, and other syndromes (Box 17-6). In later life, acute pain may be superimposed on persistent pain and in an effort to treat either, we add an iatrogenic source for new pain. An example follows:

97-year-old Helen Thomas lives alone, considers herself well, and is almost always bright and cheerful. She has had osteoarthritis for the last 30 years. Her hips ache most of the time and keep her from doing everything she wants to do, but she "does pretty good." She takes over-the-counter NSAIDs every day to take away the "sharp" pain in her hip. When walking her dog in the snow, she falls and breaks a hip. She has considerable postoperative hip pain, but she does not want to "bother the nurses." She is less talkative, is somewhat irritable, and declares that she "just wishes they would give me that pill I take at home." When the nurse conducts a thorough assessment, she finds that Ms. Thomas is slightly confused, is getting very little sleep, and has a pressure ulcer on her coccyx. She complains that her repaired hip hurts most of the time, as does her "good side" and now her "tail bone." Ms. Thomas has been prescribed Tylenol with codiene, but she takes very little of it. She is resistive to rehabilitation.

Ms. Thomas had been living with persistent pain. While she was cheerful, her pain still negatively impacted her quality of

BOX 17-4   BARRIERS TO PAIN MANAGEMENT IN OLDER ADULTS

HEALTH CARE PROFESSIONAL BARRIERS

Lack of education regarding pain assessment and management
Concern regarding regulatory scrutiny
Fears of opioid-related side effects/addiction
Belief that pain is a normal part of aging
Belief that cognitively impaired elders have less pain; lack of ability to assess pain in cognitively impaired
Personal beliefs and experiences with pain
Inability to accept self-report without "objective" signs

PATIENT AND FAMILY BARRIERS

Fear of medication side effects
Concerns related to addiction
Belief that pain is a normal part of the aging process
Belief that nothing much can be done for pain in older people
Fear of being a "bad patient" if complaining/fear of what pain may signal

HEALTH CARE SYSTEM BARRIERS

Cost
Time
Cultural bias regarding opioid use

Modified from Hanks-Bell M et al: *The Online Journal of Issues in Nursing* 9, 2004. Available at www.nursingworld.org/ojin/topic21/tpc21_6.htm; Barber JB, Gibson SJ: *Drug Safety* 32:457-74, 2009.

life. She falls and has acute pain; there was no reasonable expectation that the persistent pain in the other hip had gone away. When assessed, she reports ongoing pain but was not being given anything on a regular basis and therefore her pain was undertreated. It is reasonable to believe that the lack of pain management led to her staying in one position for long periods of time and now with a cause for iatrogenic pain, an immobility-related pressure ulcer. It is most likely that her cognitive status is being compromised by her sleeplessness, pain, and immobility. Unless there is an interruption in this cycle, Ms. Thomas will likely continue to deteriorate and lose her independence.

Pain in Elders with Cognitive Impairments

Persons with cognitive impairment are consistently untreated or undertreated for pain. Studies have shown that older adults who are cognitively impaired receive less pain medication, even though they experience the same painful conditions as elders who are cognitively intact (Herr and Decker, 2004; Herr et al., 2006a,b; Kovach et al., 2006a,b; Ware et al., 2006). Many caregivers believe that people who are cognitively impaired do not experience pain as severely as those who are cognitively intact. However, according to Herr and Decker (2004, pp. 47-48):

> There is no convincing evidence that peripheral nociceptor responses of pain transmission are impaired in people with dementia, although controversy does exist about central nervous system changes that influence or diminish interpretation of pain transmission. Those with dementia may have altered affective responses to pain, probably due to their inability to cognitively process the painful sensation in the context of prior pain experience, attitudes, knowledge, and beliefs.

BOX 17-5   FACT AND FICTION ABOUT PAIN IN THE ELDERLY

MYTH: Pain is expected with aging.
FACT: Pain is not normal with aging. The presence of pain in the elderly necessitates aggressive assessment, diagnosis, and management similar to that of persons at any age.
MYTH: Pain sensitivity and perception decrease with aging.
FACT: While an older adult may have developed excellent coping skills making it more difficult for others to observe cues for pain, there is no evidence that there is a reduction in actual pain.
MYTH: If a patient does not complain of pain, there must not be much pain.
FACT: This is erroneous in all ages but particularly in the elderly. Older patients may not report pain for a variety of reasons. They may fear the meaning of pain, diagnostic workups, or pain treatments. Depending on one's belief systems they may not want to be a bother, may believe suffering is necessary to atone for past sins, may fear addiction, or may think pain is a normal part of aging. Cognitive and communication difficulties also may make older people unable to report pain.
MYTH: A person who has no functional impairment, appears occupied, or is otherwise distracted from pain must not have significant pain.
FACT: Patients have a variety of reactions to pain. Many patients are stoic and refuse to "give in" to their pain. Over extended periods, the elderly may mask any outward signs of pain. This varies highly by culture.
MYTH: Narcotic medications are inappropriate for patients with persistent nonmalignant pain.
FACT: Opioid analgesics are often indicated in persistent nonmalignant pain.
MYTH: Potential side effects of narcotic medication make them too dangerous to use in the elderly.
FACT: Narcotics may be used safely in the elderly. Although elderly patients may be more sensitive to narcotics, this does not justify withholding narcotics and failing to relieve pain.
MYTH: People with dementia do not feel pain.
FACT: Older adults with cognitive impairment are just as likely to experience painful illnesses. They feel pain, but changes in the brain may change the way pain is processed. They may not understand or even remember their pain or may not be able to report what they feel. Changes in behavior (e.g., agitation, aggression, calling for help, sleep pattern changes, appetite changes) are common pain behaviors in cognitively impaired elders.

Adapted from Ferrell BR, Ferrell BA: Pain in the elderly. In Watt-Watson JH, Donovan MI, editors: *Pain management: nursing perspective,* St Louis, 1992.

BOX 17-6   COMMON CAUSES OF NEUROPATHIC PAIN IN OLDER ADULTS

Stroke
Diabetes
Peripheral vascular disease
Herpes zoster
Degenerative disk disease

As a result, responses to painful experiences may be different from the "typical" response of a person who is cognitively intact. It is best to practice under the "assumption that any condition that is painful to a cognitively intact person would also be painful to those with advanced dementia who cannot express themselves" (Herr et al., 2010). Research has suggested that older people with mild to moderate cognitive impairment

---

BOX 17-7   **PAIN CUES IN THE PERSON WITH COMMUNICATION DIFFICULTIES**

CHANGES IN BEHAVIOR
Restlessness and/or agitation or reduction in movement
Repetitive movements
Physical tension such as clenching teeth or hands
Unusually cautious movements, guarding

ACTIVITIES OF DAILY LIVING
Sudden resistance to help from others
Decreased appetite
Decreased sleep

VOCALIZATIONS
Person groans, moans, or cries for unknown reasons
Person increases or decreases usual vocalizations

PHYSICAL CHANGES
Pleading expression
Grimacing
Pallor or flushing
Diaphoresis (sweating)
Increased pulse, respirations, or blood pressure

BOX 17-8   **MNEMONIC FOR PAIN ASSESSMENT: PAINED OLD CART**

Pain is real (Believe the patient!)
Ask about pain regularly
Isolation (psychological and social problems)
Notice nonverbal pain signs
Evaluate pain characteristics
Does pain impair function?
Onset
Location
Duration
Characteristics
Aggravating factors
Relieving factors
Treatment previously tried

From *Aging Successfully* (newsletter of the Division of Geriatric Medicine, St Louis University School of Medicine; Geriatric Research, Education and Clinical Centers, St Louis Veterans Administration Medical Center; the Gateway Geriatric Education Center of Missouri and Illinois) 11:6, 2001.

BOX 17-9   **ADDITIONAL FACTORS TO CONSIDER WHEN ASSESSING PAIN IN THE ELDERLY**

Function: How is the pain affecting the elder's ability to participate in usual activities, perform activities of daily living, and perform instrumental activities of daily living?

   Alternative expression of pain: Have there been recent changes in cognitive ability or behavior, such as increased pacing, grimacing, or irritability? Is there an increase in the number of complaints? Are they vague and difficult to respond to? Has there been a change in sleep-wake patterns? Is the person resisting certain activities, movements, or positions?

   Social support: What are the resources available to the elder in pain? What is the role of the elder in the social system, and how is pain affecting this role? How is pain affecting the elder's relationship with others?

   Pain history: How has the elder managed previous experiences with pain? What is the perceived meaning of the past and present pain? What are the cultural factors that affect the elder's ability to express pain and receive relief?

---

can provide valid reports of pain using self-report scales, but people with more severe impairment and loss of language skills may be unable to communicate the presence of pain in a manner that is easily understood but should be treated nonetheless (Herr & Decker, 2004; Herr et al., 2006a; Kovach et al., 2006a; Ware et al., 2006).

Non-Verbal Expressions of Pain

For those with dementia who are no longer able to express themselves verbally, communication of pain usually occurs through changes in behavior, such as agitation, aggression, increased confusion, or passivity. Caregivers should be educated to be particularly alert for passive behaviors because they are less disruptive and may not be recognized as changes that may signal pain. Providing comfort to those who cannot express themselves requires careful observation of behavior and attention to caregiver reports, knowing when subtle changes have occurred, and a willingness to help (Box 17-7). In nursing homes, the certified nursing assistants play an important role in pain assessment.

Regular assessment, use of standardized tools with consistent documentation, and communication are the most important components of pain assessment (Figure 17-1). This leads to the ability to adjust the plan of care promptly, consistently, and expertly in the promotion of comfort.

PROMOTING HEALTHY AGING: IMPLICATIONS FOR GERONTOLOGICAL NURSING

Assessment

The nurse is usually the first person to hear a patient's report of pain or become aware of a person's pain, making the ability to perform a comprehensive pain assessment critical. The nurse is in a key position to work with the elder in the management of pain, be it acute or persistent. The nurse works with the whole person to find comfort.

Considering pain as the fifth vital sign is not a consideration of simply the presence or absence of pain, but the self-rating of intensity. Assessment always begins with a patient's self-report of pain and usually includes uses a Likert-type rating or Visual analog of some type. A comprehensive pain assessment includes the identification of the factors influencing the pain experience and the opportunity for comfort (Box 17-8). This is the subjective and the objective whole of what it means to have pain, be a person in pain and one who finds relief. It includes what has hurt in the past and what has helped and how the pain affects function and role (Box 17-9). Awareness of the individual's health wellness paradigm is especially important in a pain assessment (see Chapter 5). What does the pain mean? Is the pain believed to be the result of imbalance, a form of punishment, or an infection? A good pain assessment includes a determination of the cause for this pain if possible, and what has been done and can be done to treat the cause if possible. Detailed assessment pain protocols and videos are available through the Hartford Geriatric Nursing Institute at http://consultgerirn.org/topics/pain/want_to_know_more.

INITIAL PAIN ASSESSMENT TOOL

Patient's name_____   Date_____

Age _____ Room _____

Diagnosis_____   Physician_____

Nurse _____

I. LOCATION: Patient or nurse mark drawing.

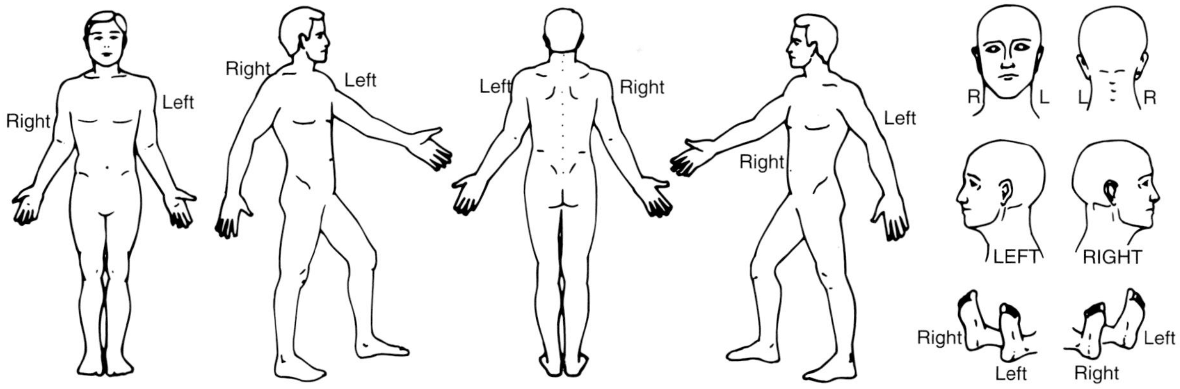

II. INTENSITY: Patient rates the pain. Scale used _____

    Present:_____
    Worst pain gets:_____
    Best pain gets:_____
    Acceptable level of pain:_____

III. QUALITY: (Use patient's own words, e.g., *prick, ache, burn, throb, pull, sharp*.) _____

IV. ONSET, DURATION VARIATIONS, RHYTHMS: _____

V. MANNER OF EXPRESSING PAIN: _____

VI. WHAT RELIEVES THE PAIN? _____

VII. WHAT CAUSES OR INCREASES THE PAIN? _____

VIII. EFFECTS OF PAIN: (Note decreased function, decreased quality of life.) _____
    Accompanying symptoms (e.g., nausea) _____
    Sleep_____
    Appetite _____
    Physical activity_____
    Relationship with others (e.g., irritability)_____
    Emotions (e.g., anger, suicidal, crying)_____
    Concentration _____
    Other _____

IX. OTHER COMMENTS: _____

X. PLAN: _____

FIGURE 17-1 Initial pain assessment tool. (From McCaffery M, Bebee A: *Pain: clinical manual of nursing practice,* St. Louis, 1989, Mosby.)

If it is reasonable to expect a person to have pain (e.g., postoperatively), it is important to assess for its presence on a regular basis. Depending on culture, the elder may not relate pain complaints unless directly asked specific questions such as, "Do you have pain now?" "Where is your pain?" "Do you have pain every day?" "Does pain keep you from sleeping at night or doing your daily activities?"

The pain assessment takes on more meaning if it is conducted during activity, such as during physical therapy or in day-to-day nursing activities. Travis and colleagues (2003) use the term iatrogenic disturbance pain (IDP) to describe a type of pain that can be caused by the care provider. The authors suggest that, in some circumstances, tasks such as application of a blood pressure cuff, transfers out of bed, bathing, and moving and

---

BOX 17-10 **SETTING PAIN GOALS**

Mrs. Henry was a 98-year-old white woman with stomach cancer. She was in remarkably good health otherwise. As her tumor enlarged so did her pain, and eventually around-the-clock morphine was needed in order for her to continue her usual activities, including baking cakes for the hospice staff! The associated constipation was controlled with a stool softener, but she also had dose-related visual hallucinations. Despite efforts to lower the dose to rid her of these, it was not possible to do so and maintain her pain relief. She finally declared, "I guess I will just have to learn to live with these puppies running around at my feet, better that then hurting. As least I know they are not real!"

---

repositioning patients in the bed may cause an unacceptable level of discomfort. Patients with severe physical limitations (e.g., contractures) and significant cognitive impairment and persons at the end of life may be particularly likely to experience IDP. Travis and colleagues (2003) suggest the use of a 5-day IDP tracking sheet for assessment and monitoring of IDP. Other suggestions provided include gentle handling, adequate staffing, appropriate lifting devices and techniques, analgesic administration before care or treatments that may cause discomfort, education of staff on proper lifting and moving techniques, and assessment of discomfort during care provision.

Pain Rating Scales

The use of rating scales, such as those found in Figures 17-2 and 17-3, have become the standard of care. A patient with persistent pain is asked to rate the "worst" and "best" pain. If the cause is something for which there is little control, such as one of the pain syndromes, a "pain" or "comfort" goal can be set (Box 17-10). The scales also serve as a basis for evaluation of the effectiveness of the pain-relieving intervention, leaving the determination of the relative painfulness to the patient and avoiding variation by the nurse. Scales have been found to be useful for persons who are cognitively intact and those with mild to moderate cognitive impairment. Scales that are currently available and tested may not be reliable for persons with delirium or more severe impairments (Herr et al., 2010).

For cognitively intact older adults, the Numeric Rating Scale (NRS) (see Figure 17-3 b), a verbally administered 0-10 numerical rating scale, may be a good first choice, especially if the patient has limited vision (Hanks-Bell et al., 2004). The Verbal Descriptor Scale (VDS) and the Pain Thermometer, an adaptation of the VDS, are also good choices and have been shown to be effective in the older adult population (Herr, 2002). The VDS includes adjectives describing pain, such as mild, moderate, severe, and worst pain imaginable. The Pain Thermometer is a diagram of a thermometer with word descriptions that show increasing pain intensities. The Faces Pain Scale (FPS) and the Faces Pain Scale-Revised (FPS-R) (Hicks et al., 2001) show a series of faces, with each depicting a different facial expression indicating level of pain. They were originally developed for children but may be effective for older adults as well, especially for persons with poorer verbal skills. However, it may be difficult to determine if pain or mood is being measured when using the FPS (Hanks-Bell et al., 2004). Both the Pain Thermometer and the FPS depend on visual acuity and may need to be enlarged for the visually impaired older person. Choice of instrument depends on the setting.

BOX 17-11 **GENERAL RECOMMENDATIONS FOR ASSESSMENT TECHNIQUES WITH NONCOMMUNICATIVE PATIENTS**

- Attempt to obtain a self-report of pain from the patient; yes/no response acceptable.
- If unable to obtain a self-report, document why it cannot be used and further observation and investigation are indicated.
- Look for possible causes of pain or discomfort; common conditions and procedures that cause pain (e.g., arthritis, surgery, wound care, history of persistent pain, constipation, lifting/moving).
- Medicate before any procedures causing discomfort.
- Observe and document patient behaviors that may indicate pain or distress or that are unusual from the person's normal patterns and responses. Behavioral observation scales may be used but should be used consistently and with proper training.
- Surrogate reports (family members, caregivers) of pain and behavior changes as well as patients' usual patterns and responses to pain and discomfort. This must be from a person who knows the patient well and should be combined with the other assessment techniques.
- If comfort measures and attention to basic needs (e.g., warmth, hunger, toileting) are not effective, attempt an analgesic trial based on the intensity of the pain and analgesic history. For mild to moderate pain, acetaminophen every 4 hours for 24 hours. If behaviors improve, continue and add appropriate non-pharmacological interventions. If behaviors continue, consider a single low-dose, short-acting opioid and observe effect. May titrate dose upward 25% to 50% if no change in behavior from initial dose. Continue to explore possible causes of behavior; observe for side effects and response.

From Herr K et al: *Pain Management Nursing* 7:44-52, 2006.

Assessment of Pain in Cognitively Impaired, Non-Verbal Older Adults

The Comprehensive Pain Assessment described above is only possible when caring for an elder who is cognitively intact or minimally to moderately impaired. For all others, an alternate approach is needed (Box 17-11; Figure 17-4). Instead the nurse and caregiver rely on the sometimes subtle and always confusing cues as to the person's needs and experiences, including pain. This has been a system fraught with potential errors as the assessment varies from nurse to nurse and shift to shift.

In 2008, a state-of-the-art review of tools for pain assessment in nonverbal patients was published following an extensive examination of the tools themselves (Herr et al., 2008). This review expanded the knowledge of nurses concerned with pain, especially for use in geriatrics, joining the practice guidelines available through the American Medical Director Association and the Center for Nursing Excellence at the University of Iowa. In 2010, Dr. Herr and colleagues completed a further analysis of the pain-behavioral assessment tools for use in the nursing home setting to enable the systematic identification of persons who are in pain but unable to say so. The Pain Assessment in Advanced Dementia Scale (PAINAD) and Pain Assessment Checklist for Seniors with Limited Ability to Communicate (PACSLAC) were recommended for use. They are complementary to the MDS-3 assessment, which is already required for use in the facilities. Due to the complexity of assessing pain in a non-verbal adult, the group recommended that both tools be used to determine the presence or absence of pain (i.e., at assessment and during monitoring of the symptom). A valuation of the intensity of the pain for that person is not possible.

Brief Pain Inventory

Date _____ / _____ / _____   Time: _____

Name: _____ _____ _____
Last   First   Middle Initial

1) Throughout our lives, most of us have had pain from time to time (such as minor headaches, sprains, and toothaches). Have you had such pain other than these everyday kinds of pain today?

1. Yes   2. No

2) On the diagram, shade the areas where you feel pain. Put an X on the area that hurts the most.

Right   Left   Left   Right

3) Please rate your pain by circling the one number that best describes your pain at its **worst** in the past 24 hours.

| 0 | 1 | 2 | 3 | 4 | 5 | 6 | 7 | 8 | 9 | 10 |
No pain   Pain as bad as you can imagine

4) Please rate your pain by circling the one number that best describes your pain at its **least** in the past 24 hours.

| 0 | 1 | 2 | 3 | 4 | 5 | 6 | 7 | 8 | 9 | 10 |
No pain   Pain as bad as you can imagine

5) Please rate your pain by circling the one number that best describes your pain on the **average.**

| 0 | 1 | 2 | 3 | 4 | 5 | 6 | 7 | 8 | 9 | 10 |
No pain   Pain as bad as you can imagine

6) Please rate your pain by circling the one number that tells how much pain you have **right now.**

| 0 | 1 | 2 | 3 | 4 | 5 | 6 | 7 | 8 | 9 | 10 |
No pain   Pain as bad as you can imagine

7) What treatments or medications are you receiving for your pain?

_____

_____

8) In the past 24 hours, how much **relief** have pain treatments or medications provided? Please circle the one percentage that most shows how much relief you have received.

| 0% | 10 | 20 | 30 | 40 | 50 | 60 | 70 | 80 | 90 | 100% |
No relief   Complete relief

9) Circle the one number that describes how, during the past 24 hours, pain has interfered with your:
A. General activity

| 0 | 1 | 2 | 3 | 4 | 5 | 6 | 7 | 8 | 9 | 10 |
Does not interfere   Completely interferes

B. Mood

| 0 | 1 | 2 | 3 | 4 | 5 | 6 | 7 | 8 | 9 | 10 |
Does not interfere   Completely interferes

C. Walking ability

| 0 | 1 | 2 | 3 | 4 | 5 | 6 | 7 | 8 | 9 | 10 |
Does not interfere   Completely interferes

D. Normal work (includes both work outside the home and housework)

| 0 | 1 | 2 | 3 | 4 | 5 | 6 | 7 | 8 | 9 | 10 |
Does not interfere   Completely interferes

E. Relations with other people

| 0 | 1 | 2 | 3 | 4 | 5 | 6 | 7 | 8 | 9 | 10 |
Does not interfere   Completely interferes

F. Sleep

| 0 | 1 | 2 | 3 | 4 | 5 | 6 | 7 | 8 | 9 | 10 |
Does not interfere   Completely interferes

G. Enjoyment of life

| 0 | 1 | 2 | 3 | 4 | 5 | 6 | 7 | 8 | 9 | 10 |
Does not interfere   Completely interferes

FIGURE 17-2 Brief pain inventory. (Copyright Charles S. Cleeland, PhD, Houston. May be duplicated for use in clinical practice.)

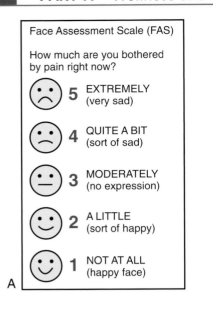

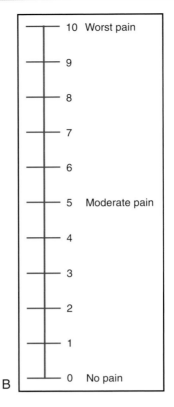

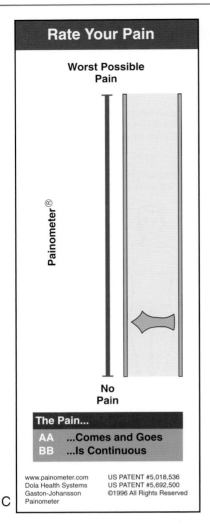

FIGURE 17-3 Examples of commonly used pain assessment scales. **A,** Face Assessment Scale (FAS). **B,** Numeric Rating Scale (NRS). **C,** The Gaston-Johansson Painometer. (**A,** Adapted from Philadelphia Geriatric Center Pain Intensity Scale. In Cramer K et al: Philadelphia College of Pharmacy proposed guidelines for the management of chronic nonmalignant pain in the elderly LTC resident, Feb 1988; Jacox A et al: Pub No 94-0592, Rockville, Md, 1994, Agency for Health Care Policy and Research [AHCPR], U.S. Department of Health and Human Services; Gaston-Johansson F et al. Nursing Home Medicine 4:325, 1996; McCaffery M: *Nursing Home Medicine* 5:143, 1997; Bridgeport, Conn, HealthCare Center Pain Assessment, created from pain assessment methodologies of the Joint Commission on Accreditation of Healthcare Organizations [JCAHO]; **B,** From Pasero C and McCaffery M: *Pain assessment and pharmacologic management*, St. Louis, 2011, Mosby. **C,** Copyright 1996 Fannie Gaston-Johansson, Dr Med Sci, RN, FAAN, Baltimore, Md. May be duplicated for use in clinical practice.)

The PAINAD is a simple, short, focused tool that can be used on a more frequent basis; it has been found to demonstrate sensitivity to change with intervention (Warden et al., 2003). Four behaviors are rated by an observer on a scale of 0 to 2: breathing independent of vocalization, negative vocalizations, facial expression, and body language and consolability. The tool is described in detail at a number of sites easily available online. It is in use in its original form internationally. The PACSLAC is a comprehensive behavioral assessment tool that may be very useful as an initial pain screen as well as an interval measure. There are four domains of observation: facial expression, activity/body movement, social/personality/mood, and physiological/sleeping/eating/vocal. The PACSLAC can serve as a guide for the care provided by the CNA in a nursing facility (Fuchs-Lachelle & Hadjistavropoulos, 2004; Herr et al., 2010).

Detailed instructions and downloads of the PACSLAC are available on-line in various formats.

Interventions: Providing Comfort

Working with the older adult in pain and achieving optimal pain management are especially challenging. Clinical manifestations are complex with multiple potential sources and sites for pain. Pain that interferes with functioning or quality of life is a problem that should be addressed. This pain may be one for which there is a reasonable certainty that relief can be found or for which some level of modulation is possible. Both take commitment and determination to achieve. The frequency of polypharmacy and the chance of interactions cause some to hesitate, increasing the potential for under-treated or un-treated pain. Finally, there is often a societal expectation that pain is a

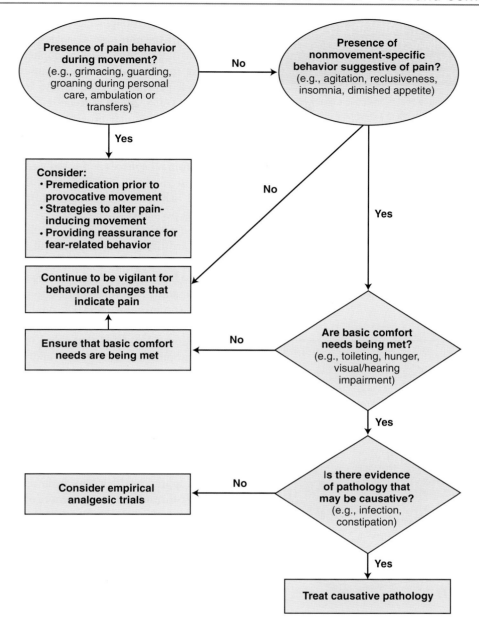

FIGURE 17-4 Algorithm for the assessment of pain in elders with severe cognitive impairment. (From Herr K, Decker S: Assessment of pain in older adults with severe cognitive impairment, *Annals of Long-Term Care* 12:46, 2004; adapted from Weiner DK, Herr K: Comprehensive interdisciplinary assessment and treatment planning: an integrative overview. In Rudy T, editor: *Persistent pain in older adults: an interdisciplinary guide for treatment,* New York, 2002, Springer.)

natural part of aging or that full relief is not possible, even when quality of life is compromised, as in the example of Mrs. Thomas earlier in the chapter. Instead, the gerontological nurse can advocate for and work with the elder and significant others to prevent needless suffering and achieve a high level of pain relief and health-related quality of life. Multiple modalities are available today to promote comfort, and when used together, pain can be relieved in most cases.

Pharmacological Interventions to Promote Comfort

In 2009, the American Geriatrics Society published an update of their original guideline for the management of persistent pain. In the document, the authors recognize the many conundrums encountered in using pharmacological interventions for pain management in the older patient but nonetheless impress

upon the reader the need to do so. They provide several overarching general principles which, when followed, can help minimize drug interactions and adverse events (Box 17-12).

Analgesics (non-opioid and opioid agents) and adjuvant medications (antidepressants, anticonvulsants, herbal preparations) have all been found to have a role in promoting comfort in older adults in pain, and while revisions are under consideration the recommended stepwise progression from WHO remains the standard of care (Figure 17-5). However, several age-related changes and several common health problems seen in late life are now recognized as cause to reconsider the uses of some of the non-opioids with some older adults (AGS, 2009). While the goal is adequate pain relief to the extent that function is preserved and quality of life maintained or returned, there is always a need to watch for medication misuse with

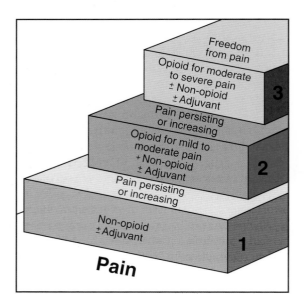

FIGURE 17-5 World Health Organization (WHO) three-step analgesic ladder. (Redrawn from World Health Organization: *Cancer pain relief*, ed 2, Geneva, 1996, WHO.)

analgesics; it is less of a concern with persistent pain in late life (Papaleontiou et al., 2010).

To achieve the highest level of pain control, it is helpful to ease the "memory of pain," especially for those whose persistent pain is intense (e.g., some neuropathic pain or cancer-related pain). This means that it is necessary to prevent the pain, not simply relieve it. The most effective way to do this is to provide around-the-clock (ATC) dosing, at the appropriate dosage; it provides a more stable therapeutic plasma level of the analgesics and eliminates the extremes of overmedication and undermedication. Additional analgesics that are prescribed on an as-needed basis (PRN) should be used freely for pain that "breaks through" the ATC management (Portenoy et al., 2006). Which medications are used and the dosing will need to be determined, but with long-acting and sustained-release formulations currently available, some level of ATC relief should be possible.

Non-opioid Analgesics. Acetaminophen (Tylenol) and NSAIDs are the non-opioid analgesics most often used for pain relief in older adults. Acetaminophen has been found to be effective for the most common causes of pain, osteoarthritis, and back pain and should always be considered a first-line approach (AGS, 2009). If acetaminophen is used for persistent pain, ATC dosing may provide adequate relief. It is not associated with gastrointestinal bleeding or adverse renal or cardiac effects. However, the maximum dose is 4 g (4000 mg) in 24 hours from **all sources** and is reduced for people with renal or hepatic dysfunction or who drink alcohol; the dose is easily reached when "extra-strength" formulations are taken at 1000 mg per tablet.

When persistent pain is of an inflammatory nature, during a short arthritic flair or in persistent rheumatoid arthritis, one of the NSAIDs may be needed. Older adults have been found to be at a higher risk for adverse drug effects from NSAIDs than younger adults, especially in persons with renal, gastric, or cardiac compromise. NSAIDs bind with proteins and may induce toxic responses in elders if serum albumin levels are low. In addition, other drugs that elders routinely take compete for the same protein receptor sites and may be displaced by the NSAID, creating unstable therapeutic effects. Not surprisingly, NSAIDs have been implicated in a significant number of hospitalizations for adverse drug reactions in older adults, especially when co-administered with aspirin (AGS, 2009; Papaleontiou et al., 2010). In some persons, non-acetylated NSAIDs (e.g., trisalicylate) may be more effective or have fewer side effects.

Two approaches that have been used to address the potentially life-threatening consequences of NSAID use is the introduction of COX-2 inhibitors and adding gastro-protective agents to the drug regimen. Cyslooxygenase-2 (COX-2) selective inhibitors (e.g., Celebrex) appear to be as effective and have fewer GI side effects. However, two others in this group were taken off the market for their risk for adverse cardiac effects. Co-administration of any of the gastric agents available (misoprostol, H2 antagonists, or proton pump inhibitors) may be helpful and reasonable, especially for persons at a higher risk for GI bleeding. However, serious concerns remain, including an alert by the U.S. Food and Drug Administration and the American Geriatrics Society.

! SAFETY ALERT

NSAID Use

In 2006, the Food and Drug Administration in the United States issued a warning regarding the concomitant use of aspirin (81 mg) and ibuprofen. When taken together, the aspirin is less cardio-protective (i.e., there is less antiplatelet effect), and the person's risk for a cardiac event increases.

For persons who take immediate-release aspirin even a single dose of ibuprofen (400 mg), the ibuprofen should be taken at least 30 minutes after or 8 hours before the aspirin. FDA: Information for Healthcare Professionals: Concomitant Use of Ibuprofen and Aspirin, 2006. Available at http://www.fda.gov/Drugs/DrugSafety/PostmarketDrugSafetyInformationforPatientsandProviders/ucm125222.htm.

In addition to the known potential for gastrointestinal distress, new findings indicate that NSAIDs may adversely affect blood pressure, renal function, and heart failure. Overall, the use of NSAIDs increases the risk for cardiac events, and then use must take these risks into consideration. The current guideline includes:

> The decision to prescribe NSAIDs in the management of persistent pain in older adults demands individualized consideration. Comorbidities, concomitant medications, and associated risk factors (including, possibly, genetics) all affect the decision to introduce such treatment. Key issues in the selection of NSAID therapy are pain amelioration, cardiovascular risk, nephrotoxicity, drug interactions, and gastrointestinal toxicity (AGS, 2009, p. 1338).

Opioid Analgesics. If long-term management of moderate to severe pain is needed, opioids may be preferred because of their lower or predictable rate of adverse reactions, especially in light of the safety concerns just noted (see also chapter 12). For most, opioids will provide relief and are the core of a multi-pronged approach. The AGS advises that their use be considered seriously and carefully when other modalities are not effective or appropriate and when they will not make the condition worse (2009). Opioids have been found to be effective for all types of pain but not for all persons (Samer et al., 2010; Schofield, 2010).

Due to a number of age-related changes, opioids may produce a greater analgesic effect, a higher peak, and a longer duration of effect; a short trial with clear goals is recommended along with careful clinical observation of effect. Sedation and impaired cognition often occur when opioid analgesics are started or doses increased. This often causes great concern from patients, families, and nurses but is only transient and may be necessary to achieve the goal of pain relief. Safety measures, such as fall precautions, are needed until the person is stabilized.

> ⚠ **SAFETY ALERT**
>
> Some medications used in younger adults, for example, meperidine (Demerol), are always contraindicated in the older adult.

Opioid treatment should begin with "as-needed" doses of short-acting medications and should be titrated based on the amount needed, response obtained, and side effects over a 24-hour period. Current recommendations are to start with the lowest anticipated effective dose, monitor response frequently, and increase dose slowly to desired effect. Once the amount of medication needed for relief in the 24-hour period has been determined, conversion is made to long-acting opioids to achieve a steady-state, ATC effect. If a change is needed from one drug to another, and the dose of active ingredient is known, then conversion resources are available so that the patient can remain pain free (search "equianalgesic"). Additional non-opioids and adjuvant medications or short-acting opioids can then be used for breakthrough PRN treatment. If PRN medications are needed regularly, the long-acting opioid dosage should be adjusted accordingly. Unfortunately, too often the titration is not done (i.e., dosages are not adjusted after the original prescription) and pain relief is inadequate, especially in the long-term care setting (Hutt et al., 2006).

Side effects of opioids are significant to older adults; they include gait disturbance, dizziness, sedation, falls, nausea, pruritus, and constipation (Shorr et al., 2007). Several of these will resolve on their own as the body develops tolerance to the drug. Some side effects may be prevented when the prescribing provider works closely with the patient and the nurse to slowly increase the dose of the drug to a point where the best relief can be obtained with the fewest side effects. Because constipation is almost universal when opioids are used, the nurse should ensure that an appropriate bowel regimen is begun at the same time as the opioids. A daily dose of a combination stool softener and mild laxative may be very helpful, and adequate fluid intake is essential. Prophylactic use of antiemetics may be helpful for associated nausea until tolerance develops.

Adjuvant Drugs. There are a number of drugs developed for other purposes that have been found to be useful in pain management, sometimes alone, but more often in combination with an analgesic; these have come to be referred to as *adjuvant drugs*. They include antidepressants, anticonvulsants, and other agents that alter neural membranes, or neural processing.

While they are used with the range of types of persistent pain, they are thought to be most effective for neuropathic pain syndromes (pain described as sharp, shooting, piercing, or burning). Tricyclic antidepressants such as amitriptyline were first found to provide some relief in postherpetic neuralgia and diabetic nephropathy, despite their higher adverse effect profiles and side effects. While the mechanism is unknown, the mixed serotonin and norepinephrine reuptake inhibitors (SNRIs) such as duloxetine (Cymbalta) and venlafaxine (Effexor) seem to be effective with fewer problems. The serotonin reuptake inhibitors (SSRIs) have not been effective in the management of physical pain (AGS, 2009).

Other Drugs. Several other products are used in attempts to control pain, depending greatly on the situation, the cause of the pain, and the mechanism of action of the agent. Corticosteroids are sometimes used for a range of inflammatory conditions and will reduce the associated pain. However, the well-known side effects and toxicity limit their use to anything but very specific circumstances or the shortest use possible. The exact mechanism of muscle relaxants is unknown, and the risk for fall-related injury is high. Topical agents (e.g., capsaicin, lidocaine patch) may have some mild to moderate local effect; skin must be intact and the area watched for signs of irritation. Several other topical agents are in development. Cannabinoids are in use but are not yet subjected to rigorous clinical trials.

Non-pharmacological Measures

While pharmacological interventions have been the mainstay of the Western model to pain management, it is now well recognized that combining pharmacological and non-pharmacological approaches is the most effective and appropriate way to control pain, especially the persistent pain common in later life and in older adults. While most approaches have been used for dozens or even thousands of years, more and more of the non-pharmacological measures are gaining acceptance by both patients and insurers such as Medicare. Several are identified here, acknowledging that whole chapters could be devoted to any one approach. The data to support the efficacy of the approaches vary.

Energy/Touch Therapies. Some say the use of touch therapies is a legacy in nursing. Over the years, different kinds of touch have been formalized to include those referred to as Healing Touch (HT), Therapeutic Touch (TT), and Reiki (see Chapter 21). A review of all of the literature and experts available through 2008 was conducted and published in the Cochrane Database. Only modest pain relief was found (So et al., 2008). The acceptability of touch by individual and culture varies considerably. Some touch may never be acceptable, such as cross-gender touch in strict Muslim or Orthodox Jewish traditions. The culturally sensitive nurse always requests permission before touching a patient.

Transcutaneous Electrical Nerve Stimulation. Transcutaneous Electrical Nerve Stimulation or TENS has been used in a variety of settings to treat a range of conditions and became very popular with both patients and health professionals. Patients often anecdotally reported that at least they were doing "something" for their chronic pain. In 2001, the state of the science related to efficacy was examined and only inconclusive evidence was found, making it impossible to support or refute this approach (Carroll et al., 2001). In 2008, the efficacy of this approach was still in question (Nnoaham & Kumbang, 2008).

Acupuncture and Acupressure. Acute pain is registered as pain impulses pass through the theoretical pain gate in the spine and register the sensation in the brain, which in turn signals the central mechanism of the brain to return counter-impulses, which close the gate. Acupuncture uses tiny needles inserted along specific meridians or pathways in the body. Acupressure is pressure applied with the thumbs or tip of the index finger at the same locations as those used in acupuncture. It is thought that acupuncture and acupressure stimulate nerve clusters that cause the gate to close more quickly or that trigger the release of the body's own opiate substances, enkephalins (endorphins). Acupuncture and acupressure have been used for thousands of years, and scientific evidence of their effectiveness in the treatment of persistent pain is growing (Vas et al., 2006; Witt et al., 2006). In some cases, Medicare and some private insurance companies will pay for the cost of acupuncture treatment from a licensed acupuncturist.

Relaxation, Meditation, and Guided Imagery. Pain is often accompanied by a strong affective component. Pain is not experienced alone, but with the emotions of anger or frustrations or despair (anxiety and depression). We now know that all of these emotional stressors stimulate the sympathetic nervous system releasing norepinephrine: the strength of the mind-body connection. The norepinephrine in turn increases the sensation of pain. Hence reducing emotional stressors lessens muscle tension and other physiological manifestations of pain. Distraction, relaxation, and meditation all enable the quieting of the mind and muscles, providing the release of tension and anxiety. Relaxation should be adjunctive to all pharmacological interventions. Meditation and guided imagery are two methods of promoting relaxation. Imagery uses the client's imagination to focus on settings full of happiness and relaxation rather than on stressful situations. Several studies using guided imagery have shown that pain perception in foot pain and abdominal pain was decreased. It was suggested that a strong image of a pain-free state effectively alters the autonomic nervous system's responses to pain (Peck & Gentili, 2008).

Music. In a review of studies of the effect of music on pain, the results were very slight but differed greatly in part due to the heterogeneity of the studies. All showed a decrease in the intensity of pain, and/or opioid requirements for those with pain who listened to music (Cepeda et al., 2006). McCaffrey and Freeman (2003) found music as a form of distraction to be helpful when dealing with pain from osteoarthritis, and Park (2010) found some relief for persons with dementia who listened to their preferred music.

Hypnosis. Hypnosis, another behavioral strategy, can be used to alter pain perception, thus blocking pain awareness; to substitute another feeling for a painful one; to displace pain sensation to a smaller body area; or to alter the meaning of pain so that it is viewed as less important and less debilitating (Peck & Gentili, 2008). Research has demonstrated that hypnotic analgesia reduces what are called "overreactions" to pain when apprehension and stress are apparent. Most of the population have some capacity for hypnosis and with training can increase their control in this area.

Activity. Activity can be helpful in several ways. It is thought that the less active an individual is, the less tolerable activity becomes. Anyone who becomes inactive may feel more general discomfort than the active person. However, some activities can stimulate pain. Use of analgesics in conjunction with activity may be necessary. The administration of an analgesic PRN medication 20 to 30 minutes before a specific activity may lessen or eliminate discomfort and fear of discomfort after the activity and greatly enhance the individual's capacity for that activity. The nurse should learn the patient's body tolerance for activity and work within those parameters.

Cognitive-Behavioral Therapy. Through cognitive-behavioral therapy (CBT), the elder learns that self-efficacy and self-care skills are both powerful mediators of pain (Tan et al., 2009). CBT is central to all other approaches to pain management. This means finding ways of coping with the circumstances in which one finds oneself to the degree possible. Through the setting of self-identified goals and treatment contracts with the nurse, the helplessness, hopelessness, and anxiety that often accompany persistent pain can be replaced with determination to expertly manage one's pain and increase the individually controlled interventions for comfort and prevention (Box 17-13) (Davis & White, 2008).

BOX 17-13   CLINICAL PEARL

The person can take the lead in his or her own pain management by keeping a journal that includes an account of pain during the day; the times, type, and dose of medication taken; its effect; and the duration of its benefit. This type of information helps establish patterns that may be useful in improving pain management by adjusting activity, providing medications appropriately, and helping the person feel useful and in control of some aspect of care and of his or her life with pain. The diary should be reviewed by the health care provider to assess the relationship between pain, medication use, and activity. A pain graph provides a visual picture of the highs and lows of the pain and provides the information needed for the appropriate adjustment of the selected intervention.

Pain Clinics

Pain clinics provide a specialized, often comprehensive and multidisciplinary approach to the management of pain that has not responded to the usual, more standard approaches as described herein. The use of such pain clinics by the elderly has been limited. However, their use should be encouraged when appropriate. The number and types of pain clinics and programs have increased as a response to continued poor pain management by general health care practice. Pain center programs may be inpatient, outpatient, or both. Pain clinics are generally one of three types: syndrome-oriented, modality-oriented, or comprehensive. Syndrome-oriented centers focus on a specific chronic pain problem, such as headache or arthritis pain. Modality-oriented centers focus on a specific treatment technique, such as relaxation or acupuncture/acupressure. The comprehensive centers tend to be larger and associated with medical centers. These centers include many services and provide a thorough initial assessment (physical, mental, psychosocial) of the person in pain. A comprehensive treatment plan is developed utilizing multiple modalities and usually a multidisciplinary team of interventionists.

The goals of pain management centers are to decrease pain intensity to a tolerable limit or eliminate it, if possible; improve functionality and activities of daily living (ADLs); increase involvement in family and social activities; decrease depression; and improve mood. This is accomplished by improving quality and frequency of assessment, improving optimal use of analgesics, assisting in minimizing analgesic adverse reactions, selecting non-pharmacological interventions, and evaluating outcomes associated with treatment. Physiological and cognitive-behavioral modalities are used to reduce or alleviate pain. The nurse should be familiar with the types of pain management clinics available in their communities to provide the patient and family with necessary information to make a knowledgeable decision in selecting a reputable center.

SUMMARY

Pain management is one in which both pharmacological and non-pharmacological interventions work in harmony. The basic approach to pain management and control is one that considers that whatever has worked in the past and been effective without causing harm should be encouraged. This is particularly applicable for older adults with a lifetime of experience at managing pain with both the approaches used in Western medicine and those learned through their cultural heritages. The nurse, the patient, and the significant others work together to find comfort for the patient. Evaluation of pain relief strategies requires repeated reassessment of the patient's status and comfort level both qualitatively and quantitatively. Qualitative indicators of better management or relief include physical indicators such as relaxation of skeletal muscles that were tense and rigid during pain. The individual no longer assumes a constricted pain posture. Behavior may reflect an increased activity level and sense of self-worth and the ability to better concentrate, focus, and increase attention span, regardless of cognitive status. The individual is better able to rest, relax, and sleep. In fact, the individual may sleep for what might seem like excessively long periods, but this is in response to the exhaustion that pain imposes on the body. Verbal indicators reflect the patient referring to the decrease in pain or the absence of pain during conversation.

Pain can be minimized through gentle handling, touch, and careful observation of the person's reaction to procedures. Use of pillows for support or body positioning, appropriate and comfortable seating and mattresses, frequent rest periods, and pacing of activities to balance activity and rest are important.

Whether the pain is brief or long-standing, the anticipated result of diagnostic procedures or surgery, or related to a terminal condition, a plan for appropriate intervention should be developed and initiated. This begins with a discussion between the nurse and prescribing provider, patient, and significant others and includes how much pain is anticipated and how long it might last, how it will be treated, what alternatives will be available if the initial treatment does not adequately relieve the pain, and what level of pain is desired by the patient.

The evaluation of pain management and relief is measured quantitatively with the same instruments used in the initial assessment for a means of comparison. Reevaluation of the frequency and intensity of pain; behavioral signs and symptoms that suggest pain; response to pharmacological and non-pharmacological interventions; and the impact of pain on mood, ADLs, sleep, and other quality-of-life measures are all included. Adjustments of treatment regimens and interventions are based on reassessment findings. Active involvement of the patient, family, and all caregivers is essential for comprehensive pain assessment, management, and evaluation. Finally, an individualized approach will optimize pain management and, in doing so, promote the health of persons at any stage of life and wellness (Box 17-14). If assessment is correct and the patient is listened to and handled gently and with care, anxiety can be controlled and interventions will prove more effective.

BOX 17-14   GUIDELINES FOR INDIVIDUALIZING PAIN MANAGEMENT

1. Use a variety of pain control measures.
2. Institute pain control measures before pain becomes severe.
3. Use around-the-clock dosing for persistent pain with careful titration to achieve relief.
4. Use the lowest dose of pharmacological interventions, but use those that provide relief and those that are least invasive first.
5. Consider patients' ideas and cultural patterns in the development of pain management care plans.
6. Encourage the patient's and family's participation in the pain management plan that is educationally, culturally, and socially appropriate.
7. Listen to how patients describe the severity of pain. Physical signs and perceived severity are not predictably related, and expressions are usually culturally mediated.
8. Be aware that patients respond differently to different pain control measures. What is effective one day may not be effective the next day.
9. Be aware that persons from minority groups and older adults have been historically undertreated for pain.
10. Assess, intervene, evaluate, and repeat frequently.

KEY CONCEPTS

- The experience of pain is multifactorial with physical, psychological, and spiritual components.
- Pain is a subjective experience that is unique to each individual.
- It is the responsibility of the health care professional to address the needs of the person in pain.
- The pain most common in later life is that which is persistent and from musculoskeletal sources.
- The undertreatment of pain in older adults, especially those in long-term care facilities and elders of color, is well documented.
- A careful assessment of the presence or absence of pain is possible regardless of the cognitive status of the person who may be in pain.
- If it is reasonable to expect a person in a particular circumstance to experience pain, it is reasonable to expect that pain is being felt by the person regardless of his or her ability to express this.

- It is never acceptable to fail to treat pain (or the expectation of pain) to the extent possible.
- Acetaminophen is recommended as the first-line approach for the pharmacological management of mild to moderate pain with a maximum of 4 gm in 24 hours.
- Around-the-clock dosing of the appropriate medication will optimize pain relief for those with persistent pain.
- The use of NSAIDs for pain relief in the older adult must be done with caution and the awareness of the increased risk for associated cardiac events.
- The use of opioids has been found to be very effective and has the potential to significantly restore function to persons with persistent pain.
- Optimal pain management incorporates both pharmacological and non-pharmacological approaches.

evolve   To access your student resources, go to *http://evolve.elsevier.com/Ebersole/TwdHlthAging*

CASE STUDY   PAIN IN ELDERS

Ms. P. was a 66-year-old diabetic and, after a stroke, had to relocate to a nursing facility. In a short time her diabetes began to have uncontrollable fluctuations. Her blood sugar ranged from 20 mEq/mL to 800 mEq/mL. Some of this was caused by erratic eating habits, almost no exercise, frequent urinary tract infections, and considerable stress related to her condition and her future. She bumped her toe while being assisted into her wheelchair after occupational therapy. In a few days, the bruise had sloughed skin, and an open sore was evident. In spite of appropriate treatment, the sore became necrotic and was debrided. Ms. P, who rarely complained, began to moan while she was sleeping and cry a lot during the day. She complained of a continuous burning sensation and said that it felt as if her toe was "on fire." One day she threw her coffee cup across the room complaining that it was not hot enough. Various pain medications were given by mouth on an inconsistent basis, but the relief she experienced was minimal. She began to beg to die. The nurses thought perhaps she was right—after all, her general condition was poor, and life held little satisfaction for her.

Based on the case study, develop a nursing care plan using the following procedure:*

- List Ms. P.'s comments that provide subjective data.
- List information that provides objective data.
- From these data, identify and state, using accepted format, two nursing diagnoses you determine are most significant to Ms. P. at this time.

- List two of Ms. P.'s strengths that you have identified from the data.
- Determine and state outcome criteria for each diagnosis. These must reflect some alleviation of the problem identified in the nursing diagnosis and must be stated in concrete and measurable terms.
- Plan and state one or more interventions for each diagnosed problem. Provide specific documentation of the source used to determine the appropriate intervention. Plan at least one intervention that incorporates Ms. P.'s existing strengths.
- Evaluate the success of the intervention. Interventions must correlate directly with the stated outcome criteria to measure the outcome success.

CRITICAL THINKING QUESTIONS

1. Discuss Ms. P.'s situation and her probable prognosis.
2. What could be done, based on the information you have, to improve Ms. P.'s condition?
3. Discuss the reasons for sporadic pain medication and inattention to the patient's signals and requests.
4. Do you think nurses are concerned about addiction in cases like Ms. P.'s?
5. In what situations do you believe addiction to pain medications is a priority concern?
6. Discuss issues of power and control related to pain management.

*Students are advised to refer to their nursing diagnosis text and identify possible or potential problems.

RESEARCH QUESTIONS

1. Do pain perceptions generally diminish as one ages?
2. What type of persistent pain do elders find most intolerable?
3. How do elders describe the pain of arthritis?
4. Do elders really fear the physical pain that may accompany dying?

5. What non-pharmacological means of pain control do elders use most frequently?
6. What non-pharmacological means of pain control are effective, and in what circumstances do they provide pain relief?

7. What are the reliable ways of assessing pain in cognitively impaired elders?
8. How can pain and pain relief be evaluated in the cognitively impaired?
9. How effective is patient-controlled analgesia (PCA) use by elders?
10. For whom and under what circumstances should the various modalities of pain management be used?
11. How does culture influence pain expression and treatment?

REFERENCES

American Geriatrics Society: Pharmacological Management of Persistent Pain in Older Persons: American Geriatrics Society Panel on the Pharmacological Management of Persistent Pain in Older Persons, *Journal of the American Geriatrics Society* 57:1331, 2009.

Arnstein P: Balancing analgesic efficacy with safety concerns in the older patient, *Pain Management Nursing* 11(2 Suppl):S11, 2010.

Campbell LC, Andrews N, Scipio C, Flores B, Feliu MH, Keefe FJ: Pain and coping in Latino populations, *Journal of Pain* 10(10):1012-1019, 2009.

Carroll D, Moore RA, McQuay HJ, et al: Transcutaneous electrical nerve stimulation (TENS) for chronic pain. *Cochrane Database of Systematic Reviews* 3:CD003222, 2001.

Cepeda MS, Carr DB, Lau J, et al: Music for pain relief. *Cochrane Database of Systematic Reviews* 19:CD004843, 2006.

Davis GC, White TL: A goal attainment pain management program for older adults with arthritis, *Pain Management Nursing* 9:171, 2008. Epub 2008 Nov 7.

Fuchs-Lachelle S, Hadjistavropoulos T: Development and preliminary validation of the pain assessment checklist for seniors with limited ability to communicate (PACSLAC), *Pain Management Nursing* 5:37, 2004. See also http://e-pacslac.com.

Hanks-Bell M, Halvey K, Paice J: Pain assessment and management in aging, *The Online Journal of Issues in Nursing* 9:1, 2004. Available at www.nursingworld.org/ojin/topic21/tpc21_6.htm.

Herr K: Chronic pain challenges and assessment strategies, *Journal of Gerontological Nursing* 28:20, 2002.

Herr K: Pain in the older adult: an imperative across all health care settings, *Pain Management Nursing* 11(2 Suppl):S1, 2010.

Herr K, Bursch H, Black B: State of the art review of tools for assessment of pain in nonverbal older adults. 2008. City of Hope Pain and Palliative Care Resource Center. Available at http.prc.coh.org/PAIN-NOA.htm

Herr K, Decker S: Assessment of pain in older adults with severe cognitive impairment, *Annals of Long-Term Care* 12:46, 2004.

Herr K, Coyne PJ, Key T, et al: Pain assessment in the nonverbal patient: position statement with clinical practice recommendations, *Pain Management Nursing* 7:44, 2006a.

Herr K, Bjoro K, Decker S: Tools for assessment of pain in nonverbal older adults with dementia: a state of the science review, *Journal of Pain and Symptom Management* 31:170, 2006b.

Herr K, Bursch H, Ersek M, et al: Use of pain-behavioral assessment tools in the nursing home: Expert consensus recommendations for practice, *Gerontological Nursing* 36:18, 2010.

Hicks CL, von Baeyer CL, Spafford PA, et al: The Faces Pain Scale—revised: toward a common metric in pediatric pain measurement, *Pain* 93:173, 2001.

Hutt E, Pepper GA, Vojir C, et al: Assessing the appropriateness of pain medication prescribing practices in nursing homes, *Journal of the American Geriatrics Society* 54:231, 2006.

International Association for the Study of Pain: Position statement: IASP Pain Terminology, 2010. Available at http://www.iasp-pain.org/AM/Template.cfm?Section=Pain_Defi...isplay.cfm&ContentID=1728.

Jansen MP: Pain in older adults. In Jansen MP, editor, *Managing pain in the older adult*, New York, 2008, Springer.

Joint Commission: Health Care Issues: Pain Management. November 12, 2009. Available at http://www.jointcommission.org/NewsRoom/health_care_issues.htm#9.

Kovach C, Logan BR, Noonan PE, et al: Effects of the Serial Trial Intervention on discomfort and behavior of nursing home residents with dementia, *American Journal of Alzheimer's Disease and Other Dementias* 21:147, 2006a.

Kovach C, Noonan PE, Schlidt AM, et al: The serial trial intervention: an innovative approach to meeting the needs of individuals with dementia, *Journal of Gerontological Nursing* 32:18, 2006b.

McCaffrey R, Freeman E: Effect of music on chronic osteoarthritis pain in older people, *Journal of Advanced Nursing* 44:517, 2003.

Nnoaham KE, Kumbang J: Transcutaneous electrical nerve stimulation (TENS) for chronic pain. *Cochrane Database of Systematic Reviews* 2008 Jul 16:CD003222.

Park H: Effect of music on pain for home-dwelling persons with dementia. *Pain Management Nursing* 11:141, 2010. Epub 2009 Sep 8.

Papaleontiou M, Henderson CR, Turner BJ, et al: Outcomes associated with opioid use in the treatment of chronic noncancer pain in older adults: A systematic review and meta-analysis, *Journal of the American Geriatrics Society* 58:1353, 2010.

Peck SDE, Gentili A: Mind-body and energy therapies. In Jansen MP, editor, *Managing pain in the older adult*, New York, 2008, Springer.

Portenoy RK, Bennett DS, Rauck R, et al: Prevalence and characteristics of breakthrough pain in opioid-treated patients with chronic cancer pain, *The Journal of Pain* 7:583, 2006.

Robinson P: Pharmacological management of pain in older persons, *The Consultant Pharmacist* 25(Suppl A):11, 2010.

Samer CF, Daali Y, Wagner M, et al: Genetic polymorphisms and drug interactions modulating CYP2D6 and CYP3A activities have a major effect on oxycodone analgesic efficacy and safety, *British Journal of Pharmacology* 160:919, 2010.

Schofield P: "It's your age": The assessment and management of pain in older adults, *Continuing Education in Anaesthesia, Critical Care & Pain* 10:93, 2010.

So PS, Jiang Y, Qin Y: Touch therapies for pain relief in adults. *Cochrane Database of Systematic Reviews* 2008 Oct 8:CD006535.

Shorr RI, Hoth AB, Rawls N: *Drugs for the geriatric patient*. St. Louis, 2007, Saunders.

Tan EP, Tan ES, Ng BY: Efficacy of cognitive behavioural therapy for patients with chronic pain in Singapore, *Annals of the Academy of Medicine, Singapore* 38:952, 2009.

Travis SS, Menscer D, Dixon SO, Turner MJ: Assessing and managing iatrogenic disturbance pain for frail, dependent adults in long-term care situations, *Annals of Long-Term Care* 11:33, 2003.

Vas J, Perea-Milla E, Mendez C, et al: Efficacy and safety of acupuncture for chronic uncomplicated pain: a randomised controlled study, *Pain* 126:245, 2006.

Warden V, Hurley AC, Volicer L: Development and psychometric evaluation of the pain assessment in advanced dementia (PAINAD) scale, *Journal of the American Medical Directors Association* 4:9, 2003. See also http://www.amda.com/publications/caring/may2004/painad.cfm.

Ware LJ, Epps CD, Herr K, et al: Evaluation of the revised faces pain scale, verbal descriptor scale, numeric rating scale, and Iowa pain thermometer in older minority adults, *Pain Management Nursing* 7:117, 2006.

Witt CM, Jena S, Brinkhaus B, et al: Acupuncture in patients with osteoarthritis of the knee or hip: a randomized, controlled trial with an additional nonrandomized arm, *Arthritis and Rheumatism* 54:3485, 2006.

Mental Health

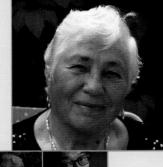

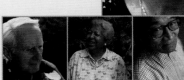

Theris A. Touhy

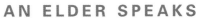 **evolve** *http://evolve.elsevier.com/Ebersole/TwdHlthAging*

A STUDENT SPEAKS

The process of aging scares me. Aging brings up emotions such as low self-esteem, powerlessness, and hopelessness. An old person has to accept the existing gap between the young and the old. I still remember telling my grandmother she was old-fashioned and out of touch. Now, I realize how rude I was to her. By the time I am about 75 years old, I will be just as depressed as some of the elderly I work with.

Rossana, age 28

AN ELDER SPEAKS

I am very irritable and quick to anger, and this is increasing as I age. I think people's strengths increase as they age, and their weaknesses do also.

Madeline, age 78

LEARNING OBJECTIVES

Upon completion of this chapter, the reader will be able to:

1. Discuss factors contributing to mental health and wellness in late life.
2. Discuss the effect of chronic mental health problems on individuals as they age.
3. List symptoms of anxiety and depression in older adults, and discuss assessment, treatment, and nursing responses.
4. Recognize elders who are at risk for suicide, and utilize appropriate techniques for suicide assessment and interventions.

5. Specify several indications of substance abuse in elders, and discuss appropriate nursing responses.
6. Evaluate interventions aimed at promoting mental health and wellness in older adults.
7. Develop an individualized nursing plan of care for an older person with depression and bipolar disorder.

Mental health is not different in later life, but the level of challenge may be greater. Developmental transitions, life events, physical illness, cognitive impairment, and situations calling for psychic energy may interfere with mental health in older adults. These factors, though not unique to older adults, often influence adaptation. However, anyone who has survived 80 or so years has been exposed to many stressors and crises and has developed tremendous resistance. Most older people face life's challenges with equanimity, good humor, and courage. It is our task to discover the strengths and adaptive mechanisms that will assist them to cope with the challenges.

What it means to be mentally healthy is subject to many interpretations and familial and cultural influences. Mental health, as with physical health, can be thought of as being on a fluctuating continuum from wellness to illness. Mental health

in late life is difficult to define because a lifetime of living results in many variations of personality, coping, and life patterns. One can say what 5-year-olds or 15-year-olds in general are like, but the same is not true for older people. Each individual becomes, the older he or she gets, more uniquely himself or herself.

Erikson et al. (1986) proposed that autonomy, intimacy, generativity, and integrity were all aspects of mentally healthy adult adaptation. Well-being in late life can be predicted by cognitive and affective functioning earlier in life. Thus, it is very important to know the older person's past patterns and life history (Chapter 6). Qualls (2002) offered the following comprehensive definition of mental health in aging: A mentally healthy person is "one who accepts the aging self as an active being, engaging available strengths to compensate for weaknesses in order to create personal meaning, maintain maximum autonomy by mastering the environment, and sustain positive relationships with others" (p. 12).

Including older adults with dementia, nearly 20% of people older than 55 years experience mental health disorders that are not part of normal aging, and these figures are expected to rise significantly in the next 25 years with the aging of the population. "The long-term consequences of military conflict and the twentieth century drug culture will add to the burden of psychiatric illnesses" (Kolanowski & Piven, 2006). Prevalence of mental health disorders may be even higher because these disorders are both underreported and not well researched, especially among racially and culturally diverse older people. The numbers of older people with mental illness will soon overwhelm the mental health system. Mental disorders are associated with increased use of health care resources and overall costs of care when compared to nondepressed older adults, regardless of chronic morbidity (Evans, 2008; Shellman et al., 2007). The most prevalent mental health problems in late life are anxiety, severe cognitive impairment, and mood disorders. Alcohol abuse and dependence is also a growing concern among older adults.

The focus of this chapter is on the differing presentation of mental health disturbances that may occur in older adults and the nursing responses important in maintaining the mental health and self-esteem of older adults at the optimum of their capacity. Readers should refer to a comprehensive psychiatric–mental health text for more in-depth discussion of mental health disorders. A discussion of cognitive impairment and the behavioral symptoms that may accompany this disorder is found in Chapter 19.

STRESS AND COPING IN LATE LIFE

Stress and Stressors

To understand mental health and mental health disorders in aging, it is important to be aware of stressors and their effect on the functioning of older people. The experience of stress is an internal state accompanying threats to self. Healthy stress levels motivate one toward growth, whereas stress overload diminishes one's ability to cope effectively. As a person ages, many situations and conditions occur that may create disruptions in daily life and drain one's inner resources or create the need for new and unfamiliar coping strategies. The narrowing range of biopsychosocial homeostatic resilience and changing environmental needs as one ages may produce a stress overload (Evans, 2008).

Effects of Stress

Much remains unknown about the connection between emotions and health and illness, but it is known that the mind and body are integrated and cannot be approached as separate entities. Stress may reduce one's coping ability and negatively impact neuroendocrine responses that ultimately impair immune function, and older adults show greater immunological impairments associated with distress or depression (Kolanowski and Piven, 2006). Research on psychoneuroimmunology has explored the relationship between psychological stress and various health conditions such as cardiovascular disease, type 2 diabetes, certain cancers, Alzheimer's disease, frailty, and

---

BOX 18-1	POTENTIAL STRESSORS IN LATE LIFE

- Abrupt internal and external body changes and illnesses
- Other-oriented concerns: children, grandchildren, spouse or partner
- Loss of significant people
- Functional impairment
- Sensory impairments
- Memory impairment (or fear of)
- Loss of ability to drive (particularly men)
- Acute discomfort and pain
- Breach in significant relationships
- Retirement (lost social roles, income)
- Ageist attitudes
- Fires, thefts
- Injuries, falls
- Major unexpected drain on economic resources (house repair, illness)
- Abrupt changes in living arrangements to a new location (home, apartment, room, or institution)

---

functional decline. The production of proinflammatory cytokines influencing these and other conditions can be directly stimulated by negative emotions and stressful experiences.

Older people often experience multiple, simultaneous stressors (Box 18-1). Some older people are in a chronic state of grief because new losses occur before prior ones are fully resolved; stress then becomes a constant state of being. Stress tolerance is variable and based on current and ongoing stressors, health, as well as coping ability. For example, if an elder has lost a significant person in the previous year, the grief may be manageable. If he or she has lost a significant person and developed painful, chronic health problems, the consequences may be quite different and can cause stress overload. In the older adult, stress may appear as a cognitive impairment or behavior change that will be alleviated as the stress is reduced to the parameters of the individual's adaptability. Regardless of whether stress is physical or emotional, older people will require more time to recover or return to prestress levels than younger people.

Any stressors that occur in the lives of older people may actually be experienced as a crisis if the event occurs abruptly, is unanticipated, or requires skills or resources the individual does not possess. Some individuals have developed through a lifetime of coping with stress, a tremendous stress tolerance, whereas others will be thrown into crisis by changes in their life with which they feel unable to cope. Important to remember is that there is great individual variability in definition of a stressor. For some, the loss of a pet canary is a major stressor; others accept the loss of a good friend with grief but without personal disorganization.

Factors Affecting Stress

Researchers concerned with the effects of stress in the lives of older people have examined many moderating variables and have concluded that cognitive style, coping strategies, social resources (social support, economic resources), personal efficacy, and personality characteristics are all significant to stress management. Social relationships and social support are particularly salient to stress management and coping. Social relationships may reduce stress and boost the immune system by providing resources (information, emotional, or tangible)

| BOX 18-2 | FACTORS INFLUENCING ABILITY TO MANAGE STRESS |

BOX 18-2 FACTORS INFLUENCING ABILITY TO MANAGE STRESS

- Health and fitness
- A sense of control over events
- Awareness of self and others
- Patience and tolerance
- Resilience
- Hardiness
- Social support
- Personal stability zones or a strong sense of self
- Beliefs and values

that promote adaptive behavioral or neuroendocrine responses to acute or chronic stressors (Holt-Lunstad et al., 2010). In fact, individuals with adequate social relationships have a 50% greater likelihood of survival compared to those with poor or insufficient social relationships, an effect comparable with quitting smoking and exceeding many known risk factors for mortality (e.g., obesity, physical inactivity).

Some factors that influence one's ability to manage stress are presented in Box 18-2. Resilience, hardiness, and resourcefulness have been associated with coping with stress and crisis and may explain the ability of some individuals to withstand stress. Kolanowski and Piven (2006) noted that while we know the qualities associated with resilience, hardiness, and resourcefulness, it is not clear if they are personality traits or processes by which the individual responds to the environment. Further research is needed to more fully understand these concepts and their relationship to positive outcomes.

Hardiness

The quality of hardiness is seen to have a protective influence against illness during stress (Kobasa, 1979). The cornerstones of hardiness are control, commitment, and challenge (Kobasa, 1979). Central to hardiness is the viewpoint that stress is a decision-making challenge and that meaning comes from making decisions. Stressful situations are seen as opportunities for growth. Life goals and a sense of purpose or meaning undergird hardiness. Factors associated with hardiness are social connectedness, confronting problems head-on, extending oneself to others, and spiritual grounding (Vance et al., 2008).

Research suggests that individuals with high levels of hardiness characteristics display higher levels of physical and mental health and age successfully. Nurses can identify hardiness characteristics in older individuals and encourage development of new hardiness resources. Vance and colleagues (2008) provide an example of an individualized program of hardiness training that focuses on specific ways to learn coping strategies for dealing with obstacles and responding with positive adaptive behaviors.

Resilience

Resilience is a concept closely related to hardiness that is associated with coping with stress and crisis. Resilience is defined as "flourishing despite adversity" (Hildon et al., 2009, p. 36). The process of resilience is characterized by successfully adapting to difficult and challenging life experiences, especially those that are highly stressful or traumatic. Resilient people "bend rather than break" during stressful conditions and are able to return

to adequate (and sometimes better) functioning after stress ("bouncing back"). Characteristics associated with resilience include: positive interpersonal relationships; a willingness to extend oneself to others; optimistic or positive affect; keeping things in perspective; setting goals and taking steps to achieve these goals; high self-esteem and self-efficacy; determination; a sense of purpose in life; creativity; humor; and a sense of curiosity. These are considered personality traits as well as ways of responding to difficult events that have been learned and developed over time (Resnick & Inguito, 2010). Older people may demonstrate greater resilience and ability to maintain a positive emotional state under stress than younger individuals. Resilience in older adults has been associated with management of chronic pain, better function, mood, enhanced cognitive capacity, quality of life, and an overall adjustment to the stressors associated with aging.

Resnick & Inguito (2010) suggest that understanding and evaluating resilience are important "so that individuals with low resilience can be identified and appropriate interventions implemented to help them overcome challenges associated with aging and engage in behaviors associated with successful aging such as exercise" (p. 2). Professional interventions and supportive services can enhance resilience. Rogerson and Emes (2008) explored the concept of resilience among frail community-dwelling older adults who participated in an adult day program. Participants identified the resources provided by the adult day program as major contributors to resilience. Resilience came in the form of functional fitness through regular physical activity, enhancing the size and quality of the social support network, and linking the participant to community resources.

Resourcefulness

Resourcefulness has also been linked to positive coping with life stressors. Resourcefulness is characterized as a "cognitive behavioral repertoire of self-control skills accompanied by a belief in one's ability to cope effectively with adversity" (Zauszniewski et al., 2007). Zauszniewski and colleagues describe a study investigating the effect of resourcefulness training (RT) for chronically ill older adults residing in assisted living facilities. RT teaches and reinforces the cognitive and behavioral skills that strengthen personal and social resourcefulness. Personal resourcefulness skills include coping strategies, problem-solving, positive self-talk, priority setting, and decision-making. Social resourcefulness skills involve assisting older people to make decisions about when and how to seek help from formal and informal sources as well as strategies to strengthen internal (self-help) and external (help-seeking) resources for maintenance of healthy functioning. Results of the study suggest that teaching resourcefulness skills is a nursing intervention that may enhance positive affect and cognition, promote independence and improve function in older adults (Zauszniewski et al., 2007).

Coping

Coping is a complex developmental and multifaceted process that develops over the lifespan. Some experts suggest that coping may be less effective in older individuals because of increased vulnerability to health problems and other stressors. Others postulate that older adults may use fewer coping styles but are just as skilled in coping as middle-aged individuals.

Coping may also contribute more to the health of older than younger individuals because older adults utilize it to optimize their resources. Further research with older adults is needed, but coping "may be an important component of optimal aging" (Yancura & Aldwin, 2008, p. 11). Box 18-3 presents some coping strategies of older adults.

Coping Strategies

Coping strategies are the stabilizing factors that help individuals maintain psychosocial balance during stressful periods. Coping strategies involve the identification, coordination, and appropriate use of personal and environmental resources to deal with stressors (Demers et al., 2009). Coping is a process that begins with appraisal of the stressor's potential impact and the tools available for dealing with it. The appraisal of the stressor as benign, threat, harm/loss, or challenge guides the choice of coping strategies (Lazarus & Folkman, 1984; Moos et al., 2006; Yancura & Aldwin, 2008). Individuals use a mixture of coping strategies depending on the situation and their skills and experience. Individuals with more personal (cognition) and environmental resources (social network) use more varied coping strategies, and this may be related to longer life expectancy (Demers et al., 2009). Types of coping strategies and their descriptions are presented in Box 18-4.

PROMOTING HEALTHY AGING: IMPLICATIONS FOR GERONTOLOGICAL NURSING

Assessment

Evans (2008) notes that most older adults manage the transitions and stresses that may accompany aging with "resilience, hardiness and resourcefulness but those with specific vulnerabilities may develop maladaptive responses and mental illness" (p. 2). Older adults who lack adequate social support or have accumulated stressors, unresolved grief, preexisting psychiatric illness, cognitive impairment, or inadequate coping resources are most vulnerable to mental health problems. Particularly at risk are older adults who have dual risk factors of life transition and loss of social support.

General issues in the psychosocial assessment of older adults involve distinguishing among normal, idiosyncratic, and diverse characteristics of aging and pathological conditions. Baseline data is often lacking from an individual's earlier years. Using standardized tools and functional assessment is valuable, but the data will be meaningless unless placed in the context of the patient's early life and hopes and expectations for the future. An understanding of past and present history, the person's coping ability, social support, and the effect of life events are all part of a holistic assessment. Careful listening to the person's life story, an appreciation of their strengths, and coming to know them in their uniqueness is the cornerstone of assessment (Chapter 6).

Assessment of mental health includes examination for cognitive function or impairment and the specific conditions of anxiety and adjustment reactions, depression, paranoia, substance abuse, and suicidal risk. Assessment of mental health must also focus on social intactness and affectual responses appropriate to the situation. Attention span, concentration, intelligence, judgment, learning ability, memory, orientation, perception, problem solving, psychomotor ability, and reaction time are assessed in relation to cognitive intactness and must be considered when making a psychological assessment. Assessment includes specific processes that are intact, as well as those that are diminished or compromised. Assessment for specific mental health concerns is discussed throughout this chapter and in Chapter 7. Assessment of cognitive function is discussed in Chapters 7 and 19.

Obtaining assessment data from elders is best done during short sessions after some rapport has been established. Performing repeated assessments at various times of the day and in different situations will give a more complete psychological profile. It is important to be sensitive to a patient's anxiety, special needs, and disabilities and vigilant in protecting the person's privacy. The interview should be focused so that attention is given to strengths and skills, as well as deficits.

Interventions

Nurses can design individualized interventions to enhance coping ability such as enhancing the characteristics of resilience, hardiness, and resourcefulness. Enhancing functional status and independence, promoting a sense of control, fostering social supports and relationships, and connecting to resources are all important nursing interventions. Practices such as meditation, yoga, exercise, as well as spirituality and religiosity, can enhance coping ability. Mind-body therapies that integrate cognitive, sensory, expressive, and physical aspects are most helpful. Reminiscence is useful in understanding the coping style of an elder, helping the elder to remember how he or she coped successfully, and how these strategies might be applied to the current situation, and enhancing self-esteem and feelings of self-worth.

FACTORS INFLUENCING MENTAL HEALTH CARE

Attitudes and Beliefs

The rate of utilization of mental health services for elders, even when available, is less than that of any other age-group. Estimates are that 63% of older adults with a mental health disorder do not receive the services they need, and only about 3% report seeing mental and behavioral health professionals for treatment (American Psychological Association, 2010). Some of the reasons for this include reluctance on the part of older people to seek help because of pride of independence, stoic acceptance of difficulty, unawareness of resources, and fear of being "put away." Stigma about having a mental health disorder ("being crazy"), particularly for older people, discourages many from seeking treatment. Ageism also affects identification and treatment of mental health disorders in older people.

Symptoms of mental health problems may be looked at as a normal consequence of aging or blamed on dementia by both older people and health care professionals. In older people, the presence of co-morbid medical conditions complicates the recognition and diagnosis of mental health disorders. Also, the myth that older people do not respond well to treatment is still prevalent. Other factors—including the lack of knowledge on the part of health care professionals about mental health in late life; inadequate numbers of geropsychiatrists, geropsychologists, and geropsychiatric nurses; and limited availability of geropsychiatric services—present barriers to appropriate diagnosis and treatment.

Availability and Adequacy of Mental Health Care

With the passage of the mental health parity legislation in July 2008, Medicare's discriminatory practice of imposing a 50% coinsurance requirement for outpatient mental health services instead of the 20% required for other medical services was changed. The reduction of this coinsurance to 20% over a period of six years will bring payments for mental health care in line with those required for all other Medicare Part B services (Centers for Medicare and Medicaid services, 2010). The passage of this legislation will significantly improve the lives of older adults by providing them with improved access to mental health care (American Association for Geriatric Psychiatry, 2008). A 190-day lifetime limit still remains on treatment in inpatient mental health facilities. Psychiatric services may be provided by a psychiatrist, psychologist, licensed clinical social worker, nurse practitioner, or geropsychiatric clinical nurse specialist. New models of providing mental health care in primary care settings, many utilizing advanced practice nurses with geropsychiatric preparation, show promise for improving access and outcomes (Arean et al., 2005; Callahan et al., 2005). However, as Evans (2008) notes, nurses will need to assist older people to access appropriate mental health services and understand reimbursement issues.

Settings of Care

Older people receive psychiatric services across a wide range of settings, including acute and long-term inpatient psychiatric units, primary care, and community and institutional settings. Nurses will encounter older adults with mental health disorders in emergency departments or in general medical-surgical units. Admissions for medical problems are often exacerbated by depression, anxiety, cognitive impairment, substance abuse, or chronic mental illness. Medical patients present with psychiatric disorders in 25% to 33% of cases, although they are often unrecognized by primary care providers. Evans (2008) suggests that nurses who can identify mental health problems early and seek consultation and treatment will enhance timely recovery. Advanced practice psychiatric nursing consultation is an important and effective service in acute care settings.

Nursing homes and, increasingly, residential care/assisted living facilities (RC/ALs), although not licensed as psychiatric facilities, are providing the majority of care given to older adults with psychiatric conditions. Estimates of the proportion of nursing home residents with a significant mental health disorder range from 65% to 91%, and only about 20% receive treatment from a mental health clinician (Grabowski et al., 2010). Nursing homes are also caring for younger individuals with mental illness, and the number of individuals with mental illness other than dementia has surpassed the dementia admissions (Splete, 2009). Medicaid beneficiaries with schizophrenia between 40 and 64 years of age are four times more likely to be admitted to a nursing home compared with Medicaid beneficiaries in the same group without a mental illness (Grabowski et al., 2010). It is often difficult to find placement for an older adult with a mental health problem in these types of facilities, and few are structured to provide best practice care to individuals with mental illness.

Residential care/assisted living facilities also have a high proportion of residents with mental health disorders. In one of the few studies of mental health in this setting, Gruber-Baldini and colleagues (2004) reported that more than 50% of residents were taking a psychotropic medication and 66% had some mental health problem indicator (medication, depression, psychosis, or other psychiatric illness). Older adults in home and community settings also experience mental health concerns and inadequate treatment. "Family caregivers of depressed home care recipients are likely to be depressed as well with 18.8% reporting high levels of distress (Ayalon et al., 2010, p. 515).

Along a range of different measures of quality, the treatment of mental illness in nursing homes and residential care facilities is substandard (Grabowski et al., 2010). Some of the obstacles to mental health care in nursing homes and RC/AL facilities

BOX 18-5 RESEARCH HIGHLIGHTS

Keeping the Bully Out: Understanding Older African Americans' Beliefs and Attitudes Toward Depression

The purpose of this qualitative study was to gain insight into older African Americans' beliefs and attitudes toward depression. 51 older African Americans from senior centers, churches, and senior-housing sites in a northeast urban setting participated in the study. Seventy percent were female and the mean age was 71.3 years. Participants were asked to describe what the word *depression* meant to them, share everything they knew about depression, as well as how they felt about someone who was depressed.

Participants viewed depression as negative ("a bully") and a sign of personal weakness that can be controlled through faith. If depression is viewed as a source of shame, individuals are not likely to share their feelings. Instead, they may present with somatic complaints and increased physical impairment rather than emotional complaints. This can lead to missed diagnoses. The belief that depression was something that one can control suggests a lack of knowledge about depression. Possible reasons for this lack of knowledge include mistrust of health care providers as well as few available community resources. Because of the strong influence of faith in keeping the bully out, older African Americans may be more comfortable discussing depression in the setting of their church rather than seeking help from medical providers.

Given the disparities in identification and treatment of depression in African Americans, as well as the lack of research in this area, findings from this study can assist nurses in understanding some of the factors contributing to disparities and enhance culturally competent care. Partnerships with churches to enhance depression education and alleviate the stigma associated with the illness, recognizing that somatic complaints and functional decline may signal depression in this population, and appreciation of the strong role of faith as a way of coping with hardship, may all be beneficial to decrease disparities in this population.

Source: Shellman J, Mokel M, Wright B: "Keeping the bully out: Understanding older African Americans' beliefs and attitudes toward depression, *Journal of the American Psychiatric Nurses Association* 13:230, 2007.

include: (1) shortage of trained personnel; (2) limited availability and access for psychiatric services; (3) lack of staff training related to mental health and mental illness; and (4) inadequate Medicaid and Medicare reimbursement for mental health services. An insufficient number of trained personnel affects the quality of mental health care in nursing homes and often causes great stress for staff.

New models of mental health care and services are needed for nursing homes and RC/AL facilities to address the growing needs of older adults in these settings. Psychiatric services in nursing homes, when they are available, are commonly provided by psychiatric consultants who are not full-time staff members and are inadequate to meet the needs of residents and staff. Suggestions for optimal mental health services in nursing homes include the routine presence of qualified mental health clinicians; an interdisciplinary and multidimensional approach that addresses neuropsychiatric, medical, environmental, and staff issues; and innovative approaches to training and education with consultation and feedback on clinical practices (Grabowski et al., 2010). Training and education of frontline staff who provide basic care to residents is essential. There is an urgent need for well-designed controlled studies to examine mental health concerns in both nursing homes and RC/ALs and the effectiveness of mental health services in improving clinical outcomes.

Cultural and Ethnic Disparities

Lack of knowledge and awareness of cultural differences about the meaning of mental health, differences in the way concerns may become apparent, the lack of culturally sensitive instruments for measuring behavioral outcomes, the lack of culturally competent mental health treatment, and limited research in this area must all be addressed in light of the rapidly increasing numbers of culturally and ethnically diverse older adults (Kolanowski & Piven, 2006). Disparities affecting mental health care in diverse populations include less access to mental health services, poorer quality of care, and underrepresentation in research. Racially, culturally, and ethnically diverse older adults are more likely than other ethnic groups to be underdiagnosed and undertreated for depression. Some identified barriers to the use of services include stigma about a mental health diagnosis, co-morbid medical problems, clinical presentation of somatization, a lack of bilingual staff, a lack of awareness of the existence of services, and difficulties with the patient-provider relationship (Ortiz and Romero, 2008; Shellman et al., 2007). Box 18-5 presents research findings on older African Americans' beliefs and attitudes toward depression. Chapter 5 discusses culture and aging in depth.

It is important to include a cultural assessment and a discussion of what culturally and ethnically diverse older adults believe about their mental health problems in all assessment situations. Culturally appropriate education about mental health concerns is also important. Research on all aspects of culture and mental health is critically needed. Improvement in mental health care for ethnically and culturally diverse older adults "requires strong and collective commitments to overcome barriers of poverty, discrimination, and prejudice, linguistic difficulty, cultural conflicts, social stigma, and a lack of culturally competent health services, and build a health care system that is equal, affordable, available, and acceptable" (Zahn, 2004, p. 3).

Gerontological nurses must advocate for better and more appropriate treatment of mental health needs for older people and should closely monitor proposals for federal and state revisions to services and budget cuts in this area. More data is needed on the mental health needs of geriatric and ethnic minority populations, and, in recognition of this need, a follow-up study to the IOM (2008) study, *The Re-tooling for an Aging America: Building the Health Care Workforce*, will be conducted.

Geropsychiatric Nursing

Geropsychiatric nursing is the master's level subspecialty within the adult-psychiatric mental health nursing field. Few educational programs focus on this specialty, and, unfortunately, few professional curricula include adequate content on mental health and aging. Increased attention to the preparation of mental health professionals specializing in geriatric care is important to improve mental health care delivery to older adults (Mellilo et al., 2005). The Geropsychiatric Nursing Collaborative, a project of the American Academy of Nursing funded by the John A. Hartford Foundation, has developed geropsychiatric nursing competency enhancements for entry and advanced practice level education and will be developing a range of training materials and learning tools to improve the current knowledge and skills of nurses in mental health care for older adults (http://hartfordign.org/education/geropsych_nursing_comp/). The geropsychiatric nursing Collaborative has produced a vidoe on the role of geropsychiatric nursing in the mental health of elder people (www.aannet.org/i4a/pages/index.cfm?pageid=4501). Kolanowski and Piven (2006) provide a comprehensive literature review of research in geropsychiatric nursing and recommendations for future directions. Increased attention to preparation of mental health professionals, as well as continued research on mental health in aging, are important initiatives to improve care delivery for the growing numbers of older adults.

MENTAL HEALTH DISORDERS

Anxiety Disorders

A general definition of anxiety is unpleasant and unwarranted feelings of apprehension, which may be accompanied by physical symptoms. Anxiety itself is a normal human reaction and part of a fear response; it is rational, within reason. Anxiety becomes problematic when it is prolonged, is exaggerated, and interferes with function.

Anxiety disorders are not considered part of the normal aging process, but the changes and challenges that older adults often face (e.g., chronic illness, cognitive impairment, emotional losses) may contribute to the development of anxiety symptoms and disorders. Many anxious older people have had anxiety disorders earlier in their lives, but late-onset anxiety is not a rare phenomenon. Anxiety disorders that occur in older people include generalized anxiety disorder (GAD), phobic disorder, obsessive-compulsive disorder, panic disorder, and posttraumatic stress disorder (PTSD). Additionally, the high prevalence of cormorbid mood-anxiety disorders suggest the importance of further investigation of the modifying influence of anxiety on depression treatment outcomes (Byers et al., 2010).

Prevalence

Epidemiological studies indicate that anxiety disorders are common in older adults; however, relatively few patients are diagnosed with these disorders in clinical practice. The occurrence of anxiety meeting the criteria for a diagnosable disorder ranges from 3.5% to 12% of older people (Flood & Buckwalter, 2009). Anxiety symptoms that may not meet the Diagnostic and Statistical Manual of Mental Disorders *(DSM-IV)* (American Psychiatric Association, 2000) criteria (subthreshold symptoms) are even more prevalent, with estimated rates from 15% to 20% in community samples, with even higher rates in medically ill populations (Ayers et al., 2006).

Byers and colleagues (2010) conducted a large-scale study of mood and anxiety disorders among older adults and reported that while prevalence rates of *DSM-IV* mood and anxiety disorders in late life tend to decline with age, the rates of anxiety disorders are as high or even higher than mood disorders. Among community-dwelling older adults aged 70 to 79, this study found an overall rate of anxiety of 19% (20% in women and 12% in men). Phobic disorders were the most prevalent individual disorder. Phobias, especially those associated with falling, generalized anxiety disorder (GAD), and posttraumatic

stress disorder (PTSD), are increasingly emerging for the first time in late life. Women have higher prevalence rates of symptoms of anxiety and coexisting depression-anxiety than men. These authors noted that anxiety disorders were prominent and pervasive in older adults even onto the oldest years (85 and over).

Anxiety symptoms and disorders are significant yet understudied conditions in older adults. Anxiety in older people is not often thought of as a serious problem, and there is little research or empirical data on anxiety in older people. Similar to other mental health problems, the diagnostic criteria and treatment methods for anxiety disorders are largely based on data from young and middle-aged adults and may not reflect the unique problems of older adults (Smith, 2005; Wetherell et al., 2005).

Older people are less likely to report psychiatric symptoms or acknowledge anxiety, and often attribute their symptoms to physical health problems. Separating a medical condition from the physical symptoms of an anxiety disorder may be difficult. The presence of cognitive impairment also makes diagnosis complicated. It is estimated that 40% to 80% of older people with Alzheimer's disease or related dementias experience anxiety-related symptoms that may be expressed with behavior, such as agitation, irritability, pacing, crying, and repetitive verbalizations (Smith, 2005) (Chapter 19).

Anxiety is frequently the presenting symptom of depression in older adults, and up to 60% of patients with a major depressive disorder also suffer from an anxiety disorder (Seekles et al., 2009). Anxiety disorders without co-morbid depression are also common (Kolanowski & Piven, 2006). Risk factors for anxiety disorders in older people include the following: female, urban living, history of worrying or rumination, poor physical health, low socioeconomic status, high-stress life events, and depression and alcoholism.

Geriatric anxiety is associated with more visits to primary care providers and increased average length of visit. Anxiety symptoms and disorders are associated with many negative consequences including decreased physical activity and functional status, substance abuse, decreased life satisfaction, and increased mortality rates (Ayers et al., 2006; Kolanowski & Piven, 2006; Wetherell et al., 2005). Unidentified or untreated anxiety disorders in older people adversely affect well-being and quality of life.

PROMOTING HEALTHY AGING: IMPLICATIONS FOR GERONTOLOGICAL NURSING

Assessment

Data suggest that approximately 70% of all primary care visits are driven by psychological factors (e.g., panic, generalized anxiety, stress, somatization) (American Psychological Association, 2010). This means that nurses often encounter anxious older people and can identify anxiety-related symptoms and initiate assessments that will lead to appropriate treatment and management. Whether symptoms represent a diagnosable anxiety disorder is perhaps less important than the fact that the individual will suffer needlessly if assessment and treatment are not addressed.

The general and pervasive nature of anxiety may make diagnosis difficult in older adults. In addition, older adults tend to deny the psychological symptoms, attribute anxiety-related symptoms to physical illness, and have co-existent medical conditions that mimic symptoms of anxiety. Some of the medical disorders that cause anxiety include cardiac arrhythmias, delirium, dementia, chronic obstructive pulmonary disease (COPD), heart failure, hyperthyroidism, hypoglycemia, postural hypotension, pulmonary edema, and pulmonary embolism.

Anxiety is also a common side effect of many drugs including anticholinergics, digitalis, theophylline, antihypertensives, beta-blockers, beta-adrenergic stimulators, corticosteroids, and over-the-counter (OTC) medications such as appetite suppressants and cough and cold preparations. Caffeine, nicotine, and withdrawal from alcohol, sedatives, and hypnotics will cause symptoms of anxiety.

Assessment of anxiety in older people focuses on physical, social, and environmental factors, as well as past life history, long-standing personality, coping, and recent events. Older people more often report somatic complaints rather than cognitive symptoms such as excessive worrying. It is important to remember that expressed fears and worries may be realistic or unrealistic, so the nurse must investigate and obtain collateral information from family or caregivers. For example, fear of leaving the home may be related to frequent falling or crime in the neighborhood. Worries about financial stability may be related to the current economic situation or financial abuse by other people.

It is important to investigate other possible causes of anxiety, such as medical conditions and depression. Diagnostic and laboratory tests may be ordered as indicated to rule out medical problems. Cognitive assessment, brain imaging, and neuropsychological evaluation are included if cognitive impairment is suspected (Chapter 19). When co-morbid conditions are present, they must be treated. A review of medications, including OTC and herbal or home remedies, is essential, with elimination of those that cause anxiety.

Few assessment instruments are designed and evaluated for older adults, and if such instruments are used, they should be weighed carefully with other data—complaints, physical exam, history, and collateral interview data (Smith, 2005). Box 18-6 presents suggested questions to identify anxiety disorders in older people.

When assessing anxiety reactions in nursing homes, look for daily disturbances, such as with staff or caregiver changes, room changes, or events over which the individual feels a lack of control or influence. By themselves, these circumstances seldom provoke an anxiety reaction, but they may be "the straw that breaks the camel's back," particularly in frail elders. Anxiety embodies an overwhelming sense of being out of control of one's life and destiny. Restoring the individual's sense of control as quickly as possible is critical. Providing a structured environment may alleviate anxiety in older people experiencing dementia. Nurses must be alert to the signs of anxiety in frail older people or those with dementia, since they may be unable to tell us how they are feeling. Carefully observing behavior and searching for possible reasons for changes in behavior or patterns are important.

Interventions

Although further research is needed to provide evidence to guide treatment, existing studies suggest that anxiety disorders in older people can be treated effectively. Treatment choices depend on the symptoms, the specific anxiety diagnosis, co-morbid medical conditions, and any current medication regimen. Nonpharmacological interventions are preferred and are often used in conjunction with medication (Smith, 2005).

Pharmacological   Research on the effectiveness of medication in treating anxiety in older people is limited. Age-related changes in pharmacodynamics and issues of polypharmacy make prescribing and monitoring in older people a complex undertaking. Antidepressants in the form of selective serotonin reuptake inhibitors (SSRIs) are usually the first-line treatment. Within this class of drugs, those with sedating rather than stimulating properties are preferred (e.g., citalopram, paroxetine, sertraline, venlafaxine).

Second-line treatment may include short-acting benzodiazepines (alprazolam, lorazepam) or mirtazapine. Treatment with benzodiazepines should be used for short-term therapy only (less than six months) and relief of immediate symptoms, but must be used carefully in older adults. Use of older drugs, such as diazepam or chlordiazepoxide, should be avoided because of their long-half lives and the increased risk of accumulation and toxicity in older people. All these medications can have problematic side effects, such as sedation, falls, cognitive impairment, and dependence. Nonbenzodiazepine anxiolytic agents (buspirone) may also be used. Buspirone has fewer side effects but requires a longer period of administration (up to four weeks) for effectiveness.

Nonpharmacological   Cognitive behavioral therapy (CBT) and relaxation training are effective psychosocial treatments for older adults with anxiety disorders or symptoms (Thorp et al., 2009). CBT is designed to modify thought patterns, improve skills, and alter the environmental states that contribute to anxiety. CBT may involve relaxation training and cognitive restructuring (replacing anxiety-producing thoughts with more realistic, less catastrophic ones), and education about signs and symptoms of anxiety. Significant decreases in anxiety and depression over time have been reported when older women participated in a course using psychoeducation and skills training (Smith, 2005). Interventions for stress management discussed earlier including meditation, yoga, and other therapies

---

BOX 18-6   SUGGESTED QUESTIONS TO IDENTIFY ANXIETY IN OLDER PEOPLE

1. Have you been concerned about or fretted over a number of things?
2. Is there anything going on in your life that is causing you concern?
3. Do you find that you have a hard time putting things out of your mind?

Other questions useful in identifying how and when physical symptoms began:

1. What were you doing when you noticed the chest pain?
2. What were you thinking about when you felt your heart start to race?
3. When you can't sleep, what is usually going through your head?

Adapted from Lang AJ and Stein MB: Anxiety Disorders: How to Recognize and Treat the Medical Symptoms of Emotional Illness, *Geriatrics*, 56(5):24-27, 31-34, 2001.

BOX 18-7   INTERVENTIONS FOR ANXIETY IN OLDER ADULTS

- Establish therapeutic relationship and come to know the person
- Listen attentively to what is said and unsaid; use a nonjudgmental approach
- Support the person's strengths and have faith in his/her ability to cope, drawing on past successes
- Encourage expression of needs, concerns, questions
- Allow and reinforce the person's personal reaction to or expression of pain, discomfort, or threats to well-being (e.g., talking, walking, other physical or nonverbal expressions); in frail elders, careful observation is important since they may not be able to adequately voice concerns and feelings; pay attention to non-verbal behavior
- Accept the person's defenses; do not confront, argue, or debate
- Help the person identify precipitants of anxiety and their reactions
- Teach the person about anxiety, symptoms, effect of anxiety on the body
- Avoid excessive reassurance; this may reinforce undue worry
- If irrational thoughts are present, offer accurate information while encouraging the expression of the meaning of events contributing to anxiety; reassure of safety and your presence in supporting them
- Intervene when possible to remove the source of anxiety
- Explain all activities, procedures, and issues in advance and ensure the person's understanding
- Encourage positive self-talk, such as "I can do this one step at a time" and "Right now I need to breathe deeply"
- Teach distraction or diversion tactics; progressive relaxation exercises; deep breathing
- Encourage participation in physical activity, adapted to the person's capabilities
- Help the person to identify anxiety-producing situations and emphasize that early interruption of the anxious response prevents escalation
- Encourage the use of community resources such as friends, family, churches, socialization groups, self-help and support groups, mental health counseling

Adapted from: Flood M, Buckwalter K: Recommendations for the mental health care of older adults: Part 1—An overview of depression and anxiety, *Journal of Gerontological Nursing* 35:26, 2009.

are also important in the treatment and management of anxiety in older people. Suggested interventions for anxiety in older adults are presented in Box 18-7.

The therapeutic relationship between the patient and the health care provider is the foundation for any intervention. Family support, referral to community resources, support groups, and sources of educational materials, are other important interventions.

Other Anxiety Disorders
Posttraumatic Stress Disorder

According to the *DSM-IV* (American Psychiatric Association, 2000), PTSD was recognized over 20 years ago as a syndrome characterized by the development of symptoms after an extremely traumatic event that involves witnessing, or unexpectedly hearing about, an actual or threatened death or serious injury to oneself or another closely affiliated person. Individuals often reexperience the traumatic event in episodes of fear and experience symptoms such as helplessness, flashbacks, intrusive thoughts, memories, images, emotional numbing, loss of interest, avoidance of any place that reminds of the traumatic event, poor concentration, irritability, startle reactions, jumpiness, and hypervigilance.

Individuals with PTSD may have ongoing sleep problems, somatic disturbances, anxiety, depression, and restlessness. Over the long term, individuals with PTSD may be impaired in work, may have maladaptive lifestyles, and do not develop close relationships. Avoidance or numbing, dissociation, intrusive symptoms, and survivor guilt seem to occur less frequently in older people as symptoms of PTSD, whereas estrangement from others may occur more often (Wetherell et al., 2005). PTSD is fairly common with a lifetime prevalence of 7% to 12% of adults, but prevalence rates among older adults have not been adequately investigated.

In the cohort of Vietnam veterans (now in the "baby boomer" cohort), PTSD prevalence is 15%. The probability of significant increases in future prevalence of PTSD is likely (Kolanowski & Piven, 2006). It occurs increasingly in women. Rape is the most likely specific trauma that will result in long-lived PTSD in women, followed by child abuse, being threatened with a weapon, being molested, being neglected as a child, and physical violence. For men, the greatest trauma is also rape, followed by abuse as a child, combat, and being molested.

PTSD has become a part of our national vocabulary and reminds us of the deep and lasting toll that war and natural disasters take. PTSD was first recognized as an outcome of overwhelmingly stressful experiences of individuals in the war in Vietnam and is now a growing concern among Gulf War and Iraq War veterans. Only recently realized is the fact that many World War II veterans have lived most of their lives under the shadow of PTSD without its being recognized.

Seniors in our care now have also experienced the Great Depression, the Holocaust, racism, and the Korean conflict—events that also may precipitate PTSD. Although they may have managed to keep symptoms under control, a person who becomes cognitively impaired may no longer be able to control thoughts, flashbacks, or images. This can be the cause of great distress that may be exhibited by aggressive or hostile behavior. There may be some association between PTSD and a greater incidence and prevalence of dementia, but further research is needed (Qureshi et al., 2010).

Older individuals who are Holocaust survivors may experience PTSD symptoms when they are placed in group settings in institutions. Bludau (2002) described this as the concept of second institutionalization. Older women with a history of rape or abuse as a child may also experience symptoms of PTSD when institutionalized, particularly during the provision of intimate bodily care activities, such as bathing. Box 18-8 provides some clinical examples of PTSD.

Assessment and Intervention. PTSD prevention and treatment are only now getting the research attention that other illnesses have received over the years. The care of the individual with PTSD involves awareness that certain events may trigger inappropriate reactions, and the pattern of these reactions should be identified when possible. Knowing the person's past history and life experiences is essential in understanding behavior and implementing appropriate interventions. An instrument to assess PTSD in older adults can be found at http://consultgerirn.org/uploads/File/trythis/try_this_19.pdf (Box 18-9).

Effective coping with traumatic events seems to be associated with secure and supportive relationships; the ability to freely

BOX 18-8   CLINICAL EXAMPLES OF PTSD IN OLDER ADULTS

ERNIE'S STORY

Ernie may have had PTSD, though it was only speculative after his suicide. On his 18th birthday, Ernie joined the U.S. Army Air Corps (precedent to our present U.S. Air Force) in 1941. He was quickly trained and sent to Burma, China, and India. During his three-year stint, Ernie survived two airplane crashes, saw several of his companions mutilated in crashes, watched the torture of captured Japanese, and witnessed the capture of some of his friends. When Ernie returned to the United States, his hair had turned from deep auburn to pure white. He retired from the service after 20 years but was never really able to work after his retirement.

Ernie's life was filled with episodes of alcoholic binges, outbursts of anger, and episodes of abusing others, all seemingly quite out of his control. One friend remained from his service days and visited him periodically until his death in 1996. Other relationships seemed to have been superficial and to have had little meaning for Ernie. On his 78th birthday, which he spent alone, Ernie shot himself. One must wonder how many of the elderly veterans of World War II, the most highly suicidal group in the United States, are suffering from PTSD.

JACK'S STORY

An 80-year-old World War II veteran resident with dementia was admitted to a large Veterans Administration (VA) nursing home. Jack's wife told the staff that he had been a high school principal who was very successful in his position. He had recurring frightening dreams throughout his life related to his war experiences, and he would always turn off the radio or TV when there were programs about World War II. Now, due to his dementia, he was unable to control his thoughts and feelings. While in the nursing home, he would become very agitated and attempt to hit other residents around him when placed in the large dayroom. The staff recognized this as a PTSD reaction from his years as a prisoner of war. They always placed him in a smaller dayroom near the nursing station away from other residents, where he remained calm and pleasant. The aggression stopped without the need for medication.

PTSD, Posttraumatic stress disorder.

BOX 18-9   EVIDENCE-BASED PROTOCOLS FOR MENTAL HEALTH DISORDERS IN OLDER ADULTS

Assessment of PTSD: http://consultgerirn.org/uploads/File/trythis/try_this_19.pdf

Assessment of depression: http://consultgerirn.org/topics/depression/want_to_know_more

Assessment of suicidal risk: http://consultgerirn.org/topics/depression/need_help_stat/

Assessment of alcohol use: http://consultgerirn.org/uploads/File/trythis/try_this_17.pdf

Detection of depression in older adults with dementia Evidence-Based Guideline: www.guideline.gov/summary.aspx?doc_id=11054&nbr=005833&string=depression+and+dementia

Evans L: *Mental health issues in aging:* http:hartfordign.org/uploads/File/gnec_state_of_science_papers/gnec_mental_health.pdf

express or fully suppress the experience; favorable circumstances immediately following the trauma; productive and active lifestyles; strong faith, religion, and hope; a sense of humor; and biological integrity. CBT with pharmacological therapy may be useful for supporting the person with PTSD, although there are no studies on the use of psychotherapy in the treatment of PTSD in older adults. Results of a small pilot study conducted by Thorp (2009) using prolonged exposure therapy suggest benefit among older veterans, and a larger study

comparing prolonged exposure therapy to relaxation training is currently being conducted. Evidence-based psycho-spiritual interventions may also be effective in the treatment of veterans with PTSD and may be more acceptable among those who have a fear of mental illness-related stigma (Bormann et al., 2008). Medication therapy is also used, and sertraline and paroxetine have U.S. Food and Drug Administration (FDA) approval to treat PTSD.

Obsessive-Compulsive Disorder

Obsessive-compulsive disorder (OCD) is characterized by recurrent and persistent thoughts, impulses, or images (obsessions) that are repetitive and purposeful, and intentional urges of ritualistic behaviors (compulsions) that improve comfort level but are recognized as excessive and unreasonable. OCD is an anxiety disorder that significantly impairs function and consumes more than one hour each day (American Psychiatric Association, 2000). Among older adults, symptoms are often not sufficient to seriously disrupt function and thus may not be considered a true disorder but rather a coping strategy. If symptoms progress to a point at which they disrupt function, the elder will need clinical attention. Recommended treatments include exercise and CBT in combination with pharmacological treatment (SSRIs), if indicated.

PARANOID SYMPTOMS IN OLDER ADULTS

The onset of true psychiatric disorders is low among older adults, but psychotic manifestations may occur as a secondary syndrome in a variety of disorders, the most common being Alzheimer's disease and other dementias, as well as Parkinson's disease. New-onset paranoid symptoms are common among older adults and can present in a number of conditions in late life. Paranoid symptoms can signify an acute change in mental status as a result of a medical illness or delirium, or they can be caused by an underlying affective or primary psychotic mental disorder. These symptoms can also manifest as a result of behavioral and psychological symptoms of dementia. Paranoia is also an early symptom of Alzheimer's disease, appearing approximately 20 months before diagnosis. Medications, vision and hearing loss, social isolation, alcoholism, depression, the presence of negative life events, financial strain, and PTSD can also be precipitating factors in paranoid symptoms (Chaudhary & Rabheru, 2008) (Box 18-10). Paranoid symptoms can present as persecutory delusions, paranoid ideation, and increased suspiciousness.

Paranoid Ideation

Paranoid ideation may manifest as mild suspiciousness and/or paranoia. The reaction is milder than delusions and the individual is in better control of their behavior and able to continue with daily activities with minimal disruption to themselves and others (Chaudhary and Rabheru, 2008).

Delusions

Delusions are beliefs that guide one's interpretation of events and help make sense out of disorder, even though they are inconsistent with reality. The delusions may be comforting or threatening, but they always form a structure for understanding

---

BOX 18-10 **POSSIBLE CAUSES OF PSYCHOSIS AND/OR PSYCHOTIC SYMPTOMS IN OLDER ADULTS**

- Schizophrenia
- Delusional disorder
- Mood disorders with psychotic features (bipolar disorder, major depression)
- Delirium
- Psychotic symptoms associated with Alzheimer's disease, vascular dementia, Lewy body disease, frontal lobe dementias
- Parkinson's disease
- Substance abuse
- Polypharmacy, medication reactions and toxicity

Data from: Mentes J, Bail J: Psychosis in older adults. In Mellilo K, Houde S, editors: *Geropsychiatric and mental health nursing*, Sudbury, Mass., 2005, Jones & Bartlett, pp. 174-175.

BOX 18-11 **CLINICAL EXAMPLES**

MAGGIE'S STORY

Maggie persistently held onto the delusion that her son was a very important attorney and was coming to force the administration to discharge her from the nursing home. Her son, a factory worker, had been dead for 10 years. The events of her day, her hopes, and her status were all organized around this belief. It is clear that without her delusion she would have felt forlorn, lost, and abandoned.

HERMAN'S STORY

Herman was an 88-year-old man in a nursing home who insisted that he must go and visit his mother. His thoughts seemed clear in other respects (often the case with people who are delusional), and one of the authors (P.E.) suspected that he had some unresolved conflicts about his dead mother or felt the need of comforting and caring. P.E. did not argue with him about his dead mother, since arguing is never a useful approach to persons with delusions. Rather, she used the best techniques she could think of to assure him that she was interested in him as a person and recognized that he must feel very lonely sometimes. He continued to say that he must go and visit his mother. When P.E. could delay his leaving no longer, she walked with him to the nurses' station and found that his 104-year-old mother did indeed live in another wing of the institution and that he visited her every day.

---

situations that otherwise might seem unmanageable. A delusional disorder is one in which conceivable ideas, without foundation in fact, persist for more than one month.

Common delusions of older adults are of being poisoned, of children taking their assets, of being held prisoner, or of being deceived by a spouse or lover. In older adults, delusions often incorporate significant persons rather than the global grandiose or persecutory delusions of younger persons. Fear and a lack of trust originating from a basis in reality may become magnified, especially when one is isolated from others and does not receive reality feedback. Many delusions related to family members and their actions or intentions occur among institutionalized older people. Some may aid in coping, whereas others may be troubling to the person. One study found that 21% of 125 new nursing home residents had delusions (Grossberg, 2000). It is always important to determine if what "appears" to be delusional ideation is, in fact, based in reality. Box 18-11 presents some clinical examples.

Hallucinations

Hallucinations are best described as sensory perceptions of a nonexistent object and may be spurred by the internal stimulation of any of the five senses. Although not attributable to environmental stimuli, hallucinations may occur as a combined result of environmental factors. Hallucinations arising from psychotic disorders are less common among older adults, and those that are generated are thought to begin in situations in which one is feeling alone, abandoned, isolated, or alienated. To compensate for insecurity, a hallucinatory experience is stimulated, often an imaginary companion. Imagined companions may fill the immense void and provide some security, but they may also become accusing and disturbing.

The character and stages of hallucinatory experiences in late life have not been adequately defined. Many hallucinations are in response to physical disorders, such as dementia, Parkinson's disease, sensory disorders, and medications. Hallucinations of older adults most often seem mixed with disorientation, illusions, intense grief, and immersion in retrospection, the origins being difficult to separate. Older people with hearing and vision deficits may also hear voices or see people and objects that are not actually present (illusions). Some have explained this as the brain's attempt to create stimulation in the absence of adequate sensory input. If illusions or hallucinations are not disturbing to the person, they do not necessitate treatment.

One older woman in a nursing home who had Alzheimer's disease and was experiencing agnosia would look in the mirror and talk to "the nice lady I see in there." "Do you want to eat or go out for a walk with me?" she would ask. It was comforting to her, and therefore she did not need medication for her "hallucination," as some would have labeled her behavior. As is the case with many disease symptoms, frail elders do not typically manifest the cardinal signs we have been taught to associate with certain physical and mental disorders. Diagnostic criteria, and often evidence-based practice guidelines, have been developed out of observation and research with younger people and may not always fit the older person. Until knowledge and research on the unique aspects of aging increase, nurses and other health care professionals are urged to individualize their assessment and treatment of older people using available guidelines specific to older people.

PROMOTING HEALTHY AGING: IMPLICATIONS FOR GERONTOLOGICAL NURSING

Assessment

The assessment dilemma is often one of determining if paranoia, delusions, and hallucinations are the result of medical illnesses, medications, dementia, psychoses, deprivation, or overload because the treatment will vary accordingly. Treatment must be based on a comprehensive assessment and a determination of the nature of the psychotic behavior (primary or secondary psychosis) and the time of onset of first symptoms (early or late). Treating the underlying cause of a secondary psychosis caused by medical illnesses, dementia, substance abuse, or delirium is a priority (Mentes & Bail, 2005).

Assessment of vision and hearing is also important since these impairments may predispose the older person to paranoia or suspiciousness. Psychotic symptoms and/or paranoid ideation also present with depression, so depression screening should also be conducted. Assessment of suicide potential is also indicated because individuals experiencing paranoid symptoms are at significant risk for harm to self.

> *"For new onset, persistent, late-life psychotic disorders not secondary to a mood disorder or general medical condition other then cognitive impairment, the differential should include dementia, delusional disorder, and very-late onset schizophrenia-like psychosis" (Chaudhary & Rabheru, 2008, p. 147).*

It is never safe to conclude that someone is delusional or paranoid or experiencing hallucinations unless you have thoroughly investigated his or her claims, evaluated physical and cognitive status, and assessed the environment for contributing factors to the behaviors.

Interventions

Frightening hallucinations or delusions, such as feeling that one is being poisoned, usually arise in response to anxiety-provoking situations and are best managed by reducing situational stress, being available to the person, providing a safe, nonjudgmental environment, and attending to the fears more than the content of the delusion or hallucination. Direct confrontation is likely to increase anxiety and agitation and the sense of vulnerability; it also may disrupt the relationship. A more useful approach is to establish a trusting relationship that is nondemanding and not too intense.

It is important to identify the client's strengths and build on them. Demonstrating respect and a willingness to listen to complaints and fears is important. It is important that the nurse be trustworthy, give clear information, and present clear choices. Do not pretend to agree with paranoid beliefs or delusions, but rather ask what is troubling to the person and provide reassurance of safety. It is important to try to understand the person's level of distress as well as how he or she is experiencing what is troubling. For institutionalized older people, other suggestions are to avoid television, which can be confusing, especially if the person awakens and finds it on or has a hearing or vision

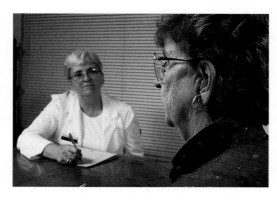

Demonstrating respect and a willingness to listen is the foundation for a caring nurse-patient relationship. From Harkreader H, Hogan MA: *Fundamentals of nursing: caring and clinical judgment*, ed 3, St Louis, 2007, Saunders.

impairment. In addition, reduce clutter in the person's room, eliminate shadows that can appear threatening. Provide glasses and hearing aids to maximize sensory input and decrease misinterpretations.

If symptoms are interfering with function and interpersonal and environmental strategies are not effective, antipsychotic drugs may be used. The newer atypical antipsychotics (risperidone, olanzapine) are preferred but must be used judiciously, with careful attention to side effects and monitoring of response. In the case of depression with psychotic features, combination therapy with an antidepressant and an atypical antipsychotic agent may be useful. In cognitively impaired individuals with paranoid ideation, there is some evidence suggesting that treatment with cognitive enhancer medications (cholinesterase inhibitors and memantine) may be of benefit. If symptoms interfere with function and safety, and non-pharmacological interventions are not effective, antipsychotic medications may be used. However, none of the antipsychotic medications are approved for use in treatment of behavioral responses in dementia. The benefits are uncertain, and adverse effects offset any advantages (Schneider et al., 2006). See Chapter 19 for further discussion of behavior and psychological symptoms in dementia and non-pharmacological interventions.

Psychoeducation, individual or group therapy, environmental and behavioral modification strategies, and supportive environments are also important treatment considerations. The presence of these symptoms contributes to caregiver burden and stress, and they are often precipitating factors to institutionalization, so caregiver support and utilization of community resources is important.

SCHIZOPHRENIA

Schizophrenia is a severe mental disorder characterized by two or more of the following symptoms: delusions, hallucinations, disorganized thinking, disorganized or catatonic behavior (called positive symptoms) and affective flattening, poverty of speech, or apathy (called negative symptoms) that cause significant social or occupational dysfunction, and are not accompanied by prominent mood symptoms or substance abuse or can be attributed to medical causes (American Psychiatric Association, 2000). The diagnostic criteria for schizophrenia are the same across the life span.

People with schizophrenia are the largest group of older people with severe mental health problems, and the numbers are expected to grow over the next decade with the increased longevity of the population. As Evans (2008) notes: "Persons living with mental illness also grow old and the changes associated with aging may further compromise a lifetime of challenged coping, thus exacerbating symptomatology and well-being" (p. 2). Although the onset of schizophrenia usually occurs between adolescence and the mid-30s, it can extend into and first appear in late life. However, 85% of older people with schizophrenia were diagnosed before age 45 (Berry & Barrowclough, 2009). Prevalence of schizophrenia in older people is estimated to be approximately 0.6%—about half of the prevalence in younger adults. Distinction is made between early-onset schizophrenia (EOS), occurring before age 40; midlife onset (MOS), between ages 40 and 60; and late onset (LOS), after age 60.

There is some suggestion that there may be neurobiologic differences between LOS and EOS, and further investigation is needed.

Patients with LOS are more likely to be women, and paranoia is the dominant feature of the illness. They tend to have a greater prevalence of visual hallucinations, less prevalence of a formal thought disorder, fewer negative symptoms, and less family history of schizophrenia. Women with LOS are also at greater risk for tardive dyskinesia, have less impairment in the areas of learning and abstraction, and require lower doses of neuroleptic medications for symptom management (Smith, 2005). Individuals with EOS who have grown older may experience fewer hallucinations, delusions, and bizarre behavior as well as inappropriate affect. Positive symptoms may wane, whereas negative symptoms tend to persist into late life (Mentes & Bail, 2005).

PROMOTING HEALTHY AGING: IMPLICATIONS FOR GERONTOLOGICAL NURSING

Interventions

Treatment for schizophrenia includes both medications and environmental interventions. Conventional neuroleptic medications (e.g., haloperidol) have been effective in managing the positive symptoms but are problematic in older people and carry a high risk of disabling and persistent side effects, such as tardive dyskinesia (TD). The abnormal involuntary movement scale (AIMS) is useful for evaluating early symptoms of TD (Chapter 7). The newer atypical antipsychotic medications (e.g., risperidone, olanzapine, quetiapine), given in low doses, are associated with a lower risk of extrapyramidal symptoms (EPS) and TD. Federal guidelines for the use of antipsychotic medications in nursing homes provide the indications for use of these medications in schizophrenia.

Other important interventions include a combination of support, education, physical activity, and CBT. Findings of a qualitative study with older persons with schizophrenia suggest that the stigma of schizophrenia may interfere with the building of trust between nurses and patients (Leutwyler & Wallhagen, 2010). These authors suggest that nurses need to provide continual respectful feedback and education to the person, be respectful of the person's time, and reduce stigmatizing perceptions of the patient to enhance trust and positive outcomes.

Families of older people with schizophrenia experience the burden of caring for a family member with a chronic disability as well as dealing with their own personal aging. Community-based support services are needed that include assistance with housing, medical care, recreation services, and services that help the family plan for the future of their relative. There are relatively few services in the community for older persons with schizophrenia. The National Alliance for the Mentally Ill (NAMI) (www.nami.org) is an important resource for clients and their families (Mentes & Bail, 2005).

Individuals with severe persistent mental illnesses such as schizophrenia form a disenfranchised group whose access to medical care has been limited, leading to greater functional declines, morbidity, and mortality, as demonstrated by statistics that individuals with schizophrenia have a life expectancy 20% lower than the general population (Davis, 2004). Schizophrenia is a costly disease both in terms of personal suffering and medical care costs. An estimated 41% of older people with schizophrenia now reside in nursing homes (Leutwyler & Wallhagen, 2010). Interventions to improve independent functioning irrespective of age and in conjunction with community services would decrease the expenses associated with institutionalization (Madhusoodanan & Brenner, 2007, p. 30).

BIPOLAR DISORDER

Bipolar disorder is not common in late life, but recurrence of remitted disease does occur. It is anticipated that with the growing number of older people, more cases will be seen. Ten percent of inpatient psychiatric admissions among older adults are for bipolar disorder. The disease occurs more often among individuals ages 60 to 64 years, with a declining incidence in older cohorts (Sherrod et al., 2010). Bipolar disorders, characterized by periods of mania and depression, often level out in late life, and individuals tend to have longer periods of depression. Mania is a more frequent cause of hospitalization than depression, but depression may account for more disability.

Similar to other psychiatric disorders in older adults, co-morbidities often mask the presence of the disorder and it is frequently misdiagnosed, underdiagnosed, and undertreated (Kennedy, 2008).

"One survey among individuals with bipolar disorder found that an astounding 69% were originally misdiagnosed and received an average of 3.5 diagnoses and saw an average of 4 physicians before an accurate diagnosis was determined. Depression was a frequent misdiagnosis and those with bipolar disorder were prescribed antidepressant medications, which inadvertently placed them at risk for manic episodes and increased risk of rapid cycling" (Sherrod et al., 2010, p. 21).

PROMOTING HEALTHY AGING: IMPLICATIONS FOR GERONTOLOGICAL NURSING

Assessment

Assessment includes a thorough physical examination and laboratory and radiological testing to rule out physical causes of the symptoms and identify co-morbidities. A medication review should be conducted since symptoms can be a side effect of medications such as antidepressants, benzodiazepines, amphetamines, prednisone, and captopril. Obtaining an accurate history from the individual, as well as the family, is important and should include assessment of symptoms associated with depression, mania, hypomania, and a family history of bipolar disorder. Episodes of mania combined with depressed features and a family history of bipolar disorder are highly indicative of the diagnosis. The genetic basis of the disease is being investigated, and two genes that influence the activity of nerve cells in

BOX 18-12   FOCUS ON GENETICS

Mental Health

Research on the genetic basis for mental health disorders such as depression, schizophrenia, and bipolar disorder, as well as Alzheimer's disease, is being conducted by the National Institute of Mental Health Center for Collaborative Genetic Studies on Mental Disorders. Information can be obtained at www.nimgenetics.org.

the brain may play a key role in an individual's risk for bipolar disorder (Box 18-12). Sherrod and colleagues (2010) provide two algorithms for the appropriate diagnosis and management of bipolar disorder, and the National Institute of Mental Health (NIMH) provides comprehensive information on the diagnosis and treatment of bipolar disorder (www.nimh.nih.gov/health/publications/bipolar-disorder/complete-index.shtml).

Interventions

Lithium, the most commonly used substance for individuals with bipolar disorders, has neurological effects that make it difficult for older people to tolerate; it also has a long half-life (more than 36 hours). Careful monitoring of blood levels and patient response is important. Recommended treatment consists of a combination of one or more mood stabilizers (e.g., lithium, valproic acid, caramazepine, lamotrigine). If the patient does not respond to these medications, atypical antipsychotic drugs are possible alternative treatments, but with the same safety warnings discussed earlier and are not to be used if dementia is suspected. Olanzapine, aripiprazole, and seroquel are all approved for the treatment of bipolar disorder and may relieve symptoms of severe mania and psychosis (www.nimh.nih.gov/publications/bipolar-disorder/complete-index.shtml). ECT may also be used when medication and/or psychotherapy are not effective.

Patient and family education and support are essential, and the family must understand that the individual is not able to control mania and irritating behaviors because of a chemical imbalance in the brain. Treatment with medication and intensive psychotherapy, CBT interpersonal and rhythm therapy (improving relationships with others and managing regular daily routines), or family-focused therapy has been reported to be effective in decreasing relapses, preventing hospitalization, and improving adherence to treatment plans (Miklowitz et al., 2007). The NIMH-funded Geriatric Bipolar (Geri-BD) trial is ongoing and will provide additional information about bipolar disease in older people. Another NIMH-funded study, The Systematic Treatment Enhancement Program for Bipolar Disorder (STEP BD) includes an older adult segment and will contribute to evidence-based treatment (Kennedy, 2008). Other resources for bipolar disorder can be found on the Evolve website.

DEPRESSION

Depression is not a normal part of aging, and studies show that most older people are satisfied with their lives, despite physical problems (National Institute of Mental Health [NIMH], 2008). To understand depression, the nurse must understand the influence of late-life stressors and changes, culture, and the beliefs older people, society, and health professionals may have about depression and its treatment.

Prevalence and Consequences

Depression is the most common mental health problem of late life and among the most treatable, but it can be life-threatening if unrecognized and untreated. The prevalence of major depression in older adults (1% to 5%) is somewhat lower than that in the general population, but minor depression and depressive symptoms are experienced by a large number of older people (Evans, 2008). One in ten older adults visiting a physician suffers from depression (http://impact-uw.org/).

Estimates of prevalence vary widely depending on the qualitative variables being considered and the definition being used. The prevalence of major depression in home care recipients ranges from 12% to 26%, but depressive symptoms are present in as many as 57% of this population. Among homebound older adults, two thirds with clinically significant depression had not received treatment (Sirey et al., 2008). For older adults in nursing homes, the prevalence of depressive symptoms may be as high as 54%, and a recent study reported that 23% were not treated and only 2.5% received some form of behavioral therapy. Depression is a major reason why older people are admitted to nursing homes (Kurlowicz & Harvath, 2008a; Morley, 2010).

Depression and illness are likely to co-occur. Becoming sick doubles the probability of becoming depressed, and becoming depressed doubles the probability of becoming sick (Thielke et al., 2010). More than 15% of older adults with chronic physical conditions are depressed, and depression has been called "the unwanted cotraveler" accompanying many medical illnesses (Byrd, 2005, p. 132). Many medications that older people may take also can also cause depression.

Depression is a major source of morbidity in older adults (Heller et al., 2010). Depression and depressive symptomatology are associated with negative consequences such as increased disability, delayed recovery from illness and surgery, excess use of health services, cognitive impairment, malnutrition, decreased quality of life, and increased suicide and non–suicide-related death (Evans, 2008; Kurlowicz & Harvath, 2008b). Depression remains underdiagnosed and undertreated, and major depressive disorder (MDD) is undiagnosed in approximately half of older persons with this disorder (Das et al., 2007).

The stigma associated with depression may be more prevalent in older people, and they may not acknowledge depressive symptoms or seek treatment. Many elders, particularly those who have survived the Great Depression, both world wars, the Holocaust, and other tragedies, may see depression as shameful, evidence of flawed character, self-centered, a spiritual weakness, and sin or retribution.

Health professionals often expect older people to be depressed and may not take appropriate action to assess for and treat depression. The differing presentation of depression in older people, as well as the increased prevalence of medical problems that may cause depressive symptoms, also contributes to inadequate recognition and treatment. Up to one in four primary care patients suffer from depression, but primary care physicians identify only one third of these patients (Chizobam et al., 2008). Even if depression is identified, only about one half of Americans diagnosed with a major depression receive treatment for it, and even fewer, about one fifth, receive treatment consistent with current guidelines (Gonzalez et al., 2010).

Ethnic and Cultural Considerations

Depression diagnosis and treatment is an even greater concern for ethnically and culturally diverse elders. African American and black Caribbeans who experience a major depressive episode are more likely to be untreated, and they experience more disabling effects than non-Hispanic whites. Mexican-American and African-American individuals with depression have the lowest rates of depression care and treatment in accordance with accepted guidelines (Gonzalez et al., 2010). Nursing home patients who are female, black, or cognitively impaired are less likely to receive treatment for depression (Byrd, 2005; Kurlowicz & Harvath, 2008a).

Results of a recent study (Heller et al., 2010) suggested that African-American women might be more reluctant to admit feelings of depression or report impairment in functioning and are more likely to continue with their normal daily routines as they had in the past when faced with adversity. African-American women might be reluctant to use words such as *depression* or *sadness,* and Heller and colleagues (2010) suggest "a good signal of a depressive state worthy of follow-up might be reluctance to describe themselves as happy or enjoying life" (p. 344). African Americans may be less knowledgeable about depression and less likely to discuss depression with mental health providers, preferring education from less traditional sources such as churches (Box 18-5). As discussed earlier in the chapter, ethnicity and cultural background affect both recognition and treatment of depression and other mental health disorders in ways not yet completely understood. With the increase in the numbers of racially, ethnically, and culturally diverse elders and evidence of disparities in health outcomes, in created attention is essential (Kurlowicz & Harvath, 2008a).

Failure to treat depression increases morbidity and mortality. There is no evidence that current evidence-based treatments for geriatric depression, such as psychotherapy, psychosocial interventions, and medications, are any less effective as people age. (Kurlowicz & Harvath, 2008a; Thielke et al., 2010). It is highly likely that nurses will encounter a large number of older people with depressive symptoms in all settings. Recognizing depression and enhancing access to appropriate mental health care are important nursing roles to improve outcomes for older people.

Etiology

The causes of depression in older adults are complex and must be examined in a biopsychosocial framework. Factors of health, gender, developmental needs, socioeconomics, environment, personality, losses, and functional decline are all significant to the development of depression in later life. Biologic causes, such as neurotransmitter imbalances or dysregulation of endocrine function, have also been proposed as factors influencing the development of depression in late life (Kurlowicz & Harvath, 2008a).

Some of the medical disorders that cause depression are cancers; cardiovascular disorders; endocrine disorders, such as thyroid problems and diabetes; neurological disorders, such as Alzheimer's disease, stroke, and Parkinson's disease; metabolic and nutritional disorders, such as Vitamin B12 deficiency and malnutrition; viral infections, such as herpes zoster and hepatitis; and advanced macular degeneration. Among patients who have suffered a cerebral vascular accident, the incidence of major depressive disorder is approximately 25%, with rates being close to 40% in patients with Parkinson's disease (Das et al., 2007).

Vascular depression is a term being used to describe a late-life depression associated with vascular changes in the brain and characterized by executive dysfunction (Thakur & Blazer, 2008). Serious symptoms of depression occur in up to 50% of older adults with Alzheimer's disease, and major depression occurs in about 25% of cases. Depression in individuals with Alzheimer's disease may be due to an awareness of progressive decline, but research suggests that there may be a biological connection between depression and Alzheimer's disease as well (Friedman et al., 2009; Kurlowicz & Harvath, 2008a; Morley, 2010).

Medications may also result in depressive symptoms including hypertensives, angiotensin-converting enzyme (ACE) inhibitors, methyldopa, reserpine, guanethidine, antidysrhythmics, anticholesteremics, antibiotics, analgesics, corticosteroids, digoxin, and L-dopa (Kurlowicz & Harvath, 2008b).

Other important factors influencing the development of depression are alcohol abuse, loss of a spouse or partner, loss of social supports, lower income level, caregiver stress (particularly caring for a person with dementia), and gender. Some psychological traits, such as neuroticism, pessimistic thinking, and being less open to new experiences, have been found to be associated with higher rates of depression and suicide (Das et al., 2007). Some common risk factors for depression are presented in Box 18-13.

Differing Presentation of Depression in Elders

The *DSM-IV* (American Psychiatric Association, 2000) provides criteria for the diagnosis of major depression, dysthymia, and minor (subsyndromal) depression. Depression can be

---

BOX 18-13   RISK FACTORS FOR DEPRESSION IN OLDER ADULTS

- Chronic medical illnesses, disability, functional decline
- Pain
- Alzheimer's disease and other dementias
- Bereavement
- Caregiving
- Female (2:1 risk)
- Lower SES
- Family history of depression
- Previous episode of depression
- Admission to long-term care or other change in environment
- Medications
- Alcohol or substance abuse
- Living alone
- Widowhood
- New stressful losses, including loss of autonomy; loss of privacy; loss of functional status; loss of independence; loss of body part; or loss of family member, roommate, or pet

SES, Socioeconomic status.

considered a syndrome consisting of an array of affective, cognitive, and somatic or physiological symptoms. Depression may range in severity from mild symptoms to more severe forms, both of which can persist over long periods. Suicidal ideation and psychotic features (delusional thinking) accompany more severe depression (Kurlowicz & Harvath, 2008a).

The *DSM-IV* criteria "do not capture symptoms distinctive of geriatric depression" (Byrd, 2005, p. 136). The criteria stipulate that for a diagnosis of major depression, dysthymia, or minor depression, the symptoms must not be the result of a medical condition or a substance (medication, alcohol). Co-morbid medical conditions are, however, the "hallmark of depression in older people and a major difference from depression in younger people" (Kurlowicz & Harvath, 2008a, p. 63).

Symptoms of depression are different in older people. Older people who are depressed report more somatic complaints, such as physical symptoms, insomnia, loss of appetite and weight loss, memory loss, or chronic pain. Somatic complaints may be even more prominent in individuals with limited education and no previous psychiatric history. The somatic complaints "are often difficult to distinguish from the physical symptoms associated with chronic physical illness" (Kurlowicz & Harvath, 2008a, p. 59). Hypochondriasis is also common, as are constant complaining and criticism, which may actually be expressions of depression.

Decreased energy and motivation, lack of ability to experience pleasure, hopelessness, increased dependency, poor grooming and difficulty completing activities of daily living (ADLs), withdrawal from people or activities enjoyed in the past, decreased sexual interest, and a preoccupation with death or "giving up" are also signs of depression in older people. Feelings of guilt and worthlessness, seen in younger depressed individuals, are less frequently seen in older people. Patients with late-life depression are also less likely to have a family history of depression than younger individuals (Das et al., 2007).

Individuals often present with complaints of memory problems, the "so-called pseudodementia (the dementia syndrome of depression) in which the patient has a memory loss and functional decline but of a generally more recent and abrupt onset than the more common progressive dementias. Making the clinical evaluation even more confusing is the strong association of depression with dementia" (Ham et al., 2007, p. 238). Depression and depressive symptoms occur frequently in individuals with dementia as well as those with mild cognitive impairment (MCI), the prevalence of depression in dementia is estimated to be around 45% (Change and Roberts, 2011), and are associated with increased mortality, reduced quality of life, increases in caregiver burden and distress, and higher rates of institutionalization (Gellis et al., 2009). It is essential to differentiate between dementia and depression, and older people with memory impairment should be evaluated for depression. Symptoms such as agitated behavior and repetitive verbalizations in persons with dementia may be a symptom of depression (Chapter 19). An evidence-based guideline for detection of depression in dementia (Brown et al., 2007; Brown et al., 2009) provides assessment tools, algorithms for detection of depression, and process and outcome monitors (see Box 18-9).

Recognition and treatment of minor (subsyndromal) depression in older adults is emerging as a significant concern. Minor depression is two to four times as common as major depression in older adults. Minor depression is associated with clinically significant distress and impairment and imposes an increased risk of developing major depression. Twenty-five percent of persons with minor depression will go on to experience a major depressive episode (Byrd, 2005).

PROMOTING HEALTHY AGING: IMPLICATIONS FOR GERONTOLOGICAL NURSING

Assessment

Both health care providers and patients have difficulty identifying signs of depression (NIMH, 2008). Assessment involves a systematic and thorough evaluation using a depression screening instrument, interview, history and physical, functional assessment, cognitive assessment, laboratory tests, medication review, determination of iatrogenic or medical causes, and family interview as indicated. Assessment for depressogenic medications and for related co-morbid physical conditions that may contribute to or complicate treatment of depression must also be included. A comprehensive guide to assessment and treatment of depression in older adults can be found in Box 18-9.

Screening of all older adults for depression should be incorporated into routine health assessments across the continuum of care—in hospitals, primary care, long-term care, home care, and community-based settings. (Kolanowski & Piven, 2006; Kurlowicz & Harvath, 2008). The Geriatric Depression Scale (GDS) was developed specifically for screening older adults and has been tested extensively in a number of settings. The GDS and other assessment tools for depression are discussed in Chapter 7.

Interventions

If depression is diagnosed, treatment should begin as soon as possible, and appropriate follow-up should be provided. Depressed people are usually unable to follow through on their own and without appropriate treatment and monitoring may be candidates for deeper depression or suicide. The most effective treatment is a combination of pharmacological therapy and psychotherapy or counseling. However, as Morley (2010) noted,

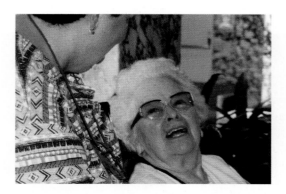

Creating hopeful environments in which meaningful activities and supportive relationships can be enjoyed is an important nursing role in the treatment of depression. From Christensen B, Kockrow E: *Foundations and adult health nursing*, ed 6, St Louis, 2011, Mosby.

"behavioral interventions are at present underused and pharmaceutical approaches are overused" (p. 302). Interventions are individualized and are based on history, severity of symptoms, concomitant illnesses, and level of disability.

Generally, a stepped care approach is recommended in which there are separate pathways for the management of mild to moderate and severe depression and the sequential application of different types of treatment, followed by monitoring progress and modifying treatment as indicated. Unutzer (2007) suggests that "there is controversy about the effectiveness of psychotherapies and antidepressant medications in patients with depression that does not meet the full diagnostic criteria for major depression. Watchful waiting may be appropriate for these patients as long as the depression is carefully tracked and treatment initiated if symptoms worsen" (p. 2274). Treatment for individuals with mild to moderate depression may involve self-help, counseling, and physical exercise. For those with severe depression, treatment would include antidepressants and psychotherapy (Seekles et al., 2009).

An interdisciplinary approach, collaborative models of care, and care management, often involving advanced practice nurses, has been successful in improving outcomes of depression as well as lowering costs of care (Unutzer et al., 2008). Services provided by psychiatric-mental health clinical nurse specialists in primary, home, and long-term care may be particularly effective in improving outcomes for depressed individuals and are well received by patients (Saur, et al., 2007; Morley, 2010).

The IMPACT (Improving Mood—Promoting Access to Collaborative Treatment for Late-Life Depression) model (Unutzer et al., 2002), an evidence-based approach for depression care and treatment in primary care, has been shown to reduce depressive symptoms at least 50% compared to usual care in a cost-effective manner (http://impact-uw.org/about/key.html). There are exciting roles for nursing since collaborative care models often use nursing care managers (Smith, 2010). Key components of the model are presented in Box 18-14.

Family and social support, education, grief management, exercise, humor, spirituality, CBT, brief psychodynamic therapy, interpersonal therapy, reminiscence, life review therapy (see Chapter 6), and problem-solving therapy have all been noted to be helpful in depression. Results of a recent study (Lauretsky et al., 2011) suggest that complementary use of a mind-body exercise, such as Tai chi chih, may provide additional improvements of clinical outcome in the pharmocological treatment of geriatric depression. Box 18-15 presents suggestions for families and professionals caring for older adults with depression.

Medications

There are more than 20 antidepressants approved by the FDA for the treatment of depression in older adults. The most commonly prescribed are the SSRIs. These agents work selectively on neurotransmitters in the brain to alleviate depression. The SSRIs are generally well tolerated in older people. Common side effects include nausea, vomiting, dizziness, drowsiness,

---

BOX 18-14   IMPACT KEY COMPONENTS

1. Collaborative care: The patient's primary care provider works with a care manager to develop and implement a treatment plan (medications and/or brief, evidence-based psychotherapy). Care manager and primary care provider consult with psychiatrist to change treatment plans based on patient response.
2. Depression Care Manager: May be a nurse, social worker or psychologist who educates the patient and family about depression, supports antidepressant therapy if appropriate, coaches patients on behavioral activation and pleasant events scheduling, offers brief (six to eight weeks) course of counseling such as problem-solving treatment, and monitors depression symptoms for treatment response.
3. Designated psychiatrist: Consults with care manager and primary care provider on care of patients who do not respond to treatments as expected.
4. Outcome measurement: Care managers measure depressive symptoms at the start of treatment as expected.
5. Stepped care: Treatment adjusted based on clinical outcomes and according to an evidence-based algorithm, aim for a 50% reduction in symptoms within 10-12 weeks. If patient is not significantly improved at 10-12 weeks after the start of a treatment plan, try a change to a different medication, addition of psychotherapy, a combination of medication and psychotherapy, or other treatments suggested by the team psychiatrist.

From IMPACT Implementation Center, University of Washington: *IMPACT Key Components.* Available at http://impact-uw.org/about/key.html. Accessed July 15, 2010.

BOX 18-15   INTERPERSONAL SUPPORT BY FAMILY AND PROFESSIONALS

- Provide relief from discomfort of physical illness.
- Enhance physical function (i.e., regular exercise and/or activity; physical, occupational, recreational therapies).
- Develop a daily activity schedule that includes pleasant activities.
- Increase opportunities for socialization and enhance social support.
- Provide opportunities for decisions and to exercise control.
- Focus on spiritual renewal and rediscovery of meanings.
- Reactivate latent interests, or develop new ones.
- Validate depressed feelings as aiding recovery; do not try to bolster the person's mood or deny his or her despair.
- Help the person become aware of the presence of depression, the nature of the symptoms, and the time limitation of depression.
- Provide an accepting atmosphere and an empathic response.
- Share yourself.
- Demonstrate faith in the person's strengths.
- Praise any and all efforts at recovery, no matter how small.
- Assist in expressing and dealing with anger.
- Do not stifle the grief process; grief cannot be hurried.
- Create a hopeful environment where self-esteem is fostered and life is meaningful.
- Assist in dealing with guilt, real or neurotic.
- Foster development of connections with others.

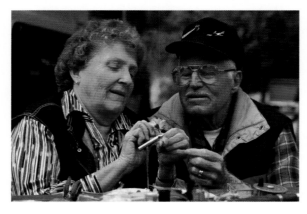

Elders enjoying an activity together. Courtesy of Corbis.

and hyponatremia. Choice of medication depends on co-morbidities, drug side effects, and the type of effect desired. People with agitated depression and sleep disturbances may benefit from medications with a more sedating effect, whereas those who are not eating may do better taking medications that have an appetite-stimulating effect. If depression is immobilizing, psychostimulants may be used.

Medications must be closely monitored for side effects and therapeutic response. Side effects can be especially problematic for older people with co-morbid conditions and complex drug regimens. It is important to carefully look for drug interactions and monitor for side effects when starting antidepressant medications. There are a wide range of antidepressant medications, and several may have to be evaluated. As with other medications for older people, doses should be lower at first and titrated as indicated while adequate treatment effect is ensured (Kurlowicz & Harvath, 2008b).

"Up to 12 weeks of treatment may be needed to elicit a full response. Only about 40% to 65% of patients have an adequate response to any given antidepressant, and trials of alternative antidepressants or combinations of antidepressants, with or without psychotherapy, are required in a substantial number of patients. Treatment should continue at full doses for at least 6-12 months after remission because recurrence rates after earlier discontinuation are as high as 70%" (Unutzer, 2007, p. 2273).

More severe depression complicated by psychosis or suicidal intent may necessitate lifelong medication therapy. Often, older people may be resistant to take medication for depression, and it is helpful to stress that while there may be circumstances precipitating the depression, the final effect is a biochemical one that medications can correct (Ham et al., 2007).

ECT is considered an excellent, safe therapy for older people with depression that is resistant to other treatments and for patients at risk for serious harm because of psychotic depression, suicidal ideation, or severe malnutrition, with efficacy rates ranging from 60% to 80% (Morley, 2010; Unutzer, 2007). ECT is much improved, but older people will need a careful explanation of the treatment since they may have many misconceptions.

SUICIDE

Elders compose only 13% of the U.S. population but account for 20% of the suicide deaths. The rate of suicide among older adults is higher than that for any other age group—and the suicide rate for persons 85 years and older is the highest of all—twice the overall national rate (Edelstein et al., 2009). Non-Hispanic white men with mild depressive disorder are five times more likely to commit suicide than the general population (Das et al., 2007). Older widowers are thought to be the most vulnerable because they have often depended on their wives to maintain the comforts of home and the social network of family and friends. Women in all countries have much lower suicide rates, possibly because of greater flexibility in coping skills based on multiple roles that women fill throughout their lives. The more children a woman has, the lower her risk of suicide. Older African Americans have a much lower

suicide rate; however, suicide rates of elderly black men are increasing, so attention must be paid to assessment in this group (Joe et al., 2006). Despite these alarming statistics, there is little research on suicide ideation and behavior among older adults.

It is important to note that recent data suggests that baby boomers appear to be driving a dramatic increase in suicide rates among middle-aged people. From 2000-2005, the suicide rate increased nearly 30% for men and women aged 50-59 with some college but no degree. High rates of substance abuse and the onset of chronic illness are among the possible factors in this rising suicide rate (Phillips et al., 2010).

In most cases, depression and other mental health problems, including anxiety, contribute significantly to suicide risk. Eighty percent of suicides are related to depression (Das et al., 2007). Common precipitants of suicide include physical or mental illness, death of a spouse or partner, substance abuse, and pathological relationships. Suicide may have some familial tendencies, with estimates that a suicide of one parent in the family is associated with a six-fold increase of suicide in the children (Kennedy, 2008). One of the major differences in suicidal behavior in the old and the young is lethality of method. Eight out of 10 suicides for men older than 65 were with firearms. Older people rarely threaten to commit suicide, they just do it.

Up to 75% of older adults who die by suicide visited a physician within one month before death; 40% visited within one week of the suicide, and 20% visited the physician on the day of the suicide (National Institute of Mental Health, 2008). However, only 44% of those visits were for mental health reasons. In a study investigating the prevalence of suicide ideation among community-dwelling older adults and the relationship between suicide ideation, major psychiatric disorder, and mental health service use, Corna and colleagues (2010) reported that only 8% of the participants reporting suicide ideation sought out any kind of "specialized" mental health care, 22.8% discussed these issues with their general health care provider, and less than 5% discussed their mental health concerns with other types of providers.

Older people with suicide ideation, or with other mental health concerns, often present with somatic complaints. The statistics suggest that opportunities for assessment of suicidal risk are present, but the need for intervention is not seen as urgent or not even recognized. Consequently, it is very important for providers in all settings to inquire about recent life events, implement depression screening for all older people, evaluate for anxiety disorders, assess for suicidal thoughts and ideas based on depression assessment, and recognize warning signs and risk factors for suicide. Behavioral clues and risk and recovery factors are presented in Box 18-16.

PROMOTING HEALTHY AGING: IMPLICATIONS FOR GERONTOLOGICAL NURSING

Assessment

Older people with suicidal intent are encountered in many settings. It is our professional obligation to prevent, whenever possible, an impulsive destruction of life that may be a response to a crisis or a disintegrative reaction. The lethality potential of

BOX 18-16 SUICIDE RISK AND RECOVERY FACTORS

RISK FACTORS AND WARNING SIGNS

Male gender
Physical illness
Functional impairment
Depression
Alcohol and substance misuse and abuse
Major loss, such as the death of a spouse or partner
History of major losses
Recent suicide attempt
History of suicide attempts
Major crises or transitions, such as retirement or relocation to an assisted living or nursing facility
Major crises in the lives of family members
Social isolation
Preoccupation with death
Poorly controlled pain
Expression of the belief that one is in the way, a burden
Giving away favorite possessions, money

RECOVERY FACTORS

A capacity for the following:
  Understanding
  Relating
  Benefiting from experience
  Benefiting from knowledge
  Accepting help
  Being loving
  Expressing wisdom
  Displaying a sense of humor
  Having a social interest
  Accepting a caring and available family
  Accepting a caring and available social network
  Accepting a caring, available, and knowledgeable professional and health network

an elder must always be assessed when elements of depression, disease, and spousal loss are evident. Any direct, indirect, or enigmatic references to the ending of life must be taken seriously and discussed with the elder.

"Suicide assessment should include a description of both sides of the suicide equation: reasons for wanting to take one's life and life affirming reasons for not doing so. Suicide assessments should include assessment of the presence of protective or resiliency factors, which complements the conventional assessment of suicide risk and the prevention of suicide" (Edelstein et al., 2009, p. 743).

The most important consideration for the nurse is to establish a trusting and respectful relationship with the person. Since many older people have grown up in an era when suicide bore stigma and even criminal implications, they may not discuss their feelings in this area. The stigma related to mental illness also affects older people's willingness to share their feelings of sadness or anxiety. It is also important to remember that in older people, typical behavioral clues such as putting personal affairs in order, giving away possessions, and making wills and funeral plans are indications of maturity and good judgment in late life and cannot be construed as indicative of

suicidal intent. Even statements such as "I won't be around long" or "I'm ready to die" may be only a realistic appraisal of the situation in old age.

If there is suspicion that the elder is suicidal, use direct and straightforward questions such as the following:

- Have you ever thought about killing yourself?
- How often have you had these thoughts?
- How would you kill yourself if you decided to do it?

! SAFETY ALERT

Always ask direct questions of the patient and family about suicide risks and suicide ideation.

Interventions

It is important to have a suicide protocol in place that clearly defines how the nurse will intervene if a positive response is obtained from any of the questions. The person should never be left alone for any period of time until help arrives to assist and care for them. Patients at high risk should be hospitalized, especially if they have current psychological stressors and/or access to lethal means. Patients at moderate risk may be treated as outpatients provided they have adequate social support and no access to lethal means. Patients at low risk should have a full psychiatric evaluation and be followed up carefully (Das et al., 2007). Box 18-9 for a protocol for suicide risk assessment. A toolkit for senior living communities for promotion of mental health and prevention of suicide is available at http://store.samhsa.gov/products/sma-4515.

Suicide is a taboo topic for most of us, and there is a lingering fear that the introduction of the topic will be suggestive to the patient and may incite suicidal action. Precisely the opposite is true. By introducing the topic, we demonstrate interest in the individual and open the door to honest human interaction and connection on the deep levels of psychological need. It is the nature of our concern and our ability to connect with the alienation and desperation of the individual that will make a difference. Working with isolated, depressed, and suicidal elders challenges the depths of nurses' ingenuity, patience, and self-knowledge.

SUBSTANCE MISUSE AND ALCOHOL USE DISORDERS

Alcohol

Substance abuse often arises in old age as a coping mechanism to deal with loss, anxiety, depression, boredom, or pain associated with chronic illness. Misuse of alcohol and prescription medications appears to be a more common problem among older adults than abuse of illicit drugs. However, illicit drugs, such as cocaine and heroin, are becoming more prevalent with the aging of the baby boomer generation, who have a greater lifetime history of substance abuse (Evans, 2008). Estimates are that the number of adults over age 50 with substance abuse problems will double by 2020. In 2020, approximately 50% of individuals ages 50 to 74 will be in a high-risk group (use of alcohol and marijuana before age 30) compared with less than 9% in 1999 (Substance Abuse and Mental Health Services Administration, 2010). The most common type of substance-use disorder is heavy drinking (Naegle, 2008). Alcohol-related problems in the elderly often go unrecognized, although the residual effects of alcohol abuse complicate the presentation and treatment of many chronic disorders of older people.

The current *DSM-IV* (American Psychiatric Association, 2000) criteria for abuse (failure to fulfill major role obligations at work, school, or home; substance use in physically hazardous situations; substance-related legal problems; or recurrent social or interpersonal problems) was developed and validated on young and middle-aged adults and may not adequately describe consequences of alcohol use in older adults (Finfgeld-Connett, 2004). In the general population, alcohol abuse is readily recognized because of social or work problems; however, elders may live alone and not come under scrutiny at work. They may easily hide their drinking.

Although alcohol use generally declines with age, the misuse and abuse of alcohol is a growing concern among older adults and is expected to increase with the aging of the population (Kirchner et al., 2007). The exact extent of alcohol abuse is not known, but a recent study reported that more than one third of drinkers over age 60 consume amounts of alcohol that are excessive or potentially harmful in combination with certain diseases or medications they may be taking. Men age 65 and over have a higher prevalence of unhealthy drinking than women (Epstein et al., 2007; Merrick et al., 2008).

Up to 50% of nursing home patients have a history of alcohol abuse, and hospital admissions for alcohol-related problems may be equal to admission rates for myocardial infarction (Masters, 2003). The actual prevalence of alcohol-related hospitalizations is most likely greater than reported, and many studies have shown that older adults are less likely to receive a primary diagnosis of alcoholism than are younger adults (Culberson, 2006a).

Most severe alcohol abuse is seen in people ages 60 to 80 years, not in those older than 80 years. Two thirds of elderly alcoholics are early-onset drinkers (alcohol use began at age 30 or 40), and one third are late-onset drinkers (use began after age 60). Late-onset drinking may be related to situational events such as illness, retirement, or death of a spouse and includes a higher number of women (Finfgeld-Connett, 2005).

Gender Issues

While men (particularly older widowers) are four times more likely to abuse alcohol than women but prevalence in women may be underestimated. The number and impact of older female drinkers is expected to increase over the next 20 years as the disparity between men's and women's drinking decreases (Epstein et al., 2007). Women of all ages are significantly more vulnerable to the effects of alcohol misuse, including drug interactions, physical injury from alcohol-related falls and accidents, cognitive impairment, and liver and heart disease. Older women are more susceptible to the effects of alcohol since they have less body water than men, less mean muscle mass, and lower levels of the enzyme that breaks down alcohol. Even low-risk drinking levels (no more than one standard drink/day) can be hazardous for older women (Epstein et al., 2007). Older women also experience unique barriers to detection of and treatment for alcohol problems. Health care providers often assume that older women do not drink problematically, so they do not screen for this. Often, alcohol abuse in women is undetected until the consequences are severe (Epstein et al., 2007).

Drug Effects

Many drugs that elders use for chronic illnesses cause adverse effects when combined with alcohol. Alcohol interacts with at least 50% of prescription drugs (Naegle, 2008). Medications that interact with alcohol include analgesics, antibiotics, antidepressants, antipsychotics, benzodiazepines, H2 receptor antagonists, nonsteroidal antiinflammatory drugs (NSAIDs), and herbal medications (echinacea, valerian). Acetaminophen taken on a regular basis, when combined with alcohol, may lead to liver failure. Alcohol diminishes the effects of oral hypoglycemics, anticoagulants, and anticonvulsants. All older people should be given precise instructions regarding the interaction of alcohol with their medications.

Other effects of alcohol in older people include urinary incontinence, which results from rapid bladder filling and diminished neuromuscular control of the bladder; gait disturbances from alcohol-induced cerebellar degeneration and peripheral neuropathy; depression and suicide; sleep disturbances and insomnia; and dementia or delirium. Elders who drink to excess are susceptible to cognitive decline, physical decline, functional decline, and increased risk for injury.

Physiology

Older people develop higher blood alcohol levels because of age-related changes (increased body fat, decreased lean body mass and total body water content) that alter absorption and distribution of alcohol (Culberson, 2006a). Reduced liver and kidney function slow alcohol metabolism and elimination. A decrease in the gastric enzyme alcohol dehydrogenase results in slower metabolism of alcohol and higher blood levels for a longer time. Risks of gastrointestinal ulceration and bleeding may be higher in older people because of the decrease in gastric acidity that occurs in aging (Letizia & Reinboltz, 2005).

PROMOTING HEALTHY AGING: IMPLICATIONS FOR GERONTOLOGICAL NURSING

Assessment

Screening for alcohol and drug use (prescription or illicit) should be part of health visits for people over age 60, but screening is not routinely conducted in primary, acute, or long-term care settings (Evans, 2008; Kolanowski & Piven, 2006). Reasons for the low rates of alcohol detection among older adults by health care professionals include poor symptom recognition, inadequate knowledge about screening instruments, lack of age-appropriate diagnostic criteria for abuse in older people, and ageism. Alcohol-related problems may be overlooked in older people because they do not disrupt their lives or are not clearly linked to physical disorders. Health care providers may also be pessimistic about the ability of older people to

BOX 18-17   SIGNS AND SYMPTOMS OF POTENTIAL ALCOHOL PROBLEMS IN OLDER ADULTS

Anxiety
Irritability (feeling worried or "crabby")
Blackouts
Dizziness
Indigestion
Heartburn
Sadness or depression
Chronic pain
Excessive mood swings
New problems making decisions
Lack of interest in usual activities
Falls
Bruises, burns, or other injuries
Family conflict, abuse
Headaches
Incontinence
Memory loss
Poor hygiene
Poor nutrition
Insomnia
Sleep apnea
Social isolation
Out of touch with family or friends
Unusual response to medications
Frequent physical complaints and physician visits
Financial problems

Adapted from National Institute on Alcohol Abuse and Alcoholism: Older adults and alcohol problems, Participant Handout, 2005. Available at www.niaaa.nih.gov. Accessed July 9, 2008; Geriatric Mental Health Foundation: Substance abuse and misuse among older adults: prevention, recognition and help, 2006. Available at www.gmhfonline.org. Accessed July 8, 2008.

change long-standing problems (Naegle, 2008). Finfgeld-Connett (2004) reported that 37% of primary care physicians overlooked alcohol abuse among older women because "it is one of the few pleasures they have left" (p. 32).

Alcoholism is a disease of denial and not easy to diagnose, particularly in older people with psychosocial and functional decline from other conditions that may mask decline caused by alcohol. Early signs such as weight loss, irritability, insomnia, and falls may not be recognized as indicators of possible alcohol problems and may be attributed to "just getting older." Box 18-17 presents signs and symptoms that may indicate the presence of alcohol problems in older adults.

The possible health benefits of alcohol in moderation have been reported in the literature (reduced risk of coronary artery disease, ischemic stroke, Alzheimer's disease, and vascular dementia). As a result, older people may not perceive alcohol use as potentially harmful, but clinically significant adverse effects can occur in some individuals consuming as little as two to three drinks per day over an extended period. Because of the increased risk of adverse effects from alcohol use, the National Institute on Alcohol Abuse and Alcoholism (NIAAA) has recommended that individuals over age 65 limit alcohol consumption to no more than one standard drink per day. The Substance Abuse and Mental Health Services Administration (SAMSHA) recommends a maximum of two drinks on any drinking occasion (holidays or other celebrations) and somewhat lower limits for women. Health professionals must share information with older people about safe drinking limits and the deleterious effects of alcohol intake.

Alcohol users often reject or deny the diagnosis, or they may take offense at the suggestion of it. Feelings of shame or disgrace may make elders reluctant to disclose a drinking problem. This may be especially true among ethnically or culturally diverse older women from a background in which alcohol use is highly discouraged (Finfgeld-Connett, 2004). Families of older people with substance abuse disorders, particularly their adult children, may be ashamed of the problem and choose not to address it. Health care providers may feel helpless over alcoholism or uncomfortable with direct questioning or may approach the person in a judgmental manner. Many of the traditional ways of dealing with alcoholism emphasize a confrontational or punitive approach that may have "little impact on a person who views him or herself at the final stage of life" (Naegle, 2008, p. 207). A caring and supportive approach that provides a safe and open atmosphere is the foundation for the therapeutic relationship. It is always important to search for the pain beneath the behavior.

Culberson (2006b) suggests that a simple question—"Have you had a drink containing alcohol within the past 3 months?"—be included in an assessment to identify clients in whom further screening is indicated. This may be followed by administration of a screening instrument such as the Michigan Alcoholism Screening Test—Geriatric Version (MAST-G) (available at http://consultgerirn.org/uploads/File/trythis/try_this_17.pdf) (see Box 18-9) or the CAGE (Cut, Annoyed by others, feel Guilty, need Eye opener) Questionnaire (Evans, 2008; Naegle, 2008). Assessment of depression is also important. Alcohol and depression screenings should be offered routinely at health fairs and other sites where older people may seek health information and should be included as part of the annual assessment of all older adults. Screening should be done both before prescribing any new medications that may interact with alcohol and as needed after life-changing events (Epstein et al., 2007).

Interventions

Alcohol problems affect physical, mental, spiritual, and emotional health. Interventions must address quality of life in all of these spheres and be adapted to meet the unique needs of the older adult (Box 18-18). Abstinence from alcohol is seen as the desired goal, but a focus on education, alcohol reduction, and reducing harm is also appropriate. Increasing the awareness of older adults about the risks and benefits of alcohol consumption in the context of their own situation is an important goal (Merrick et al., 2008). Treatment and intervention strategies include cognitive-behavioral approaches, individual and group counseling, medical and psychiatric approaches, referral to Alcoholics Anonymous, family therapy, case management and community and home care services, and formalized substance abuse treatment. Treatment outcomes for older people have been shown to be equal to or better than those for younger people (Naegle, 2008).

Unless the person is in immediate danger, a stepped-care intervention approach beginning with brief interventions followed by more intensive therapies, if necessary, should be used.

BOX 18-18 ADAPTING ALCOHOL TREATMENT INTERVENTIONS FOR OLDER ADULTS

- Ensure treatment by staff experienced in working with older people.
- Accommodate for vision, hearing, and other functional impairments.
- Provide easy access and transportation if needed.
- Address issues older adults tend to face such as loss, grief, and health problems.
- Include relevant topics to older adults such as worries about the future of independent living, grandparenting, retirement, and fixed income.
- Consider using life review and reminiscence techniques.
- Use a respectful rather than confrontational approach.
- Slow the pace of treatment.
- Use case management and interdisciplinary approaches.
- Address spiritual needs.
- Tailor treatment to level of cognitive function.
- Provide opportunities for interesting activities and socialization opportunities that don't involve drinking.
- Focus on strengths and past coping skills used during hard times.
- Demonstrate faith in the person's ability to change, and avoid ageist attitudes.
- Consider groups designed for women only, since their needs are different.

Adapted from: Epstein E, Fischer-Elber K, Al-Otaiba Z: Women, aging, and alcohol use disorders, co-published simultaneously in *Journal of Women & Aging* 19:31, 2007; Malatesta V, editor: *Mental health issues of older women: a comprehensive review for health care professionals*, Florence, Ken, 2007, Routledge.

Brief interventions may range from one meeting to four or five short sessions. Brief intervention is a time-limited, patient-centered strategy focused on changing behavior and assessing patient readiness to change. Sessions can range from one meeting of 10 to 30 minutes to 4 or 5 short sessions. The goals of brief intervention are to (1) reduce or stop alcohol consumption, and (2) facilitate entry into formalized treatment if needed. Research results indicate that this type of intervention, with counseling by nurses in primary care settings, is effective for reducing alcohol consumption, and older people may be more likely to accept treatment given by their primary care provider (Culberson, 2006b; Jalbert et al., 2008).

Long-term self-help treatment programs for elders show high rates of success, especially when social outlets are emphasized and cohort supports are available. A significant concern is the lack of programs designed specifically for older people, particularly older women, whose concerns are very different from those of a younger population who abuse drugs or alcohol. Only 7% of substance abuse treatment facilities in the United States in 2006 reported that they have a specific program on group designed specifically for older adults (Han et al., 2006). Health status, availability of transportation, and mobility impairments further may limit access to treatment.

Epstein and colleagues (2007) suggest the development of treatment sites in senior centers, and assisted living facilities. A telemedicine-based collaborative care model using nursing care management may be another alternative (Fortney et al., 2007). Additional information on late-life addictions can be found in the Substance Abuse Among Older Adults Treatment Improvement Protocol (TIP), available at www.samhsa.gov. Videos about Problem Drinking in Older Adults are available at http://nihseniorhealth.gov/videolist.html (See evolve resources).

Acute Alcohol Withdrawal

When there is significant physical dependence, withdrawal from alcohol can become a life-threatening emergency. Detoxification should be done in an inpatient setting because of the potential medical complications and because withdrawal symptoms in older adults can be prolonged. Older people who drink are at risk of experiencing acute alcohol withdrawal if admitted to the hospital for treatment of acute illnesses or emergencies. All patients admitted to acute care settings should be screened for alcohol use and assessed for signs and symptoms of alcohol-related problems. Older people with a long history of consuming excess alcohol, previous episodes of acute withdrawal, and/or a history of prior detoxification are at increased risk of acute alcohol withdrawal (Letizia & Reinboltz, 2005).

Symptoms of acute alcohol withdrawal vary but may be more severe and last longer in older people. Minor withdrawal (withdrawal tremulousness) begins 6 to 12 hours after a patient has consumed the last drink. Symptoms include tremor, anxiety, nausea, insomnia, tachycardia, and increased blood pressure and frequently may be mistaken for common problems in older adults. Major withdrawal is seen 10 to 72 hours after cessation of alcohol intake, and symptoms include vomiting, diaphoresis, hallucinations, tremors, and seizures (Letizia & Reinboltz, 2005).

Delirium tremens (DTs) is the term used to describe alcohol withdrawal delirium; it usually occurs 24 to 72 hours after the last drink but may occur up to 10 days later. DTs occur in 5% of patients with acute alcohol withdrawal and is considered a medical emergency, with a mortality rate from respiratory failure and cardiac arrhythmia as high as 15%. Other signs and symptoms include confusion, disorientation, hallucinations, hyperthermia, and hypertension. The Clinical Institute Withdrawal Assessment (CIWA) scale is recommended as a valid and reliable screening instrument (www.pubs.niaa.nih.gov) (Letizia & Reinboltz, 2005).

Recommended treatment is the use of short-acting benzodiazepines at one half to one third the normal dose around the clock or as needed during withdrawal. Disulfiram use in older adults to promote abstinence is not recommended because of the potential for serious cardiovascular complications. The use of oral or intravenous alcohol to prevent or treat withdrawal is not established.

The CIWA aids in medication adjustments. Other interventions include assessing mental status, monitoring vital signs, and maintaining fluid balance without overhydrating. Calm and quiet surroundings, no unnecessary stimuli, consistent caregivers, frequent reorientation, prevention of injury, and support and caring are additional suggested interventions. Nutritional assessment is indicated, as well as addition of a multivitamin containing folic acid, pyridoxine, niacin, vitamin A, and thiamine (Letizia & Reinboltz, 2005).

Other Substance Abuse Concerns

A more common concern seen among older people is the misuse of prescription and OTC medications. Drug misuse is defined as use of a drug for reasons other than those for which it was prescribed. Older people are prescribed more than 33% of all prescription drugs, and the nonmedical use of prescription drugs is increasing in people over age 60. The negative effects of polypharmacy are often increased by an older person's use of alcohol (Naegle, 2008). Dependence on sedative, hypnotic, or anxiolytic drugs, often prescribed for anxiety or insomnia, and taken for many years with resulting dependence, is especially problematic for older women, who are more likely than men to receive prescriptions for these drugs (Epstein et al., 2007; Kolanowski & Piven, 2006). Benzodiazepines represent 17% to 23% of drugs prescribed to older adults (Morgan et al., 2005). Opiates are ranked second only to benzodiazepines among abused prescription drugs in the older adult population (Naegle, 2008). Increases in illness and mortality are associated with misusing prescription and nonprescription medications, although this is not considered a disorder by the *DSM-IV*. Chapter 11 discusses appropriate assessment and treatment of insomnia, and anxiety treatment was discussed earlier in this chapter.

Some of the reasons for the abuse of psychoactive prescription medications may be inappropriate prescribing and ineffective monitoring of response and follow-up. In many instances, older people are given prescriptions for benzodiazepines or sedatives because of complaints of insomnia or nervousness, without adequate assessment for depression, anxiety, or other conditions that may be causing the symptoms. Older people may not be informed of the side effects of these medications, including interactions, with alcohol, dependence, and withdrawal symptoms. More importantly, conditions such as anxiety and depression may not be recognized and treated appropriately.

Risk, prevention, assessment, and treatment of alcohol and substance abuse have not been sufficiently studied among older people. Diagnostic criteria to identify alcohol and prescription drug misuse among older adults, particularly older women and culturally and ethnically diverse elders, also need further investigation. Nurses in contact with older adults in institutionalized and community settings must be competent in assessment for mental health disorders as well as in screening, assessment, and counseling about the use of alcohol and prescribed, illicit, and OTC drug use. Providing education to older people and their families and referring to specialists and community resources are also important nursing roles and essential to "best practices" (Naegle, 2008, p. 661).

---

evolve To access your student resources, go to *http://evolve.elsevier.com/Ebersole/TwdHlthAging*

KEY CONCEPTS

- The prevalence of mental health disorders is expected to increase significantly with the aging of the baby boomers.
- Mental health disorders are underreported and underdiagnosed among older adults. Somatic complaints are often the presenting symptoms of mental health disorders, making diagnosis difficult.
- The incidence of psychotic disorders with late-life onset is low among older people, but psychotic manifestations can occur as secondary symptoms in a variety of disorders, the most common being Alzheimer's disease. Psychotic symptoms in Alzheimer's disease necessitate different assessment and treatment than long-standing psychotic disorders.
- Anxiety disorders are common in late life, and re-establishing feelings of adequacy and control is the heart of crisis resolution and stress management.
- PTSD is finally being recognized in older adults who have been subjected to extremely traumatic events.

- Depression is the most common emotional disorder of aging and likewise the most treatable. Unfortunately, it is often neglected or assumed to be a condition of aging that one must "learn to live with." An important nursing intervention is screening for depression.
- Suicide is a significant problem among older men. Assessment of suicidal intent is important especially in light of loss. Many come to be seen by the health care professional with physical complaints shortly before they commit suicide.
- Substance abuse, particularly alcohol, and misuse of prescription drugs are often underrecognized and undertreated problems of older adults, particularly older women. Screening and appropriate assessment and intervention are important in all settings.
- Further research is needed to fully understand the cultural and ethnic differences in mental health concerns, as well as appropriate assessment and treatment in culturally and ethnically diverse older people.

CASE STUDY   BIPOLAR DISORDER

Myra is a 71-year-old white woman who was admitted to the geropsychiatry inpatient unit for alcohol abuse and noncompliance with her lithium, which had been prescribed for a diagnosed bipolar disorder. Myra's primary mode of coping with her depression and mood swings has been to drink alcohol, meet abusive men, and play bingo. However, when she stops taking her dose of lithium, she begins to have flights of ideas, argues with her daughters, and tries to pick up men in her apartment complex. After seeing her at home, you discover that she has a long history of being physically abused by her husband, now deceased for eight years, and has been living with one daughter who also has emotionally and physically abused her, causing her to be hospitalized. Myra's ability to test reality is compromised because of years of denial and low self-esteem. She says, "I used to have lots of times when I felt really good in between the depressions. Now I feel depressed most of the time." She tells you that her daughters harass her and interfere in her life. Your goals as a community-based nurse are to facilitate her independence (being able to live in her own apartment), to assist her with medication compliance, and to intervene with Myra to improve relationships with her daughters. Home visits are approved through Medicare for two months after hospital discharge.

Based on the case study, develop a nursing care plan using the following procedure*:

Continued

CASE STUDY—CONT'D

- List Myra's comments that provide subjective data.
- List information that provides objective data.
- From these data, identify and state, using accepted format, two nursing diagnoses you determine are most significant to Myra at this time. List two of Myra's strengths that you have identified from the data.
- Determine and state outcome criteria for each diagnosis. These criteria must reflect some alleviation of the problem identified in the nursing diagnosis and must be stated in concrete and measurable terms.
- Plan and state one or more interventions for each diagnosed problem. Provide specific documentation of the sources used to determine the appropriate intervention. Plan at least one intervention that incorporates Myra's existing strengths.
- Evaluate the success of the intervention. Interventions must correlate directly with the stated outcome criteria to measure the outcome success.

CRITICAL THINKING QUESTIONS

1. How will you evaluate Myra's ability to live independently?
2. What particular strategies are necessary to meet the goals of the nursing care plan?
3. Given that Myra's primary coping strategy is drinking alcohol, how will you facilitate her sobriety and help her deal with stress?
4. How much involvement with Myra's daughters do you believe is necessary to assist with her transition back into her own apartment?
5. Given the limited number of visits covered by Medicare, what information does Myra need to provide self-care? In other words, the nurse must be teaching Myra how to live independently after discharge from home health care. What does Myra need to know?
6. Discuss the meanings and the thoughts triggered by the student's and the elder's viewpoints expressed at the beginning of the chapter. How do these vary from your own experience?

*Students are advised to refer to their nursing diagnosis text and identify possible or potential problems.

CASE STUDY — DEPRESSIVE DISORDER WITH SUICIDAL THOUGHTS

Jake had cared for his wife Emma during a long and painful illness until she died four years ago. He found that alcohol provided a way to cope with the stress. Within a year after her death, Jake met a lady to whom he was very attracted, and a few months later she moved in with him. Jake managed to move his things around until some space was made for her personal items, but neither of them was very comfortable with this. He really did not like to move his things from their usual place and, because her allotted space was so small, she felt like an intruder. He collected guns, and she shuddered when she saw them. He was an avid fan of John Wayne movies, and she preferred going to the symphony. He liked meat and potatoes, and she was a vegetarian. She also disapproved of his increasing reliance on alcohol. The blending of two such different lifestyles proved difficult. In a few months she moved out, and Jake blamed himself. He said over and over, "I should have done more for her. I'm not good for anything anymore." His friends began to pull away from him, just when he needed them most, because he seemed to talk of nothing but his various aches, pains, and pills and his general discouragement with life. Jake's consumption of alcohol increased markedly. He had some health problems: a mild heart failure, a lack of exercise, dairy products gave him diarrhea, he was somewhat obese, and his knees were painful most of the time. He routinely visited his allergist, his internist, his orthopedist, and his cardiologist. However, it seemed the more he went to these specialists, the worse he felt. He was taking several medications, and each time he saw one of his clinicians, he came away with another prescription. No one asked about his drinking, and he never mentioned it. He awoke one morning feeling very dizzy, so he went to his internist later in the day. He began to share the litany of his discomforts, and the physician reminded him that at 76 years of age he could not expect to always feel in top shape.

When he returned from seeing the physician, Jake called his daughter and surprised her by saying he had just decided he would take a week off and go to Hawaii to see if the sun and sand would revive him. Jake was not usually impulsive. His daughter, fortunately, was a psychiatric nurse and was concerned about the change in his behavior.

Based on the case study, develop a nursing care plan using the following procedure*:

- List Jake's comments that provide subjective data.
- List information that provides objective data.
- From these data, identify and state, using accepted format, two nursing diagnoses you determine are most significant to Jake at this time. List two of Jake's strengths that you have identified from the data.
- Determine and state outcome criteria for each diagnosis. These criteria must reflect some alleviation of the problem identified in the nursing diagnosis and must be stated in concrete and measurable terms.

- Plan and state one or more interventions for each diagnosed problem. Provide specific documentation of the source used to determine the appropriate intervention. Plan at least one intervention that incorporates Jake's existing strengths.
- Evaluate the success of the intervention. Interventions must correlate directly with the stated outcome criteria to measure the outcome success.

CRITICAL THINKING QUESTIONS

1. Discuss the variations in symptoms of depression in the old and the young.
2. Describe some of the reasons that elders are more vulnerable to depression than younger people are.
3. Describe a time when you were depressed and the feelings you had. What did you do about it?
4. Given the situation in this case, discuss what your thoughts would be if you were Jake's daughter.
5. Given his daughter's background, what are her responsibilities in this case?
6. What is the responsibility of a student nurse in the case of suspected suicidal thoughts?
7. Would you address the possibility of suicidal thoughts if you were the nurse in the physician's office? When and how would you take on this task?
8. What action should be taken for Jake's protection?
9. Would you expect that Jake is still grieving over the death of his wife? What are your thoughts about this situation?
10. What are the clues or indications that an elder is thinking of committing suicide?
11. What are some of signs of suicidal intent in young adults? How are these signs different from those of elders?
12. Under what conditions do you think a person has a right to take his or her life?
13. What are your thoughts about Jake's use of alcohol?
14. Do you think suicide is a sign of weakness or strength?
15. Do you agree or disagree with the following statements based on the evidence about depression and suicide in older adults?
    - Normally older people feel depressed much of the time.
    - Older people are more likely than young people to admit to depression.
    - Most older people talk about suicide but rarely try to kill themselves.
    - Depression of the elderly is helped by medications.
    - Depression may be the cause of forgetfulness.
    - Depression in the elderly is often linked with illness and alcoholism.

*Students are advised to refer to their nursing diagnosis text and identify possible or potential problems.

RESEARCH QUESTIONS

1. What is the prevalence of mental health disorders in community-dwelling older adults? What mental health care is nursing able to provide in the home?
2. How common is alcohol abuse a strategy of self-care used by the older adult with emotional concerns?
3. What types of interventions are most appropriate for older adults with alcohol or drug abuse problems?
4. Is psychiatric home care a more cost-effective alternative than institutional care?
5. In what circumstances are antidepressants useful in grief reactions.
6. What are the cardinal symptoms of depression in the oldest-old?
7. How many physicians consider or evaluate for the presence of depression in elders who see them for physical complaints?
8. What are the most reliable tools for identifying depression in cognitively intact and cognitively impaired elders?
9. What is the meaning of depression in older people of different cultures and ethnicity?
10. What type of mental health assessment and interventions are culturally appropriate for diverse older people?

REFERENCES

American Association for Geriatric Psychiatry: Action alert: Medicare parity, 2008. Available at http://capwiz.com/aagp/issues/alert/?alertid=11593391. Accessed July 30, 2008.

American Psychiatric Association: *Diagnostic and statistical manual of mental disorders (DSM-IV)*, ed 4, Washington, DC, 2000, The Association.

American Psychological Association: Growing mental and behavioral health concerns facing older Americans. Available at www.apa.org. about/gr/issues/aging/growing-concerns.aspx. Accessed August 1, 2010.

Arean P, Ayalon L, Hunkeler E, et al: Improving depression care for older minority patients in primary care, *Medical Care* 43:381, 2005.

Ayalon L, Fialová D, Areán PA, et al: Challenges associated with the recognition and treatment of depression in older recipients of home care services, *International Psychogeriatrics* 22:514, 2010.

Ayers C, Loebach J, Wetherell E, et al: Treating late-life anxiety, *Psychiatric Times* 23:1, 2006. Available at www.psychiatrictimes.com/display/article/10168/46976?pageNumber=1. Accessed June 27, 2008.

Berry K, Barrowclough C: The needs of older adults with schizophrenia: implications for psychological interventions, *Clinical Psychology Review* 29:68, 2009.

Bludau J: Second institutionalization: impact of personal history on patients with dementia, *Caring Ages* 3:3, 2002.

Bormann J, Thorp S, Wetherell J, et al: A spirituality based group intervention for combat veterans with posttraumatic stress disorder: feasibility study, *Journal of Holistic Nursing* 26:109, 2008.

Brown E, Raue P, Halpert K: Evidence-based guideline: Detection of depression in older adults with dementia, *Journal of Gerontological Nursing* 35:11, 2009.

Brown E, Raue P, Halpert K: Detection of depression in older adults with dementia. In M.G. Titler (series editor), *Series on evidence-based practice for older adults*. Iowa City: The University of Iowa Gerontological Nursing Interventions Research Center, Research Translation and Dissemination Core, 2007.

Byers A, Yaffe K, Covinsky K, et al: High occurrence of mood and anxiety disorders among older adults, *Archives of General Psychiatry* 67:489, 2010.

Byrd E: Nursing assessment and treatment of depressive disorders of late life. In Mellilo K, Houde S, editors: *Geropsychiatric and mental health nursing*, Sudbury, Mass., 2005, Jones & Bartlett.

Callahan C, Kroenke K, Counsell S, et al: Treatment of depression improves physical functioning in older adults, *Journal of the American Geriatrics Society* 53:367, 2005.

Centers for Medicare and Medicaid Services: Medicare and your mental health benefits. Available at http://www.medicare.gov/Publications/Pubs/pdf/10184.pdf. Accessed August 1, 2010.

Chang C, Roberts B: Strategies for feeding patients with dementia, *A American Journal of Nursing* 111(4), 2011.available at ajnonline.com (May 15, 2011).

Chaudhary M, Rabheru K: Paranoid symptoms among older adults, *Geriatrics and Aging* 11:143, 2008.

Chizobam A, Bazargan M, Hindman D, et al: Depression symptomatology and diagnosis: Discordance between patients and physicians in primary care settings, *BioMed Central Family Practice* 9, 2008. Available at http://www.biomedcentral.com/1471-2296/9/1/abstract. Accessed July 17, 2008.

Corna L, Cairney J, Streiner D: Suicide ideation in older adults: relationship to mental health problems and service use, *The Gerontologist*, 50(6):785-797, 2010.

Culberson J: Alcohol use in the elderly: beyond the CAGE. Part 1 of 2: prevalence and patterns of problem drinking, *Geriatrics* 61:23, 2006a.

Culberson J: Alcohol use in the elderly: beyond the CAGE. Part 2 of 2: screening instruments and treatment strategies, *Geriatrics* 61:20, 2006b.

Das B, Greenspan M, Muralee S, et al: Late-life depression: a review, *Clinical Geriatrics* 15:35, 2007.

Davis B: Assessing adults with mental disorders in primary care, the nurse practitioner, *American Journal of Primary Health Care* 29:19, 2004.

Demers L, Robichaud L, Gelinas I, et al: Coping strategies and social participation in older adults, *Gerontology* 55:233, 2009.

Edelstein B, Heisel M, McKee D, et al: Development and psychometric evaluation of the Reasons for Living—Older Adults Scale: A suicide risk assessment inventory, *The Gerontologist* 49:736, 2009.

Epstein E, Fischer-Elber K, Al-Otaiba Z: Women, aging, and alcohol use disorders, *Journal of Women & Aging* 19:31, 2007.

Evans L: Mental health issues in aging. 2008. The Hartford Institute for Geriatric Nursing. Available at http://hartfordign.org/uploads/File/gnec_state_of_science_papers/gnec_mental_health.pdf.

Erikson EH, Erikson JM, Kivnick HQ: *Vital involvement in old age: the experience of old age in our time*, New York, 1986, WW Norton.

Finfgeld-Connett DL: Treatment of substance misuse in older women: using a brief intervention model, *Journal of Gerontological Nursing* 30:31, 2004.

Finfgeld-Connett DL: Self-management of alcohol problems among older adults, *Journal of Gerontological Nursing* 31:51, 2005.

Flood M, Buckwalter K: Recommendations for the mental health care of older adults: Part 1—An overview of depression and anxiety, *Journal of Gerontological Nursing* 35:26, 2009.

Fortney J, Pyne J, Edlund M, et al: A randomized trial of telemedicine-based collaborative care for depression, *Journal of General Internal Medicine* 22:1086, 2007.

Friedman M, Kennedy G, Williams K: Cognitive camouflage—how Alzheimer's can mask mental illness, *Aging Well* 2:16, 2009.

Gonzalez H, Vega W, Williams D, et al: Depression care in the United States: Too little too few, *Archives of General Psychiatry* 67:37, 2010.

Grabowski D, Aschbrenner K, Tome V, et al: Quality of mental health care for nursing home residents: A literature review, *Medical Care Research and Review*, published on-line March 11, 2010, doi 10.1177/1077558710362538. (website): http://mcr.sagepub.com/content/early/2010/03/11/1077558710362538. Accessed August 6, 2010.

Grossberg GT: Diagnosis and treatment of late-life psychosis in the elderly, *Long-Term Care Forum* 1:7, 2000.

Gruber-Baldini A, Boustani M, Sloane P, et al: Behavioral symptoms in residential care/assisted living facilities: prevalence, risk factors, and medication management, *Journal of the American Geriatrics Society* 52:1610, 2004.

Ham R, Sloane R, Warshaw G, et al: *Primary care geriatrics: A case-based approach*, ed 5, St Louis, 2007, Mosby.

Han B, Gfroerer J, Swindle J, Penne M: Substance abuse disorder among older adults in the US in 2010, *Addiction* 104:88-96, 2009.

Heller K, Viken R, Swindle R: Screening for depression in African American and Caucasian older women, *Aging & Mental Health* 14:339, 2010.

Hildon Z, Montgomery S, Blane D, et al: Examining resilience of quality of life in the face of health-related and psychosocial adversity at older ages: What is "right" about the way we age? *The Gerontologist* 50:36, 2009.

Holt-Lunstad J, Smith T, Layton J: Social relationships and mortality risk: A meta-analytic review, *Public Library of Science Medicine* 7:2, 2010.

Institute of Medicine: Retooling for an aging America: Building the healthcare workforce, 2008. Available at http://www.iom.edu/Reports/2008/Retooling-for-an-Aging-America-Building-the-Health-Care-Workforce.aspx. Accessed June 7, 2010.

Jalbert J, Quilliam B, Lapane K: A profile of concurrent alcohol and alcohol-interactive prescription drug use in the US population, *Journal of General Internal Medicine* 23:1318, 2008.

Joe S, Baser R, Breeden G et al: Prevalence of and risk factors for lifetime suicide risks among blacks in the United States, *Journal of the American Medical Association* 296:2112, 2006.

Kennedy GJ: Bipolar disorder in late life: depression, *Primary Psychiatry* 15:30, 2008.

Kirchner J, Zubritsky C, Cody M, et al: Alcohol consumption among older adults in primary care, *Journal of General Internal Medicine* 22:92, 2007.

Kobasa SC: Stressful life events, personality, and health: An inquiry into hardiness, *Journal of Personality and Social Psychology* 37:1, 1979.

Kolanowski A, Piven M: Geropsychiatric nursing: The state of the science, *Journal of the American Psychiatric Nurses Association* 12:75, 2006.

Kurlowicz L, Harvath T: Depression. In Capezuti E, Swicker D, Mezey M, et al., editors: *Evidence-based geriatric nursing protocols for best practice*, ed 3, New York, 2008a, Springer.

Kurlowicz L, Harvath T: *Depression: nursing standard of practice protocol*, New York, 2008b, Hartford Institute for Geriatric Nursing. Available at www.consultgerirn.org. Accessed August 5, 2010.

Lavretsky H, Alstein L, Olmstead R, Ercoli L, et al: Complementary Use of Tai Chi Chih Augments Escitalopram Treatment of Geriatric Depression, *American Journal of Geriatric Psychiatry* March 6, 2011.

Lazarus R, Folkman S: *Stress appraisal and coping*, New York, 1984, Springer.

Letizia M, Reinboltz M: Identifying and managing acute alcohol withdrawal in the elderly, *Geriatric Nursing* 26:176, 2005.

Leutwyler H, Wallhagen M: Understanding physical health of older adults with schizophrenia: building and eroding trust, *Journal of Gerontological Nursing* 36:38, 2010.

Madhusoodanan S, Brenner R: Caring for the chronically mentally ill in nursing homes, *Annals of Long-Term Care* 15:29, 2007.

Masters J: Moderate alcohol consumption and unappreciated risk for alcohol-related harm among ethnically diverse urban-dwelling elders, *Geriatric Nursing* 24:155, 2003.

Mellilo K, Hoff L, Huff M: Geropsychiatric nursing as a subspecialty. In Mellilo K, Houde S, editors: *Geropsychiatric and mental health nursing*, New York, 2005, Springer.

Mentes J, Bail J: Psychosis in older adults. In Mellilo K, Houde S, editors: *Geropsychiatric and mental health nursing*, Sudbury, Mass., 2005, Jones & Bartlett.

Merrick E, Hodgkins D, Garnick D, et al: Unhealthy drinking patterns in older adults: prevalence and associated characteristics, *Journal of the American Geriatrics Society* 56:214, 2008.

Miklowitz DF, Otto MW, Frank E, et al: Psychosocial treatments for bipolar depression: A 1-year randomized trial from the Systematic Treatment Enhancement Program (STEP), *Archives of General Psychiatry* 64:419, 2007.

Moos R, Brennan P, Schutte K, et al: Older adults' coping with negative life events: common processes of managing health, interpersonal, and financial/work stressors, *International Journal of Aging and Human Development* 62:39, 2006.

Morgan B, White D, Wallace A: Substance abuse in older adults. In Mellilo K, Houde S, editors: *Geropsychiatric and mental health nursing*, Sudbury, Mass., 2005, Jones & Bartlett.

Morley J: Depression in nursing home residents, *Journal of the American Medical Directors Association* 5:301, 2010.

Naegle M: Substance misuse and alcohol use disorders. In Capezuti E, Swicker D, Mezey M, et al., editors: *Evidence-based geriatric nursing protocols for best practice*, ed 3, New York, 2008, Springer.

National Institute of Mental Health: How do older adults experience depression? 2008. Available at www.nimh.nih.gov. Accessed October 2, 2008.

Ortiz I, Romero L: Cultural implications for assessment and treatment of depression in Hispanic elderly individuals, *Annals of Long-Term Care* 16:45, 2008.

Phillips J, Robin A, Nugent C, Idler E: Understanding recent changes in suicide rates among middle-aged: period or cohort effects, *Public Health Reports*, 125(5):680-688, 2010.

Qualls S: Defining mental health in later life, *Generations* 26:9, 2002.

Qureshi S, Kimbrell T, Pyne J, et al: Greater prevalence and incidence of dementia in older veterans with posttraumatic stress disorder, *Journal of the American Geriatrics Society* 58:1627, 2010.

Resnick B, Inguito P: The resilience scale: psychometric properties and clinical applicability in older adults, *Archives of Psychiatric Nursing* 2010 (in press). Available at www.sciencedirect.com

Rogerson M, Emes C: Fostering resilience within an adult day program, *Activities, Adaptation & Aging* 32:1, 2008.

Saur C, Steffens D, Harpole L, et al: Satisfaction and outcomes of depressed older adults with psychiatric clinical nurse specialists in primary care, *Journal of the American Psychiatric Nurses Association* 13:62, 2007.

Schneider LS, Tariot P, Dagerman K, et al: Effectiveness of atypical antipsychotic drugs in patients with Alzheimer's disease, *New England Journal of Medicine* 355:1525, 2006.

Seekles W, van Straten A, Beekman A, et al: Stepped care for depression and anxiety: from primary care to specialized mental health care: a randomized controlled trial testing the effectiveness of a stepped care program among primary care patients with mood or anxiety disorders, *BMC Health Services Research* 9:90, 2009. Available at www.biomedcentral.com/1472-6963/9/90. Accessed August 5, 2010.

Shellman J, Mokel M, Wright B: "Keeping the bully out": understanding older African Americans' beliefs and attitudes toward depression, *Journal of the American Psychiatric Nurses Association* 13:230, 2007.

Sherrod T, Quinlan-Colwell A, Lattimore T, et al: Older adults with bipolar disorder: guidelines for primary care providers, *Journal of Gerontological Nursing* 36:20, 2010.

Simrey J, Bruce M, Carpenter M, Booker D: Depression symptons and suicided ideation among older adults receiving home delivering meals, *International Journal of Geriatic Psychiatry*, 23(12):1306-1311, 2008.

Smith M: Nursing assessment and treatment of anxiety in late life. In Mellilo K, Houde S, editors: *Geropsychiatric and mental health nursing*, Sudbury, Mass., 2005, Jones & Bartlett.

Smith M: Collaborative care models for late-life depression and anxiety: roles for nurses, *Journal of Gerontological Nursing* 36:3, 2010.

Splete H: Mentally ill eclipse residents with dementia, *Caring for the Ages* 10(12):11, 2009.

Thakur M, Blazer D: Depression in long-term care, *Journal of the American Medical Directors Association* 9:82, 2008.

Thielke S, Diehr P, Unutzer J: Prevalence, incidence, and persistence of major depressive symptoms in the Cardiovascular Health Study, *Aging & Mental Health* 14:168, 2010.

Thorp S, Ayers C, Nuevo R, et al: Meta-analysis comparing different behavioral treatments for late-life anxiety, *American Journal of Geriatric Psychiatry* 17:105, 2009.

Unutzer J, Katon W, Callahan C, et al: Long-term cost effects of collaborative care for late-life depression, *American Journal of Managed Care* 14:95, 2008.

Unutzer J: Late-life depression, *New England Journal of Medicine* 357:2269, 2007.

Unutzer J, Katon W, Callahan C, et al: Collaborative care management of late-life depression in the primary care setting, *Journal of the American Medical Association* 288:2836, 2002.

Substance Abuse and Mental Health Services Administration: Substance abuse by older adults: estimates of future impact on the treatment system. Available at www.oas.samsha.gov. Accessed August 12, 2010.

Wetherell J, Maser J, Balkom A: Anxiety disorders in the elderly: outdated beliefs and a research agenda, *Acta Psychiatrica Scandinavica* 111:401, 2005 (editorial).

Vance D, Struzick T, Masten J: Hardiness, successful aging, and HIV: implications for social work, *Journal of Gerontological Social Work* 51:260, 2008.

Yancura L, Aldwin C: Coping and health in older adults, *Current Psychiatry Reports* 10:10, 2008.

Zauszniewski J, Bekhet A, Lai C, McDonald P, Musil C: Effects of teaching resourcefulness and acceptance of affect, behavior, and cognition of chronically ill elders, *Issues in Mental Health Nursing* 28:575-592, 2007.

Cognitive Impairment

Theris A. Touhy

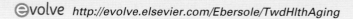

evolve *http://evolve.elsevier.com/Ebersole/TwdHlthAging*

A STUDENT SPEAKS

I imagine I am in my late eighties and my husband and I live with our daughter. I am experiencing an unpleasant physical change; I am losing my memory. I can sharply remember all details about events that happened a long time ago but often fail to recall what happened two hours ago. Although this situation scares me and I wonder what will happen if my family gets tired of my forgetfulness, I remind myself that I live with the people who love and care for me very much and will not desert me when I need them the most.

Tatyana, age 30

AN ELDER SPEAKS

It has been quite a relief to be in this retirement community . . . everyone here forgets names and words, and I don't feel alone when I'm forgetful.

Liz, age 84

LEARNING OBJECTIVES

On completion of this chapter, the reader will be able to:

1. Discuss concepts related to cognition and memory in later life.
2. Differentiate between delirium, dementia, and depression.
3. Discuss nursing interventions for prevention and treatment of delirium.
4. Identify potential risk and modifying factors for the development of dementia.
5. Discuss the different types of dementia and appropriate diagnosis.

6. Describe nursing models of care for persons with dementia.
7. Discuss common concerns in care of persons with dementia and nursing responses.
8. Discuss strategies to enhance quality of life for caregivers of persons with dementia.
9. Develop a nursing care plan for an individual with cognitive impairment.

This chapter focuses on cognition in aging, the diseases that affect cognition, and nursing care of older adults with cognitive impairment. We remain oriented to the healthy aging model while we examine each of the states of mentation in late life as having the potential for comfort and pleasures. All elders are deserving of active nursing intervention to maintain the highest practicable level of function and quality of life.

We have artificially separated cognitive function from mental health, though they are in most ways interdependent. The mind is in some ways limited by the capacities of the brain, yet just as in medicine, there is a danger of evaluating the person by the measured and tested efficiency of cells and organs. Nowhere is this more important than in examining the cognition of older people. Citing John Morris, professor of neurology at Washington University in St. Louis, Crowley (1996) says that if brain

function becomes impaired in old age, it is a result of disease, not aging.

Cognitive health and health promotion activities to maintain brain health are discussed in Chapter 2; cognitive assessment instruments in Chapter 7; and communication with persons experiencing cognitive impairment in Chapter 6.

ADULT COGNITION

Cognition is the process of acquiring, storing, sharing, and using information. Components of cognitive function include language, thought, memory, executive function, judgment, attention, and perception (Desai et al., 2010). The determination of intellectual capacity and performance has been the focus of a major portion of gerontological research. Cognitive functions may remain stable, or decline with increasing age. The cognitive functions that remain stable include attention span, language skills, communication skills, comprehension and discourse, and visual perception. The cognitive skills that decline are verbal fluency, logical analysis, selective attention, object naming, and complex visuospatial skills.

Early studies about cognition and aging were cross-sectional rather than longitudinal and were often conducted with older adults who were institutionalized or had coexisting illnesses. It has been generally believed that cognitive function declines in old age because of a decreased number of neurons, decreased brain size, and diminished brain weight. Although these losses are features of aging, they are not consistent with deteriorating mental function, nor do they interfere with everyday routines. Neuron loss occurs mainly in the brain and spinal cord and is most pronounced in the cerebral cortex. The neuronal dendrites atrophy with aging, resulting in impairment of the synapses and changes in the transmission of the chemical neurotransmitters dopamine, serotonin, and acetylcholine. This causes a slowing of many neural processes. However, overall cognitive abilities remain intact.

The aging brain maintains resiliency or the ability to compensate for age-related changes. The old adage "use it or lose it" applies to cognitive as well as physical health. Stimulating the brain increases brain tissue formation, enhances synaptic regulation of messages, and enhances the development of cognitive reserve (CR). CR is based on the concept of neuroplasticity, which is the capacity of the brain to change in response to various stimuli, such as daily stressors and activities. Neuroplasticity was once thought to decrease with age, but current literature suggests that cognitive performance can be enhanced with mental stimulation. Maximizing the potential benefits of brain plasticity and CR requires engaging in challenging cognitive, sensory, and motor activities, as well as meaningful social interactions, on a regular basis throughout life.

High CR may allow the individual to continue to learn and adapt to changing stimuli, despite the presence of age-related changes. CR is probably set early in the first two to three decades of life, and stimulating environments, education, and healthy lifestyles throughout life appear to enhance cognitive reserve. CR affects the ability of the adult brain to sustain normal function in the face of significant disease or injury. Brain diseases and injuries may be less apparent in those with greater CR because they are able to tolerate lost neurons and synapses (Desai et al., 2010; Yevchak et al., 2008). For example, individuals who attained more years of education may have high levels of Alzheimer's disease pathology, but few, if any, clinical symptoms.

There are many myths about aging and the brain that may be believed by both health professionals and older adults. It is important to understand cognition and memory in late life and dispel the myths that can have a negative effect on wellness and may, in fact, contribute to unnecessary cognitive decline (Box 19-1).

The cognitive development of older people is often measured against the norms of young or middle-aged people, which may not be appropriate to the distinctive characteristics of older adults. In addition, most tests of cognitive ability were designed to test young children, and most do not address cultural or

---

BOX 19-1	MYTHS ABOUT AGING AND THE BRAIN

MYTH: People lose brain cells every day and eventually just run out.
FACT: Most areas of the brain do not lose brain cells. Although you may lose some nerve connections, it can be part of the reshaping of the brain that comes with experience.
MYTH: You can't change your brain.
FACT: The brain is constantly changing in response to experiences and learning, and it retains this "plasticity" well into aging. Changing our way of thinking causes corresponding changes in the brain systems involved, that is, your brain believes what you tell it.
MYTH: The brain doesn't make new brain cells.
FACT: Certain areas of the brain including the hippocampus (where new memories are created) and the olfactory bulb (scent-processing center) regularly generate new brain cells.
MYTH: Memory decline is inevitable as we age.
FACT: Many people reach old age and have no memory problems. Participation in physical exercise, stimulating mental activity, socialization, healthy diet, and stress management help maintain brain health. The incidence of dementia does increase with age, but when there are changes in memory, older people need to be evaluated for possible causes and receive treatment.
MYTH: There is no point in trying to teach older adults anything since "you can't teach an old dog new tricks."
FACT: Basic intelligence remains unchanged with age, and older adults should be provided with opportunities for continued learning. Minimizing barriers to learning, such as hearing and vision loss, and applying principles of geragogy enhance learning ability.

Adapted from American Association of Retired Persons: Myths about aging and the brain, 2007. Accessed January 5, 2010, from http://www.aarp.org/health/brain-health/info-2006/myths_about_aging_and_the_brain.html.

---

ethnic differences. Other reasons have been advanced for the variations of intellectual performance of the older adult being tested (Box 19-2). Therefore, these tests may have little relevance for the daily function of older people. Intelligence in old age is dynamic, and certain abilities change and even improve with age.

Fluid and Crystallized Intelligence

Fluid intelligence (often called native intelligence) consists of skills that are biologically determined, independent of experience or learning. It is associated with flexibility in thinking, inductive reasoning, abstract thinking, and integration. Fluid intelligence "enables people to identify and draw conclusions about complex relationships" (Miller, 2008, p. 187). Crystallized intelligence is composed of knowledge and abilities that the person acquires through education and life. Measures of crystallized intelligence include verbal meaning, word association, social judgment, and number skills. Older people perform more poorly on performance scales (fluid intelligence), but scores on verbal scales (crystallized intelligence) remain stable. This is known as the classic aging pattern (Hooyman and Kiyak, 2011). The tendency to do poorly on performance tasks may be related to age-related changes in sensory and perceptual abilities as well as psychomotor skills. Speed of cognitive processing and slower reaction time also affect performance.

Late adulthood is no longer seen as a period when growth has ceased and cognitive development halted; rather it is seen as a life stage programmed for plasticity and the development of unique capacities. Older people do maintain their ability to

BOX 19-2 COMPLEXITIES OF ACCURATELY ASSESSING INTELLECT IN OLD AGE

- The old are most frequently compared with college students, whose chief occupation is proving their intellectual capacity.
- Young adults are in the habit of being tested and have developed test wisdom, a skill never developed by the older adult or one that has grown rusty with disuse.
- Test material may not be relevant to the world of older adults, especially those of different cultures.
- The ability to concentrate is inversely related to anxiety.
- Intellectual function declines differentially. The old are assumed deficient in encoding during learning, storing information for retention, and/or speed of retrieving stored information.
- Older people always perform more slowly than younger people in tasks involving neuromuscular learning because of slower reaction time and an increase in cautious behavior.
- Older people often perform poorly on test items because they are less likely to guess and more likely not to answer any items that seem ambiguous to them.

- Cautiousness has often been described as the reason older adults do not perform as well as younger people in memory tasks. Other personality traits, such as less impulsiveness and greater emotional stability, also seem to influence how well older people perform on memory tests.
- Older people may have difficulty focusing attention and ignoring irrelevant stimuli.
- Subject attrition in longitudinal studies of older adults shows evidence of the survival of the intellectually superior.
- No evidence suggests general slowing of central nervous system activity in old age as had been commonly presumed and reported by researchers.
- Intellectual performance relying on verbal functions shows little or no decline with age, but speeded tests using nonverbal psychomotor functions show a great decline.
- Social cognition and social context are related in terms of the function of older adults. Older adults who maintain the best cognitive function are also those with a high social interactional level.

understand situations and learn from new experiences. These findings are significant to satisfaction in late life, because the capacity for effective lifestyle management and one's cognitive resources contribute to adaptation and enjoyment. Chapter 6 discusses learning in later life and presents effective teaching-learning strategies.

Memory

Memory is defined as the ability to retain or store information and retrieve it when needed. Memory is a complex set of processes and storage systems. Three components characterize memory: immediate recall; short-term memory (which may range from minutes to days); and remote or long-term memory. Biological, functional, environmental, and psychosocial influences affect memory development throughout adulthood. Recall of newly encountered information seems to decrease with age, and memory declines are noted in connection with complex tasks and strategies. Even though some older adults show decrements in the ability to process information, reaction time, perception, and capacity for attentional tasks, the majority of functioning remains intact and sufficient.

Familiarity, previous learning, and life experience compensate for the minor loss of efficiency in the basic neurological processes. In unfamiliar, stressful, or demanding situations, however, these changes may be more marked. Normal older adults may complain of memory problems, but their symptoms do not meet the criteria for mild cognitive impairment (MCI) or dementia. The term *age-associated memory impairment (AAMI)* has been used to describe memory loss that is considered normal in light of a person's age and educational level. This may include a general slowness in processing, storing, and recalling new information, and difficulty remembering names and words. However, these concerns can cause great anxiety in older adults who may fear dementia. Many medical or psychiatric difficulties (depression, anxiety) also influence memory abilities, and it is important for older adults with memory complaints to have a comprehensive evaluation.

Cognitive stimulation and memory training may be helpful for cognitively intact older adults, as well as for those with cognitive impairment (Camp and Skrajner, 2004; Yevchak et al.,

2008). Cognitive stimulation and memory training techniques include mnemonics (strategies to enhance coding, storage, and recall), internal and external aids, reasoning and speed-of-processing training, cognitive games (e.g., Scrabble, chess, crossword puzzles), and spaced retrieval techniques. Many games and aids are available that may be useful to enhance memory and stimulate cognitive function. Continued attention to diet, exercise, cardiovascular risk factors, and meaningful activities are also important to brain health (Chapter 2 and Table 19-3).

Cognitive Impairment

Cognitive impairment (CI) is a term that describes a range of disturbances in cognitive functioning, including disturbances in memory, orientation, attention, and concentration. Other disturbances of cognition may affect intelligence, judgment, learning ability, perception, problem solving, psychomotor ability, reaction time, and social intactness.

Cognitive Assessment

An older person with a change in cognitive function needs a thorough assessment to identify the presence of specific pathological conditions. Pathological conditions causing impairment of cognition include delirium, dementia, and depression. The literature reveals that both physicians and nurses in all settings routinely fail to appropriately assess an individual's cognitive functioning. Pathological conditions are often undiagnosed, reversible causes not identified, and opportunities for early intervention missed. As a result, the person experiences greater impairment and functional decline (Braes et al., 2008).

Some of the reasons for this include the complexity of cognitive assessment and the existence of several conditions with similar symptoms (dementia, depression, delirium) (Table 19-1). Other reasons include the often atypical symptom presentation in older adults and the belief, on the part of health care professionals as well as older people, that alterations in cognitive functioning are part of the "normal" aspects of aging (Braes et al., 2008; Evans, 2007; Fletcher, 2008). Older people may be diagnosed with dementia as a result of an occurrence of confusion or altered mental status without a comprehensive evaluation. Older adults should be routinely and regularly

TABLE 19-1	DIFFERENTIATING DELIRIUM, DEPRESSION, AND DEMENTIA		
CHARACTERISTIC	**DELIRIUM**	**DEPRESSION**	**DEMENTIA**
Onset	Sudden, abrupt	Recent, may relate to life change	Insidious, slow, over years and often unrecognized until deficits obvious
Course over 24 hours	Fluctuating, often worse at night	Fairly stable, may be worse in the morning	Fairly stable, may see changes with stress
Consciousness	Reduced	Clear	Clear
Alertness	Increased, decreased, or variable	Normal	Generally normal
Psychomotor activity	Increased, decreased, or mixed Sometimes increased, other times decreased	Variable, agitation or retardation	Normal, may have apraxia or agnosia
Duration	Hours to weeks	Variable and may be chronic	Years
Attention	Disordered, fluctuates	Little impairment	Generally normal but may have trouble focusing
Orientation	Usually impaired, fluctuates	Usually normal; may answer "I don't know" to questions or may not try to answer	Often impaired; may make up answers or answer close to the right thing or may confabulate but tries to answer
Speech	Often incoherent, slow, or rapid; may call out repeatedly or repeat the same phrase	May be slow	Difficulty finding word, perseveration
Affect	Variable but may look disturbed, frightened	Flat	Slowed response, may be labile

Modified from Sendelbach S, Guthrie PF, Schoenfelder DP: Acute confusion/delirium, *J Gerontol Nurs* 35(11):11-18, 2009.

assessed for cognitive function in all settings, and nurses must have the skills to recognize cognitive impairment and monitor cognitive functioning. "Assessment of cognitive function is the first and most critical step in a cascade of strategies to prevent, reverse, halt, or minimize cognitive decline" (Braes et al., 2008, p. 42). (Chapter 7 discusses assessment tools used to evaluate cognitive function).

DELIRIUM

Dementia, delirium, and depression have been called the three *D's* of cognitive impairment because they occur frequently in older adults. These important geriatric syndromes are not a normal consequence of aging, although incidence increases with age. Because cognitive and behavioral changes characterize all three *D's*, it can be difficult to diagnose delirium, delirium superimposed on dementia (DSD), or depression. Inability to concentrate, with resulting memory impairment and other cognitive dysfunction, can occur in late-life depression. The term pseudodementia has been used to describe the cognitive impairment that may accompany depression in older adults (Chapter 18).

Delirium is characterized by an acute or subacute onset, with symptoms developing over a short period of time (usually hours to days). Symptoms tend to fluctuate over the course of the day, often worsening at night. Symptoms include disturbances in consciousness and attention and changes in cognition (memory deficits, perceptual disturbances). Perceptual disturbances are often accompanied by delusional (paranoid) thoughts and behavior (Evans and Kurlowicz, 2007).

In contrast, dementia typically has a gradual onset and a slow, steady pattern of decline without alterations in consciousness (Voyer et al., 2010). Knowledge about cognitive function in aging and appropriate assessment and evaluation are keys to differentiating these three syndromes. Table 19-1 presents the clinical features and the differences in cognitive and behavioral characteristics in delirium, dementia, and depression. The accepted criteria for a diagnosis of delirium are presented in the Diagnostic and Statistical Manual of Mental Disorders (American Psychiatic Association, 2000).

Etiology

The development of delirium is a result of complex interactions among multiple causes. Delirium results from the interaction of predisposing factors (e.g., vulnerability on the part of the individual due to predisposing conditions, such as cognitive impairment, severe illness, and sensory impairment) and precipitating factors/insults (e.g., medications, procedures, restraints, iatrogenic events). While a single factor, such as an infection, can trigger an episode of delirium, several co-existing factors are also likely to be present. A highly vulnerable older individual requires a lesser amount of precipitating factors to develop delirium (Inouye et al., 1999; Voyer et al., 2010).

The exact pathophysiological mechanisms involved in the development and progression of delirium remain uncertain, and further research is needed to understand its neuropathogenesis. Delirium is thought to be related to disturbances in the neurotransmitters in the brain that modulate the control of cognitive function, behavior, and mood. Irving and Foreman (2006) note that "there is growing evidence of cholinergic failure as a common pathway in delirium" (p. 122). The causes of delirium are potentially reversible; therefore accurate assessment and diagnosis are critical. Delirium is given many labels: acute confusional state, acute brain syndrome, confusion, reversible dementia, metabolic encephalopathy, and *toxic psychosis*.

Incidence and Prevalence

Delirium is a prevalent and serious disorder that occurs in elders across the continuum of care. Estimates are that delirium may affect up to 42% of hospitalized older adults and as many as 87% of older adults in intensive care units (ICUs) (Cole and McCusker, 2009; Marcantonio et al., 2010; Sweeny et al., 2008). Older people who have undergone surgery and those with dementia are particularly vulnerable to delirium. The prevalence of delirium is as high as 65% after orthopedic surgery, particularly hip fracture repair (Rigney, 2006). Among older people experiencing cardiac surgery, as many as 20% to 25% experience delirium, affecting even those without any documented preoperative cognitive impairments (Clarke et al.,

2010). A 16% delirium rate in patients newly admitted to subacute care has been reported. More than 50% of these patients are still delirious one month after admission (Marcantonio et al., 2010). Delirium is associated with increased morbidity, mortality, and institutionalization, independent of age, co-existing illnesses, or illness severity (Witlox et al., 2010).

The incidence of delirium superimposed on dementia (DSD) ranges from 22% to 89% (Tullmann et al., 2008). Older patients with dementia are three to five times more likely to develop delirium, and it is less likely to be recognized and treated than is delirium without dementia. DSD is associated with high mortality among hospitalized older people (Bellelli et al., 2008). Changes in the mental status of older people with dementia are often attributed to underlying dementia, or "sundowning," and not investigated. This is particularly significant since about 25% of all older hospitalized patients may have Alzheimer's disease or another dementia (Voelker, 2008). Delirium can accelerate the trajectory of cognitive decline in individuals with Alzheimer's disease. Further research is needed to determine whether prevention of delirium may delay cognitive decline in individuals with Alzheimer's disease (Fong et al., 2009). Despite its prevalence, DSD has not been well investigated, and there are only a few relevant studies in either the hospital or community setting.

Recognition of Delirium

Delirium is a medical emergency and one of the most significant geriatric syndromes (Waszynski and Petrovic, 2008). However, it is often not recognized by physicians or nurses. Studies indicate that delirium is unrecognized in 66% to 84% of patients (Pisani et al., 2006; Balas et al., 2007). A comprehensive review of the literature suggested that "nurses are missing key symptoms of delirium and appear to be doing superficial mental status assessments" (Steis and Fick, 2008, p. 47). Factors contributing to the lack of recognition of delirium among health care professionals include inadequate education about delirium, a lack of formal assessment methods, a view that delirium is not as essential to the patient's well-being in light of more serious medical problems, and ageist attitudes (Kuehn, 2010a; Waszynski and Petrovic, 2008). Failure to recognize delirium, identify the underlying causes, and implement timely interventions contributes to the negative sequelae associated with the condition (Tullmann et al., 2008; Kuehn, 2010a).

Dahlke and Phinney (2008) investigated interventions nurses use to assess, prevent, and treat delirium, as well as the challenges and barriers nurses face in caring for patients with delirium in the acute care setting. The authors concluded that cognitive changes in older people are often labeled confusion by nurses and physicians, are frequently accepted as part of normal aging, and are rarely questioned. If the nurse believed that confusion was normal in older adults, he or she would be less likely to recognize symptoms of delirium as a medical emergency necessitating their attention and intervention. Confusion in a child or younger adult would be recognized as a medical emergency, but confusion in older adults may be accepted as a natural occurrence, "part of the older person's personality" (p. 46).

In the Dahlke and Phinney study, nurses reported that caring for patients with delirium was seen as "annoying, frustrating and not interesting" (2008, p. 45). Nurses expressed that the care of older patients with delirium interfered with what was perceived as the "real work" of caring for a medical or surgical patient. Insufficient knowledge and inadequate time and resources also influenced appropriate care. The authors conclude that nurses are faced with the predicament of fitting care for older adults into a system that does not recognize the unique needs of this population. Clearly, education and attitudes about older people must be addressed if we want to improve care outcomes for the growing number of older adults who will need care.

Risk Factors for Delirium

The risk of delirium increases with the number of risk factors present. The more vulnerable the individual, the greater the risk. The multifactorial model for delirium (MMD), developed by Inouye and Charpentier (1996), can be used to guide identification of risk factors in hospitalized older adults. In the first study examining the use of this model in long-term care, Voyer and colleagues (2010) report that the MMD is relevant among this population and can be used to prevent delirium and improve care outcomes in this setting.

Identification of high-risk patients, risk factors, prompt and appropriate assessment, and continued surveillance are the cornerstones of delirium prevention. More than 35 potential risk factors have been identified for delirium. Among the most predictive are immobility, functional deficits, use of restraints or catheters, medications, acute illness, infections, alcohol or drug abuse, sensory impairments, malnutrition, dehydration, respiratory insufficiency, surgery, and cognitive impairment. Unrelieved or inadequately treated pain significantly increases the risk of delirium (Irving and Foreman, 2006). Medications account for 22% to 39% of all delirium, and all medications, particularly those with anticholinergic effects and any new medications, should be considered suspect. Invasive equipment, such as nasogastric tubes, intravenous (IV) lines, catheters, and restraints, also contribute to delirium by interfering with normal feedback mechanisms of the body (Box 19-3).

Clinical Subtypes of Delirium

Delirium is categorized according to the level of alertness and psychomotor activity. The clinical subtypes are hyperactive, hypoactive, and mixed. Box 19-4 presents the characteristics of each of these clinical subtypes. In non-ICU settings, approximately 30% of delirium is hyperactive, 24% hypoactive, and 46% is mixed. Because of the increased severity of illness and the use of psychoactive medications, hypoactive delirium may be more prevalent in the ICU. Although the negative consequences of hyperactive delirium are serious, the hypoactive subtype may be missed more often and is associated with a worse prognosis because of the development of complications such as aspiration, pulmonary embolism, pressure ulcers, and pneumonia. Increased hospital stays, longer duration of delirium, and higher mortality have been associated with hypoactive delirium.

Consequences of Delirium

Delirium has serious consequences and is a "high priority nursing challenge for all nurses who care for older adults" (Tullmann et al., 2008, p. 113). Delirium results in significant

BOX 19-3   PRECIPITATING FACTORS FOR DELIRIUM

- Total number of medications >6
- Pharmacological agents, especially narcotics, anticonvulsants, psychotropics, anticholinergics, hypnotics, anxiolytics
- Hypoxemia and metabolic disturbances
- Infection, especially respiratory and urinary tract
- Dehydration, with and without electrolyte disturbances
- Electrolyte imbalances
- Volume overload
- Intravenous catheter complications
- Prolonged bleeding
- Transfusion reaction
- New pressure ulcer
- Emergency admission or admission from a long-term care facility
- Prolonged emergency room stay (>12 hours)
- Withdrawal syndromes (alcohol and sedative-hypnotic agents)
- Major medical and surgical treatments (especially hip fracture)
- Nutritional deficiencies
- Dementia
- Circulatory disturbances (congestive heart failure [CHF], myocardial infarction [MI], cerebrovascular accident [CVA])
- Anemia
- Pain (either unrelieved or inadequately treated)
- Sensory deficits
- Social isolation, lack of family contact
- Retention of urine and feces
- Use of invasive equipment
- Use of restraint or immobilizing device
- Prolonged immobility
- Functional deficits
- Depression
- Sensory overstimulation or understimulation
- Abrupt loss of a significant person
- Multiple losses in a short span of time
- Move to a radically different environment (hospitalization, nursing home)

BOX 19-4   CLINICAL SUBTYPES OF DELIRIUM

HYPOACTIVE DELIRIUM
"Quiet or pleasantly confused"
Reduced activity
Lack of facial expression
Passive demeanor
Lethargy
Inactivity
Withdrawn and sluggish state
Limited, slow, and wavering vocalizations

HYPERACTIVE DELIRIUM
Excessive alertness
Easy distractibility
Increased psychomotor activity
Hallucinations, delusions
Agitation and aggressive actions
Fast or loud speech
Wandering, nonpurposeful repetitive movement
Verbal behaviors (yelling, calling out)
Removing tubes
Attempting to get out of bed

MIXED
Unpredictable fluctuations between hypoactivity and hyperactivity

distress for the patient, his or her family and significant others, and nurses. Delirium is associated with increased length of hospital stay and hospital readmissions, increased services after discharge, and increased morbidity, mortality, and institutionalization, independent of age, co-existing illnesses, or illness severity (Witlox et al., 2010).

Recent research indicates that delirium is associated with lasting cognitive impairment and psychiatric problems. While the majority of hospital inpatients recover fully from delirium, a substantial minority will never recover or recover only partially. Patients with delirium that remains unresolved at discharge should be screened again at three months and followed closely. The persistence of delirium after discharge may interfere with the ability to manage chronic conditions and contribute to poor outcomes (Cole and McCusker, 2009). Screening all older adults before they leave the hospital may help to identify those in need of specific transitional care (Chapter 16) with more frequent follow up after hospitalization (Lindquest et al., 2011). Further research is needed to determine the reasons for the long-term poor outcomes, whether characteristics of the delirium itself (subtype or duration) influence prognosis, and how the long-term effects might be decreased.

PROMOTING HEALTHY AGING: IMPLICATIONS FOR GERONTOLOGICAL NURSING

Assessment

Several instruments can be used to assess the presence and severity of delirium. To detect changes, it is very important to determine the person's usual mental status. If the person cannot tell you this, family members or other caregivers who are with the patient can be asked to provide this information. If the patient is alone, the responsible party or the institution transferring the patient can provide this information by phone. Do not assume the person's current mental status represents his or her usual state, and do not attribute altered mental status to age alone or assume that dementia is present. All older patients, regardless of their current cognitive function, should have a formal assessment to identify possible delirium when admitted to the hospital (Box 19-5).

The MMSE-2 is considered a general test of cognitive status that helps identify mental status impairment. Although the MMSE-2 alone is not adequate for diagnosing delirium, it represents a brief, standardized method to assess mental status and can provide a baseline from which to track changes (see also Chapter 7). Several delirium-specific assessment instruments are available, such as the Confusion Assessment Method (CAM) (Inouye et al., 1990) and the NEECHAM Confusion Scale (Neelon et al., 1996). The CAM-ICU is another instrument specifically designed to assess delirium in an intensive care population and has recently been validated for use in critically ill, nonverbal patients who are on mechanical ventilation (Ely et al., 2001; Rigney, 2006).

Assessment using the MMSE-2, CAM, and NEECHAM should be conducted on admission to the hospital, throughout the hospitalization for all patients identified at risk for delirium, and for all patients who exhibit signs and symptoms of delirium or develop additional risk factors (Steis and Fick, 2008). Results of a study (Waszynski and Petrovic, 2008) suggested that the CAM was useful in identifying delirium in hospitalized adults, and nurses found it very helpful in identifying changes in cognitive functioning. As a result of these findings, the CAM was made a customary part of the daily flow sheet.

Once a patient is identified as having delirium, reassessment should be conducted every shift. Documenting specific objective indicators of alterations in mental status rather than using the global, nonspecific term confusion will lead to more appropriate prevention, detection, and management of delirium and its negative consequences. Findings from assessment using a validated instrument are combined with nursing observation, chart review, and physiological findings. Delirium often has a fluctuating course and can be difficult to recognize, so assessment must be ongoing and include multiple data sources.

Interventions

Nonpharmacological   Intervention begins with prevention. An awareness and identification of the risk factors for delirium and a formal assessment of mental status are the first-line interventions for prevention. Balas and colleagues (2007) suggest that "nurses make multiple decisions throughout the day that can potentially enhance or diminish the likelihood that their patients will experience delirium" (p. 152). Nurses play a pivotal role in the identification of delirium, and it is imperative that they accurately report patients' mental status to the medical team so that causative factors can be identified and treated (Irving and Foreman, 2006).

Because the etiology of delirium is multifactorial, "for an intervention strategy to be effective, it should target the multifactorial origins of delirium with multicomponent interventions that address more than one risk factor" (Rosenbloom-Brunton et al., 2010, p. 23). Multidisciplinary approaches to prevention of delirium seem to show the most promising results, but continued research is needed to evaluate what type of approach has the most beneficial effect in specific clinical settings. The current disease model of delirium care is not effective (Dahlke and Phinney, 2008).

A well-researched multidisciplinary program of delirium prevention in the acute care setting, the Hospital Elder Life Program (HELP) (Inouye et al., 1999; Bradley et al., 2005; Rubin et al., 2006), focuses on managing six risk factors for delirium: cognitive impairment, sleep deprivation, immobility, visual impairments, hearing impairments, and dehydration. The program is used in more than 60 hospitals in the United States and internationally. Patient outcomes with the use of this model include a 40% reduction in the incidence of delirium, a 67% reduction in rates of functional decline, and significant cost savings in both hospitals and long-term care facilities. Most of the interventions can be considered quite simple and part of good nursing care.

The Family-HELP program, an adaptation and extension of the original HELP program, trains family caregivers in selected protocols (e.g., orientation, therapeutic activities, vision and hearing). Initial research demonstrates that active engagement of family caregivers in preventive interventions for delirium is feasible and supports a culture of family-oriented care (Rosenbloom-Brunton et al., 2010).

Examples of interventions in the HELP program include the following: offering herbal tea or warm milk instead of sleeping medications, keeping the ward quiet at night by using vibrating beepers instead of paging systems, using silent pill crushers, removing catheters and other devices that hamper movement as soon as possible, encouraging mobilization, assessing and managing pain, and correcting hearing and vision deficits. Fall risk reduction interventions, such as bed and chair alarms, low beds, reclining chairs, volunteers to sit with restless patients, and keeping routines as normal as possible with consistent caregivers, are other examples of interventions. Further information on the Elder Life Program can be found at http://elderlife.med.yale.edu/public/public-main.php. Box 19-6 presents suggested interventions for delirium.

Another innovative approach is the delirium doula. Borrowing the concept of a "doula" from maternity care, this concept was designed by student nurses who had completed a maternity placement where doulas were used. The proposed role of the delirium doula would include providing support, adjusting the environment to meet the patient's behavior or needs, and assisting the patient to get help when required (Balas et al., 2004; Balas et al., 2007; Irving and Foreman, 2006; Sweeny et al., 2008).

A commonly used intervention for patients with delirium in acute care is the use of "sitters" or "constant observers (COs)." Costs associated with this practice can be very high, and data indicate that the use of sitters or COs does not consistently decrease the incidence of unsafe patient behavior in the patient with delirium. Nor do they assist in identifying causes of delirium or identifying appropriate interventions. Sweeny and colleagues (2008) report on the implementation of a multicomponent, evidence-based alternative to COs for care of patients with delirium in an acute care hospital. The program focused on fall risk–reduction strategies, as well as assessment of delirium using the CAM, and a protocol for intervention. Results suggest that costs associated with COs decreased from $1.5 million to $250,000 in 2 years with no change in the use of restraints or the incidence of falls.

Pharmacological   Pharmacological interventions to treat the symptoms of delirium may be necessary if patients are in danger of harming themselves or others, or if nonpharmacological interventions are not effective. However, pharmacological

---

BOX 19-6   SUGGESTED INTERVENTIONS TO PREVENT DELIRIUM

- Know baseline mental status, functional abilities, living conditions, medications taken, alcohol use.
- Assess mental status using Mini-Mental State Exam-2 (MMSE-2), Confusion Assessment Method (CAM), or NEECHAM Confusion Scale, and document.
- Correct underlying physiological alterations.
- Compensate for sensory deficits (e.g., hearing aids, glasses, dentures).
- Encourage fluid intake (make sure fluids are accessible).
- Avoid long periods of giving nothing orally.
- Explain all actions with clear and consistent communication.
- Avoid multiple medications, and avoid problematic medications.
- Be vigilant for drug reactions or interactions; consider onset of new symptoms as an adverse reaction to medications.
- Avoid use of sleeping medications; use music, warm milk, or noncaffeinated herbal tea to alleviate discomfort.
- Attempt to find out why behavior is occurring rather than simply medicating for it (e.g., need to toilet, pain, fear, hunger, thirst).
- Avoid excessive bed rest; institute early mobilization.
- Encourage participation in care for activities of daily living (ADLs).
- Minimize the use of catheters, restraints, or immobilizing devices.
- Use least restrictive devices (mitts instead of wrist restraints, reclining geri-chairs with tray instead of vest restraints).
- Hide tubes (stockinette over intravenous [IV] line), or use intermittent fluid administration.
- Activate bed and chair alarms.
- Place the patient near the nursing station for close observation.
- Assess and treat pain.
- Pay attention to environmental noise.
- Normalize the environment (provide familiar items, routines, clocks, calendars).
- Minimize the number of room changes and interfacility transfers.
- Do not place a delirious patient in the room with another delirious patient.
- Have family, volunteer, or paid caregiver stay with the patient.

BOX 19-7   COMMUNICATING WITH A PERSON EXPERIENCING DELIRIUM

- Know the person's past patterns.
- Look at nonverbal signs, such as tone of voice, facial expressions, and gestures.
- Speak slowly.
- Be calm and patient.
- Face the person and keep eye contact; get to the level of the person rather than standing over him or her.
- Explain all actions.
- Smile.
- Use simple, familiar words.
- Allow adequate time for response.
- Repeat if needed.
- Tell the person what you want him or her to do rather than what you don't want him or her to do.
- Give one-step directions; use gestures and demonstration to augment words.
- Reassure of safety.
- Keep caregivers consistent.
- Assume that communication and behavior are meaningful and an attempt to tell us something or express needs.
- Do not assume that the person is unable to understand or is demented.

Caring for patients with delirium can be a challenging experience. Patients with delirium can be difficult to communicate with, and disturbing behaviors such as pulling out IV lines or attempting to get out of bed disrupt medical treatment and compromise safety. It is important for nurses to realize that behavior is an attempt to communicate something and express needs. The patient with delirium feels frightened and out of control. The calmer and more reassuring the nurse is, the safer the patient will feel. Box 19-7 presents some communication strategies that are helpful in caring for people experiencing delirium.

DEMENTIA

In contrast to delirium, which is usually a reflection of an acute physiological disturbance or severe depression that may affect cognition, dementia is an irreversible state that progresses over years and causes memory impairment and loss of other intellectual abilities severe enough to cause interference with daily life. Degenerative dementias include Alzheimer's disease (AD), Parkinson's disease dementia (PDD), dementia with Lewy bodies (DLB), and frontotemporal lobe dementias (FTDs). Alzheimer's disease (AD) accounts for 50% to 70% of all dementia cases. Vascular cognitive impairment (VCI) encompasses several syndromes: vascular dementia; mixed primary neurodegenerative disease and vascular dementia; and cognitive impairment of vascular origin that does not meet the dementia criteria. Increasing evidence suggests that most dementias have neurodegenerative (most commonly AD) and vascular features, and these seem to act synergistically (Desai et al., 2010).

Other less commonly occurring dementias are Creutzfeldt-Jakob disease (CJD) (subacute spongiform encephalopathy); and human immunodeficiency virus (HIV)–related dementia. Normal pressure hydrocephalus (NPH) causes a dementia characterized by ataxic gait, incontinence, and memory

interventions should not replace thoughtful and careful evaluation and management of the underlying causes of delirium. Pharmacological treatment should be one approach in a multicomponent program of prevention and treatment. Research on the pharmacological management of delirium is limited, but it has been suggested that "with increased understanding of the neuropathogenesis of delirium, drug therapy could become primary to the treatment of delirium" (Irving and Foreman, 2006, p. 122). A few studies have suggested that use of dexmedetomidine as a sedative or analgesic may reduce the incidence or duration of delirium (Kuehn, 2010b).

Ozbolt and colleagues (2008) conducted a literature review of the use of antipsychotics for treatment of delirious elders and concluded that the atypical antipsychotics demonstrate similar rates of efficacy to haloperidol for the treatment of delirium and have a lower rate of extrapyramidal side effects. Further research is needed since no double-blind placebo trials exist. Short-acting benzodiazepines are often used to control agitation but may worsen mental status. In ICU patients with delirium, lorazepam has been identified as an independent risk factor for developing delirium (Pandharipande et al., 2006). Psychoactive medications, if used, should be given at the lowest effective dose, monitored closely, and reduced or eliminated as soon as possible so that recovery can be assessed.

TABLE 19-2   TYPES OF DEMENTIA AND TYPICAL CHARACTERISTICS

TYPE OF DEMENTIA	CHARACTERISTICS
Alzheimer's disease	Most common type of dementia accounting for 60% to 80% of cases. Hallmark abnormalities are deposits of the protein fragment beta-amyloid (plaques) and twisted strands of the protein tau (tangles). Difficulty remembering names and recent events, difficulty expressing oneself with words, spatial cognition problems, impaired reasoning and judgment, apathy, and depression are often early symptoms. Language disturbances may also be a presenting symptom. Later symptoms include impaired judgment; disorientation; behavior changes; and difficulty speaking, swallowing, and walking.
Vascular dementia (also known as multi-infarct or poststroke dementia or vascular cognitive impairment (VCI))	Second most common type of dementia. Impairment is caused by decreased blood flow to parts of the brain due to a series of small strokes that block arteries. Symptoms often overlap with AD, although memory may not be as seriously affected.
Mixed dementia	Characterized by the hallmark abnormalities of AD and another type of dementia, most commonly vascular dementia but also other types such as dementia with Lewy bodies. Mixed dementia is more common than previously thought. Neurodegenerative changes occur along with vascular changes.
Parkinson's disease dementia (PDD)	Later onset of dementia, at least one year after onset of parkinsonian features. Hallmark abnormality is Lewy bodies (abnormal deposits of the protein alpha-synuclein) that form inside the nerve cells of the brain.
Dementia with Lewy bodies	Pattern of decline similar to AD, including problems with memory and judgment as well as behavior changes. Alertness and severity of cognitive symptoms may fluctuate daily. Visual hallucinations, muscle rigidity, and tremors are common. Exhibit a sensitivity to neuroleptic drugs, so these medications should be avoided.
Creutzfeldt-Jakob disease (CJD) and vCJD (transmissible spongiform encephalopathy)	A rapidly fatal and rare form of dementia characterized by tiny holes that give the brain a "spongy" appearance under a microscope. May be hereditary, occur sporadically, or occur through transmission from infected individuals. Failing memory, behavioral changes, lack of coordination, visual disturbances. vCJD (bovine spongiform encephalopathy/mad cow disease). Occurs in younger patients and may be caused by contaminated feed.
Frontotemporal dementia	Involves damage to brain cells, especially in the front and side regions of the brain. Symptoms include change in personality and behavior and difficulty with language. Pick's disease, characterized by Pick's bodies in the brain, is one form of frontotemporal dementia.
Normal pressure hydrocephalus	Caused by buildup of fluid in the brain without corresponding increase in CSF pressure. Symptoms include difficulty walking (ataxic gait), memory loss, incontinence. Can sometimes be corrected with surgical installation of a shunt to drain excess fluid.

Data from: 2010 Alzheimer's Disease Facts and Figures, Overview of Alzheimer's Disease. Available at www.alz.org. Accessed September 28, 2010.

impairment. This disease is reversible and treated with a shunt that diverts cerebrospinal fluid away from the brain (Alzheimer's Association, 2010a; Desai et al., 2010; Kamat et al., 2010) (Table 19-2).

Different types of dementia have different symptom patterns and distinguishing microscopic brain abnormalities. The symptoms of dementia also overlap and can be further complicated by co-morbid medical conditions. Accurate diagnosis is important, since treatment and prognosis vary. The rate of diagnosis of dementia is quite low despite advances in technology and knowledge about the different types and causes of dementia. In some studies, as many as 75% of patients with moderate to severe dementia and more than 95% of those with mild impairment escape diagnosis in the primary care setting. Clearly, education of both professionals and the community is needed so that more timely diagnosis and treatment can be initiated (Stefanacci, 2008). The diagnosis of dementia is complex, and it is essential that older people with symptoms of cognitive impairment receive specialized assessment to determine the causes so that treatment can be tailored appropriately.

Incidence and Prevalence

Dementia is one of the most disabling and burdensome of chronic health conditions. The growing worldwide epidemic of dementia has frightening implications for the health of older people and their families and the health and societal costs associated with the disease. Healthy People 2020 has added a new topic on dementia with the goal of reducing the morbidity and costs associated with the condition and of maintaining and enhancing the quality of life for persons with dementia, including Alzheimer's disease (U.S. Department of Health and Human Services, 2010). The cost of care for someone with dementia is three times more than for those who do not have the disease (Hall et al., 2009). It is estimated that the cost of caring for a single person with Alzheimer's is $56,800 a year, the bulk of that borne by the family (shriver report, 2010).

In 2010, the total estimated worldwide costs of dementia were $604 billion. The costs of dementia are set to soar with an estimated 85% increase by 2030. The economic impact on families is insufficiently appreciated. About 70% of the costs occur in Western Europe and North America. The World Alzheimer's Report 2010 suggests that if dementia were a company, it would be the world's largest by annual revenue exceeding Wal-Mart ($414 billion) and Exxon Mobil ($311 billion) (Alzheimer's Disease International, 2010).

Alzheimer's Disease

Alzheimer's disease (AD), the most common form of dementia, was first described by Dr. Alois Alzheimer in 1906. In the United States, about 5.4 million people age 65 and older and 200,000 individuals younger than age 65 have AD. If current trends continue, by the year 2050, the prevalence of AD is expected to quadruple unless medical breakthroughs identify ways to prevent or more effectively treat the disease. AD is the sixth leading cause of death and the nation's third most expensive medical condition.

In the absence of any new effective treatments for AD, the cumulative costs of AD care will exceed $20 trillion in today's dollars by 2050. These costs include a 600% increase in Medicare costs and a 400% increase in Medicaid costs. One factor contributing to the soaring cost projections is that nearly half of the individuals with AD would be in the later stages of the disease when more expensive around-the-clock care is often necessary (Alzheimer's Association, 2010a).

While the ultimate goal is to discover a treatment that can prevent or cure AD, even modest improvements in treatment can have a huge impact. The Alzheimer's Association (2010b) has published future cost trajectories for AD if a hypothetical treatment is found to delay onset by five years, or a new treatment is discovered to slow the progression of the disease. A hypothetical intervention that delayed the onset of AD by five years would result in a 57% reduction in the number of AD patients and reduce projected Medicare costs of AD by half. The current lifetime risk of AD for a 65-year-old is estimated to be at 10.5%. A screening instrument for AD pathology (with 90% sensitivity and specificity) and a treatment that slows progression by 50% would reduce that risk to 5.7% (Alzheimer's Association, 2010b).

The hypothetical treatments would result in substantial positive outcomes for people with AD, and for the nation as a whole, even if the outcomes were well short of a cure. "These scenarios are similar in assumptions and results to what has already been achieved in other diseases, including stroke, heart disease, some cancers, and HIV/AIDS, where there has been a substantial societal commitment to overcome these diseases" (p. 17). AD has been called an unfolding natural disaster that requires immediate and substantial research investments (Alzheimer's Association, 2010a).

Types of Alzheimer's Disease

AD is characterized by the development of neuronal intracellular neurofibrillary tangles consisting of the protein tau and extracellular deposits of amyloid-β (Aβ) peptides in fibril structures, the loss of connections between nerve cells in the brain, and the death of these nerve cells (Mattsson et al., 2009). These changes in the brain develop slowly over many years of pathology accumulation. At the same time, some people have the brain changes associated with AD and yet do not show symptoms of dementia.

AD has two types: early-onset dementia (EO-D) and late-onset dementia. EO-D is a rare form, affecting only about 5% of all people who have AD. It develops between the ages of 30 and 60 years. This form of AD can result from gene mutations on chromosomes 21, 14, and 1, and each of these mutations causes abnormal proteins to be formed. Mutations on chromosome 21 cause the formation of abnormal amyloid precursor protein (APP). A mutation on chromosome 14 causes abnormal presenilin 1 to be made, and a mutation on chromosome 1 leads to abnormal presenilin 2. Mutations in the presenilin 1 gene account for 30% to 70% of EO-D. These mutations cause an increased amount of beta-amyloid protein, the major component of AD plaques, to be formed (National Institute on Aging, 2011).

The autosomal dominant inheritance pattern means that offspring in the same generation have a 50/50 chance of developing EO-D if one of their parents had it. Even if only one of these mutated genes is inherited from a parent, the person will almost always develop early-onset AD. Predictive genetic testing, with appropriate precounseling and postcounseling, may be offered to at-risk individuals with an apparent autosomal-dominant inheritance of AD. Adult children with a family history of EO-AD, especially children who have a history of both parents having EO-D, may also benefit from genetic counseling (Desai et al., 2010) (Box 19-8).

Most cases of AD are the late-onset form, developing after the age of 60 years. The mutations seen in EO-D are not involved in this form of the disease. This disorder does not clearly run in families, and late-onset AD is probably related to variations in one or more genes in combination with lifestyle and environmental factors. The apolipoprotein E (APOE) gene, found on chromosome 19, has been extensively studied as a risk factor, and a particular variant of this gene, the e4 allele, seems to increase a person's risk for developing late-onset AD.

The inheritance pattern of late-onset AD is uncertain. People who inherit one copy of the APOE e4 allele have an increased risk of developing the disease; those who inherit two copies are at even greater risk. Not all people with AD have the e4 allele, and not all people who have the e4 allele will develop the disease. A blood test is available that can identify which APOE alleles a person has, but screening for APOE4 in asymptomatic individuals in the general population is not recommended. At this time, the APOE test is useful for studying AD risk in large groups of people but not for determining one person's specific risk. Using an approach called a genome-wide association study, four to seven other AD risk-factor genes have been identified (Desai et al., 2010; National Institute on Aging, 2011).

Research

The focus of research on AD is on the interaction between risk-factor genes and lifestyle or environmental factors. Increasing evidence strongly points to the potential risk roles of vascular risk factors (VRFs) and disorders (e.g., midlife obesity, dyslipidemia, hypertension, cigarette smoking, obstructive sleep apnea, diabetes, and cerebrovascular lesions) and the potential protective roles of psychosocial factors (e.g., higher education, regular exercise, healthy diet, intellectually challenging leisure activity, and active socially integrated lifestyle) in the

TABLE 19-3	RISK FACTORS AND PROTECTIVE FACTORS FOR ALZHEIMER'S DISEASE: POTENTIAL MECHANISMS

FACTOR	RISK	POTENTIAL MECHANISMS
Advanced age	Increased risk	Possible decreased brain reserves
Sex	Females have increased risk	Living longer and loss of neuroprotective effects of estrogen
Family history	Increased risk	APP, presenilin-1, presenilin-2 mutations may result in oversecretion of amyloid β (Aβ) in familial AD APOE4 allele increases risk of sporadic (late-onset) AD
Depression	Increased risk	May decrease brain reserves/transmitters
High-fat and cholesterol diet	Increased risk	Increased neuroinflammation; possible increased substrate for APP
CRP (C-reactive protein)	Increased risk	Increased neuroinflammation
Homocysteine	Increased risk	Increased oxidative stress, free radical toxicity, increased atherosclerotic sequelae
Smoking	Increased risk	Accelerated cerebral atrophy, perfusional decline, and white matter lesions
Diabetes mellitus	Increased risk	Impaired glucose uptake in neuronal cells, decreased blood supply due to small-vessel disease
Hyperlipidemia	Increased risk	Increased Aβ accumulation
Genetic	Increased risk	Mutations of presenilin-1, presenilin-2, APP
Hypertension	Increased risk	Decreased cerebral blood flow/cerebral ischemia, white matter lesions
Head trauma	Increased risk	Not fully understood; possible blood-brain barrier disruption
Obesity	Increased risk	Hyperlipidemia and hypertension and via their mechanisms described earlier
Mediterranean diet	Decreased risk	Decreased neuroinflammation, decreased oxidative stress, decreased Aβ_{42} toxicity
Increased education	Decreased risk	Education may increase neural connections
Increased mental activity	Decreased risk	Cognitive reserve model in which people cope better and can generate more neurons during their lifetime
Increased physical activity	Decreased risk	Increased cerebral blood flow, increased brain-derived neurotrophic factor

From Kamat S, Kamat A, Grossberg G: *Clinics in Geriatric Medicine* 26:113, 2010.

pathogenesis and clinical manifestations of dementia (especially AD and VCI). Head trauma is also considered a risk factor. In a study of professional football players, those with a history of three or more concussions were five times more likely to develop mild cognitive impairment than those without concussions (Ghetu et al., 2010).

"There are many modifiable risk and protective factors for dementia. It is important that we educate at-risk patients and family members of those with dementia about the importance of addressing modifiable risk factors as early as possible so as to potentially delay or decrease the risks of developing dementias such as AD. Truly, prevention is the wave of the future in the dementia arena" (Kamat et al., 2010, p. 20).

Table 19-3 presents risk factors and protective factors for AD.

Diagnosis

In 2011, new diagnostic criteria that better reflect the full continuum of Alzheimer's disease from its earliest effects to its eventual impact on mental and physical function, were published by the National Institute on Aging (NIA) and the Alzheimer's Association. The recommendations are discussed in detail in several recent publications (Jack et al., 2011; Albert et al., 2011; Sperling et al., 2011; McKhann et al., 2011). The original diagnostic guidelines for AD were developed in 1984 and have not been revised since that time. These original guidelines were the first to address the disease and described only later stages, when symptoms of dementia are already evident.

The new guidelines describe the earliest preclinical stages of the disease, mild cognitive impairment, and dementia due to Alzheimer's pathology. The new guidelines also address the use of imaging and biomarkers in blood and spinal fluid that may help determine whether changes in the brain and those in body fluids are due to Alzheimer's disease. Biomarkers are increasingly being used in the research setting to detect onset

of the disease and to track progression, but cannot yet be used routinely in clinical diagnosis without further testing and validation. The guidelines call for removing age restrictions for the onset of AD; include updated criteria to distinguish Alzheimer's dementia from other forms of cognitive impairment; and expand symptoms beyond memory impairment to difficulty expressing oneself with words, spatial cognition problems, and impaired reasoning and judgment. The overall goal of the new guidelines is to provide standards for research and practice that advance the field farther in the direction of early detection and treatment.

Three distinct stages of Alzheimer's disease are proposed: preclinical, mild cognitive impairment (MCI), and Alzheimer's dementia.

Preclinical. The preclinical stage, for which the guidelines only apply in a research setting, describes a phase in which brain changes, including amyloid buildup and other early nerve cell changes, may already be in process. At this point, significant clinical symptoms are not yet evident. In some people, amyloid buildup can be detected with positron emission tomography (PET) scans and cerebrospinal (CSF) analysis, but it is unknown what the risk for progression to Alzheimer's dementia is for these individuals. However, use of these imaging and biomarker tests at this stage are recommended for research only. The biomarkers are still being developed and standardized and are not ready for use by clinicians in general practice. With further research on biomarkers, as set forth in the new guidelines, it may be possible to predict who is at risk for the development of MCI and Alzheimer's dementia, and who would benefit most as interventions are developed.

Mild Cognitive Impairment. The guidelines for MCI are also largely for research, although they clarify existing guidelines for MCI for use in a clinical setting. In MCI, there would be evidence of concern about a change in cognition, in comparison to the person's prior level. Declines in performance in one or more cognitive domains would be greater than expected for the patient's age and educational background. Memory problems are enough to be noticed and measured, but do not compromise a person's function. People with MCI may or may not progress to Alzheimer's dementia.

Alzheimer's Dementia. These criteria apply to the final stage of the disease, and are most relevant for health care providers and patients. They outline ways clinicians should approach evaluation of the cause and progression of cognitive decline. The guidelines expand the concept of Alzheimer's dementia beyond memory loss as its most central characteristic. A decline in other aspects of cognition, such as word-finding, vision/spatial issues, and impaired reasoning or judgment may be the first symptom to be noticed. At this stage, biomarker test results may be used in some cases to increase or decrease the level of certainty about a diagnosis of Alzheimer's dementia and to distinguish Alzheimer's dementia from other dementias.

Cultural Differences

African Americans are about twice as likely to have AD as whites, and Hispanics are about 1.5 times more likely than whites. There does not appear to be any known genetic factor for these differences. The higher incidence of hypertension and diabetes in these populations may increase the risk of AD (Alzheimer's Association, 2010a). Research is limited on cultural disparities in the incidence of dementia, as well as the influence of culture and ethnicity on the recognition and interpretation of cognitive changes and the assessment, diagnosis, and treatment of AD and other dementias (Tappen et al., 2010).

Further research is needed to understand how individuals from racially and culturally diverse groups view dementia and how cultural beliefs about disease etiology and symptoms influence diagnosis, treatment, and help-seeking behaviors (Neary and Mahoney, 2005; Hargrave, 2006; Williams et al., 2010). Studies have shown that African Americans may view dementia as a "normal consequence of aging, a form of mental illness, or manifestation of culture-specific physical syndromes" (e.g., "worriation" or "spells"). These health beliefs may lead to normalizing or minimizing symptoms, promote denial, and delay help-seeking behaviors (Hargrave, 2006, p. 37).

Hispanics may attribute the etiology of dementia to a "lack of balance in one's lifestyle, punishment for bad behavior, or mental illness (locos) or a temporary state of nervous, or nervousness" (Neary and Mahoney, 2005, p. 169). However, recent studies suggest that limited knowledge about dementia is a more significant deterrent to recognizing its symptoms and seeking assessment and treatment (Hargrave, 2006; Neary and Mahoney, 2005). Development of culturally and linguistically appropriate sources of information about dementia is important (Neary and Mahoney, 2005). The Diversity Toolbox, prepared by the Alzheimer's Association (www.alz.org/professionals_and_researchers_caring_for_diverse_populations.asp) is an important resource for nurses and other health professionals working with culturally and racially diverse older adults.

Treatment

Individuals with cognitive impairment require ongoing monitoring of disease progression and response to therapy as well as regular health maintenance and health promotion interventions. "Successful treatment of AD and its symptoms is likely to be just as complex as its etiology" (Kolanowski et al., 2010, p. 215). Assessment should occur at least every six months after diagnosis or any time there is a change in behavior or increase in the rate of decline. Assessment should include daily functioning, cognitive status, co-morbid medical conditions, behavioral symptoms, medications, living arrangement, and safety.

Beginning at the time of diagnosis and continuing through the course of the disease, ongoing assessment of the individual's decision-making capacity is essential. Health care surrogates should be determined and wishes for palliative and end-of-life care determined. In early stages, individuals usually retain their decision-making capacity and should be involved in all discussions.

Caregivers of individuals with dementia also need ongoing assessment, attention to physical and emotional health, support, and education, and this should begin with the diagnosis. Access to a knowledgeable provider who can follow them throughout the course of the illness is essential and leads to improved outcomes and less distress (Hain et al., 2010). Collaborative care management programs for the treatment of AD, often led by advanced practice nurses, have been shown to improve quality of care, decrease the incidence of behavioral and psychological symptoms of dementia, and decrease caregiver stress (Callahan et al., 2006; Duru et al., 2009). Chodosh and colleagues (2007) reported that adherence to guideline-recommended dementia care was less than 40%, so continued attention to effective care management models is important. Nurses can play a significant role in the development and implementation of such models. Issues related to caregiving are discussed later in the chapter.

Pharmacological. Current treatment guidelines recommend CI therapy as first-line treatment in patients with mild to moderate AD, and these medications may also be prescribed for MCI and the vascular dementias. The currently available cholinesterase inhibitors (CIs) are donepezil, galantamine, and rivastigmine. These medications work by blocking acetylcholinesterase. They have similar efficacy and side effects. The most common side effects with the CIs are nausea and diarrhea. Recommendations should start at low doses with slow titration to decrease side effects. Rivastigmine (Exelon) is now available in a patch that may be more convenient to use, may have fewer side effects, and provides a consistent day-long dose.

No published study directly compares these drugs. Because they work in a similar way, it is not expected that switching from one of these drugs to another will produce significantly different results. However, a person may respond better to one drug than another. Treatment with these drugs should be started on diagnosis or after six months of AD symptoms with effectiveness reassessed every six months. Dosage of these medications should be reduced gradually when discontinuing to prevent rapid decompensation (Hall et al., 2009). Memantine, an N-methyl-D-aspartate receptor antagonist, is also approved for moderate AD and may be used either alone or in conjunction with a CI. Memantine is now available in a once-a-day dose (Memantine XR). Results of a recent study assessing the clinical trials' evidence for memantine's efficacy in mild Alzheimer's disease suggest that evidence is lacking for a benefit of this medication in mild AD and meager evidence for its efficacy in moderate AD. Further trials are needed to assess the potential for memantine either alone, or added to CIs, in mild and moderate AD (Schneider et al., 2011). At this time, there is insufficient evidence to support the use of antioxidant therapy with vitamin E, gingko biloba, estrogen, or NSAIDs (Desai et al., 2010).

Medication therapy is directed toward the symptoms of AD and does not affect the neuronal decline that will eventually produce severe disability. The medications are aimed at slowing, not reversing, cognitive decline. Data from clinical trials and meta-analyses indicate that there is a small, statistically significant benefit on cognition, activities of daily living, and behavior with the use of these medications. Patients and family members must be provided with realistic expectations from pharmacological therapy (Segal-Gidan, 2010). Patients with Lewy body disease may show more dramatic improvements in cognitive status than those with AD taking a cholinesterase inhibitor (Hall et al., 2009).

Depression frequently accompanies dementia, and it is important to assess for depression and treat if present, or it will cause excess disability. Selective serotonin reuptake inhibitors, serotonin/norepinephrine reuptake inhibitors, noradrenergic reuptake inhibitors, or norepinephrine/dopamine reuptake inhibitors can be used, and selection of the medication depends on the symptom presentation of depression (Hall et al., 2009) (Chapters 9 and 18).

Delaying both disease onset and progression would significantly reduce the burden of AD, particularly in the late stages of the disease. Positive effects on the behavioral manifestations of AD have also been shown with CI therapy, suggesting that cholinergic mechanisms, among other neurotransmitters, are involved in the manifestation of some behavioral and psychological symptoms of dementia (Figiel and Sadowsky, 2008). A number of drugs are being investigated for treatment and prevention of Alzheimer's disease. A major area of focus is on drugs that prevent or reduce beta amyloid buildup (National Institute on Aging, 2010).

PROMOTING HEALTHY AGING: IMPLICATIONS FOR GERONTOLOGICAL NURSING

Nurses provide direct care for people with dementia in the community, hospitals, and long-term care facilities. They also work with families and staff, teaching best practice approaches to care and providing education and support. With the rising incidence of dementia, nurses will play an even larger role in the design and implementation of evidence-based practice and provision of education, counseling, and supportive services to individuals with dementia and their caregivers (Teri et al., 2008).

Person-Centered Care

Irreversible dementias such as Alzheimer's disease have no cure, and although new medications offer hope for improved function, the most important treatment for the disease is competent and compassionate person-centered care. "Since Alzheimer's affects mind and personality, as well as physical function, there is a great danger that the person can become obscured by the

disease, defined by symptoms rather than by her or his unique spirit and continuing sense of self" (Sifton, 2001, p. iv). Person-centered care looks beyond the disease and the tasks we must perform to the person within and our relationship with them. The focus is not on what we need to do to the person but on the person himself or herself and how to enhance well-being and quality of life.

Gerontological nurses know that the person, not the disease, is always the focus of care, and they practice from a belief that the person with dementia is still a whole person, someone who can think, feel, learn, grow, and be in a relationship (Touhy, 2004). "The person with dementia is not an object, not a vegetable, not an empty body, not a child, but an adult, who, given support, might exercise choices and respond to a respectful approach" (Woods, 1999, p. 35). Person-centered care fosters abilities, supports limitations, ensures safety, enhances quality of life, prevents excess disability, and offers hope. Care for persons with dementia is more than keeping their bodies alive, safe, and clean; performing tasks; and managing behavior—the care must also nourish their souls (Touhy, 2004).

Person-centered care is care that establishes connections and a sense of security; respects and appreciates the person; and supports the person's need to love and be loved, to be known and accepted, to give and to share, and to be productive and successful (Bell and Troxel, 2001). The culture change movement in the nation's nursing homes is grounded in the concept of person-centered care and quality of life (Kolanowski et al., 2010) (Chapter 16).

Despite a growing body of evidence on the importance of person-centered care and therapeutic work with people with dementia, the emphasis in the literature and in practice continues to be on the care of the body (bathing, feeding) and the management of aggressive and problematic behavior. "Despite the emphasis on individualized care and culture change, for many staff, the goal of care hasn't changed: control of behavior is still a priority" (Kolanowski et al., 2010, p. 216).

The emphasis on the decline associated with the disease, the catastrophic behaviors, and the loss of humanness promotes despair, hopelessness, and fear on the part of professional caregivers, patients, and families (Touhy, 2004). Special skills and attitudes are required to nurse the person with dementia, and caring is paramount. It is not an area of nursing that "just anyone can do" (Splete, 2008, p. 11). Williams and colleagues (2005) provide a comprehensive set of nurse competencies to improve dementia care.

Nutrition, ADLs, maintenance of health and function, safety, communication, behavioral changes, caregiver needs and support, and quality of life are the major care concerns for patients, families, and staff who care for people with dementia. Mary Opal Wolanin, a gerontological nursing pioneer, suggested that nurses are not as interested in the neurofibrillary tangles in the brain as they are in trying to smooth out the environmental and relational tangles the person experiences.

The overriding goals in caring for older adults with dementia are to maintain function and prevent excess disability, structure the environment and relationships to maintain stability, compensate for the losses associated with the disease, and create a therapeutic milieu that nurtures the personhood of the individual and maintains quality of life. Box 19-9 presents an

| BOX 19-9 | GENERAL NURSING INTERVENTIONS IN CARE OF PERSONS WITH DEMENTIA |

BOX 19-9 GENERAL NURSING INTERVENTIONS IN CARE OF PERSONS WITH DEMENTIA

- Address safety
- Structure daily living to maximize remaining abilities
- Monitor general health and impact of dementia on management of other medical conditions
- Support advance care planning and advanced directives
- Educate caregivers in the areas of problem-solving, resource access, long range planning, emotional support, and respite

From Evans L: Complex care needs in older adults with common cognitive disorders. Available at http://hartfordign.org/uploads/File/gnec_state_of_science_papers/gnec_dementia.pdf. Accessed October 14, 2010.

overview of general nursing intervention principles in the care of persons with dementia. Box 19-5 presents evidence-based resources that nurses will find helpful in designing care for persons with dementia.

Three common care concerns for people with moderate to late-stage dementia are discussed in the remainder of this chapter: behavior concerns, ADL care, and wandering. Nutrition is discussed in Chapter 14, and communication is discussed in Chapter 6. Caregiving for persons with dementia is discussed later in the Chapter 22.

Behavior Concerns and Nursing Models of Care

Behavior and psychological symptoms of dementia (BPSD) may present in as many as 90% of individuals at some point in the disease trajectory. BPSD are symptoms of disturbed perception, thought content, mood, and behavior and may include anxiety, depression, hallucinations, delusions, aggression, screaming, restlessness, agitation, and resistance to care (Dettmore et al., 2009; Kolanowski et al., 2010). BPSD symptoms cause a great deal of distress to the person and the caregivers and often precipitate institutionalization. For formal caregivers in institutions, caring for older people with BPSD symptoms is positively associated with physical and psychological caregiver burden as well (Miyamoto, Tachimori, Ito, 2010).

Several nursing models of care are helpful in recognizing and understanding the behavior of individuals with dementia and can be used to guide practice and assist families and staff in providing care from a more person-centered framework. The Progressively Lowered Stress Threshold model (PLST) and the Need-driven Dementia-compromised Behavior model (NDDB) focus on "the close interplay between person, context, and environment. These models propose that behavior is used to communicate or express, in the best way the person has available, unmet needs (physiological, psychosocial, disturbing environment, uncomfortable social surroundings) and/or difficulty managing stress as the disease progresses" (Evans, 2007, p. 7).

The Vulnerability Framework, derived from research in nursing homes, builds on the person, context, and environment interaction and adds the element of time. Findings of this study suggest that care providers in nursing homes were aware of interventions that modify the state (i.e., the person) and space (i.e., the environment), but time (perceived and real) poses significant barriers to implementation of nonpharmacological interventions for BPSD (Kolanowski et al., 2010).

The PLST Model The progressively lowered stress threshold (PLST) model (Hall and Buckwalter, 1987; Hall, 1994) was one of the first models used to plan and evaluate care for people with dementia in every setting. The PLST model categorizes symptoms of dementia into four groups: (1) cognitive or intellectual losses, (2) affective or personality changes, (3) conative or planning losses that cause a decline in functional abilities, and (4) loss of the stress threshold, causing behaviors such as agitation or catastrophic reactions. Symptoms such as agitation are a result of a progressive loss of the person's ability to cope with demands and stimuli when the person's stress threshold is exceeded. Five common stressors that may trigger these symptoms are fatigue; change of environment, routine, or caregiver; misleading stimuli or inappropriate stimulus levels; internal or external demands to perform beyond abilities; and physical stressors such as pain, discomfort, acute illness, and depression.

Using this model, care is structured to decrease the stressors and provide a safe and predictable environment. Positive outcomes from use of the model include improved sleep; decreased sedative and tranquilizer use; increased food intake and weight; increased socialization; decreased episodes of aggressive, agitated, and disruptive behaviors; increased caregiver satisfaction with care; and increased functional level (DeYoung et al., 2003; Hall and Buckwalter, 1987). Box 19-10 presents the principles of care derived from the PLST model.

Need-Driven Dementia-Compromised Behavior Model The need-driven, dementia-compromised behavior (NDB) model (Kolanowski, 1999; Richards et al., 2000; Algase et al., 2003) is a framework for the study and understanding of behavioral symptoms of dementia. All behaviors have meaning and are a form of communication, particularly as verbal communication becomes more limited. The NDB model proposes that the behavior of persons with dementia carries a message of need that can be addressed appropriately if the person's history and

BOX 19-10 PRINCIPLES OF CARE DERIVED FROM PLST MODEL

1. Maximize functional abilities by supporting all losses in a prosthetic manner.
2. Establish a caring relationship, and provide the person with unconditional positive regard.
3. Use behaviors indicating anxiety and avoidance to determine appropriate limits of activity and stimuli.
4. Teach caregivers to try to find out causes of behavior and to observe and evaluate verbal and nonverbal responses.
5. Identify triggers related to discomfort or stress reactions (factors in the environment, caregiver communication).
6. Modify the environment to support losses and promote safe function.
7. Evaluate care routines and responses on a 24-hour basis, and adjust plan of care accordingly.
8. Provide as much control as possible; encourage self-care, offer choices, explain all actions, do not push or force the person to do something.
9. Keep environment stable and predictable.
10. Provide ongoing education, support, care, and problem solving for caregivers.

Adapted from Hall GR, Buckwalter KC: *Archives of Psychiatric Nursing* 1:399, 1987.

habits, physiological status, and physical and social environment are carefully evaluated (Kolanowski, 1999). Rather than behavior being viewed as disruptive, it is viewed as having meaning and expressing needs. Behavior reflects the interaction of background factors (cognitive changes as a result of dementia, gender, ethnicity, culture, education, personality, responses to stress) and proximal factors (physiological needs such as hunger or pain, mood, physical environment [e.g., light, noise]) with social environment (e.g., staff stability and mix, presence of others) (Richards et al., 2000).

Optimal care is provided by manipulating the proximal factors that precipitate behavior and by maximizing strengths and minimizing the limitations of the background factors. "Caregivers must first identify and address the unmet need(s) that come from both sets of factors rather than control the behavior by extinguishing the call for help with sedating drugs" (Dettmore et al., 2009). For instance, sleep disruptions are common in people with dementia. If the person is not getting adequate sleep at night, agitated or aggressive behavior during the day may signal the need for more rest. Interventions to modify proximal factors interfering with sleep, such as noise, frequent awakenings during the night, and daytime boredom, can help meet the need for rest and sleep and decrease agitation or aggression.

Assessment   It is essential to view all behavior as meaningful and an expression of needs. The focus must be on understanding that behavioral expressions communicate distress, and the response is to investigate the possible sources of distress and intervene appropriately. There are many possible reasons for BPSD. After ruling out medical problems (e.g., pneumonia, dehydration, impaction, infection/sepsis, fractures, pain, or depression) as a cause of behavior, continued assessment to identify why distressing symptoms are occurring is important (Evans, 2007). Conditions such as constipation or urinary tract infections can cause great distress for cognitively impaired older people and may lead to marked changes in behavior (e.g., agitation, falls, refusal of care), so careful assessment is important. Pain is a frequent cause of aggressive behavior (striking out, resistance to care), and, after careful assessment of other possible causes, treatment with a trial of analgesics should be considered (Hall et al., 2009) (Chapter 17).

Fear, discomfort, unfamiliar surroundings and people, illness, fatigue, depression, need for autonomy and control, caregiver approaches, communication strategies, and environmental stressors are frequent precipitants of behavioral symptoms. "For the individual with late-stage dementia, a good deal of their discomfort comes from non-physiological sources, for example, from difficulty sorting out and negotiating everyday life activities" (Kovach et al., 1999, p. 412). Hall and colleagues suggest that "caregivers may not understand that behaviors are a symptom of the disease, much as pain would be expected with a malignancy. Understanding what triggers behavior is important. What may appear as hallucinations or delusions to the caregiver might be misinterpretations by the person of a television program, family photographs, or images reflected in a mirror. In these cases, it is much safer to turn off the television, remove photographs from the area, or cover a mirror than to place the patient on an antipsychotic medication" (Hall et al., 2009, pp. 40, 41). Box 19-11 presents precipitating factors for BPSD.

> ## BOX 19-11   CONDITIONS PRECIPITATING BEHAVIORAL SYMPTOMS IN PERSONS WITH DEMENTIA
>
> - Communication deficits
> - Pain or discomfort
> - Acute medical problems
> - Sleep disturbances
> - Perceptual deficits
> - Depression
> - Need for social contact
> - Hunger, thirst, need to toilet
> - Loss of control
> - Misinterpretation of the situation or environment
> - Crowded conditions
> - Changes in environment or people
> - Noise, disruption
> - Being forced to do something
> - Fear
> - Loneliness
> - Psychotic symptoms
> - Fatigue
> - Environmental overstimulation or understimulation
> - Depersonalized, rushed care
> - Restraints
> - Psychoactive drugs

Putting yourself in the place of the person with dementia and trying to see the world from his or her eyes will help you understand their behavior. Questions of what, where, why, when, who, and what now, are important components of the assessment of behavior. Box 19-12 presents a framework for asking questions about the possible meanings and messages behind observed behavior. Use of a behavioral log over a two- to three-day period to track when the behavior occurs, the circumstances, and the response to interventions is recommended and required in skilled nursing facilities. The Behave-AD, the Cohen-Mansfield Agitation Inventory, and the Neuropsychiatric Inventory for Nursing Homes, are examples of reliable instruments that can be used in assessment (Dettmore et al., 2009).

Interventions   All evidence-based guidelines endorse an approach that begins with comprehensive assessment of the behavior and possible causes followed by the use of nonpharmacological interventions as a first line of treatment (American Geriatrics Society, American Association for Geriatric Psychiatry, 2003; Benoit et al., 2006; Lyketsos et al., 2006). Despite these recommendations, psychotropic medications to treat BPSD are often the first-line response. This is of serious concern in light of the side effects of such medications. None of these medications are approved for use in treatment of behavioral responses in dementia (Kuehn, 2010b; Schneider et al., 2006).

In nursing homes, Kolanowski et al., (2010) suggest that "nurses continue to request and physicians continue to prescribe psychotropic drugs for the majority of residents with BPSD" (p. 215). Several authors suggest that insufficient staffing in nursing homes; time; emphasis on controlling residents rather than understanding; lack of interdisciplinary team approaches and family involvement; and inadequate education and research about behavior and use of nonpharmacologic interventions contribute to less than optimal practice

BOX 19-12   FRAMEWORK FOR ASKING QUESTIONS ABOUT THE MEANING OF BEHAVIOR

WHAT?
What is being sought? What is happening? Does the behavior have a physical or emotional component or both? What are the person's responses? What would be done if the person was 20 years old instead of 80? What is the behavior saying? What is the emotion being expressed?

WHERE?
Where is the behavior occurring? Environmental triggers?

WHEN?
When does the behavior most frequently occur? After what (e.g., activities of daily living [ADLs], family visits, mealtimes)?

WHO?
Who is involved? Other residents, caregivers, family?

WHY?
What happened before? Poor communication? Tasks too complicated? Physical or medical problem? Person being rushed or forced to do something? Has this happened before and why?

WHAT NOW?
Approaches and interventions (physical, psychosocial)?
Changes needed and by whom?
Who else might know something about the person or the behavior or approaches?
Communicate to all and include in plan of care.

Adapted from Hellen C: *Alzheimer's disease: activity focused care,* Boston, 1998, Butterworth-Heinemann; Ortigara A. *Alzheimer's Care Quarterly* 1:91, 2000.

(Dettmore et al., 2009; Kolanowski et al., 2010). Often these drugs are prescribed" in response to frustration and helplessness on the parts of both caretakers and loved ones alike (Dettmore et al., 2009, p. 14).

Pharmacological approaches may be considered in addition to nonpharmacological approaches if there has been a comprehensive assessment of reversible causes of behavior; the person presents a danger to self or others; nonpharmacological interventions have not been effective; and the risk/benefit profiles of the medications have been considered (Dettmore et al., 2009; Kolanowski et al., 2010). If psychotropic medications are used, the person must be monitored closely for extrapyramidal signs, orthostasis, somnolence, and neuroleptic malignant syndrome. Strict federal regulations monitor the use of psychotropic medications in skilled nursing facilities (Chapter 9).

Less is known about care approaches for BPSD in community-dwelling older people with dementia, but behavior and communication problems are common sources of ongoing stress as well as precipitants to nursing home placement. In a recent study exploring what matters most to family caregivers of persons with mild to moderate dementia, participants struggled with behavior problems, such as aggression and delusions. In the words of one participant: "It isn't that I want to get rid of the man. If it was a physical thing, my God I'd feed and wash him and do everything but I don't know how to handle this." (Hain et al., 2010). Clearly more research is needed to fully understand BPSD and effective interventions in both institutional and home settings.

Nonpharmacological Approaches   Nonpharmacological approaches are resident-centered and include interventions such as meaningful activities, validation therapy, social contact (real or simulated), animal-assisted therapy, exercise, sensory stimulation, reminiscence, Montessori-based activities, environmental design (e.g., special care units, homelike environments, gardens, safe walking areas), changes in mealtime and bathing environments, consistent staffing assignments, bright light therapy, aromatherapy, massage, music, relaxation, distraction, and nonconfrontational interaction (Dettmore et al., 2009; Evans, 2007; Edgerton and Richie, 2010; Kolanowski et al., 2010; Holliday-Welsh et al., 2009; Smith et al., 2009).

There is a large amount of literature on nonpharmacological interventions, and these approaches are recommended in the culture change movement. In general, these interventions have shown promise for improving quality of life for persons with dementia despite a lack of rigorous evaluation. Sensory enhancement/relaxation methods, such as bright light therapy, music therapy, Snoezelen (a relaxation technique popular in Europe), and massage, have been studied most extensively, and there is good evidence for their effectiveness (Box 19-13).

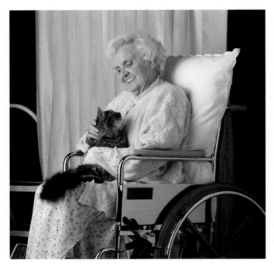

A nursing home resident enjoying pet therapy. (Courtesy of Corbis.)

BOX 19-13   RESEARCH HIGHLIGHTS

Massage in the Management of Agitation in Nursing Home Residents with Cognitive Impairment

This study examined the potential of massage to reduce wandering, verbally agitated and abusive behavior, physically agitated and abusive behavior, socially inappropriate/disruptive behavior, and resistive care behavior in cognitively impaired nursing home residents. The type of massage used in the study was effleurage, which uses gliding or sliding movements with light to moderate pressure over the skin in a smooth, continuous manner. Primary areas of the body massaged were the upper extremities, including the head, shoulders, and hands. The massage was provided by a physical therapy assistant trained in massage techniques. Massage was associated with significant improvement in wandering, verbally agitated/abusive behavior, physically agitated/abusive behavior, and resistive care behavior.

Massage is an accessible, easily learned intervention that is effective in controlling some types of agitation in cognitively impaired older adults and should be further studied as a nonpharmacological intervention that can be used by formal and informal caregivers.

From Holliday-Welsh D, Gessert C, Renier C: *Geriatric Nursing* 30:108, 2009.

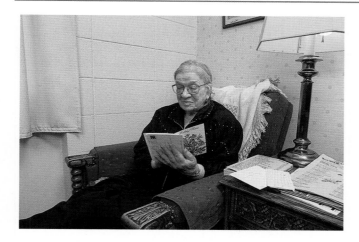

Meaningful activities provide cognitive stimulation. (From Sorrentino SA, Gorek B: *Mosby's textbook for long-term care assistants*, ed 5, St. Louis, 2007, Mosby.)

Therapeutic activities are important in enhancing function and quality of life for individuals with dementia in both institutional, community, and home settings. In nursing facilities, there should be opportunities for participation in meaningful and enjoyable individual and group therapeutic activities that are available across the 24-hour day. Activities should be tailored to the personality traits, interests, and abilities of the individual (Hill et al., 2010; Smith et al., 2010). Recreational specialists often develop and administer these programs, but trained staff, family members, and volunteers can also be utilized to enhance programming activities. The NEST (Needs, Environment, Stimulation, and Technique) approach provides over 80 therapeutic protocols for therapeutic activities consistent with the NDB model of dementia care (Buettner and Fitzsimmons, 2009). While socialization and stimulation activities are very important, development of therapeutic interventions to maintain and promote health and optimal functioning of persons with dementia need continued research (see Chapter 2).

Providing Care for Activities of Daily Living

The losses associated with dementia interfere with the person's communication patterns and ability to understand and express thoughts and feelings. Perceptual disturbances and misinterpretations of reality contribute to fear and misunderstanding. Often, bathing and the provision of other ADL care, such as dressing, grooming, and toileting, are the cause of much distress for both the person with dementia and the caregiver.

Bathing   Bathing and care for ADLs, particularly in nursing homes, can be perceived as an attack by persons with dementia who may respond by screaming or striking out. A rigid focus on tasks or institutional care routines, such as a shower three mornings each week, can contribute to the distress and precipitate distressing behaviors. Being touched or bathed against one's will violates the trust in caregiver relationships and can be considered a major affront (Rader and Barrick, 2000). The behaviors that may be exhibited by the person with dementia are not deliberate attacks on caregivers by a violent person. The message is, in the words of Rader and Barrick (2000, p. 49), "Please find another way to keep me clean, because the way you are doing it now is intolerable."

To care effectively for older adults with dementia, nurses and other caregivers need to try to put themselves in the place of the person with dementia and try to see the world from his or her eyes. The following paragraph will illustrate:

> You are asleep in the chair at home when suddenly you are awakened by a person you have never seen before trying to undress you. Then he or she puts you naked into a hard, cold chair and wheels you down a hallway. Suddenly cold water hits you in the face and the person is touching your private areas. You don't understand why the person is trying to do this to you. You are embarrassed, frightened, cold, and angry. You hit and scream at this person and try to get away.

Family members and nurses caring for people with dementia must understand that they are the ones who must change their behavior, reactions, and approaches because the person with dementia cannot do this. Education to teach caregivers how to interact with persons with dementia during direct care show efficacy for aggression and resistive behavior. Using appropriate communication strategies, explaining all actions before doing, not pushing or forcing people who are resistant, providing positive feedback, paying attention to body posture and facial expressions, using gestures, demonstration, one-step directions, staying calm and pleasant, providing warmth and comfort, and allowing appropriate time for response are some general suggested techniques to enhance ADL care interactions.

In research in nursing homes, Rader and Barrick (2000) have provided comprehensive guidelines for bathing people with dementia in ways that are pleasurable and decrease distress. Asking the question "What is the easiest, most comfortable, least frightening way for me to clean the person right now?" guides the choice of interventions (Rader and Barrick, 2000, p. 42). Suggested interventions to make bathtime more pleasurable and safer include knowing the person's lifetime bathing routines and preferences; providing care only when the person is receptive; respecting refusals to participate in care; explaining all actions; realizing that a bath is not an essential intervention; encouraging self-care to the extent possible; making bathrooms and shower areas warm, comfortable, and safe; being attentive to pain and discomfort; and using alternative bathing methods, such as a towel bath or sponge bath (Rader et al., 2006). Additional resources related to bathing older adults can be found on the Evolve website.

Another innovative approach being investigated in Sweden is caregiver singing and the use of background music during ADL care in nursing homes. Caregivers play and sing familiar songs during care routines. When compared to usual care practices, this approach enhanced the expression of positive moods and emotions, increased the mutuality of communication, and reduced aggression and resistive care behaviors (Götell et al., 2010) http://www.dementiacaresinging.com/. While further systematic intervention studies are needed, music therapy is recognized as an evidence-based intervention with positive outcomes in dementia care (Gerdner, 2010) (Chapter 24).

Wandering

Wandering associated with dementia is one of the most difficult management problems encountered in home and institutional settings. Wandering is considered a behavioral problem of dementia that involves "cognitive impairment affecting abstract thinking, language, judgment, and spatial skills; disorientation and difficulty relating to the environment; low social interaction, pacing or increased motor activity, and aimless or purposeful motor activity that causes a social problem such as getting lost, leaving a safe environment, or intruding in inappropriate places" (Futrell et al., 2010, p. 6).

Wandering is a complex behavior and is not well understood. There is a need for more research on wandering as well as interventions for this behavior. Some research indicates that there may be a relationship between certain types of wandering and different presentations of dementia (Dewing, 2006). People with dementia who wander may have more visuospatial impairments, anxiety and depression, and a history of a prior active lifestyle.

Wandering presents safety concerns in all settings. Wandering behavior affects sleep, eating, safety, the caregiver's ability to provide care, and interference with the privacy of others. The behavior can lead to falls, elopement (leaving the home or facility), injury, and death (Futrell et al., 2010; Rowe et al., 2010). The stimulus for wandering arises from many internal and external sources. Wandering can be considered a rhythm, intrinsically and extrinsically driven. The following excerpts about wandering from an article by Laurenhue (2001) provide a great deal of insight into this concern from the person's perspective:

> "Wandering and restlessness is one of the by-products of Alzheimer's disease . . . When the darkness and emptiness fills my mind, it is totally terrifying . . . Thoughts increasingly haunt me. The only way I can break the cycle is to move" (Davis, 1989, p. 96).
>
> "Very often, I wander around looking for something which I know is very pertinent, but then after awhile I forget all about what it was I was looking for. When I'm wandering around, I'm trying to touch base with—anything, actually. If anything appeared I'd probably enjoy it, or look at it or examine it and wonder how it got there. I feel very foolish when I'm wandering around not knowing what I'm doing and I'm not always quite sure how to do any better. It's not easy to figure out what the heck I'm looking for" (Henderson, 1998, p. 24).

Wandering behaviors can be predicted through careful observation and knowing the person's patterns. For example, if the person with dementia starts wandering or trying to leave the home around dinnertime every day, meaningful activities such as music, exercise, and refreshments can be provided at this time. Research suggests that wandering may be less likely to occur when the person is involved in social interaction. There are also several instruments to assess risk for wandering, and Futrell and colleagues (2010) developed an evidence-based protocol for wandering. Environmental interventions, such as camouflaging doorways, providing enclosed outdoor gardens and paths for walking, and electronic bracelets that activate alarms

---

BOX 19-14   INTERVENTIONS FOR WANDERING OR EXITING BEHAVIORS

- Face the person, and make direct eye contact (unless this is interpreted as threatening).
- Gently touch the person's arm, shoulders, back, or waist if he or she does not move away from a door or other exit.
- Call the person by his or her formal name (e.g., Mr. Jones).
- Listen to what the person is communicating verbally and nonverbally; listen to the feelings being expressed.
- Identify the agenda, plan of action, and the emotional needs the agenda is expressing.
- Respond to the feelings expressed, staying calm.
- Repeat specific words or phrases, or state the need or emotion (e.g., "You need to go home, you're worried about your husband").
- If such repetition fails to distract the person, accompany him or her and continue talking calmly, repeating phrases and the emotion you identify.
- Provide orienting information only if it calms the person. If it increases distress, stop talking about the present situations. Do not "correct" the person or belittle his or her agenda.
- At intervals, redirect the person toward the facility or the home by suggesting, "Let's walk this way now" or "I'm so tired, let's turn around."
- If orientation and redirection fail, continue to walk, allowing the person control but ensuring safety.
- Make sure you have a backup person, but he or she should stay out of eyesight of the person.
- Have someone call for help if you are unable to redirect. Usually the behavior is time limited because of the person's attention span and the security and trust between you and the person.

Adapted from Rader J, Doan J, Schwab M: *Geriatric Nursing* 6:196, 1985.

---

at exits, are also used. There are a number of assistive technology devices and programs that can enhance the safety of persons who wander (Chapter 13). Box 19-14 presents other suggested interventions.

Wandering behavior may also result in people with dementia going outside and getting lost, a phenomenon studied by Rowe (2003). The Alzheimer's Association estimates that 60% of people with dementia will wander and become lost in the community at some point (www.alz.org/living_with_alzheimers_wandering_behaviors.asp). Conclusions from Rowe's (2003) research, a retrospective review of the records of Safe Return (a nationwide federally funded identification program of the Alzheimer's Association), advised that all people with dementia should be considered capable of becoming lost. Caregivers must prevent people with dementia from leaving homes or care facilities unaccompanied, register the person in the Safe Return program, and have a plan of action in case the person does become lost. Rowe also suggests that police must respond rapidly to requests for searches, and the general public should be informed about how to recognize and assist people with dementia who may be lost (2003). Box 19-15 presents specific recommendations from this study.

CAREGIVING FOR PERSONS WITH DEMENTIA

More than 70% of persons with dementia live at home, and family and friends provide nearly 75% of their care. Nearly 15 million people provide care for a loved one with AD or another

BOX 19-15 RECOMMENDATIONS TO AVOID PEOPLE WITH DEMENTIA GETTING LOST

- Do not leave the person with dementia alone in the home.
- Secure the environment so that the person cannot leave by himself or herself while the caregiver is asleep or busy.
- If the person lives in a nursing facility, keep in a supervised area; do frequent checks; use bed, chair, and door alarms and Wanderguard bracelets; identify potential wanderers by special arm bands; and disguise doorways.
- Place locks out of reach, hide keys, and lock windows.
- Consider motion detectors or home security systems that alert when doors are opened.
- Register the person in the Safe Return program of the Alzheimer's Association, and ensure that the person wears the Safe Return jewelry or clothing tags at all times.
- Register with the Silver Alert system if available.
- Let neighbors know that a person with dementia lives in the neighborhood.
- Prepare a search-and-rescue plan in case the person becomes lost.
- Keep copies of up-to-date photos ready for distribution to searchers, police, hospitals, and the media.
- Conduct a search immediately if the person becomes lost.
- Call the local law enforcement agency and the Safe Return program to report the missing person.
- If the person is not found within 6 to 12 hours (or sooner depending on weather conditions), search any wooded areas or fields near where the person was last seen. People with dementia may not seek help or respond to calls and may try to hide from searchers; search in an organized manner with as many searchers as possible.

Adapted from Rowe MA: *American Journal of Nursing* 103:32, 2003.

form of dementia, amounting to 17 billion hours or more than $202 billion in unpaid care. The $202 billion is on top of the $183 billion estimate for Alzheimer's care expected to be delivered in 2011 by health care workers in home, hospital, and long term care facilities an increase of $11 billion over a year ago (Alzheimer's Association, 2011). These caregivers provide more hours of help than caregivers of other older people and experience more adverse consequences to their physical and mental health. Caregivers of persons with dementia have lower self-rated health scores; display fewer health-promoting behaviors; and have higher depression and anxiety rates, higher morbidity and mortality rates, sleep problems, and higher numbers of illness-related symptoms (Alzheimer's Association, 2010a; Elliott et al., 2010).

The Shriver Report: A Woman's Nation Takes on Alzheimer's (2010) (http://www.shriverreport.com/) provides some concerning statistics about the impact of Alzheimer's disease and Alzheimer's caregiving on women in the United States. Almost two thirds of Americans with Alzheimer's disease are women, and women compose 60% of the unpaid caregivers for family members with the disease. There are 10 million women who either have Alzheimer's disease or are caring for someone with the disease. One third of these female caregivers are caring for both children and family members at the same time. Moreover, women experience a greater incidence of depression, cardiovascular disease, and obesity—factors linked to the risk developing Alzheimer's disease. The rising

epidemic of Alzheimer's disease is a women's health issue that requires the attention of nurses and other health care professionals as well as the development of adequate community services and support programs.

More than 60% of Alzheimer's and dementia caregivers rate the emotional stress of caregiving as very high; one-third report symptoms of depression (Alzheimer's association, 2011). Factors that influence the stress of caregiving include grief over the multiple losses that occur, the physical demands and duration of caregiving (up to 20 years), and resource availability. The deleterious effects of caregiving in dementia are intensified when the care recipient demonstrates behavioral disturbances and impairments in ADLs and IADLs. While most of the research has centered on psychological problems, the relationship between caregiving and physical health needs further investigation (Alzheimer's Association, 2010a; Elliott et al., 2010).

The NINR studies, Resources for Enhancing Alzheimer's Caregiver Health (REACH 1 and 11) found that active skills training interventions were more effective at relieving caregiver burden and depression than more passive techniques, such as providing information. REACH interventions provided a series of 12 training interventions (9 in-home and 3 by telephone) over 6 months to teach caregivers about Alzheimer's disease and the skills to manage troublesome behaviors, maintain social support, reframe negative emotions, manage stress, and enhance their own healthy behaviors. Outcomes suggest that the intervention reduced depression and burden and improved quality of life (Elliott et al., 2010; Mittelman et al., 2007).

Grief is a major dimension of caregiving for persons with dementia, beginning on the day of diagnosis and continuing long after the death of the person. "Losses come in smaller steps such as the day the doctor told her that her husband should not drive, the moment when he asked her his daughter's name, and the most excruciating, his placement in residential care" (Peterson, 2006, p. 15). Losses are ongoing in dementia and include the loss of relationship, loss of a previous lifestyle, loss of independence, and loss of a confidante. The concept of anticipatory grief is used to describe the grief process and has a significant influence on quality of life for persons with dementia and their caregivers (Ross and Dagley, 2009; Hain et al., 2010). Often, caregivers do not recognize grief and do not seek help. An inventory to assess grief in caregivers (Marwit and Meuser, 2002) may be useful in both practice and research, and grief counseling should be included in caregiver intervention programs.

Most research has focused on caregiving in the late stages of dementia and on the "burden" of caregiving. Many authors suggest that the "concept of burden alone does not adequately explain the complexities of caregiving for an older person with dementia" (Suwa, 2002, p. 5). Warmth, pleasure, comfort, spiritual growth, self-transcendence, and other positive dimensions of caregiving have also emerged in qualitative studies (Acton, 2002; Farran et al., 2004). In the study by the Alzheimer's Foundation of America (2008), 77% of survey participants reported that they had become stronger than they thought; 64% believed that they had become more compassionate as a result of caregiving; and 59% said they feel closer to the patient since they began caring for them. Further research is needed to help us understand how we can extend caring to both the caregiver and the person with dementia in ways that maintain personhood, enhance relationships, promote quality of life, and balance the stresses with the joys.

Special Considerations for Caregiving in Mild Cognitive Impairment, Early-Stage Dementia, and Early-Onset Dementia

Mild Cognitive Impairment and Early-Stage Dementia

To date, the preponderance of research and intervention programs for caregivers has been directed toward persons and their families living with later stages of dementia and has focused on preparing caregivers to cope with issues such as behavior problems, incontinence, ADL care, and nursing home placement. Many of the issues addressed are not relevant to those with EO-D, MCI, or mild stages of dementia; will not be of interest to them in the future; and can be frightening and misleading as well (Blieszner and Roberto, 2010; Hain et al., 2010).

Areas of concern for caregivers of persons with MCI and early-stage dementia center less on personal care needs and more on communication, behavior, and relationships. Some of the issues identified in research include dealing with loss, frustration, anger, balancing care of self with care for the person with dementia, reorienting themselves to a different life, uncertainty about the future, changes in the couple relationship, difficulties in communication, and doing the best job they can to ensure that the person with dementia receives the best care and life is as pleasurable as possible for them and for the person with dementia (Blieszner and Roberto, 2010; Hain et al., 2010) (Box 19-16).

Additionally, individuals with MCI, EO-D, or mild dementia are aware of their diagnosis and need opportunities to share their feelings and needs and receive support as well. Research must include the voices of those experiencing the health challenge of dementia. For individuals with EO-D and those with MCI and early-stage dementia, interventions that help both the person and his or her caregiver to deal with changing roles, stress, frustration, loss, communication difficulties, and the couple relationship are particularly needed (Hain et al., 2011; Keady et al., 2007).

Family members of persons with early-onset dementia and those in earlier stages of dementia often struggle in the caregiving role with little help or support and are already experiencing a need for support services, particularly for social and psychological support (Hain et al., 2010). Problems appearing early in the caregiving trajectory have long-term implications for psychosocial outcomes, such as burden and depression. Early intervention is important, and use of services such as respite, housekeeping, and day programs not only help in meeting daily demands but may also promote closer relationships and improved cognitive and functional outcomes (Norton et al., 2009). The importance of a proactive approach, with interventions offered at the beginning of the care trajectory, rather than a reactive approach, is being noted in the literature and treatment guidelines (Ducharme et al., 2009).

BOX 19-16   RESEARCH HIGHLIGHTS

What Matters Most to Family Carers of People with Mild to Moderate Dementia

Interviews were conducted with 10 family carers (7 spouses and 3 adult children) of individuals with mild to moderate dementia to explore what matters most to family carers of people with mild to moderate dementia. Participants were recruited from a Memory and Wellness Center and the interview took place as part of a free GNP consultation offered at the Center. Questions posed included the following: Tell me more about having your loved one diagnosed with mild to moderate dementia; What matters most to you right now?; What support and/or information, if any, do you need now?; Describe what you think your future will be like as a carer of someone with mild to moderate dementia?; What are some of your future hopes and dreams?

Findings reinforced the complexity of the carer role, which is plagued with emotional ambiguity as people experience both the rewards and challenges of caregiving. The participants reported difficulty knowing where to turn for advice and guidance, particularly when related to handling behavior problems. Participants often tried to do it alone and were unaware of the type of resources available, how they worked, or how to access them. They described many stresses but felt guilty for getting angry or frustrated, and they missed the activities they used to do. They were living day to day, afraid of the future, and trying to reorient themselves to a different life and make it as pleasurable as possible for both them and the person with dementia. Their affection and commitment to the loved one made them determined to fight and do their best.

The early stage of dementia may be the most crucial time to intervene and establish a health care provider-patient/family partnership. Support for caregivers should begin at the time of initial diagnosis and continue throughout the disease trajectory because needs vary according to the level of dementia. The study lays the groundwork for further exploration of the efficacy of a GNP consultation as an intervention to determine what matters most to carers of persons with mild to moderate dementia, mutual goal setting, and the development of individualized strategies to support carers on their journey.

Source: Hain, D, Touhy T, Engstrom G: *Alzheimer's Care Today* 11:162, 2010.

Early-Onset Dementia

Persons with EO-D are a growing subpopulation of persons with dementia, and the knowledge base for diagnosis, treatment, and interventions is just beginning to develop. There are some model programs, but generally there is a lack of services and programs for this group, and the majority of resources are designed for an older population. With the growing numbers of persons with EO-D, the disease is being recognized as a significant clinical and social problem. Caregivers of persons with EO-D report higher levels of burden and poorer emotional well-being than those reported by caregivers with late-onset dementia (Rose et al., 2010; Werner et al., 2009).

Rose and colleagues (2010) identified the following themes from case study analysis to describe the challenges associated with EO-D for individuals and their families: 1) coping with the stigma associated with dementia; 2) lack of access to services and benefits that are reserved for those who are older; 3) loss of income, work roles, and related benefits during prime working years; 4) loneliness and isolation for both the person with dementia and his or her family members; 5) difficulties in meeting the safety needs of someone who is physically able; 6) challenges in finding appropriate long-term care placement in facilities or day center programs designed for and populated primarily for older adults; and 7) difficulties that caregivers may experience when working while caring for a family member or for small children while caring for a spouse with EO-D.

Additionally, changes in the relationship with partners and other family members and anxiety and burden associated with the development of the disease by first-degree at-risk relatives of persons with EO-D are major concerns. Individuals with EO-D and their families experience a double economic strain because they often lose their income while at the same time not being eligible for financial assistance. EO-D is not categorized as a disability or terminal illness and does not qualify younger patients to receive the same benefits as those available to younger persons (Werner et al., 2009). Rose and colleagues (2010) offer suggestions for interventions to meet the needs of individuals with EO-D and their caregivers.

Continued research is needed to develop programs and services that address the differential needs of caregivers and

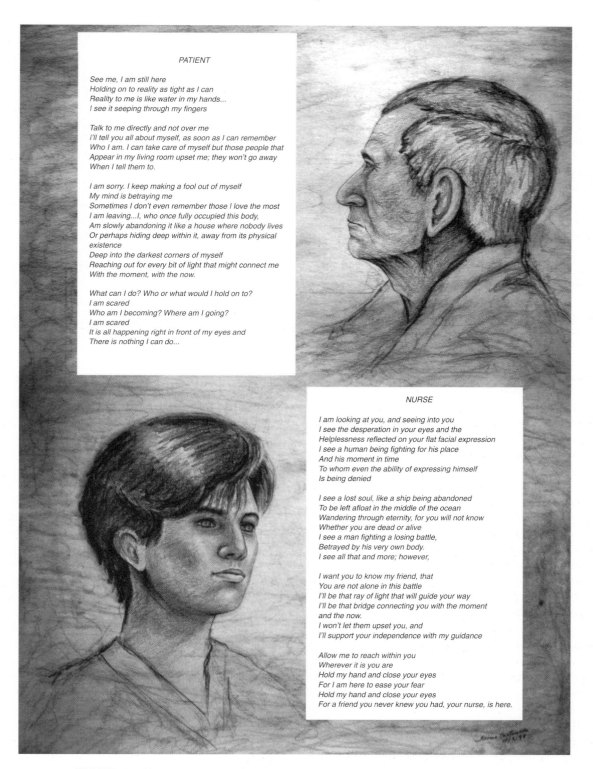

PATIENT

See me, I am still here
Holding on to reality as tight as I can
Reality to me is like water in my hands...
I see it seeping through my fingers

Talk to me directly and not over me
I'll tell you all about myself, as soon as I can remember
Who I am. I can take care of myself but those people that
Appear in my living room upset me; they won't go away
When I tell them to.

I am sorry. I keep making a fool out of myself
My mind is betraying me
Sometimes I don't even remember those I love the most
I am leaving...I, who once fully occupied this body,
Am slowly abandoning it like a house where nobody lives
Or perhaps hiding deep within it, away from its physical existence
Deep into the darkest corners of myself
Reaching out for every bit of light that might connect me
With the moment, with the now.

What can I do? Who or what would I hold on to?
I am scared
Who am I becoming? Where am I going?
I am scared
It is all happening right in front of my eyes and
There is nothing I can do...

NURSE

I am looking at you, and seeing into you
I see the desperation in your eyes and the
Helplessness reflected on your flat facial expression
I see a human being fighting for his place
And his moment in time
To whom even the ability of expressing himself
Is being denied

I see a lost soul, like a ship being abandoned
To be left afloat in the middle of the ocean
Wandering through eternity, for you will not know
Whether you are dead or alive
I see a man fighting a losing battle,
Betrayed by his very own body.
I see all that and more; however,

I want you to know my friend, that
You are not alone in this battle
I'll be that ray of light that will guide your way
I'll be that bridge connecting you with the moment
and the now.
I won't let them upset you, and
I'll support your independence with my guidance

Allow me to reach within you
Wherever it is you are
Hold my hand and close your eyes
For I am here to ease your fear
Hold my hand and close your eyes
For a friend you never knew you had, your nurse, is here.

FIGURE 19-1 Nurse and person. (Copyright © 1998 by Jaime Castaneda, Lake Worth, Fla.)

individuals with dementia based on stage of illness and type of dementia. Evidence is accumulating that caregiver intervention programs that include bundled interventions, such as individual and group modalities for both the person with dementia and the caregiver—as well as combined groups, education, counseling, support group participation, opportunities to discuss individual concerns with health professionals, care management, and the continuous availability of telephone support—may be the most effective (Mittelman et al., 2007). Continued research and development of programs of support and services for individuals with MCI, early stage dementia, and EO-D and their caregivers is a priority, as is continued evaluation of the effectiveness of interventions in practice.

NURSING ROLES IN THE CARE OF PERSONS WITH DEMENTIA

Caregiving for someone with dementia by family members, or formal caregivers, requires exquisite skills, knowledge of evidence-based practice, and a deep knowing of the person. Rader and Tornquist (1995) reflect on the knowledge required and provide a view of caregiving roles that is quite useful and understandable for all caregivers. The author has found that nursing assistants and family caregivers can truly relate to the practical wisdom in these words.

Magician role: To understand what the person is trying to communicate both verbally and nonverbally, we must be a magician who can use our magical abilities to see the world through the eyes, the ears, and the feelings of the person. We know how to use tricks to turn an individual's behavior around or prevent it from occurring and causing distress.

Detective role: The detective looks for clues and cues about what might be causing distress and how it might be changed. We have to investigate and know as much about the person as possible to be a good detective.

Carpenter role: By having a wide variety of tools and selecting the right tools for the job, we build individualized plans of care for each person.

Jester role: Many people with dementia retain their sense of humor and respond well to the appropriate use of humor. This does not mean making fun of but rather sharing laughter and fun. "Those who love their work and do it well employ good doses of humor as part of the care of others as well as for self-care" (Rader and Barrick, 2000, p. 42). The jester spreads joy, is creative, energizes, and lightens the burdens (Rader and Barrick, 2000; Laurenhue, 2001).

Figure 19-1 presents a nursing situation that one nurse experienced in caring for a patient with dementia who was being admitted to a nursing home. Written from the perspective of the nurse and his knowing of the patient, the story provides insight into important nursing responses, such as person-centered care, therapeutic communication, and establishing meaningful relationships. It is a lovely example of expert gerontological nursing for older adults with dementia and a fitting way to end this chapter.

evolve   To access your student resources, go to *http://evolve.elsevier.com/Ebersole/TwdHlthAging*

█ KEY CONCEPTS

- Nurses must advocate for thorough assessment of any elder who appears to be experiencing cognitive decline and inability to function in important aspects of life.
- Delirium results from the interaction of predisposing factors (e.g., vulnerability on the part of the individual due to predisposing conditions such as cognitive impairment, severe illness, and sensory impairment) and precipitating factors/insults (e.g., medications, procedures, restraints, iatrogenic events). Delirium is characterized by an acute onset, fluctuating levels of consciousness, and frequent misperceptions and illusions. It often goes unrecognized and is attributed to age or dementia. People with dementia are more susceptible to delirium. Knowledge of risk factors, preventive measures, and treatment of underlying medical problems is essential to prevent serious consequences.
- Medications and pain are frequently the causes of delirious states in older people.
- Irreversible dementias follow a pattern of inevitable decline accompanied by decreased intellectual function, personality changes, and impaired judgment. The most common of these is Alzheimer's disease.
- Alzheimer's disease has been the subject of enormous research in attempts to understand the causes. There is growing evidence that Alzheimer's disease starts many years before symptoms appear, and attention to risk and modifying factors is receiving increased attention. Research is continuing in attempts to discover ways to protect against or halt the progress of the disease.
- Individuals with cognitive impairment respond best to calmness and patience, adaptations of communication techniques, and environments and relationships that enhance function, support limitations, ensure safety, and provide opportunities for a meaningful quality of life. Because cognitively impaired persons may be unable to express their feelings and needs in ways that are easily understood, the gerontological nurse must always try to understand the world from their perspective.
- Families provide most of the care for persons with dementia, and while many gain satisfaction from this, they experience more adverse consequences to their physical and mental health than caregivers of other older adults. Caregiving for persons with MCI, early-stage dementia, and EO-D presents different challenges and needs than caregiving in late-stage dementia, and more research is needed.

CASE STUDY COGNITIVE IMPAIRMENT

William was 69 years old and had been a successful builder until his retirement from business 4 years ago. His wife, Caroline, of 30 years was a high school teacher. Their marriage had been minimally gratifying, but both enjoyed their work and had felt they led a full and satisfying life. They had no children but had developed a large social network over the years; most were friends who were in some way work related. Six months ago William began to seem restless; he was easily angered and embarrassed himself and his wife several times by being verbally abusive during a social function with their friends. William was also less careful about his grooming. Because he had always been most meticulous about his appearance, his wife was quite alarmed that he seemed not to notice or care. After returning from one particularly exhausting vacation trip, William became enraged when he thought someone had stolen his wallet. He ignored his wife's efforts to calm him and became even angrier. Later his wife found his wallet in an inner suit jacket pocket. He ordinarily kept his wallet in the back pocket of his trousers. His wife began to feel anxious and frightened of him, though he had never physically abused her. She urged him to see the physician for a "general checkup" but was not surprised that he refused. She went to the physician for tranquilizers to quell her anxiety. He gave her a prescription for Prozac and sent her on her way. Her nurse-neighbor dropped by one day and found her in tears saying, "I just can't stand it anymore. William is not like himself. We used to have such fun and now he is angry all the time." As the nurse-neighbor, how would you help Caroline and William?

Based on the case study, develop a nursing care plan using the following procedure*:
- List William's comments that provide subjective data.
- List information that provides objective data.

- From these data, identify and state, using accepted format, two nursing diagnoses you determine are most significant to William at this time. List two of William's strengths that you have identified from data.
- Determine and state outcome criteria for each diagnosis. These must reflect some alleviation of the problem identified in the nursing diagnosis and must be stated in concrete and measurable terms.
- Plan and state one or more interventions for each diagnosed problem. Provide specific documentation of the source used to determine the appropriate intervention. Plan at least one intervention that incorporates William's existing strengths.
- Evaluate the success of the intervention. Interventions must correlate directly with the stated outcome criteria to measure the outcome success.

CRITICAL THINKING QUESTIONS

1. What memory aids might you suggest for a person who is complaining of memory problems?
2. What are some of the differences between delirium, dementia, and depression?
3. What nursing interventions will assist in preventing delirium in the hospitalized elder?
4. Identify several signs of early dementia.
5. How can Alzheimer's disease be diagnosed accurately?
6. Discuss some specific interventions to promote comfort during bathing for persons with dementia.
7. What type of communication techniques would be helpful in assisting with ADL activities for a person with dementia?

* Students are advised to refer to their nursing diagnosis text and identify possible or potential problems.

RESEARCH QUESTIONS

1. What barriers do nurses encounter in recognizing delirium in hospitalized older adults?
2. How does delirium experienced in the hospital affect care outcomes for older people who are discharged home?
3. How do cognitive stimulation programs affect the function of older adults with dementia?
4. What types of programs can be developed to enhance the health of older adults with dementia?
5. Do educational programs for informal and formal caregivers of older persons with dementia improve understanding and management of behavioral problems?
6. What are the primary care concerns of family caregivers of older adults in the home setting?
7. What type of support and services are most needed by caregivers of persons with MCI, early-stage dementia, and EO-D?

REFERENCES

Acton G: Self-transcendent views and behaviors: exploring growth in caregivers of adults with dementia, *Journal of Gerontological Nursing* 28:22, 2002.

Algase DL, Beel-Bates C, Beattie ERA: Wandering in long-term care, *Annals of Long-Term Care* 11:33, 2003.

Alzheimer's Association (2010a): 2010 Alzheimer's Facts and Figures. Available at www.alz.org/ alzheimers_disease_facts_figures.asp. Accessed October 7, 2010.

Alzheimer's Association (2010b): Changing the trajectory of Alzheimer's disease: A national imperative. Available at http://www.alz.org/ alzheimers_disease_trajectory.asp. Accessed October 7, 2010.

Alzheimer's Association (2010c): Preclinical Alzheimer's Disease Workgroup, 2010. Available at www.alz.org/research/diagnostic_ criteria/. Accessed September 29, 2010.

Alzheimer's Association: Fact sheet: Alzheimer's disease facts and figures, March 2011. Available at: http://www.alz.org/index.asp accessed May 17, 2011.

Alzheimer's Disease International: World Alzheimer Report 2010: The global economic impact of dementia. Available at http:// www.alz.org/documents/national/World_ Alzheimer_Report_2010.pdf. Accessed October 7, 2010.

Alzheimer's Foundation of America: I CAN: Investigating caregivers' attitudes and needs, 2008. Available at www.alzfdn.org. Accessed January 20, 2008.

American Geriatrics Society, American Association for Geriatric Psychiatry: The American Geriatrics Society and American Association for Geriatric Psychiatry recommendations for policies in support of quality mental health care in nursing homes, *Journal of the American Geriatrics Society* 51:1299, 2003.

American Psychiatric Association: *Diagnostic and statistical manual of mental disorders, DSM-IV-TR*, Washington, DC, 2000, The Association.

Balas MC, Gale M, Kagan SH: Delirium doulas: an innovative approach to enhance care for critically ill older adults, *Critical Care Nurse* 24:36, 2004.

Balas B, Gale M, Kagan S: Delirium in older patients in surgical intensive care units, *Journal of Nursng Scholarship* 39(2):147-154, 2007.

Bell V, Troxel D: Spirituality and the person with dementia: a view from the field, *Alzheimer's Care Quarterly* 2:31, 2001.

Bellelli G, Frisoni GB, Turco R, et al: Delirium superimposed on dementia predicts 12-month survival in elderly patients discharged from a postacute rehabilitation facility, *The Journals of Gerontology Series A: Biological Sciences and Medical Sciences* 63:1124, 2008.

Benoit M, Arbus C, Blanchard F, et al: Professional consensus on the treatment of agitation, aggressive behavior, oppositional behavior and psychotic disturbances in dementia, *Journal of Nutrition, Health & Aging* 10:410, 2006.

Blernow K, Zetterberg H: Is it time for biomarker-based diagnostic criteria for prodormal Alzheimer's disease? *Alzheimer's Research & Therapy* 2:8, 2010.

Blieszner R, Roberto K: Care partner responses to the onset of mild cognitive impairment, *The Gerontologist* 50:11, 2010.

Bradley EH, Webster TR, Baker D, et al: After adoption: sustaining the innovation: a case study of disseminating the Hospital Elder Life Program, *Journal of the American Geriatrics Society* 53:1455, 2005.

Braes T, Millisen K, Foreman M: Assessing cognitive function. In Capezuti E, Swicker D, Mezey M, et al., editors, *Evidence-based geriatric nursing protocols for best practice*, ed 3, New York, 2008, Springer.

Buettner L, Fitzsimmons S: *N.E.S.T. (Needs, environment, stimulation, techniques): interdisciplinary dementia practice guidelines.* State College, PA, 2009, Venture Publishing.

Callahan C, Boustani M, Unversagt F, et al: Effectiveness of collaborative care for older adults with Alzheimer's disease in primary care, *Journal of the American Medical Association* 295:2148, 2006.

Camp C, Skrajner J: Resident-assisted Montessori programming (RAMP): training persons with dementia to serve as activity group leaders, *Gerontologist* 44:426, 2004.

Chodosh J, Mittman B, Connor K, et al: Caring for patients with dementia: how good is the quality of care? Results from three health systems, *Journal of the American Geriatrics Society* 55:1260, 2007.

Clarke S, McRae M, Del Signore S, Schubert M, Styra R: Delirium in older cardiac surgery patients, *Journal of Gerontological Nursing* 36(11):34-45, 2010.

Cole M, McCusker J: Improving the outcomes of delirium in older hospital inpatients, *International Psychogeriatrics* 21:613, 2009.

Crowley SL: Aging brain's staying power, *AARP Bulletin* 37:1, 1996.

Dahlke S, Phinney A: Caring for hospitalized older adults at risk for delirium: the silent, unspoken piece of nursing practice, *Journal of Gerontological Nursing* 34:41, 2008.

Davis R: *My journey into Alzheimer's disease*, Wheaton, Ill, 1989, Tyndale House Publishers.

Desai A, Grossberg G, Chibnall J: Healthy brain aging: A road map, *Clinics in Geriatric Medicine* 26:1, 2010.

Dettmore D, Kolanowski A, Boustani M: Aggression in persons with dementia: use of nursing theory to guide clinical practice, *Geriatric Nursing* 30:8, 2009.

Dewing J: Wandering into the future: reconceptualizing wandering "A natural and good thing," *International Journal of Older People Nursing* 1:239, 2006.

DeYoung S, Just G, Harrison R: Decreasing aggressive, agitated, or disruptive behavior participation in a behavior management unit, *Journal of Gerontological Nursing* 28:22, 2003.

Ducharme F, Beaudet L, Legault A, et al: Development of an intervention program for Alzheimer's family caregivers following diagnostic disclosure. *Clinical Nursing Research* 18:44, 2009.

Duru O, Etther S, Vassar S, et al: Cost evaluation of a coordinated care management intervention for dementia, *American Journal of Managed Care* 15:521, 2009.

Edgerton E, Richie L: Improving physical environments for dementia care: making minimal changes for maximum effect, *Annals of Long-Term Care* 18:43, 2010.

Elliott A, Burgio L, DeCoster J: Enhancing caregiver health: findings from the resources for enhancing Alzheimer's caregiver health II intervention, *Journal of the American Geriatrics Society* 58:30, 2010.

Ely EW, Margolin R, Francis J, et al: Evaluation of delirium in critically ill patients: validation of the Confusion Assessment Method for the intensive care unit (CAM-ICU), *Critical Care Medicine* 29:1370, 2001.

Evans L: Complex care needs in older adults with common cognitive disorders, Section A: Assessment and management of dementia, 2007. Available at http://hartfordign.org/uploads/File/gnec_state_of_science_papers/gnec_dementia.pdf. Accessed October 10, 2010.

Farran C, Loukissa D, Lindeman D, et al: Caring for self while caring for others: the two-track life of coping with Alzheimer's disease, *Journal of Gerontological Nursing* 30:38, 2004.

Figiel G, Sadowsky C: A systematic review of the effectiveness of rivastigmine for the treatment of behavioral disturbances in dementia and other neurological disorders, *Current Medical Research and Opinion* 24:157, 2008.

Fletcher K: Dementia. In Capezuti E, Swicker D, Mezey M, et al., editors: *Evidence-based geriatric nursing protocols for best practice*, ed 3, New York, 2008, Springer.

Fong T, Jones R, Marcantonio E, et al: Delirium accelerates cognitive decline in Alzheimer's disease, *Neurology* 72:1570, 2009.

Futrell M, Mellilo K, Remington R: Evidence-based guideline: Wandering, *Journal of Gerontological Nursing* 36:6, 2010.

Gerdner L: Individualized music for elders with dementia, *Journal of Gerontological Nursing* 36:7, 2010.

Ghetu M, Bordelon P, Langan R: Diagnosis and treatment of mild cognitive impairment. *Clinical Geriatrics* 18:30, 2010.

Gotell E, Brown S, Ekman SL: Communicating through caregives singing during morning care situations, *Scandanavian Journal of Caring Sciences*, published online June 21, 2010.

Hain D, Touhy T, Sparks M, Engstrom G: Hearing the whole story: interventions for individuals and couples living with early-stage dementia. Unpublished manuscript, 2011.

Hain D, Touhy T, Engstrom G: What matters most to carers of people with mild to moderate dementia as evidence for transforming care, *Alzheimer's Care Today* 11:162, 2010.

Hall GR: Caring for people with Alzheimer's disease using the conceptual model of progressively lowered stress threshold in the clinical setting, *Nursing Clinics of North America* 29:129, 1994.

Hall GR, Buckwalter KC: Progressively lowered stress threshold: a conceptual model for care of adults with Alzheimer's disease, *Archives of Psychiatric Nursing* 1:399, 1987.

Hall G, Gallagher M, Dougherty J: Integrating roles for successful dementia management, *The Nurse Practitioner* 34:35, 2009.

Hargrave R: Caregivers of African-American elderly with dementia: a review and analysis, *Annals of Long-Term Care* 14:36, 2006.

Henderson C: *Partial view: an Alzheimer's journal*, Dallas, 1998, Southern Methodist Press.

Hill N, Kolanowski A, Kurum E: Agreeableness and activity engagement in nursing home residents with dementia, *Journal of Gerontological Nursing* 36:45, 2010.

Holliday-Welsh D, Gessert C, Renier C: Massage in the management of agitation in nursing home residents with cognitive impairment, *Geriatric Nursing* 30:108, 2009.

Hooyman N, Kiyak H: *Social Gerontology: A multidisciplinary perspective*, Boston, 2011, Allyn & Bacon.

Inouye SK, van Dyck CH, Alessi CA, et al: Clarifying confusion: the confusion assessment: a new method for detection of delirium, *Annals of Internal Medicine* 113:941, 1990.

Inouye S, Charpentier P: Precipitating factors for delirium in hospitalized elderly persons: predictive model and baseline vulnerability, *Journal of the American Medical Association* 275:852, 1996.

Inouye SK, Bogardus ST Jr, Charpentier PA, et al: A multicomponent intervention to prevent delirium in hospitalized older patients, *New England Journal of Medicine* 340:669, 1999.

Irving K, Foreman M: Delirium, nursing practice and the future, *International Journal of Older People Nursing* 1:121, 2006.

Kamat S, Kamat A, Grossberg G: Dementia risk prediction: Are we there yet? *Clinics in Geriatric Medicine* 26:113, 2010.

Keady J, Williams S, Hughes-Roberts J: "Making mistakes": Using co-constructed inquiry to illuminate meaning and relationships in the early adjustment to Alzheimer's disease: A single case study approach. *Dementia* 6:342, 2007.

Kolanowski AM: An overview of the Need-Driven Dementia—Compromised Behavior Model, *Journal of Gerontological Nursing* 25:7, 1999.

Kolanowski A, Fick D, Frazer C, et al: It's about time: use of nonpharmacological interventions in the nursing home, *Journal of Nursing Scholarship* 42:214, 2010.

Kovach C: Assessment and treatment of discomfort for people with late-stage dementia, *Journal of Pain and Symptom Management* 18(6):412-419, 1999.

Kuehn B: Delirium often not recognized or treated despite serious long-term consequences, *Journal of the American Medical Association* 304:389, 2010a.

Kuehn B: Questionable antipsychotic prescribing remains common despite serious risks, *Journal of the American Medical Association* 303:1582, 2010b.

Laurenhue K: Each person's journey is unique, *Alzheimer's Care Quarterly* 2:79, 2001.

Lindquist LA, Go L, Fleisher J, Jain N, Baker N: Improvements in cognition following hospital community dwelling seniors, *Journal of General Internal Medicine* 2011 Mar 4. DOI: 10.1007/s11606-011-1681-1.

Lyketsos CG, Colenda CC, Beck C, et al: Position statement of the American Association for Geriatric Psychiatry regarding principles of care for patients with dementia resulting from Alzheimer disease, *American Journal of Geriatric Psychiatry* 14:561-573, 2006.

Marcantonio E, Bergmann M, Kiely D, et al: Randomized trial of a delirium abatement program for postacute skilled nursing facilities, *Journal of the American Geriatrics Society* 58:1019, 2010.

Marwit S, Meuser T: Development and initial validation of an inventory to assess grief in caregivers of persons with Alzheimer's disease, *Gerontologist* 42:751, 2002.

Mattsson N, Zetterberg H, Hansson O, et al: CSF biomarkers and incipient Alzheimer disease in patients with mild cognitive impairment, *Journal of the American Medical Association* 302:385, 2009.

Miller C: *Nursing for wellness in older adults*, Philadelphia, 2008, Wolters Kluwer-Lippincott Williams & Wilkins.

Miyamoto Y, Tachimori H, Ito H: Formal caregiver burden in dementia: impact of behavioral and psychological symptoms of dementia and activities of daily living, *Geriatric Nursing* 31(4):246-253, 2010.

Mittelman MS, Roth DL, Clay OJ, et al: Preserving health of Alzheimer caregivers: impact of a spouse caregiver intervention. *American Journal of Geriatric Psychiatry* 15:780, 2007.

National Institute on Aging: Alzheimer's disease medication fact sheet. Available at www.nia.nih.gov/Alzheimer's/Publications/medicationsfs.htm. Accessed May 15, 2011.

Neary S, Mahoney D: Dementia caregiving: the experiences of Hispanic/Latino caregivers, *Journal of Transcultural Nursing* 16:163, 2005.

Neelon VJ, Champagne MT, Carlson JR, et al: The NEECHAM confusion scale: construction, validation and clinical testing, *Nursing Research* 45:324, 1996.

Norton M, Piercy K, Rabins P, et al: Caregiver-recipient closeness and symptom progression in Alzheimer disease: the Cache County dementia progression study. *The Journals of Gerontology, Series B. Psychological Sciences and Social Sciences* 64:560, 2009.

Ozbolt L, Paniagura M, Kaiser R: Atypical antipsychotics for the treatment of delirious elders, *Journal of the American Medical Directors Association* 9:19, 2008.

Pandharipande P, Shintani A, Peterson J, et al: Lorazepam is an independent risk factor for transitioning to delirium in intensive care unit patients, *Anesthesiology* 104:21, 2006.

Peterson B: Grief and dementia, *Aging Today* 5:13, 2006.

Pisani M, Araujo K, Van Ness P, et al: A research algorithm to improve detection of delirium in the intensive care unit, *Critical Care* 10:R121, 2006.

Rader J, Barrick A, Hoeffer B, et al: The bathing of older adults with dementia, *American Journal of Nursing* 106:40, 2006.

Rader J, Barrick A: Ways that work: bathing without a battle, *Alzheimer's Care Quarterly* 1:35-49, 2000.

Rader J, Tornquist E: *Individualized dementia care*, New York, 1995, Springer.

Richards K, Lambert C, Beck C: Deriving interventions for challenging behaviors from the need-driven dementia-compromised behavior model, *Alzheimer's Care Quarterly* 1:62, 2000.

Rigney T: Delirium in the hospitalized elder and recommendations for practice, *Geriatric Nursing* 27:151, 2006.

Rose K, Palmer J, Richeson N, et al: Care considerations for persons with early-onset dementia: A case analysis, *Alzheimer's Care Today* 11:151, 2010.

Rosenbloom-Brunton D, Henneman E, Inouye S: Feasibility of family participation in a delirium prevention program for hospitalized older adults, *Journal of Gerontological Nursing* 36:22, 2010.

Ross A, Dagley J: An assessment of anticipatory grief as experienced by family caregivers of individuals with dementia, *Alzheimer's Care Today* 10:8, 2009.

Rowe MA: People with dementia who become lost, *American Journal of Nursing* 103:32, 2003.

Rowe MA, Kairalla JA, McCrae CS: Sleep in dementia caregivers and the effects of a nighttime monitoring system, *Journal of Nursing Scholarship* 42:338, 2010.

Rubin FH, Williams J, Lescisin D, et al: Replicating the Hospital Elder Life Program in a community hospital and demonstrating effectiveness using quality improvement methodology, *Journal of the American Geriatrics Society* 54:969, 2006.

Schneider LS, Tariot PN, Dagerman KS, et al: Effectiveness of atypical antipsychotic drugs in patients with Alzheimer's disease, *New England Journal of Medicine* 355:1525, 2006.

Schneider LS, Dagerman KS, Higgins JP, McShane R: Lack of evidence for the efficacy of memantine in mild Alzheimer disease, *Archives of Neurology* online published online April 22, 2011. DOI:10.1001/archneurol.2011.69.

Segal-Gidan F: Alzheimer's management from diagnosis to late stage. Available at www.clinicaladvisor.com/alzheimer's-management-from-diagnosis-to-late-stage/printarticle/173456. Accessed September 29, 2010.

Shriver M, The Alzheimer's Association: The Shriver Report: A Woman's Nation Takes on Alzheimer's. Available at http://www.shriverreport.com/. Accessed October 15, 2010.

Sifton C: Life is what happens while we are making plans, *Alzheimer's Care Quarterly* 2:iv, 2001.

Smith M, Kolanowski A, Buettner L, et al: Beyond bingo: meaningful activities for persons with dementia in nursing homes, *Annals of Long-Term Care* 17:22, 2009.

Splete H: Nurses have special strategies for dementia, *Caring for the Ages* 9:11, 2008.

Stefanacci R: Evidence-based treatment of behavioral problems in patients with delirium, *Annals of Long-Term Care* 16:33, 2008.

Steis M, Fick D: Are nurses recognizing delirium? *Journal of Gerontological Nursing* 34:40, 2008.

Suwa S: Assessment scale for caregiver experience with dementia, *Journal of Gerontological Nursing* 28:5, 2002.

Sweeny S, Bridges S, Wild L, et al: Care of the patient with delirium, *American Journal of Nursing* 108:72CC, 2008.

Tappen R, Rosselli M, Engstrom G: Evaluation of the functional activities questionnaire (FAQ) in cognitive screening across four American ethnic groups, *The Clinical Neuropsychologist* 24:646, 2010.

Teri L, McKenzie G, LaFazia D, et al: Improving dementia care in assisted living residences: addressing staff reactions to training, *Geriatric Nursing* 30:153, 2008.

Touhy T: Dementia, personhood and nursing: learning from a nursing situation, *Nursing Science Quarterly* 17:43, 2004.

Tullmann D, Mion LC, Fletcher K, et al: Delirium prevention, early recognition and treatment. In Capezuti E, Swicker D, Mezey M, et al., editors, *Evidence-based geriatric nursing protocols for best practice*, ed 3, New York, 2008, Springer.

U.S. Department of Health and Human Service, Office of Disease Prevention and Health Promotion: *Healthy People 2020 Frameworks: Phase 1 report: recommendations for the framework and format of Healthy People 2020* (2010). Available at http://www.healthypeople.gov. Accessed December 2010.

Voyer P, Richard S, Doucet L, et al: Examination of the multifactorial model of delirium among long-term care residents with dementia, *Geriatric Nursing* 31:105, 2010.

Voelker R: Programs ease hospitalization experience for patients with dementia, *CNS Senior Care* 7:17, 2008.

Waszynski C, Petrovic K: Nurse's evaluation of the confusion assessment method: a pilot study, *Journal of Gerontological Nursing* 34:49, 2008.

Werner P, Stein-Shvachman I, Korczyn AD: Early onset dementia: clinical and social aspects, *International Psychogeriatrics* 21:631, 2009.

Williams C, Hyer K, Kelly A, Leger-Krall S, Tappen R: Development of nurse competencies to improve dementia care, *Geriatric Nursing* 26(2):98-102, 2005.

Williams C, Tappen R, Rosselli M, Keane F, Newlin K: Willingness to be screened and tested for cognitive impairment: cross-cultural comparison, *American Journal of Alzheimer's Disease and Other Dementias* 26(2):160-166, 2010.

Witlox J, Eurelings L, deJonghe J, et al: Delirium in elderly patients and the risk of postdischarge mortality, institutionalization, and dementia: A meta-analysis, *Journal of the American Medical Association* 304:443, 2010.

Woods B: Dementia challenges assumptions about what it means to be a person, *Generations* 13:39, 1999.

Yevchak A, Loeb S, Fick D: Promoting cognitive health and vitality: A review of clinical implications, *Geriatric Nursing* 29:302, 2008.

Economic, Legal, and Ethical Issues

Kathleen Jett

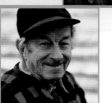

ⓔvolve *http://evolve.elsevier.com/Ebersole/TwdHlthAging*

A STUDENT SPEAKS

We went on a home visit with our preceptors today. I could hardly stand it. The house was filthy and so was he. The nurse said that he was not taking care of himself but that he had always been that way. I don't know why they can't make him go to a nursing home so someone can take care of him!

Evelyn, age 21

AN ELDER SPEAKS

When I was growing up, life was hard. We were so poor we couldn't do much but to hold on tight. When I was lucky I could get work plowing a field for $1 an acre. You work hard and you make do. There were not such things as going to a doctor or hospital; you did the best you could and pray you don't get sick. . . . Then when I turned 65 I got a little check from the government and a red, white, and blue insurance card [Medicare card]. The check isn't much, about $521 a month [SSI], but you know I consider myself blessed and much better off than ever before. And now I don't worry about my health; I will be taken care of, praise the Lord.

Aida at 74 in 1994

LEARNING OBJECTIVES

On completion of this chapter, the reader will be able to:

1. Explain how health care is financed in the United States.
2. Briefly explain the history of Social Security and some of the anticipated challenges.
3. Compare the types of health care services available under Medicare.
4. Describe the differing levels of decisional capacity and their implications in gerontological nursing.
5. Differentiate the types of elder mistreatment.
6. Identify persons at risk for abuse or neglect.
7. Describe strategies that may be used to minimize the risk for elder mistreatment.
8. Identify the nurse's legal responsibility in his or her own home state when neglect or abuse is suspected.
9. Describe the role of the nurse-advocate in relation to legal, health, and economic issues of concern to the older adult.

FINANCE IN LATE LIFE

Before the industrial revolution of the late 1800s, persons in most countries and cultures worked until they were no longer physically able to do so. In many cases the "work" of the individual changed with time and as capabilities diminished, and it did not cease until shortly before death. Family members and the community provided care when necessary (Bohm, 2001). It was not until the rigors of industrial work that opportunities disappeared for those with declining abilities. In the mid-1800s, the term *retire* was defined as "withdraw from service" but changed to mean "no longer fit for service" in the early 1900s. Care became less available as whole families joined the urban workforce. Congregate living, including nursing homes, and

Social Security as a form of ongoing income for eligible workers were created as a result of the social changes of the time.

In the early 1900s, almshouses and poor houses emerged to provide care for frail indigent persons who did not have family available or able to care for them (see Chapter 1). Most of these facilities were supported by charitable organizations. Later, the government became involved, and when the primary population in almshouses was the elderly, many essentially became public nursing institutions. In some places the law supported the use of public monies for a formerly private purpose (care of the elderly), and local governments were authorized to purchase land and erect facilities for the care of the elderly and could tax its citizens to maintain them. In the early 1900s, it was determined that the care of indigent elderly could be construed to be a public responsibility. Because the concept of personal responsibility continued to exist, poor persons who were admitted to care facilities were required to contribute any property they owned that could be used to help pay for the care and maintenance provided.

Social Security

Considered by many to be one of the most successful federal programs, Social Security was established in 1935 in the depths of the Great Depression. The primary function of the program was to provide monetary benefits to older retired workers and was viewed as a means to prevent or minimize the dependency of older members on younger members of society (Weinberger, 1996).

Social security and a number of programs that followed were set up as "age-entitlement" programs. This meant that an individual could receive the benefits simply because of their age and regardless of their need. In other words, the monetary support is available to those persons at a certain age regardless of their personal resources. The benefits, however, were and still are limited to American citizens and legal residents older than a certain age, or who are totally and permanently disabled and have paid into the Social Security program, or who are married to someone who has done so. Social Security is a major source of income for those who are 65 and over (Figure 20-1).

The program has been managed on what is called a pay-as-you-go system. Payroll taxes on a percentage of income are collected from employees and employers and are immediately distributed to beneficiaries (retirees and the disabled or eligible spouses) in the form of income and health services. Social Security funds, although individually deposited by employers and employees, are not reserved for any one individual. No one has an account set aside in his or her name. All funds that are not immediately paid out to beneficiaries are "borrowed" by the federal government for regular operating expenses. The

government converts the borrowed funds into government bonds, reflecting the debt of the government to Social Security, and places these in a "trust fund" watched over by the trustees of the fund. However, no funds are specifically identified to pay back those monies borrowed from the Social Security Trust Fund (Weinberger, 1996). Details of the changing status of Social Security (and Medicare) are provided to the public annually and may be accessed at www.ssa.gov/OACT/TR/index.html (Trustees, 2010a).

The amount of income one will receive at the time of retirement and each year thereafter depends on the age at retirement and the amount of contributions. The return is not of the investments specifically but on a calculation based on the number of "credits" paid into the system. The amount needed for a credit increases automatically each year. For example, in 2010 workers received a credit for each $1090 earned up to 4 in any one year. In general, a person has to have earned 40 credits to take advantage of the benefits of Social Security. For the current cohort of older adults, this calculation has been most beneficial to white men, who are more likely to have worked the most consistently and at higher salaries than all other groups of workers. A cost-of-living adjustment (COLA) increase had occurred each year there was a corresponding increase in the Consumer Price Index. However, due to the down turn in the U.S. economy there was no COLA in 2011. In 2010, the average Social Security benefit was $1164 for the 57 million recipients with a maximum Social Security benefit of $2346 and a minimum of $0 (Social Security Administration [SSA], 2010).

At the time of its inception, the system was constructed to transfer funds from those believed to be relatively well off (workers) to those believed to be relatively and uniformly poor (retirees). As long as the amount of contributions from workers exceeds that paid to beneficiaries, the program, as designed, can exist, or remain solvent. The combination of the increasing number of beneficiaries, the decreasing number of workers (in proportion to the beneficiaries), and the intangible nature of the "trust fund" has resulted in concern that the program will cease to exist in the near future—a potential threat to the future incomes of retirees who have spent their lives paying into a system that may not be available to them in their later years. The extent of this threat has been hotly debated in recent years. While the depth of the concern varies from year to year, in 2010 it was anticipated that Social Security expenditures exceeded tax credits due in part to the economic recession at the time. Despite deep concern, a solution has not been found. One attempt in 1983 to delay the problem has been implemented by raising the age of "retirement." The age at which one becomes eligible for Social Security benefits is increasing slowly and will transition to 67 years old for those born in 1960 or after.

Supplemental Security Income

Not all older persons living in the United States have Social Security benefits adequate to provide even the most basic necessities of life. This is true especially for persons who have spent their lives employed in the agriculture industry or as domestic workers and have been paid very low wages, often on a cash basis. Supplemental Security Income (SSI) was established in 1965 by Title XIX of the Social Security Act. SSI provides for a minimum level of economic support to persons age 65 and over,

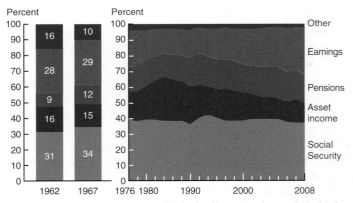

NOTE: A married couple is age 65 and over if the husband is age 65 and over or the husband is younger than age 55 and the wife is age 65 and over. The definition of "other" includes, but is not limited to, public assistance, unemployment compensation, workers compensation, alimony, child support, and personal contributions. Reference population: These data refer to the civilian noninstitutionalized population.
SOURCE: Social Security Administration, 1963 Survey of The Aged, and 1968 Survey of Demographic and Economic Characteristics of the Aged; U.S. Census Bureau, Current Population Survey, Annual Social and Economic Supplement, 1977-2009.

FIGURE 20-1 Sources of income for married couples and nonmarried people who are age 65 and over, percent distribution, selected years 1962-2008. (Redrawn from Federal Interagency Forum on Aging-Related Statistics: *Older Americans 2010: Key indicators of well-being*, Washington DC, 2010, U.S. Government Printing Office.)

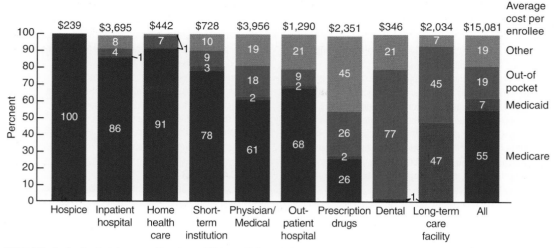

NOTE: "Other" refers to private insurance, Department of Veterans Affairs, and other public programs.
Reference population: These data refer to Medicare enrollees.
SOURCE: Centers for Medicare and Medicaid Services, Medicare Current Beneficiary Survey.

FIGURE 20-2 Sources of payment for health care services for Medicare enrollees age 65 and over, by type of service, 2006. (Redrawn from Federal Interagency Forum on Aging-Related Statistics: *Older Americans 2010: Key indicators of well-being*, Washington DC, 2010, U.S. Government Printing Office.)

blind, or disabled regardless of their earning power in early life or when capable of working. SSI either provides "total support" or supplements a low Social Security benefit. In 2010, the SSI federal benefit for approximately 7 million people was a maximum of $674 per month for a single person and $1011 for a couple, although some states supplement this amount to some extent (SSA, 2010).

Other Late Life Income

Finally, financing late life may include private retirement or pension plans. Individuals may pay into the plans themselves (e.g., IRAs) or through their employers (e.g., 401K accounts). The private retirement, pension funds, or a combination of these are invested in private sector financial instruments (e.g., stocks, bonds, or real estate holdings) or perhaps in government treasury notes. Those funds are held for the beneficiary and may become part of his or her estate if the beneficiary dies before collecting the pension. Some private retirement annuities provide for several choices for receipt of funds after retirement. The retiree could elect to take his or her pension based on his or her own life only or based on the retiree's and a spouse's life. In other words, a person may set up a plan so that he or she receives all or most of the benefit during his or her lifetime rather than providing for any survivor benefit. Notification of the potential survivor of such a choice is not always required (Hooyman and Kiyak, 2008). The amount received is actuarially determined based on the life expectancy of one or two beneficiaries and whether a guaranteed minimum number of years are selected.

PAYING FOR HEALTH CARE

Economic factors are always a consideration in the delivery of health care, regardless of who pays for it. In most countries across the globe, health care is a universal entitlement. That is, some level of health care is available to all persons either living

in or working in the country; health care is considered a right. In these settings, health care providers are considered workers alongside of others in the service sector. The universal services are supported to a large extent by payroll taxes in most cases, which can be significant. The insurance risk is shared among all citizens. Although these plans have significant benefits, challenges have also been encountered, such as long waits for elective or non-urgent procedures and rationing of other types of services. As the population in a particular country prospers, a "second tier" of care develops that can be purchased. That is, some of the services that are more limited in the country's plan can be purchased if one can afford to do so and an outside provider can be found.

In the United States, health care has always been a purchased service—not a right (Figure 20-2). It is primarily purchased either directly or indirectly through an insurance plan of some kind with the cost of the plan directly proportional to the benefits provided. The federal government purchases the majority of care through its insurance plans (Medicare, Railroad Medicare, Medicaid, and TRICARE) or provides it directly through the Veterans Administration. State governments are also significantly involved through the shared Medicaid plan and in public and mental health services. The major insurance plan available to older adults living in the United States is Medicare. Persons without insurance purchase all health care in an "out-of-pocket" manner. They are expected to pay whatever the charge is for a received service. Although the number of uninsured persons is expected to increase each year, most elders fall under one of the safety nets of Medicare, Medicaid, or both.

Medicare

History

In 1934, President Franklin D. Roosevelt appointed the Committee on Economic Security (CES) to craft a Social Security bill. The original report included a health insurance plan, but because of much opposition to it, Roosevelt deferred the health

---

BOX 20-1   FUNDAMENTALS OF ORIGINAL MEDICARE PARTS A AND B*

MEDICARE PART A

Medicare Part A is designed primarily to partially cover the costs of inpatient hospital care and other specialized care as listed below:

- Acute hospitalization coverage, through a prospective payment system, includes costs of semiprivate rooms, meals, nursing services, operating and recovery room, intensive care, drugs, laboratory and radiology fees, blood products, and other necessary medical services and supplies. There is a deductible for days 1 to 60. This is repeated any time the person is rehospitalized after 60 days. After 60 days, there is a daily co-pay that increases over time. There is no coverage after 150 days. Deductibles and co-pays increase every year. The deductibles and co-pays are either paid out-of-pocket or by Medicaid or Medigap policies.
- Nursing home care is covered by Medicare only if the person had been in an acute care setting for 3 days before the admission and only as long as a skilled service is needed and for a maximum of 100 days. While the facility is paid on a prospective payment system similar to the acute care setting, for the patients, the first 20 days are covered at 100%, and for days 21 to 100 a substantial daily co-pay is required. There is no coverage if skilled care is not continuously needed.
- Home health care may be covered by Medicare (also prospective payment) on an intermittent and/or part-time basis for skilled nursing care, physical therapy, and rehabilitative services. The person must be ill enough to be

considered homebound. Custodial care is not covered. Medicare pays 80% of the approved amount for durable medical equipment and supplies.

- Hospice care is provided for terminally ill persons expected to live less than six months who elect to forgo traditional medical treatment for the terminal illness. Medicare pays for all but limited co-pays for outpatient drugs and inpatient care. Hospice Medicare replaces Medicare Parts A and B for all costs associated with the terminal condition.
- Inpatient psychiatric care is a limited number of days in a lifetime; partial payment; other limitations apply.

MEDICARE PART B

Medicare Part B is designed to cover some of the costs associated with outpatient or ambulatory services. Deductibles and co-pays are required in most cases:

- Physician and nurse practitioner services, including some prescribed supplies and diagnostic tests.
- Physical, occupational, and speech therapy for the purpose of rehabilitation
- Limited durable medical equipment.
- Clinical laboratory services fully covered if deemed medically necessary after a deductible.
- Outpatient hospital treatment, blood, and ambulatory surgical services.
- Preventive services (many with no co-pay or deductible).
- Diabetic supplies (excluding insulin and other medications).

*See www.cms.gov for the latest information about covered services and associated costs. These are all subject to change.

---

insurance part of the bill to avoid losing Social Security (see earlier discussion) (Corning, 1969). The American Medical Association opposed any national program of health insurance, believing it to be "socialized medicine," and made efforts to prevent its implementation (Goodman, 1980). Fortune magazine polled the American public in 1942 and found that 76% of those polled opposed government-financed medical care (Cantril, 1951).

In the early 1960s, President Lyndon Johnson recognized that the numbers of older persons, those with serious disabilities, and poor children were increasing significantly and that often these vulnerable groups were without access to needed health services. Although opposition continued, Johnson proposed amendments (Title XVIII and Title XIX) to the Social Security Act to address these social problems. In Senate and House hearings, some legislators described the amendments as steps that would continue to destroy independence and self-reliance and would tax the poor and middle class to subsidize the health care of the wealthy (Twight, 1997).

Nonetheless, legislation was passed in 1965 and 1966 to expand the Social Security system by establishing Medicare, Railroad Medicare (for retired railroad workers), and Medicaid. Medicaid's criteria included income and asset restrictions. In a short time after implementation of these plans, millions more persons could receive health care, and the costs for the services escalated rapidly. Prescription drug coverage in the form known as Medicare Part D was not added until U.S. President George W. Bush's administration in 2006. The Affordable Care Act of the Obama administration (2010) contained a number of provisions with potential impact designed to improve health care services for older adults. These provisions are expected to be enacted over a period of years, however significant changes remain possible due to opposition to the legislation (AARP, 2010).

Overview

Medicare is an insurance plan for persons who are age 65, blind, or totally disabled, including those with end-stage renal disease. It combines the age-entitlement Medicare A with purchased B (Original Plan), C (Advantage Plans), and D (Prescription Plan). When one enrolls in Medicare, one selects the type of coverage and the premiums as one does with any other insurance plan. Medicare Part A was created to cover the costs of hospital and limited nursing home care (Box 20-1). Medicare Parts B & C were created as a purchasable and affordable voluntary insurance plan that covered outpatient and health care provider services in the forms of (1) fee-for-service, (2) preferred provider, and (3) managed care plan. Medicare Part D is a prescription drug plan.

Like Social Security, Medicare Part A was designed as a pay-as-you-go system; that is, taxes collected from employers and employees are used for payment of current Medicare beneficiaries and are not placed in a fund earmarked for taxpayers' future medical expenses. Of the costs of Medicare Part B, Part C, and Part D, 75% comes from the general revenue of the federal government. The remainder comes primarily from the beneficiaries themselves in the form of premiums and co-pays.

Persons enrolled in Medicare pay a monthly premium for components B through D, usually deducted directly from their Social Security income. As of January 1, 2007, this premium is based on income as reported to the Internal Revenue Service. In the Original Medicare B and most other purchased plans, the patient is responsible for paying premiums to the insurer and is required to make a co-pay when services are received; in this way, the patient is sharing the cost. In the Medicare Advantage Plans (Medicare C), the patient is assigned to specific providers and vendors who have entered into a prior (prospective) agreement with the insurer about services provided and patient co-pays. These plans were created in an attempt to control the skyrocketing costs associated with the fee-for-service model. With the Medicare Advantage Plans, a provider or health care system receives a flat capitated rate from Medicare for each potential recipient of care. Within pre-established guidelines, all medically necessary services must be provided by that provider or health care system.

Medicare is administered by the Centers for Medicare and Medicaid Services (CMS) and is a part of the Department of Health and Human Services, a special entity created to improve the administration of the programs. In 2009, nearly 47 million persons were covered by some part of Medicare with total expenditures of $509 billion (CMS, 2009). In 2010, major changes in Medicare were made into law through the Affordable Care Act (ACA). Through roughly 165 provisions, the ACA will reduce costs by decreasing payment rate while at the same time reducing fraud and increasing coverage for preventive services and research (Trustees, 2010b). The impact of these changes remains to be seen.

Medicare Part A

Medicare Part A is a hospital insurance plan covering acute care and acute and short-term rehabilitative care and some costs associated with hospice care and home health care under certain circumstances. Those qualified automatically receive a Medicare card (red, white, and blue) indicating Medicare Part A coverage when he or she becomes eligible to receive Social Security income. Those who have not paid an adequate amount into the U.S. Social Security system may be eligible to purchase Part A coverage for a monthly fee ($450 per month in 2011). Coverage begins the first day of the month of eligibility. The coverage and co-payments vary by setting under the original fee-for-service plans. When acute care is needed, the co-payments can be quite high, especially for stays of over 60 days. The initial deductible is $1132 (as of 2011) with no co-insurance until day 91 when it is $283 per day for days 61 to 90 each benefit period. After the 90th day, a person begins using "lifetime reserve days"—up to 90 at $566 per day (CMS, 2011).

Rehabilitative care, usually provided in skilled nursing facilities, is paid for only if it occurs within a set time from a hospital discharge and as long as the patient requires what is called skilled care (only that which is provided by a licensed nurse or physical or occupational therapist). Medicare Part A will pay 100% of the first 20 days of a nursing home stay, with a co-pay of up to $141.50 per day for days 21 to 100 and no coverage after that (CMS, 2011). At any time the person no longer needs skilled care, Medicare coverage stops. Medicare does not cover additional charges that may be incurred during a long-term care stay, such as incontinence supplies or laundry.

Home health care under Medicare must consist of medically-necessary part time or intermittent skilled nursing, physical therapy, or speech-language pathology or a continuing need for occupational therapy. It must be provided at the written direction of a physician and through a certified agency. Ongoing supervision can be provided by either a physician or a nurse practitioner. The person receiving the care must be home-bound. It must be provided through a home health care and for the purposes of active rehabilitation as seen in the nursing home setting. There are no co-payments for home health care and

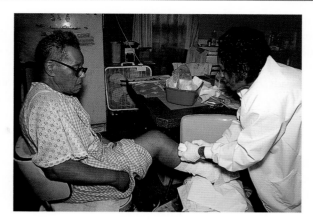

(Wound care is usually a "covered service" under Medicare Part A when provided by a registered nurse in a person's home and all other requirements are met. From Lewis SM, Heitkemper MM, Dirksen SR, et al: Medical-surgical nursing: assessment and management of clinical problems, ed 7, St Louis, 2007, Mosby.)

limited co-pays for hospice care. When the assistance needed is limited to personal care or medication supervision, it is not covered by Medicare at all. There is not co-pay for these services but a 20% co-pay for any durable medical equipment that may be needed, such as hospital beds or oxygen equipment.

Hospice services (see Chapter 23) are usually provided in the home; for which there are no co-pays or deductibles. If short term respite or inpatient stays are necessary for the comfort of the patient or family support there is a 5% co-pay.

Medicare Part B

In the 7 months surrounding a person's 65th birthday (from 3 months before), all persons who are eligible for Medicare Part A **must** select and apply for Part B or Part C (see below) through the Social Security Administration (www.socialsecurity.gov). Medicare Part B covers the costs associated with the services provided by physicians; nurse practitioners; outpatient services (e.g., laboratory services); qualified physical, speech, and occupational therapists. Beginning in 2011, most deductibles and other cost-sharing of preventive care has been removed, and the one-time-only wellness checkup has been replaced with an annual covered exam (Whitehouse, n.d.).

Medicare Part B is often referred to as "Original Medicare," based on a traditional fee-for-service arrangement wherein the charge was individually determined by the provider and payment due at the time services rendered. At this time, there are two models for reimbursement—one in which the provider "accepts assignment" or accepts the fees set by Medicare or does not. Under the latter system providers may bill patients directly, and the patients in turn "file" or request reimbursement from their insurance company (e.g., Medicare, AARP, etc.) for whatever portion they are eligible for. If assignment is accepted, the patient cannot be billed any more than the difference between what the provider is reimbursed (about 80% for physicians and 85% of physicians rate for NPs) and the "allowable" charges; charges are determined on an annual basis by CMS and vary regionally. A provider who does not accept assignment may charge the patient up to 15% above the allowable charge. A combination of an increasing number of wealthy elders and fewer primary care providers has spawned a new industry of "boutique" services, including physician practices. For an additional "membership" or "convenience" or "surcharge," the patient has heretofore unknown access to his or her choice of health care services and providers.

The advantages of the Original Medicare Plan include choice and access. Participants can seek the services of any provider they choose and do so without a referral. While the numbers are diminishing, providers all over the United States accept Medicare, and participants can change providers as often as desired. With the Original Medicare Plan, the patient is responsible for an annual deductible, co-pays, coinsurance charges, and a monthly premium. In 2011, this was $115.40 a month for persons with incomes of $85,000 or less as an individual or $170,000 or less as a family. The premiums rise gradually to $369.10 with incomes up to $214,000 individual and $428,000 family. The annual deductible was $162 (CMS, 2011).

Medicare Part C

Otherwise referred to as Medicare Advantage Plans (MAPs), Medicare Part C uses a prospective payment plan and include traditional health maintenance organizations (HMOs) and managed care plans. All traditional services covered by Medicare Part A and Part B must be provided, and additional services, co-pays, and deductibles are predetermined. Medicare Advantage Plans may or may not also provide prescription drug benefits; if so, they are referred to as MAP-PDs. Not all MAPs are offered at all locations in the United States. Those that have been granted *Medicare per capita waivers* cannot refuse applicants based on pre-existing health conditions. MAP premiums vary in price depending on location and range of services. The elder is referred to the Medicare website for more information or a counselor available through senior organizations (www.medicare.gov).

MAPs may provide a cost savings to the member as well as extra benefits. In most cases, a member of the plan pays no premium. However, special rules must be followed, and the member may be charged extra co-pays for additional services. The member is also restricted to certain providers and hospitals. There are fewer out-of-pocket costs unless an individual decides to see a provider or to seek a service without a referral or outside the system to which he or she has subscribed; such services are usually not covered at all. Referrals are required for all services other than that of the primary health care provider. The negative aspects of MAPs are the access barriers to services beyond primary care, such as specialists and high-tech procedures and treatments.

MAPs differ from other plans in that they are expected to emphasize preventive medicine, comprehensive care, periodic physical examinations, and immunizations. The best of these plans are complete health care systems with highly trained physicians, nurse practitioners, and nurses working out of single or regional and completely equipped medical centers. Some HMOs provide extensive health education services, support groups, and telephone support services to homebound patients. The supplemental services offered may save the participant a considerable amount in the costs of medications, assistive devices, and professional consultation charges.

The premium is in the form of a "capitated" payment. The MAP receives a set amount on a monthly or quarterly basis regardless of service use for each member enrolled and regardless of the amount of care given. All necessary care must be provided from this amount. The MAP assumes all of the liability for costs incurred for the care of the member based on the plan. This model has created abuses and horror stories in which elders were denied needed treatments to save money for the corporate providers. Patient protection laws now allow consumers to lodge complaints and initiate legal action against these abuses. The Center for Patient Advocacy supported a much-needed bill that became law in October 1999 (www.biapa.org). This law allows appeals when a MAP denies care, guarantees access to specialists when needed, ensures that health-related decisions are made by health care providers rather than bureaucrats, and holds the plans legally accountable for medical decisions that cause harm.

Medicare Part D

In 2003, the Medicare Modernization Act established a prescription drug benefit for eligible recipients of Medicare, known as Medicare Part D; the plan was implemented on January 1, 2006. It is an elective prescription drug plan (PDP) with associated out-of-pocket premiums and co-payments. All persons with either Medicare Part A or Medicare Part B are eligible to voluntarily purchase a Medicare Part D PDP. Help with the costs associated with Medicare Part D is available for persons with low incomes (below 150% of the poverty level) and those who receive Medicaid. For persons with both Medicare and Medicaid (called "dual eligibles"), the new plan wasn't voluntary and replaced the former drug benefit under Medicaid. Dually eligible persons who did not choose a plan are arbitrarily assigned to a PDP.

The PDPs established under Medicare Part D are all commercial plans that have contractual arrangements with CMS. To be included as an option, the company must agree to follow the rules set forth by CMS and change as directed. With the agreement to provide the minimum level of benefits established by Medicare Part D regulations, the plan is deemed "credible" by the CMS and becomes accepted as equivalent (Stefanacci, 2006). Like other insurance plans, once enrolled in either Medicare Part D or another credible PDP, a person cannot change a plan until the next open enrollment period except under special circumstances. These circumstances include those who are admitted to, reside in, or are discharged from a skilled nursing facility and persons with dual-eligibility. Different than other plans, if the person does enroll in Medicare Part D at the same time as enrolling in Medicare Part B, late enrollment penalties are charged. Persons can change their plans during the "open enrollment" periods each year.

Most PDPs are set up in a similar way. Deductibles, co-pays, gaps, and limits are dependent on the premiums paid, ranging from about $25 to about $100 with an annual deductible of $250. After the person had spent $250, the PDP covered 75% of the cost of the approved drugs up to $2000, with a 25% co-pay (Medicare paid $1500, the person paid $500). The next $2850 in costs was paid directly by the individual (called the "donut hole"). When the total costs for approved drugs reached $5100 ($3600 out-of-pocket), the PDP paid 95% (5% co-pay) of all drug costs for the rest of the year. The premiums and co-pay amounts are expected to change annually and vary greatly from plan to plan. The deductible and donut-hole are repeated yearly. More than 8 million elders reached this "donut hole" or gap in 2007. The Affordable Care Act of 2010 attempted to address this, first with a rebate of $250 when the hole is reached, and beginning in 2011, pharmaceutical companies agreed to institute a 50% discount on brand name drugs purchased during that time (Whitehouse, n.d.). Although most PDPs have donut holes, a person may elect a plan with lower co-pays or broader drug coverage for a higher monthly premium (CMS, 2010).

Nurses, nurse practitioners, physicians, pharmacists, and community volunteers spend hours helping beneficiaries enroll at appropriate times and select the insurance plans that best meet their needs. This sometimes onerous task can be instrumental in promoting healthy aging.

Supplemental Insurance/Medigap Policies

Because of the potentially high co-payments associated with Medicare, persons who are able to do so often purchase supplemental insurance plans. These feature standard benefits, and generally several different policies are available from which to select in each state. Persons searching for an appropriate plan can be referred to the Medicare website for their state or can request a printed copy of the standard plans (available at www.medicare.gov). Plans referred to as Medigap cover only the deductibles and part of the co-insurance amounts based on Medicare-approved amounts contracted with providers.

Other sources of insurance coverage are through employee benefit offices (e.g., covered under COBRA) or organizations such as the American Association of Retired Persons (AARP). Physicians and nurse practitioners who agree to accept the Medicare assignment amount can collect the uncovered percentage (e.g., 20%) from the secondary insurance. In some parts of the country (and for some persons), alternative health plans for older adults are available, such as Indian Health Services for anyone who is a documented member of one of the Indian Nations or Medicare Railroad or care through demonstration programs or Programs of All Inclusive Care for the Elderly (PACE) (see Chapter 16).

Care for Veterans

The Veterans Health Administration (VA) system has long held a leadership position in gerontological research, medical care, and extended care. In fact, a great deal of the research that guided gerontologists in earlier years was generated through the VA system, as were innovations in care. In addition, the majority of geriatric fellowships have been provided through VA hospitals. The VA system has been a forerunner of the various continua of care providers now in place. Since early on, this system provided VA-run nursing homes, home care and community-based programs, respite care, blindness rehabilitation, mental health, and numerous other services in addition to acute medical/surgical provisions.

At the current time, about 12 million World War II and Vietnam era veterans and their dependents may be eligible for health care services through veteran's hospital networks. In the past, veteran's hospitals and services were available on an as-needed basis for anyone who had served in the uniformed services at any time. It was not necessary for individuals to use

their Medicare benefits. However, this system has undergone significant change. One of the first changes that veterans noted was restrictions placed on the use of veteran's hospitals and services. Instead of coverage of any health problems, priorities were set for those problems that were in some way deemed "service connected"; in other words, the health care problem had to be linked to the time the person was on active duty.

Veterans older than age 65 are now expected to obtain and use Medicare for their non–service-connected health problems, with the responsibilities for co-pays and deductibles the same as for other beneficiaries. An outcry among veterans and veteran groups resulted in the development of a free Medigap policy known as TRICARE for Life (TFL).

TRICARE for Life

TRICARE is a Medigap policy provided by the Department of Defense for Medicare-eligible beneficiaries ages 65 and older and their dependents or widows or widowers older than age 65. This plan requires that the person enroll in both Medicare Part A and Part B and pay the premiums for Part B. As a Medigap policy, TFL covers those expenses not covered by Medicare, such as co-pays and prescription medicines. Dependent parents or parents-in-law may be eligible for pharmacy benefits if they turned age 65 on or after April 1, 2001, and are enrolled in Medicare Part B. For more information about this, see www.tricare.osd.mil.

Medicaid

Medicaid is a health insurance program jointly funded by federal and state governments using tax dollars collected into the general funds of each. It provides health services for low-income children, pregnant women, those who are permanently disabled, and persons age 65 and older. For elders with low incomes, Medicaid usually covers all Medicare premiums, co-pays, and deductibles and may provide additional health benefits. Persons who are dually eligible are frequently required to be enrolled in MAP-PD plans.

Medicaid was created in 1965 as part of Title XIX of the Social Security Act at the same time as Medicare. It makes payments for health care provided to Medicaid recipients directly to health care providers. Because it is a joint program, CMS administers the program at the federal level, and a state agency administers at each state level. Eligibility for Medicaid is determined by the state and is based on income and assets, categorical need, and lack of ability to afford, even with Medicare, the medical care required.

Federal law requires states to provide a certain minimum level of service, and states may add other coverage such as prescription drugs (now replaced by Medicare Part D), vision care, dentures, prostheses, case management, and other medical or rehabilitative care provided by a licensed health care practitioner. In most cases, Medicaid covers more services than Medicare, including custodial care in nursing homes and preventive care with no co-pays or deductibles; however, this is highly variable both by state and year and depends on the state's fiscal health and political priorities.

If institutional long-term care is needed, a single adult without a dependent child but with a low income (less than approximately $1200 per month and few assets) is required to contribute all but $35 of his or her monthly income to partially cover the actual costs of care. The difference between the person's contribution and Medicaid's allowable charge is paid by a combination of state and federal revenues. This ensures that the neediest disabled adults are cared for. Persons with incomes above the limit set by the state are not eligible for assistance with health care expenses under Medicaid.

For a person who requires the financial support of Medicaid for a nursing home stay and has a spouse who is able to remain in the community, Congress enacted provisions in 1988 to protect him or her from "spousal impoverishment." Only one half of the combined value of the household goods, automobile, and burial funds are counted as belonging to the patient and used for calculation of any support eligibility. The remainder of the assets belongs to the spouse in the community up to a set amount ($109,560 in 2009).

Because some people who believed they would soon need nursing home care transferred funds to become eligible for Medicaid and avoid using their own funds for that care, laws have been enacted to preclude ineligible persons from defrauding government programs. Some transfers are permitted, such as to a spouse or a disabled, dependent child. Any other transfer (i.e., to another person or to a trust) is considered an improper transfer and will be invalid for the purpose of qualifying for Medicaid. When a person applies for Medicaid, a "look-back period" determines if funds have been transferred that would normally be available to the applicant. Transfers to recipients other than a trust have a look-back period determined by the state (e.g., 36 months); transfers to a trust have a look-back period of 60 months. If transfers were made, Medicaid support will not begin until the costs incurred and paid equal the amount of the transfer. For example, an income-eligible person, who transfers $100,000 and is in a nursing home where the monthly rate is $4000, would be ineligible for Medicaid for 25 months ($4000 × 25 months = $100,000). This is known as "spend-down." These regulations attempt to ensure that individuals pay what they can for the care they need but still provides a safety net when funds are exhausted.

The majority of the Medicaid funds are used to provide long-term nursing home care for older and disabled adults. The federal government has attempted to slow the flow of Medicaid monies to pay for nursing home and other care for the non-poor by a series of laws enacted to require people to pay as much as they can from their own funds. Examples include the following (Teske, 2000):

- The 1993 Omnibus Budget Reconciliation Act (OBRA) permitted states to recover the costs of nursing home care from a deceased person's estate.
- The 1996 Health Insurance Portability and Accountability Act (HIPAA) reduced the allowable methods of hiding or transferring monies before needing or entering long-term care.
- The 1997 Balanced Budget Act targeted lawyers and other estate planners, holding them responsible for attempting to circumvent laws that required persons to pay for their own long-term care.

Long-Term Care Insurance

Some persons are electing to purchase additional insurance (long-term care insurance [LTCI]) for their potential long-term

---

BOX 20-2   QUESTIONS TO CONSIDER WHEN REVIEWING A LONG-TERM CARE INSURANCE POLICY

What type of long-term care insurance is it?
What services does it cover e.g., custodial care?
What does it not cover?
   Diagnoses?
   Locations of care?
What does it cost?
   Does this change?
How are premiums paid?
   When are the premiums paid?

---

care needs. Ideally, these policies would cover the expenses related to co-pays for long-term care and coverage for what is called custodial care or help with day-to-day needs (as opposed to skilled care). Traditionally, these policies were limited to care in long-term care facilities and provided a flat-rate reimbursement to residents for their costs. However, these policies are becoming more creative and innovative and may, under some circumstances, cover home care costs instead of or in addition to care in long-term care facilities. Many plans are being marketed. Even the American Nurses Association (ANA) has a plan available to ANA members (www.nursingworld.org).

The purchaser is cautioned to read the policy carefully and understand all the details, limitations, and exclusions, such as if the plan covers the amount and type of service that the person would desire if it were to be needed (Box 20-2). They may have a benefit period or a lifetime. The benefit period may be in days or in dollars spent. Particular concerns are related to Alzheimer's disease because many policies exclude these individuals from home benefits and include very limited institutional benefits. The best LTCI packages are those that have been negotiated by a large employer or state organization or association. It is also advisable to have the elder or family member check consumer reports of the particular insurance company and its reliability before applying for a policy. Additional information can be obtained from the Department of Health and Human Services at www.longtermcare.gov.

LEGAL AND ETHICAL ISSUES IN GERONTOLOGICAL NURSING

In the day-to-day practice of caring for older adults, the gerontological nurse may face questions that are often ethical in nature but with legal components; especially when the individual is medically, physically, or cognitively frail. Decision making related to end-of-life issues is addressed in Chapter 23. Herein, decision making from a process perspective is considered—specifically, consideration of decision-making capacity. If the person's capacity is questioned, legal protection may be needed. While the nurse (unless also an attorney) cannot provide any legal advice, it is imperative for her or him to be cognizant of several key legal issues frequently encountered in the work of gerontological nursing. And finally, elder mistreatment is addressed, both the technical details of risk

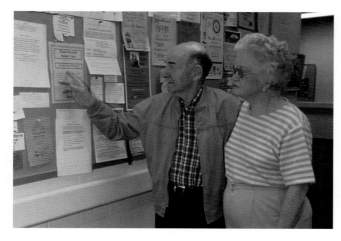

(Information about legal and other resources is available at many public settings such as libraries and community centers. From Lewis SM, Heitkemper MM, Dirksen SR, et al: *Medical-surgical nursing: assessment and management of clinical problems, (single volume)*, ed 7, St Louis, 2007, Mosby; courtesy of Rick Brady, Riva, MD.)

BOX 20-3 QUESTIONS OF INFORMED CONSENT

Mr. Brown was an 84-year-old African-American man who was hospitalized for complications of advanced diabetes. He was scheduled for a bilateral orchiectomy the next morning. When the geriatric clinical nurse specialist stopped by to see him, she found him to be pleasant and in good spirits. He was also moderately to profoundly hard of hearing and had limited reading skills and visual acuity. A copy of his surgical consent was at the bedside with an "X" on the signature line. Mr. Brown's glasses were on his bedside table, and his hearing aids were reportedly home. Mr. Brown was given a stethoscope to wear and speaking into the bell, asked if he had any questions about what he had consented to. He replayed that it was "just something he needed for his sugar." Through our "listening device," we explained the procedure that was planned. He became noticeably upset and immediately withdrew his consent until he could find out more about his alternatives and prognosis.

---

factors and the ethical stress when a victim declines the nurse's assistance.

Decision Making

Consent is a concept that arises from the ethical principles of human self-determination and **autonomy**. In the health care situation, consent refers to accepting or refusing care and treatments and is expressed in the legal doctrine of **informed consent.** In most circumstances the consent is implied, such as when the person ingests a medication provided to him or her or cooperates with a dressing change. At other times, a more structured approach is used with very specific required steps, such as when a patient gives informed consent prior to a surgical procedure or to participate in research. State law generally specifies the extent of information to be disclosed and the circumstances in which it is provided (e.g., prior to any sedating medications). In older adults, attention must also be paid to ensure that any special needs, such as sensory deficits, are addressed to assure that both the legal and ethical principles of informed consent are met (Box 20-3). Most courts have upheld the requirements of providing information that a reasonable health care provider would disclose in the same or similar

---

BOX 20-4 DAX'S CASE

In 1973, a young man named Donald "Dax" Cowart was severely burned in a flash fire. He lost both of his ears and eyes, his nose, and skin over 65% to 68% of his body. During many years of hospitalization, he repeatedly begged to be allowed to refuse further excruciatingly painful treatment. However, at the time, the prevailing ethical principles in health care were paternalism and beneficence—in that others were empowered to make the health care decisions deemed best for us. Years after the accident, Mr. Cowart continues to maintain that he should have had a right to refuse treatment, even if it meant his death. This case became part of the national ethical conversations influencing the change to health care based on the ethical principles of autonomous consent and patient self-determination (search "Dax's Case").

---

circumstances or that which a reasonable client would consider material to his or her decision. Consent for research participation is a more detailed and extensive process, because treatments provided in such circumstances may not necessarily directly benefit the participant. Research with the very frail and those with changing levels of consciousness has been difficult and has limited the advancement of science in some areas.

Informed consent is only possible due to the presumption that adults are competent, a legal term indicating that he or she has decision-making capacity. **Competence** is presumed when one achieves the legal age of "adult." Decisional capacity to consent is presumed of all adults regardless of age unless legally declared otherwise. That is, one remains competent until a judge has adjudicated one to lack capacity; the procedure used when this is questioned is determined by state statutes.

While the provider has a responsibility to inform, the individual must make decisions. Decisional capacity is an individual's ability to understand the problem, the options, the decision made, and consequences of the decision, that is, appreciate its possible risks and benefits (Carroll, 2010). The person then makes a decision within the context of his or her own health values and needs (Box 20-4).

In day-to-day gerontological practice with frail elders, it is important to artificially differentiate between *competence* (the legal term) and *capacity* (the functional term). While the person may still be legally competent, does he or she have the capacity to understand at the level needed for the decision at hand? Deciding which foods to accept is very different from deciding to undergo a surgical procedure. He or she may have no or limited capacity for one type of decision but full capacity for another. Magid and colleagues (2006) suggest that decisional capacity be considered three-dimensional: the risk for the treatment (high or low), the benefit of the treatment (high or low), and the patient's decision (accept or refuse). It is widely accepted that the higher the risk and the lower the benefit, the more important that the patient be the one to make the decision.

Clearly, the determination of capacity is on a continuum from the most simple to the most complex, and with the latter it is more likely that legal protections may be needed to protect the person and ensure that decision making, as needed, can be done in a manner in which the person would want if the person were able. These options include powers of attorney, conservatorship, and guardianship. It is important that the nurse understand the differences among the options and the meaning of each.

Powers of Attorney

A power of attorney (POA) is a legal document and device in which one person (principle) designates another person (e.g., family member, friend) to act on his or her behalf. The appointed person becomes known as the attorney-in-fact or agent. The two main types are a general POA and a durable POA. The agent named in a general POA usually represents the principle in ways that are indicated in the document, for example, in matters of business, but not to make decisions related to health care. A general POA is no longer in effect if the principle becomes incapacitated, but it does continue in the durable POA.

A health care power of attorney is needed for health care decisions. The attorney-in-fact appointed in a durable health care POA usually has rights and responsibilities to make health-related decisions for persons when they are unable to make them for themselves. The appointed person is a *proxy* or health care surrogate. A health care surrogate is expected to use "substituted judgment" in making decisions; that is, the decision is expected to be that which the person would have made for herself or himself if able to do so and not what the surrogate would make for herself or himself in the same situation. Therefore, it is always advisable that the choice of the surrogate is someone who is willing to uphold the wishes of the person or holds similar values. Whether the health care surrogate is allowed to make end-of-life decisions is determined by state statutes.

Powers of attorney are in effect only at the specific request of the elder or, in the case of the durable power of attorney, in the event that he or she is unable to act on his or her own behalf. As soon as the person regains abilities, the POA is no longer in force unless the individual requests it to continue. The elder retains all of the rights and responsibilities afforded by usual law. This is the least restrictive form of assistance with decision making for persons with impaired capacity. An important aspect of the power of attorney is that persons who are given decision-making rights are those who have been chosen by the elder rather than a court.

Guardians and Conservators

Guardians and conservators are individuals, agencies, or corporations who have been appointed by the court to have care, custody, and control of a disabled person and manage his or her personal or financial affairs (or both). Such a disability often includes an inability to make informed decisions about personal matters and lack of capacity to provide for one's physical health and safety, including, but not limited to, health care, food, shelter, and personal hygiene.

Whereas a conservator is the person appointed to control the finances of the ward, the person appointed to be responsible for the person is usually called the guardian. The conservator or guardian continues in that role until the court rescinds the order and in no other way. Each state is slightly different in how this is handled. In many, the ward, as a person without any legal standing, is unable to petition the courts to have his or her rights restored.

In some states, limits are set according to the degree of protection needed. Total dependency means the person cannot meet basic needs for survival and is unable to manage the environment in any self-sustaining way. Some dependency means the person may be able to manage certain challenges of life; health or judgment may interfere with management of other needs. In the latter situation, a limited guardian may be appointed to protect the person in very specific ways.

The appointments of a guardian or conservator are made at court hearings in which someone demonstrates the incapacity of the elder. Often the elder is not present. The elder is declared incapacitated (formerly called incompetent). The elder is then considered a ward, and all legal rights are lost. All decision making is the legal right and responsibility of the conservator or guardian. As with an attorney-in-fact, substituted judgment is expected to form the basis of decision making.

The guardian, who replaces the attorney-in-fact if present, must take custody of the ward, establish safe shelter, provide for care and maintenance, provide appropriate consent for medical or other professional care, manage financial resources carefully, protect and ensure the rights of the ward, and file an annual report with the appointing court (Nacev and Rettig, 2002). Whether the guardian can make end-of-life decisions depends on the structure of the guardianship and state law.

A guiding principle in guardianships is to accomplish the care and protection needed in the least restrictive way; this is not so different from the care nurses provide in long-term care and home care situations. The law supports the idea that a person has a right to as much autonomy as he or she can manage without sacrificing safety.

There are considerable pros and cons in the use of conservatorships and guardianships, including high risk for exploitation by the conservator. These should be considered only in extreme cases. Nurses working with older adults and their families can encourage the use of advanced planning, including the appointments of health care surrogates and powers of attorney as alternatives that are less restrictive, noting that the definitions and rules vary from state to state.

ELDER MISTREATMENT

Elder mistreatment is a complex phenomenon that includes elder abuse, exploitation, and neglect. While the exact definition varies somewhat, it always means harm that is caused by someone in a caregiving or trust relationship. Mistreatment of older frail and vulnerable adults is found in all socioeconomic, racial, and ethnic groups in the United States and across the globe. It can be seen in any configuration of family and in every setting. It is one of our most unrecognized and underreported social problems today. Elder mistreatment may be intentional, accidental, episodic, or recurrent. It always warrants further assessment. However, unlike children, it requires the permission of the elder unless he or she is not able to speak for himself or herself.

In recognition of the escalating problem of elder mistreatment, countries are busy defining the problem and implementing plans for prevention. Federal definitions of elder abuse, neglect, and exploitation appeared for the first time in the 1987 Amendments to the Older Americans Act. These definitions were provided in the law only as guidelines for identifying the problems and not for enforcement purposes. The specific definitions of elder abuse or mistreatment are now defined by state law and vary considerably from one jurisdiction to another. In 1992, the U.S. Congress passed the Family Violence Prevention and Services Act mandating an analysis of the problem and the Vulnerable Elder Rights Protection Act. In December 2001, the first National Summit on Elder Abuse in the United States was held to identify future directions in the protection of abused elders. Since that time, there has been a global awareness of the problem with countries working for solutions. The National Center for Elder Abuse (NCEA) provides detailed information on the state of elder abuse and related laws and activities (see www.ncea.aoa.gov).

In some cases, defining mistreatment is becoming more difficult as our countries become more diverse. Cultural differences are numerous in the identification and definition of abuse (Malley-Morrison et al., 2006). Given our diverse society, this must be considered. For example, Moon (2001) examined the attitudes toward elder abuse, the tolerance of abuse, and the tendency to blame the victims in a group of first-generation Chinese, Japanese, Korean, and Taiwanese Americans. None of the respondents were in favor of reporting suspected or known abuse or of outside intervention, and their tolerance for abuse was associated with victim blaming. The Korean Americans were also significantly more tolerant of financial exploitation than the other groups.

Just how much mistreatment is occurring is almost impossible to ascertain. The best available estimates may be between 1 and 2 million Americans at least age 65, or 4% to 6% (NCEA, 2005; Post et al., 2010). However, up to 80% of actual mistreatment may be unreported (Meiner, 2011). In a recent cross-sectional study of abuse among community-dwelling women older than age 55, nearly one half reported having experienced some type of abuse, and many of them reported repeated abuse (Fisher and Regan, 2006). Usually victims are unwilling or afraid to report the problem because of shame, embarrassment, intimidation, or fear of retaliation. The abuser may be the only caregiver available to the elder, and reporting or complaining could leave the elder without care at all (Box 20-5).

Most abuse occurs in the home setting, where the majority of caregiving occurs. Most abusers are spouses or adult children. The majority (84%) of the documented cases are among white elders (Meiner, 2011). The incidence of elder abuse is expected to increase with the increase in numbers of persons in need of care, the increased conflicting demands on the caregiver's time, and the increased pressure to report suspicions of abuse.

The most common types of mistreatment are financial exploitation and physical, psychological, and sexual abuse. Medical abuse is also seen, wherein the person is subjected to unwanted treatments or procedures, or medical neglect in which desired treatment is withheld. A particular problem in the elderly is pain under-treatment which can be considered a form of medical neglect (Lewis, 2006). Caregiver neglect implies that the caregiver has not met his or her obligation to the elder for whom he or she is recognized as responsible and includes abandonment (Fulmer, 2002). Self-neglect means that a person is not caring for herself or himself in the manner in which most peers would. In all cases, the vulnerable person is harmed.

Abuse

Abuse is intentional and may be physical, psychological, or sexual and always violates a person's rights (NCEA, 2007) (Box 20-6). When the abuser or neglectful person is a recognized caretaker (e.g., a family member, friend, nurse), the caretaker is subject to tort litigation; that is, he or she can be sued for the injuries to the elderly person and may have to pay monetary damages. If the abuse or neglect is of such a nature that it rises to a criminal act or if the abuse has to do with theft or conversion of property or money, the caretaker is subject to criminal prosecution. Many states have reporting statutes that require certain persons, including nurses, who become aware of abuse, neglect, or exploitation to report it to appropriate authorities. Who that authority is can be found in state laws (NCEA, 2010).

Physical Abuse

Physical abuse is the use of physical force that may result in bodily injury, physical pain, or impairment. It includes, but is not limited to, acts of violence such as striking (with or without an object), hitting, beating, pushing, shoving, shaking, slapping, kicking, pinching, and burning. The inappropriate use of chemical and physical restraints, force-feeding, and physical punishment of any kind also are examples of physical abuse. Any unexpected injury, bruise, or change in behavior of the elderly person may be a sign that requires further investigation. Bruises that are the result of physical abuse are most likely found on the face, the lateral aspect of the arm, and the posterior torso, and are larger (>5 cm). Frequently, the person will not be

---

BOX 20-5   WOMEN AND ABUSE

A study conducted by Bonnie Fisher and Saundra Regan examined the types of abuse, repeated abuse, and the experiences of multiple abuse by women over age 60. Those who responded to a telephone survey consisted of 842 women living in the community. Almost one half of the women had experienced some type of abuse since age 55; many of these reported repeated abuse. The abused women were more likely than the non-abused women to complain of health problems, including bone and joint problems, digestive problems, depression or anxiety, chronic pain, high blood pressure, or heart problems.

Data from Fisher BS, Regan SL: *Gerontologist* 46:200, 2006.

BOX 20-6   TYPES OF ELDER MISTREATMENT*

Physical abuse: The use of physical force that may result in bodily injury, physical pain, or impairment.

Sexual abuse: Nonconsensual sexual contact of any kind with an elderly person, including with those persons unable to give consent.

Emotional or psychological abuse: The infliction of anguish, pain, or distress through verbal or nonverbal acts, including intimidation or enforced social isolation.

Medical abuse: Subjecting a person to unwanted medical treatments or procedures; medical neglect occurs when a medically necessary and desired treatment is withheld.

Financial or material abuse or exploitation: The illegal or improper use of an elder's funds, property, or assets.

Neglect: The refusal or failure to fulfill any part of a person's previously agreed obligation or duties to an elder dependent on the person for care or assistance.

Abandonment: The desertion of an elder by an individual who had assumed the responsibility of providing care or assistance.

*Elder mistreatment implies that the recipient of the mistreatment is in a situation or condition in which the ability to protect oneself is limited in some way. Otherwise the actions are more accurately described as domestic violence, sexual assault, or fraud.

able to explain or offer a reasonable explanation for the injury (Wiglesworth et al., 2009).

Psychological/Emotional Abuse

Emotional or psychological abuse includes but is not limited to verbal assaults, insults, threats, intimidation, humiliation, and harassment. Psychological abuse is the infliction of anguish, pain, or distress through verbal or nonverbal acts. Treating an older person like a child; isolating the person from his or her family, friends, or regular activities; and enforced social isolation are examples of psychological abuse. This type of abuse may be a deliberate effort to dehumanize the person, sometimes to mitigate the guilt of providing poor care or abusing the person emotionally.

Sexual Abuse

Sexual abuse is nonconsensual sexual contact of any kind with another person, regardless of age. Sexual contact with a person incapable of giving consent is also considered sexual abuse. It includes but is not limited to unwanted touching and all types of sexual assault or battery, such as rape, sodomy, coerced nudity, and sexually explicit photographing. Nurses and other health care providers may observe injuries from rough or forceful sexual activity. However, sometimes injury may not be present but certain behaviors may be revealing. Fear of certain persons, resistance to necessary touch in the genital area, or reports of sexual contact cannot be ignored.

Financial or Material Exploitation

Financial or material exploitation is the illegal or improper use of another's funds, property, or assets. Exploitation may be accomplished by force, such as demanding that the person sign checks or other documents with the threat of withholding care. It can also be done with stealth through deceit, misrepresentation, or fraud, such as cashing a person's checks without authorization or permission, forging a signature, or misusing or stealing an older person's money or possessions. Also, conservatorship, guardianship, or POA can be improperly used.

Whereas other forms of abuse have external signs, it is often difficult to detect financial exploitation. Care is costly, and much of the person's assets may be gone before it is noted that far more has been used than seems to be needed. Changes in banking practices, failure to pay medical or other care bills, unexpected changes in a will, and finding personal valuable items missing are all evidence of possible financial exploitation and should be reported to the state department on aging or similar agency.

Undue Influence

Undue influence is often used as a means of achieving financial or material exploitation. As described by Quinn (2002, p. 11):

> Undue influence is the substitution of one person's will for the true desires of another. . . . Undue influence takes place when one person uses his or her role and power to exploit the trust, dependency or fear of another to gain psychological control over the weaker person's decision-making, usually for financial gain.

Undue influence may occur in an insidious way because the victim is often isolated from friends and family and convinced that the only one who cares is the caretaker. Perhaps a younger person, for instance, attempts to defraud a lonely widow or widower of assets through romance and marriage. In these cases, intervention is difficult because the victim has developed trust and reliance on the abuser and has usually entered into the relationship voluntarily. Undue influence may be exerted on the elder, and a companion or home care provider will manage to convince the elder to transfer assets and even the deed to the home. These situations are being examined more carefully in the courts, and some states are activating legal protections against undue influence (Quinn, 2002; Quinn and Tomita, 2003). Quinn has developed guidelines for nurses attempting to identify signs of undue influence (Box 20-7).

Neglect

Neglect is the most common form of elder mistreatment and may be at the hands of a caregiver or oneself. Neglect of self and

---

BOX 20-7	SIGNS AND SYMPTOMS OF UNDUE INFLUENCE

- Actions inconsistent with his or her life history. Actions run counter to the person's previous long-time values and beliefs.
- Makes sudden changes with regard to financial management. Examples include cashing in insurance policies or changing titles on bank accounts or real property.
- Elder changes his or her will and previous disposition of assets.
- Elder is taken to practitioners different from those he or she has always trusted. Examples include bankers, stockbrokers, attorneys, physicians, and realtor.
- Elder is systematically isolated from or is continually monitored with others who care about him or her.
- Someone suddenly moves into the person's home, or the elder is moved into someone's home under the guise of providing better care.
- Someone attempts to get income checks directed differently from the usual arrangement.
- Documents are suddenly signed frequently as the elder nears death.
- A history of mistrust exists in the elder's family, especially with financial affairs, and the elder places unusual trust in newfound acquaintances.

- Someone promises to provide lifelong care in exchange for property on the elder's death.
- Statements of the elder and the alleged abuser vary concerning the elder's affairs or disposition of assets.
- A power imbalance exists between the parties in matters of finances or health.
- Someone shows unfairness to the weaker party in a transaction. The stronger person unduly benefits by the transaction.
- The elder is never left alone with anyone. No one is allowed to speak to the elder without the alleged abuser having a way of finding out about it.
- Unusual patterns arise in the elder's finances. For instance, numerous checks are written out to "cash," always in round numbers, and often in large amounts.
- The elder reports meeting a "wonderful new friend who makes me feel young again." The elder then becomes suspicious of family and begins to avoid family gatherings.
- The elder is pressed into a transaction without being given time to reflect or contact trusted advisors.

From Quinn M: *Geriatric Nursing* 23:11, 2002.

neglect by caretakers are often difficult to define because they are intertwined with energy, lifestyle, and resources. Nurses must be cautious in setting specific boundaries around neglect. However, when basic needs go unmet, intervention may be required. Physical neglect is the most common and obvious occurrence and may be indicated by a person's failure to thrive, untreated medical conditions (medical neglect), badly neglected grooming, malnutrition, and dehydration.

Caregiver Neglect

Neglect is passive abuse not characterized by physical violence. Caregiver neglect is seen as an act of omission or withholding needed goods and services such as food, medication, medical treatment, and personal care necessary for the well-being of the frail elder. It also includes behavior that ignores the person's obvious needs even though the caretaker is present.

Neglect by a caregiver may occur for many reasons. Sometimes it is the result of caregiver stress, the result of feeling overwhelmed by the responsibilities of caregiving. Or it can be active neglect that is deliberate and malicious (Quinn and Tomita, 2003). However, some acts of neglect occur because of incompetence, unawareness of importance of the neglected care, no legal requirement to give such care, unavailability of resources, or exhaustion. The caregivers' own frailty and advanced age are often mitigating factors. Passive neglect—simply ignoring or not attending to needs—is most prevalent.

Self-Neglect

Elder self-neglect is a behavior of the individual person. It is usually a function of a person's diminished physical or mental capacity that threatens his or her own health or safety. Self-neglect generally manifests itself in an older person as a refusal or failure to provide himself or herself with adequate safety, food, water, clothing, shelter, personal hygiene, or health care. Self-neglect may be associated with increasing severity of physical or mental impairments but may also reflect a lifestyle of alcoholism and drug abuse (Quinn and Tomita, 2003). However, in some situations, a mentally competent person who understands the consequences of his or her decisions makes a conscious and voluntary decision to engage in acts that threaten his or her health or safety as a matter of personal choice. It is an ethical and legal question as to how much health care professionals should intervene in these situations unless it can definitely be determined that the person lacks decision-making capacity or competence.

Risk Factors

Elder abuse requires an abuser, an elder, and the context of caregiving or trust. There are multiple risk factors for one to be or become an abuser or abused. Persons who are abusing alcohol or other substances, have emotional or mental illnesses, or have a history of abusing or being abused are more likely to be abusers, as are caregivers who are exhausted and frustrated (Box 20-8). Wang and colleagues (2006) found that in Taiwan, abusers were most likely to be younger women with higher levels of education and higher levels of burden. The abuser is usually the caregiver but may also be the care recipient. Caregivers, be they informal (e.g., spouses) or formal (e.g., nursing assistants), may be subjected to verbal and physical abuse by the

---

BOX 20-8   A TYPICAL ABUSED ELDER AND ABUSER

ABUSED
White woman
Single
Over 75
Dependent on a caregiver for shelter and food
Incontinent
Frail or have an illness or mental disability

ABUSERS
Family member
Middle-aged or older
Daughter or son of the elder
Low self-esteem
Impaired impulse control

POSSIBLE ABUSER BEHAVIOR
Aggression
Defensive or increasingly resentful attitude toward the elder
Blames the victim for an injury
Treats the elder like a child
Caregiver shows new affluence while withholding food or medication from the elder

Data from Nies MA, McEwan M: *Community/public health nursing: promoting the health of populations,* ed 6, 2011, Saunders.

---

person for whom they are caring. This may be a lifelong pattern that intensifies in the current situation.

Although any person can be abused, women are at particular risk. The typical abused elder is a white, 75-year-old woman who lives alone and is frail, confused, or depressed (Lantz, 2006). The risk for abuse is intensified if the person has been abused in the past or if his or her behavior is considered aggressive, combative, or provocative; that is, the person is viewed as overly demanding or unappreciative (Harrell et al., 2002). The level of dependency is also a factor; the more dependent the elder, the more vulnerable he or she is to being abused. However, in Wiglesworth's study, the abused were functioning at a fairly high level (2009). Men or women who had abused the caregiver earlier in life may be at risk for retaliation. Because both the majority of caregiving and the majority of abuse occur within the family, this is the context. Caregiver/care recipient relationships that were conflicted earlier in life will continue to be so. Dyer and colleagues (2000) found that individuals older than age 75 who are diagnosed with depression or dementia are the most likely to be mistreated. Victims were most likely to be female and living in a household with family members. In their study of those who had been physically abused to the point of bruising, Wiglesworth and colleagues (2009) found the majority to be white women over age 76, not necessarily demented, and with the ability to do some activities for themselves and in the household. Many used assistive devices to ambulate. The abusers were predominately (86.6%) family members.

Abuse and exploitation can also occur in the situation of a hired caregiver. When a number of providers are giving care, monitoring becomes especially difficult. Situations of potential formal caregiver abuse include those in which there is inadequate supervision of patient care, poor coordination of services, inadequate staff training, theft and fraud, drug and alcohol abuse by staff, tardiness and absenteeism, unprofessional and criminal conduct, and inadequate record keeping. The nurse should pay particular attention to the caregiver who is alone, with no support from others and no opportunities for respite. The abuse may be a lifelong pattern in which the victim has always felt somewhat at fault and will remain in the situation.

PROMOTING HEALTHY AGING: IMPLICATIONS FOR GERONTOLOGICAL NURSING

Nurses are expected to provide safety and security to the persons under their care, to the best possible extent. When caring for vulnerable elders, it also may mean wrestling with difficult and problematic legal and ethical issues in the provision of care. This may mean assessing the person's decision-making capacity (Box 20-9) or contacting protective services when there is evidence of potential abuse.

As noted, unless otherwise adjudicated (declared by the courts), each individual has presumed capacity to control his or her life, including what happens to his or her body, that is, the autonomous legal and ethical right to determine what treatments are received or not. This has received a significant amount of legal support through the passage of the Patient Self-Determination Act of the 1980s and HIPAA of 1997. The dilemma occurs when the person's capacity to make health care decisions is called into question. This is not a question of preference or question of the person's taste or values in his or her choices, but in the ability to understand the problem at hand, the choice made, and it consequences. It is always necessary to determine whether the appearance of incapacity is truly one of impairment or whether it is inconsistent with the preferences, expectations, or values of the nurse, caregiver, or potential health care surrogate and therefore interpreted as lack of capacity (Torke et al., 2010).

The nurse is expected to work toward preserving the individual's integrity, independence, dignity, and assets to the best possible extent. In some situations, this results in conflict. While working in a nursing facility, one of the authors (K.J.) regularly heard from previously distant or uninvolved relatives of somewhat impaired elders. These relatives would declare that they were the "power of attorney" and therefore had the right to override an individual's apparent decisions or choices or would insist on access to the person's medical and health information. In such a situation, several nursing actions are recommended. First, the nurse should clarify the issues at hand and the conflicts that may be presented. Second, the nurse can work with other professionals to conduct an assessment of gross measures of the elder's capacity, including knowledge of and confidence in the person making the POA claim while realizing that these are clinical judgments and do not replace court decisions or legal action. Third, if, in the clinical judgment of the health care team, the elder may have limitations in some decision-making capacity, the nurse must clarify the type of POA that is held (if it is regular or durable) and, if applicable, respond accordingly. This would include obtaining a copy of the document for the patient's record and having it reviewed by an attorney for authenticity and applicability. Health information can be released only to persons approved by the patient, through permission or the written permission, such as that indicated on a POA.

On the other hand, if the nurse is presented with proof that the patient has been adjudicated to have limited or no capacity, the guardian indeed is the decision maker and sole representative of the patient or resident. The guardian is then the person who will decide who has access to the patient's information. The facility in which the person resides will need to have its own legal consultation in determining the authority of the documents and in guiding the health care team in any specific directions in any legal documents. However, as an advocate, the nurse still has a responsibility to protect the patient from neglect or exploitation from all sources, including guardians. Nurses who are consulted by clients about legal issues should not attempt to provide legal advice but, instead, should refer their clients to an attorney, preferably one who is certified by the National Elder Law Foundation (www.nelf.org). The state or local bar association is able to assist nurses and their clients with this information.

When working with frail and vulnerable elders, nurses must always be vigilant in their sensitivity to the potential for abuse, observing for signs and symptoms in all their interactions with vulnerable elders. In addition to the obvious physical signs (Box 20-10), the nurse looks for more subtle signals. Is there an unusual delay between the beginning of a health problem and when help is sought? Are appointments often missed without reasonable explanations? Are the histories given by the elder and

---

BOX 20-9   EVIDENCE-BASED PRACTICE

DECISION-MAKING IN OLDER ADULTS WITH DEMENTIA

See http://consultgerirn.org/uploads/File/trythis/try_this_d9.pdf by Ethel L. Mitty, EdD, RN.
See also Healthcare Decision Making: Nursing Standard of Practice Protocol: Health Care Decision Making at http://consultgerirn.org/topics/treatment_decision_making/want_to_know_more by Ethel L. Mitty, EdD, RN and Linda Farber Post, JD, MA, BSN.

BOX 20-10   SIGNS OF AND RESPONSES TO ELDER MISTREATMENT

SIGNS AND SIGNALS

Slapping, bruising, striking (with or without an object), burning, shaking; inappropriate use of physical restraints; force feeding
Unwanted touching; all sexual assault or battery
Verbal assaults; insults or threats; intimidations or humiliation; treating like an infant; isolating from family, friends, or regular activities; giving "the silent treatment"
Being dropped off at a hospital, nursing facility or institution, or shopping center

NURSING INTERVENTIONS

Thorough assessment with precise documentation (including photographic documentation taken before the victim is washed or treated)
Collection and preservation of any and all physical evidence (e.g., dirty or bloody clothing, bandages, sheets)
Social services consultation
If the elder is in immediate danger, consider implementing a safety plan (e.g., hospital admission)
Mandatory report to the appropriate state agency and/or law enforcement on the suspicion of abuse or neglect

Modified from Jarvis C: *Physical examination and health assessment,* ed 5, Saunders, 2008; Lewis SM, Heitkemper MM, Dirksen SR, et al: *Medical-surgical nursing (single volume): assessment and management of clinical problems,* ed 7, St Louis, 2007, Mosby.

the caregiver inconsistent? Also, behavioral indications may suggest an abusive situation. Does the caregiver do all of the talking in a situation, even though the elder is capable? Does the caregiver appear angry, frustrated, or indifferent while the elder appears hesitant or frightened? Is the caregiver or the care recipient aggressive toward one another or the nurse?

If abuse is suspected, a full and specialized assessment should be done, including a determination of the safety of the victim and the desires of the victim if competent. Assessment of mistreatment involves several components, and an evidence-based tool is also available (Box 20-11 and Figure 20-3). Because of the sensitive nature of such an assessment, specialized training is recommended for all gerontological nurses (Fulmer and Greenberg, 2008).

The nurse's response to potential abuse or neglect of the vulnerable may be mandated. In most jurisdictions in the United States, nurses have a legal responsibility to protect the vulnerable, be they children, persons with disabilities, or elders with limited physical or cognitive capacity. However, here more than in any other situation is it imperative for the nurse to have at least a working knowledge of the laws that protect vulnerable elders.

Mandatory Reporting

In most states and U.S. jurisdictions, licensed nurses are "mandatory reporters," that is, persons who are required to report suspicions of abuse to the state, usually to a group called Adult Protective Services (APS). Failure to report suspicions may result in civil and/or criminal penalties (Meiner, 2011). The standard for reporting is one of reasonable belief; that is, the nurse must have a reasonable belief that a vulnerable person either has been or is likely to be abused, neglected, or exploited. Actual knowledge is not required (Meiner, 2011). Usually these reports are anonymous. If the nurse believes the elder to be in immediate danger, the police should be notified. How the nurse accomplishes this varies with the work setting. In hospitals and nursing homes, this is often reported first internally to the facility social worker. In the home care setting, the report is made to the nursing supervisor. It would be very unusual for the nurse not to go through his or her employer. However, the nurse who is a neighbor, friend, or privately paid caregiver may be under obligation to make the report directly. In the nursing home or licensed assisted living facility, the nurse has the additional resource of calling the state long-term care ombudsman for help.

In each state, ombudsmen are either volunteers or paid staff members who are responsible for acting as advocates for vulnerable elders in institutions (www.ltcombudsman.org). All reports, either to the state ombudsman or to APS, will be investigated. A unique aspect of elder abuse compared with child abuse is that the physically frail but mentally competent adult can refuse assessment and intervention and often does. Abused but competent elders cannot be removed from harmful situations without their permission, much to the frustration of the nurse and other health care providers.

Prevention of Abuse

In the ideal situation, gerontological nurses are alert to potential mistreatment of vulnerable elders and take steps to prevent the occurrence of abuse or neglect. In some situations, the abuse may be preventable, and in others, it is less likely to be preventable. If the abuse is the result of psychopathological conditions, especially if the situation is long-standing, the nurse probably cannot prevent the abuse. However, nurses can make sure that the potential victims know how to get help if it is needed and the resources that are available to them, and nurses can provide support and encouragement that it is possible to leave the situation. The nurse can also work with the elder, caregiver, and community supports to increase the exposure of the elders to others.

If the abusive behavior is learned or a response to stress, the situation may be subject to change. Learned abuse, theoretically, can be unlearned and may respond to a close working relationship with a mentoring professional who can demonstrate positive problem solving and new ways of managing difficult situations.

If the abuse is based in the stress of the caregiving situation, nurses can be very proactive and help all involved take action to lessen the stress. This may include finding respite services, changing the situation entirely (giving permission to the caregiver to give up the role), referring to support groups for expression of frustrations and peer support, teaching people how to use crisis hotlines, professional consultation, victim support groups, victim volunteer companions, and, above all, thoughtful and compassionate care for the victim and the perpetrator (Quinn and Tomita, 2003; Pillemer and Wolf, 1986). See Box 20-12 for tips on the prevention of elder mistreatment.

Finally, for elders who become incapacitated, legal protection may be necessary. Gerontological nurses can become familiar with the laws that specifically affect older adults in their state. This can be done by speaking with an elder law attorney or selecting continuing education programs to update knowledge in the field of client legal protections. Once informed of the laws affecting frail elders, nurses are in a position to assist elders and family members in seeking legal representation when necessary and in selecting the approach that will solve the problems in the least restrictive manner possible. Although initiating these interventions is usually the responsibility of the social worker and enacted by lawyers and judges, the nurse should understand the basic concepts and the types of legal protection for elders and other incapacitated persons.

BOX 20-12 **TIPS FOR THE PREVENTION OF ELDER MISTREATMENT**

- Make professionals aware of potentially abusive situations.
- Educate the public about normal aging processes.
- Help families develop and nurture informal support systems.
- Link families with support groups.
- Teach families stress management techniques.
- Arrange comprehensive care resources.
- Provide counseling for troubled families.
- Encourage the use of respite care and day care.
- Obtain necessary home health care services.
- Inform families of resources for meals and transportation.
- Encourage caregivers to pursue their individual interests.

1. General Assessment	Very Good	Good	Poor	Very Poor	Unable to Assess
a. Clothing					
b. Hygiene					
c. Nutrition					
d. Skin integrity					

Additional Comments:

2. Possible Abuse Indicators	No Evidence	Possible Evidence	Probable Evidence	Definite Evidence	Unable to Assess
a. Bruising					
b. Lacerations					
c. Fractures					
d. Various stages of healing of any bruises or fractures					
e. Evidence of sexual abuse					
f. Statement by elder re: abuse					

Additional Comments:

3. Possible Neglect Indicators	No Evidence	Possible Evidence	Probable Evidence	Definite Evidence	Unable to Assess
a. Contractures					
b. Decubiti					
c. Dehydration					
d. Diarrhea					
e. Depression					
f. Impaction					
g. Malnutrition					
h. Urine burns					
i. Poor hygiene					
j. Failure to respond to warning of obvious disease					
k. Inappropriate medications (under/over)					
l. Repetitive hospital admissions due to probable failure of health care surveillance					
m. Statement by elder re: neglect					

Additional Comments:

4. Possible Exploitation Indicators	No Evidence	Possible Evidence	Probable Evidence	Definite Evidence	Unable to Assess
a. Misuse of money					
b. Evidence of financial exploitation					
c. Reports of demands for goods in exchange for services					
d. Inability to account for money/property					
e. Statement by elder re: exploitation					

Additional Comments:

5. Possible Abandonment Indicators	No Evidence	Possible Evidence	Probable Evidence	Definite Evidence	Unable to Assess
a. Evidence that a caretaker has withdrawn care precipitously without alternate arrangements					
b. Evidence that elder is left alone in an unsafe environment for extended periods without adequate support					
c. Statement by elder re: abandonment					

Additional Comments:

6. Summary	No Evidence	Possible Evidence	Probable Evidence	Definite Evidence	Unable to Assess
a. Evidence of abuse					
b. Evidence of neglect					
c. Evidence of exploitation					
d. Evidence of abandonment					

Additional Comments:

FIGURE 20-3 Abuse and neglect assessment. (Reprinted from *Journal of Emergency Nursing*, 10(3). Fulmer, T., Street, S., & Carr, K. Abuse of the elderly: Screening and detection, pp. 131-140. Copyright 1984, with permission from The Emergency Nurses Association)

Advocacy

An advocate is one who maintains or promotes a cause; defends, pleads, or acts on behalf of a cause for another; fights for someone who cannot fight; and often gets involved in getting someone to do something he or she would not otherwise do.

Topics for advocacy can include protection of specific rights (e.g., promoting the least restrictive residential alternative for another), finding the best nursing home, or testifying at the judicial appointment of a conservator. Other areas of advocacy include the rights of medical patients, the right to have in-home supportive services, and maintenance of government benefits, such as veterans' benefits, Medicare, Social Security (SS) and Supplemental Security Income (SSI), and food stamps. Advocates function in various arenas: with their own and other disciplines within their own agencies, with other agencies, with physicians, with families, with neighbors and community representatives, with professional organizations, with legislators, and with courts.

Nurses act as advocates when they support the person as a free agent who has autonomy in the health care situation. In a health care situation, advocacy is acting for or on behalf of another in terms of pleading for and supporting the best interests of that other person with respect to choice, provision, and refusal of health care. However, situations occur in the care of older adults when the elder is either not strong enough or does not have the mental capacity to exert measures to protect his or her own interests. When this occurs, the nurse's role is to ensure that not only the person is protected but that his or her voice, when he or she can or could express himself or herself, is not lost.

evolve To access your student resources, go to *http://evolve.elsevier.com/Ebersole/TwdHlthAging*

KEY CONCEPTS

- The Social Security system in the United States provided a guaranteed income for persons who have paid a requisite amount into the system earlier in their lives.
- Both the Social Security and the Medicare insurance programs are based on a "pay-as-you-go" arrangement with persons, with funds from current workers used to support current retirees.
- Social Security provides an income to the majority of those retired persons in the United States.
- Medicare is a near universal health insurance plan for persons who are age 65, blind, permanently disabled, or with end-stage renal disease.
- Medicare is composed of parts A, B, C, and D. There is no premium for Medicare Part A, hospitalization. There are considerable differences between Parts B and C, one of which must be selected at the age of eligibility.
- Medicaid provides coverage for the out-of-pocket medical expenses for poor Medicare beneficiaries.
- Informed consent is based on the ethical principle of autonomy, which requires the capacity to understand a situation, the choices one has, and the consequences of a decision.
- In the health care setting, an individual may be legally competent but have diminished or varying levels of capacity to make health-related decisions.
- Varying levels of protection are available to protect persons with diminished capacity and to assure that his or her voice is still heard.
- Elder mistreatment is an umbrella term that covers abuse, neglect, exploitation, and abandonment.
- The nurse has a legal responsibility in most states to report suspected mistreatment of frail or disabled elders.

CASE STUDY   ELDER ABUSE

Mrs. Henry, 87 years old, is admitted to the medical/surgical floor of a community hospital with a fractured right orbit and ruptured eye globe. Her husband attends to her with care and concern, trying to anticipate her needs. He is active and appears much younger than his stated age of 85. The emergency department report states the cause of the injury as "fall at home." Although Mrs. Henry is alert and oriented, she appears very thin, frail, and withdrawn. Her husband also voices concern that she seems confused at times. When the gerontological clinical nurse specialist arrives to do a basic intake, she reports to the nurses that she is concerned that Mrs. Henry has been abused. Her husband answers all the questions posed to his wife, and, as he does so, Mrs. Henry seems to withdraw even further from both him and the staff. Mr. Henry does not leave his wife's side for hours. Finally he leaves for a quick cup of coffee, and the nurse who had been providing care quickly goes into the room and asks Mrs. Henry what happened. She begins to cry and says that her husband hit her. She is immediately offered shelter and protection. She declines, saying that she has nowhere else to go but back home and that she will be okay. The husband returns to find the nurse talking to his wife privately and immediately gathers up her things, and they leave the hospital against medical advice.

Based on the case study, develop a nursing care plan using the following procedure*:
- List Mrs. Henry's comments that provide subjective data.

- List information that provides objective data.
- From these data, identify and state, using accepted format, two nursing diagnoses you determine are most significant to Mrs. Henry at this time. List two of Mrs. Henry's strengths that you have identified from the data.
- Determine and state outcome criteria for each diagnosis. These must reflect some alleviation of the problem identified in the nursing diagnosis and must be stated in concrete and measurable terms.
- Plan and state one or more interventions for each diagnosed problem. Provide specific documentation of the source used to determine the appropriate intervention. Plan at least one intervention that incorporates Mrs. Henry's existing strengths.
- Evaluate the success of the intervention. Interventions must correlate directly with the stated outcome criteria to measure the outcome success.

CRITICAL THINKING QUESTIONS
1. Identify the risk factors for elder abuse in this situation.
2. Provide the subjective data suggesting abuse.
3. Provide the objective data suggesting abuse in this situation.
4. Describe the nurse's legal responsibility to Mrs. Henry at this time.
5. Why might Mrs. Henry believe she has no options?
6. Describe the next step the nurse will take on the departure of this patient.

*Students are advised to refer to their nursing diagnosis text and identify possible or potential problems.

RESEARCH QUESTIONS

1. What do elders find most helpful about Medicare? What do they find least helpful?
2. How would elders like to see Medicare changed?
3. What are elders' thoughts and attitudes about managed care?
4. Who do elders most frequently contact when they need legal and economic advice?
5. How many elders feel secure about their economic future?
6. What are the current average out-of-pocket costs for elder health care?
7. How do elders feel about the rationing of health care based on age or survivability?
8. Are the poverty-inducing effects of widowhood and retirement different in specific ways in various ethnic groups?
9. What are the prevalent attitudes of the elderly persons with whom you are acquainted regarding their economic future?
10. What are your responsibilities in reporting elder abuse in your state?
11. Are shelters available to frail elders who are attempting to escape from abuse?

REFERENCES

American Association of Retired Persons: How health care reform will affect health care quality and delivery of services, 2010. Available at http://assets.aarp.org/rgcenter/ppi/health-care/fs197-health.pdf.

Bohm D: Striving for quality in American nursing homes, *DePaul Journal of Health Care Law* 4:317, 2001.

Cantril H: *Public opinion 1935-1946*, Princeton, NJ, 1951, Princeton University Press.

Carroll DW: Assessment of capacity for medical decision-making. *Journal of Gerontological Nursing* 36:47, 2010.

Centers for Medicare and Medicaid Services: *Medicare and you, 2010*, Baltimore, 2010, The Centers.

Centers for Medicare and Medicaid Services: *Medicare and you, 2011*, Baltimore, 2011, The Centers.

Centers for Medicare and Medicaid Services: Medicare enrollment—national trends, 2009. Available at http://www.cms.gov/MedicareEnRpts/Downloads/HISMI2009.pdf.

Corning P: *The evolution of Medicare: from idea to law, research report No 29*, Washington, DC, 1969, U.S. Department of Health, Education and Welfare, Social Security Administration, Office of Research and Statistics, U.S. Government Printing Office.

Dyer CB, Pavlik VN, Murphy KP, et al: The high prevalence of depression and dementia in elder abuse and neglect, *Journal of the American Geriatrics Society* 48:205, 2000.

Fisher BS, Regan SL: The extent and frequency of abuse in the lives of older women and their relationships with health outcomes, *Gerontologist* 46:200, 2006.

Fulmer T, Greenberg S: Elder abuse and neglect assessment, 2008. Available at http://consultgerirn.org/topics/elder_mistreatment_and_abuse/want_to_know_more#item_6 .

Goodman JC: *The regulation of medical care: is the price too high? Cato public policy research monograph No 3*, San Francisco, 1980, Cato Institute.

Harrell R, Toronjo CH, McLaughlin J, et al: How geriatricians identify elder abuse and neglect, *American Journal of the Medical Sciences* 323:34, 2002.

Hooyman NR, Kiyak HA: *Social gerontology: a multidisciplinary perspective*, ed 8, New York, 2008, Pearson.

Lantz MS: Elder abuse and neglect: help starts with recognizing the problem, *Clinical Geriatrics* 14:10, 2006.

Lewis M: Pain. In Meiner S, Lueckenotte A, editors: *Gerontologic nursing*, ed 3, St Louis, 2006, Mosby.

Lewis SM, Heitkemper MM, Dirksen SR, et al: *Medical surgical nursing: assessment and management of clinical problems*, ed 7, 2007, Mosby.

Magid M, Dodd ML, Bostwick JM, et al: Is your patient making the "wrong" treatment choice? *Journal of Family Practice* 5:13, 2006.

Malley-Morrison K, Nolido N, Chawla S: International perspectives on elder abuse: five case studies, *Educational Gerontology* 32:1, 2006.

Meiner S: Legal and ethical issues. In Meiner S, editor: *Gerontologic nursing*, ed 4, St Louis, 2011, Mosby.

Moon A: Elder mistreatment among four Asian American groups: an exploratory study on tolerance, victim blaming, and attitudes toward their party intervention. *Journal of Gerontological Social Work* 36:153, 2001.

Nacev AN, Rettig J: A survey of key issues in Kentucky elder law, *Northern Kentucky Law Review* 29(1):139, 2002.

National Center on Elder Abuse: State Directory of Helplines, Hotlines, and Elder Abuse Prevention Resources. Last modified June 15, 2010. Available at http://www.ncea.aoa.gov/NCEAroot/Main_Site/Find_Help/State_Resources.aspx.

Pillemer KA, Wolf RS: *Elder abuse: conflict in the family*, Dover, Me, 1986, Auburn House.

Post L, Page C, Conner T, et al: Elder abuse in long-term care: Types, patterns and risk factors. *Research on Aging* 32:323, 2010.

Quinn M: Undue influence and elder abuse: recognition and intervention strategies, *Geriatric Nursing* 23:11, 2002.

Quinn M, Tomita SK: *Elder abuse and neglect: causes, diagnoses and intervention strategies*, ed 3, New York, 2003, Springer Series on Social Work.

Social Security Administration: Understanding Supplementary Security Income Home Page, 2010. Available at http://www.ssa.gov/ssi/text-understanding-ssi.htm.

Stefanacci R: How to help your patients choose the right prescription drug plan, *Annals of Long-Term Care* 14:17, 2006.

Teske R: How to cope with the coming crisis in long-term care, Heritage Lecture #658, April 2000. Available at www.heritage.org/Research/HealthCare/h1658.cfm.

Trustees: OASDI Trustees report, 2010a. Available at http://www.ssa.gov/OACT/TRSUM/index.html.

Trustees: 2010 Annual Report of the Boards of Trustees of the Federal Hospital Insurance and Federal Supplementary Insurance Trust Funds, 2010b. Available at http://www.cms.gov/ReportsTrustFunds/downloads/tr2010.pdf.

Torke AM, Moloney R, Siegler M, Abalos A, Alexander GC: Physicians' view on the importance of patient preferences in surrogate decision-making, *J Am Geriatr Soc* 58(3):533-538, 2010.

Twight C: Medicare's origin: the economics and politics of dependency, *Cato Journal* 16:1997.

Wang JJ, Lin JN, Lee FP: Psychologically abusive behavior by those caring for the elderly in domestic context, *Geriatric Nursing* 27:284, 2006.

Weinberger M: *Social Security: facing the facts*, Washington, DC, 1996, Cato Project on Social Security privatization. Available at www.socialsecurity.org/pubs/ssps/ssp3.html.

Whitehouse: Health Reform for American Seniors. The Affordable Care Act Gives America's Seniors Greater Control Over Their Own Health Care, n.d. Available at http://www.whitehouse.gov/sites/default/files/rss_viewer/health_reform_seniors.pdf.

Wiglesworth A, Austin R, Corona M, et al: Bruising as a marker of physical elder abuse, *Journal of the American Geriatrics Society* 57:1191, 2009.

Intimacy and Sexuality

Theris A. Touhy

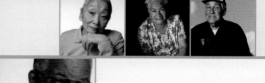

evolve *http://evolve.elsevier.com/Ebersole/TwdHlthAging*

A STUDENT SPEAKS

I'm sorry but I cannot imagine my grandparents having sexual intercourse or being interested in information about sexual health. I never thought much about sexuality and older people but, I must say, I do hope that I will have a fulfilling sexual life when I am old.

Jennifer, age 21

AN ELDER SPEAKS

These early morning hours are terribly lonely . . . that's when I have such a longing for someone who loves me to be there just to touch and hold me . . . and to talk to. **Sister Marilyn Schwab (From Schwab M: *A gift freely given: the personal journal of Sister Marilyn Schwab, Mt Angel, Ore, 1986, Benedictine Sisters.*)**

LEARNING OBJECTIVES

On completion of this chapter, the reader will be able to:

1. Discuss touch and intimacy as integral components of sexuality.
2. Discuss the therapeutic benefits of touch for older people.
3. Discuss the physiological, social, and psychological factors that affect the older adult's sexual function.
4. Describe the various approaches to sexuality assessment that may reduce nurse-client anxiety in discussing a sensitive area.
5. Identify the risks to sexual integrity.
6. Discuss interventions that foster sexual integrity.
7. Develop a plan of care for an elder to promote sexual health.

TOUCH

Touch is the first of our senses to develop and provides us with our most fundamental means of contact with the external world (Gallace and Spence, 2010). It is the oldest, most important, and most neglected of our senses. Touch is 10 times stronger than verbal or emotional contact. All other senses have an organ on which to focus, but touch is everywhere. Touch is unique because it frequently combines with other senses. An individual can survive without one or more of the other senses, but no one can survive and live in any degree of comfort without touch.

In the absence of touching or being touched, people of all ages can become sick and become touch starved. "Touch is experienced physically as a sensation as well as affectively as emotion and behavior. The interaction of touch affects the autonomic, reticular, and limbic systems, and thus profoundly affects the emotional drives" (Kim and Buschmann, 2004, p. 35).

The human yearning for physical contact is embedded in our language in such figurative terms as "keep in touch," "handle with care," and "rubbed the wrong way." We will focus on touch as an overt expression of closeness, intimacy, and sexuality. We believe an individual must recognize the power of touch and its intimacy to fully comprehend sexuality. Touch and intimacy are integral parts of sexuality, just as sexuality is expressed through intimacy and touch. Together, touch and intimacy can offer the older adult a sense of well being. Throughout life, touch provides emotional and sensual knowledge about other individuals—an unending source of information, pleasure, and pain.

We love and are loved by virtue of our skin sensation and appearance. How our skin is arranged affects others' willingness to touch us. Even though beauty is said to be only skin deep, skin is significant. The wrinkled skin of the old person shows the beautiful lines of hard work and experience. Old hands

409

and old faces tell much of the bearer's capacity for intimacy. Sensations of old skin, clean, dry, and powdered or cologned, linger in the remote memories of many individuals who were held by a grandmother or grandfather. These features provide our foundation for intimacy with the old.

Response to Touch

The Touch model proposed by Hollinger and Buschmann (1993) proposes that attitudes toward touch and acceptance of touch affect the behaviors of both caregivers and patients. Two types of touch occur during the nurse-patient relationship: procedural and non-procedural. Procedural touch (task-oriented or *instrumental touch*) is physical contact that occurs when a particular task is being performed. Non-procedural touch (expressive physical touch) does not require a task but is affective and supportive in nature, such as holding a patient's hand.

Nurses should recognize the influence of their own personality, cultural expectations, and early exposure to touching. Everyone has definite feelings and opinions about touch based on his or her own life experience. "Individuals learn the boundaries of tactual communication culturally" (Kim and Buschmann, 2004, p. 37). Touch only if it is comfortable, and do not assume that a person likes or wants to be touched (Rheaume and Mitty, 2008). Individuals quickly discern the discomfort of another if touch is not an integral part of behavior. It is important to remember that the comfort of touching depends on the location of touch, the situation, social status, culture, and age.

A test of the person's readiness to be touched is to initiate a hand clasp or handshake. The person can feel the tension or the welcoming relaxation that occurs. Some people respond warmly to a firm touch and others to a light or casual touch. Useful information may be obtained through a handshake. Does the individual grasp firmly or hesitate? Does he or she relinquish quickly or hold on? Are the fingers intertwined or held together? Is the hand limp, passive, or responsive, or is it tremulous, sweaty, or cold?

Fear of Touching

Often a nurse will touch in a condescending way (a pat on the head or a tweak of the toe) or in a circumscribed nursing treatment. Of all health care professionals, nurses have the most frequent opportunities to provide gentle, reassuring, renewing touch. The intimacy of the nurse-patient contacts may influence a nurse to be overly circumspect. However, the use of touch involves risk and may be misinterpreted by the nurse or patient. Stirring sexual feelings, if that is a response to gentle touching, is a human response and need not frighten.

Nurses sometimes respond negatively to a breach in the "status" of touch. A status system of touch exists that is significant to health care. A person of higher status may touch an individual of an inferior status, but the reverse is discouraged. Similarly, name familiarity may be used by an individual in a superior position but is greatly resented if the lower-ranking person presumes the same liberty. Because this notion is embedded in many hierarchical structures, treating everyone with respect regarding their name and propensity for touch is prudent. Instant familiarity is seldom useful. It should not be surprising when a patient reciprocates with the same level of intimacy as the nurse initiates. Therapeutic, caring touch by the

nurse is a potent healing intervention. It is important that touching be done with respect regarding the person's comfort and with the nurse's intention of providing a comforting and healing modality within the nurse-patient relationship.

Touch Zones

Hall (1969) identifies different categories of touching—expanding or contracting zones around which every individual extends the sensory experience of touching, smelling, hearing, and seeing. The categories of touching include the intimate, vulnerable, consent, and social zone (Figure 21-1). Entering the zone of intimacy, which is identified as being in an area within an arm's length of the individual's body and is the space used for comforting, protecting, and lovemaking, is part of the nurse's function. The vulnerable zone is highly sexually charged and will be protected. The most intimate area, the genitalia, is the most personally protected area of the body and causes the most stress and anxiety when approached, touched, or viewed by the caregiver. The consent zone requires the nurse to seek out or ask permission to touch or initiate procedures to these areas. The social zone includes the areas of the body that are the least sensitive or embarrassing to be touched and that do not necessarily require permission to be handled.

Illness, confinement, and dependency seen in institutionalization are stresses on the intimate zone of touch. Just as caregivers enter a room without knocking, so they often intrude into the intimate circle of touch without asking. A person's need for privacy and personal space is strongly related to acceptance and response to touch. If the need for privacy and distance is great, touch should be used judiciously. The parameters of the intimate zone of touch are examined in this chapter to emphasize the importance of understanding behavior that might occur when the nurse enters this arena.

Touch Deprivation

Montagu (1986) noted that "tactile hunger" becomes more powerful in old age when other sensuous experiences are diminished and direct sexual expression is often no longer possible or available. Furthermore, Montagu believes the cause of illness

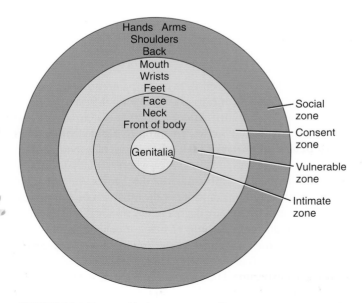

FIGURE 21-1 Zones of intimacy or sexuality.

may be greatly influenced by the quality of tactile support received. Do older people suffer touch deprivation? Many elders do if they are separated from caring others. Older men, in particular, may find it hard to reach out to others for comforting and caring touch. The previous lifestyles of these men often discouraged touch, except in the intimacy of sexual contact, which may no longer be available to them (Montagu, 1986). Older women are allowed considerably more freedom to touch, although they may lack the opportunity. Studies have shown that older women have reduced access to nonsexual intimacy, such as greeting someone with a hug or kiss or playing or cuddling with a grandchild (Waite et al., 2009). Since older women are more often widowed, reduced access to these other forms of nonsexual intimacy can further deprive them of warm and loving contact.

In the cases of the isolated or institutionalized older person, higher death rates are more related to the quality of human relationships than they are to the degree of cleanliness, nutrition, and physical disabilities on which we focus. Sansone and Schmitt (2000) noted that older people in nursing homes experience touch every day as they are bathed, dressed, toileted, fed, and positioned. The type of touch they desire is not task-oriented touch but "gentle, patient, conscious touch of another person that says to them, 'I'm here, I care, you are important to me.' It's the kind of touch that goes beyond routine and bonds one human being with another" (p. 304).

Adaptation to Touch Deprivation

People can survive extreme sensory deprivation as long as the sensory experiences of the skin are maintained. An outstanding feature of touch according to Ackerman (1995) is that it does not have to be performed by a person or other living thing. Some sustenance or peace for the old may be gained from the self-contained stimulation of a rocking chair or slowly stroking an animal's fur or wearing something that provides sensory stimulation.

Music, perceived through the skin as well as the ears, may be another source of touch stimulation that is self-induced. Skin touched by the vibrations of music is enveloped and caressed. Music and dancing seem to be two important mechanisms of enjoyment of older people (Chapter 24). In later years, older adults often return to dancing after decades of ignoring the pleasurable activity. Perhaps this desire is a response to the need for more touch.

Therapeutic Touch

Touch is a powerful healer and a therapeutic tool that nurses can use to satisfy "touch hunger" of older people. Nursing has recognized the importance of touch and has the social sanctions to touch the body in the intimate and personal care of a person, an opportunity too often not fully used for the betterment of the older person's adaptation to environment and location in time and space. Touch can serve as a means of providing sensory stimulation, reducing anxiety, relieving physical and psychological pain, and comforting the dying, as well as sexual expression.

Kreiger's experiments with therapeutic touch (1975) demonstrate physiological and psychological improvement in patients who are exposed to consistent "doses" of touch.

BOX 21-1 RESEARCH HIGHLIGHTS

Effects of Slow-Stroke Back Massage and Hand Massage on Relaxation in Older People

Massage is a traditional nursing intervention and a part of early nursing history. Yet, few studies have examined the benefits of massage for older people. The authors conducted a review of the psychological and physiological effects of slow-stroke back massage and hand massage with older people. Twenty-one studies were reviewed, and the most common protocols were 3-minute slow-stroke back massage and 10-minute hand massage. Overall, statistically significant improvements in physiological and psychological indicators provide support for the use of slow-stroke back massage and hand massage with older people in clinical practice across settings. Outcomes of these forms of massage included reduction of anxiety, increased relaxation, and reduction in verbal aggression and aggressive behaviors in individuals with dementia.

Nurses can be educated in the knowledge and skill to administer these techniques into practice and educate caregivers on their use. Slow-stroke back massage and hand massage for relaxation may be an effective alternative to pharmacological therapy in reducing stress and improving quality of life for older people.

From Harris M, Richards K: *Journal of Clinical Nursing* 19:917, 2010.

"Hands-on healing and energy based interventions have been found in cultures throughout history, dating back at least 5000 years" (Wang and Hermann, 2006, p. 34). "Laying on of the hands" and the power of touch to heal had largely disappeared with the scientific revolution. The phenomenon has reemerged as healing touch and therapeutic touch movements. A growing body of research supports the healing power of touch, and Energy Field, Disturbed is an approved nursing diagnosis (Wang and Hermann, 2006, p. 34). Many nurses have learned how to perform therapeutic and healing touch and use these modalities in their practice with people of all ages. Positive outcomes of interventions utilizing touch in nursing homes, particularly with people with dementia and agitated behaviors, have been reported (Box 21-1). Further research on the use of touch with older people is needed. Touch is a powerful tool to promote comfort and well-being when working with elders.

INTIMACY

Although intimacy is often thought of in the context of sexual performance, it encompasses more than sexuality and includes five major relational components: commitment, affective intimacy, cognitive intimacy, physical intimacy, and interdependence (Youngkin, 2004). "Intimacy is from a Greek work meaning 'closest to; inner lining of blood vessels'" (Steinke, 2005, p. 40). It is a warm, meaningful feeling of joy. Intimacy includes the need for close friendships; relationships with family, friends, and formal caregivers; spiritual connections; knowing that one matters in someone else's life; and the ability to form satisfying social relationships with others (Steinke, 2005).

Youngkin (2004) points out that older people may be concerned about changes in sexual intimacy but "social relationships with people important in their lives, the ability to interact intellectually with people who share similar interests, the supportive love that grows between human beings (whether romantic or platonic), and physical nonsexual intimacy are equally—and in many instances more—important than the physical intimacy of direct sexual relations. All of these facets of intimate life are integrally woven into the fabric of aging, along with other influences that can make life rewarding" (p. 46). Intimacy needs change over time, but the need for intimacy and satisfying social relationships remains an important component of healthy aging.

SEXUALITY

Sexuality is defined as a central aspect of being human and encompasses sex, gender identities and roles, sexual orientation, eroticism, pleasure, intimacy, and reproduction (World Health Organization, 2004). As a major aspect of intimacy, sexuality includes the physical act of intercourse, as well as many other types of intimate activity. It includes components such as sexual desire, activity, attitudes, body image, and gender-role activity (Zeiss and Kasl-Godley, 2001). Sexuality provides the opportunity to express passion, affection, admiration, and loyalty. It can also enhance personal growth and communication. Sexuality also allows a general affirmation of life (especially joy) and a continuing opportunity to search for new growth and experience.

Sexuality, similar to food and water, is a basic human need, yet it goes beyond the biological realm to include psychological, social, and moral dimensions (Waite et al., 2009) (Figure 21-2). The constant interaction among these spheres of sexuality work to produce harmony. The linkage of the four dimensions composes the holistic quality of an individual's sexuality.

The social sphere of sexuality is the sum of cultural factors that influence the individual's thoughts and actions related to interpersonal relationships, as well as sexuality related to ideas and learned behavior. Television, radio, literature, and the more traditional sources of family, school, and religious teachings combine to influence social sexuality. The belief of that which constitutes masculine and feminine is deeply rooted in the individual's exposure to cultural factors (Chapter 5).

The psychological domain of sexuality reflects a person's attitudes, feelings toward self and others, and learning from experiences. Beginning with birth, the individual is bombarded with cues and signals of how a person should act and think about the use of "dirty words" or body parts. Conversation is self-censored in the presence of or in discussion with certain people. The moral aspect of sexuality, the "I should" or "I shouldn't," makes a difference that is based in religious beliefs or in a pragmatic or humanistic outlook.

The final dimension, biological sexuality, is reflected in physiological responses to sexual stimulation, reproduction, puberty, and growth and development. Because of the interrelatedness, these dimensions affect each other directly or indirectly whenever an aspect of sexuality is out of harmony.

Sexuality is a vital aspect to consider in the care of the older person regardless of the setting. Sexuality exists throughout life in one form or another in everyone. All older people have a need to express sexual feelings, whether the individuals are healthy and active or frail. Sexuality is linked with the person's personality and identity and has a significant role in promoting better life adaptation.

Acceptance and Companionship

Sexuality validates the lifelong need to share intimacy and have that offering appreciated. Sexuality is love, warmth, sharing, and touching between people, not just the physical act of coitus. Margot Benary-Isbert, in her book *The Vintage Years* (1968), expresses the essence of sexuality most eloquently (p. 200):

> Let us not forget old married couples who once shared healthy and happy days as they now share the unavoidable limitations of old age and grow even closer together in love and patience. When they exchange a smile, a glance, one can guess that they still think each other beautiful and loveable.

Femininity and Masculinity

Males and females possess characteristic behavioral traits, which Jung refers to as the anima (female) and animus (male). Past social pressures did not often allow the appearance of sensitivity, gentleness, and sentimentality in most men. Men were

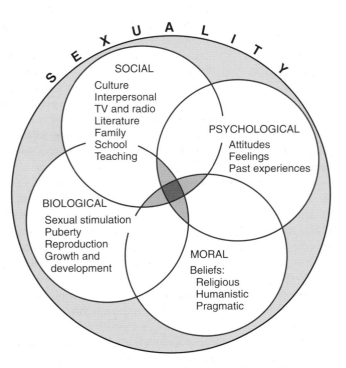

FIGURE 21-2   Interrelationship of dimensions of sexuality.

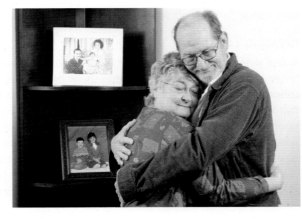

Love and affection are important to older persons. (From Sorrentino SA, Gorek B: *Mosby's textbook for long-term care assistants*, ed 5, St Louis, 2007, Mosby.)

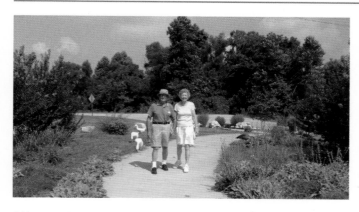

Older couples enjoy love and companionship. (From Monahan FD, Sands JK, Neighbors M, et al: *Phipps' medical-surgical nursing: health and illness perspectives,* ed 8, St Louis, 2007, Mosby.)

expected to be strong, to be in control of situations, and to handle their emotions. On the other hand, women were not viewed as aggressive or the major decision makers.

Often seen and perpetuated among older adults are socially accepted standards characteristic of masculine and feminine behavior, which reflect male and female role models dominant in their formative years. Jung's work has shown this view to be so, indicating that strong attitude types (male and female) and roles and functions associated with these attitudes are developed as adaptations of the person to the demands of the environment.

Man believed that repressing his feminine traits was virtuous; and woman, until recently, repressed her animus. Both men and women, however, are not consciously aware that they possess the opposite sexual identity. Goldblatt (1972) contends that neither gonads nor chromosomal sex is a determinant of sexual behavior. Money and Tucker (1975), in their work *Sexual Signatures,* believe that social stimulation provides gender identity and limits the individual's concept of self. In essence, society expects men to be men and women to be women.

In the latter part of life, self-knowledge deepens. People tend to discover traits in their nature that were previously suppressed or heretofore remained in the unconscious. At this time, the emergence of the anima (in men) and animus (in women) may be seen. Jung identified this experience as the expression of the psyche that in the first half of life was turned inward. In late life, directed outward, this expression becomes indicative of the capacity for fuller living. Men become more comfortable with tenderness, "more dependent on the marriage for their sense of well-being, and more willing to accommodate for the sake of preserving peace" (Huyck, 2001, p. 11). Women become more assertive and self-confident. The person's ability to accord his or her other nature its due recognition will enhance sexuality.

SEXUAL HEALTH

The World Health Organization defines sexual health as a state of physical, emotional, mental, and social well-being related to sexuality (2004). Sexual health is a realistic phenomenon that includes four components: personal and social behaviors in agreement with individual gender identity; comfort with a range of sexual role behaviors and engagement in effective interpersonal relations with both sexes in a loving relationship or long-term commitment; response to erotic stimulation that produces positive and pleasurable sexual activity; and the ability to make mature judgments about sexual behavior congruent with one's beliefs and values. "Sexual health, as with physical health, is not simply the absence of sexual dysfunction or disease, but, rather a state of sexual well-being that includes a positive approach to a sexual relationship and anticipation of a pleasurable experience without fear, shame, or coercion" (Rheaume and Mitty, 2008, p. 342).

These interpretations speak of the multifaceted nature of the biological, psychosocial, cultural, and spiritual components of sexuality and imply that sexual behavior is the capacity to enhance self and others. Sexual health is individually defined and wholesome if it leads to intimacy (not necessarily coitus) and enriches the involved parties.

Factors Influencing Sexual Health
Expectations

A large number of cultural, biological, psychosocial, and environmental factors influence the sexual behavior of older adults. The older person may be confronted with barriers to the expression of his or her sexuality by reflected attitudes, health, culture, economics, opportunity, and historic trends. Factors affecting a person's attitudes on intimacy and sexuality include family dynamics and upbringing and cultural and religious beliefs (Chapter 5). Older people often internalize the broad cultural proscriptions of sexual behavior in late life that hinder the continuance of sexual expression. Much sexual behavior stems from incorporating other people's reactions. Older people do not feel old until they are faced with the fact that others around them consider them old. Similarly, older adults do not feel asexual until they are continually treated as such.

American society continues to struggle with open acceptance of sexual expression for the young but continues to remain hostile to the attempts of older people to do the same. Sexual interest and activity in older adults are sometimes regarded as deviant behavior and described in such terms as "dirty old man," "lecher," and "old biddy." The same activity attempted by a younger person would be viewed as appropriate. An often quoted statement by Alex Comfort (1974) sums it up nicely: "In our experiences, old folks stop having sex for the same reasons they stop riding a bicycle—general infirmity, thinking it looks ridiculous, no bicycle." Box 21-2 presents some of the myths about sexuality in older people that may be held by older people themselves and by society in general.

Redefinitions

Sexuality in the older person shifts its focus from procreation to an emphasis on companionship, physical nearness, intimate communication, and a pleasure-seeking physical relationship. Some researchers have coined the phrase "from procreation to recreation," which refers to this change in sexual emphasis.

Activity Levels

For both heterosexual and homosexual individuals, research supports that liberal and positive attitudes toward sexuality, greater sexual knowledge, satisfaction with a long-term

BOX 21-2 SEXUALITY AND AGING WOMEN: COMMON MYTHS

- Masturbation is an immature activity of youngsters and adolescents, not older women.
- Sexual prowess and desire wane during the climacteric, and menopause is the death of a woman's sexuality.
- Hysterectomy creates a physical disability that results in the inability to function sexually.
- Sex has no role in the lives of the elderly, except as perversion or remembrance of times past.
- Sexual expression in old age is taboo.
- The elderly are too old and frail to engage in sex.
- The young are considered lusty and virile; the elderly are considered lecherous.
- Sex is unimportant or over in the lives of the elderly.
- Elderly women do not wish to discuss their sexuality with professionals.

relationship or a current intimate relationship, good social networks, psychological well-being, and a sense of self-worth are associated with greater sexual interest, activity, and satisfaction. Both early studies of sexual behavior in older adults, and more recent ones, indicate that men and women remain sexually active and find their sexual lives satisfying. Determinants of sexual activity and functioning include the interaction of each partner's sexual capacity, motivation, conduct, and attitudes, as well as the quality of the dyadic relationship (Waite et al., 2009). Patterns of sexual activity in earlier years are the major predictor of sexual activity in later life, and individuals with higher levels of sexual activity in middle age show less decline with advanced age (Kennedy et al., 2010).

The National Social Life, Health, and Aging Project (NSHAP) is a national probability survey of 3005 men and women between ages 57 and 85 that is focused on intimate social relationships, including marriage, social ties, and sexuality. The central hypothesis of the study is that individuals with high-quality intimate social and sexual relationships will age better in terms of health and well-being than those with poor-quality relationships or those who lack social relationships (Lindau et al., 2007; Lindau and Gavrilova, 2010; Suzman, 2009). Findings from this survey revealed that about three quarters of individuals ages 57 to 85 are married or living with a partner and three quarters of those are sexually active. The prevalence of sexual activity declined with age: 73% of people between ages 57 and 64 reported being sexually active; 53% of those between ages 65 and 74; and 26% of those between ages 75 and 85.

Sexual activity was closely tied to overall health, and people whose health was rated as excellent or very good were nearly twice as likely to be sexually active as those who rated their health as poorer. The most common reason for sexual inactivity among those with a partner was the male partner's health. Men are more sexually active than women, most likely because women live longer and may not have a partner. Women, especially those not in a relationship, were more likely than men to report lack of interest in sex (Lindau et al., 2007; Lindau and Gavrilova, 2010).

Cohort and Cultural Influences

The era in which a person was born influences attitudes about sexuality. Women in their 80s today may have been strongly influenced by the prudish, Victorian atmosphere of their youth and may have experienced difficult marital adjustments and serious sexual problems early in their marriages. Sexuality was not openly expressed or discussed, and this was a time when "pleasurable sex was for men only; women engaged in sexual activity to satisfy their husbands and to make babies" (Rheaume and Mitty, 2008, p. 344). These kinds of experiences shape beliefs and knowledge about sexual expression as well as comfort with sexuality, particularly for older women. It is important to come to know and understand the older person within his or her social and cultural background and not make judgments based on one's own belief system.

The next generation of older people ("baby boomers") has experienced other influences, including more liberal attitudes toward sexuality, the women's movement, a higher number of divorced adults, the human immunodeficiency virus (HIV) epidemic, and increased numbers of gay and lesbian couples, that will affect their views and attitudes as they age. The baby boomers and beyond, as they find themselves experiencing sexuality beyond the age they had assigned to their elders, may alter current perceptions.

Most of what is known about sexuality in aging has been gained through research with well-educated, healthy, white older adults. Further research is needed among culturally, socially, and ethnically diverse older people; those with chronic illness; and gay, lesbian, and bisexual older people. Suzman (2009) suggests the importance of early life experiences in understanding aging and sexual patterns, an area missing when studies focus on experiences after age 65 only.

Biological Changes with Age

Acknowledgement and understanding of the age changes that influence sexual physiology, anatomy, and the stages of sexual response may partially explain alteration in sexual behavior to accommodate these changes and facilitate continued pleasurable sex. Characteristic physiological changes during the sexual response cycle do occur with aging, but these vary from individual to individual depending on general health factors. The changes occur abruptly in women starting with menopause but more gradually in men, a phenomenon called *andropause* (Kennedy et al., 2010). The "use it or lose it" phenomenon also applies here: the more sexually active the person is, the fewer changes he or she is likely to experience in the pattern of sexual response. Changes in the appearance of the body (wrinkles, sagging skin) may also affect the older person's security about his or her sexual attractiveness (Arena and Wallace, 2008). Table 21-1 summarizes physical changes in the sexual response cycle.

Older people who do not understand the physical changes that affect sexual activity become concerned that their sex life is approaching its natural conclusion with the onset of menopause or, for men, when they discover a change in the firmness of their erection or the decreased need for ejaculation with each orgasm or when the refractory period is extended between episodes of intercourse. A major nursing role is to provide information about these changes, as well as appropriate assessment and counseling within the context of the individual's needs.

TABLE 21-1	PHYSICAL CHANGES IN SEXUAL RESPONSES IN OLD AGE
FEMALE	**MALE**
Excitation Phase	
Diminished or delayed lubrication (one to three minutes may be required for adequate amounts to appear)	Less intense and slower erection (but can be maintained longer without ejaculation)
Diminished flattening and separation of labia majora	Increased difficulty regaining an erection if lost
Disappearance of elevation of labia majora	Less vasocongestion of scrotal sac
Decreased vasocongestion of labia minora	Less pronounced elevation and congestion of testicles
Decreased elastic expansion of vagina (depth and breadth)	
Breasts not as engorged	
Sex flush absent	
Plateau Phase	
Slower and less prominent uterine elevation or tenting	Decreased muscle tension
Nipple erection and sexual flush less often	No color change at coronal edge of penis
Decreased capacity for vasocongestion	Slower penile erection pattern
Decreased areolar engorgement	Delayed or diminished erectal and testicular elevation
Labial color change less evident	
Less intense swelling or orgasmic platform	
Less sexual flush	
Decreased secretions of Bartholin glands	
Orgasmic Phase	
Fewer number and less intense orgasmic contractions	Decreased or absent secretory activity (lubrication) by Cowper gland before ejaculation
Rectal sphincter contraction with severe tension only	Fewer penile contractions
	Fewer rectal sphincter contractions
	Decreased force of ejaculation (approximately 50%) with decreased amount of semen (if ejaculation is long, seepage of semen occurs)
Resolution Phase	
Observably slower loss of nipple erection	Vasocongestion of nipples and scrotum slowly subsides
Vasocongestion of clitoris and orgasmic platform	Very rapid loss of erection and descent of testicles shortly after ejaculation
	Refractory time extended (time required before another erection ranges from several to 24 hours, occasionally longer)

Adapted from Kennedy G, Martinez M, Garo N: *Primary Psychiatry* 17:21, 2010.

SEXUAL DYSFUNCTION

Sexual dysfunction is defined as impairment in normal sexual functioning and can have many causes, both physical and psychological. Sexual disorders in older people have not been well studied, but generally, the following four categories are described: hypoactive sexual desire disorder; sexual arousal disorder; orgasmic disorder; and sexual pain disorders (Arena and Wallace, 2008).

Male Dysfunction

Erectile dysfunction (ED) is the most prevalent sexual problem in men. In the NSHAP study, ED was reported by 31% of men ages 57 to 65 and by about 44% of those over age 65 (Waite et al., 2009). ED is defined as the inability to achieve and sustain an erection sufficient for satisfactory sexual intercourse in at least 50% or more attempts. When discussing ED with older men, it is important to provide education about normal age-related changes as well. Older men require more physical penile stimulation and a longer time to achieve erection, and the duration of orgasm may be shorter and less intense (Rheaume and Mitty, 2008).

An erection is governed by the interaction among the hormonal, vascular, and nervous systems. A problem in any of these systems can cause ED. Of course, multiple causes exist for this problem in older men. Nearly one third of ED is a complication of diabetes. Alcoholism, medications, depression, and prostate cancer and treatment are also causes of ED in older men. The new nerve-sparing microsurgical techniques used for prostatectomies often spare erectile function. Anxiety and relationship issues are additional causes of ED, and, as Rheaume and Mitty (2008) note, some men may have widower's syndrome (difficulty achieving erection because they harbor guilt about pursuing a sexual relationship after the death of their spouse). Testosterone levels have little to do with ED but can have a major effect on libido (sexual desire).

The use of phosphodiesterase inhibitors (PE5s) such as sildenafil (Viagra), vardenafil (Levitra), and tadalafil (Cialis) has revolutionized treatment for ED regardless of cause. Some have commented that this can be called "the Viagratization of the older population." Contraindications to the use of these medications include nitrate therapy, heart failure with low blood pressure, certain antihypertensive regimens, and other medications and cardiovascular conditions. See Chapter 9 for further discussion of contraindications and side effects.

Before the availability of these medications, intracavernosal injections with the drugs papaverine and phentolamine, vasoactive agents that reduce resistance of arteriolar and cavernosal smooth muscle tissue of the penis, were used. Penile implants of the semirigid, adjustable-malleable, or hinged and inflatable types are available when impotence does not respond to other treatments or is irreversible. The hinged and inflatable types, which are inserted in the testicular area, are the most popular. Another alternative is the vacuum pump device, which works by creating a vacuum that draws blood into the penis, causing an erection. Vacuum pumps are available in manual and battery-operated versions and may be covered by Medicare if deemed medically necessary (Rheaume and Mitty, 2008).

Female Dysfunction

Female dysfunction is considered "persistent impediment to a person's normal pattern of sexual interest, response, or both" (Kaiser, 2000, p. 1174). Female sexual function can be influenced by factors such as culture, ethnicity, emotional state, age, and previous sexual experiences, as well as age-related changes in sexual response. For heterosexual women, frequency of intercourse depends more on the age, health, and sexual function of the partner or the availability of a partner rather than on their own sexual capacity. Postmenopausal changes in the urinary or genital tract as a result of lower estrogen levels can make sexual activity less pleasurable (Rheaume and Mitty, 2008). Dyspareunia, resulting from vaginal dryness and thinning of the vaginal tissue, occurs in one third of women older than age 65. In many instances, using water-soluble lubricants such as K-Y, Astroglide, Slip, and HR lubricating jelly during foreplay or intercourse can resolve the difficulty. Topical low-dose estrogen creams, rings, or pills that are introduced into the vagina may also help to plump tissues and restore lubrication, with less absorption than oral hormones (Kennedy et al., 2010; Rheaume and Mitty, 2008).

Women can experience arousal disorders resulting from drugs such as anticholinergics, antidepressants, and chemotherapeutic agents and from lack of lubrication from radiation, surgery, and stress. Orgasmic disorders also may result from drugs used to treat depression. Unlike ED, studies of vascular insufficiency are less clear in women with sexual dysfunction. Prolapse of the uterus, rectoceles, and cystoceles can be surgically repaired to facilitate continued sexual activity. Urinary incontinence (UI) is another condition that may affect sexual activity for both men and women. Appropriate assessment and treatment are important because many causes of UI are treatable (see Chapter 11 for a discussion of UI).

ALTERNATIVE SEXUAL LIFESTYLES: LESBIAN, GAY, BISEXUAL, AND TRANSGENDER

It is difficult to estimate the number of LGBT individuals over age 65, and underidentification and undercounting occurs as a result of stigma in identifying oneself in this group (Services and Advocacy for Gay, Lesbian, Bisexual, and Transgender Elders [SAGE] and Movement Advancement Project [MAP], 2010). However, The National Gay and Lesbian Task Force's Aging Initiative estimates that about 3 million Americans over age 65 are lesbian, gay, bisexual, or transgender (LGBT), and this figure is likely to double by 2030 (Gelo, 2008). Lesbians will likely be overrepresented in these numbers, reflecting both general population trends and the decimation wrought by HIV/AIDS, which disproportionately affected gay men (SAGE and MAP, 2010). Gay and lesbian older people face the "double stigma" of being both old and homosexual, with lesbians facing the triple threat of being women, elderly, and having a different sexual orientation (Agronin, 2004).

Whereas discrimination in health and social systems affects gays and lesbians of all ages, gay and lesbian elders may be even more at risk for discrimination as a result of lifelong experiences with marginalization and oppression. LGBT older adults are much less likely than their heterosexual peers to access needed health and social services or identify themselves as gay or lesbian to health care providers (SAGE and MAP, 2010). Gay and bisexual men may have more chronic conditions, suffer greater psychological distress and even the more affluent and educated may be uninsured (Wallace et al., 2011).

Recently published reports (American Society on Aging and MetLife, 2010; Institute of Medicine, 2011; SAGE and MAP, 2010) have added to the body of knowledge about aging LGBT individuals. However, there is still a lack of knowledge as well as research. Reasons for this include difficulties in studying the LGBT population because of differences in self-identification, societal attitudes, and a lack of support for research with this population (Blando, 2001). Research has been conducted primarily with middle class white gay men and lesbians in urban areas. Even less is known about bisexual and transgender older people.

The Institute of Medicine Report (2011), The Health of Lesbian, Gay, Bisexual and Transgender People: Building a Foundation for Better Understanding, recommends that the National Institutes of Health (NIH) encourage research to include sexual and gender minorities explicitly in their samples using the NIH policy on the inclusion of women and racial and ethnic minorities in clinical research as a model. The United States Department of Health and Human Services (HHS) has announced recommendations to address lesbian, gay, bisexual, and transgender health care issues including a commitment to collecting LGBT health data through federally funded surveys, guidance to states regarding access to federal welfare programs for LGBT families and protection of same-sex partner's assets when his or her family uses Medicaid for long-term care, and expanded outreach regarding the range of HHS funding opportunities for organizations that serve the LGBT community (U.S. Department of Health and Human Services, 2011). In 2010, HHS funded the nation's first national technical assistance resource center to support public and private organizations serving the unique needs of LGBT older adults.

Older LGBT individuals are as diverse as the remainder of the heterosexual elder population. Many age successfully, are healthy, and are active with satisfied lives. Some are coupled, have children, and are open about their sexual orientation, and some are not. Some of these individuals have only recently "come out"; others have been "out" most of their lives; and some find themselves isolated in the larger society. Older gay and lesbian individuals are more likely to have kept their relationships hidden than those who grew up in the modern day gay liberation movement. Transgender and bisexual individuals are less likely to "be out" (American Society on Aging and MetLife, 2010).

Because lesbian and gay individuals are denied legal marriage except in a handful of states that acted only very recently on the issues, most LG adults over age 60 are single. Gay and bisexual men over age 50 are twice as likely to live alone as heterosexual men of the same age, while older lesbian and bisexual women are about one third more likely to live alone.

Approximately one third of the lesbians "come out" after age 50. Many lesbians married, raised children, divorced, and lead double lives (Butler and Lewis, 2002). In the case of transgender people, medical providers for many years required candidates for sex reassignment surgery to divorce their spouses, move to a new place, and construct a false personal history consistent with their new gender expression. These practices resulted in transgender people losing even more of their social and personal support systems than might otherwise have been the case (SAGE and MAP, 2010).

Health care providers may assume that their LGBT patients are heterosexual and neglect to obtain a sexual history, discuss sexuality, or be aware of their particular medical needs. Providers receive little education and training in the needs of this population and may lack sensitivity when caring for older LGBT individuals (Gelo, 2008). Sensitivity is of utmost importance when attempting to obtain a health history. Using open-ended questions such as "Who is most important to you?" or "Do you have a significant other?" is much better than asking "Are you married?" This form of the question allows the nurse to look beyond the rigid category of family. Euphemisms are frequently used for a life partner (e.g., roommate, close friend). Asking individuals if they consider themselves as primarily heterosexual, homosexual, or bisexual is also better. This question conveys recognition of sexual variety. An older lesbian woman in a health care situation may refer to herself indirectly by saying "people like us." Nurses need to become more aware of these nuances and try to understand the fear of discovery that is apparent in the older gay man and lesbian woman. These elders are of a generation in which they were, and may still be, closeted because of the homophobic experiences they had throughout their younger years.

Better support and care services for LGBT individuals by care providers should include working through homophobic attitudes and discomfort discussing sexuality, learning about special issues facing older gay men and lesbians, and becoming aware of the gay and lesbian resources in the community. LGBT elders living in metropolitan areas may find organizations particularly designed for them, such as Senior Action in a Gay Environment (SAGE); New Leaf Outreach to Elders (formerly GLOE, San Francisco); and the Lesbian and Gay Aging Issues Network (LGAIN). Additional resources can be found on the Evolve website.

Finally, facilities or agencies already in the community need to be assessed from the perspective of the client, patient, or resident who may be gay, lesbian, bisexual, or transgender. Ninety-six percent of America's social service and caregiving agencies for older adults offer no services specifically designed for LGBT older adults, and 46% of them indicated that LGBT older people would be unwelcome at senior centers if their sexual orientation were known (Gelo, 2008). Medicare has finalized new rules to require equal visitation rights for all hospital patients, including a visitor who is a same-sex domestic partner. Programs to increase awareness of the needs of LGBT elders and reduce discrimination are necessary especially in light of the anticipated increase in older LGBT individuals.

Chapter 22 also provides further discussion of relationship and family issues of elder LGBT individuals.

INTIMACY AND CHRONIC ILLNESS

Chronic illnesses and their related treatments may bring many challenges to intimacy and sexual activity. Steinke (2005), in an excellent article discussing intimacy needs and chronic illness, suggests that although some research has been done on the effects of myocardial infarction on sexual function, less information is available for patients with heart failure, implantable cardioverter-defibrillators (ICDs), hypertension, arthritis, chronic pain, or chronic obstructive pulmonary disease (COPD).

Often, patients and their partners are given little or no information about the effect of illnesses on sexual activity or strategies to continue sexual activity within functional limitations. Timing of intercourse (mornings or when energy level is highest), oral or anal sex, masturbation, appropriate pain relief, and different sexual positions are all strategies that may assist in continued sexual activity. If pain due to arthritis is a concern, taking pain medications or a warm bath prior to lovemaking may be helpful. "Side-by-side, back-to-belly (spoon) or the cross-wise sex position with one partner supine and the other on his or her side require less flexion of hip and knee and these positions may reduce the pressure of body weight associated with the missionary position" (Kennedy et al., 2010, p. 26). Table 21-2 presents other suggestions for individuals with chronic illness.

For individuals with cardiac conditions, manual stimulation (masturbation) may be an alternative that can be used early in the recovery period to maintain sexual function if the practice is not objectionable to the patient. Studies show that masturbation is less taxing on the heart and makes less oxygen demand. Although self-stimulation is steeped in myth and fear, masturbation is a common and healthy practice in late life. Individuals without partners or those whose spouses are ill or incapacitated find that masturbation is helpful. As children, today's older population was discouraged from practicing this pleasurable activity with stories of the evils of fondling a person's own genitals. In the NSHAP study, more than 50% of male participants and 25% of female participants acknowledged masturbating, regardless of whether or not they had a sexual partner (Lindau et al., 2007). Masturbation provides an avenue for resolution of sexual tensions, keeps sexual desire alive, maintains lubrication and muscle tone of the vagina, provides mild physical exercise, and preserves sexual function in individuals who have no other outlet for sexual activity and gratification of their sexual need.

One couple, who had long sustained a satisfactory sexual relationship, was unable to imagine engaging in the alternative modes of sexual expression (cunnilingus, mutual masturbation, and repositioning) suggested when the wife developed severe osteoarthritis. The old gentleman brought the worn and dog-eared illustrative pamphlet back to the nurse in the health clinic. "She just won't go for it, nurse!" In such cases, the most well-meant advice may not be useful. To resolve such incompatible needs, the nurse may best counsel the most sexually active and liberal partner in ways to achieve orgasm while still remaining sexually comforting for the other partner.

Tabloski (2010) provides age-appropriate illustrations of coital positions for older people with cardiovascular disease that

TABLE 21-2	CHRONIC ILLNESS AND SEXUAL FUNCTION: EFFECTS AND INTERVENTIONS	
CONDITION	**EFFECTS/PROBLEMS**	**INTERVENTIONS**
Arthritis	Pain, fatigue, limited motion Steroid therapy may decrease sexual interest or desire	Advise patient to perform sexual activity at time of day when less fatigued and most relaxed Suggest use of analgesics and other pain-relief methods before sexual activity Encourage use of relaxation techniques before sexual activity such as a warm bath or shower, application of hot packs to affected joints Advise patient to maintain optimum health through a balance of good nutrition, proper rest, and activity Suggest that he or she experiment with different positions, use pillows for comfort and support Recommend use of a vibrator if massage ability is limited Suggest use of water-soluble jelly for vaginal lubrication
Cardiovascular disease	Most men have no change in physical effects on sexual function; one fourth may not return to pre–heart attack function; one fourth may not resume sexual activity Women do not experience sexual dysfunction after heart attack Fear of another heart attack or death during sex Shortness of breath	Encourage counseling on realistic restrictions that may be necessary Instruct patient and spouse on alternative positions to avoid strain Suggest that patient avoid large meals several hours before sex Advise patient to relax; plan medications for effectiveness during sex
Cerebrovascular accident (stroke)	Depression May or may not have sexual activity changes Often erectile disorders occur; decrease in frequency of intercourse and sexual relations Change in role and function of partners Decreased physical endurance, fatigue Mobility and sensory deficits Perceptual and visual deficits Communication deficit Cognitive and behavioral deficits Fear of relapse or sudden death	Encourage counseling Instruct patient to use alternative positions Suggest use of a vibrator if massage ability is limited Suggest use of pillows for positioning and support Suggest use of water-soluble jelly for lubrication Instruct patient to use alternative forms of sexual expression
Chronic obstructive pulmonary disease (COPD)	No direct impairment of sexual activity although affected by coughing, exertional dyspnea, positions, and activity intolerance Medications may lead to erectile difficulties	Encourage patient to plan sexual activity when energy is highest Instruct patient to use alternative positions Advise patient to plan sexual activity at time medications are most effective Suggest use of oxygen before, during, or after sex, depending on when it provides the most benefit
Diabetes	Sexual desire and interest unaffected Neuropathy and/or vascular damage may interfere with erectile ability; about 50% to 75% of men have erectile disorders; a small portion have retrograde ejaculation Some men regain function if diagnosis of diabetes is well accepted, if diabetes is well controlled, or both Women have less sexual desire and vaginal lubrication Decrease in orgasms/absence of orgasm can occur; less frequent sexual activity; local genital infections	Recommend possible candidates for penile prosthesis Instruct patient to use alternative forms of sexual expression Recommend immediate treatment of genital infections
Cancers Breast	No direct physical affect; there is a strong psychological effect: loss of sexual desire, body-image change, depression/reaction of partner	Encourage individual or group counseling
Most other cancers	Men and women may lose sexual desire temporarily Men may have erectile dysfunction; dry ejaculation; retrograde ejaculation Women may have vaginal dryness, dyspareunia Both men and women may experience anxiety, depression, pain, nausea from chemotherapy, radiation, hormone therapy, and nerve damage from pelvic surgery	

can be used in teaching. Steinke (2005) also provides specific suggestions and teaching plans that will be very useful for nurses working with older people for sexual counseling after myocardial infarction and for older people with CHF, COPD, ICDs, and hypertension.

INTIMACY AND SEXUALITY IN LONG-TERM CARE FACILITIES

Research is needed on sexuality in residential care facilities and nursing homes, but surveys suggest that a significant number of older people living in these settings might choose to be sexually active if they had privacy and a sexual partner (Messinger-Rapport et al., 2003). Intimacy and sexuality among residents includes the opportunity to have not only coitus but also other forms of intimate expressions, such as hugging, kissing, hand holding, and masturbation. Wallace (2003) commented that the sexual needs of older adults in long-term care facilities should be addressed with the same priority as nutrition, hydration, and other well-accepted needs. The institutionalized older person has the same rights as non-institutionalized elders to engage in or refrain from sexual activity.

Nursing homes are required by federal regulation to allow married spouses to share a room if they desire, but no other requirements related to sexual activity in nursing homes exist. However, what about unmarried individuals in intimate relationships or gay and lesbian partners? In research with older gay and lesbian individuals and their families (Brotman et al., 2003), participants reported being terrified of going into care facilities and having to hide their relationships or lose their partners and friends. One lesbian couple, who had been living together for several decades, was separated by health care professionals and family members who were not aware of the nature of their partnership. Another partner in a lesbian relationship changed her last name to her partner's so that they would be taken for sisters and put in the same room.

Privacy is a major issue in nursing homes that can prevent fulfillment of intimacy and sexual needs. Suggestions for providing privacy and an atmosphere accepting of sexual activity include the availability of a private room, not interrupting when doors are closed and sexual activity is taking place, allowing residents to have sexually explicit materials in their rooms, and providing adaptive equipment, such as siderails or trapezes and double beds. In one facility where one of the authors (T.T.) worked, the staff would assist one of the female residents to be freshly showered, perfumed, and in a lovely nightgown when she and her partner wanted to have sexual relations.

Attitudes about intimacy and sexuality among long-term care staff and, often, family members may reflect general societal attitudes that older people do not have sexual needs or that sexual activity is inappropriate. Families may have difficulty understanding that their older relative may want to have a new relationship. Caregivers often view residents' sexual acts as problems rather than as expressions of the need for love and intimacy. Reactions may include disapproval, discomfort, and embarrassment, and caregivers may explicitly or implicitly discourage or deny intimacy needs.

Staff, family, and resident education programs to promote awareness, provide education on sexuality and intimacy in later life, involve residents in discussions of sexuality, and discuss interventions to respond to residents' needs are important in long-term care settings. Staff education should include the opportunity to discuss personal feelings about sexuality, changes associated with aging, the impact of diseases and medications on sexual function, as well as role playing and skill training in sexual assessment and intervention. Rheaume and Mitty (2008) suggest the use of the Sexual Dysfunction Trivia Game (Skinner, 2000) and the Staff Attitudes about Intimacy and Dementia (SAID) (Kamel and Hajjar, 2003) in staff education programs and policy development. Additional resources that may be helpful in education programs can be found on the Evolve website.

INTIMACY, SEXUALITY, AND DEMENTIA

Intimacy and sexuality remain important in the lives of persons with dementia and their partners throughout the illness. Intimacy and sexuality may "serve as a nonverbal form of communication and intimacy when other cognitive skills and functions have declined" (Agronin, 2004, p. 13). As dementia progresses, particularly in persons living in long-term care facilities, intimacy and sexuality issues may present challenges, especially regarding the impaired person's ability to consent to sexual activity, and require accurate assessment and documentation.

Determination of a cognitively impaired person's ability to consent to participation in a sexual activity involves concepts of voluntary participation, mental competence, and an understanding of the risks and benefits. It is important for the person to understand the potential physical risks but also the "psychological risks including risk of loss through transfer, death, or discharge of his or her partner" (Messinger-Rapport et al., 2003, p. 52).

> *"A resident with dementia might be mistaking another person for his or her spouse and begin exhibiting unwelcome intimate behavior toward that person. On the other hand, sexual expression between residents could indicate development of a new relationship, as beautifully depicted in the 2007 movie with Julie Christie, Away from Her. More recently, former Supreme Court Justice Sandra Day O'Connor poignantly described the relationship between her husband, who had Alzheimer's disease, and another resident in a residential care setting"* (www.usatoday.com/news/nation/2007-11-12-court_N.htm) *(Rheaume and Mitty, 2008, p. 348).*

The Hebrew Home for the Aged in Riverdale, New York, initiated model sexual policies in 1995 that have been used to develop a guide for long-term care facilities for intimacy, sexuality, and sexual behavior for older people with dementia. These guidelines can be found at www.fhs.mcmaster.ca/mcah/cgec/toolkit.pdf.

Inappropriate sexual behavior (exposing oneself, masturbating in public, or making inappropriate sexual advances or sexual comments) may also occur in long-term care settings. These behaviors are most distressing to staff and to other residents. Rheaume and Mitty (2008) suggest that an interdisciplinary sexual assessment to determine the underlying need that the person is expressing and how it might be addressed is important. These kinds of behavior may be triggered by unmet intimacy needs or may be symptoms of an underlying physical problem, such as a urinary tract or vaginal infection.

Encouraging family and friends to touch, hug, kiss, and hold hands when visiting may help to meet touch and intimacy needs and decrease inappropriate sexual behavior. Also, allowing the person to stroke a pet or hold a stuffed animal may be helpful. Aggressive or violent behavior may require limit setting, working with the resident and family, providing for sexual expression in a non-harmful manner, and pharmacological treatment if indicated (Messinger-Rapport et al., 2003). Staff will need opportunities for discussion and assistance with interventions.

HIV/AIDS AND OLDER ADULTS

Nearly 25% of people with HIV in the United States are over age 50. Predictions are that this figure could rise to 50% by 2015. Between 2003 and 2007, the annual estimated number of individuals age 50 and older living with AIDS increased more than 60% (Population Reference Bureau, 2009). The racial/ethnic disparities in HIV/AIDS among older people parallel trends among all age groups. Rates of HIV/AIDS among older African Americans are 12 times higher than for Caucasian older people, and the rates for Hispanic older adults are 5 times as high compared to Caucasian older adults (Emlet et al., 2009).

Women older than age 60 make up one of the fastest-growing risk groups, and the rise in cases in women of color over age 50 has been especially steep. Most got the virus from sex with infected partners (National Institute on Aging [NIA], 2009). In the last decade, AIDS cases in women over age 50 are reported to have tripled, while heterosexual transmission rates in this age group may have increased as much as 106% (HIV Wisdom for Older Women, 2010).

The incidence of HIV in older people is rising faster among the older population than it is in those 24 years of age and younger. Incidence is expected to continue to increase as more individuals become infected later in life, and those who were infected in early adulthood live longer as a result of advances in disease treatment. The compromised immune system of an older individual makes him or her even more susceptible to HIV or AIDS than a younger person. AIDS in older adults has been called the "Great Imitator" because many of the symptoms such as fatigue, weakness, weight loss, and anorexia are common to other disease conditions and may be attributed to normal aging. Older adults with HIV may also be at more risk for cognitive decline and may be misdiagnosed with Alzheimer's disease (AD) instead of AIDS. Dementia associated with AIDS is rapid in onset as opposed to the slow, progressive decline with AD. In addition, the idea that elders are not sexually active limits physicians' and other care providers' objectivity to recognize HIV-AIDS as a possible diagnosis.

Contrary to popular belief, HIV/AIDS in the older adult population is not the result of blood transfusions alone, nor is it confined to the homosexual population. Older adults are sexually active and at risk for HIV/AIDS and other sexually transmitted diseases. People older than age 50 are about one sixth as likely to use condoms during sex. Older women who are sexually active are at high risk for HIV/AIDS (and other sexually transmitted

infections) from an infected partner, resulting, in part, from normal age changes of the vaginal tissue—a thinner, drier, friable vaginal lining that makes viral entry more efficient.

Lack of awareness about HIV in older people often results in late diagnosis and treatment. Older people may have the virus for years before being tested. By the time of diagnosis, the virus may be in the late stages (NIA, 2009). Older adults are also at higher risk of HIV-medication toxicity (Vance et al., 2009). Mortality rates are higher for older adults with HIV, and survival time after diagnosis is shorter (Population Reference Bureau, 2009).

In general, elders lack adequate knowledge about HIV/AIDS and believe that it "just does not happen in my generation." This view places elders at high risk for HIV and AIDS. Further, older people may have limited access to HIV tests and age-appropriate information. Only 16% of older adults over age 65 have been tested for HIV, compared to 40% of those ages 50 to 64, 61% of those ages 30 to 49, and 54% of people ages 18 to 29 (University of Connecticut Health Center, 2010). Older adults, especially older women, have also not been included in research and drug trials on HIV/AIDS.

In 2010, Medicare began covering HIV screening for beneficiaries who are at increased risk or who request it. The CDC has also revised HIV-screening recommendations to include provisions for testing adults age 65 and older. In addition to screening for HIV, assessment and screening for other sexually transmitted infections (gonorrhea, chlamydia, syphilis, trichomonas, human papillomavirus [HPV]) should also be a part of primary care for sexually active elders. If symptoms of another disease such as herpes arise, testing should occur as well.

Educational materials and programs aimed at older adults need to be developed that include information about what HIV/AIDS is and how it is and is not transmitted, the need to use condoms for protection when engaging in sexual activity, symptoms of which to be aware, and the treatments that are available. Jane Fowler, director of the National HIV Wisdom for Older Women program (WOW), suggests that HIV/AIDS educational campaigns and programs are not targeted to older individuals and asks, "How often does a wrinkled face appear on a prevention poster?" (HIV Wisdom for Older Women, 2010). Only 15 out of 50 states have HIV publications for older adults.

Physicians, nurse practitioners, and other health professionals need to increase their knowledge of HIV in older adults and become comfortable taking a complete sexual history and talking about sex with older adults. In addition, the myth that elders do not engage in sexual activity must be put to rest. An innovative program in Broward County, Florida, the Seniors HIV Intervention Project (SHIP), educates seniors as educators and peer counselors to deliver educational workshops on HIV/AIDS in churches, condominiums, and other community sites. A group of older adults at the Michael-Ann Russell Jewish Community Center in Miami Beach, Florida, produced an animated Claymation video in which the figures openly talk about using condoms and getting checked for HIV and STDs (http://growingbolder.com/media/health/sex/a-sexy-affair-241582.html#content_tabs). Additional resources with specific information about HIV and older people that can be used in prevention and education can be found on the Evolve website.

PROMOTING HEALTHY AGING: IMPLICATIONS FOR GERONTOLOGICAL NURSING

Nurses have multiple roles in the area of sexuality and older people. The nurse is a facilitator of a milieu that is conducive to the older person asking questions and expressing his or her sexuality. The nurse has the responsibility to help maintain the sexuality of older people by offering opportunity for discussion. Some older people remain or want to remain sexually active, whereas others do not see this as an important part of their life. Nurses should open the door to discussions of sexual concerns in a nonjudgmental manner, helping those who want to continue to be sexually active, and making it clear that stopping sex is an acceptable option for others (Lindau et al., 2007). The nurse should be an educator and provide information and guidance to older people who need it.

Assessment

To assist and support older people in their sexual needs, nurses should be aware of their own feelings about sexuality and their attitudes toward intimacy and sexuality in older people (single, married, and homosexual). Only after confronting one's own attitudes, values, and beliefs can the nurse provide support without being judgmental. Rarely are sexual histories elicited from the older adult. Physical examinations often do not include the reproductive system unless it is directly involved in the present illness. However, when questions about sexual issues are asked or when the older adult is examined, the nurse needs to be particularly cognizant of the era and culture in which the individual has lived to understand the factors affecting conduct.

Older persons should be asked about their sexual satisfaction, because they may not mention it voluntarily. Anticipation of problems in older individuals' sexual experiences can ward off anxiety, misconceptions, and an arbitrary cessation of sexual pleasure. Validation of the normalcy of sexual activity or a discussion of the physiological changes that occur either with age or the effects by altering the routine or interfering with sexual activity.

By altering the routine or interfering with physical condition or medications that are associated with poor sexual health and functioning, screening for HIV/AIDS and other sexually transmitted diseases, and education about safe sexual practices are also important. and education about safe sexual practices are also important. Because of professionals' discomfort discussing sexuality or lack of knowledge about sexuality in older people, medications are often prescribed to both older men and women without attention to the sexual side effects. If medications that affect sexual function are necessary, adjustment of doses, use of alternative agents, and prescription of antidotes to reverse the sexual side effects are important. For a complete listing of medications that can affect sexual functioning and suggestions for management, see http://www.netdoctor.co.uk/menshealth/feature/medicinessex.htm. Counseling may also be needed for

the older person to adapt to natural physiological changes and image-altering surgical procedures. The nurse may also be a consultant and counselor to others who give care to older people.

The PLISSIT model (Annon, 1976) is a helpful guide for discussion of sexuality. A Nursing Standard of Practice Protocol: Sexuality in Older Adults (Arena and Wallace, 2008) and a video illustrating the use of the PLISSIT model are available at www.consultgerirn.org (Box 21-3). Youngkin (2004) provides suggestions for use of the PLISSIT model with older people:

- **Permission:** Obtain permission from the client to initiate sexual discussion. Allow the person to discuss concerns related to sexual issues, and gather information about what might have changed in the person's life to affect sexual needs and response. Questions such as the following can be used: "What concerns or questions do you have about fulfilling your sexual needs?" or "In this era of HIV and other sexually transmitted infections, I ask all my patients about sexual practices and concerns. Are there any questions I can answer for you?"
- **Limited Information:** Provide the limited information to function sexually (Wallace, 2003b). Offer teaching about the normal age-associated changes that affect sexual performance or how illness may affect sexuality. Encourage the person to learn more about the concern from books and other sources.
- **Specific Suggestions:** Offer suggestions for dealing with problems such as lubricants for atrophic vaginitis; use of condoms to prevent sexually transmitted infections; proper use of ED medications; how to communicate sexual and other needs; ways to increase comfort with coitus or ways to be intimate without coital relations.
- **Intensive Therapy:** Refer as appropriate for complex problems that require specialist intervention.

Box 21-4 provides other suggestions for assessment, from the perspective of the older adult.

Interventions

Interventions will vary depending on the needs identified from the assessment data. Following a comprehensive assessment, interventions may center on the following categories: 1) education regarding age-associated change in sexual function; 2) compensating for age-associated changes; 3) effective management of acute and chronic illness affecting sexual function; 4) removal of barriers associated with fulfilling sexual needs; and 5) special interventions to promote sexual health in cognitively impaired older adults (Arena and Wallace, 2008). Education about prevention of HIV and STDs is also important in sexually active older adults.

In summary, the nurse has a variety of roles in ensuring the sexuality of older people: facilitator, educator, consultant, counselor, and advocate. Sexuality is an amalgamation of biological, psychological, and social moral elements that affect pleasure, adaptation, and a general feeling of well-being in older people.

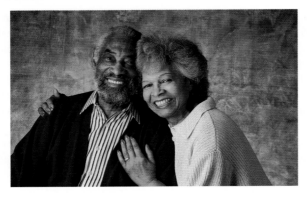

Sexuality is an important need in late life and affects pleasure, adaptation, and a general feeling of well-being. (Copyright © Getty Images.)

BOX 21-3 PLISSIT MODEL

P Permission from the client to initiate sexual discussion
LI Providing the Limited Information needed to function sexually
SS Giving Specific Suggestions for the individual to proceed with sexual relations
IT Providing Intensive Therapy surrounding the issues of sexuality for the clients (may mean referral to specialist)

Compiled from Annon J: *Journal of Sex Education and Therapy* 2:1, 1976; Wallace M: *Dermatology Nursing* 15:570, 2003; Youngkin EQ: *Advance for Nurse Practitioners* 12:45, 2004.

BOX 21-4 GUIDELINES FOR HEALTH CARE PROVIDERS IN TALKING TO OLDER ADULTS ABOUT SEXUAL HEALTH

HEALTH CARE PROVIDERS SHOULD SPEND TIME WITH OLDER ADULTS
- Be available to discuss the subject.
- Give us your full attention.
- Allow time to ask questions.
- Take time to answer questions.
- Health care providers should use clear and easy-to-understand words.
- Use plain, everyday language.
- Explain medical terms in plain English.
- Give explanations or answers to questions in simple terms.

HEALTH CARE PROVIDERS SHOULD HELP OLDER ADULTS FEEL COMFORTABLE TALKING ABOUT SEX
- Help us to break the ice.
- Make us feel comfortable in asking questions.
- Offer permission to express feelings and needs.
- Do not be afraid or embarrassed to discuss sexuality problems.

HEALTH CARE PROVIDERS SHOULD BE OPEN-MINDED AND TALK OPENLY
- Do not assume there are no concerns.
- Be open.
- Ask direct questions about sexual activity and attitudes.
- Discuss sexual concerns freely.
- Answer questions honestly.
- Just talk about it.
- Do not evade sexual concerns.
- Be willing to discuss sexual problems.
- Probe sexual concerns if elder wishes.

HEALTH CARE PROVIDERS SHOULD LISTEN
- Be prepared to listen.
- Listen so we feel you are interested in our problems.
- Let us talk.

HEALTH CARE PROVIDERS SHOULD TREAT OLDER ADULTS WITH A RESPECTFUL AND NONJUDGMENTAL ATTITUDE
- See us as individuals with sexual needs.
- Accept us for what we are: gay, straight, bisexual.
- Be nonjudgmental.
- Show genuine concern and respect.

HEALTH CARE PROVIDERS SHOULD ENCOURAGE DISCUSSION
- Make opportunities for one-to-one discussion.
- Provide privacy.
- Promote candid discussion.
- Provide discussion groups to ask questions.
- Develop support groups.

HEALTH CARE PROVIDERS CAN GIVE ADVICE OR SUGGESTIONS
- Provide information.
- Offer to find solutions and alternatives to given situations.
- Provide explicit pamphlets; explain sexual positions, lubrication.
- Discuss old taboos.
- Give suggestions of ways to help solve sexual problems.

HEALTH CARE PROVIDERS NEED TO UNDERSTAND THAT SEX IS NOT JUST FOR THE YOUNG
- Try to eliminate the idea that sex and love are just for younger people.
- Acknowledge that sexual impulses are healthy and do not disappear as individuals age.
- Treat older adults as normal sexual beings and not as asexual elderly people.
- Recognize that sex can improve—can become even better when one is older.

ⓔvolve   To access your student resources, go to *http://evolve.elsevier.com/Ebersole/TwdHlthAging*

KEY CONCEPTS

- Touch provides sensory stimulation, reduces anxiety, and provides pain relief, comfort, and sexual expression.
- The absence of touch, a powerful sense, threatens survival.
- Sexuality is love, sharing, trust, and warmth, as well as physical acts. Sexuality provides an individual with self-identity and affirmation of life.

- Sexual activity continues in old age, though adaptations are needed for the age-related changes of the male and female genital systems.
- Generally speaking, medications, ill health, and lack of a partner affect sexual activity.
- Further research is needed to promote knowledge and understanding of the sexual health of LGBT older adults.
- AIDS awareness and the practice of safe sex among older adults are still lacking. Health professionals, too, do not consider older adults at risk for AIDS, even though the incidence

of AIDS in the older population is rapidly increasing. Finding appropriate services for the older adult with AIDS may prove difficult.

- The major role of the nurse in enhancing the sexual health of older adults in the community or in long-term care settings is education and counseling about sexual function; adaptations for age-related changes and chronic conditions; prevention of HIV/AIDS and STDs in sexually active older adults; and the maintenance of sexuality for the older adult's health, well-being, and pleasure.

CASE STUDY   SEXUALITY IN LATE LIFE

George was a 70-year-old man who had been widowed for 6 years. He lived alone in a lovely home in the hills of San Francisco. His many friends tried to introduce him to a lady who would be attractive to him, but they were unaware of his real concerns. Although George was attracted to young, energetic women, often barely older than his daughters, he was justifiably cautious regarding their sincere attraction to him because he had a considerable estate. In addition, his sexual desire was waning and his capacity for sexual performance was unpredictable. One thing George expressed fairly frequently was, "I don't like demands made on me." To further complicate the picture, George had begun to take medication to reduce his benign prostatic hypertrophy (BPH) that had become increasingly troublesome. The medication further reduced his sexual desire. In addition, George's sleep pattern was disturbed by the need to arise three or four times each night to void. George came to the clinic for follow-up evaluation of his BPH, and, while talking with the nurse, he began crying uncontrollably, much to his embarrassment and the nurse's surprise because George had always seemed to be a rather solid and stoic fellow who was reluctant to discuss feelings.

Based on the case study, develop a nursing care plan using the following procedure*:

- List George's comments that provide subjective data.
- List information that provides objective data.

- From these data, identify and state, using accepted format, two nursing diagnoses you determine are most significant to George at this time. List two of George's strengths that you have identified from the data.
- Determine and state outcome criteria for each diagnosis. These criteria must reflect some alleviation of the problem identified in the nursing diagnosis and must be stated in concrete and measurable terms.
- Plan and state one or more interventions for each diagnosed problem. Provide specific documentation of the sources used to determine the appropriate intervention. Plan at least one intervention that incorporates George's existing strengths.
- Evaluate the success of the intervention. Interventions must correlate directly with the stated outcome criteria to measure the outcome success.

CRITICAL THINKING QUESTIONS

1. How would you begin discussing sexuality with George?
2. What are the factors that may be underlying George's sexual distress?
3. Discuss BPH and its prevalence and usual effects.
4. With a partner, role-play and demonstrate your interpersonal interaction with George in this situation.
5. What resources or recommendations would you suggest for George?

*Students are advised to refer to their nursing diagnosis text and identify possible or potential problems.

RESEARCH QUESTIONS

1. What do women find are the most troubling changes in their sexuality as they grow older?
2. What do men find are the most troubling changes in their sexuality as they grow older?
3. What are the differences in sexual feelings and expression in the 60-year-old, the 70-year-old, the 80-year-old, and the 90-year-old individual?
4. What are the chronic disorders that most affect sexual performance of men and women, and how are individuals affected?
5. How many individuals older than age 60 have ever been given the opportunity to provide a thorough sexual history?
6. What community and health resources are available to meet the needs of LGBT older adults?
7. What is the knowledge level about HIV/AIDS for people older than age 65?

REFERENCES

Ackerman D: *A natural history of the senses,* New York, 1995, Vantage Books.

Agronin M: Sexuality and aging: an introduction, *CNS Long-Term Care* Summer:12, 2004.

American Society on Aging and MetLife: Still out, still aging. Available at http://www.asaging. org/constituent_groups/lain/. Accessed September 20, 2010.

Annon J: The PLISSIT model: a proposed conceptual scheme for behavioral treatment of sexual problems, *Journal of Sex Education and Therapy* 2:1, 1976.

Arena J, Wallace M: Issues regarding sexuality. In Capezuti E, Swicker D, Mezey M, et al: *Evidence-based geriatric nursing protocols for best practice,* New York, 2008, Springer.

Benary-Isbert M: *The vintage years,* New York, 1968, Abingdon Press.

Blando J: Twice hidden: older gay and lesbian couples, friends and intimacy, *Generations* xxv:87, 2001.

Brotman S, Ryan B, Cormier R: The health and social service needs of gay and lesbian elders

and their families in Canada, *Gerontologist* 43:192, 2003.

Butler R, Lewis M: *The new love and sex after 60,* New York, 2002, Ballantine Books.

Comfort A: Sexuality in old age, *Journal of the American Geriatrics Society* 22:440, 1974.

Emlet C, Gerkin A, Orel N: The graying of HIV/AIDS: Preparedness and needs of the aging network in a changing epidemic, *Journal of Gerontological Social Work* 52:803, 2009.

Gallace A, Spence C: The science of interpersonal touch: An overview, *Neuroscience and Biobehavioral Reviews*, 34:246, 2010.

Gelo F: Invisible individuals—LGBT elders, *Aging Well* 1:36, 2008.

Goldblatt R: Factors influencing sexual behavior, *Journal of the American Geriatrics Society* 20:49, 1972.

Institute of Medicine, National Academies: *The Health of Lesbian, Gay, Bisexual, and Transgender People: Building a Foundation for Better Understanding* (2011). Available at http://www.iom.edu/Reports/2011/The-Health-of-Lesbian-Gay-Bisexual-and-Transgender-People.aspx. Accessed May 12, 2011.

Hall ET: *The hidden dimensions*, Garden City, NY, 1969, Doubleday.

HIV Wisdom for Older Women: Things you should know about HIV and older women, 2010. Available at http://www.hivwisdom.org/facts.html. Accessed September 20, 2010.

Hollinger, LM, Buschmann MT: Factors influencing the perception of touch by elderly nursing home residents and their health caregivers, *Journal of Gerontological Nursing* 21:37, 1993.

Huyck M: Romantic relationships in later life, *Generations* xxv:9, 2001.

Kaiser FE: Sexual dysfunction in men; sexual dysfunction in women. In Beers MH, Berkow R, editors: *The Merck manual of geriatrics*, ed 3, Whitehouse Station, NJ, 2000.

Kamel H, Hajjar R: Sexuality in the nursing home, part 2: managing abnormal behavior—legal and ethical issues, *Journal of the American Medical Directors Association* 4:203, 2003.

Kennedy G, Martinez M, Garo N: Sex and mental health in old age, *Primary Psychiatry* 17:21, 2010.

Kim EJ, Buschmann MBT: Touch-stress model and Alzheimer's disease: using touch intervention to alleviate patients' stress, *Journal of Gerontological Nursing* 30:33, 2004.

Kreiger D: Therapeutic touch: the imprimatur of nursing, *American Journal of Nursing* 75:784, 1975.

Lindau S, Schumm L, Laumann E, et al: A study of sexuality and health among older adults in the United States, *New England Journal of Medicine* 357:762, 2007.

Lindau S, Gavrilova N: Sex, health, and years of sexually active life gained due to good health: evidence from two US population based cross sectional surveys of ageing, *British Medical Journal* 340, 2010. Available at http://www.bmj.com/cgi/content/full/340/mar09_2/c810. Accessed September 20, 2010.

Messinger-Rapport BJ, Sandhu SK, Hujer ME: Sex and sexuality: is it over after 60? *Clinical Geriatrics* 11:45, 2003.

Money J, Tucker P: *Sexual signatures: being a man or woman*, Boston, 1975, Little, Brown.

Montagu A: *Touching: the human significance of the skin*, ed 3, New York, 1986, Harper & Row.

National Institute on Aging: HIV/AIDS and older people, 2009. Available at http://www.nia.nih.gov/healthinformation/publications/hiv-aids.htm. Accessed September 20, 2010.

Population Reference Bureau/Today's research on aging: HIV/AIDS and older adults in the United States, 18, 2009.

Rheaume C, Mitty E: Sexuality and intimacy in older adults, *Geriatric Nursing* 29:342, 2008.

Sansone P, Schmitt L: Providing tender touch massage to elderly nursing home residents: a demonstration project, *Geriatric Nursing* 21:303, 2000.

Services and Advocacy for Gay, Lesbian, Bisexual, and Transgender Elders (SAGE) and Movement Advancement Project: Improving the lives of LGBT older adults. Available at https://sageusa.org/resources/resource_view.cfm?resource=183. Accessed September 20, 2010.

Skinner KD: Creating a game for sexuality and aging: the sexual dysfunction trivia game, *Journal of Continuing Education in Nursing* 31:185, 2000.

Steinke E: Intimacy needs and chronic illness, *Journal of Gerontological Nursing* 31:40, 2005.

Suzman R: The National Social Life, Health, and Aging Project: An introduction, *The Journals of Gerontology Series B: Psychological Sciences and Social Sciences* 64B:i5, 2009.

Tabloski PA: *Clinical handbook for gerontological nursing*, ed 2. Upper Saddle River, NJ, 2010, Pearson Prentice Hall.

United States Department of Health and Human Services: *U.S. Department of Health and Human Services recommended actions to improve the health and well-being of lesbian, gay, bisexual, and transgender communities* (2011). Available at http://www.hhs.gov/secretary/about/lgbthealth.html. Accessed May 12, 2011.

University of Connecticut Health Center: Medicare to help with screening for HIV in older Americans. Available at http://today.uchc.edu/headlines/2010/jan10/hiv.html. Accessed September 20, 2010.

Vance D, Childs G, Moneyham L, et al: Successful aging with HIV, *Journal of Gerontological Nursing* 35:19, 2009.

Waite L, Laumann E, Das A, et al: Sexuality: measures of partnerships, practices, attitudes, and problems in the National Social Life, Health and Aging Study, *Journals of Gerontology Series B: Psychological Sciences and Social Sciences* 64B:156, 2009.

Wallace M: Best practices in nursing care to older adults: sexuality, *Dermatology Nursing* 15:570, 2003.

Wallace SP, Cochran SD, Durazo EM, Ford CL: *The health of aging lesbian, gay and bisexual adults in California*. Los Angeles CA: UCLA Center for Health Policy Research, 2011. Available at http://www.chis.ucla.edu. Accessed May 12, 2011.

Wang K, Hermann C: Pilot study to test the effectiveness of healing touch on agitation in people with dementia, *Geriatric Nursing* 27:34, 2006.

World Health Organization: Sexual health: A new focus for WHO, 2004, Progress in Reproductive Health Research. Available at www.who.int/en/. Accessed September 20, 2010.

Youngkin EQ: The myths and truths of mature intimacy, *Advance for Nurse Practitioners* 12:45, 2004.

Zeiss A, Kasl-Godley J: Sexuality in older adults' relationships, *Generations* xxv:18, 2001.

Relationships, Roles, and Transitions

Theris A. Touhy

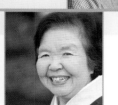

evolve http://evolve.elsevier.com/Ebersole/TwdHlthAging

A STUDENT SPEAKS

I'm really worried about retirement! That is ridiculous at my age, but I keep reading and hearing about Social Security and Medicare running out of money for the baby boom generation. Those are my parents! What about me? **Joseph, age 30**

AN ELDER SPEAKS

I thought when my children left home that my most important job was done. But they came home again and again, and then my mother-in-law came to live with us. Finally, the kids were really on their own and married, so now I take care of the grandchildren while they both work to make ends meet. I just pray daily that my husband will remain healthy. I don't think I could deal with one more thing. **Esther, age 64**

LEARNING OBJECTIVES

On completion of this chapter, the reader will be able to:

1. Explain the issues involved in adapting to transitions and role changes in later life.
2. Discuss changes in family structure and functions in society today.
3. Examine family relationships in later life.
4. Identify the range of caregiving situations and the potential challenges and opportunities of each.
5. Discuss nursing responses with older adults experiencing caregiver roles or other transitions.

This chapter examines the various relationships, roles, and transitions that are characteristic in later life. Important roles of older adults include that of spouse, partner, parent, grandparent, great-grandparent, sibling, friend, mentor, and caregiver. The role functions of these relationships shift as societal norms and economics change. Biomedical technology, political agendas, social expectations, and worldwide economic fluctuations are continually changing the face of aging. Even more changes are expected as the first wave of baby boomers enters young-old age. The major concerns of this group are adequate health care coverage, the preservation of Social Security, and caregiving demands. This major change in the aging landscape is only one of many massive social changes that have altered the patterns of work, family, and kinship structures in recent decades.

The chief concerns in this chapter are the impact of these numerous changes on the quality of life and the range of possibilities for elders in their most important affiliations. Individuals live longer, families are smaller, more women work, and caregiving has become a normative life experience. Thus social change and individual need continue to change the nature of the life course and affiliative inclinations.

LATER LIFE TRANSITIONS

Role transitions that occur in late life include retirement, grandparenthood, widowhood, and becoming a caregiver or recipient of care. These transitions may occur predictably or may be imposed by unanticipated events. Retirement is an example of a predictable event that can and should be planned long in advance, although for some, it can occur unexpectedly as a result of illness, disability, or being terminated from a job. To the degree that an event is perceived as expected and occurring at the right time, a role transition may be comfortable and even welcomed. Those persons who must retire "too early" or are widowed "too soon" will have more difficulty adapting than those who are at an age when these events are expected.

The speed and intensity of a major change may make the difference between a transitional crisis and a gradual and comfortable adaptation. Most difficult are the transitions that incorporate losses rather than gains in status, influence, and opportunity. The move from independence to dependence and becoming a care recipient is particularly difficult. Conditions that influence the outcome of transitions include personal meanings, expectations, level of knowledge, preplanning, and emotional and physical reserves. Cohort, cultural, and gender differences are inherent in all of life's major transitions. Those transitions that make use of past skills and adaptations may be less stressful. The ideal outcome is when gains in satisfaction and new roles offset losses.

Retirement

Retirement, as we formerly knew it, has changed. Retirement is no longer just a few years of rest from the rigors of work before death. It is a developmental stage that may occupy 30 or more years of one's life and involve many stages. The transitions are blurring, and the numerous patterns and styles of retiring have produced more varied experiences in retirement. With recent events that have seriously threatened pension security and portability, as well as a declining economy, more older people are remaining in the workforce. Forty-four percent of retirees work for pay at some point after retirement (see Chapter 1, Figure 1-7). Some do so because of economic need, whereas others have a desire to remain involved and productive. Obviously, health and financial status affect decisions and abilities to work or engage in new work opportunities. The baby boomers increasingly face the prospect of working longer, and 33% of this generation do not own assets and have little in savings or projected retirement income beyond Social Security. Eighty-three percent of baby boomers intend to keep working after retirement (Hooyman & Kiyak, 2011).

Retirement Planning

Current research suggests that retirement has positive effects on life satisfaction and health, although this may vary depending on the individual's circumstances. Predictors of retirement satisfaction are presented in Box 22-1. Decisions to retire are often based on financial resources, attitude toward work, family roles and responsibilities, the nature of the job, access to health insurance, chronological age, health, and self-perceptions of ability to adjust to retirement (Box 22-2). Retirement planning is advisable

---

BOX 22-2   ISSUES IN RETIREMENT POTENTIAL

1. Financial need versus resources
2. Employability
3. Rewards derived from employment
   - Wages sufficient for needs and morale
   - Satisfaction level, possibility for resolution of job frustrations
   - Meaning of job, contact with friends, source of prestige
4. Psychosocial characteristics—attitudes toward retirement
   - Attitudes of significant others (advising? directing?)
   - Strength of work ethic
   - Effect of retirement on prestige
5. Personality factors
   - Time orientation (past, present, future)
   - Active versus passive in planning
   - Rationalism versus fatalism as life stance
   - Type-A versus type-B personality (hard-driving, easy-going)
   - Inner-directed versus other-directed (enjoyment of self or need for high level of external motivation)
6. Level of information about retirement
   - Planning programs on job, adult education, or community programs
   - Awareness of friends and family who have retired and how influenced by them
7. Pressures to retire
   - Compulsory, age discriminatory
   - Unemployment (how long?)
   - Job retrogression (being moved down the ladder)
   - Skill obsolescence (opportunities for developing other skills?)
   - Peer pressure (organized or informal)
   - Employer pressure (reduced incentives to continue work, increased incentives to retire)
   - Family pressure (spouse's working status)
   - Health, discomfort, or disability interfering with job performance and dependability

---

BOX 22-1   PREDICTORS OF RETIREMENT SATISFACTION

- Good health
- Functional abilities
- Adequate income
- Suitable living environment
- Strong social support system characterized by reciprocal relationships
- Decision to retire involved choice, autonomy, adequate preparation, higher-status job prior to retirement
- Retirement activities that offer an opportunity to feel useful, learn, grow, and enjoy oneself
- Positive outlook, sense of mastery, resilience, resourcefulness
- Good marital relationship if married
- Sharing similar interests to spouse/significant other

Data from Hooyman N, Kiyak H: *Social gerontology: A multidisciplinary perspective*, ed 9, Boston, 2011, Allyn & Bacon.

---

during early adulthood and essential in middle age. However, people differ in their focus on the past, present, and future and their realistic ability to "put away something" for future needs. Retirement preparation programs are usually aimed at employees with high levels of education and occupational status, those with private pension coverage, and government employees. Thus the people most in need of planning assistance may be those least likely to have any available, let alone the resources for an adequate retirement. Individuals who are retiring in poor health, culturally and racially diverse persons, and those in lower socioeconomic levels may experience greater concerns in retirement and may need specialized counseling. These groups are often neglected in retirement planning programs.

Working couples must plan together for retirement. Decisions will depend on their career goals, shared future interests, and the quality of their interpersonal relationship. The following are some questions one must weigh when deciding to retire or continue working:

- What do I want to do?
- Who needs me, and what are my best opportunities?
- What am I best able to do?
- What is the meaning of my life?
- What should my life accomplish or contribute?
- Am I financially secure for the rest of my life if I live 30 or more years?
- Can I afford to completely retire from paid work?

Retirement education plans are supplied through employers, group lectures, individual counseling, books. DVDs, and Internet resources. However, at this juncture and in light of the many hazards experienced by pre-retirees, planning is often insufficient. Many individuals have very high expectations for the final third of their lives. Although federal laws encourage increased participation in company-sponsored 401(k) plans, many of these plans are unreliable and rates of return have diminished considerably. The continued availability of Social Security is of great concern to current and future retirees (Chapter 20).

The adequacy of retirement income depends not only on work history but also on marital history. The poverty rates of older women are excessively high. Couples who had previous marriages and divorces may have significantly lower economic resources available than those in first marriages. Child support, divorce settlements, and pension apportionment to ex-spouses may have diminished retirement income. This problem is an ever-increasing impediment to retirement because, among couples presently approaching retirement age, fewer than half are in a first marriage. Policies have been based on the traditional lifelong marriage, and this is no longer appropriate.

Special Considerations in Retirement

Retirement security depends on the "three-legged stool" of Social Security pensions, savings, and investments (Stanford and Usita, 2002). Older people with disabilities, those who have lacked access to education or held low-paying jobs with no benefits, and those not eligible for Social Security are at economic risk during retirement years. Culturally and racially diverse older persons, women—especially widows and those divorced or never married—immigrants, and gay and lesbian men and women often face greater challenges related to adequate income and benefits in retirement. Unmarried women, particularly African Americans, face the most negative prospects for retirement now and for at least the next 20 years (Hooyman and Kiyak, 2011).

Inadequate coverage for women in retirement is common because their work histories have been sporadic and diverse. Women are often called on to retire earlier than anticipated because of family needs. Whereas most men have always worked outside the home, it is only within the past 30 years that this has been the expectation of women. Therefore large cohort differences exist. Traditionally, the variability of women's work histories, interrupted careers, the residuals of sexist pension policies, Social Security inequities, and low-paying jobs created hazards for adequacy of income in retirement. The scene is gradually changing in many respects, but the gender bias remains.

Basing retirement calculations on gender and projected survival statistics is now illegal, though until the early 1980s, women were allotted less pension income based purely on their expected longevity compared with men. Although this is no longer in force, women who retired 20 or 25 years ago remain penalized because of gender. Older women are likely to have several years of no earnings calculated into the averages that determine the amount of their Social Security benefits. Some women find that they will receive more if their Social Security benefits are calculated on their husband's earnings; this may be true even though widowed or divorced. The Social Security

Administration must be contacted regarding these matters because many variables must be considered.

Barriers to equal treatment for LGBT couples include job discrimination, unequal treatment under Social Security, pension plans, and 401(k) plans. LGBT couples are not eligible for Social Security survivor benefits, and unmarried partners cannot claim pension plan rights after the death of the pension plan participant. These policies definitely place LGBT elders at a disadvantage in retirement planning.

PROMOTING HEALTHY AGING: IMPLICATIONS FOR GERONTOLOGICAL NURSING

Successful retirement adjustment depends on socialization needs, energy levels, health, adequate income, variety of interests, amount of self-esteem derived from work, presence of intimate relationships, social support, and general adaptability. Nurses may have the opportunity to work with people in different phases of retirement or participate in retirement education and counseling programs (Box 22-3). Talking with clients older than age 50 about retirement plans, providing anticipatory guidance about the transition to retirement, identifying those who may be at risk for lowered income and health concerns, and referring to appropriate resources for retirement planning and support are important nursing interventions.

It is important to build on the strengths of older adults' life experiences and coping skills and to provide appropriate counseling and support to assist older people to continue to grow and develop in meaningful ways during the transition from the work role. In ideal situations, retirement offers the opportunity to pursue interests that may have been neglected while fulfilling other obligations. However, for too many older people, retirement presents challenges that affect both health and well-being, and nurses must be advocates for policies and conditions that allow all older people to maintain quality of life in retirement.

Death of a Spouse

Losing a partner after a long, close, and satisfying relationship is the most difficult adjustment one can face, aside from the loss of a child. The loss of a spouse is a stage in the life course that can be anticipated but seldom is. Seventy-six percent of women over age 85 are widowed compared with 38% of men (Federal Interagency Forum on Aging, 2010). "Spousal bereavement is associated with significant distress, which has multifactorial ramifications for physical and mental health outcomes assessment" (Minton and Barron, 2008, p. 45). The death of a life partner is essentially a loss of self. The mourning is as much for

BOX 22-3	PHASES OF RETIREMENT

Remote: Future anticipation with little real planning
Near: Preparation and fantasizing regarding retirement
Honeymoon: Euphoria and testing of the fantasies
Disenchantment: Letdown, boredom, sometimes depression
Reorientation: Developing a realistic and satisfactory lifestyle
Stability: Personal investment in meaningful activities
Termination: Loss of role resulting from illness or return to work

oneself as for the individual who has died. A core part of oneself has died with the partner, and even with satisfactory grief resolution, that aspect of self will never return. Even those widows and widowers who reorganize their lives and invest in family, friends, and activities often find that many years later they still miss their "other half" profoundly.

With the loss of the intimate partner, several changes occur simultaneously that involve social status, economics, and self-image. Individuals who have been self-confident and resilient seem to fare best. The transitional phase of grief, if handled appropriately, leads to the confirmation of a new identity, the end of one stage of life and the beginning of another (Chapter 23). Seldom in life is there such an abrupt and distinct breach that creates intense pain but offers the opportunity for the emergence of a new identity.

Gender differences are found in the literature on widowhood. Bereaved husbands may be more socially and emotionally vulnerable. Suicide risk is highest among men over age 80 who have experienced the death of a spouse. Widowers adapt more slowly than widows to the loss of a spouse and often remarry quickly. Loneliness and the need to be cared for is a factor influencing widowers to seek out new partners. Association with family and friends, being members of a church community, and continuing to work or engage in activities can all be helpful in the adjustment period following the death of a wife. Common bereavement reactions of widowers are listed in Box 22-4 and should be discussed with male clients.

PROMOTING HEALTHY AGING: IMPLICATIONS FOR GERONTOLOGICAL NURSING

Assessment

Nurses working with the bereaved will need to review Lindemann's classic grief studies to understand the initial somatic responses of the bereaved (Lindemann, 1944). Feelings of the bereaved one are not orderly or progressive; they are conflicted, ambivalent, suicidal, full of rage, and often suspicious. Widows and widowers may exhibit personality disorganization that would be considered mentally aberrant or frankly psychotic under other circumstances. Some people handle grief with less apparent decompensation. Grief reactions must be accepted as personally valid and useful evidences of healing. DeVries (2001) discusses the signs of ongoing bonds and connections with the deceased (e.g., dreaming of the deceased, ongoing daily communication, "checking in") that persist long after death and

counsels professionals to reexamine the idea that there is a timetable for "resolution" of grief. There are several tools that can be used to assess aspects of the bereavement process including coping, grief symptomatology, personal growth, continuing bonds, and health risk assessment (Minton and Barron, 2008).

Interventions

Nurses will interact with bereaved older people in many settings. Knowing the stages of transition to a new role as a widow or widower will be useful in determining interventions, although each individual is unique in this respect. Individuals respond to losses in ways that reflect the nature and meaning of the relationships as well as the unique characteristics of the bereaved. Patterns of adjustment are presented in Box 22-5. With adequate support, reintegration can be expected in two to four years. People with few familial or social supports may need professional help to get through the early months of grief in a way that will facilitate recovery. To support the grieving person, it is necessary to extend one's own self to reconnect the severed person with a world of warmth and caring. No one nurse or family member can accomplish this task alone. Hundreds of small, caring gestures build strength and confidence in the grieving person's ability and willingness to survive. Additional information about dying, death, and grief can be found in Chapter 23.

BOX 22-4   COMMON WIDOWER BEREAVEMENT REACTIONS

- Search for the lost mate
- Neglect of self
- Inability to share grief
- Loss of social contacts
- Struggle to view women as other than wife
- Erosion of self-confidence and sexuality
- Protracted grief period

BOX 22-5   PATTERNS OF ADJUSTMENT TO WIDOWHOOD

STAGE ONE: REACTIONARY
(First Few Weeks)
Early responses of disbelief, anger, indecision, detachment, and inability to communicate in a logical, sustained manner are common. Searching for the mate, visions, hallucinations, and depersonalization may be experienced.
Intervention: Support, validate, be available, listen to individual talk about mate, reduce expectations.

STAGE TWO: WITHDRAWAL
(First Few Months)
Depression, apathy, physiological vulnerability occur; movement and cognition are slowed; insomnia, unpredictable waves of grief, sighing, and anorexia occur.
Intervention: Protect individual against suicide, monitor health status, and involve in support groups.

STAGE THREE: RECUPERATION
(Second Six Months)
Periods of depression are interspersed with characteristic capability. Feelings of personal control begin to return.
Intervention: Support accustomed lifestyle patterns that sustain and assist individual to explore new possibilities.

STAGE FOUR: EXPLORATION
(Second Year)
Individual begins new ventures, testing suitability of new roles; anniversaries, holidays, birthdays, and date of death may be especially difficult.
Intervention: Prepare individual for unexpected reactions during anniversaries. Encourage and support new trial roles.

STAGE FIVE: INTEGRATION
(Fifth Year)
Individual will feel fully integrated into new and satisfying roles if grief has been resolved in a healthy manner.
Intervention: Assist individual to recognize and share own pattern of growth through the trauma of loss.

RELATIONSHIPS IN LATER LIFE

The classic study of Lowenthal and Haven (1968) has been reviewed in detail and elaborated many times since its inception. The importance of caring relationships and the presence of a confidante as a buffer against "age-linked social losses" is demonstrated in the study. Maintaining a stable intimate relationship was more closely associated with good mental health and high morale than was a high level of activity or elevated role status. Individuals seem able to manage stresses if some relationships are close and sustaining. Increasingly evident is that a caring person may be a significant survival resource. Frequently nurses become the caring other in an older person's life, especially among elders living in nursing homes (Touhy, 2001). Social bonding increases health status through as yet undetermined physiological pathways, though studies in psychoneuroimmunology are giving us clues. Social support is related to psychological and physical well-being, and participation in meaningful social activities is also a modifying factor that may offset the risk of dementia.

This segment of the chapter familiarizes the reader with relationships as experienced in old age within generations and between generations. A network of kin, friends, and acquaintances can sustain the older adult and give life meaning. We might use the analogy of a tree that withstands storms and drought through an extensive root system, which provides stability and nourishment that may be helpful; such is old age. The ground around the tree must be tended to keep it thriving. We may find ourselves best caring for older people by caring for those who are important to them.

Primary relationships are intimate associations that provide a strong sense of sharing and belonging; these are the deep roots of our tree analogy. Relationships that are more formal, impersonal, superficial, and circumstantial are often time limited, sometimes intense but with a tendency to dissipate. These relationships are the surface network of roots that extend outward in many directions and are sustained by their profusion but wither with neglect or insignificance. Thus the primary network may need professional strengthening to bear the increasing demands.

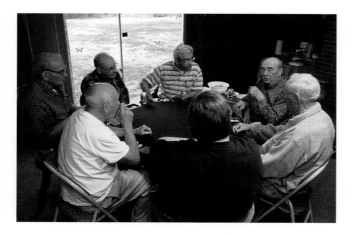

Friends play an important role in the lives of older adults. (From Lewis SM et al: *Medical-surgical nursing: assessment and management of clinical problems,* ed 6, St Louis, 2004, Mosby; courtesy of Rick Brady, Riva, MD.)

Friendships

Friends are often a significant source of support in late life. The majority of older people live with others, but the incidence of older people living alone is increasing, especially after age 75 when 23% of men and 50% of women live alone. Those living alone are most likely to be women, elders of color, the oldest-old, low-income older adults, and those in rural areas. The number of friends may decline, but the majority of older adults have at least one close friend with whom they maintain close contact, share confidences, and can turn to in an emergency (Hooyman and Kiyak, 2011). Friendships are often sustaining in the face of overwhelming circumstances. Friends provide the critical elements of satisfactory living that families may not, providing commitment and affection without judgment. Personality characteristics between friends are compatible because the relationships are chosen and caring is shared without obligation. Trust, demonstrations of caring, and mutual problem solving are important aspects of the friendships.

Friends may share a lifelong perspective or may bring a totally new intergenerational viewpoint into one's life. Late-life friendships often develop out of changing situations, such as shared tenancies, relocation to retirement or assisted living communities, widowhood, and involvement in volunteer pursuits. As desires and pursuits change, some friendships evolve that the person never would have considered in his or her youth. Friends function in many ways: (1) act as surrogate kin, (2) ease the loneliness of widowhood, and (3) validate one's generational viewpoint.

Considering the obvious importance of friendship, it seems to be a neglected area of exploration and a seldom considered resource for professionals working with older people. Because close friendships have such influence on the sense of well-being of elders, anything done to sustain them or assist in building new friendships and social networks will be helpful. Generally, women tend to have more sustaining friendships than men do, and this factor contributes to resilience, a characteristic linked to successful aging (Hooyman and Kiyak, 2011). Nurses may include in their assessment questions about older individuals' friendships and their importance and availability. Linking older adults to resources for social participation and meaningful activities is also an important intervention.

Mentoring Relationships

Professionals and, in some other situations, other older adults may develop intense reciprocal relationships with younger adults, and vice versa. These relationships often have an intimacy that is similar to that of parent and offspring. For some older people a relationship may fill a need for offspring who were never produced. In some cases, these relationships may be more satisfactory because the inherent generational expectations are attenuated by the absence of obligation. Elder retired academics often become involved with young neophyte students and professionals, the elder benefiting from fresh ideas and the younger from the wisdom of the elder. When the relationship is not one of mentoring, it may be a replacement of the idealized parent or grandparent who is no longer or was never available. "Catherine was the great-grandmother I never knew." "Priscilla was a model of gracious aging." "Mary Opal was a mentor and a surrogate mother."

FAMILIES

The idea of family evokes strong impressions of whatever an individual believes the typical family should be. Because everyone comes from a family, these impressions have powerful symbolic meanings. However, in today's world, the definition of family is in a state of flux. As recently as 100 years ago, the norm was the extended family made up of parents, their grown children, and the children's children, often living together and sharing resources, strengths, and challenges. As cities grew and adult children moved in pursuit of work, parents did not always come along, and the nuclear family evolved. The norm in the United States became two parents and their two children, or at least that was the norm in what has been considered mainstream America. This pattern was not as common, nor is it yet, in many families of color, especially living in what are called "ethnic neighborhoods," where the extended family is still the norm. Today, only about 23.5% of U.S. households are composed of nuclear families.

A decrease in fertility rates has reduced family size, and American families are smaller today than ever before (2.6 people in the nuclear family). A delay in the age of childbearing is more common, with the average age of first births now 25 years, and first births to women over 35 increasing nearly 8 times since 1970. The high divorce and remarriage rate results in households of blended families of children from previous marriages and the new marriage. Single-parent families, blended families, gay and lesbian families, childless families, and fewer families altogether are common.

Multigenerational families have grown by approximately 60% since 1990 (Hooyman & Kiyak, 2011). Growth of multigenerational households has accelerated during the economic downturn. From 2008 to 2010, the number of multigenerational households increased from 5.3% to 6.1% (American Association of Retired Persons (AARP), 2011). Older people without families, either by choice or circumstance, have created their own "families" through communal living with siblings, friends, or others. Indeed, it is not unusual for childless persons residing in long-term care facilities to refer to the staff as their new "family."

Family members, however they are defined, form the nucleus of relationships for the majority of older adults and their support system if they become dependent. A longstanding myth in society is that families are alienated from their older family members and abandon their care to institutions. Nothing could be farther from the truth. Family relationships remain strong in old age, and most older people have frequent contact with their families. Most older adults possess a large intergenerational web of significant people, including sons, daughters, stepchildren, in-laws, nieces, nephews, grandchildren, and great-grandchildren, as well as partners and former partners of their offspring. As discussed later in the chapter, families provide the majority of care for older adults. Changes in family structure will have a significant impact on the availability of family members to provide care for older people in the future.

As families change, the roles of the members or expectations of one another may change as well. Grandparents may assume parental roles for their grandchildren if their children are unable to care for them; or grandparents and older aunts and uncles

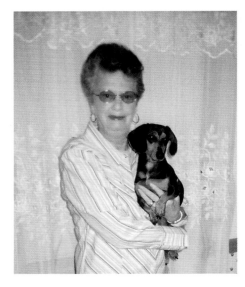

Pets are a part of the family and are particularly beneficial to older adults. They provide companionship, comfort, and caring. (From Monahan F et al: *Phipps' medical-surgical nursing: health and illness perspectives,* ed 8, St Louis, 2006, Mosby.)

may assume temporary caregiving roles while the children, nieces, and nephews work. Adult children of any age may provide limited or extensive caregiving to their own parents or aging relatives who become ill or impaired. A spouse or a sibling may become a caregiver as well. This caregiving may be temporary or long term.

Close-knit families are more aware of the needs of their members and work to resolve problems and find ways to meet the needs of members, even if they are not always successful. Emotionally distant families are less available in times of need and have greater potential for conflict. If the family has never been close and supportive, it will not magically become so when members grow older. Resentments long buried may crop up and produce friction or psychological pain. Long-submerged conflicts and feelings may return if the needs of one family member exceed those of the others. In coming to know the older adult, the gerontological nurse comes to know the family as well, learning of their special gifts and their life challenges. The nurse works with the elder within the unique culture of his or her family of origin, present family, and support networks, including friends.

Types of Families
Traditional Couples

The marital or partnered relationship in the United States is a critical source of support for older people, and nearly 55% of the population age 65 and older is married and lives with a spouse. Although this relationship is often the most binding if it extends into late life, the chance of a couple going through old age together is exceedingly slim. Women over age 65 are three times as likely as men of the same age to be widowed. Men who survive their spouse into old age ordinarily have multiple opportunities to remarry if they wish. Even among the oldest-old, the majority of men are married (Federal Interagency Forum on Aging, 2010). A woman is less likely to have an opportunity for remarriage in late life.

In late marriages or remarriage, developing an intimate, sharing relationship between individuals who have had 75 or 80 years of separate experiences often brings conflicting ideologies into the new relationship and can be an enormous challenge. Older people who remarry usually choose someone they have previously known and with whom they share similar backgrounds and interests. Often, older couples live together but do not marry because of economic and inheritance reasons.

The needs, tasks, and expectations of couples in late life differ from those in earlier years. Some couples have been married more than 60 or 70 years. These years together may have been filled with love and companionship or abuse and resentment, or anything in between. However, in general, marital status (or the presence of a long-time partner) is positively related to health, life satisfaction, and well-being. For all couples, the normal physical and sociological circumstances in late life present challenges. Some of the issues that strain many of these relationships include (1) the deteriorating health of one or both partners, (2) limitations in income, (3) conflicts with children or other relatives, (4) incompatible sexual needs, and (5) mismatched needs for activity and socialization.

Divorce. In the past, divorce was considered a stigmatizing event. Today, however, it is so common that a person is inclined to forget the ostracizing effects of divorce from 60 years ago. Divorced and separated (including married with spouse absent) older persons represented only 11.8% of all older persons in 2006 (Administration on Aging, 2008). However, this percentage has increased since 1980, when approximately 5.3% of the older population were divorced or separated with the spouse absent. There are large generational and individual differences in expectations from marriage, but older couples are becoming less likely to stay in an unsatisfactory marriage. Health care professionals must avoid making assumptions and be alert to the possibility of marital dissatisfaction in old age. Nurses should ask, "How would you describe your marriage?"

Long-term relationships are varied and complex, with many factors forming the glue that holds them together. Marital breakdown may be more devastating in old age because it is often unanticipated and may occur concurrently with other significant losses. Health care workers must be concerned with supporting a client's decision to seek a divorce and with assisting him or her in seeking counseling in the transition. A nurse should alert the client that a divorce will bring on a grieving process similar to the death of a spouse and that a severe disruption in coping capacity may occur until the client adjusts to a new life. The grief may be more difficult to cope with because no socially sanctioned patterns have been established, as is the case with widowhood. In addition, tax and fiscal policies favor married couples, and many divorced elderly women are at a serious economic disadvantage in retirement.

Nontraditional Couples

As the variations in families grow, so do the types of coupled relationships. Among the types of couples we see today are lesbian, gay, bisexual, and transgender (LGBT) couples. Although the number of LGBT people of any age has remained elusive, an estimated 3 million Americans over age 65 are LGBT with projections that this figure is likely to double by 2030 (Gelo, 2008). Many LGBT individuals are raising children, either alone or as part of a couple. Although these couples are less often seen in the aging population, they are still there but may not be obvious because of long-standing discrimination and fear. It is important to recognize that there are considerable differences in the experiences of younger LGBT individuals when compared to those who are older. Older LGBT individuals did not have the benefit of antidiscrimination laws and support for same-sex partners. They were also more likely to keep their sexual orientation and relationships "hidden."

Many older LGBT individuals have been part of a live-in couple at some time during their life, but as they age, they are more likely to live alone. Some may have developed social networks of friends, members of their family of origin, and the larger community but many lack support. Organizations that serve these communities need to enhance outreach and support mechanisms to enable these individuals to maintain independence and age safely and in good health (Wallace et al, 2011). The continued legal and policy barriers faced by LGBT elders contribute to the challenges for those in domestic partnerships as they age. Recent HHS recommendations addressing these issues may improve access to benefits in the future (U.S. Department of Health and Human Services, 2011) (See Chapter 19). Healthy People 2020 includes a new section on LGBT health and efforts to improve health and address health disparities (U.S. Department of Health and Human Services, 2010).

Increasing numbers of same-sex couples are choosing to have families, and this will call for greater understanding of these "new" types of families, young and old. The majority of research has involved gay and lesbian couples, and much less is known about bisexual and transgender relationships. Much more knowledge of cohort, cultural, and generational differences among age groups is needed to understand the dramatic changes in the lives of gay and lesbian individuals in family lifestyles. The National Resource Center of Lesbian, Gay, Bisexual, and Transgender Aging has a new portal focused on caregiving resources for LGBT caregivers (http://www.lgbtagingcenter.org/resources/resources/CFM?t=1). Chapter 21 discusses the health concerns of LGBT older adults in more detail.

Elders and Their Adult Children

In adulthood, relationships between the generations become increasingly important for most people. Older parents enjoy being told about the various activities and successes of their offspring, and these adult children begin to see aspects of themselves that are and have developed from their parents. At times, the relationships may become strained because the younger adults are more concerned with their own spouses, partners, and children. The parents are no longer central to their lives, though offspring may be central to the lives of their parents. The most difficult situations occur when the elder parents are openly critical or judgmental about the lives of their offspring. In the best of situations, adult children shift to the role of friend, companion, and confidant to the elder, a concept known as filial maturity.

Most older people see their children on a regular basis, and even children who do not live close to their older parents maintain close connections, and "intimacy at a distance" can occur (Hooyman and Kiyak, 2011; Silverstein and Angelli, 1998). Approximately 50% of older people have daily contact with their adult children; nearly 80% see an adult child at least once a week; and more than 75% talk on the phone at least weekly with an adult child (Administration on Aging, 2008).

By and large, elders and their children have relationships that are reciprocal in nature and characterized by affection and mutual support. These relationships are both the most important and potentially the most conflicted. Family resources are shared from birth and usually in some way until and after death. These resources may be tangible, such as money, belongings, and housing. Intangible resources may include advice, support, guidance, and day-to-day assistance with life. Elders provide a family history perspective, models for growing old, assistance with grandchildren, a sense of continuity, and a philosophy of aging. The older family members often serve as kin-keepers. Kin-keeper is a term used to denote a family member who arranges get-togethers, develops the family history and rituals, and in other ways promotes solidarity and unity among the kin.

Consider the example of Grandma Daisy, who always merited a special visit from any of the kin in her vast northwestern network. A pioneer settler in her small community, she knew the names, ages, and whereabouts of the children and spouses and the grandchildren and spouses of all of her eight children. They seldom saw one another but always felt a connecting link through Grandma Daisy. When she died at age 94, a great portion of the family history and sense of solidarity died with her. She was a true kin-keeper.

Never Married Older Adults

Approximately 4% of older adults today have never married. Older people who have lived alone most of their lives often develop supportive networks with siblings, friends, and neighbors. Never-married older adults may demonstrate resilience to the challenges of aging as a result of their independence and may not feel lonely or isolated. Furthermore, they may have had longer lifetime employment and may enjoy greater financial security as they age. Single older adults will increase in the future because being single is increasingly more common in younger years (Hooyman and Kiyak, 2011).

Grandparents

The role of grandparenting, and increasingly great-grandparenthood, is experienced by most older adults. Eighty percent of those over age 65, and 51% of those ages 50 to 64, have grandchildren. There are approximately 80 million grandparents in the United States today, spanning ages 30 to 110, with grandchildren that range from newborns to retirees. Fifty percent of grandparents are under age 60, and some will experience grandparenthood for more than 40 years (Livingston and Parker, 2010; Legacy Project, 2010). Sixty-eight percent of individuals born in 2000 will have four grandparents alive when they reach 18; and 76% will have at least one grandparent at age 30 (Hooyman and Kiyak, 2011).

Great-grandparenthood will become more common in the future in light of projec-tions of a healthier aging. However, with changing family structures and fewer individuals choosing not to marry or have children, there may be fewer grandchildren in the future. Gender and lineage are greatly influential in the meaning of grandparenthood. There is a great matrilineal

advantage in grandparenting relationships, but the role of grandfathers is also significant in the lives of many children. This area needs further study.

As the term implies, the "grands" are a step beyond parents in their concerns, exposure, and responsibility. The majority of grandparents derive great emotional satisfaction from their grandchildren. Historically, the emphasis has been on the progressive aging of the grandparent as it affects the relationship with the grandchild, but little has been said about the effects of the growth and maturation of the grandchild on the relationship. Many young adults who have had close contact with their grandparents report that this relationship was very meaningful in their lives. Growing numbers of adult grandchildren are assisting in caregiving for frail grandparents.

The age, vitality, and proximity of both grandchild and grandparent produce a kaleidoscope of possible activities and interactions as both progress through their aging processes. Approximately 80% of grandparents see a grandchild at least monthly, and nearly 50% do so weekly. Geographic distance does not significantly affect the quality of the relationship between grandparents and their grandchildren. The Internet is increasingly being used by distant grandparents as a way of staying involved in their grandchildren's lives and forging close bonds (Hooyman and Kiyak 2011).

Younger grandparents typically live closer to their grandchildren and are more involved in child care and recreational activities (Box 22-6). Older grandparents with sufficient incomes may provide more financial assistance and other types of instrumental help. The need for support for adult children and grandchildren has the potential to increase during current economic conditions and may pose significant financial concerns for older people (American Association of Retired Persons, 2010). More than 60% of grandparents report taking care of their grandchildren on a regular basis, and 13% are primary caregivers. This phenomenon is discussed later in the chapter.

Siblings

Late-life sibling relationships are poorly understood and have been neglected by researchers. As individuals age, they often have more contact with siblings than they did in the years when

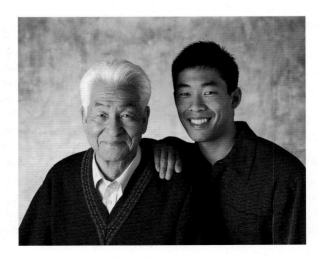

Grandparenting is an important role for elders. (Copyright © Getty Images.)

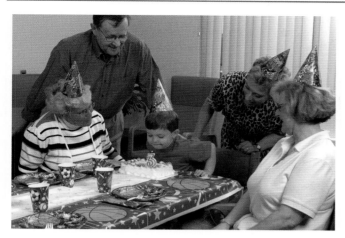

Grandparents take part in family activities. (From Sorrentino SA, Gorek B: *Mosby's textbook for long-term care assistants*, ed 5, St Louis, 2007, Mosby.)

BOX 22-6	**A GRANDMOTHER AS SEEN BY AN 8-YEAR-OLD CHILD**

"A grandmother is a woman who has no children of her own. That is why she loves other people's children."

"Grandmothers have nothing to do. They are just there: when they take us for a walk they go slowly, like caterpillars along beautiful leaves. They never say, 'Come on, faster, hurry up!'"

"Everyone should try to have a grandmother, especially those who don't have a TV."

From *Ageing in Focus*, March 2006.

---

family and work demands were more pressing. About 80% of older people have at least one sibling, and they are often strong sources of support in the lives of never married older persons, widowed persons, and those without children. For many elders, these relationships became increasingly important because they have a long history of memories and are of the same generation and similar backgrounds. Sibling relationships become particularly important when they are part of the support system, especially among single or widowed elders living alone.

The strongest of sibling bonds is thought to be the relationship between sisters. When blessed with survival, these relationships remain important into late old age. In some remarkable cases, such as the Delaney sisters, the two personalities complement each other and function well together in coping with the demands of independent living at great old age. Bessie (age 101 years) was feisty and abrupt, whereas Sadie (age 103 years) did what was needed with quiet determination (Delaney and Delaney, 1993). Of course, much has to do with age differences, place in the family, and personality. Service providers should inquire about sibling relationships of past and present *significance*. Consider the following:

I remember the days when I detested Buddy, especially in our adolescence, but he is the only one still alive who has been a part of my entire life. Now, when we reflect on our divergent paths it is with a mixture of pleasure and poignancy. When our parents, other siblings, and mates died, we held each other together. Others call him Joe, but he will always be my Buddy.

The loss of siblings has a profound effect in terms of awareness of one's own mortality, particularly when those of the same gender die. When an elder reaches the age of the sibling who died, the reaction can be quite disruptive. Not only is grieving activated, but also rehearsal for one's own death may occur. In some cases in which an elder sibling survives younger ones, there may be not only a deep grief but also pangs of guilt: "Why them and not me?"

Other Kin

Interaction with collateral kin (i.e., cousins, aunts, uncles, nieces, nephews) generally depends on proximity, preference, and the general availability of primary kin. The quality of relationships varies but is still a potential source of joy, support, assistance, or conflict. Maternal kin (related through female bloodlines) may be emotionally closer than those in one's paternal line (Jett, 2002). These relatives may provide a reservoir of kin from which to find replacements for missing or lost intimate relationships for single or childless people as they grow older.

Fictive Kin

Fictive kin are non-blood kin who serve as "genuine fake families," as expressed by Virginia Satir. These non-relatives become surrogate family and take on some of the instrumental and affectional attributes of family. Fictive kin are important in the lives of many elders, especially those with no close or satisfying family relationships and those living alone or in institutions. Fictive kin includes both friends and, often, paid caregivers. Primary care providers, such as nursing assistants, nurses, or case managers, often become fictive kin. Professionals who work with older people need to recognize the instrumental and emotional support, as well as the mutually satisfying relationships, that occur between friends, neighbors, and other fictive kin who assist dependent older adults.

FAMILY CAREGIVING

There are four kinds of people in the world: those who have been caregivers, those who are currently caregivers, those who will be caregivers, and those who will need caregivers (Rosalynn Carter as quoted by Mary Lund, 2005, p. 152).

Family caregiving has become a normative experience (similar to marriage, working, or retirement) for many of America's families and cuts across racial, ethnic, and social class distinctions. Gerontological nurses are most likely to encounter elders with their family and friends in situations relating to caregiving of some kind. Family members and other unpaid caregivers provide 80% of care for older adults in the United States. More than 65 million people, nearly 29% of the U.S. population, provide care for a chronically ill, disabled, or aged family member or friend during any given year. Caregivers are present in one of every five households, and seven out of ten caregivers are caring for loved ones over 50 years old. Informal caregivers may also include friends, paid and unpaid workers, or volunteers in the home, but current trends suggest that the use of paid, formal care by older persons with disabilities in the community has been decreasing, while their sole reliance on family caregivers has been increasing (National Family Caregivers Association [NFCA], 2010).

Approximately 66% of family caregivers are women, and the typical family caregiver is a 49-year-old woman caring for a widowed mother who does not live with her. Middle-aged caregivers, "the sandwich generation," often struggle to balance the demands of work and parenting with caregiving for an older relative. Caregiving can also present financial burdens, and women who are family caregivers are 2.5 times more likely than non-caregivers to live in poverty. Even though generally considered a women's issue, in more and more cases, male caregivers, including those other than spouses (e.g., brothers, nephews, sons), are assuming a full range of caregiving roles. Thirty-nine percent of caregivers are men, and this area needs further research to uncover their special needs and challenges. Additionally, 1.4 million children ages 8 to 18 provide care for an adult relative, and 73% are caring for a parent or grandparent. This is another area that requires more investigation (Centers for Disease Control and Prevention [CDC] and the Kimberly-Clark Corporation, 2008; NFCA, 2010; Ostwald, 2009).

Caregivers spend an average of 20 hours per week providing care for their loved ones, and the value of these services is estimated to be $375 billion annually—more than twice as much as is spent on home care and nursing home care combined, and exceeding Medicaid long-term care spending in all states. Without family caregivers, the present level of long-term care could not be sustained. Supporting family caregivers and their ability to provide care at home or in the community is crucial to our long-term care system.

Caregiving is considered a major public health issue, and attention to the physical and mental health of caregivers is receiving increased attention. The aging of the population, medical advances, shorter hospital stays, limited discharge planning by hospitals, and expansion of home care technology will increase the demand for family caregivers in the future. It is estimated that the number of family caregivers will increase by 85% from 2000 to 2050. However, the number of family members who are available to provide care will decrease substantially in that same time period (CDC and the Kimberly-Clark Corporation, 2008). Recruitment and retention of all levels of health care workers for long-term care services is also a significant problem. The Institute of Medicine Report (2008) states that "unless action is taken immediately, the health care workforce will lack the capacity (in both size and ability) to meet the needs of older patients in the future" (p. 23).

Impact of Caregiving

Although caregiving is a means to "give back" to a loved one and can be a source of joy in the giving, it is also stressful. Caregivers are considered to be "the hidden patient" (Schulz and Beach, 1999, p. 2216). Family caregiving has been associated with increased levels of depression and anxiety, poorer self-reported physical health, compromised immune function, and increased mortality (CDC and the Kimberly-Clark Corporation, 2008).

Caregiving is a very complex issue, and assuming a caregiving role is "a time of transition that requires a restructuring of one's goals, behaviors, and responsibilities. It requires

---

BOX 22-7   SUGGESTIONS TO REDUCE CAREGIVER STRESS

To reduce caregiver stress, nurses are advised to use all means and resources at their disposal to do the following:
- Restore a sense of control and effectiveness in the situation.
- Reinforce any social supports that are available to the caregiver.
- Find opportunities for group participation with other caregivers.
- Advise routine times of respite, and assist caregiver in finding respite sources.

Schmall and colleagues suggest the following*:
- Tailor programs and services to the unique situation of caregiver and care recipient.
- Urge the caregiver to take care of self.
- Encourage caregiver to maintain activities important to his or her well-being.
- Allow the caregiver to express negative and angry feelings they may have about the care recipient and the caregiving experience.
- Encourage the caregiver's efforts to use all available resources and assistance.
- Include all directly involved parties in decisions about care.
- Praise whatever is being done well, and encourage letting go of things that have not gone well.

*Schmall VL, Stiehl R: Coping with caregiving: *How to manage stress when caring for older relatives*, Corvallis, OR, 2003, Pacific Northwest Extension. Available at http://extension.oregonstate.edu/catalog/PDF/PNW/PNW315.pdf.

---

taking on something new but it is also about loss—of what was and what could have been. There is the emotional pain of seeing a parent or spouse become physically or cognitively incapacitated. Caregivers experience the whole range of human emotions: guilt, anger, frustration, exhaustion, anxiety, fear, grief, sadness, love, and the not-to-be underestimated satisfaction of having done a good job" (Lund, 2005, p. 152).

Whereas not all caregivers experience consequential stress, the circumstances that are more likely to cause problems with caregiving include competing role responsibilities (e.g., work, home), advanced age of the caregiver, high-intensity caregiving needs, insufficient resources, poor self-reported health, living in the same household with the care recipient, dementia of the care recipient, and prior relational conflicts between the caregiver and care recipient (Box 22-7). In addition, appraisal, coping responses, and social support have been reported to be significant predictors of stress in the caregiving role. Lack of adequate long-term care services and financial difficulty have been reported to be the most consistent predictors of health and psychosocial outcomes (Robison et al., 2009). Caregivers of persons with dementia may experience even greater emotional and physical stress than other caregivers. Caregiving for older people with Alzheimer's disease and other dementias presents some unique challenges and is discussed in Chapter 19.

Cultural differences have been reported in caregiving burden and stress, and further research is needed in light of the increasing numbers of racially and culturally diverse elders and their unique needs. Some studies suggest that perceived caregiver stress and burden may be less in African-American caregivers as a result of the use of more cognitive and emotion-focused coping strategies and reliance on faith and spirituality. However the effect of caregiving on physical health in this population is often overlooked and may be significant. Culturally diverse caregivers are also reported to rely less on formal support and have more available informal support networks to assist in caregiving. Some of these findings may be attributed to inadequate outreach to these populations as a result of our belief that "they take care of their own," as well as a lack of culturally competent formal services (Pinquart and Sorenson, 2005; Skarupski et al., 2009; Siefert et al., 2008).

The positive benefits of caregiving have been given more attention in recent years, but further research is needed to help understand what factors influence how caregivers perceive the experience. Positive benefits of caregiving may include enhanced self-esteem and well-being, personal growth and satisfaction, and finding or making meaning through caregiving. Most attention in caregiving research has been given to the caregiver and less to the care recipient or to the relationship between the caregiver and care recipient.

Patricia Archbold and colleagues studied caregiving as a role and examined how the relationships between the caregiver and care recipient (mutuality) and the preparation of the caregiver (preparedness) influence reactions to caregiving (Archbold et al., 1990). Caregivers who have a positive relationship with the care recipient experience less stress and find caregiving more meaningful. Nursing interventions to assist in preparing the caregiver for the caregiving role, particularly at the time of discharge from the hospital, also seem to prevent or reduce role strain. Further research is needed to understand the complexities of the caregiving and care receiving role and provide a theory base for nursing interventions. Boxes 22-8 and 22-9 present some suggestions for caregivers.

Spousal Caregiving

Spouses provide a great deal of caregiving, and 80% of persons who live with spouses with disabilities provide care for them. Of family caregivers over age 60, spouses provide the most care. Many may have significant health problems that are neglected in deference to the greater needs of the incapacitated partner. The disabled spouse may need physical care that is beyond the

---

BOX 22-8   CAREGIVER NEEDS

- Finding time for myself
- Keeping the person I care for safe
- Balancing work and family responsibilities
- Managing emotional and physical stress
- Finding easy and satisfying activities to do with the care recipient
- Learning how to talk to physicians
- Making end-of-life decisions
- Moving or lifting the care recipient; bathing and dressing
- Managing the challenging behaviors of the care recipient
- Negotiating health care and home and community-based services
- Managing complex medication schedules or high-tech medical equipment
- Choosing a home health agency, assisted living or skilled nursing facility
- Managing incontinence or toileting problems
- Finding non-English educational material

From Curry L, Walker C, Hogstel MO: *Geriatric Nursing* 27:166, 2006; Family Caregiver Alliance: Caregiver assessment: principles, guidelines and strategies for change, Report from a National Consensus Development Conference (vol 1), San Francisco, 2006, The Alliance.

BOX 22-9   SUGGESTIONS FOR CAREGIVERS

- Educate yourself about the disease or medical condition
- Find a health care professional who understands the disease
- Consult with other experts to help plan for the future (legal, financial)
- Tap your social resources for assistance
- Find a confidante
- Take time for relaxation and exercise
- Use community resources
- Maintain your sense of humor
- Explore religious beliefs and spiritual values
- Set realistic goals

From U.S. Department of Health and Human Services Administration on Aging, National Family Caregiver Support Program Resources: Taking Care of Yourself. Available at www.aoa.gov. Accessed June 28, 2007.

---

capabilities of the spousal caregiver. Spousal caregivers provide more intensive, time-consuming care than other family caregivers, as much as 56 hours of care per week on average. They also are less likely to receive assistance from other family members. Older spouses are at greater risk for negative consequences and often take on greater burdens than they can reasonably handle and wait longer for outside help, using formal services as a last resort. Spousal caregivers are more prone to loneliness, depression, increased risk of stroke (particularly among African-American male caregivers), and have a 63% greater chance of dying than people of the same age who are not caring for spouses (Ostwald, 2009). More wives than husbands provide care, but this is expected to change as life expectancy for men increases.

Older spouses caring for disabled partners also face many role changes. Older women may need to learn to drive, manage money, or make decisions by themselves. Male caregivers may need to learn how to cook, shop, do laundry, and provide personal care to their wives. Spousal caregivers also deal with the added responsibilities of caregiving while at the same time dealing with the anticipated loss of their spouse. Nurses should be alert to situations in which health care personnel may be able to provide supports and resources that make it possible for an individual to assume new responsibilities without being totally overwhelmed. Adult day programs, respite care services, or periodic assistance from a home health aide or homemaker may make it possible for the couple to continue to live together. It is important to pay attention to the physical and mental health needs of the caregiver as well as the care recipient.

Aging Parents Caring for Developmentally Disabled Children

Although we tend to think of caregivers as middle-aged adults caring for elders, an unknown number of elders are caring for their middle-aged children who are physically and mentally disabled. Earlier in the past century, these developmentally disabled children usually died before reaching adulthood; now, with improved care, they are surviving. For the first time in history, individuals with developmental disabilities are outliving their parents.

With increased survival, these adults with developmental disabilities are also at risk for developing chronic illness and will need more care and services. For example, individuals with

Down's syndrome are more likely to develop dementia. Often, the burden of caring for a developmentally disabled child has been carried by parents for their entire adult life and will end only with the death of the parent or the adult child. Parental caregivers who are aging face changes in their financial resources and health that affects their continued caregiving ability.

A major worry is how their child will be cared for if they develop a debilitating illness or when they die. The phenomenon of an aging parent caring for an aging child is beginning to receive attention by both organizations for aging and organizations for developmentally disabled individuals. The Planned Lifetime Assistance Network (PLAN), available in some states through the National Alliance for the Mentally Ill, provides lifetime assistance to individuals with disabilities whose parents or other family members are deceased or can no longer provide for their care (www.nami.org). The Alzheimer's Association and other aging organizations offer education and support programs for both parents and their developmentally disabled adult children in some communities. There is a continued need for more community-based care and housing for developmentally disabled adults who are aging (Hooyman and Kiyak, 2011).

Grandparents Raising Grandchildren

In recent years, more grandparents have become, by default, the primary caregivers of grandchildren because the parents are unable to provide the care needed as a result of child abuse, teen pregnancy, imprisonment, joblessness, military deployment, drug and alcohol addictions, illness, death, and other social problems. Over two million grandparents are providing primary care (custodial grandparents) for grandchildren in the United States. In the United States, 1 out of every 10 children lives with a grandparent, and 41% of those children are being raised primarily by that grandparent. More than two thirds of grandparent primary caregivers are younger than 60 years, and 62% are female. Nearly one in five are living below the poverty line (Livingston and Parker, 2010; Smith et al., 2008). The phenomenon of grandparents serving as primary caregivers is more common among African Americans and Hispanics than whites, but the increase in grandparent primary caregiving across the last decade has been much more pronounced among whites (a 19% increase) (Livingston and Parker, 2010).

Grandparents raising grandchildren is a global phenomenon as well. Although the number of children being raised by grandparents in the United States is significantly high, it is much less than the millions of children in Africa and other developing countries who are raised by grandparents or other relatives. Grandparents in these developing countries face great challenges in providing basic subsistence for their grandchildren, and often for themselves. The Grandmother Project (http://www.grandmotherproject.org/) is a U.S. nonprofit organization working to strengthen the leadership role of grandmothers in improving health for women and children in Laos, Senegal, Mali, Uzbekistan, and Albania. Outcomes of the project include greater confidence among grandmothers, increased community respect for elder women, and improvements in advice to young women on pregnancy, infant feeding, and neonatal health.

Research is lacking related to the physical and mental health consequences of grandparents raising grandchildren, and no clear data are available on the effect of grandparent caregiving on health status (Smith et al., 2008). For many, it is a life-changing decision to dedicate one's life to raising a child at a time in life when one may be looking forward to more leisure and less responsibility. The unexpected career of caregiving for grandchildren and the "off timing" of this family role transition contributes to the challenges faced (Musil et al., 2010).

Often, crisis situations precipitate the decision, and time for preparation is not available. In many cases, grandparents assume care so that their grandchildren's care is not taken over by the public care system (delBene, 2010). As with other types of caregiving, there are both blessings and burdens. Grandparents who are caregivers report that it provides a sense of purpose that keeps them going, and, in some cases, children raised solely by grandparents fare better than those in single-parent families (Roe and Minkler, 1998-1999). The experience of children who have been raised by a grandparent also needs to be investigated.

For many grandparents, however, economic, health, and social challenges associated with caregiving may include limited income and financial support through the welfare system, lack of informal support systems, loss of leisure and social activities in retirement, and shame or guilt related to their children's inability to parent. Too often, both the children and their grandparents are in need of help. Approximately twice as many children cared for by a custodial grandparent have emotional or behavioral problems compared to those in two-parent families. Physical and mental stressors are also greater when grandparents are raising a chronically ill or special-needs child (delBene, 2010; Hooyman and Kiyak, 2011) (Box 22-10). Routine screening and monitoring of the psychological distress of primary care grandparents and offering support, advice, and referral to reduce stressors is important (Smith et al., 2009).

Primary care grandparents with a network of social support seem to experience less negative consequences, but instrumental supports such as assistance with child rearing and finances are often lacking. Resourcefulness has been found to be a

---

🔔 BOX 22-10   RESEARCH HIGHLIGHTS

Grandmothers and Caregiving to Grandchildren: Continuity, Change, and Outcomes

This study examined transitions in caregiving and how the experience of becoming a primary caregiver to grandchildren or having adult children and grandchildren move in or out affects the well-being of the grandmother. Data were collected from 485 grandmothers who participated in the longitudinal study and mailed in questionnaires every 12 over 24 months. The Resiliency Model of Family Stress, Adjustment and Adaptation was the conceptual framework for the study.

Grandmothers raising grandchildren reported the most stress, intrafamily strain, and perceived problems in family functioning, the worst physical health and more depressive symptoms, and the least reward and subjective support. Physical health and stress increased over time. Findings suggest that transitions into a primary grandparent role may be ideal times to provide supportive counseling and anticipatory guidance. The physical and mental health and physical function of primary grandmothers should be monitored and supported during grandparent caregiving. Resourcefulness training may be an effective approach to enhance stress management and improve quality of life.

Source: Musil C, Gordon N, Warner C, et al: *The Gerontologist.* First published online: August 19, 2010.

BOX 22-11 EMPOWERMENT GRANDPARENT PROGRAM: SUGGESTED EDUCATION TOPICS

- Introduction to empowerment
- Children and self-esteem
- Communicating with children
- Dealing with behavior problems
- Talking about sex, HIV, and drugs
- Dealing with loss
- Addressing a child's grief and loss
- Navigating the service system
- Legal and entitlement issues
- Developing advocacy skills
- Getting your message across
- What did we learn?

Source: Cox C: *Social Work* 47:45, 2002.

BOX 22-12 SUGGESTED NURSING INTERVENTIONS WITH GRANDPARENT CAREGIVERS

- Early identification of at-risk grandparents
- Comprehensive assessment of physical, psychosocial, and environmental factors affecting those in the caregiving role for grandchildren
- Anticipatory guidance and counseling about child growth and development and other child-raising issues
- Referral to resources for support, counseling, and financial assistance
- Advocacy for policies supportive of grandparents who have assumed a caregiving role

significant predictor of mental health in studies of primary grandmothers, and interventions to enhance resourcefulness may be helpful (Musil et al., 2009; 2010) (see Chapter 18). Education and training programs and support groups are valuable resources that should be available in communities. Nurses can be instrumental in developing and conducting these types of interventions. The empowerment model of training, developed by Cox (2002), resulted in strengthening parenting skills, self-efficacy, and problem-solving skills in a group of African-American grandparents. The program also resulted in the development of the participants into community peer educators to further empower the communities in which they live (Box 22-11). Other suggestions for nursing interventions with older adults providing primary care to their grandchildren are presented in Box 22-12.

The U.S. government has recognized that increasing numbers of older adults are raising grandchildren, great-grandchildren, and other younger relatives. The Temporary Assistance for Needy Families Program (TANF) provides assistance but is limited to benefits for the child only. No funds are provided for financial support of the grandparent or for child care. Legal options for primary care grandparents include guardianship, custody, adoption, and informal and formal foster parenthood (Hooyman and Kiyak, 2011). However, there is a continued need to develop services that support grandparents as sole caregivers and that attend to the physical and mental health of primary care (custodial) grandparents. In October 2000,

Congress enacted the National Family Caregiver Support Program (NFCSP) under the Older Americans Act. This program provides support services, education and training, counseling, and respite care. Nurses can refer the grandparents to their local area agency on aging to inquire about available resources. Additional resources related to grandparents can be found on the Evolve website.

Long-Distance Caregiving

Because of the increasing mobility of today's society, more children move away from home for education or employment and do not return home. When the parent needs help, it must be provided "long distance." This is perhaps one of the most difficult situations, and it presents unique challenges. The usual impulse is to want to move the elder into the family's home or to a more accessible location for the family, but this may not be best for an elder or for the family. Many factors must be considered, and family communication is essential. Box 22-13 presents factors to consider when planning to add an older person to the household. Plans and alternatives should be discussed before emergency events and may prevent the need for hasty decisions.

Conferring with a geriatric care manager in advance of any evidence of problems may forestall the need to move the parent into the adult child's home. Issues that need to be considered include identifying a local person who will be available quickly in emergency situations; identifying reliable individuals or services that will provide daily monitoring if necessary; identifying acceptable facilities for assisted living if that becomes necessary; determining which family member is most likely to be free to travel to the elder if needed; and being sure that legalities regarding advance directives, a will, and power of attorney (for health care and financial) have been established.

A profession and industry have emerged to assist the geographically distant family member to ensure that an older relative will be cared for. This profession is made up of geriatric care managers, some of whom are nurses or social workers. A care manager can be hired to do everything a family member would do if able, from being available in an emergency, to helping with estate planning, to making arrangements for a move to a nursing home. Often care managers know of resources that can assist the elder to remain independent and yet assure the family that safety and other needs are being met. These services are available primarily to those who are able to pay for them because they are not covered by private insurance, Medicare, or any public agencies. Although these services are expensive, they are far less expensive than alternative living arrangements or institutional placement.

Similar services may be available for persons with very low incomes by asking the local area agency on aging about local "Community Care for the Elderly" programs. Some states also have nursing home diversion projects to provide home support to those who would otherwise qualify for Medicaid coverage for nursing home care. When incomes are too high to qualify for Medicaid and too low to pay for private care managers, the persons and their families must do the best they can. Long-distance care then depends on the goodness of neighbors, local friends, and apartment managers and frequent trips by the long-distance caregiver to the elder.

BOX 22-13   PLANNING TO ADD AN OLDER PERSON TO THE HOUSEHOLD

QUESTIONS YOU NEED TO ASK

- What are the needs of the new member and of the family?
- Where will space be allotted for the new member?
- How will the new member be included in existing family patterns?
- How will responsibilities be shared?
- What resources in the community will assist in the adjustment phase?
- Is the environment safe for the new member?
- How will family life change with the added member, and how does the family feel about it?
- What are the differences in socialization and sleeping patterns?
- What are the older person's strong needs and expectations?
- What are the older person's skills and talents?

MODIFICATIONS YOU NEED TO MAKE

- Arrange semiprivate living quarters if possible.
- Regularly schedule visits to other relatives to give each family time for respite and privacy.
- Arrange adult day health programs and senior activities for the older person to help keep contact with members of his or her own generation. Consider how the older person will feel about giving up familiar surroundings and friends.

DISCUSS POTENTIAL AREAS OF CONFLICT

- Space: especially if someone has given up his or her space to the older relative.
- Possessions: older people may want to move possessions into house; others may not find them attractive or may insist on replacing them with new things.

- Entertaining: times when old and young feel the need or desire to exclude the other from social events.
- Responsibilities and chores: the older person may feel useless if he or she does nothing and may feel in the way if he or she does something; young persons may feel that their position is usurped or may be angry if they wait on the parent.
- Expenses: increased cost of home maintenance, food, clothing, and recreation may not be shared appropriately.
- Vacations: whether to go together or alone; young persons may feel uneasy not taking the older person out and may feel resentful if they must.
- Child rearing: disagreement over child-rearing policies.
- Child care: grandparental babysitting may be welcomed by family and resented by older person, or, if not allowed, older person may feel lack of trust in capability.

DECREASE AREAS OF CONFLICT BY DOING THE FOLLOWING

- Respect privacy.
- Discuss space allocations.
- Discuss elderly person's furnishings before move.
- Make it clear in advance when social events include everyone or exclude someone.
- Make clear decisions about household tasks; all should have responsibility geared to ability.
- Have the older person pay a share of expenses and maintain a separate phone to reduce strain and increase feelings of independence.

PROMOTING HEALTHY AGING: IMPLICATIONS FOR GERONTOLOGICAL NURSING

Nurses are often the primary care providers and care managers for elders and their families both in the home and in the institutional setting. The nurse monitors progress and manages chronic disorders of the elder within the context of the family.

Assessment

Family Assessment   A comprehensive assessment of the elder includes assessment of the family: Who are the members? What is the family history? What are their usual roles and their strengths, contributions, and deterrents to the function of the family unit? Assessing the family's needs and strengths, as well as its sources of stress, particular methods of coping, meaning of caregiving, cultural values, support system, and family dynamics, will help the nurse know the family and design responses that may strengthen the family unit.

Often, nurses see families in times of crisis when an older family member needs care. It is important to encourage the expression of feelings from all involved family members, as well as the older person, and maintain a nonjudgmental attitude. It is important for the nurse to be aware of his or her vision of what a "family" should be and what a "family" should do. Our values should not enter into assessment and intervention with clients. Meiner (2011, p. 113) reminds us that we should not "label families as 'dysfunctional.' It is necessary to identify the strengths within each family and to build on those strengths while recognizing the family's limitations in providing support

and caregiving." Thus, the nurse's role is to teach, monitor, and strengthen the family system so as to maintain health and wellness of the entire family structure.

A mutually constructed, written assessment of a family's needs and coping capacities can be both comprehensive and specific and becomes a document of the family's strengths in times of stress. Including the family in the discussion of the outcome of the assessment is recommended for all settings, especially in long-term care facilities and home care. Table 22-1 presents a family assessment.

Caregiver Assessment   Family members who assume the caregiving role, as just discussed, experience both stressors and benefits. The stresses, expectations of future needs and problems, and the positive aspects of the caregiving situation should be explored. Caregiver assessment includes how the family member can help the care recipient and how the health care team can help the person providing care. In light of the physical and emotional stressors often associated with the caregiving role, nurses need to monitor the physical and emotional health of both the caregiver and the care recipient and provide support as necessary. A partnership model, combining the "nurse's professional expertise with the caregiver's knowledge of the family member, is recommended" (Schumacher et al., 2006, p. 47). A Nursing Standard of Practice Protocol: Family Caregiving (Messecar, 2008) is available at http://consultgerirn.org/topics/family_caregiving/want_to_know_more. Box 22-14 presents a research-based model to guide nursing interventions with caregivers.

Principles to guide caregiver assessment include the following: (1) caregiver assessment should include the needs and preferences of both the care recipient and the family caregiver;

TABLE 22-1	FAMILY SUPPORT SYSTEM ASSESSMENT*
Size	Number in extended family who are accessible
	Number of daughters who are accessible
	Number of sons who are accessible
	Number of grandchildren, nephews, nieces, confidants, siblings
Ability	Economic status of each:
	Poverty
	Lower middle
	Middle
	Upper middle
	Wealthy
Willingness	Frequency of involvement:
	Monthly
	Weekly
	Daily
	Constant
Functions	Contributions to elderly member:
	Money
	Chores
	Transportation
	Listening and psychological support
	Functional assistance
Deterrents	Other demands:
	Work
	Travel
	Adolescent children
Recent stresses	Poor health
	Job change
	Moves
	Deaths

*The strengths and limitations of the family or possible dysfunctional aspects can be assessed in a superficial but helpful manner by using the Family APGAR (Smilkstein G, Ashworth C, Montano D: *Journal of Family Practice* 15:303, 1982).

BOX 22-14	NURSING ACTIONS TO CREATE AND SUSTAIN A PARTNERSHIP WITH CAREGIVERS

- Surveillance and ongoing monitoring
- Coaching: helping caregivers apply knowledge and develop skills
- Teaching: providing information and instruction
- Fostering partnerships: fostering communication and collaboration between the caregiver and the care recipient and between them and the nurse
- Providing psychosocial support: attending to psychosocial well-being
- Rescuing: providing a safety net by stepping in to provide direct care and making clinical decisions
- Coordinating: orchestrating the work of other health care team members and the activities of the caregiver

Data from Eilers J, Heermann JA, Wilson ME, et al: *Oncology Nursing Forum* 32:849, 2005; Schumacher K, Beck CA, Marren JM: *American Journal of Nursing* 106:40, 2006.

TABLE 22-2	RECOMMENDED DOMAINS AND CONSTRUCTS OF CAREGIVER ASSESSMENT

DOMAINS	CONSTRUCTS
Context	Caregiver relationship to care recipient
	Physical environment (home, facility)
	Household status (e.g., number in home)
	Financial status
	Quality of family relationships
	Duration of caregiving
	Employment status (work/home/volunteer)
Caregiver's perception of health and functional status of recipient	Activities of daily living (ADLs) (e.g., bathing, dressing)
	Instrumental activities of daily living (IADLs) (e.g., managing finances, using the telephone)
	Psychosocial needs
	Cognitive impairment
	Behavioral problems
	Medical tests and procedures
Caregiver values and preferences	Caregiver/care recipient willingness to assume/accept care
	Perceived filial obligation to provide care
	Culturally based norms
	Preferences for scheduling and delivering care and services
Well-being of the caregiver	Self-rated health
	Health conditions and symptoms
	Depression or other emotional distress (e.g., anxiety)
	Life satisfaction/quality of life
Consequences of caregiving	Perceived challenges:
	Social isolation
	Work strain
	Emotional and physical health
	Financial strain
	Family relationship strain
	Perceived benefits:
	Satisfaction of helping family member
	Developing new skills and competencies
	Improved family relationships
Skills/abilities/ knowledge to provide recipient with needed care	Caregiving confidence and competencies
	Appropriate knowledge of medical care tasks (e.g., wound care)
Potential resources that caregiver could choose to use	Formal and informal helping network and perceived quality of social support
	Existing or potential strengths (e.g., what is presently going well)
	Coping strategies
	Financial resources (health care and service benefits, entitlements such as Veteran's Affairs, Medicare)
	Community resources and services (caregiver support programs, religious organizations, volunteer agencies)

From Recommended Domains and Constructs, p. 16, Family Caregiver Alliance, 2006: Caregiver assessment: principles, guidelines and strategies for change, Report from a National Consensus Development Conference (vol 1), San Francisco, The Alliance. www.caregiver.org.

(2) caregiver assessment should reflect culturally competent practice; (3) caregiver assessment should be multidimensional and conducted with an interprofessional approach; and (4) caregiver assessment should result in a plan of care developed collaboratively with the caregiver that specifies the provision of services and intended measurable outcomes (Family Caregiver Alliance, 2006). Table 22-2 presents the components of caregiving assessment. Several validated caregiver assessment instruments are available, including the Preparedness for Caregiving Scale and the Mutuality Scale (Archbold et al., 1992), the Caregiver Strain Index developed by Robinson (1983), and the Modified Caregiver Strain Index (http://consultgerirn.org/topics/family_caregiving/want_to_know_more) (Figure 22-1).

Interventions

Research over the past several decades has provided a wealth of information on interventions to support caregivers and improve their health and well-being. The Centers for Disease Control

Directions: Here is a list of things that other caregivers have found to be difficult. Please put a checkmark in the columns that apply to you. We have included some examples that are common caregiver experiences to help you think about each item. Your situation may be slightly different, but the item could still apply.

	Yes, On a Regular Basis=2	Yes, Sometimes =1	No=0
My sleep is disturbed (For example: the person I care for is in and out of bed or wanders around at night)	_____	_____	_____
Caregiving is inconvenient (For example: helping takes so much time or it's a long drive over to help)	_____	_____	_____
Caregiving is a physical strain (For example: lifting in or out of a chair; effort or concentration is required)	_____	_____	_____
Caregiving is confining (For example: helping restricts free time or I cannot go visiting)	_____	_____	_____
There have been family adjustments (For example: helping has disrupted my routine; there is no privacy)	_____	_____	_____
There have been changes in personal plans (For example: I had to turn down a job; I could not go on vacation)	_____	_____	_____
There have been other demands on my time (For example: other family members need me)	_____	_____	_____
There have been emotional adjustments (For example: severe arguments about caregiving)	_____	_____	_____
Some behavior is upsetting (For example: incontinence; the person cared for has trouble remembering things; or the person I care for accuses people of taking things)	_____	_____	_____
It is upsetting to find the person I care for has changed so much from his/her former self (For example: he/she is a different person than he/she used to be)	_____	_____	_____
There have been work adjustments (For example: I have to take time off for caregiving duties)	_____	_____	_____
Caregiving is a financial strain	_____	_____	_____
I feel completely overwhelmed (For example: I worry about the person I care for; I have concerns about how I will manage)	_____	_____	_____

[Sum responses for "Yes, on a regular basis" (2 pts each) and "yes, sometimes" (1 pt each)]

Total Score =

FIGURE 22-1 Modified Caregiver Strain Index. (From Thornton, M., & Travis, S.S. (2003). Analysis of the reliability of the Modified Caregiver Strain Index. *The Journal of Gerontology, Series B, Psychological Sciences and Social Sciences*, 58(2), p. S129. Copyright © The Gerontological Society of America. Reproduced by permission of the publisher.)

and Prevention provide extensive information about putting evidence-based programs into practice (http://www.cdc.gov/aging/caregiving/assuring.htm). As part of the Affordable Health Care Act, $68 million in grants are to be awarded to states, territories, tribal, and community-based organizations to help older people and their caregivers better understand and navigate their health and long-term care options.

Intervention programs should include risk assessment, education about caregiving and stress, caregiver health and home safety, support groups, linkages to ongoing telephone or e-mail support, counseling, resource identification, and stress management. Linking caregivers to community resources, such as respite care, adult day programs, and financial support resources, are important. Respite care allows the caregiver to take a break from caregiving for various periods of time. Respite care may be provided in institutions, in the home, or in other community settings. Nurses should be aware of respite care resources in their communities and the local Area Agency on Aging can provide information on respite care and other caregiver services. These interventions, when available, can alleviate much of the stress of caregiving.

With many caregivers trying to balance caregiving responsibilities while still working, educational programs offered in the workplace can be beneficial for both the caregiver and the employer (Curry et al., 2006). Box 22-15 presents suggested topics for programs Chapter 29 dicusses caregiving for individuals with dementia. Additional resources related to caregiver education and support programs can be found on the Evolve website.

Interventions with caregivers must always consider the great variability in family structures, resources, traditions, and history. The range of adaptations is enormous, and the goal is always to restore the balance of the system to the greatest extent possible and support caregivers in their caring. The family can be visualized as a mobile with many parts, and when one part is touched,

---

BOX 22-15   TOPICS FOR WORKPLACE CAREGIVER ASSISTANCE PROGRAMS

- Normal and healthy aging
- Communicating effectively with older adults
- Medication use
- Caring for the caregiver
- Specific health information
- Community resources
- Supplemental services
- Housing and long-term care options
- Medicare, Medigap, and other insurance (e.g., long-term care)
- Support groups
- End-of-life and legal information (e.g., advance directives)

From Curry L, Walker C, Hogstel MO: *Geriatric Nursing* 27:166, 2006.

---

each part shifts to regain the balance. The intrusion of professionals in a family system will temporarily unbalance the system and may provide an opportunity to restore the balance in a healthier manner, sometimes by adding an element or increasing the weight of one or decreasing the weight of another.

When the nurse works with a family from a different culture that may have rituals and routines unfamiliar to him or her, the nurse needs to be particularly careful to respect these differences. The nurse can work with the family to make the best use of their strengths, whatever they may be. Each family member can be valued for what he or she brings to the situation.

"Family members must not be allowed to 'fail' while providing care; a nurse should be available to step in when demands of the situation exceed family members' capabilities. And the nurse should be prepared to step back when the family's support is what's needed" (Schumacher, 2006, p. 48).

---

evolve   To access your student resources, go to *http://evolve.elsevier.com/Ebersole/TwdHlthAging*

KEY CONCEPTS

- Roles define individual and societal expectations of function.
- Ability to successfully negotiate transitions and develop new and gratifying roles depends on personal and environmental supports, timing, clarity of expectations, personality, and degree of change required.
- Numerous patterns of retirement exist, and therefore retirement per se cannot be viewed categorically.
- Pre-retirement planning and post-retirement follow-up significantly affect positive adaptation to the transition.
- Elders and their family members carry a long history. Current family dynamics must be understood within the context of family history.

- Loss of a spouse is the role change that has the greatest potential for life disruption, and nursing support can make a significant positive difference in the transition.
- Widowers are a neglected group in the literature and in the service arena. These men are particularly vulnerable to physical and mental stress.
- Family members and other unpaid caregivers provide 80% of care for older adults in the United States.
- Caregiving activities are one of the most major social issues of our time as well as a significant public health problem.
- Grandparents are increasingly assuming primary caregiving roles with grandchildren.

CASE STUDY RETIREMENT

Sandy was a professor at a small, private college in a metropolitan area. Although she had taught nursing for 25 years and loved her work, it had been a demanding year, and she was very tired. A rumor had recently circulated that the college was in trouble financially. Some of the most affluent alumni could no longer be counted on for gifts and endowments because the football coach had not produced a winning team for several years. Because the tuition was becoming exorbitant, the college had recently lost some students to one of the three state college campuses within driving distance of the city. The trustees of the college, in a move to cut expenses, offered an incentive to professors who were willing to retire early; an extra year of service credit was presented for every six years worked. Sandy was only 55 years old but thought that the 4 years of extra credit would bring her near the minimum retirement age for Social Security (an error, of course, because her age did not change with her service credit). Rather impulsively, Sandy decided to accept the offer after telling colleagues, "Well, you know how I love to travel. Why wait until I'm too old to enjoy retirement? Why don't you think about the offer, too? This is a once-in-a-lifetime opportunity." Near the end of the academic year, the celebrations began: recognition, plaques, expressions of gratitude from students, and envy from her associates. The send-off was wonderful. In the summer, Sandy withdrew her savings and booked a cruise to the Greek islands. The journey was lovely, and she enjoyed every moment. Sandy began to feel depressed when she got off the ship but knew it was only because the elegant cruise was over. However, as fall came around, Sandy began to feel more depressed. Most of her friends were teachers, and they were all back at work. Sandy briefly thought of going to Pittsburgh to visit her sister but decided against the idea because she and her sister had really never been very compatible. Then Sandy was hit with some of the realities of early retirement: she was unable to withdraw any of her considerable tax-deferred savings before she was 59 and a half years of age without significant penalty, her health insurance coverage was considerably less comprehensive after retirement, her colleagues were all busy, and she was very bored. Then the real blow fell. The college, in desperation, had dipped into the retirement funds to remain solvent, and the retirees' pensions were now at risk. Sandy's sister, who was a nurse, called to announce that she wanted to come and stay a few days while she attended a conference in the city. When she arrived, Sandy overwhelmed her with the litany of woes. If you were Sandy's sister, what would you do?

Based on the case study, develop a nursing care plan using the following procedure*:
- List Sandy's comments that provide subjective data.
- List information that provides objective data.
- From these data, identify and state, using accepted format, two nursing diagnoses you determine are most significant to Sandy at this time. List two of Sandy's strengths that you have identified from the data.
- Determine and state outcome criteria for each diagnosis. These criteria must reflect some alleviation of the problem identified in the nursing diagnosis and must be stated in concrete and measurable terms.
- Plan and state one or more interventions for each diagnosed problem. Provide specific documentation of the source used to determine the appropriate intervention. Plan at least one intervention that incorporates Sandy's existing strengths.
- Evaluate the success of the intervention. Interventions must correlate directly with the stated outcome criteria to measure the outcome success.

CRITICAL THINKING QUESTIONS

1. Identify several important family and social roles that elder members of your family fulfill.
2. What are the factors to consider in role transitions, and how can transitions be made smoother?
3. What factors must be considered in the decision to retire?
4. Discuss the differences you would expect in adaptation to retirement between an individual who retired because of ill health and one who retired because he or she desired to do so.
5. How do you think retirement differs for men and women?
6. Describe what you think would be an ideal retirement.
7. Plan specific ways in which you would present a retirement seminar to workers in a computer microchip factory.
8. Explain the major issues in adaptation to a major role change, such as retirement and widowhood.
9. Discuss how you think an individual can prepare for widowhood.
10. Discuss the meanings and the thoughts triggered by the young person's and elder's viewpoints expressed at the beginning of the chapter. How do these vary from your own experience?

*Students are advised to refer to their nursing diagnosis text and identify possible or potential problems.

RESEARCH QUESTIONS

1. What are the challenges associated with older people working longer?
2. What are the patterns of adaptation of widowers? How do the patterns differ for young-old and old-old?
3. Who divorces in later life and for what reasons?
4. What are the differences between grandparenting and great-grandparenting?
5. Are there differences in the experience of primary grandparent caregivers based on ethnicity, race, and culture?
6. How do adults who were raised by grandparents view this experience?
7. Do interventions to improve the physical health of caregivers relate to less reported stress and improved health outcomes?
8. What are the reactions of elders to the care given by their offspring?

REFERENCES

Administration on Aging: Profile of Older Americans, Washington, DC, 2008.

American Association of Retired Persons: Grandparents increasingly fill need as caregivers. Available at http://www.aarp.org/relationships/grandparenting/news-09-2010/grandparents_increasingly_fill_need_as_caregivers.html. Accessed October 18, 2010.

American Association of Retired Person Public Policy Institute: Fact sheet: multigenerational householder are increasing, Fact sheet 221, April 2011.

Archbold PG, Stewart BJ, Greenlick MR, et al: Mutuality and preparedness as predictors of caregiver role strain, *Research in Nursing and Health* 13:375, 1990.

Archbold PG, Stewart BJ, Greenlick MR, et al: The clinical assessment of mutuality and preparedness in family caregivers to frail older people. In Funk SG, Tornquist EM,

Champagne MT et al., editors: *Key aspects of elder care: managing falls, incontinence, and cognitive impairment*, New York, 1992, Springer.

Centers for Disease Control and Prevention and the Kimberly-Clark Corporation: *Assuring Healthy Caregivers, A Public Health Approach to Translating Research into Practice: The RE-AIM Framework*. Neenah, WI, 2008, Kimberly-Clark Corporation. Available at www.cdc.gov/aging/caregiving/assuring.htm. Accessed October 16, 2010.

Cox C: Empowering African American Custodial Grandparents, *Social Work* 47:45, 2002.

Curry LC, Walker C, Hogstel MO: Educational needs of employed family caregivers of older adults: evaluation of a workplace project, *Geriatric Nursing* 27:166, 2006.

Delaney S, Delaney E: *Having our say: the Delaney sisters' first 100 years*, New York, 1993, Kodansha International.

DelBene S: African American grandmothers raising grandchildren: A phenomenological perspective of marginalized women, *Journal of Gerontological Nursing* 36:32, 2010.

deVries B: Grief: intimacy's reflection, *Generations* 25:75, 2001.

Family Caregiver Alliance: *Caregiver Assessment: Principles, Guidelines and Strategies for Change*. Report from a National Consensus Development Conference (Vol. I). San Francisco: The alliance, 2006.

Federal Interagency Forum on Aging: Older Americans 2010: Key indicators of well-being. Available at http://www.agingstats.gov/agingstatsdotnet/Main_Site/Data/2010_Documents/Docs/OA_2010.pdf. Accessed October 16, 2010.

Gelo F: Invisible individuals—LGBT elders, *Aging Well* 1:36, 2008.

Hooyman N, Kiyak H: *Social gerontology: A multidisciplinary perspective*, ed 9, Boston, 2011, Allyn & Bacon.

Institute of Medicine: Retooling for an aging America: Building the healthcare workforce, 2008. Available at http://www.iom.edu/Reports/2008/Retooling-for-an-Aging-America-Building-the-Health-Care-Workforce.aspx. Accessed June 7, 2010.

Jett KF: Making the connection: seeking and receiving help by elderly African Americans, *Qualitative Health Research* 12:373, 2002.

Legacy Project: Fast facts on grandparenting and intergenerational mentoring. Available at www.legacyproject.org/specialreports/fastfacts.html. Accessed October 16, 2010.

Lindemann E: Symptomatology and management of acute grief, *American Journal of Psychiatry* 101:141, 1944.

Livingston G, Parker K: Since the start of the great recession, more children raised by grandparents. Available at http://pewresearch.org/pubs/1724/sharp-increase-children-with-grandparents-caregivers. Accessed October 16, 2010.

Lowenthal MF, Haven C: Interaction and adaptation: intimacy as a critical variable, *American Sociological Review* 33:20, 1968.

Lund M: Caregiver, take care, *Geriatric Nursing* 26:152, 2005.

Meiner S: *Gerontological nursing*, ed 4, St Louis, 2011, Mosby.

Messecar D: Family Caregiving: Nursing Standard of Practice Protocol, Hartford Institute for Geriatric Nursing, Want to Know More, January 2008. Available at http://consultgerirn.org/topics/family_caregiving/want_to_know_more. Accessed November 7, 2010.

Minton M, Barron C: Spousal bereavement assessment: A review of bereavement-specific measures, *Journal of Gerontological Nursing* 34:34, 2008.

Musil C, Warner C, Zauszniewski J, et al: Grandmother caregiving, family stress and strain, and depressive symptoms, *Western Journal of Nursing Research* 31:389, 2009.

Musil C, Gordon N, Warner C, et al: Grandmothers and caregiving to grandchildren: continuity, change, and outcomes over 24 months, *The Gerontologist*. First published online: August 19, 2010.

National Family Caregivers Association: Caregiving statistics. Available at http://www.thefamilycaregiver.org/about_nfca/. Accessed October 16, 2010.

Livingston G, Parker K: Since the start of the great recession, more children raised by grandparents. Available at http://pewresearch.org/pubs/1724/sharp-increase-children-with-grandparent-caregivers. Accessed October 16, 2010.

Ostwald S: Who is caring for the caregiver? Promoting spousal caregiver's health, *Family and Community Health* 32:S5, 2009.

Pinquart M, Sorensen S: Ethnic differences in stressors, resources, and psychological outcomes of family caregiving: a meta-analysis, *Gerontologist* 45:90, 2005.

Robinson B: Validation of a Caregiver Strain Index, *Journal of Gerontology* 38:344, 1983.

Robison J, Fortinsky R, Kelppinger A, et al: A broader view of family caregiving: effects of caregiving and caregiver conditions on depressive symptoms, health, work, and social isolation, *Journals of Gerontology Series B: Psychological Sciences and Social Sciences* 64B:768, 2009.

Roe KM, Minkler M: Grandparents raising grandchildren: challenges and responses, *Generations* 22:25, 1998-1999.

Schulz R, Beach SR: Caregiving as a risk factor for mortality: the caregiver health effects study, *Journal of the American Medical Association* 262:2215, 1999.

Schumacher K, Beck CA, Marren JM: Family caregivers: caring for older adults, working with their families, *American Journal of Nursing* 106:40, 2006.

Siefert M, Williams A, Dowd M, et al: The caregiving experience in a racially diverse sample of cancer family caregivers, *Cancer Nursing* 31:399, 2008.

Silverstein M, Angelli J: Older parents' expectations of moving closer to their children, *Journal of Gerontology* 53B:S153, 1998.

Skarupski K, McCann J, Bienias J, et al: Race differences in emotional adaptation of family caregivers, *Aging & Mental Health* 13:715, 2009.

Smith G, Palmieri P, Hancock G, et al: Custodial grandmothers' psychological distress, dysfunctional parenting, and grandchildren's adjustment, *International Journal of Aging & Human Development* 67:327, 2008.

Stanford P, Usita P: Retirement: who is at risk? *Generations* 26:45, 2002.

Touhy TA: Nurturing hope and spirituality in the nursing home, *Holistic Nursing Practice* 15:45, 2001.

U.S. Department of Health and Human Service, Office of Disease Prevention and Health Promotion: *Healthy People 2020 Frameworks: Phase 1 report: recommendations for the framework and format of Healthy People 2020* (2010). Available at http://www.healthypeople.gov. Accessed December 2010.

CHAPTER

23

Loss, Death, and Palliative Care

Kathleen Jett

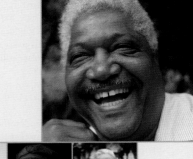

evolve *http://evolve.elsevier.com/Ebersole/TwdHlthAging*

A STUDENT SPEAKS

When I started nursing school I was so afraid that I would have to take care of someone who was dying—or maybe even died! Then I found out that to share that time before death with a person is a special privilege.   **Ana, age 20**

AN ELDER SPEAKS

When we were in our 60s, my friends and I met over cards, went on trips, and experienced all of the joys of retirement. We didn't have much time to worry about aches and pains. In our 70s we had less time to play because we were busy visiting one another in the hospital or in nursing homes. In our 80s we met frequently again, but it was usually at our friends' funerals, leaving little time for cards or travel. Now that I am in my 90s, hardly any of my friends are still alive; you know it gets kind of lonely, so you just have to make new younger friends!   **Theresa, age 93**

LEARNING OBJECTIVES

On completion of this chapter, the reader will be able to:

1. Compare and contrast the needs of elders in response to varying types of losses.
2. Differentiate different types of grief and the needs of the griever.
3. Discuss the attributes of the nurse that are needed to provide the highest quality of care to those experiencing loss or death.
4. Discuss the benefits and limitations of the available conceptual frameworks for dying and grieving.
5. Identify aspects of palliative care in which there is a special need to work within the cultural boundaries.
6. Develop interventions that will enhance coping and the reestablishment of equilibrium within the family.
7. Differentiate among the types of advance directives, and explain the role and responsibilities of the nurse as they relate to each of them.
8. Determine the legal status of Death with Dignity laws for the state in which the nurse practices.
9. Discuss the pros and cons of active and passive euthanasia.

LOSS, GRIEF, AND BEREAVEMENT

Loss, dying, and death are universal, incontestable events of the human experience. With age, the number of losses increases. Some of these are associated with the normal changes with aging, such as the loss of flexibility in the joints, and some are related to the normal changes in everyday life and life transitions, such as moving and retirement. Other losses are those of loved ones through death. Some deaths are considered normative and expected, such as that of older parents. The death of adult children or grandchildren is considered non-normative and always unexpected.

Regardless of that which is lost, each one has the potential to trigger grief and the process we call bereavement or *mourning*. Only the person facing the loss can determine its meaning. The terms *grief, bereavement,* and *mourning* are commonly used interchangeably. However, grief is an individual's response to a loss. Bereavement is an active and evolving process as one copes with grief. Mourning includes those behaviors used to incorporate the loss into one's life. Mourning behaviors are influenced by social norms and defined in cultural norms that proscribe the appropriate ways of both reacting to the loss and coping with it, such as wearing black in many traditions or covering the mirrors and windows and "sitting shiva" in Jewish traditions.

Although there are well-defined cultural expectations in response to loss through death, no guidelines exist for behavior when the loss is of another type. For example, there is a loss of autonomy when one can no longer care for oneself, the loss of the long-time companionship of a pet, or perhaps even self-esteem as one copes with physical changes.

One loss and its accompanying grief may be superimposed on others such as relocation, a shrinking support network, economic changes, or role change. This phenomenon can lead to a continual state of grieving, known as bereavement overload. No sooner has the individual begun to grieve for one loss, and then another occurs, and so forth. When the losses accumulate in quick succession, the griever may become incapacitated and require careful and skilled support and guidance.

This chapter addresses grief as a response to loss, the needs of the person with life-limiting conditions, and the provision of palliative care. Loss is considered broadly to include anything that has meaning to the person. The purpose of this chapter is to provide gerontological nurses the basic information needed to promote effective grieving and good and appropriate deaths. It further provides a background to palliative care.

GRIEF WORK

Researchers have tried for years to understand the grieving process, resulting in a number of proposed models and theories to explain and predict the human response. Elisabeth Kübler-Ross is best known for describing what have become known as the [emotional] stages of dying (1969). Other notable theorists looked specifically at the grieving process; these include Rando (1995), Worden (2009), Corr (2000), and Doka (1989). The models evolved between the 1960s and 1990s and strongly influence what nurses, physicians, other health care professionals, and society in general have been taught about grieving and dying. Although intended to describe physical death and related grief, we propose that these same models can be applied to grieving of any of the losses in the lives of older adults that are considered significant or meaningful, from anticipating the loss of self to that of others.

A Loss Response Model

Regardless of the theorist, grief is described as a process that has a beginning with physical and psychological manifestations; a middle, when the griever's day-to-day functioning may be affected; and an end, when the individual emerges refocused and has adjusted to the loss. Influenced by esteemed psychiatrist Avery Weisman (1979) and building on the work of thanatological scholars and that of the nurse Barbara Giacquinta (1977), a systems approach is proposed to both understand the grieving process and design nursing interventions to provide comfort and support to those who have experienced or are experiencing a loss. In the Loss Response Model, the family and the person as grievers are viewed as a system that strives to maintain equilibrium (Figure 23-1). A systems approach lends itself to an understandable and usable model of the grieving process from which nursing interventions are easily developed.

From the perspective of this model, when loss occurs within the system, the impact is experienced as a state of disequilibrium. The system is in chaos; either the person or family

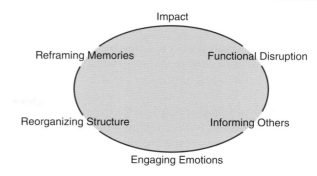

FIGURE 23-1 The loss response model. (Adapted from Giacquinta B: Helping families face the crisis of cancer, *American Journal of Nursing* 77:1585, 1977.)

members are acutely grieving and functional disruption ensues (that is, the usual patterns of the system are disturbed), with the result that dysfunction interferes with usual day-to-day activities. The loss seems unreal. The first step toward reestablishing equilibrium is to attempt to make sense of the chaos. The family or individual then searches for meaning: why did this happen to us? How will we survive the loss? If an elder is responding to the loss of a child or a grandchild, thoughts of "why wasn't it me?" are common. The next step toward equilibrium is movement toward integration of the loss. The griever(s) informs others. Each time the story is repeated, the loss becomes more real, and the system begins movement toward a new steady state. Informing others involves engaging emotions that may have been previously withheld or subdued because of the shock of the impact. The engagement of emotions serves as the threads upon which the system can be stabilized. The expression of emotions can release energy that can be used to reorganize the family structure. As roles change, adaptation and accommodation are necessary. Someone else steps in to perform the roles of the person who is now unable to do so is absent. For example, when the elder patriarch dies, the eldest son may step up and assume some of his father's roles and responsibilities. Finally, if the system is to survive, it will need to redefine itself. One of the ways that it does this is by reframing its memories. Families accept that family portraits and reunions are still possible, just different from how they were before the loss, or they accept that a person can still be vital, active, and important even after the loss of the ability to drive a car, to walk unassisted, or to live alone.

Types of Grief

Grieving takes enormous amounts of physical and emotional energy. It is the hardest thing anyone can do and may be especially hard for those who are accumulating losses, as one does with aging, or face multiple losses at the same time, such as following a catastrophic event. The most common types of grief are anticipatory, acute, chronic, and complicated. Another type, disenfranchised or unspeakable grief, may be occurring and hidden but nonetheless can be quite significant.

Anticipatory Grief

Anticipatory grief is the response to a real or perceived loss before it occurs—a dress rehearsal, so to speak. One observes grief in preparation for a potential loss, such as loss of belongings (e.g., selling a home), moving (e.g., into a nursing home), or knowing that a body part or function is going to change (e.g., a mastectomy), or in anticipation of the death of a loved one. Behaviors that may signal anticipatory grief include preoccupation with the particular loss, unusually detailed planning, or a sudden change in attitude toward the thing or person to be lost.

If the loss is certain but the timing is either uncertain or it does not occur when or as expected, those awaiting the loss may become irritable or impatient, not because they want the loss to occur but in response to the emotional ups and downs of the waiting. Glaser and Strauss (1968) describe what they call an interruption in the sentimental order of a nursing unit when this occurs—no one quite knows how to behave. Family and friends as well as professional grievers, such as nurses, usually deal much more easily with known losses at a known time or in a set manner (Glaser and Strauss, 1968). Some individuals feel more in control of the situation because anticipatory grief facilitates planning and preparation for death by saying good-byes in special ways (Zilberfein, 1999).

Anticipatory grief also can result in the phenomenon of premature detachment from an individual who is dying or detachment of the dying person from the environment. Pattison (1977) calls this premature withdrawal of others *sociological death* and premature withdrawal from loved ones prior to death *psychological death*. In either case, the person who is dying is no longer involved in day-to-day activities of living and essentially suffers a premature death.

Acute Grief

Acute grief is a crisis. It has a definite syndrome of somatic and psychological symptoms of distress that occur in waves lasting varying periods of time. These symptoms may occur every time the loss is acknowledged, others are informed, or another person offers condolences. Preoccupation with the loss is a phenomenon similar to daydreaming and is accompanied by a sense of unreality. Depending on the situation, feelings of self-blame or guilt may be present and manifest themselves as hostility or anger toward usual friends, depressive signs, or withdrawal.

It is often difficult for persons who are acutely grieving to accomplish their usual activities of daily living or meeting other responsibilities *(functional disruption)*. Even if the tasks are accomplished, the person may complain of feeling distracted, restless, and "at loose ends." Common, simple activities, such as dressing, that normally take a few minutes may take much longer. Deciding which clothing to wear may seem too complex a task. Fortunately, the signs and symptoms of acute grief do not last forever, or none of us could survive. Acute grief will be the most intense in the months immediately after the loss, with the intensity of feelings lessening over time. Acute grief is experienced at a national or global level after catastrophic events, such as the attack of the World Trade Centers in New York City or the Indonesian tsunami.

Chronic Grief

Grieving takes time, sometimes much longer than anyone anticipates. In most cases, the acute grief comes to some resolution as memories are reframed. For many, there is a lingering sadness

---

BOX 23-1 SHADOW GRIEF

I was browsing through an art show and saw several beautiful carved, wooden birds. My mother collected them, and I knew she would like them. I turned to point them out to her. But she wasn't there, but for that fleeting moment it felt as if she was at my side. Only she had died about 10 years earlier. I stopped and thought about how much I loved her and how much I wished I could be sharing that moment with her. Then I moved on to the next booth, and she was gone.

Kathleen Jett

---

referred to as shadow grief (Horacek, 1991). It may temporarily inhibit some activity but is considered a normal response. The intermittent pain of grief may be triggered by anniversary dates (birthdays, holidays, anniversaries) or by sensory stimuli, such as the smell of perfume, a color, or a sound (Box 23-1). For the survivors of major tragedies, war, or crime, the "shadows" may never completely go away. Persons may deal with this response to their loss in many different ways. Each year, individuals visit the Vietnam War Memorial in Washington, D.C., to remember and leave items that connect them to those who have died. Similarly, individuals make pilgrimages to the Wailing Wall in Jerusalem, praying and placing prayer papers in the crevices of the wall. In Mexico, the annual holiday "Day of the Dead" is a time when people visit the graves of their family members, leave food, grieve anew, and feel a renewed sense of connection with those who have died before them. These practices may instead be considered healthy and restorative for those who participate. Other chronic grief is a form of complicated grieving.

Complicated Grief

Some chronic grief is more than that of shadow and crosses over the boundary to what we call complicated grief. It has been thought that complicated grief begins with chronic, uncomplicated grief but that obstacles interfere with its evolution toward adjustment, so that the *reestablishment of equilibrium* is distrubed. The memories resist being reframed for many months and even years. Issues of guilt, anger, and ambivalence toward the individual who has died are factors that will impede the grieving process until these issues are resolved. Reactions are exaggerated and memories are experienced as recurrent acute grief—repeatedly, months and years later. Signs of possible complicated grief include excessive and irrational anger, outbursts in social settings, and insomnia that lingers for an extended time or surfaces months or years later. The grief may also trigger a major depressive episode. Cognitive difficulties that accompany a major depressive episode may be misinterpreted as dementia in the very frail and result in inappropriate treatment. This type of grief requires the professional intervention of a grief counselor, a psychiatric nurse practitioner, or a psychologist who is skilled in helping grieving elders (Corless, 2006).

Disenfranchised Grief

The person whose loss cannot be openly acknowledged or publicly mourned experiences what is called *disenfranchised* or *unspeakable grief*. The grief is socially disallowed or unsupported (Doka, 1989). The person does not have a socially recognized right to be perceived or function as a bereaved person. In other words, a relationship is not recognized; the loss is not sanctioned; or the griever is not recognized. Disenfranchised grief has frequently been associated with domestic partnerships (e.g., same-sexed partner) and marriages (e.g., bi-racial), in which the family of the deceased does not acknowledge the partner, or in secret relationships (e.g., extra-marital), in which the involved party cannot tell others of the meaning or depth of the attachment. Disenfranchised grief can also occur in situations of family discord, in which a member of the family is considered the "black sheep." An unspeakable grief may follow a suicide or death due to AIDS. The person in late life can experience disenfranchised grief when family or friends do not understand the full meaning, for example, of a retiree's retirement, the death of a pet, or gradual losses caused by chronic conditions. Families coping with a member who has Alzheimer's disease may also experience disenfranchised grief when others perceive the death of the elder as a blessing and fail to support the griever or caregiver who has struggled for years with anticipatory grief and now must cope with the actual death.

Factors Affecting Coping with Loss

In the language of the *Loss Response Model*, coping with loss is the ability to move from a state of chaos and disequilibrium to one of reorder, equilibrium, and peace. Many factors affect the ability to cope with loss and grief (Box 23-2).

Psychiatrist Avery Weisman found that those who are more likely to effectively deal with loss are "good copers" (1979, p. 42-43). These are individuals or families who have experience with the successful management of crisis. They are resourceful, and they are able to draw on techniques that have worked in the past. These individuals or families do the following:

- Avoid avoidance
- Confront realities, and take appropriate action
- Focus on solutions
- Redefine problems
- Consider alternatives
- Have good communication with others
- Seek and use constructive help
- Accept support when offered
- Can keep up their morale

In other words, the persons who cope with loss most effectively are those who can acknowledge the loss and try to make sense of it. They can maintain composure, use generally good judgment, and can remain optimistic without denying the loss. Good copers seek guidance when it is needed.

On the contrary, those who cope less effectively have few, if any, of these abilities. They tend to be more rigid, pessimistic, and demanding, and they experience emotional extremes. They are more likely to be dogmatic and expect perfection from themselves and others. Ineffective copers are also more likely to live alone, socialize little, and have few close friends or have an ineffective support network. They may have a history of mental illness, or they may have guilt, anger, and ambivalence toward the individual who has died or that which has been lost. Those at risk for pathological grief will more likely have unresolved past conflicts or be facing the loss at the same time as other secondary stressors. They will have fewer opportunities as a result of the loss. They are the elders who are most in need of the expert interventions of grief counselors and skilled gerontological nurses.

PROMOTING HEALTHY AGING: IMPLICATIONS FOR GERONTOLOGICAL NURSING

Loss, grief, and death are parts of the lives of all and occur with increasing frequency as one ages. The goal of the gerontological nurse is not to prevent grief but to support those who are grieving and coping with loss. Although the acute emotions associated with loss will go away, the potential long-term detrimental effects can be ameliorated. While promoting healthy aging, the nurse works with grieving elders as part of the normal workday; this is both a privilege and a responsibility. It is one of the few areas in nursing in which small actions can make

---

BOX 23-2 FACTORS INFLUENCING THE GRIEVING PROCESS

PHYSICAL
Number of concurrent medical conditions
Use of sedatives (delays, does not lessen grief)
Nutritional state, if inadequate, reduces the ability to cope or meet demands of daily living; Inadequate rest can lead more quickly to mental and physical exhaustion
Exercise, if inadequate, limits emotional outlet; may increase aggressive feelings, tension, and anxiety

PSYCHOLOGICAL
Unique nature and meaning of loss
Individual coping behavior, personality, and mental health
Individual level of maturity and intelligence
Previous experience with loss or death
Social, cultural, ethnic, religious, or philosophic background
Sex-role conditioning
Immediate circumstances surrounding loss
Timeliness of the loss
Perception of preventability (sudden vs. expected)

Perceived importance of the loss or relationship to that which is lost
Number, type, and quality of secondary losses
Presence of concurrent stresses or crises

SOCIAL
Individual support systems and the acceptance of assistance of its members
Individual sociocultural, ethnic, religious, or philosophic background
Educational, economic, and occupational status
Ritual

SPECIFIC TO DYING AND DEATH (IN ADDITION TO THE ABOVE)
Role that the deceased occupied in family or social system
Amount of unfinished business
Perception of deceased's fulfillment in life
Immediate circumstances surrounding death
Length of illness before death
Anticipatory grief and involvement with dying patient

From Beare PG, Myers JL: *Adult health nursing*, ed 3, St Louis, 1998, Mosby.

BOX 23-3 ASSESSMENT OF THE DYING PATIENT AND FAMILY

PATIENT
Age
Gender
Coping styles and abilities
Social, cultural, ethnic background
Previous experience with illness, pain, deterioration, loss, grief
Mental health
Lifestyle
Fulfillment of life goals
Amount of unfinished business
The nature of the illness (death trajectory, problems particular to the illness, treatment, amount of pain)
Time passed since diagnosis
Response to illness
Knowledge about the illness or disease
Acceptance or rejection of the diagnosis
Amount of striving for dependence or independence
Feelings and fears about illness
Comfort in expressing thoughts and feelings and how much is expressed
Location of the patient (home, hospital, nursing home)
Relationship with each member of the family and significant other since diagnosis
Family rules, norms, values, and past experiences that might inhibit grief or interfere with a therapeutic relationship

FAMILY
Family makeup (members of family)
Developmental stage of the family
Existing subsystems
Specific roles of each member
Geographic proximity

CHARACTERISTICS OF THE FAMILY SYSTEM
How flexible or rigid
Type of communication
Rules, norms, expectations
Values, beliefs
Quality of emotional relationships
Dependence, interdependence, freedom of each member
How close to or disengaged from the dying member
Established extrafamilial interactions
Strengths and vulnerabilities of the family
Style of leadership and decision-making
Unusual methods of problem solving, crisis resolution
Family resources (personal, financial, community)
Current problems identified by the family
Quality of communication with the caregivers
Immediate and long-range anticipated needs

From Hess PA: Loss, grief, and dying. In Beare P, Myers J: *Adult health nursing*, ed 3, St Louis, 1998, Mosby.

---

a large difference in the quality of life for the persons to whom we provide care.

Assessment

The goal of the grief assessment is to differentiate those who are likely to cope effectively from those who are less likely so that appropriate interventions can be planned (Box 23-3). A grief assessment is based on knowledge of the grieving process. Data are obtained through observation of behavior of the individual in the context of gender and culture (Goldstein et al., 2004).

A thorough grief assessment includes questions about spiritual or existential needs, such as recent significant life events, and the relationship to that which has been or will be lost. How many other stressful or demanding events or circumstances are going on in the griever's life? Information about concurrent life stresses will help determine the intensity of support needed and the risk for complicated grieving. The nurse determines what stress management techniques are normally used and if they have been helpful (e.g., talking it out) or detrimental (e.g., substance abuse) in the past. Are usual support systems available? Was the griever's identity closely tied to that which is lost, such as a lifelong athlete who is faced with never walking again? If the loss is of a partner, how was the relationship? The loss of an abusive or controlling partner may liberate the survivor, who may feel guilty for not feeling the amount of grief they or others expect. For many older women who depended on their spouses financially, death may leave them impoverished, significantly complicating their grief. A survivor may be suddenly homeless after the loss of a domestic partner in jurisdictions in which such relationships are unrecognized. Knowing more about the loss and the effect of the loss on the elder's life will enable the nurse to construct and implement appropriate and caring responses.

Interventions

Therapeutic communication, a basic nursing skill, is the cornerstone of gerontological nursing, end-of-life care, and palliative care. This includes knowing what to say and when to listen. At all times, communication begins with gently establishing rapport. Nurses introduce themselves and explain their roles (e.g., charge nurse, staff nurse, medication nurse) and the time they will be available.

Loss Response Model

If it is the time of *impact* (e.g., just after a new serious diagnosis, at the death of a family member, or as a new but resistant resident of a long-term care facility), nurses can provide support and a safe environment ensuring that basic needs, such as meals or rest, are met. While it is tempting to give advice at this time, it is more therapeutic to provide a grieving person permission to express feelings. The nurse can soften the despair by fostering reasonable hope, such as, "You will make it through one moment at a time, and I will be here to help."

Nurses observe for functional disruption and offer support and direction in the immediate postcrisis period. They may have to help the family figure out what needs to be done immediately and find ways to do it—the nurse either offers to complete the task or finds a friend or family member who can step in so the disruption does not have any deleterious effects and movement toward equilibrium is possible.

As grievers search for meaning, they may need help finding what they are looking for and spend time talking it out. Sometimes what they are looking for is information about a disease, a situation, or a person, and the nurse can assist in obtaining the information whenever possible. Talking it out requires active listening when grievers are trying to make sense of the loss and find meaning in it, questioning their values, and constructing new ones to account for the change in their reality.

The expressions of grief and emotion, be they moments of panic or hysteria, and sharing them with others help make the grief less frightening. The nurse can help the person "feel it out." Feeling it out is a cathartic experience. In many instances, the nurse facilities the griever's expressions of hurt, anger, crying, and so forth. The nurse may have to say, "It's okay to [have whatever feelings the griever has]." Sometimes it is a spiritual search and help is in the form of finding a resource or a place of peace, such as the chapel. Often, what is needed most is someone to listen to the existential and unanswerable questions, the "whys" and "hows."

Sometimes nurses offer to inform others for the grievers, thinking that this is something that will help. Because it usually is therapeutic for grievers to talk to others about the losses, nurses should refrain from helping in this way. Instead, the nurse can offer to find a phone number or hold the griever's hand during the conversation or just "be there" when the news is being shared. In this way, the nurse provides support when the griever's emotions engage.

As the person or family moves toward equilibrium after a loss, be it a death, a move from home to a nursing home, or other change with meaning, the nurse can help the person reorganize this new life. The nurse talks with the elder about what was most valued about living at home and what habits were comforting and finds ways to incorporate these in a new way to the new environment. For example, if the person always had a cup of tea before bed but now does not have access to a kitchen, "cup of tea at h.s." can become part of the individualized plan of care.

For the cycle of grieving to reach some level of resolution, new memories are needed. The grandmother who had always hosted her eldest daughter's birthday party can still do that even if she is now a resident in a long-term care facility. When the nurse has the information about this important ritual, he or she can help the person reserve a private space within the facility, send out invitations, and have the birthday party as always but now reframed as it is catered by the facility in the elder's new "home."

Reminiscence is often helpful in creating new memories (see Chapter 6). Listening to the story, endlessly repeated, is difficult to do. The story is likely to change with each retelling as new memories or perspectives develop. Reminiscence is a means by which denial can fall by the wayside and allow reality of the loss to filter slowly into the conscious mind. Reminiscence helps the griever acknowledge that the loss is indeed real and that life can go on, even though the future may be experienced in a different way.

By incorporating the loss and putting the deceased into the life story in a new way (re-forming the story), energy can be invested in all other relationships that exist or may come to be. Drawing out anecdotes and vignettes of the relationship helps the griever keep control over the story of his or her life and reframe it into a new, updated memory. Encourage the griever to talk and tell the story of the relationship as it had been.

The nurse's role is also as an advocate who displays the behavioral qualities of responsiveness, authenticity, commitment, and competence, that is, caring (Krohn, 1998) (Table 23-1).

TABLE 23-1	CARING BEHAVIORS
BEHAVIOR	**CARING ACTION**
Advocacy	Extend oneself to find proper help
	Work to grant reasonable requests
Authenticity	Sharing feelings appropriately
	Honesty
	Use of healing touch
Responsiveness	Be available
	Interact verbally
	Provide comfort
	Provide privacy
	Be nonjudgmental
Commitment and presence	Grooming
	Quiet for talking
	Time
	Presence
Competence	Perform tasks consistently
	Radiate self-assurance in care giving
	Teach simply and completely
Give positive meaning to another's life	Listen
	Touch*
	Point out reactions to family
	Praise when appropriate
	Help them gain a sense of control

From Krohn B: *Geriatric Nursing* 19:276, 1998.
*The appropriateness of the use of touch varies greatly by culture (see Chapter 5).

Countercoping

Weisman (1979) described the work of health care professionals related to grief as "countercoping." Although he was speaking of working with people with cancer, it is equally applicable to working with people who are grieving for other losses. "Countercoping is like counterpoint in music, which blends melodies together into a basic harmony. The patient copes; the therapist [nurse] countercopes; together they work out a better fit" (Weisman, 1979, p. 109). Weisman suggests four specific types of interventions or countercoping strategies: (1) clarification and control, (2) collaboration, (3) directed relief, and (4) cooling off.

Clarification and Control. The nurse helps elders cope with loss and dying by helping them confront the loss by getting or receiving information, considering alternatives, and finding a way to make the grief manageable. The nurse helps persons resume control by encouraging them to avoid acting on impulse.

Collaboration. The nurse collaborates by encouraging the griever to share stories with others and repeat the stories as often as is necessary as he or she "talks it out" in the way described above. The nurse as a collaborator is more directive than usual; it may be acceptable to say, "No, this is not a good time to make any major decisions."

Directed Relief. Some temporary directed relief may be necessary, especially during acute grief. Catharsis may be helpful. In many instances, the nurse encourages the griever to cry or otherwise express feelings, such as hurt or anger. The nurse may have to say something like, "Expressing your feelings is important." Activity may also be recommended as a natural extension of feelings. Intense physical activity gives one some control over emotions. In some cultures, people may tear their clothes or cut their hair. There are numerous ways of acting out feelings—from throwing things, to taking a walk, to busying oneself with tasks, to expressing feelings through creative works.

Cooling Off. From time to time, the griever might need to be encouraged to temporarily avoid processing the loss through diversions that worked in the past during times of stress, especially when things need to be done or decisions need to be made. The nurse may need to suggest new tactics. "Cooling off" also means encouraging the person to modulate emotional extremes and to think about ways to make sense of the loss, to build a new sense of self-esteem after the loss, and to reestablish life patterns.

At all times, active listening is preferable to giving advice. When listening, the nurse soon discovers that it is not the actual loss that is of utmost concern but, rather, the fear associated with the loss. If the nurse listens carefully to both the stated and the implied, expressions such as the following may be heard: "How will I go on?" "What will I do now?" "What will become of me?" "I don't know what to do." "How could he (she) do this to me?" Because the nurse knows that there will be some resolution, such comments may seem exaggerated or melodramatic, but to the one who is grieving, there seems to be no end to the pain. The person who is actively grieving cannot yet look ahead or know that the despair and other feelings will resolve. Like good copers, good gerontological nurses must be flexible, practical, resourceful, and abundantly optimistic.

DYING AND DEATH

A major question arises when considering dying and death in late life. When is a person with multiple chronic or repeated acute or progressive health problems considered to be "dying"? Although sometimes confused with the onset of acute, treatable health problems, the consensus is that irreversible physical deterioration is the prime indicator of dying. However, other, more subtle cues may be present. An approaching death is also suspected when coded communication is used by the individual, such as saying good-bye instead of the usual goodnight, giving away cherished possessions as gifts, urgently contacting friends and relatives with whom the person has not communicated for a long time, and direct or symbolic premonitions that death is near. Anxiety, depression, restlessness, and agitation are behaviors that are frequently categorized as manifestations of confusion or dementia but, in reality, may be responses to the inability to express feelings of foreboding and a sense of life escaping one's grasp.

Many people have said that death is not the problem; it is the dying that takes the work. This is true for all involved: the person, the loved ones, the professional caregivers such as the nurses, and, especially in long-term care facilities, the nursing assistants.

Before the 1900s, most women and men died at home. Women died during childbirth, and men died of unknown causes. During times of war, most men died in battle or from battle-associated injuries. The life expectancy at birth in 1900 was 46.3 years for men and 48.3 years for women (United States). Now both men and women live well into their 70s and beyond (see Chapter 1). While most people prefer to die at home, they still most often die in acute and long-term care settings, although the number of home deaths is increasing.

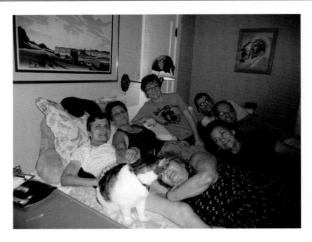

Kathy (bottom left) surrounded by her life boat, about 4 weeks before her death, family, friends, caregivers all. (Photo by Patty Getford.) Age 60.

Dying is both a challenging life experience and a private one. How one deals with dying is often a reflection of the way the person has handled earlier losses and stressors. Most people probably die as they have lived. Although not all older adults have had fulfilling lives or have a sense of completion, transcendence, or self-actualization, their deaths at the age or after that of their parents are considered normative. If the dying process is particularly long or the death occurs after a painful illness, we may rationalize it or view it as relief, at least in part. Death at a younger age or as the result of trauma or catastrophe is viewed as tragic and sometimes incomprehensible. After 9/11, no one rationalized the deaths of the older victims as a relief; all deaths were considered an unacceptable loss of human potential.

Conceptual Model for Understanding the Dying Process

As models have been proposed to explain the grieving process, so have they been proposed for the process of dying. One of the most well-known has been that of Elisabeth Kübler-Ross, MD. In her book *On Death and Dying* (1969), she reported observations of predominately middle-aged in-patients on the psychiatric ward where she did her psychiatry residency. She proposed the stages of dying as denial, anger, bargaining, depression, and acceptance. Nurses and many others have tried to help the dying work through denial to achieve acceptance before their deaths. However, we have come to realize that the "stages" are actually types of emotional reactions to dying that people experience and not a step-wise model at all.

The Living-Dying Interval

Whereas physically we may begin dying early in life as proposed by the theories of aging, in personal terms, dying begins at a moment called the "crisis knowledge of death" (Pattison, 1977, p. 44) and ends at the moment of physiological death. Pattison (1977) calls the time between these two points the living-dying interval, made up of the acute, chronic, and terminal phases. The chronological time of the living-dying interval is accordion-like because of remissions and exacerbations in the terminal diagnosis; it may last days, weeks, months, or years. The manner in which one faces dying is an expression of personality, circumstances, illness, and culture.

The crisis knowledge of death occurs when someone receives the information that he or she will not live as long as previously anticipated. Certainly it would appear that the more the discrepancy between the previously believed length of life and the newly projected length of life, the more the adjustment and perhaps the intensity of acute grief.

The point of crisis is a moment in time that is followed by an acute phase. It is usually the peak time of stress and anxiety as the life and future of the individual and the family is thrown into disequilibrium. Crisis intervention is most effective here because the individual, family, and caregivers are struggling to come to terms with the knowledge. A significant amount of anticipatory grieving may be observed.

Because no one can live with a crisis indefinitely, most of the dying time is spent in the chronic phase. During this time, the dying and those about them are forced to resume some sense of normalcy. Bills still need to be paid, dishes still need to be washed, and life can still be lived. The challenge for persons with terminal diagnoses and their families is to work toward living while dying and not dying while dying. Entertainment, work, and relationships can be maintained as normally as the individual's condition permits. Life goes on despite the anticipation of its end. Physical signs and symptoms and indicators of spiritual distress can be adequately addressed (Table 23-2).

The terminal phase is reached when the speed of the physical dying is accelerated and the dying person no longer has the energy to maintain the activities of everyday life. The terminal phase is ushered in by withdrawal or turning away from the outside world in response to internal body signals that tell the dying person to conserve energy. The focus then turns to preserving energy and completing life's journey. In some cultures, this period is called the "death watch" and is associated with proscribed rituals. It is especially important for the nurse to understand and respect the cultural expectations of his or her patients at this time (Goldstein et al., 2004).

The living-dying interval can reflect an integrated or disintegrated experience (Pattison, 1977). The interval is integrated when each new crisis occurs, is dealt with effectively, and the quality of life while dying is preserved. The interval is disintegrated if one crisis tumbles onto the next one without any effective resolution; the quality of life while dying is compromised (Figure 23-2). Martocchio (1982) describes living-dying patterns as peaks and valleys, descending (stepwise) plateaus, and progressive downward slopes. The patterns may be singular or in combination and may or may not be related to the pathological parameters of the disease.

Theories suggest that any approach to coping with dying should consider a basic understanding of all dimensions and all the individuals involved and tasks associated with each phase of living-dying. The approach should foster empowerment by emphasizing the options available while the person lives on,

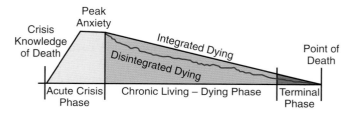

FIGURE 23-2 The living-dying interval. (From Pattison EM: *The experience of dying*, Englewood Cliffs, NJ, 1977, Prentice-Hall.)

TABLE 23-2	SIGNS AND SYMPTOMS ASSOCIATED WITH THE TERMINAL PHASE OF THE LIVING-DYING INTERVAL: NURSING INTERVENTIONS	
PHYSICAL	**RATIONALE**	**INTERVENTION**
Coolness	Diminished peripheral circulation to increase circulation to vital organs	Socks, light cotton blankets or warm blankets if needed; *do not use electric blanket*
Increased sleeping	Conservation of energy	Respect need for increased rest; inquire as to their wishes regarding timing of companionship
Disorientation	Metabolic changes	Identify self by name before speaking to patient; speak softly, clearly, and truthfully
Fecal and/or urinary incontinence	Increased muscle relaxation	Change bedding as needed; use bed pads; *avoid indwelling catheters*
Noisy respirations	Poor circulation of body fluids, immobilization, and the inability to expectorate	Elevate the head with pillows, or raise the head of the bed, or both; gently turn the head to the side to drain
Restlessness	Metabolic changes and relative cerebral anoxia	Calm the patient by speech and action; reduce light; gently rub back, stroke arms, or read aloud; play soothing music; *do not use restraints*
Decreased intake of food and fluids	Body conservation of energy for function	Provide nutrition within limits expressed by patient or in advance directive Semi-solid liquids easiest to swallow. Protect mouth and lips from the discomfort of dryness
Decreased urine output	Decreased fluid intake and decreased circulation to kidney	None
Altered breathing pattern	Metabolic and oxygen changes	Elevate the head of bed; speak gently to patient
EMOTIONAL OR SPIRITUAL	**PRESUMED RATIONALE**	**INTERVENTION**
Withdrawal	Prepares the patient for release and detachment and letting go	Continue communicating in a normal manner using a normal voice tone; identify self by name; give permission to die
Vision-like experiences of dead friends or family; religious vision	Preparation for transition	Accept the reality of the experience for the person; reassure them that the feeling is normal
Restlessness	Tension, fear, unfinished business	Listen to patient express his or her fears, sadness, and anger. Facilitate completion of business if possible
Unusual communication	Signals readiness to let go	Say what needs to be said to the dying patient; kiss, hug, cry with him or her as appropriate

From Hess PA: Loss, grief, and dying. In Beare P, Myers J: *Adult health nursing*, ed 3, St Louis, 1998, Mosby.

emphasizing participation or shared aspects of coping with dying (interpersonal network), and providing guidance for care providers and helpers.

The Family

Older adults of today are usually members of multigenerational families. Although members may be geographically distant, in many cases some degree of filial tie exists. When an elder becomes seriously or terminally ill and cannot uphold his or her role or obligation, the family balance or dynamics are significantly altered (functional disruption). For example, new arrangements are needed when an elder who has been providing child care or help with meal preparation is no longer able to do so. This change may cause considerable familial distress; as will the need for elder care when day-to-day help seems impossible due to work needs and schedules. Even the elderly person who is single and relies on friends and neighbors finds a change in the relationships. Depending on the role the individual has in the family/friend constellation, problems often begin at the time of diagnosis or shortly thereafter. Roles and traits of the person who is now considered to be dying may create adjustment difficulties in the soon-to-be survivors, whether they are partners, spouses, adult children, or grandchildren. Adult children often begin to see their own mortality through the death of their parent with the re-forming and reframing of a new family order.

The idea that family members can remain involved with the dying person can be a constant conflict as they anticipate and plan for life without the dying family member. This change requires enormous energy by family members who are already burdened with their own anticipatory grief, daily living, and, in many cases, raising their own children and possibly grandchildren. A number of adaptive tasks may facilitate healthy resolution of the loss of a family member (see Chapter 22).

Family members have to separate their own identities from that of the patient and learn to tolerate the reality that another family member will die while they live on. The ability of the family to support, love, and provide intimacy may lead to exhaustion, impatience, anger, and a sense of futility if the patient's dying is prolonged. Family members may be at different points in grief than the patient is, which can hinder communication between the patient and family. As the illness worsens, physical disability increases, or the patient's needs intensify, so may the family members' feelings of helplessness and frustration.

Responding to the effects of grief requires acknowledging feelings that surface during the dying process. Coming to terms with the reality of the impending loss means that family members must go through many emotional responses in achieving acceptance of the loved one's approaching death as observed by Kübler-Ross. Because people are "supposed to" die in old age according to social norms, the grief responses may not be exceptionally intense; on the other hand, many filial relationships that seem superficial can result in very deep and acute grief responses.

The family may feel extremely pressured during the final days of a relative's life and need the support of the nurse. They may feel caught between experiencing the present and remembering the patient as he or she was, between pushing for more interventions with the potential to extend the dying or letting life take its course, and occasionally wanting to retreat because

of a discordant relationship with the patient. Families frequently feel guilt-ridden if they believe they are thinking more about their needs than those of the dying patient, yet their day-to-day needs and responsibilities are a reality.

Despite the family's grief and pain, they must give the patient permission to die; let the loved one know that it is all right to let go and leave. This gesture is the last act of love and dignity that the family can offer the dying patient. Occasionally, no family is available to say, "It's okay to let go." The task then falls to the nurse who has developed a meaningful relationship with the patient through care.

PROMOTING A GOOD DEATH: IMPLICATIONS FOR GERONTOLOGICAL NURSING

The needs of the dying are like threads in a piece of cloth. Each thread is individual but necessary to the integrity and completeness of the fabric. If one thread is pulled, it touches the other threads, affecting the fabric's appearance, the thread placement, and the stability of the piece. When one need is unmet, it will affect all others because they are all interwoven. Separating the physical, psychological, and spiritual needs of the dying in late life in order to identify specific interventions and approaches is difficult because of their interconnection.

The responsibility of the nurse is to provide safe conduct as the dying and their families navigate through unknown waters to a good and appropriate death. It is one that a person would choose if choosing were possible (Box 23-4). A good and appropriate death is one in which one's needs are met for as long as possible, and life retains meaning. There are several ways to approach an understanding of the needs of persons who are dying and the responsibilities of the nurse in the promotion of a healthy death (Figure 23-3). The following is an approach proposed by Weisman from his work with cancer patients.

Interventions
The 6 Cs Approach

Weisman (1979) identified six needs of the dying: care, control, composure, communication, continuity, and closure (the 6 Cs). The importance of each to the person is influenced by his or

BOX 23-4	INDICATORS OF AN APPROPRIATE AND GOOD DEATH

- Care needed is received, and it is timely and expert.
- One is able to control one's life and environment to the extent that is desired and possible and in a way that is culturally consistent with one's past life.
- One is able to maintain composure when necessary and to the extent desired.
- One is able to initiate and maintain communication with significant others for as long as possible.
- Life continues as normal as possible while dying with the added tasks that may be needed to deal with and adjust to the inevitable death.
- One can maintain desirable hope at all times.
- One is able to reach a sense of closure in a way that is culturally consistent with one's practices and life patterns.

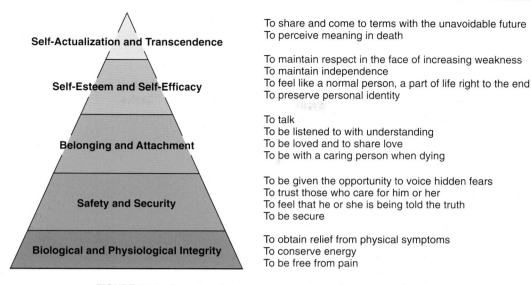

Self-Actualization and Transcendence

To share and come to terms with the unavoidable future
To perceive meaning in death

Self-Esteem and Self-Efficacy

To maintain respect in the face of increasing weakness
To maintain independence
To feel like a normal person, a part of life right to the end
To preserve personal identity

Belonging and Attachment

To talk
To be listened to with understanding
To be loved and to share love
To be with a caring person when dying

Safety and Security

To be given the opportunity to voice hidden fears
To trust those who care for him or her
To feel that he or she is being told the truth
To be secure

Biological and Physiological Integrity

To obtain relief from physical symptoms
To conserve energy
To be free from pain

FIGURE 23-3 Hierarchy of the dying person's needs, based on Maslow.

her background, culture, experiences, religious and philosophical orientation, the prior degree of life involvement, and perhaps gender. His approach can provide a framework for promoting health while experiencing a loss.

Care

The dying person should have the best care possible; this means freedom from pain, conservation of energy, expert management of symptoms, and support at all times. There are a number of symptoms that are commonly found among persons who are dying. These include dyspnea, fatigue, pain, and others that are more specific to the cause of death. Pain management for the person with a terminal illness requires the nurse to use a double standard. The chronic pain associated with dying is not going to stop and usually requires a regimen of narcotic and adjuvant drug therapy administered around the clock and on time, not just as requested by the patient. Narcotic addiction need not be a concern to the nurse caring for the dying; relief of pain is paramount (see Chapter 17 for a detailed discussion of pain management).

Pain goes beyond physical to psychological, induced by depression, anxiety, fear, and other unresolved emotional concerns that are just as strong and just as real. When emotional needs are not met, the total pain experience, physical and psychological, may be exacerbated or intensified. Medication alone cannot relieve this pain. Instead, empathetic listening and allowing the dying person to verbalize what is on his or her mind are important interventions that must be based on the energy level of the one who is dying. If tears and sadness are present, silence and possibly touch are worth more than words can convey. Gentleness of touch, closeness, and sitting near the person may be appropriate if within the boundaries of cultural appropriateness.

Diversional activity can sometimes ease pain: a backrub to relieve tension, a foot massage, radio or television, or exposure to art and music. If hearing is impaired, an amplifier close to the patient's ear may help. If vision is impaired, talking books or a volunteer reader can be found. In many instances,

psychological pain can be relieved if the person feels safe and has someone close by to converse, to listen, and to be with.

Dying requires much energy to cope with the physical assault of illness on the body and the spiritual and emotional unrest that dying initiates. Care also means helping the person conserve energy. How much can the individual do without becoming physically and emotionally taxed? What activities of daily living are most important for the person to do independently? How much energy is needed for the patient to talk with visitors or staff without becoming exhausted? Only the person who is dying can answer these questions, and the nurse can advocate for the person to be given the opportunity to do so; in doing so, the patient is able to remain in better control and maintain composure. By meeting the needs for freedom from pain and conservation of energy, the nurse has already begun to intervene on maximizing quality of life.

Control

While proceeding along the living-dying interval, one often feels that control over his or her life has been lost. The person is in the process of losing everything he or she has ever known or would ever know. The potential loss of identity, independence, and control over bodily functions can lead to a sense of loss of control and threatened self-esteem. The person may begin to feel ashamed, humiliated, and like a "burden." Control is the need to remain in a collaborative role relating to one's own living and dying and as active a participant in the care as desired. The nurse can help the person meet these needs by taking every opportunity to return the control to the person and, in doing so, bolster self-esteem. Essential to the facilitation of self-esteem is the premise that the values of the patient must figure significantly in the decisions that will affect the course of dying. Whenever possible, the nurse can have the person decide when to groom, eat, wake, sleep, and so on. The nurse never has the right to determine the activities of the individual, especially relating to visitors and how time is spent.

Composure

Dying is an emotional activity—for the dying and for those around them. The need for composure is that which enables the person to modulate emotional extremes within cultural norms as is appropriate. This is not to avoid the sadness; this is to have moments of relief. The nurse may use many of the "countercoping" techniques previously discussed to help persons maintain composure as they desire.

Communication

The need for communication is broad, from the need for information to make decisions to the need to share information. Although the type and content of communication that is acceptable to the person vary by culture, the nurse has a responsibility to ensure that the dying person has an opportunity for the communication he or she desires.

Communication includes auditory, visual, and tactile stimulation to appropriately nurture and foster quality of life while dying. Verbal and nonverbal communication are necessary to convey positive messages. Hand-holding, placing an arm around the shoulder, or sitting on the edge of the bed as culturally appropriate conveys to the dying person that the nurse or caregiver is available to listen.

In a classic study of terminal illness in the hospital, Glaser and Strauss (1963) identified four types of communication: *closed awareness, suspected awareness, mutual pretense,* and *open awareness.* Each of these influenced the work on the hospital unit. Closed awareness is described as "keeping the secret." Hospital staff and the family and friends know that the patient is dying, but the patient does not know it or knows and keeps the secret as well. Generally, caregivers invent a fictitious future for the patient to believe in, in hopes that it will boost the patient's morale. Although this happens less today with the legislation related to patients' rights, it still occurs. In suspected awareness, the patient suspects that he or she is going to die. Hints are bandied back and forth, and a contest ensues for control of the information.

Mutual pretense is a situation of "let's pretend." Everyone knows the patient is dying, but the patient, family, friends, nurses, and physicians do not talk about it—real feelings are kept hidden, and too often, so are questions. Open awareness acknowledges the reality of approaching death. The patient, family, friends, nurses, and physicians openly acknowledge the eventual death of the patient. The patient may ask, "Will I die?" and "How and when will I die?" The patient becomes resigned to dying, and the family grieves with the patient rather than for the patient. The nurse can encourage open awareness whenever possible while respecting the patient's cultural patterns and behaviors. It is essential to note that what is said and to whom is culturally determined. Talking about dying or death may be considered taboo, and speaking to the wrong person may be very inappropriate.

Continuity

The need for continuity is fulfilled by preserving as normal a life as possible while dying; by transcending the present, continuity helps to maintain self-esteem. Often a dying patient can feel shut off from the rest of the world at a time when he or she is still capable of being involved and active in some way. Providing stimuli such as photographs and mementos, enabling the individual to stay at home, or enabling individuality or other culturally appropriate experiences in the institutional setting engenders continuity and self-esteem. Self-esteem and dignity complement each other. Dignity involves the individual's ability to maintain a consistent self-concept.

Loneliness is the result of a loss of continuity with one's life and a diminution of one's concept of self and results in spiritual or existential distress. The nurse may ask about the person's life and those things most valued and work with the family and the patient or resident on a plan to remain engaged in as many of the activities and past roles as long as possible. A father who watches a certain ballgame with his son every Sunday can continue to do this regardless of the need to be in a hospital, a nursing home, or an in-patient hospice unit. If the person is bed-bound at home, it may be more practical to have the bed in a central area rather than in a distant room. Treating the dying elderly person as an intelligent adult, holding a hand, or putting an arm around a shoulder, if culturally acceptable, says, "I care" and "You're not alone" and "You are important."

Yet some prefer some time alone and have valued solitude (Box 23-5). This too can be respected as a way of enhancing the continuity of a long life. The nurse can find out the personal and cultural preferences and values of the person and work toward honoring these.

Closure

The need for closure is the need for the opportunity for reconciliation, transcendence, and self-actualization, the highest of Maslow's Hierarchy of Needs (Maslow, 1943). Reminiscence is one way of putting one's life in order, to evaluate the pluses and minuses of life. It is a means of resolving conflicts, giving up possessions, and making final good-byes. Learning to say "good-bye" today leaves open the possibility of many more "hellos."

BOX 23-5   MEDITATION COPING

Mrs. Herbert was a spry 76-year-old white woman. She was the sole caregiver of her husband with mid-stage Alzheimer's disease. The hospital had arranged for her husband to share a room with her while her diagnostic tests were completed and her symptoms stabilized before she went home. She had just been diagnosed with metastatic breast cancer, with a terminal diagnosis. The nurses thought that she was becoming increasingly irritable and agitated after her initial calmness. As an advanced practice nurse on an oncology unit, I was called to assess Mrs. Herbert and recommend a treatment plan. We talked for awhile—about her life, her plans for the future, and her usual coping. She explained that she had everything under control and had already made arrangements for homecare in the process of planning for the eventual long-term care needs of her husband. As she started to cry, she said, "It's just so hard with my life disrupted here. Every morning for years I have meditated for 30 minutes. My husband respects my need for quiet, and afterward I think I can do anything! I have not been able to meditate since I have been here; the nurses and staff are always coming in my room or calling on the room's intercom—I can't find any moments of peace!" The nurses and I worked out a plan with Mrs. Herbert. Every morning between 6:00 and 6:30 am, she would not be disturbed. A "Do Not Disturb" sign would be placed on the intercom at the nurses' station and on her door. A noticeable change was seen in just a few days; Mrs. Herbert was calmer and coping well again. She was most appreciative to "have my life back again."

Kathleen Jett

Pain and other symptoms that are not well cared for may interfere with this reconciliation, making appropriate interventions by the nurse especially important.

For some, closure means coming to terms with their spiritual selves, with the Great Spirit, Jesus, God, Allah, or Buddha—of that which has meaning to the person. If the patient has existential or spiritual needs, arranging for pastoral care may be offered but should never be done without the person's permission. The nurse can foster transcendence by providing patients with the time and privacy for self-reflection and an opportunity to talk about whatever they need to talk about, especially about the meanings of their lives and the meanings of their deaths.

The fabric of needs of the dying person comprise the six Cs. The influence of communication and control is omnipresent in the other needs; without them, the cloth will fray and attempts to meet the needs will be limited.

Spirituality

In 2009, a group of experts in palliative care gathered to come to a consensus on spiritual care as a dimension of palliative care (National Consensus Project, 2009). This meeting was driven in part by discovery that while addressing the spiritual needs of persons who are dying had long been an expectation of providers of hospice and palliative care, too often these needs were still not being met (Puchalski et al., 2009). Resurgence in effort has begun to address what some call the most basic of all needs.

Recommendations for many aspects of care resulted from the Consensus Project. Among these was the responsibility of all members of the health care team to be sensitive to spiritual needs and, when identified, assure that they are addressed. A special note was made that while attention to spiritual needs is an essential component of compassionate care, it is still necessary for the professional to maintain appropriate boundaries and refrain from any appearance of proselytizing.

The spiritual dimension of persons who are dying deals with the transcendental or existential relationship between the dying person and another—between the person and his or her god or the person and significant others. Signs of spiritual distress while dying include expressions of hopelessness, meaninglessness, guilt, despair, all of which can emerge indirectly through anxiety, depression, or anger. Interventions may involve calling their choice of a religious leader; sharing spiritual readings that are consistent with their beliefs, meditative poems, and music of the person's choice; obtaining religious articles such as amulets, a Bible, or a rosary; or praying. The nurse is cautioned that these interventions must be consistent with the culture and wishes of the patient and not expressions of the nurse's belief system.

Hope

Hope is expectancy of fulfillment, an anticipation, or relief from something. Hope is based on the belief of the possible, support of meaningful others, a sense of well being, overall coping ability, and a purpose in life. Erickson equates hope with integrity; it is also comparable to Maslow's self-actualization. Hope empowers, generates courage, motivates action and achievement, and can strengthen physiological and psychological functioning. Hope involves faith and trust. Hope can be classified as desirable or expectational (Pattison, 1977). Expectational hope sounds like "I hope to get better" or "I hope my children get

here in time." If this hope is a reflection of expectations that are not realistic, they can increase stress for the person and caregiver. However, this hope can be modified without being lost. In desirable hope, the wishes are something that would be appreciated if it were to occur without the fixed expectation that it will or must occur. The nurse can respond to the comment "I hope I get better" from someone who is rapidly declining with "That would be really great; in the meantime, there is so much we can do for you such as keep you comfortable."

Nurses seldom recognize the small things they do, routinely and unconsciously, to impart hope. The act of helping with grooming conveys a quiet belief that the person matters. Pain relief and comfort measures reinforce the recognition of an individual's needs and reinforce the value of the person.

The Family

The nurse is often present and supporting the family at the moment of death and in the moments preceding it. Regardless of the age of the surviving family members, as spouse, partner, children, or friends, they too have needs and nurses have a responsibility to care for them. This may be in the form of directed relief and other interventions that promote equilibrium. Nursing interventions that promote health at the time of loss include actions that empower the family to cope with the death in a manner consistent with their traditions. In a small ethnography, Herbert and colleagues (2007) found that family caregivers most needed prognostic information and were unlikely to ask for this. Hearing from the provider what the death would "look like" was a key ingredient the families found missing.

PALLIATIVE CARE

According to the World Health Organization, palliative care is "an approach to care which improves the quality of life of patients and their families facing life-threatening illness, through the prevention, assessment and treatment of pain and other physical, psychological and spiritual problems" (World Health Organization, 2010). As gerontological nurses routinely care for elders who have life-limiting conditions, such as Alzheimer's disease or Parkinson's disease, palliative care is potentially part of day-to-day practice. Palliative care is appropriate any time that the reduction of suffering is the primary goal. This may be the situation when curative treatments are no longer effective, such as with cancer or HIV, or end-stage heart or pulmonary disease. It may also be appropriate when an individual with multiple co-morbid conditions or a proxy on his or her behalf chooses to forgo aggressive treatment of any new health problem (Box 23-6). Finally, palliative care is now being considered appropriate when provided simultaneously with curative care. For example, Ms. Jones has a history of heart disease, COPD, and diabetes. She had adapted to her resultant functional limitations fairly well. However, she contracts the flu, followed by influenza-related pneumonia. Both she and her family know that with the combination of new and chronic diseases she is at a greater risk for death than someone without co-morbidities. She asks that her infection is treated to the best possible extent, but otherwise she elects palliative care—the focus on quality of life, comfort always, and cure when possible.

BOX 23-6   NO MORE TREATMENT PLEASE

Mrs. Rossario was an 86-year-old widow with no children. Her only living relative was a brother, with whom she was very close. She was a patient in our practice and arrived at the nursing home, while I was doing my rounds as a nurse practitioner. When I arrived at her room, I found her skin to be very pale and fragile, with a translucent appearance. Her face was round and puffy from intense steroid therapy, an attempt to dry the secretions in her lungs. She had been in the hospital with acute congestive heart failure six times already, and it was only May. She was completely lucid and looked me straight in the eye and stated clearly that she wanted no further treatment of any kind for her heart failure. She knew that without it she would die in a short period of time, perhaps hours. Her only question was if we could make it as comfortable as possible. With her brother at her side, we reviewed what would happen in the next few hours and assured them that we would do everything possible to keep her comfortable. We made sure that we had scopolamine, morphine, and Ativan on hand for her. With all medications stopped, she became restless and grimaced. We gave her the morphine and Ativan, and she relaxed and was more comfortable. She died with her brother at her side three hours later.

Kathleen Jett

The nursing staff should not be surprised when she refuses ventilator assistance should she deteriorate.

Whereas initially palliative care was the specialty of community-based hospices (see below), specialized units and staff are now seen in long-term care and acute care facilities. In facilities without specialized units or for persons who cannot or do not choose to move, more and more settings have interdisciplinary palliative care consultation teams to work with the patient, family, and regular health care providers, including nurses. Palliative care can be provided regardless of setting and by anyone sharing these goals and skills. The national Hospice and Palliative Care Nurses Association provides the latest Core Competencies, Statements on the Scope and Standards of Hospice and Palliative Care for Advanced Practice, Registered, Practical Nurses and Nurses Aids (see www.hpna.org).

Providing Palliative Care through Hospice

More than 40 years ago, Dame Cicely Saunders decided to find a way to reduce the suffering of those nearing death, first as a nurse and later as a physician. She established Saint Christopher's Hospice in London. The model for modern day hospice is based on the medieval concept of hospitality in which a community assists the traveler at dangerous points along his or her journey. It returns nursing to its roots—as humane, compassionate care, an ideal that has been the basis of nursing for centuries. The dying are indeed travelers—travelers along the continuum of life—and the community consists of friends, family, and specially prepared people to care—the hospice team. The philosophy of hospice care is that "the last stages of life should not be seen as defeat, but rather as life's fulfillment. It is not merely a time of negation, rather an opportunity for positive achievement . . ." (Ulrich, 1978, p. 20).

The hospice movement, as it came to be known, began in the United States in about 1971. Hospice programs started out as small, free-standing organizations with support of the community through donations and volunteer effort. While most are still free-standing (50%), many are now affiliated with hospitals (31%) and home health agencies (19%) (Egan and Labyak, 2006). Hospice services are now provided through both non-profit and for-profit organizations. Hospice care may be provided at home, in assisted living facilities, in hospice "residences," and in palliative care units in acute care hospitals. The variations in origins and style reflect the particular needs of the community, the style of leadership, funding sources, political forces, and available resources for health and social services in the community in which they are established.

Hospice programs provide comprehensive and interdisciplinary care to persons with prognoses of six months or less. At a minimum, services include medical, nursing, nursing assistant, chaplain, social work, and volunteer support. Potential services may also include massage, music, art, pet therapy, and other non-pharmacological interventions to promote comfort and quality of life. Hospices provide care not only to the dying but also to their families and friends through support groups and other bereavement services before and after the deaths. Services are usually available to individuals and families regardless of ability to pay because of the generous support of donors and volunteers. It is now a "covered service" under Medicare and a number of other insurance plans including Medicaid.

The majority of hospice care is provided in people's homes to support an identified informal caregiver. The home becomes the primary center of care, and it is provided by family members or friends, who are taught basic care, including diet, exercise, and medication management needed to care for the dying individual with intermittent visits from the hospice staff. The support of the interdisciplinary hospice team is available 24 hours a day as needed. Volunteers as members of the team are a unique aspect of care; chores are performed, and friendship and companionship are provided to the patient and family. When interventions require the presence of an LPN or RN at least half of the time and at least eight hours per day, the patient may be transferred to a facility of some kind for what is called "continuous care." Once stabilized, the person returns home. Inpatient care is also provided for periods of up to five days to provide the caregiver relief or respite (Egan and Labyak, 2006). Under a Medicare-qualified hospice program, every effort is made to keep the patient out of the acute care setting for the needs of the specified terminal condition. This does not prohibit one from receiving acute care for other treatable conditions.

The unprecedented contribution of hospice continues to be the reestablishment of control for the dying person. Through both pharmacological and non-pharmacological means, control of pain and other symptoms can often be accomplished without denying the patient full alertness and the ability to communicate to others. This gift, so to speak, allows addressing all of Weisman's Six Cs (see discussion earlier in the chapter). The crux of accomplishing this end is the anticipation of symptoms and intervention by the caregiver before problems occur. Both hospice and other palliative care programs support and guide the family in patient care and ensure safe passage* for the patient, that he or she will not die alone, and that the family will not be abandoned. Bereavement services for the family extend for a period of time on an emergency and regular basis after the death of the patient. Life is made as meaningful as possible.

---

*Or in a manner consistent with his or her traditions and wishes (e.g., alone, in privacy).

BOX 23-7 SKILLS NEEDED FOR THE PRACTICE OF PALLIATIVE/ END-OF-LIFE CARE

The nurse should be able to:
- Talk to patients and families about dying.
- Be knowledgeable about symptom control and pain-control techniques (opioid dosing and other pharmacological interventions).
- Provide comfort-oriented nursing interventions.
- Provide palliative treatments.
- Recognize physical changes that precede eminent death.
- Deal with own feelings.
- Deal with angry patients and families.
- Be knowledgeable and deal with the ethical issues in administering end-of-life palliative therapies.
- Be knowledgeable, and inform patients about ADs.
- Be knowledgeable of the legal issues in administering end-of-life palliative care.
- Be adaptable and sensitive to religious and cultural perspectives.
- Explain the meaning of hospice.

Modified from White KR, Coyne PJ, Patel UB: *Journal of Nursing Scholarship* 33:147, 2001, Sigma Theta Tau International.
ADs, Advance directives.

BOX 23-8 SUMMARY OF HOSPICE PHILOSOPHY AND PRINCIPLES

- Hospice is a philosophy, not a facility, one in which the primary focus is on palliative care.
- Hospice affirms life, not death.
- Hospice strives to maximize present quality of living.
- Hospice offers palliative care to all people and their family members, regardless of age, gender, nationality, race, creed, or sexual orientation, who are coping with a life-threatening illness, dying, death, and bereavement.
- The hospice approach offers care to the patient and family as a unit.
- Hospice programs make service available on a 24-hour-a-day, 7-day-a-week basis without interruption, even if the patient care setting changes.
- Participants in hospice programs give special attention to supporting each other.
- Hospice is holistic care.
- A highly qualified, specially trained team of hospice professionals and volunteers work together to meet the physiological, psychological, social, spiritual, and economic needs of the patient and family facing terminal illness and bereavement.
- Hospice offers a safe, coordinated program of palliative and supportive care, in a variety of settings, from the time of admission through bereavement, with the focus of keeping the terminally ill patient in his or her home as long as possible.
- Hospice offers continuing care and ongoing support to bereaved survivors after the death of someone they love.
- Hospice is accountable for the appropriate allocation and utilization of its resources to provide optimum, culturally competent care consistent with patient and family needs and desires.
- Hospice has an organized governing body that has complete and ultimate responsibility for the organization. The governing body entrusts the hospice administrator with overall management responsibility for operating hospice, including planning, organizing, staffing, and evaluating the organization and its services.
- Hospice is committed to continuous assessment and improvement of the quality and efficiency of its services.

Data from Hospice Standards of Practice, National Hospice and Palliative Care Organization, 2000.

Nursing practice and hospice incorporate the mind-body continuum. Nursing is considered the cornerstone of hospice care. The nurse provides much of the direct care and functions in a variety of roles: as staff nurse giving direct care, as coordinator implementing the plan of the interdisciplinary team, as executive officer responsible for research and educational activities, and as advocate for the patient and hospice in the clinical and political arena (Box 23-7).

Palliative Care in the Long-Term Care Setting

Although it is not uncommon for residents of long-term care facilities to die, the provision of directed palliative care is very limited (Stillman et al., 2005). Research has indicated that advance care planning and terminal pain management are inadequate, and support of the grieving family may be nonexistent (Stillman et al., 2005, p. 259). Studies have also found that the care of residents with hospice services and those who are identified as dying in the general population may receive similar care, but a conclusion has not been reached (Munn et al., 2006).

Philosophically, most nurses believe that palliative care has the potential to increase the comfort for long-term care residents while they are dying. Some facilities have special palliative care units or rooms that are staffed with specially trained nurses, but this is the exception (Kayser-Jones et al., 2005). In most cases, those identified as terminally ill remain in their own rooms. In other cases, the local hospice programs have nurses and staff dedicated to working with the residents of select nursing facilities. When a resident in a long-term care facility is enrolled in a formal hospice program, either within or beyond the facility (with visits by staff to the facility), the person has access to considerably more services than routine residents or patients.

Regardless of who provides palliative care, it is expected to be based on the principles derived from the American Geriatrics Society or those established by the American Nurses Association and the National Hospice and Palliative Care Organization (NHPCO) (www.nhpco.org) (Box 23-8). The NHPCO is committed to developing education in the hospice concept and promoting appropriate legislation, regulation, and reimbursement.

Recently, a variety of intervention studies have been conducted to increase the use of hospice in long-term care settings. For example, Stillman and colleagues (2005) used an educational intervention to teach palliative care approaches with some increase in the comfort level and knowledge of the staff. Another intervention study demonstrated that those facilities that identified and trained a "Palliative Care Leadership Team" increased the number of referrals to hospice, improved pain management, and increased the number of advance care planning discussions (Hanson et al., 2005).

DECISION MAKING AT THE END OF LIFE

Who makes end-of-life decisions has been the subject of research, debate, and federal legislation. The individual adult is generally recognized as the decision maker. However, this assumption is based on a Euro-American or Western perspective. Persons who are from non-Western traditions place less emphasis on the individual and more on the needs of the family or community (Blackhall et al., 1995; Mazanec and Panke, 2006). The nurse is obligated to know legal restrictions related to decision making and then work with the elder and the family on how these are consistent with their cultural patterns and needs related to the circumstances that may occur at the end of life.

Decision making about life-prolonging procedures when death is inevitable is a legal, ethical, medical, and professional issue faced by gerontological nurses in their day-to-day work. The blurring of the lines between living and dying results from technological advances, the ambivalence of whether death is to be fought or accepted, and the dilemma brought about by medical technologies. Decision making at the end of life has become increasingly complex because most people die in advanced age from chronic illnesses. In other words, they die over a period of years, slowly declining from degenerative conditions such as Alzheimer's disease, Parkinson's disease, and heart failure.

Advance Directives

Although people have always had opinions about their wishes, in the past these were made in the context of the prevailing use of the principle of paternalism, that is, reliance on the physician to make the right decision for them as they would make for their own children. With the movement away from paternalism and toward the value of autonomy, patients' involvement in treatment-related decisions became the norm. Since December 1991, hospitals, nursing homes, home health agencies, and hospices and enrollees of HMOs have been required to provide patients with information about their rights to make their own health care decisions, accept or refuse treatment, and complete an advance directive. The Patient Self-Determination Act (PSDA) recognized an advance directive (AD) as a morally and, in some jurisdictions, legally binding document in which adults could express their wishes regarding end-of-life decisions for some future time when they were unable to do so for themselves (see http://www.abanet.org/aging/toolkit/home.html). The ADs of today may be as limited to decisions regarding the use of resuscitative orders or as detailed as decisions about dialysis, antibiotics, tube feedings, and so on. The AD also allows the persons to appoint a proxy or surrogate. This is a designated other adult of their choice to speak for him or her and make decisions if the patient is unable to do so. As the proxy is selected by the individual, the legal assumption is that a designated person has more authority than the next-of-kin.

An AD can be revoked only by the individual, either verbally or in writing. The person may also indicate revocation by tearing, burning, or destroying the document, preferably in front of witnesses. Directives may also be amended; formal language is not necessary, and one can add items in writing or cross out unwanted passages (but only the creator of the document may do so). If the person becomes incompetent, revocation is no longer possible, and the last statement of wishes stands.

Two common forms of ADs are known as living will (LW) and durable power of attorney for health care (DPAHC), also called advance health care directive (AHCD). A living will is restricted to representing a person's wishes specific to the condition of a terminal illness and only after he or she has been so diagnosed and cannot speak for herself or himself. An LW is not the same as a do-not-resuscitate (DNR) order, which is a medical directive to health care professionals and is not a personal directive. The DNR order should never be written without a discussion of the implications with the patient and/or proxy.

In contrast, a DPAHC appoints a person, called a health care surrogate, to speak for the other in all matters of health care should he or she be unable to do so for themselves (not to be confused with the power of attorney discussed in Chapter 20). However, in some states the surrogate appointed in a DPAHC cannot make decisions related to withdrawal of life support, at which time both the DPAHC and LW are needed. Both the proxy and the health care surrogate are expected to make the decisions for the person that he or she would make if able to do so, using what is known as substituted judgment. Although advance directives are considered morally binding, they are legally binding only when declared so in state statutes.

All agencies that receive Medicare and Medicaid funds are mandated to disseminate PSDA information to their clients and inquire as to the existence of the same (American Bar Association, n.d.). Hospitals and long-term care facilities are responsible for providing written information at the time of admission about the individual's rights under law to refuse medical and surgical care and the right to record this in an AD. Both HMOs and home health agencies are required to do the same at the time of enrollment or initiation of services. Providers (e.g., physicians, nurse practitioners, and physician assistants) are encouraged but not obligated to provide this same information to their patients.

The exact format and signature requirements (e.g., notary) for advance directives including living wills vary from state to state. There are several clearinghouses of related information, including www.fivewishes.com or the Caring Connections website (http://www.caringinfo.org/stateaddownload), wherein persons can obtain information relevant to their state, and forms can be ordered or downloaded. Nurses should know the details of AD requirements in the state, country, or other jurisdiction in which they practice. The nurse should also be familiar with the AD form or forms used by the organization in which he or she is employed.

Barriers to Completing Advance Directives

While the concept of advance planning is not new and the PSDA has been in effect since 1991, the number of persons with completed directives remains low. This is especially true for elders from minority groups. Even if informed of the availability of hospice services, many African Americans do not elect to use the service. African Americans and Hispanic Americans have reported that a formal advance directive was not necessary due to the confidence that family members knew of their wishes already (Demons and Velez, 2006). Others have found that barriers to completing advance directives range from lack of knowledge or discomfort of the providers to limited language proficiency at the location of care. Community British nurses reported lack of resources, lack of public awareness, and difficulties talking about death as barriers to implementing advance care planning (Seymour et al., 2010). The majority (84%) of participants in a study designed to increase the number of persons who completed advance planning felt that it was irrelevant to their personal needs. In another study of a multiethnic, multilingual inpatient population, 369 patients were asked if their physicians had discussed advanced care decision making with them. Only 41% reported conversations, and the finding was across education, age, ethnic, and language groups (Kulkarni et al., 2010). In some groups the family is the decision maker of care issues, not the patient; enforcing the PSDA may be in direct conflict family's collective culture (see Chapter 5). Interpreters, used to assist the health care professional with explanations to their non–English-speaking patients, may not facilitate a clear translation of an AD because of cultural beliefs surrounding death or anticipation of poor health.

PROMOTING HEALTHY AGING: IMPLICATIONS FOR GERONTOLOGICAL NURSING

Although the nurse cannot provide legal information, he or she does serve as a resource person ready to answer many of the questions people have about end-of-life decision making and care. The nurse must consider the factors previously discussed and must attempt to ensure that patients are informed of their rights related to the PSDA in a culturally sensitive manner. The nurse may be responsible to inquire about the presence of an existing advance directive, to offer and explain the option, and to ensure that any existing directive still reflects the person's wishes. The nurse also is responsible for ensuring that existing or newly created advance directives are available in the appropriate locations in the medical record.

The nurse can help the elder to understand interventions (e.g., CPR, intubations, artificial nutrition) and their consequences. In providing this information, the nurse must avoid injecting personal bias into the discussion. The gerontological nurse is an impartial advocate for the patient regardless of the setting but is particularly important in the long-term care environment (Kayser-Jones, 2002). There, the nurse advocates for the self-determination of all patients to the best possible extent, even those with limited cognitive functioning.

The nurse acts as a patient advocate by bringing family members, elders, and prescribing providers together to discuss the difficult issues addressed in executing a directive or to simply discuss the elder's wishes. The nurse may also be the one who obtains the appropriate AD form for the elder who is well or ill. Research has suggested that if health care providers valued advance planning and were able to find the time for related discussions, the number of living wills and other documents would increase (Schickedanz et al., 2009).

No one can think of all possible contingencies that might require decisions with life-limiting conditions. The use of values assessment may help clarify what the elder holds important in his or her life and how this relates to his or her desires for health care and quality of life. Does the elder want measures to be taken to prolong life at all costs, or does he or she wish for a natural death? What are the boundaries in which suffering can be minimized? Are there any persons the elder feels comfortable with who can act as a proxy and will ensure that the elder's wishes will be carried out? Answers to these

questions are helpful in the promotion of an appropriate and good death. Before a directive is completed, the family and support persons should discuss whether those who are to be involved are comfortable with the decisions and will adhere to the directive. For elders without family, the nurse may become a sounding board, but he or she must take care to not influence the outcome.

Approaching Death

In 1991, the Supreme Court in the United States reviewed the case of *Cruzan v. State of Missouri* and confirmed a person's right to refuse unwanted treatment. No distinction was made between withholding and withdrawing the treatment. Later, case law characterized tube feeding and intravenous as medical treatments (also referred to as *artificial sustenance*) and therefore could be refused as well. Nonetheless, questions remained. These "rights" have not always been granted, and questions have been raised regarding the relationship between patients' wishes and the responsibilities and activities of health care providers. These questions were brought to the forefront by the work of Dr. Kevorkian, a proponent and practitioner of physician-assisted suicide and more recently with the hearings of what were referred to as the "death panels" in the early Obama administration in the United States.

The newer questions relate to death that is directly or indirectly hastened. Physician-assisted suicide, euthanasia, terminal sedation, and double effect are all concepts that are part of these moral and legal conversations. Legislative actions have come under the umbrella term of *Death with Dignity* and have been considered in at least 14 states and a number of countries worldwide. In 2010, the U.S. Supreme Court heard two cases regarding physician responsibility (Death with Dignity National Center [DDNC], 2010a).

Physician-Assisted Suicide

The potential for a person's ultimate control of their dying rose to a state and later a Supreme Court level. In 1994 and again in 1997, voters in Oregon (U.S.A.) passed the Death with Dignity Law legalizing a person's right to end his or her life in very specific circumstances.* While a physician may prescribe a lethal dose of a medication, neither physicians nor nurses are permitted to administer it. The voters in Washington State passed the right-to-die Initiative 1000 in 2008 with a 59% to 41% margin (Goldstein, 2008). The rule making followed that of Oregon with similar requirements.† In both states, persons requesting assisted suicide must be informed of alternatives and counseling to ensure that the person is fully informed regarding the risks of such actions. Between 1997 and 2009, 460 patients

---

*(1) competent adult, (2) prognosis of <6 months to live, (3) is judged to be mentally competent (4) one written and two oral requests at 15-day intervals (5) 15-day waiting period (6) certification by two physicians of the diagnosis, prognosis, competency, and voluntary nature of the request.

†(1) competent adult, free of depression (2) prognosis of <6 months to live, (3) request both verbal and in writing, repeated in 15 days, (4) two witnesses to request; one must not be an heir, related or employed by the health-care facility caring for the patient.

had used prescription medication to hasten their death in Oregon. In both states, the majority had cancer and were over 65 and almost exclusively white (DDNC, 2010b). Since Washington's law was enacted on March 5, 2009, 36 of the 63 people who received prescriptions have used the law to hasten their deaths (DDNC, 2010c). It is anticipated that some of these persons had been "waiting" for the law and therefore may represent a "backlog," and the annual number may decrease in future years.

At the same time, the number of persons referred to palliative care programs increased. The impact of the Death with Dignity law has led to the establishment of universal hospice availability and an increase in providers' knowledge of pain and symptom management in Oregon. Between 1997 and 2003, only 57 per 100,000 persons were reported to have committed suicide. This number amounts to only one seventh of 1% of all deaths. Eighty-nine percent of all persons who ingested a lethal dose of a medication were receiving hospice care.

Terminal Sedation or Sedation to Relief

In 1997, the U.S. Supreme Court declared that while citizens had no constitutional right to physician-assisted suicide, sedation for symptom relief may be appropriate regardless of the dose required. Referred to as *terminal sedation*, but more accurately described as *palliative sedation*, or relief of refractory symptoms (e.g., pain, nausea and vomiting, dyspnea) by whatever means necessary, even if doing so results in a hastened death. The effect of an action with the intention for comfort despite the potential for death as a result of the action is known as the *double effect*. The intention must be to relieve the suffering, and treatment is to that extent only. The intent is relief rather than death. Active euthanasia wherein the goal is death instead of relief, remains illegal everywhere except under special circumstances in the Netherlands and Belgium.

PROMOTING HEALTHY DYING WHILE AGING: IMPLICATIONS FOR GERONTOLOGICAL NURSING

Nurses are professional grievers. We invest time and caring, and if working with older adults, especially those who are frail and in acute and long-term care settings, we repeatedly experience the death of patients and residents. Some consider the death of a patient as a failure—they have "lost" the person they cared for. However, when it is a good death, it can be viewed as a professional success because the nurse provided safe conduct for the dying elder and gently cared for the survivors (Table 23-3). We can use the reminders of our own mortality as motivation to live the best we can with what we have. Nurses can seek support and support each other. As grievers, we too may need to tell the story of the dying person to those professionals around us, either in formal or informal support groups; and we need to listen to our colleagues' stories.

Caring for older adults requires knowledge of the grieving and dying processes as well as skills in providing relief of symptoms or palliative care. However, it is also acknowledged that working daily with the grieving or dying is an art. The development of the art necessitates inner strength. The nurse needs to have spiritual strength—strength from within. This does

TABLE 23-3   NURSING CARE PLAN FOR SURVIVORS

NURSING DIAGNOSIS	EXPECTED OUTCOMES	INTERVENTIONS
Loneliness, Social Isolation Related to Loss		
Manifestations: teariness, crying, sleep disturbance, weight gain, compulsive eating, weight loss, anorexia, fatigue, confusion, forgetfulness, withdrawal, disinterest, indecisiveness, inability to concentrate, guilt feelings; displays feelings of detachment, inferiority, rejection, alienation, emptiness, isolation; unable to initiate social contacts; seeks attention	Short-term and intermediate goals: The survivor will: Develop or use immediate support systems Express feelings of security Exhibit meaningful social relationships Show decreasing signs of depression Long-term goal: The survivor will: Demonstrate readiness to build a new life as a single person	Attempt to develop a therapeutic relationship through touch, empathy, and listening. Listen to perceived feelings. Help person realize that grief is a painful but normal transitional process. Encourage relationships with other persons as support systems. Encourage balance between linking phenomena (mementos, photographs, clothes, furniture) associated with the deceased and the bridging phenomena (new driving skills, evening classes, new job). Program for counseling if appropriate. Refer to appropriate agencies as needed.
Anxiety Related to Increased Legal, Financial, and Decision-Making Responsibilities		
Manifestations: anger, nervousness, palpitations, increased perspiration, face flushing, dyspnea, urinary frequency, nausea, vomiting, restlessness, apprehension, panic, fear, headache	Short-term and intermediate goals: The survivor will demonstrate adequate decision-making skills in financial and legal matters as evidenced by: Seeking legal aid as needed Writing or calling appropriate agencies Formulating a realistic budget Long-term goals: The survivor will: Cope and deal with legal, financial, and decision-making responsibilities with only a moderate degree of anxiety Make rational decisions about single life	Assist in obtaining attorney if necessary. Encourage contact of Social Security and spouse's employer to ensure receipt of all benefits. Encourage contact of insurance agencies if applicable. Discourage immediate decision-making regarding assets (e.g., home, investments). Encourage seeking of advice from individuals who are trusted. Contact proper social agencies if indigent or in need. Assist in seeking employment if health permits and client so desires. Offer alternatives for decision making. Refer to any other proper community agencies that offer needed assistance.

Adapted from Alexander J, Kiely J: *Geriatric Nursing* 7:85, 1986.

not mean that the nurse must have a specific religious orientation or affiliation but, rather, that he or she has a positive belief in self, a connection to others, and a belief that life has meaning. The effective nurse has developed a personal philosophy of life and of death. Although this may change over time and cannot be assumed to be held by anyone else, one's beliefs about life and death will help the nurse through difficult times. Emotional maturity allows the nurse to deal with disappointment and postponement of immediate wants or desires. Maturity means that the nurse can reach out for help for self when needed. Finally, to provide comfort to grieving persons, nurses must be comfortable with their own lives or at least be able to set aside their own sadness and grief while working with that of others.

It is always important to remember that some nurses are unable to care for the dying because of their own unresolved conflicts and should not be expected to function in these situations. This may be a temporary situation associated with events in the nurse's life or something deeper, such as a traumatic experience in the death of a loved one. The nurse should recognize his or her limitations and should defer care to another nurse more able. In doing so, the nurse gives the most compassionate care possible.

evolve   To access your student resources, go to *http://evolve.elsevier.com/Ebersole/TwdHlthAging*

KEY CONCEPTS

- Grief is an emotional and behavioral response to loss.
- Many theories provide a framework within which to practice palliative care.
- Grief has a beginning, a middle, and an end during which the needs of the griever change.
- Persons who are at risk for complicated grieving should receive specialized and skilled supportive care.
- The individual's response to loss and grieving is similar to how he or she has dealt with other stressors in life.
- An individual is living until he or she has died; the nurse works with the elder and significant others to maintain as high a quality of life as possible before, during, and after the loss or death.
- Hope is empowering; when appropriate to the situation, it can generate courage and resilience.

- Palliative care is that which focuses on comfort rather than cure.
- Hospice is a specific highly interprofessional approach to the provision of palliative care.
- Palliative care can be provided regardless of setting.
- Advance directives allow an individual control over life and death decisions by written communication and allow an appointed person to be his or her spokesperson when he or she is not able to communicate desires personally.
- Oregon is the first state in the United States to legalize assisted suicide in tightly controlled situations. As a result of the law, the care of the dying has improved.

CASE STUDY   COPING WITH DYING

Jesse was simply unable to believe that his wife was dying. The physician told Jesse that Jeannette was in the early stages of multiple myeloma, and that she might die in less than a year or she might have remissions and live another decade. Jesse and his wife had worked hard all their lives and raised two sons. Now they were both retired and financially secure and thought the best years of their lives were ahead of them. However, both Jesse and Jeannette were the type who approached a problem head on. They gathered all the relevant material they could find about multiple myeloma and assiduously studied it. Jeannette said that she did not want to mention her problem to others because she thought that she was unable to deal with "their piteous cancer looks." She also stressed that she expected to have long remissions and to live to be 75 years of age, at least. So why trouble friends and family? As a result of her decision, Jesse was unable to share his fear and grief because he had promised to respect Jeannette's wishes in that regard. She began a series of chemotherapeutic drugs, and friends began to notice her lethargy. They began to worry about her, but she insisted, "I'm just fine." Six months passed with a steady downward course in Jeannette's condition. Her sons began to suspect she had a malignancy, and one son, Rob, asked outright, "Are you hiding a serious illness from us?" She denied it, but Rob also noticed that Jesse was withdrawing into himself and that he was drinking more than usual. Rob knew something was wrong but was at a loss. When Rob went to the family physician for his annual checkup, the office nurse said, "Oh, Rob, how is your mother doing?"

Discuss your rationale and feelings as the office nurse, and determine a plan of action that seems appropriate at this time. Develop a long-range plan of care for this family.

Based on the case study, develop a nursing care plan using the following procedure*:

- List Jeannette's comments that provide subjective data.
- List information that provides objective data.
- From these data, identify and state, using accepted format, two nursing diagnoses you determine are most significant to Jeannette at this time. List two of Jeannette's strengths that you have identified from the data.
- Determine and state outcome criteria for each diagnosis. These criteria must reflect some alleviation of the problem identified in the nursing diagnosis and must be stated in concrete and measurable terms.
- Plan and state one or more interventions for each diagnosed problem. Provide specific documentation of the sources used to determine the appropriate intervention. Plan at least one intervention that incorporates Jeannette's existing strengths.
- Evaluate the success of the intervention. Interventions must correlate directly with the stated outcome criteria to measure the outcome success.

CRITICAL THINKING QUESTIONS

1. Considering the situation and the current regulations about the protection of patient privacy, how would you respond to the son's next question if you were the nurse?
2. As a nurse, how could you promote communication within this family to help them move toward open awareness?
3. What is your priority in attending to the needs of Jesse? Of Jeannette?

*Students are advised to refer to their nursing diagnosis text and identify possible or potential problems.

RESEARCH QUESTIONS

1. Explore your responses to being given a terminal diagnosis. What coping mechanisms work for you?
2. With which level of awareness approach would you be most comfortable? As a nurse? As a patient?
3. If you believe that you are able, discuss your grief process when you dealt with the loss of someone special in your life.
4. Practice with a partner several methods that you will use to introduce the topic of dying with a client who is critically ill and is not expected to live.
5. Describe how you would deal with a dying person and his or her family when these family members are especially protective of each other.
6. Discuss and strategize how you would bring up the topic of advance directives.
7. What advance directive is legally recognized in your state?
8. Explore with family and friends their thoughts on completing an advance directive.
9. What nursing actions do you consider assisted suicide?

REFERENCES

American Bar Association: Law for Older Americans. Heath Care Directives, n.d. Available at http://www.abanet.org/publiced/practical/patient_self_determination_act.html.

Blackhall LJ, Murphy ST, Frank G, et al: Ethnicity and attitudes toward patient autonomy, *Journal of the American Medical Association* 274:820, 1995.

Corr CA, Nabe CM, Corr DM: *Death and dying, life and living,* ed 3, Stamford City, Conn, 2000, Wadsworth.

Corless IB: Bereavement. In Ferrell BR, Coyle N: *Textbook of palliative nursing,* ed 2, NY, 2006, Oxford University Press, pp. 531-544.

Demons JL, Velez R: Geriatrics and end-of-life care. In Satcher D, Pamies RJ, *Multicultural medicine and health disparities,* New York, 2006, McGraw-Hill.

Death with Dignity National Center: Death with dignity around the U.S, 2010a. Available at http://www.deathwithdignity.org/2009/06/16/death-dignity-around-us. Accessed June 26, 2010.

Death with Dignity National Center: 2009 Summary of Oregon's Death with Dignity Act, 2010b. Available at http://www.deathwithdignity.org/media/uploads/OregonYear12Report.pdf. Accessed June 26, 2010.

Death with Dignity National Center: A careful reading of the reports indicates Oregon & Washington laws are safe & rarely used, 2010c. Available at http://www.deathwithdignity.org/2010/03/24/careful-reading-reports-indicates-oregon-washington/. Accessed June 26, 2010.

Doka KJ: Disenfranchised grief. In Doka KJ, editor: *Disenfranchised grief: recognizing hidden sorrow,* Lexington, Mass, 1989, Lexington Books.

Egan KA, Labyak MJ: Hospice palliative care: A model for quality end-of-life care. In Ferrell BR, Coyle N: *Textbook of palliative nursing,* ed 2. NY, 2006, Oxford University Press.

Giacquinta B: Helping families face the crisis of cancer, *American Journal of Nursing* 77:1585, 1977.

Glaser B, Strauss A: *Awareness of dying,* Chicago, 1963, AVC.

Glaser BG, Strauss AL: *Time for dying,* Chicago, 1968, Aldine.

Goldstein C, Anapolsky E, Park J, et al: Research guiding practice related to cultural issues at end of life care, *Geriatric Nursing* 25:58, 2004.

Goldstein J: Washington passes Initiative 1000, legalizing physician-assisted suicide. *The Wall Street Journal* Health Blog, November 5, 2008. Available at http://blogs.wsj.com/health/2008/11/05/washington-passes-initiative-1000-legalizing-physician-assisted-suicide. Accessed June 26, 2010.

Hanson LC, Reynolds KS, Henderson M, et al: A quality improvement intervention to increase palliative care in nursing homes, *Journal of Palliative Medicine* 8:576, 2005.

Herbert RS, Schultz R, Copeland V, et al: What questions do family caregivers want to discuss with health care providers in order to prepare for the death of a loved one? An ethnographic study of caregivers of patients at end of life. *Journal of Palliative Care Medicine* 11:476, 2007.

Horacek BJ: Toward a more viable model of grieving and consequences for older persons, *Death Studies* 15:459, 1991.

Kayser-Jones J: The experience of dying: an ethnographic nursing home study, *Gerontologist* 42(special no. 3):11, 2002.

Kayser-Jones J, Chan J, Kris A: A model long-term care hospice unit: care, community and compassion, *Geriatric Nursing* 26:16, 64, 2005.

Krohn B: When death is near, helping families cope, *Geriatric Nursing* 19:276, 1998.

Kübler-Ross E: *On death and dying,* New York, 1969, MacMillan.

Kulkarni SP, Karliner LS, Auerbach AD, et al: Physician use of advance care planning discussions in diverse hospitalized population. *Journal of Immigrant and Minority Health,* 2010 Jul 18 [ePub ahead of print]. Available at http://www.ncbi.nlm.nih.gov/pubmed/20640919.

Martocchio BC: *Living while dying,* Bowie, Md, 1982, RJ Brady.

Mazanec P, Panke JT: Cultural considerations. In Ferrell BR, Coyle N: *Textbook of palliative nursing,* ed 2. NY, 2006, Oxford University Press, 623-634.

Maslow AH: A theory of human motivation. *Psychological Review* 50:370, 1943.

Munn JC, Hanson LC, Zimmerman S, et al: Is hospice associated with improved end-of-life care in nursing homes and assisted living facilities? *Journal of the American Geriatrics Society* 54:490, 2006.

National Consensus Project: Clinical Practice Guidelines for Quality Palliative Care, 2nd ed, 2009. Available at http://www.nationalconsensusproject.org/Guidelines_Download.asp.

Pattison EM: The experience of dying. In Pattison EM, editor, *The experience of dying.* Englewood Cliffs, NJ, 1977, Prentice-Hall.

Puchalski C, Ferrell B, Virani R, et al: Improving the quality of spiritual care as a dimension of palliative care; The report of the consensus conference, *Journal of Palliative Care* 12:885, 2009.

Rando TA: Grief and mourning: Accommodating to loss. In Wass H, Neimyer RA, editors. *Dying—Facing the facts.* Philadelphia, 1995, Taylor & Francis, 211-241.

Schickedanz AD, Shillinger D, Landefeld CS, et al: A clinical framework for improving the advance care planning process: Start with patients' self-identified barriers, *Journal of the American Geriatrics Society* 57:31, 2009.

Seymour J, Almack K, Kennedy S: Implementing advance care planning: a qualitative study of community nurses' views and experiences. *BMC Palliative Care,* April 8, 9:4, 2010. Published online 2010 April 8. doi: 10.1186/1472-684X-9-4.

Stillman D, Strumpf N, Capezuti E, et al: Staff perceptions concerning barriers and facilitators to end-of-life care in nursing homes, *Geriatric Nursing* 26:259, 2005.

Ulrich LK: The challenge of hospice care, *Bulletin: American Protestant Hospital Association* 21:6, 1978.

Weisman A: *Coping with cancer.* New York, 1979, McGraw-Hill.

Worden JW: *Grief counseling and grief therapy: a handbook for mental health practitioners,* ed 4, New York, 2009, Springer.

World Health Organization: WHO definition of palliative care, 2010. Available at http://www.who.int/cancer/palliative/definition/en.

Zilberfein F: Coping with death: anticipatory grief and bereavement, *Generations* xxxiii:69, 1999.

Self-Actualization, Spirituality, and Transcendence

Priscilla Ebersole and Theris A. Touhy

Special thanks to Priscilla Ebersole, the original author of this chapter for her foundational and very wise contributions.

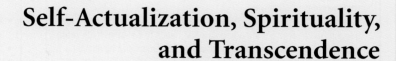

evolve *http://evolve.elsevier.com/Ebersole/TwdHlthAging*

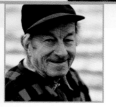

A STUDENT SPEAKS

Well, I always went to church with my parents when I was a child, but it was really boring. Now, I sometimes go with my grandmother to make her happy. I see how important it is to her, and I wonder if it will be important to me when I get really old. I'm just too busy right now.

Lori, age 22

AN ELDER SPEAKS

This is a real problem! I have three children and don't want them to squabble over my things when I'm gone. I would like it if they would each choose something special that would remind them of me, but every time I bring it up they cut me off and won't talk about it. I know there will be a big fight over the piano!

Mabel, age 74

LEARNING OBJECTIVES

On completion of this chapter, the reader will be able to:

1. Provide a comprehensive definition of self-actualization and identify several qualities of self-actualized elders.
2. Discuss the nursing role in relation to the self-actualization of elders.
3. Describe several evidences of transcendence as experienced by older people.
4. Specify various types of creative self-expression and their positive impact on health, illness, and quality of life among older adults.

5. Understand the meaning of spirituality in the lives of older people and discuss nursing responses to facilitate spiritual well-being.
6. Define the concept of legacy and name several types of legacies and what the nurse can do to facilitate their expression.

Self-actualization, spirituality, and *transcendence* are vague, ambiguous terms that mean whatever the theorist thinks. These expressions also serve as umbrella terms for other conditions and situations that are addressed throughout this chapter. These terms overlap a great deal, but we have attempted to tease out the meanings for the reader, knowing that the perception of the reader will cast a particular interpretation that we may not have thought or intended. These conditions are ineffable, within the awareness of the individual but often inexpressible. Why, if these concepts are so obscure, do we include them as the final chapter in a text for nurses working with elders? Because these concepts are the life tasks of aging, seldom fully approached earlier. Concerns of the young are to become established as adults; middle-aged persons are overwhelmed with the requirements of success and survival.

Older people are more in touch with their inner psychological life than at any other point in the life cycle (Cohen, 2006). Ferreting out the reason for being and the meaning of life is the concern of elders. "As people age, confronting mortality is part of it, but as things change, they begin to recognize who they are and who they aren't, the strengths they have and haven't. They begin to think about the value and meaning of life. Tending to look more inwards rather than outwards often happens when we are 45 to 50, but there's a screaming need for it when we reach 85 or 90" (www.agingwellmag.com/news/septstory1.shtml). An understanding of the developmental phases in the second half of life assists in understanding the journey toward self-actualization (Box 24-1).

Nurses will likely see numerous older people who are apparently not seeking any of these esoteric states of existence and

463

<table>
<tr><td>

BOX 24-1   **DEVELOPMENTAL PHASES IN THE SECOND HALF OF LIFE**

</td><td>

BOX 24-2   **TRAITS OF SELF-ACTUALIZED PEOPLE**

</td></tr>
<tr><td>

- **Midlife reevaluation:** Early 40s to late 50s and characterized by seriously confronting the sense of one's own mortality and thinking about time remaining instead of time gone by. A catalyst for uncovering unrealized creative sides of ourselves.
- **Liberation:** Mid 50s to mid 70s and characterized by a sense of personal freedom to speak one's mind and do what needs to be done. With retirement comes a new experience of personal liberation and having time to experiment with something different.
- **Summing-up:** Late 60s to the 80s and beyond and characterized by the desire to find larger meaning in the story of one's life and to deal with unresolved conflicts and unfinished business. Motivation to give of the wisdom accrued throughout life, share lessons and fortunes through autobiography and personal storytelling, philanthropy, community activism, and volunteerism.
- **Encore:** Any time from the late 70s to the end of life and characterized by the desire to restate and reaffirm major themes in one's life and explore new variations on those themes or further attend to unfinished business or unresolved conflicts and a desire to live well until the end.

</td><td>

- Time competent: The person uses past and future to live more fully in the present.
- Inner directed: The person's source of direction depends on internal forces more than on others.
- Flexible: The person can react situationally, without unreasonable restrictions.
- Sensitive to self: The person is responsive to his or her own feelings.
- Spontaneous: The person is able and willing to be themself.
- Values self: The person accepts and demonstrates strengths as a person.
- Accepts self: The person approves of self, in spite of weaknesses or deficiencies.
- Positively views others: The person sees both the bad and the good in others as essentially good and constructive.
- Positively views life: The person sees the opposites of life as meaningfully related.
- Acceptance of aggressiveness: The person is able to accept own feelings of anger and aggressiveness.
- Capable of intimate contact: The person is able to develop warm interpersonal relationships with others.

</td></tr>
</table>

From: Cohen G: Research on creativity and aging: the positive impact of the arts on health and illness, *Generations* 30(1):7-15, 2006.

have never tried to cultivate their deepest inner nature. We live in a mechanistic, scientifically based culture in which cultivation of immeasurable states of being have not been necessarily regarded or regarded at all. The dramatic increase in the population of older people has been considered a problem to be solved in an era of dwindling resources rather than a resource to enrich society. Attempting to sort, dissect, and classify everything is a hazard of our society. Despite all the human efforts for the past millenia, we have not been able to completely grasp or dissect the human soul. Therefore, with effrontery and apologies, we will devote the last chapter to just that! I have many times approached this subject incorrectly by asking individuals what it is like to be old. Now that I am old, what it is like seems too concrete. What is the meaning of this stage of life? Every nurse must ask this question of his or her older clients, friends, and parents. Do not ask on your way out the door. For many people, this notion will take some pondering. For some, it will open the door of their later lives just a crack. Others will be enlightened and will teach you a great deal.

SELF-ACTUALIZATION

Self-actualization is the highest expression of one's individual potential and implies inner motivation that has been freed to express the most unique self or the "authentic person" (Maslow, 1959, p. 3). The crux of self-actualization is defining life in such a way as to allow room for continual discovery of self. A critical consideration in developing self-actualization is an underlying sense of mastery and a sense of coherence in the life situation. This effort depends to a large extent on individual attributes, as well as self-esteem. In this unit, we hope to expose the nurse to the myriad evidences of self-actualization in old age and suggest ways in which the nurse can assist older people in seeking their own unique way of living and growing. The focus is on nursing actions that may encourage elders to seek new possibilities within themselves.

Characteristics of the Self-Actualized

In old age, threats to self-esteem are strong if value is measured only by attainment, containment, power, and influence. Ethics, values, humor, courage, altruism, and integrity flourish in people who continue to grow toward self-actualization. Numerous other attributions can be mentioned. We focus only on those qualities that seem most pertinent to the older people that health care professionals are serving (Box 24-2).

Courage

Courage is the quality of mind or spirit that enables a person to conquer fear and despair in the face of difficulty, danger, pain, or uncertainty. We believe that facing a long, painful, and restricted existence requires the highest level of courage. An older man with diabetes, amputations, and failing vision sits in his room at the retirement home, looking out the window for hours each day, for weeks, months, and years. Yet, he retains his positive spirit and love of life. This is courage. An older lady crippled with arthritis attends her ailing spouse, who no longer recognizes her. This is courage.

When asking older people how they keep going day by day, various answers are given. No one has ever said to me, "It is because I am courageous." Older people need to be told. A gold star can be given to people who have lived and survived the long battle of living many years filled with both joy and pain. Memorials are made for people who die in battle, but few monuments are raised to those who courageously wake every morning with no great purpose or challenge to push them out of bed. Believing that older people are unable to be self-actualized unless they are energetic, healthy, and wealthy is a mistake. The capacity of the spirit to find meaning in existence is often remarkable. Nurses may ask, "What sustains you in your present situation?"

Altruism

A high degree of helping behaviors is present in many older people. The very old will remember the Great Depression and the altruism that kept people physically and spiritually alive. Neighbor helped neighbor long before the government came to the rescue. Apparently, a sense of meaning in life is strongly tied to survival and is derived from the conviction of, in some way, being needed by others. Many nurses are in the field because of altruistic motives and can understand the importance of assisting others. This idea might be discussed with the elder.

Volunteering often involves new role development and endeavors that expand one's awareness. When volunteer services are considered as a means of personal enrichment and an expression of altruism, it is important for the elder to augment some latent interest areas and launch into pursuits perhaps unavailable earlier because of time constraints or other commitments. Nurses may question elders about latent interests and talents that they may want to cultivate.

Humor

Metcalf (1993) explains humor: originating in the Latin root *humor*, meaning fluid and flexible, able to flow around and wear away obstacles. In the same way that water sustains our life and well-being, humor sustains our mental well-being. Cousins (1979) and many other researchers have recognized the importance of humor in recovery from illness. The physiological effects of humor stimulate production of catecholamines and hormones and increase pain tolerance by releasing endorphins.

Elders often initiate humor, and, in our seriousness, we may overlook the dry wit or, worse, perceive it as confusion. Older people are not a humorless group and frequently laugh at themselves. Objections to jokes about old age seem to emanate from the young far more than the old. Perhaps the old, from the vantage point of a lifetime, can more clearly see human predicaments. Ego transcendence (Peck, 1955) allows one to step back and view the self and situation without the intensity and despair of the egocentric individual.

Continuous Moral Development

The moral development of mankind, on an individual and collective basis, has been of interest to philosophers and religious leaders throughout history. The driving forces of morality are love (Plato) and intellect (Aristotle).

Kohlberg's refinements of his original theories have focused on the evidence, derived from autobiographies, that in maturity, transformations of moral outlook take place. Kohlberg posited old age as a seventh stage of moral development that goes beyond reasoning and reaches awareness of one's relative participation in universal morality. This stage of moral development involves identification with a more enduring moral perspective than that of one's own life span (Kohlberg and Power, 1981). This effort involves moral expansion and the exemplary impact of the fully developing elder on the following generations, born and unborn. We have come to believe that these exemplary lives may be the most important function of elders as we decry the honor and recognition given to individuals who seem to have little integrity or reliability. Each individual carries a mass of motivations and desires. Some people

are stunted, and some will flourish. Youngsters must have models of honorable, truthful, and honest elders if we hope to cultivate these qualities in society and human experience.

Self-Renewal

Self-renewal is an ongoing process that ideally continues through adult life as one becomes self-actualized (Hudson, 1999). According to Hudson, self-renewal involves the following:

- Commitment to beliefs
- Connecting to the world
- Times of solitude
- Episodic breaks from responsibility
- Contact with the natural world
- Creative self-expression
- Adaptation to changes
- Learning from down times

Collective Self-Actualization

The collective power of self-actualized older people has already brought about many changes in society. Power is a term describing the capacity of an individual or group to accomplish something, to take command, to exert authority, and to influence. The self-actualized older person is powerful and confident. Power is the gateway to resources and recognition.

The age-equality movement, older citizens returning to school, and the revolution of older people in movements such as the Gray Panthers have produced major changes in the status and recognition of older people. Gray Panthers recognize that issues of aging are not narrow or exclusive but, rather, are representative of human rights for people of all ages. Maggie Kuhn (1979), founder of the Gray Panthers, died in 1995 at the age of 89, but her beliefs and followers survive. Kuhn perceived that the issues confronting older people are not those of self-interest. As "elders of the tribe," the old should seek "survival of the tribe" (Kuhn, 1979, p. 3).

WISDOM

Wisdom is an ancient concept that has historically been associated with the elders of a society. Wisdom represents the pinnacle of human development and can be compared to Maslow's self-actualization or Erickson's ego integrity. In many cultures, older people are respected for their years of experience and are awarded the role of wise elder in political, judicial, cultural, and religious systems (Ardelt, 2004; Hooyman & Kiyak, 2011).

Over the last two decades, there has been renewed interest in the concept of wisdom and the capacity of the aging brain to develop unique capacities (Ardelt, 1997, 2000, 2003, 2004, Baltes 1991; Baltes and Smith, 2003, 2008). Many skills improve with age but are not identified on standard cognitive screens, and certain testing conditions have exaggerated age-related declines in cognitive performance (Chapter 19). The bulk of research has focused on cognitive declines and strategies to help older people find ways to overcome cognitive failings (Helmuth, 2003). Because of this emphasis, research on cognitive capacities in aging and possible ways to stimulate wisdom has been limited (Ardelt, 2004).

Moving beyond Piaget's formal operational stage of cognitive development, adult development theories propose a more

---

BOX 24-3 **DIMENSIONS OF WISDOM**

- Cognitive: Knowledge and acceptance of the positive and negative aspects of human nature; the limits of knowledge, and of life's unpredictability and uncertainties; a desire to know the truth and comprehend the significance and deeper meaning of experiences, phenomena and events
- Reflective: Being able to perceive phenomena and events from multiple perspectives; self-awareness, self-examination, self-insight; absence of subjectivity and projections (e.g., the tendency to blame other people or circumstances for one's own situation, decisions, or feelings)
- Affective: Sympathetic and compassionate love for others; positive emotions and behaviors toward others

From: Ardelt M: Wisdom as expert knowledge system: a critical review of a contemporary operationalization of an ancient concept, *Human Development* 47:257-285, 2004.

---

advanced cognitive stage, the postformal operational stage. In this stage, individuals develop the skills to view problems from multiple perspectives, utilize reflection, and communicate thoughtfully in complex and emotionally challenging situations (Parisi et al., 2009). Recent neuroimaging research has suggested that changes in the brain, once seen only as compensation for declining skills, are now thought to indicate development of new capacities. These changes include using both hemispheres more equally than younger adults, greater density of synapses, and more use of the frontal lobes, which are thought to be important in abstract reasoning, problem solving, and concept formation (Hooyman and Kiyak, 2011; Grossmann et al., 2010).

Characteristics of wisdom. One does not become wise simply because one grows old. Nor is wisdom achieved simply because of an accumulation of life experiences. Parisi and colleagues (2009) noted that "after centuries of trying to understand what it means to be wise, there is still considerable debate about the essential components of wisdom, how it is acquired, and how it is activated" (p. 868). Most agree that the achievement of wisdom is a developmental process that requires the ability to "integrate experiences across time and utilize these experiences in a reflective manner" (Parisi et al, 2009, p. 867).

Maturity, integrity, generativity, the ability to overcome negative personality characteristics such as neuroticism or self-centeredness, superior judgment skills in difficult life situations, the ability to cope with difficult challenges in life, and a strong sense of the ultimate meaning and purpose of life are also associated with wisdom (Ardelt, 2004) (Box 24-3). The renewed emphasis on wisdom and other cognitive capabilities that can develop with age provides a view of aging that reflects the history of many cultures and provides a much more hopeful view of both aging and human development.

Paths to growing older and wiser can be fostered throughout life. Viewing older people as resources for younger people and our society places the reason for and the immense value of aging at the center of focus. This is in contrast to the view of aging as inevitable decline, personal diminishment, disengagement from life, and a drain on society. Nursing too must turn to the wise leaders who came before us as we chart our course for the future (Chapter 1). Priscilla Ebersole, one of the geriatric nursing pioneers and co-author of this chapter, shares her reflections on wisdom from the perspective of her 83 years (Box 24-4).

With the prospect of longer and healthier lives, older people are looking for more meaningful and challenging ways to foster

---

BOX 24-4 **REFLECTIONS ON WISDOM: PRISCILLA EBERSOLE, GERIATRIC NURSING PIONEER**

In thinking about wisdom, I wonder what it is and if we ever achieve anything near that in one lifetime. I now have more questions about life than I have answers.

Where are we in the process of human evolution? We seem to be consumed with speed and technical wonders. What about the extrasensory perceptions and amazing coincidences that seemingly arise randomly? Are we still primitives?

Dying: doesn't it present more questions? I have become immunized as so many I love have preceded me, but it would be wonderful to know how much time I have—or would it?

How can one develop true compassion? I have flashes of it but find I still have many judgmental feelings about many persons and events. Is this not practical?

How can I learn more from others? I am rather trapped in my own skin and imperfections.

Is it true that our hormones really affect us so much? Yes, undoubtedly I have become much more aggressive with the almost total loss of estrogen. Do I care?

Is the search for prolongevity a worthy goal? Only when one is healthy and has something to offer the world. But, really, what is healthy? Only function? Mind health?

Does history really teach us anything? Though we seem to repeat so much of it yet pondering it and our roots remains significant for me.

And what about the universe, both macro and micro of which we really still know so little? Pondering and wondering, I will never know even a bit of all I wish.

Yet, becoming old is *becoming* as life seems to hold many lifetimes in one. There are so many challenges and circumstances that change one's perspective and beliefs. One begins to feel a part of and connected to every living thing; Aunt Laura expressed it well. The youth and elders in one's lifetime are so significant in one's philosophy. Grandchildren and great grandchildren open new vistas of thought and opportunities to redo some of the faltering actions of parenthood.

Catherine, my friend who died at 106, taught me more about aging than any experience in my life. She still giggled like a school girl as she told me of some amusing event in her life.

---

continued growth and contribute to society. Programs such as Foster Grandparents, the Experience Corps, and the Sage-ing Guild are examples of this new view. Further resources can be found on the Evolve website.

CREATIVITY

Creativity is a bridge between the growing self and the transcending of self. Creativity may be the transit mechanism between self-actualization (the reaching of one's highest potential) and the step beyond, to transcend the limitations of ego. "Creativity has always been at the heart of our experience as human beings . . . this need for creativity never ends" (Perlstein, 2006, p. 5). American culture has neglected to recognize the innate creativity in elders who are too often viewed as debilitated, in need of medical attention, and the focus of societal problems. Recently, our understanding of aging has expanded to a view that older people possess unique strengths and wisdom. Promoting health in aging is more than targeting problems and developing interventions for health promotion and disease prevention. Aging is potential as well as problems. A focus on creativity and aging and the positive impact of the arts on health, illness, and quality of life is gaining importance in our understanding of health and well-being among older adults (Cohen, 2006).

The National Center for Creative Aging, established in 2001, is dedicated to fostering the relationship between creative expression and quality of life for older people. The *Beautiful Minds: Finding Your Lifelong Potential* campaign is a new initiative from the Center that focuses on raising awareness of people who are keeping their minds beautiful and the actions people can take to maintain the brain. Research suggests that there are four dimensions to brain health: the nourished mind, the socially connected mind, the mentally active mind, and the physically active mind. These dimensions stress the importance of healthy diet, social engagement, cognitive stimulation, and physical activity to brain health (www.creativeaging.org).

The Creativity and Aging Study is the first formal experimental study investigating the "influence of professionally conducted, participatory arts programs on the general health, mental health, and social activities of older people" (Cohen, 2006, p. 11). Preliminary results indicate that participation in the arts programs has positive effects on physical health, independence, and morale of participants when compared with a control group (Cohen, 2006).

Products of creativity are less important than creative attitudes. Curiosity, inquisitiveness, wonderment, puzzlement, and craving for understanding are creative attitudes. Much of the natural creative imagination of childhood is subdued by enculturation. In old age, some people seem able to break free of excessive enculturation and again express their free spirit when practical matters no longer demand their sole attention.

Creativity is often considered in terms of the arts, literature, and music. A truly self-actualized person may express creativity in any activity. Breaking through the habitual or traditional mode into authentic expression of self is creativity, whether it is through cooking, cleaning, planting, poetry, art, or teaching. Creative expression does not necessarily mean that the older person has to create a work of art. Subtler ways of expressing creativity are present even in the frailest of older people. Consider Priscilla Ebersole's description of Catherine at 100 years old and living in a nursing home:

> Catherine was self-actualized and creative to the best possible extent. Her physical constraints were enormous: she had no material assets, her range of activity was limited to her small cubicle in a skilled nursing facility, and her body was frail. However, her spirit was strong, and she knew and used her potential. Catherine's creativity was expressed at each meal when she rearranged, mixed, and added to her food. She carefully chopped a pickle and sprinkled it on her cottage cheese and added a little honey to her applesauce. Each meal was a small adventure. Several friends would visit regularly and bring Catherine small items she enjoyed. They could always count on being entertained with creatively embroidered tales of the past. The gifts they brought were always used in extraordinary ways. A scarf might be tied around her head. Powder, perfume, books, and other things would be bartered for favors from staff members or given as gifts. Her radio brought news of the day interspersed with classical music. Catherine created a milieu in which she enjoyed life and maintained her self-esteem. That she was self-actualized was never in doubt. Her artistry overflowed in myriad small gestures.

Creative Arts for Older Adults

Maximizing the use of self in the later years in unique ways might be termed creative self-actualization. Many individuals will need the stimulus of an interested person to uncover latent interests and talents. Other people will need encouragement to try new avenues of self-expression—some will be fitting for them and others not. Several ideas are presented here for nurses working with older people who may need an introduction to creative use of leisure time.

Many aspects of the developmental needs of older people are met by artistic expressions. Among these achievements are (1) conflict resolution, (2) clarification of thoughts and feelings, (3) creation of balance and an inner order, (4) a sense of being in control of the external world, (5) creation of something positive from defeating experiences or in the face of paralyzing depression, (6) artistic communication as an integral part of human experience, and (7) the sustenance of human integrity. Wikstrom (2004, p. 30) suggests that art and aesthetics "help individuals know themselves, become more alive to human conditions, provide a new way of looking at themselves and the world, and offer opportunities for participation in new visual and auditory experiences." Each person has a private, symbolic, feeling world that can be brought out by certain expressive activities.

Ideas for developing creative activities with older people are presented in Box 24-5.

Creative Expression Through Theater, Dance, Music, and Poetry

Endowment grants are available to ensure the continued contributions of elders as artists, teachers, mentors, students, volunteers, patrons, and consumers of the arts. Some of the programming grants have supported drama groups, storytelling, dance, and singing. These activities are designed for older people of all levels of ability; some are teachers and mentors, some are entertainers, and some are participants, purely for the joy of living.

Theater

Stagebridge, based in San Francisco, is the oldest senior theater stage company. Stagebridge performers adapt popular children's books about grandchildren (*Grandparent Tales*) around the world with multicultural casts ranging in age from 10 to 80 years. Other programs include a performing arts camp and presentations to nursing students to enhance sensitivity and knowledge about care of older people (www.stagebridge.com).

Dance

Rhythms infiltrate life on every level from individual cellular functions to the constantly expanding and contracting universe. Unseen and unfelt oscillating waves surround us. Felt waves—pulsating, vibrating, and undulating—stimulate us. These waves are intrinsic to existence and may somewhat explain the healing power of music, poetry, and repetitive movement. Life itself is an ongoing dance. In many countries, song, dance, and poetic history flow as naturally as breath and are inextricably interwoven in daily existence.

BOX 24-5   **IDEAS FOR DEVELOPING CREATIVE ABILITIES**

ART

Using oil pastels, create a drawing that represents self, or select three colors you like and three colors you dislike, using all six colors to create a self-portrait.

Draw a representation of your world.

Create a collage or mobile out of an assortment of materials and pictures that can represent subjects, such as the self, part of self you like or dislike, or the family.

In small groups, use clay to create an art piece or a statement.

MUSIC

Play a variety of music; focus discussion on imagery and any feelings that the music evokes.

Discuss or have clients bring in music that elicits feelings of sadness, happiness, and so on.

Show a picture (can be cut from a magazine), and ask members to see if they can imagine the sounds that might go with the picture.

Express self or group through dance and movement to select music.

MOVEMENT

Create a movement to fit the way you are feeling while introducing self to group.

Have members stand and initiate a slow, swaying motion (good exercise with which to end the group session).

Have members mirror each other's movements, such as hands or the entire body, creating a duet.

IMAGERY

Use guided fantasies and imagery to facilitate stress reduction and relaxation, awareness, the power of one's own healing capability, and self-expression through symbols and symbolisms.

WRITING

Encourage journals or diaries; set a group time available to write and share ideas.

In small groups, create a group poem.

Read selected poems or stories as a group, and then share reactions and feelings from the readings.

Create a book to be distributed to group consisting of a collection of members' writings.

Dance is not only an enjoyable social activity for many older people, but it also provides the benefits of physical activity in an enjoyable form with measurable increases in quality of life, improved balance, and mobility (Krampe et al., 2010). The physical benefits of dance include promoting head and trunk movement, shifting the center of gravity in every direction from the axis of support, and improving cardiopulmonary function.

Krampe and colleagues (2010) conducted a pilot study investigating the use of a specific type of therapeutic dance, the Lebed Method, with frail older people at a PACE Center. The Lebed Method, originally developed for women with lymphedema, combines low-impact dance with upbeat participant-specific music. Results included positive trends in the functional status of the participants, including improvement in balance and gait. Further research is needed, but the intervention shows promise for improving balance and gait and reducing fall risk. Many community centers and adult day programs for older people are incorporating dance into their activity programs, and this modality holds promise for enhancing movement, decreasing fall risk, and contributing to socialization and enjoyment.

Music

Music is a familiar and universal experience. Tonal or rhythmic music can be an inward experience or an outward expression. As such, music is adaptable to each individual. Music therapy is an individual music program prescribed by a professional music therapist to bring about desirable changes in behavior. However, the use of music listening in a clinical situation does not require special knowledge of music and is considered a safe, simple, low-cost, and evidence-based intervention nurses can use independently to improve the environment of older adults and enhance well-being (McCaffrey, 2008; Witzke et al., 2008).

The self-determined use of music as a means of enjoyment and personal expression can be achieved by listening, meditating, improvising, relaxing, moving to music, creative dancing, composing, learning new songs, studying music history, rhythmic patterning, mastering an instrument, building an instrument, or in any other manner an individual chooses to adapt music toward self-fulfillment. Music can be a comforting, structured expression, a therapeutic tool, or it can provide the opportunity for creative and imaginative self-expression. People with dementia often respond to music, moving to the rhythms and singing the words to old songs, even when their verbal communication skills are quite impaired.

The therapeutic benefits of music for older people have been well described and include comfort and pain relief, improved cognition and reduced acute confusion after knee or hip surgery, decreased anxiety and stress, improved food consumption, decreased agitation in older adults with dementia, and decreased need for physical and chemical restraints (Gerdner, 2000, 2005; Hicks-Moore, 2005; McCaffrey, 2008; McCaffrey and Freeman, 2003; McCaffrey and Good, 2000; McCaffrey and Locsin, 2006; Twiss et al., 2006; Witzke et al., 2008). An evidence-based guideline, *Individualized Music for Elders with Dementia* (Gerdner, 2010) (www.guideline.gov) can be used by nurses to better understand the use of music with older adults with dementia. This guideline also has a consumer version for family caregivers. Additionally, an interactive online continuing education module for nurses to learn more about individualized music interventions is provided through Sigma Theta Tau International and the John A. Hartford Foundation (Gerdner, 2010).

Poetry

Music and poetic expression are similar in rhythmic beauty. Traditionally, poetry has been judged and categorized by its rhythmic meter. However, modern poetry may have style and quality without a categorical rhythm. Older people enjoy the traditional patterns, rhyming qualities, and free verse. Many people who never thought of themselves as poets have discovered a talent for poetic expression.

Killick (1997, 2000, 2008) has done beautiful work with poetry writing with persons who have dementia. Killick (2005) has said that "people with dementia can often find a real solace and satisfaction and a creativity in speaking in this way and having it recognized as being of value because they're so used to being put down" (www.bbc.co.uk/radio4/youandyours/transcript_2005_46_fri_02.shtml). Koch (1977) wrote a delightful book explaining the way he began poetry groups with older individuals who did not think of themselves as poets.

Reading for Self-Development

Reading is an ageless activity, and some older people prefer the individual, passive involvement in reading to group activities. Group reading and discussion can also be enjoyable, as demonstrated in the Great Books discussion groups that meet routinely in many libraries. When an array of books is available, many older people find them sustaining. Books extend boundaries imposed by physical limitations, allow exploration into untouched areas of thought, and enrich the individual. For many older people, reading has been a major pleasure throughout life and, common as it seems, should not be underestimated as a form of self-discovery and self-actualization. Many libraries have developed creative programs to serve older people. Some of these include talking books for the visually impaired, large-print books and magazines, and a 24-hour audio reader service through a closed-circuit radio station.

Creative Arts and People with Dementia

Creative and expressive activities are not limited to the cognitively intact elder. Art, poetry, dance, music, drama, and storytelling activities are therapeutic interventions that offer great value to people with dementia. According to Bastings (2006, p. 17):

> To people with dementia, the arts bring tools that enable them to express themselves and their vision of the world. The arts operate on an emotional level, one needn't have control of rational language to write a poem, create a dance, or take a photograph. Where rational language and factual memory have failed people with dementia, the arts offer an avenue for communication and connection with caregivers, loved ones, and the greater world.

The National TimeSlips Project (Bastings, 2006) is an example of a creative storytelling program designed for people with dementia (see Chapter 6). Arts for Alzheimer's, Arts for the Aged, and the Age Exchange Theater are other examples of creative arts programs for people with dementia. At the Louis and Anne Green Memory and Wellness Center in the Christine E. Lynn College of Nursing at Florida Atlantic University, the "Artful Memories" program provides opportunities for individuals with mild to moderate dementia to learn techniques of artistic creation and expression in artistic media in a supportive and nonjudgmental environment. Works created are on display at the Center and have been made into calendars as well (Figure 24-1). Participants have derived a great deal of pleasure, pride, stimulation, and camaraderie from the time spent creating art. The arts offer people with dementia the opportunity for expression of feelings, connections, and joy and hold tremendous promise to improve the quality of life for people with dementia (Bastings, 2006). Additional resources

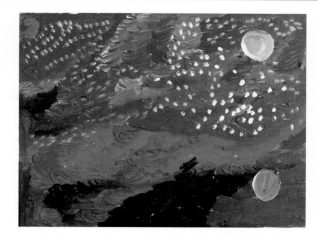

FIGURE 24-1 Artwork created by Frances Hope Goldstein in the Florida Atlantic University (FAU) Louis and Anne Green Memory and Wellness Center "Artful Memories" program.

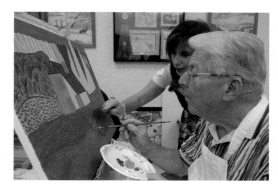

Artful Memories Program (Photo Courtesy of Florida Atlantic University, Louis and Anne Green Memory and Wellness Center.)

related to creative arts for people with dementia can be found on the Evolve website.

RECREATION

Recreation is akin to creation. The wisdom of regularly scheduled periods of recreation and recuperation following creative acts can be traced to early Jewish writings and the creation story. If God needed time to rest and recuperate, we certainly do. Inherent in creative acts is time for renewal, time for re-creation. Burnout and boredom are companions of monotony and shorten the perceived life span by emptiness and vanished time. A change of scene or companions may be exhilarating. Retreats from routine to periods of recreation are important as are retreats following intensive efforts.

An important point is that the lower four levels of need must be met to some degree before one is ready for recreation and creative acts. The individual struggling with feelings of insecurity needs predictable routines. Nurses need to assess readiness (in terms of needs met) for challenge, change, and creative expression. Many intricate plans for recreation and creative expression fail because (1) the individual is focusing energy on meeting needs at a more basic level or (2) the individual has

BOX 24-6   RESOURCES THAT CAN ENHANCE RECREATIONAL ACTIVITIES AND PROGRAMS

- Local florists may present a flower show or provide a flower-arranging activity.
- Police/fire departments may give safety presentations.
- Local religious leaders may lead readings and discussions of religious/philosophical works.
- Craft suppliers may give demonstrations.
- Local pharmacists may give talks on medication use.
- Clothing stores can sponsor fashion shows.
- Bakeries may give demonstrations of pastry decoration.
- Beauty supply houses may give makeup demonstrations.
- Travel agencies may present slide shows.
- Librarians may institute great book discussions or other activities.
- Students from community colleges may provide numerous educational events and activities.
- Garden clubs or horticultural groups may provide gardening classes.
- Collector's clubs may talk about collecting stamps, antiques, coins, or memorabilia.
- Historical societies may give tours to historic places of interest.
- Whenever possible, events should be planned as field trips to the sites of the locals involved because trips add elements of additional interest, stimulation, and involvement in the community at large.

not been consulted about his or her particular interests or talents.

Group activities often provide a sense of belonging, body integration, and better function, but they do not necessarily supply self-esteem or the opportunity for self-actualization. Self-esteem grows out of individual accomplishments and personal recognition. Self-actualization flows from confidence and a milieu in which self-expression is cultivated and valued. Resources that can enhance recreational activities and programs are presented in Box 24-6.

BRINGING YOUNG AND OLD TOGETHER

Larson (2006) suggests that intergenerational programs can "help older and younger people look beyond their generational stereotypes and know each other (body, mind, and spirit)" (p. 39). Intergenerational programs can be those in which older people assist younger people (tutoring, mentoring, child care, foster grandparent programs); those in which younger people assist older people (social visits, meal assistance); and those in which younger and older people serve together. Benefits of intergenerational programs for younger people include increased self-esteem and self-worth, improved behavior, increased involvement and success in school work, and a sense of historical and personal continuity. For older people, contact with younger people can promote life satisfaction, decrease isolation, help develop new skills and insights, promote fulfillment, establish new and meaningful relationships, and provide a sense of meaning and purpose (Larson, 2006). Examples of such programs include the Elders Share the Arts, Roots and Branches Theatre Company and the Liz Lerman Dance Exchange (www.danceexhange.org).

Recognizing the developmental significance of contact between the generations, some long-term care facilities have included children in their milieu in various ways:

- As residents (children with profound developmental disabilities or severe neurological disabilities): Elders rock, stroke, and cuddle these children, providing stimulation for both.
- As a service to employees (day care centers for children of employees): Elders sometimes assist in the care and special programs for the children, such as reading stories or teaching basic skills (tying shoes, telling time).
- In adopt-a-grandparent programs: One child affiliates with one institutionalized person with periodic visits, cards, and inclusion of the grandparent in some special family events.

Nurses in the community may want to explore potential intergenerational experiences that may be of interest to their older clients. Area Agencies on Aging can provide information on intergenerational programs that are available in the community. Although we recommend intergenerational contact when desired by the older person, certain pitfalls must be considered. Contacts with the very young, energetic child must be brief, or else the elder is likely to be exhausted, and the benefits will decrease. In intergenerational programs, young people need consistent supervision, support, and training in the developmental aspects of old age. Similarly, elders will also benefit from education and support in understanding developmental tasks of children, as well as effective methods of intergenerational communication.

PROMOTING HEALTHY AGING: IMPLICATIONS FOR GERONTOLOGICAL NURSING

In this unit, we have considered what aging can be and that the last years can truly actualize the most unique capacities of older people. Our functions as nurses who value self-actualization are (1) to continually spur our clients to ask, "What is possible and suitable for me?" and (2) to assist them in finding appropriate resources and, when needed, assist in implementing activities toward self-actualization. The nature of self-actualization is self-determination and direction. Nurses are ancillary to the process but may be needed to stir the beginnings of the search. In doing so, we may move forward with our own search.

Self-actualization implies that one actualizes the potential of self through various mechanisms. We have mentioned only a few of these mechanisms in a somewhat cursory manner, knowing that these individually instituted actions have a force of their own and that once activated go far beyond the professionals' involvement. Activities such as yoga, focused meditation, the discipline of karate, and other forms of centered concentration are segued into spirituality and transcendence.

SPIRITUALITY

Spirituality is a rather indescribable need that drives individuals throughout life to seek meaning and purpose in their existence. Spirituality is difficult to define, though many people have tried. We can observe the body and we can imagine the mind in operation and measure intelligence, but there is no computerized tomography (CT) scan of the spirit (Bell and

Troxel, 2001). Understanding spirituality is far more elusive than learning about the pathology associated with disease and illness.

Spirituality has been defined as a "quality of a person derived from the social and cultural environment that involves faith, a search for meaning, a sense of connection with others, and a transcendence of self, resulting in a sense of inner peace and well-being" (Delgado, 2007, p. 230). The spiritual aspect of people's lives transcends the physical and psychosocial to reach the deepest individual capacity for love, hope, and meaning. Erickson's concept of ego integrity and Maslow's concept of self-actualization seem closely related to development of a spiritual self.

Aging as a biological process has been studied extensively. Less attention has been paid to the study of aging as a spiritual process. As people age and move closer to death, spirituality may become more important. Declining physical health, loss of loved ones, and a realization that life's end may be near often challenge older people to reflect on the meaning of their lives. Spiritual belief and practices often play a central role in helping older adults cope with life challenges and is a strength in the lives of older adults (Hodge et al., 2010). Nursing studies of spirituality and aging indicate that spirituality increases in importance (Lowry and Conco, 2002), is a source of hope (Touhy, 2001a), aids in adaptation to illnesses such as arthritis (Potter and Zauszniewski, 2000), and has a positive influence on quality of life in chronically ill older adults (O'Brien, 2003). The ultimate goal for promoting spirituality is to support and enhance quality of life.

Spirituality must be considered a significant factor in understanding healthy aging. Rowe and Kahn's (1998) model of successful aging includes active engagement in life, minimal risk and disability, and high cognitive and physical function. Crowther and colleagues (2002) maintain that spirituality must be the fourth element of the model and is interrelated with all of the others. Spirituality may be particularly important to healthy aging in "historically disadvantaged populations who display remarkable strength despite adversities in their lives" (Hooyman and Kiyak, 2005, p. 213). The ultimate goal for promoting spirituality is to support and enhance quality of life. Spiritual well-being may be considered the ability to experience and integrate meaning and purpose in life through connectedness with self, others, art, music, literature, nature, or a power greater than oneself (Gaskamp et al., 2006).

Spirituality and Religion

Distinguishing between religion and spirituality is a concern for many health professionals. Religious beliefs and participation in religious obligations and rites are often the avenues of spiritual expression, but they are not necessarily interchangeable. "Religion can be described as a social institution that unites people in a faith in God a higher power, and in common rituals and worshipful acts. A god, divinity, and/or soul is always included in the concept" (Strang and Strang, 2002, p. 858). Each religion involves a particular set of beliefs. Spirituality is a broader concept than religion and encompasses a person's values or beliefs, search for meaning, relationships with a higher power, with nature, and with other people. The concept of spirituality is found in all cultures and societies.

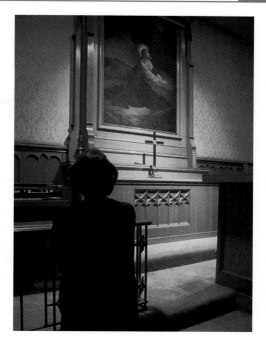

Prayer. (From Lewis SM et al: *Medical-surgical nursing: assessment and management of clinical problems,* ed 7, St Louis, 2007, Mosby.)

For some people, particularly older people, formalized religion helps them feel fulfilled. The majority of older adults describe themselves as both spiritual and religious (Hodge et al., 2010). Gerontologists appreciate the significance of religion and spirituality in promoting the well-being of elders.

"Although aging changes can affect the body and the mind, there is no evidence that the spirit succumbs to the aging process, even in the presence of debilitating physical and emotional illness" (Heriot, 1992, p. 23). For some older people, particularly those who are frail or cognitively impaired, meeting spiritual needs may be a greater challenge than for healthier elders. Functional decline and dependence can threaten the sense of identity and connection with others and the world, thus causing a loss of spirit (Leetun, 1996; Touhy 2001b). The spiritual aspect transcends the physical and psychosocial to reach the deepest individual capacity for love, hope, and meaning. The spiritual person can rise above that which is humanly expected in a situation. For example, a dying elder in great pain who was being cared for by Dr. Ebersole said: "This is so hard for you." That he was able to see beyond himself at that time was difficult to believe.

PROMOTING HEALTHY AGING: IMPLICATIONS FOR GERONTOLOGICAL NURSING

Assessment

Patients welcome a discussion of spiritual matters and want health professionals to consider their spiritual needs. The older person may have a pressing need to talk about philosophy and spiritual development. Private time for prayer, meditation, and reflection may be needed. Nurses may neglect to explore this issue with elders because religion and spirituality may not seem the high priority. The client should be assured that religious longings and rituals are important and that opportunities will be made available as desired. Nurses need to be knowledgeable and respectful about the rites and rituals of varying religions, cultural beliefs, and values (see Chapter 5). Religious and spiritual resources, such as pastoral visits, should be available in all settings where older people reside. It is important to avoid imposing one's own beliefs and to respect the person's privacy on matters of spirituality and religion (Touhy and Zerwekh, 2006).

Spiritual care entails assisting patients to find a sense of meaning and reconciliation with others and with a transcendent reality, while encouraging patients to strengthen their spiritual life as they choose. Nurses may not lead individuals to soul growth and acceptance when facing illness and disability but may have the privilege of accompanying them on the journey. If spiritual growth is the primary focus of the older person, clergy will be best suited to work with the person. Reflection, feedback, comfort, and affirmation are all a part of being with the elder, providing the supports that release energy for spiritual seeking.

An emphasis on spirituality in nursing is not new; nursing has encompassed the spiritual from its origin. The science of nursing was not seen as separate from the art and spirit of the discipline. Florence Nightingale's view of nursing was derived from her spiritual philosophy, and she considered nursing a spiritual experience, "intrinsic to human nature, our deepest and most potent resource for healing" (Macrae, 1995, p. 8). Many nursing theories address spirituality, including those of Neuman, Parse, and Watson (Martsolf and Mickley, 1998). Nursing and medicine are beginning to reclaim some of the essential healing values from their roots.

The essence of being spiritual is being whole or holistic, and attention to the spiritual needs of patients is a critical dimension of holistic nursing care. Yet surveys with practicing nurses suggest that most have had little, if any, education in spiritual care. Many nurses view spiritual nursing responses in religious terms and may feel that spirituality is a religious matter better left to clergy and religious leaders. Heriot (1992) suggested that nurses need to understand care of the human spirit both within and outside the context of religion. "Incorporating spirituality into the caring dimension of nursing requires a sensitivity to the many ways in which spirituality may be experienced and thus expressed" (Dyson et al., 1997, p. 1186).

Goldberg (1998) asserted that the connection in the nurse-patient relationship is central to spiritual care but that most nurses are "carrying out spiritual interventions at an unconscious level" (p. 840). She called for education and research to help nurses become more aware of the importance of connection and use of self in relationships as ways of bringing the elements of spiritual care into conscious awareness.

An evidence-based guideline for promoting spirituality in the older adult (Gaskamp et al., 2006) provides a framework for spiritual assessment and interventions. The guideline identifies older adults who may be at risk for spiritual distress and who might be most likely to benefit from use of the guideline (Box 24-7). Spiritual distress or spiritual pain is "an individual's perception of hurt or suffering associated with that part of his or her person that seeks to transcend the realm of the

---

BOX 24-7   IDENTIFYING ELDERS AT RISK FOR SPIRITUAL DISTRESS

- Individuals experiencing events or conditions that affect the ability to participate in spiritual rituals
- Diagnosis and treatment of a life-threatening, chronic, or terminal illness
- Expressions of interpersonal or emotional suffering, loss of hope, lack of meaning, need to find meaning in suffering
- Evidence of depression
- Cognitive impairment
- Verbalized questioning or loss of faith
- Loss of interpersonal support

Data from Gaskamp C, Sutter R, Meraviglia M, et al: *Journal of Gerontological Nursing* 32:8, 2006.

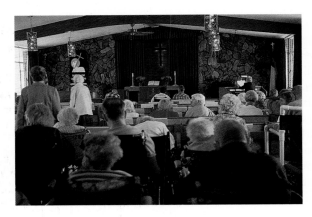

Residents attend a religious service at a nursing center. (From Sorrentino SA, Gorek B: *Mosby's textbook for long-term care assistants,* ed 5, St Louis, 2007, Mosby.)

---

material. Spiritual distress is manifested by a deep sense of hurt stemming from feelings of loss or separation from one's God or deity, a sense of personal inadequacy or sinfulness before God and man, or a pervasive condition of loneliness" (Gaskamp et al., 2006, p. 9).

The person experiencing spiritual distress is unable to experience the meaning of hope, connectedness, and transcendence. Spiritual distress may be manifested by anger, guilt, blame, hatred, expressions of alienation, turning away from family and friends, inability to enjoy, and inability to participate in religious activities that have previously provided comfort.

A spiritual history opens the door to a conversation about the role of spirituality and religion in a person's life. People often need permission to talk about these issues. Without a signal from the nurse, patients may feel that such topics are not welcome or appropriate.

There are formal spiritual assessments, but open-ended questions can also be used to begin dialogue about spiritual concerns (Box 24-8). Simply listening to patients as they express their fears, hopes, and beliefs is important. Spiritual assessments are intended to elicit information about the core spiritual needs and how the nurse and other members of the health care team can respond to them. These include the Faith, Importance/Influence, Community and Address (FICA) Spiritual History (Puchalski and Romer, 2000) and the Brief Assessment of Spiritual Resources and Concerns (Koenig and Brooks, 2002; Meyer, 2003) (Box 24-9). The Joint Commission requires

BOX 24-8	QUESTIONS TO BEGIN DIALOGUE ABOUT SPIRITUAL CONCERNS

- Tell me more about your life.
- What has been most meaningful in your life?
- To whom do you turn when you need help?
- What brings you joy and comfort?
- What are you most proud of?
- How have you found strength throughout your life?
- What are you hopeful about?
- Is spiritual peace important to you? What would help you achieve it?
- Is your religion or God significant in your life? Can you describe how?
- Is prayer or meditation helpful?
- What spiritual or religious practices bring you comfort?
- Are there religious books or materials that you want nearby?
- What are you afraid of right now?
- What do you wish you could still do?
- What are your concerns at this time for the future?
- What matters most to you right now?

Adapted from Touhy T, Zerwekh J: Spiritual caring. In Zerwekh J: *Nursing care at the end of life: palliative care for patients and families,* Philadelphia, 2006, FA Davis; Hospice of the Florida Suncoast, 2001.

BOX 24-10	SPIRITUAL NURSING RESPONSES

- Relief of physical discomfort, which permits focus on the spiritual
- Creating a peaceful environment
- Comforting touch, which fosters nurse-patient connection
- Authentic presence
- Attentive listening
- Knowing the patient as a person
- Listening to life stories
- Sharing fears and listening to self-doubts or guilt
- Fostering forgiveness and reconciliation
- Validating the person's life and assuring them they will be remembered
- Sharing caring words and love
- Encouraging family support and presence
- Fostering connections to that which is held sacred by the person
- Praying with and for the patient
- Respecting religious traditions and providing for access to religious objects and rituals
- Referring the person to a spiritual counselor

Sources: Gaskamp C, Sutter R, Meraviglia M, et al: *Journal of Gerontological Nursing* 32:8, 2006; Touhy T, Zerwekh H: Spiritual caring. In Zerwekh J: *Nursing care at the end of life: palliative care for patients and families,* Philadelphia, 2006, FA Davis.

BOX 24-9	BRIEF ASSESSMENT OF SPIRITUAL RESOURCES AND CONCERNS

Instructions: Use the following questions as an interview guide with the older adult (or caregiver if the older adult is unable to communicate).

- Does your religion/spirituality provide comfort or serve as a cause of stress? (Ask to explain in what ways spirituality is a comfort or stressor).
- Do you have any religious or spiritual beliefs that might conflict with health care or affect health care decisions? (Ask to identify any conflicts.)
- Do you belong to a supportive church, congregation, or faith community? (Ask how the faith community is supportive.)
- Do you have any practices or rituals that help you express your spiritual or religious beliefs? (Ask to identify or describe practices.)
- Do you have any spiritual needs you would like someone to address? (Ask what those needs are and if referral to a spiritual professional is desired.)
- How can we (health care providers) help you with your spiritual needs or concerns?

From Gaskamp C, Sutter R, Meraviglia M, et al: *Journal of Gerontological Nursing* 32:8, 2006, p. 10. Adapted from Meyer CL: *Dissertation Abstracts International* 55:2158B, UMI No 9428614, 2003; Koenig HG, Brooks RG: *Public Policy & Aging Report* 12:13, 2002.

spiritual assessments in hospitals, nursing homes, home care organizations, and many other health care settings providing services to older adults. The process of spiritual assessment is more complex than completing a standardized form and must be done within the context of the nurse-patient relationship.

For older people with cognitive impairment, information about the importance of spirituality and religious beliefs can be obtained from family members (Gaskamp et al., 2006). Nurses often see cognitive impairments as obstacles or excuses to providing spiritual care to people with dementia (Heriot, 1992). Nurturing mind, body, and spirit is part of holistic nursing, and nurses must provide opportunities to all elders, no matter how impaired, to live life with meaning, purpose, and hope (Touhy, 2001a).

Spiritual Responses

The caring relationship between nurses and persons nursed is the heart of nursing that touches and supports the spirit. Knowing persons in their complexity, responding to that which matters most to them, identifying and nurturing connections, listening with one's being, using presence and silence, and fostering connections to that which is held sacred by the person are spiritual nursing responses that arise from within the caring, connected relationship (Touhy, 2001b). Suggestions for spiritual care interventions are presented in Box 24-10.

Nurturing the Spirit of the Nurse

"Because spiritual care occurs over time and within the context of relationship, probably the most effective tool at the nurse's disposal is the use of self" (Soeken and Carson, 1987, p. 607). Thinking about what gives your own life meaning and value helps in developing your spiritual self and assists you in being able to offer spiritual support to patients. Examples of activities include finding quiet time for meditation and reflection; keeping your own faith traditions; being with nature; appreciating the arts; spending time with those you love; and journaling (Touhy and Zerwekh, 2006). Giving your patient the best spiritual care stems from taking care of your own spiritual needs first. Find ways to nourish your own spirit. Nurses often do not take the time to do so and become dispirited. This is especially true for nurses who work with dying patients and experience grief and loss repeatedly. Having someone to talk to about feelings is important. Practicing compassion for oneself is essential to authentic practice of compassion for others (Touhy and Zerwekh, 2006) (Box 24-11).

Know that caring for an aging body is the least of the work with the elderly. "Limiting care to the physical needs denies elders the opportunity to live out their life with meaning, purpose, and hope" (Touhy, 2001a, p. 45). Recognizing the primacy of the spirit is essential. Some very spiritual individuals

---

BOX 24-11 **PERSONAL SPIRITUALITY QUESTIONS FOR REFLECTION FOR NURSES**

- What do I believe in?
- How do I find purpose and meaning in my life?
- How do I take care of my physical, emotional, and spiritual needs?
- What are my hopes and dreams?
- Who do I love, and who loves me?
- How am I with others?
- What would I change about my relationships?
- Am I willing to heal relationships that trouble me?

Source: Touhy T, Zerwekh J: Spiritual caring. In Zerwekh J: *Nursing care at the end of life: palliative care for patients and families*, Philadelphia, 2006, FA Davis.

BOX 24-12 **RESEARCH HIGHLIGHTS**

Spirituality and Health

This qualitative study examined health and spirituality in 10 women living in a rural senior high-rise apartment setting. Range of ages of the participants was from 69 to 85 years (M = 76.5 years). Four were widowed; one was separated; three were single; and two were divorced. Six considered themselves Protestant, and four considered themselves Catholic.

A demographic questionnaire was administered, and semi-structured interviews were conducted. A broad opening question was asked: "What is the meaning of living?" This was followed by broad questions asking the participants to describe the experience of health and spirituality. If spirituality was included in responses, participants were asked: "What does spirituality mean to you?" and "What life experiences brought you to your conclusions about spirituality?"

Three themes were identified: (1) health is functional; (2) spirituality is a personal relationship with a Higher Power or God; and (3) death is a part of nature for which one is never prepared. All of the participants described spirituality as a personal relationship with a Higher Power operationalized by faith, prayer, keeping busy, and having family support. Theme clusters around spirituality included: (1) coping is keeping busy, using prayer, and having faith; (2) God has the Higher Power but individuals also have some control; and (3) beauty is in nature, colors, and inner beauty.

Participants' perceptions of spirituality were consistent with those found in the literature. While most did not regularly attend church services at this time in their life, praying and reading Bible scriptures were important to their spiritual life. Spirituality was described as a way of coping. Appreciation of the interconnectedness of health and spirituality and the use of spirituality as a coping mechanism with life events and the effects of chronic illness is important in the lives of many elders and should be included in assessment, care planning, and education of nurses. Opportunities for prayer, worship, scripture, or religious readings should be made available to those for whom this is important. Further research is needed with larger samples and diverse populations, as well as elders of other religious or non-religious backgrounds.

Data from Knestrick J, Lohri-Posey B: *Journal of Gerontological Nursing* 31:44, 2005.

---

are unable to articulate their knowing. Therefore, do not negate that aspect of an individual's experience because it is not expressed verbally. Realizing that biopsychosocial aspects of aging are all shards of the spirit will integrate every aspect of your work in gerontological nursing. The results of a nursing study on spirituality and health are presented in Box 24-12.

Faith Community Nursing

Faith community nursing (FCN) is a specialty practice for professional nursing with established scope and standards of practice (American Nurses Association, 2005). The focus of faith community nursing is "the protection, promotion and optimization of health and abilities, prevention of illness and injury, and responding to suffering in the context of values, beliefs and practices of a faith community" (ANA, 2005, p. 1). FCN was originally known as *parish nursing*, but the name was changed to Faith Community Nursing to reflect the broader scope of the practice and the full range of faiths (Dyess et al., 2009; Dyess and Chase, 2010).

In a literature review of the current state of research for FCN, Dyess, Chase and Newlin (2009) noted that FCN began 20 years ago and is widely implemented today in many faith communities in the United States and in multiple countries around the world. These authors suggest that FCN can assist in bridging the gaps in care in the current health care system, contribute to a reduction in acute health care costs, promote health and disease prevention, and integrate faith with health care to promote positive health outcomes. Models of care such as those implemented in FCN may be particularly relevant to meeting the health maintenance needs and spiritual needs of older people with chronic illness living in the community (Dyess and Chase, 2010). Further research is needed to understand the role of faith, religion, or spirituality within the practice of FCN, the diversity of beliefs and faith systems, and the impact on individual and community health outcomes through FCN interventions (Dyess et al., 2009). However, as these authors note: "The faith community is an ideal place to study the relationship between religion and health" (p. 197).

Nurses who are involved in religious organizations can also be advocates for increasing the attention given to the health needs of older people. Nurses may even spearhead particular services to older people, such as peer counseling, health screening activities, day care, home visitation programs, and respite for families. Many religious organizations reach out to homebound elders in their community by offering visits from clergy or church members, involvement in prayer circles, and other activities to maintain connection with their faith community. Communities nationwide have organized interfaith volunteer services to provide in-home services for isolated frail elders. Many of these efforts have been organized and supported by the Robert Wood Johnson Foundation, and the national Faith Based Initiative also provides support for faith-based programs.

TRANSCENDENCE

Transcendence is the high-level emotional response to religious and spiritual life and finds expression in numerous rituals and modes of cosmic consciousness. Rituals provide a means of connecting with everyone through the ages who have observed like rituals. These modes of thinking and feeling are sometimes unfamiliar to individuals who are immersed in the necessary materialistic concerns of young adulthood, yet moments do occur throughout life when one is deeply aware of being part of a larger scheme. Although some of the material in this chapter may be obscure, it is the springboard for learning to appreciate the full life cycle. The privilege of briefly walking alongside an elder on the last great journey can be truly inspiring.

Transcending is roused by the desire to go beyond the self as delimited by the material and the concrete aspects of living, to expand self-boundaries and life perspectives. "Transcendence involves detachment and separation from life as it has been lived to experience a reality beyond oneself and beyond what can be seen or felt" (Touhy and Zerwekh, 2006, p. 229). Creative thought and actions are vehicles of both self-actualization and self-transcendence, the bridge to universal expression and existence. Self-transcendence is generally expressed in five modes: creative work, religious beliefs, children, identification with nature, and mystical experiences (Reed, 1991). This section of the chapter deals with various mechanisms by which one transcends the purely physical limitations of existence.

Some people may use asceticism, self-denial, and rigorous rituals to reach the peaks of human experience; many others find more prosaic approaches just as effective. The thesis of Maslow's writings is that mystic, sacred, and transcendent experiences frequently arise from the ordinary elements of one's life (Maslow, 1970). Planting and harvesting, one of the most persistent interests of elders, is the "substance of things hoped for, the evidence of things not seen" (Hebrews 11:1). Gardening, reading, holding an infant, dealing with loss, and numerous other normal events have elements of mystery.

With each death of a loved one, throughout life, one is reborn to a slightly altered state. When deaths of significant others abound in the later years, elders must be given opportunity to express how they personally have been altered by the loss. We can speculate that with each personal loss, one moves slightly closer to the universal and away from the individual until, toward the end, one feels an affiliation with all living things—animal, plant, and mineral. Some of the old have achieved a state of existence that transcends the limits of the failing body.

Gerotranscendence

The theory of gerotranscendence (Tornstam, 1994, 1996, 2005) (Chapter 3) theorizes that human aging brings about a general potential for gerotranscendence, a shift in perspective from the material world to the cosmic and, concurrent with that, an increasing life satisfaction. Tornstam found in a survey of 912 Danish elders that shifts in cosmic awareness and ego transcendence were accompanied by satisfaction and a lesser need for social activity. The higher the level of transcendence, the more internal were the sources of satisfaction. Gerotranscendence is conceptualized as a metamorphosis, an alteration in conception of time, space, life, death, and self. Tornstam says, "Simply put, gerotranscendence is a shift in metaperspective, from a mid-life materialistic and rational vision to a more cosmic and transcendent one, accompanied by an increase in life satisfaction" (Tornstam, 1996, p. 38).

Indices of gerotranscendence are summarized in Box 24-13. Gerotranscendence is thought to be a gradual and ongoing shift that is generated by the normal processes of living, sometimes hastened by serious personal disruptions. An understanding of transcendence and the unique characteristics of this transformation in older people is important to the continued growth and development of older people.

> **BOX 24-13 CHARACTERISTICS OF INDIVIDUALS WITH A HIGH DEGREE OF GEROTRANSCENDENCE**
>
> - Have high degrees of life satisfaction
> - Engage in self-controlled social activity
> - Experience satisfaction with self-selected social activities
> - Social activities not essential to their well-being
> - Midlife patterns and ideals no longer prime motivators
> - Demonstrate complex and active coping patterns
> - Have greater need for solitary philosophizing
> - May appear withdrawn when engaged in inner development
> - Have accelerated development of gerotranscendence fomented by life crises
> - Feel shifts in perception of reality

Achieving Transcendence
Time Transcendence

Life as experienced ordinarily involves the chronological passage of time. Some types of conscious experience alter our time perception, but the unconscious destroys time. Therefore the release of the unconscious transcends the limitations of time that conscious life experience generally imposes on us. If we conquer time, we conquer annihilation and the dimensions of time that lie within the mind. Recognizing the importance of time perception, particularly in old age, is a fertile field to explore more fully. Influences on time perception include age, imminent death, level of activity, emotional state, outlook on the future, and the value attached to time. Conclusions from studies of older people generally support the view that elders perceive time as passing quickly and favor the past over the present or the future.

Peak Experiences

A peak experience is when one momentarily transcends the self through love, wisdom, insight, worship, commitment, or creativity. These experiences are the extraordinary events in one's life that clearly demonstrate self-actualization and personal authenticity. Peak experience is the time when restrictive boundaries seem to vanish, and one feels more aware, more complete, more ecstatic, or more concerned for others. Peak experiences include many modes of transcending one's ordinary limitations. Spiritual and paranormal experiences, creative acts, courage, and humor may all produce peak experiences.

The ability to embrace the possibility of every potential behavior as native to self instills compassion and a sense of oneness with the world. Keeping oneself open to transcendence involves finding the places in which such experiences can break through: soul-stirring concerts, sunrises, sunsets, or raging storms on mountaintops (Kimble, 1993). Each individual seeks states of being in which he or she feels part of a larger whole.

Meditation

Many types and rituals of meditation have flourished in Western societies in the past two decades. Some methods of meditation have been used for thousands of years in Eastern cultures. Whatever the method, the goal is to quiet the mind and center

---

BOX 24-14   BENEFITS OF MEDITATION

- Increased measured intelligence
- Increased short-term and long-term recall
- Decreased anxiety, depression, and irritability
- Greater perceived self-actualization (realization of potential)
- Better mind-body coordination
- Increased perceptual awareness
- Normalization of blood pressure
- Relief from insomnia
- Normalization of weight

---

oneself. When the mind slows, the body relaxes and less oxygen and nutrients are needed. Mindfulness meditation can decrease pain, improve sleep, and enhance well-being and quality of life (Morone et al., 2008). Meditation may also improve cognitive function.

Results of a recent pilot study (Newberg et al., 2010) using a form of meditation (Kirtan Kriya) suggest that a specific meditation performed daily for eight weeks increased brain activity in areas central to memory and improved cognition in individuals experiencing memory impairment. Other benefits of meditation are presented in Box 24-14. These benefits are all significant to older people. The fact that we see the polar opposites of these benefits so frequently attests to the stress level of many older citizens, which might be reduced through meditation.

Effective meditation requires approximately 20 minutes of focusing on a sound, a thought, or an image. Practicing two or more times daily will bring calmness, better health, and higher energy levels in its wake. Although meditation can be accomplished in any setting, a place with few distractions is helpful. People who meditate with consistency often begin to be aware of a transcendent state of being.

Nurses may introduce the values of meditation to older adults and serve as guides in the beginnings of such activities. Chanting psalms, reciting poetry by rote, praying, saying the rosary, practicing yoga, and playing a musical instrument are all mechanisms of release and renewal that may bring one into higher states of awareness.

Hope as a Transcendent Mechanism

Hope is the belief in the future and the expectation of fulfillment. Hope is the anchor that sustains life in the most difficult times and in the face of doubts and ennui. Some level of hope must be maintained to survive and to die in peace. Hope embodies desires and expectations and the limitless possibilities of humans in all times and places—present, past, and future. For many elders, hope is a major means of coping, and those who lose hope lose the capacity and desire for survival.

In a study of variables influencing hope among a group of institutionalized elders, differences were not significant in the level of hope based on age, gender, marital status, education, length of stay, self-report of physical and mental health, functional ability, and social support. Spirituality emerged as the only significant predictor of hope in the study. To be able to maintain hope in the face of losses, both physical and emotional, requires deep inner strength and faith in something greater than self. Tapping into and supporting these strengths are important nursing interventions (Touhy, 2001a).

Hope is a powerful force against despair and helps patients and families journey through difficult times. At the end of life, hope is not just associated with cure but extends beyond a physical nature to that of a social, psychological, and spiritual nature. "Because we have declared limits on treatment or cure does not mean that we have pronounced the limits of human potential. Patients are invited to open themselves to new targets of hope, to draw on strengths not yet experienced" (Jevne, 1993, p. 126).

O'Connor (1996) enumerates the critical aspects of hope: (1) the presence of an inner human energy, (2) positive expectations for the future, (3) motivation for action, and (4) formulations of meaningful, realistic goals. O'Connor further states that a person without hope has no goals or expectations for the future. All practicing nurses have observed how a small goal or hope for the future can sustain an elder. The grandson's graduation from college, the daughter's return from her travels, even a birthday may keep an elder alive until the event is safely fulfilled.

Central to the instillation of hope is the caring relationship between nurses and patients. Nursing responses that instill hope foster harmony, healing, and wholeness (Watson, 1988). Caring relationships characterized by unconditional positive regard, encouragement, and competence help patients feel loved and cared about, thus inspiring hope. A patient's hope for cure may change to a hope for freedom from pain, day-to-day experiences to enjoy precious moments of life, time to accomplish life goals before life is over, sharing love with family and friends, relief of suffering, death with dignity, and eternal life (Matzo, 2001, Touhy and Zerwekh, 2006). Nurses may foster hope by doing the following:

1. Presenting honestly the limits of human knowledge
2. Controlling symptoms and providing comfort
3. Encouraging patient and family to become involved in positive experiences that transcend the current situation
4. Determining significant aspects of the individual's life
5. Fostering spiritual processes and finding meaning
6. Exploring beliefs and values of the elder
7. Promoting connection and reconciliation
8. Providing opportunities for prayer, meditation, scripture reading, clergy visits, and religious rituals, if meaningful for the elder

Other hope-promoting experiences are presented in Box 24-15.

Transcendence in Illness

Serious illnesses influence how one perceives the meaning of life. A distinct shift in goals, relationships, and values often occurs among people who have survived life-threatening episodes. A heightened awareness of beauty and of caring relationships may occur, but a long period of emotional "splinting" may be necessary while recovering from the psychic wound of body betrayal. Newman (1994) contends that disease can be a manifestation of health as one confronts the crisis and as it reveals special meanings.

Steeves and Kahn (1987) found from their work in hospice care that certain conditions facilitate the search for meaning in illness, noting the following:

- Suffering must be bearable and not all-consuming if one is to find meaning in the experience.

BOX 24-15   HOPE-PROMOTING ACTIVITIES

- Feel the warmth of the sun.
- Share experiences children are having.
- See the crystal blue of the sky.
- Enjoy a garden or fresh flowers.
- Savor the richness of black coffee at breakfast.
- Feel the tartness of grapefruit to wake up the taste buds.
- Watch the activities of an animal in a tree outside the window.
- Benefit from each encounter with another person.
- Write messages to grandchildren, nieces, or nephews.
- Study a favorite painting.
- Listen to a symphony.
- Build highlights into each day such as meals, visits, Bible reading.
- Keep a journal.
- Write letters.
- Make a tape recording of your life story.
- Have hope objects or symbols nearby.
- Share hope stories.
- Focus on abilities, strengths, and past accomplishments.
- Encourage decision making about daily activities; foster a sense of control.
- Extend caring and love to others.
- Appreciate expressions of caring concern.
- Renew loving relationships.

Adapted from Jevne R: *Humane Medicine* 9:121, 1993; Miller, J: Coping with chronic illness: overcoming powerlessness, Philadelphia, 1983, FA Davis; Touhy T, Zerwekh J: Spiritual caring. In Zerwekh J: *Nursing care at the end of life: palliative care for patients and families,* Philadelphia, 2006, FA Davis.

- A person must have access to and be capable of perceiving objects in the environment. Even a small window on the world may be sufficient to match the limited energy one has to attend.
- One must have time that is free of interruption and a place of solitude to experience meaning.
- Clean, comfortable surroundings and freedom from constant responsibility and decision making free the soul to search for meaning.
- An open, accepting atmosphere in which to discuss meanings with others is important.

Accompanying someone in his or her grief and quest for meaning in painful events is a privilege nurses are often given. This spiritual intimacy means being willing to suffer with another, and both the nurse and the client will reap the benefits. One of the great rewards of working with older clients is observing and participating as they turn suffering into a spiritual event.

Sister Rosemary Donley (1991) defines the nursing role in the spiritual search of suffering individuals as compassionate accompaniment, meaning entering into another's reality and quietly, attentively sharing the experience. "Nurses need to be with people who suffer, to give meaning to the reality of suffering, and, in so far as possible, to remove suffering and its causes. Here lies the spiritual dimensions of health care" (Donley, 1991, p. 180). The challenge is to find meaning and some purpose in the affliction that, unchallenged, entwines and chokes identity.

LEGACIES

A legacy is one's tangible and intangible assets that are transferred to another and may be treasured as a symbol of

BOX 24-16   EXAMPLES OF LEGACIES

- Oral histories
- Autobiographies
- Written histories
- Shared memories
- Taught skills
- Works of art and music
- Publications
- Human organ donations
- Endowments
- Objects of significance
- Tangible or intangible assets
- Personal characteristics, such as courage or integrity
- Bestowed talents
- Traditions and myths perpetuated
- Philanthropical causes
- Progeny children and grandchildren
- Methods of coping
- Unique thought: Darwin, Einstein, Freud, Nightingale, and others

immortality. The purpose of legacies is to supersede death. Courage, wisdom, and insights that we perceive in our elders become part of their legacy. The desire for meaning and immortality seems to be the basic motivation for leaving a legacy. Extending one's authentic self to others can be an important activity in the last years. Throughout life, shared experiences provide satisfaction, but in the last years this exchange allows one to gain a clearer perspective on how his or her movement on earth has had impact.

Older people must be encouraged to identify that which they would like to leave and who they wish the recipients to be. This process has interpersonal significance and prepares one to leave the world with a sense of meaning. A legacy can provide a transcendent feeling of continuation and tangible or intangible ties with survivors. Legacies are the evidence of this process.

Legacies are manifold and may range from memories that will live on in the minds of others to bequeathed fortunes. Box 24-16 is a partial list of legacies. The list is as diverse as individual contributions to humanity. Erikson's seventh stage of man identifies the generative function as the main concern of the adult years and the last stage (eighth) as that of reviewing with integrity or despair that which one has accomplished. Legacies are generative and are identified and shared best as one approaches the end of life. This activity reinforces integrity.

Types of Legacies
Autobiographies and Life Histories

Oral histories are an approach to immortality. As long as one's story is told, one remains alive in the minds of others. Doers leave their products and live through them. Powerful figures are remembered in fame and infamy. The quiet, unobtrusive person survives in the memory of intimates and in family anecdotes. Everyone has a life story.

Autobiographies and recorded memoirs can serve a transcendent purpose for people who are alone—and for many who are not. Nurses can encourage older people to write, talk, or express in other ways the meaning of their lives. The human experience and the poignant anecdotes bind people together and validate the uniqueness of each brief journey in this level of awareness and the assurance that one will not be forgotten. Dying patients can express and order their memories through audiotapes, CDs, videotapes, or DVDs, which are then bequeathed to families if the older person desires. Sharing one's personal story creates bonds of empathy, illustrates a point, conveys some of the deep wisdom that we all have, and connects us with our deepest human consciousness. "It is only when people who have loved and cared for us reach the end of life that we see the full gift we have received from them. By leaving us their reminiscences, their spirits can continue in our lives as a living memorial" (Grudzen and Soltys, 2000, p. 8). See Chapter 6 for additional discussion of storytelling, reminiscence, and life review.

Creation of Self Through Journaling

Through the personal journal, one can, in thoughtful reflection, discover meaning and patterns in daily events. The self becomes a coherent story with successive revisions as old events are reread and perceived in new contexts. The journals of elders provide rich descriptions of the interior lives of the authors. May Sarton (1984) and Florida Scott-Maxwell (1968) are two of the best-known authors. The study of these journals and of the journals of less-known and less articulate elders assists nurses in understanding the inner experience of older people and, perhaps, their own.

Collective Legacies

Each person is a link in the chain of generations (Erikson, 1963) and as such may identify with generational accomplishments. An old man may think of himself as a significant part of a generation that survived the Great Depression. A middle-aged man may identify with the generation that walked on the moon. The years of youthful idealism are impressed in one's memory by the political or ideological climate of the time. This time is the stage when one searches for a fit in the larger society.

The importance of collective legacies to nurses lies in how they use this knowledge. For instance, the nurse may ask, "Who were the great men of your time?" "Which ones were important to you?" "What events of your generation changed the world?" "What were the most important events you experienced?" Mentioning certain historic events and asking about individual reactions are sometimes helpful.

Childless individuals are becoming more prevalent with each passing generation, and they must find a way to outlive the self through a legacy. Many people choose a social legacy. Florence Nightingale would be one such person, with the grand legacy she left to nurses.

Legacies Expressed Through Other People

One's legacy can be expressed in many ways through the development of others in a teaching or learning situation or through mentorship, patronage, shared talents, organ donations, and genetic transmission. Some creative works and research are legacies left to successive generations for continued modification and growth. In other words, one's legacy may be a product of his or her own brought to fruition through someone else who may also become an intermediary to later developments. Thus people and generations are tied in sequential progress. Some examples may illustrate this type of legacy:

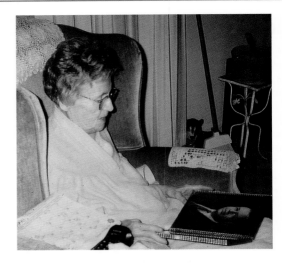

Widow reflecting on her deceased husband's legacy. (From Black JM, Hawks JH: *Medical-surgical nursing: clinical management for positive outcomes,* ed 7, St Louis, 2005, Saunders.)

- An older man cried as he talked of his grandson's talent as a violinist. Both the man and his grandson shared their love for violin, and the grandfather believed that he had genetically and personally contributed to his grandson's development as an accomplished musician.
- A professor emeritus spoke of visiting his son in a distant state and hearing him expound ideas that had been partially developed by the professor and his father before him.
- People who amass a fortune and allocate certain funds for endowment of artists, scientific projects, and intellectual exploration are counting on others to complete their legacy.

A legacy that can be converted into some tangible form can be gratifying to the older person, ensuring that it will not be readily dismissed or forgotten. The following vehicles can convey legacies:

- Summation of life work
- Photograph albums, scrapbooks
- Written memoirs
- Taped memoirs (video or audio)
- Artistic representations
- Memory gardens
- Mementos
- Genealogies
- Recorded pilgrimages

Living Legacies

Many older people wish to donate their bodies to science or donate body parts for transplant. This mechanism is a means to transcend death. Parts of the body keep another person alive, or, in the case of certain diseases, the deceased body may provide important information leading to preventive or restorative techniques in the future. Donation of body parts in old age may not be encouraged because they are often less viable than those from younger people. Nonetheless, older bodies are welcome for use as cadavers. People who are interested in providing such a legacy should be encouraged to call the nearest university biomedical center and obtain more information. The nurse then has a postmortem obligation to the client to assist in carrying out his or her wishes.

Property and Assets

Wealth may be viewed as a means toward power more often than transcendence; therefore some older people are often reluctant to disperse material goods before their death. Some elders use the future legacy as a means to exert power and control over offspring. One man said, "So long as I have that bankroll, they've got to treat me with respect" (Lustbader, 1996). The power to exert influence, to punish, and to reward is often bound up in an anticipated estate distribution.

Estates can be planned in certain ways that are decidedly advantageous for the planner, as well as the recipient, in terms of control, avoidance of lengthy probate proceedings, and taxation. Because the laws are complex and ever-changing, using the services of an estate planner would be advisable. The nurse's responsibility regarding wills may be limited to advising older people to obtain legal counsel while they are healthy and competent and plan how they would like to distribute their worldly goods.

Personal Possessions

Possessions carry more meaning as time passes; individuals change, but the possession remains much the same. A possession is a way of symbolically hanging on to individuals who are gone or times that are past. For some people, keeping personal possessions is a means of hanging on to the self that is changing with time. Cherished possessions passed on through several generations may have achieved meaning through the close family member to whom they belonged. One's personally significant items become highly charged with memories and meaning, and transferring them to friends and kin can be a tender experience. Personal possessions should never be dispersed without the individual's knowledge. Because of the uncertainty of late life lucidity, these issues should be discussed early with older individuals.

People who are approaching death must be given the opportunity to distribute their important belongings appropriately to those who they believe will also cherish them. Nurses may encourage elders to plan the distribution of their significant items carefully. Deciding when and how best these possessions should be given is often difficult. Some people choose to distribute possessions before dying. In these cases, nurses often need to help family members accept these gifts, appreciating the meaning and recognizing the significance.

Certain questions allow the older person to consider a legacy if he or she is ready to do so. For example:

- What is the meaning to you of your life experience right now?
- Have you ever thought of writing an autobiography?
- If you were able to leave something to the younger generation, what would it be?
- Have you ever thought of the impact your generation has had on the world?
- What has been most meaningful in your life?
- What possessions have special meaning for you? Who else is interested in them?
- Do you see some of your genetic traits emerging in your grandchildren?

These suggestions should stimulate ideas for spontaneous statements, which are revealing in an interpersonal context.

PROMOTING HEALTHY AGING: IMPLICATIONS FOR GERONTOLOGICAL NURSING

"The responsibility of the nurse is not to make people well, or to prevent their getting sick, but to assist people to recognize the power that is within them to move to higher levels of consciousness" (Newman, 1994, p. xv). In this chapter, we have examined methods of expanding one's limited existence by developing the authentic self, transcendent self, spiritual self, and several mechanisms used to establish immortality through a legacy. These areas often become major issues in the latter part of life, and the nurse will find it a revealing, absorbing, and challenging task to be a part of this effort. An important point is that some people may avoid any such interest or concern, particularly when angry, in pain, or denying their own mortality. Nurses need not push the individual to accomplish this task but should be available to assist the person and family members.

The basic mysteries of life elude scientific researchers, yet they are the essence of existence with meaning. Remembering, feeling, dreaming, worshipping, and grasping one's connection to the universe are the realities of the human spirit. Being old is not the centrality of the self—spirit is. Spirit synthesizes the total personality and provides integration, energizing force, and immortality. Nurses who care for older people have a great privilege in being able to accompany them on the final journey of their life. It calls for a nurse who is willing to enter into meaningful spirit-sharing relationships. Taking advantage of these opportunities will enrich our nursing, our inner selves, and the spiritual well-being of the elders whom we nurse. Such relationships have the potential to enhance inner harmony and healing. There may be no greater goal in caring for elders than helping a person see a life well lived and meaningful to themselves and others, thus providing hope that life's journey was not in vain.

As gerontological nursing scholar Sarah Gueldner (2007) so eloquently stated:

"We must help each older adult to continue to experience and express the passions that, over a lifetime, have become who they are. Older adults should continue to make their unique and precious contributions to society, and we must not fail to take note of it in even the frailest and quietest of individuals. We must give them voice and time on the center stage of life and help them connect with each other and with society in a way that fosters appreciation of the traits, talents, and memories that still define their being" (p. 4).

As we close this book, our hopes are that we have provided you with the knowledge to care for elders with competence and compassion and that you will find as much joy and fulfillment as we have in our nursing of older adults.

KEY CONCEPTS

- Self-actualization is a process of developing one's most authentic self. Maslow thought of self-actualization as the pinnacle of human development.
- Self-actualized individuals embody qualities of courage, humor, high moral development, and seeking to learn more about themselves and others.
- Opportunities for pursuing interests will assist individuals in developing latent talents, expressing their creativity, and rising beyond daily concerns.
- Groups working toward societal humanitarian advancement may accomplish collective actualization.
- Creativity emanates from people who are self-actualized and may be expressed in mundane activities, as well as the arts, music, theater, and literature.
- Transcending the material and physical limitations of existence through ritual and spiritual means is an especially important aspect of aging.
- Gerotranscendence is a theory proposed by Tornstam that implies a natural shift in concerns that occurs in the aging process. Elders are thought to spend more time in reflection, to spend less on materialistic concerns, and to find more satisfaction in life. This effort is an attempt to define aging not by the standards of young and middle adulthood but as having distinctive characteristics of its own.
- Illnesses that occur have the potential for altering one's fundamental beliefs and hopes. Nurses must give elders the opportunity to discuss the meanings of an illness. Some people find that these experiences bring new insights; others are angry. Empathic nurses will provide a sounding board while the elder makes sense of an illness within a satisfactory framework.
- Nurses need not neglect discussing spirituality with elders. Elders will respond only if it has significance for them.
- Spiritual nursing interventions emanate from the caring relationship between the older person and the nurse. The most important tool at the nurses' disposal is the use of self.

CASE STUDY   SELF-ACTUALIZATION, SPIRITUALITY, AND TRANSCENDENCE

Melba had no children but had numerous nieces and nephews, though she did not feel particularly close to any of them. She had been a nursing instructor at a community college and had enjoyed her students but had not developed a sustained relationship with any of them after they had completed her courses. At her level of nursing education, the opportunity for mentorship was lacking, though she had occasionally taken students under her wing and arranged special experiences that they particularly desired. Because she had taught several courses each year, Melba never really developed a strong affiliation to a specialty but considered herself a pediatric nurse. She had not made any major contributions to the field in terms of research or publications; a few reviews, continuing education workshops, and some nursing newsletters had really been the extent of her work outside of that which was required. Melba's husband died in 1988, and she had felt very much alone since that time, especially after her retirement three years ago. Before her husband's death, Melba had been too busy to think about the ultimate meaning of all her years of teaching and wifely activities. With time on her hands, she began to wonder what it all meant. Had she done anything meaningful? Had she really made a difference in anything or in anyone's life? Was anyone going to remember her in any special way? So many questions were making her morose. She had never been a religious person, though her husband had been a devout Catholic. He had believed that God had a purpose for him in life, and though he was not always able to understand what it might be, he seemed to have a sense of satisfaction. She began to wonder if she should go to church—would that make her feel less depressed?

One Sunday morning, Melba had decided to attend her neighborhood Catholic church, but on her way out she slipped on the icy walkway and sustained bilateral Colles' fractures. After a brief emergency room visit for assessment, immobilization of the wrists, and medications, Melba was sent back home with an order for home health and social service assessment on the following day. Of course, she had extreme difficulty managing the most basic self-care while keeping her wrists immobilized and was very dejected. When the home health nurse arrived the next morning, to Melba's amazement, it was a former student who had graduated four years previously. Melba was more chagrined than pleased and greeted her with, "Oh, I hate to have you see me so helpless. I've been feeling so useless, and, now with these wrists, I am totally useless." If you were the home health nurse, how would you begin working with Melba, knowing that your visits would be limited to just a few?

Based on the case study, develop a nursing care plan using the following procedure*:

- List Melba's comments that provide subjective data.
- List information that provides objective data.
- From these data, identify and state, using accepted format, two nursing diagnoses you determine are most significant to Melba at this time. List two of Melba's strengths that you have identified from the data.
- Determine and state the outcome criteria for each diagnosis. These must reflect some alleviation of the problem identified in the nursing diagnosis and must be stated in concrete and measurable terms.
- Plan and state one or more interventions for each diagnosed problem. Provide specific documentation of the sources used to determine the appropriate intervention. Plan at least one intervention that incorporates Melba's existing strengths.
- Evaluate the success of the intervention. Interventions must correlate directly with the stated outcome criteria to measure the outcome success.

CRITICAL THINKING QUESTIONS

1. Discuss the meanings and the thoughts triggered by the student's and elder's viewpoints as expressed at the beginning of the chapter. How do they vary from your own experience?
2. How do nursing students learn about spirituality and spiritual nursing interventions?
3. What activities might be helpful in developing your own sense of spirituality?
4. How does culture affect one's concept of spirituality?
5. How can nurses enhance spiritual care, self-actualization, and transcendence of self among elders?

*Students are advised to refer to their nursing diagnosis text and identify possible or potential problems.

RESEARCH QUESTIONS

1. Who makes out wills and when?
2. What are the motivating differences between gifts during life and those after one's death?
3. What is the perspective of older people related to spiritual assessment and interventions by nurses?
4. Can nurses describe spiritual interventions they use with older people?
5. How do nurses recognize aspects of gerotranscendence?
6. What aspects of intergenerational programs are enjoyed by younger and older individuals?

REFERENCES

American Nurses Association: *Faith community nursing: scope and standards of practice*, Silver Springs, MD, Nursesbooks.org, 2005.

Ardelt M: Wisdom and life satisfaction in old age, *Journal of Gerontology: Psychological Sciences*, 52B:15-27, 1997.

Ardelt M: Antecedents and effects of wisdom in old age: a longitudinal perspective on aging well, *Research on Aging* 22:360-394, 2000.

Ardelt M: Wisdom as expert knowledge system: a critical review of a contemporary operationalization of an ancient concept, *Human Development* 47:257-285, 2004.

Ardelt M: Empirical assessment of a three-dimensional wisdom scale, *Research on Aging* 25(3):275-324, 2003.

Baltes P: The many faces of human ageing: toward a psychological culture of old age, *Psychological Medicine* 21:837-854, 1991.

Baltes P, Smith J: New frontiers in the future of aging: from successful aging of the young old to the dilemmas of the fourth age, *Gerontology* 49:123-125, 2003.

Baltes P, Smith J: The fascination of wisdom: its nature, ontogeny, and function, *Perspectives on Psychological Science* 3:56-62, 2008.

Bastings A: Arts in dementia care: "This is not the end ... it's the end of the chapter," *Generations* 30:16, 2006.

Bell V, Troxel D: Spirituality and the person with dementia: a view from the field, *Alzheimer's Care Quarterly* 2:31, 2001.

Blues A, Zerwekh J: *Hospice and palliative care nursing*, Orlando, Fla, 1984, Grune & Stratton.

Cohen G: Research on creativity and aging: the positive impact of the arts on health and illness, *Generations* 30:7, 2006.

Cousins N: *Anatomy of an illness*, New York, 1979, WW Norton.

Crowther MR, Parker MW, Achenbaum WA, et al: Rowe and Kahn's model of successful aging revisited: positive spirituality—the forgotten factor, *Gerontologist* 42:613, 2002.

Delgado C: Sense of coherence, spirituality, stress and quality of life in chronic illness, *Journal of Nursing Scholarship* 39(3):229-234, 2007.

Donley R: Spiritual dimensions of health care: nursing's mission, *Nursing & Health Care* 12:178, 1991.

Dyess S, Chase S: Caring for adults with a chronic illness through communities of faith, *International Journal for Human Caring* 14(4):38-44, 2010.

Dyess S, Chase S, Newlin K: State of research for faith community nursing 2009, *Journal of Religion and Health* 49:188, 2009.

Dyson J, Cobb M, Forman D: The meaning of spirituality: a literature review, *Journal of Advanced Nursing* 26:1183, 1997.

Erikson EH: *Childhood and society*, ed 2, New York, 1963, WW Norton.

Gaskamp C, Sutter R, Meraviglia M, et al: Evidence-based guideline: promoting spirituality in the older adult, *Journal of Gerontological Nursing* 32:8, 2006.

Gerdner L: Individualized music for elders with dementia, *Journal of Gerontological Nursing* 36:7, 2010.

Gerdner L: An individualized music intervention for agitation, *Journal of the American Psychiatric Nurses Association* 3:177, 2000.

Gerdner L: Use of individualized music by trained staff and family: translating research into practice, *Journal of Gerontological Nursing* 3:22, 2005.

Goldberg B: Connection: an exploration of spirituality in nursing care, *Journal of Advanced Nursing* 27:836, 1998.

Grossmann I, Na J, Varnum M, Park D et al: Reasoning about social conflicts improves into old age, *Proceedings of the National Academy of Science*, published online before print April 5, 2010, doi: 10.1073/pnas.1001715107, *PNAS* April 5, 2010. Available at www.pnas.org/cgi/doi/10.1973/pnas.1001715107. Accessed January 29, 2011.

Gruden M, Soltys FG: Reminiscence at end of life: celebrating a living legacy, *Dimensions* 7(3): 4, 5, 8, 2000.

Gueldner S: Sustaining expression of identity in older adults, *Journal of Gerontological Nursing* 33:3, 2007.

Hebrews 11:1 *Holy Bible*, Chicago, 1964, John A Dickson.

Helmuth L: The wisdom of the wizened, *Science* 299:1300-1302, 2003.

Heriot C: Spirituality and aging, *Holistic Nursing Practice* 7:22, 1992.

Hicks-Moore S: Relaxing music at mealtime in nursing homes: effects on agitation patients with dementia, *Journal of Gerontological Nursing* 31:26, 2005.

Hodge D, Bonifas R, Chou R: Spirituality and older adults: ethical guidelines to enhance service provision, *Advances in Social Work* 11:1, 2010.

Hooyman N, Kiyak A: *Social gerontology: a multidisciplinary perspective*, Boston, 2005, Pearson.

Hudson F: The adult years: mastering the art of self-renewal. San Francisco, 1999, Jossey-Bass.

Jevne R: Enhancing hope in the chronically ill, *Humane Medicine* 9:121, 1993.

Killick J: *You are words*, London, 1997, Hawker Publications.

Killick J: *Openings*, London, 2000, Hawker Publications.

Killick J: Dementia, You and yours transcript, 2005. Available at www.bbc.co.uk/radio4/youandyours/transcript_2005_46_ri_02.shtml.

Killick J: *Dementia Diary*. London, 2008, Journal of Dementia Care.

Kimble M: A personal journey of aging: the spiritual dimension, *Generations* 17(2):27, 1993.

Koch K: *I never told anybody*, New York, 1977, Random House.

Koenig HG, Brooks RG: Religion, health and aging: implications for practice and public policy, *Public Policy & Aging Report* 12:13, 2002.

Kohlberg L, Power C: Moral development, religious thinking and the question of a seventh stage. In Kohlberg L, editor: *The philosophy of moral development*, vol 1, San Francisco, 1981, Harper & Row.

Koepke D as quoted in Bernstein A: Spirituality and aging: looking at the big picture. Available at http://www.agingwellmag.com/news/septstory1.shtml. Accessed July 31, 2010.

Krampe J, Rantz M, Dowell L, et al: Dance-based therapy in a program of all-inclusive care for the elderly, *Nursing Administration Quarterly* 34:156, 2010.

Kuhn M: Advocacy in this new age, *Aging* 3:297, Jul/Aug 1979.

Larson R: Building intergenerational bonds through the arts, *Generations* 30:38, 2006.

Leetun M: Wellness spirituality in the older adult, *The Nurse Practitioner* 21:60, 1996.

Lowry LW, Conco D: Exploring the meaning of spirituality with aging adults in Appalachia, *Journal of Holistic Nursing* 20:388, 2002.

Lustbader W: Conflict, emotion and power surrounding legacy, *Generations* 20:54, 1996.

Macrae J: Nightingale's spiritual philosophy and its significance for modern nursing, *Image—The Journal of Nursing Scholarship* 27:8, 1995.

Martsolf D, Mickley J: The concept of spirituality in nursing theories: differing world views and extent of focus, *Journal of Advanced Nursing* 27:294, 1998.

Maslow A: Creativity in self-actualizing people. In Anderson H, editor: *Creativity and its cultivator*, New York, 1959, Harper & Row.

Maslow A: *Religions, values and peak-experiences*, New York, 1970, Viking Press.

Matzo M: End-of-life care nurses should help patients live fully, inspire hope, *American Nurse*, September-October:1-4, 2001.

McCaffrey R: Music listening: Its effect in creating a healing environment, *Journal of Psychosocial Nursing* 46:39, 2008.

McCaffrey R, Freeman E: Effect of music on chronic osteoarthritis pain in older people, *Journal of Advanced Nursing* 44:517, 2003.

McCaffrey R, Locsin R: The effect of music on pain and acute confusion in older adults undergoing hip and knee surgery, *Holistic Nursing Practice* 20:218, 2006.

McCaffrey R, Good M: The lived experience of listening to music while recovering from surgery, *Journal of Holistic Nursing* 18:378, 2000.

Metcalf CW: *Lighten up*, Niles, Ill, 1993, Nightingale Conant (audiotapes).

Meyer CL: How effectively are nurse educators preparing students to provide spiritual care? *Dissertation Abstracts International* 55:2158B, UMI No 9428614, 2003.

Morone N, Lynch C, Greco C, et al: "I felt like a new person," The effects of mindfulness meditation on older adults with chronic pain: qualitative narrative analysis of diary entries, *Journal of Pain* 9:841, 2008.

Newman MA: *Health as expanding consciousness*, ed 2, New York, 1994, National League for Nursing Press.

Newberg AB, Wintering N, Khalsa DS, et al: Meditation effects on cognitive function and cerebral blood flow in subjects with memory loss: A preliminary study, *Journal of Alzheimer's Disease* 20:April 2010, doi:10.3233/JAD-2010-1391.

O'Brien ME: *Spirituality in nursing: standing on holy ground*, Boston, 2003, Jones & Bartlett.

O'Connor P: Hope: a concept for home care nursing, *Home Care Provider* 1:175, 1996.

Parisi J, Rebok G, Carlson M, Fried L, et al: Can the wisdom of aging be activated and make a difference socially? *Educational Gerontology* 35:867-879, 2009.

Peck R: Psychological developments in the second half of life. In Anderson J, editor: *Psychological aspects of aging*, Washington, DC, 1955, American Psychological Association.

Perlstein S: Creative expression and quality of life: a vital relationship for elders, *Generations* 30:5, 2006.

Potter ML, Zauszniewski J: Spirituality, resourcefulness, and arthritis impact on health perception of elders with rheumatoid arthritis, *Journal of Holistic Nursing* 18:311, 2000.

Puchalski C, Romer A: Taking a spiritual history allows clinicians to understand patients more fully, *Journal of Palliative Medicine* 3:129, 2000.

Reed PG: Toward a nursing theory of self-transcendence: deductive reformulation using developmental theories, *ANS. Advances in Nursing Science* 13:64, 1991.

Rowe JW, Kahn RL: *Successful aging*, New York, 1998, Pantheon–Random House.

Sarton M: *At seventy: a journal*, New York, 1984, WW Norton.

Scott-Maxwell F: *The measure of my days*, New York, 1968, Alfred A Knopf.

Soeken K, Carson V: Responding to the spiritual needs of the chronically ill, *Nursing Clinics of North America* 22:604, 1987.

Steeves R, Kahn D: Experience of meaning in suffering, *Image—The Journal of Nursing Scholarship* 19:114, 1987.

Strang S, Strang P: Questions posed to hospital chaplains by palliative care patients, *Journal of Palliative Medicine* 5:857, 2002.

Tornstam L: Gerotranscendence: a theoretical and empirical exploration. In Thomas LE, Eisenhandler SA, editors: *Aging and the religious dimension*, Westport, Conn, 1994, Greenwood Publishing Group.

Tornstam L: Gerotranscendence: a theory about maturing into old age, *Journal of Aging and Identity* 1:37, 1996.

Tornstam L: *Gerotranscendence: a developmental theory of positive aging*, New York, 2005, Springer.

Touhy T: Nurturing hope and spirituality in the nursing home, *Holistic Nursing Practice* 15:45, 2001a.

Touhy T: Touching the spirit of elders in nursing homes: ordinary yet extraordinary care, *International Journal of Human Caring* 6:12, 2001b.

Touhy T, Brown C, Smith C: Spiritual caring: end of life in a nursing home, *Journal of Gerontological Nursing* 31:27, 2005.

Touhy T, Zerwekh J: Spiritual caring. In Zerwekh J, editor: *Nursing care at the end of life: palliative care for patients and families*, Philadelphia, 2006, FA Davis.

Twiss E, Seaver J, McCaffrey R: The effects of music listening on older adults undergoing cardiovascular surgery, *Nursing in Critical Care* 11:224, 2006.

Watson J: *Nursing: human science and human care*, New York, 1988, National League for Nursing.

Wikstrom B: Older adults and the arts, *Journal of Gerontological Nursing* 30:30, 2004.

Witzke J, Rhone R, Backhaus D, et al: How sweet the sound: research evidence for the use of music in Alzheimer's dementia, *Journal of Gerontological Nursing* 34:45, 2008.

Page numbers followed by "f" indicate figures, "t" indicate tables, and "b" indicate boxes.

483